MANUAL OF INTENSIVE CARE MEDICINE

WITH ANNOTATED KEY REFERENCES

MANUAL OF INTENSIVE CARE MEDICINE

WITH ANNOTATED KEY REFERENCES

Third Edition

Edited by
Richard S. Irwin, M.D.
Professor of Medicine
University of Massachusetts Medical School;
Director, Pulmonary, Allergy,
and Critical Care Medicine
UMass Memorial Health Care
Worcester, Massachusetts

James M. Rippe, M.D.
Associate Professor of Medicine (Cardiology)
Tufts University School of Medicine,
Boston, Massachusetts;
Director
The Center for Clinical
and Lifestyle Research
Shrewsbury, Massachusetts

This edition is based on *Irwin and Rippe's Intensive Care Medicine,* Fourth Edition, edited by Richard S. Irwin, Frank B. Cerra, and James M. Rippe.

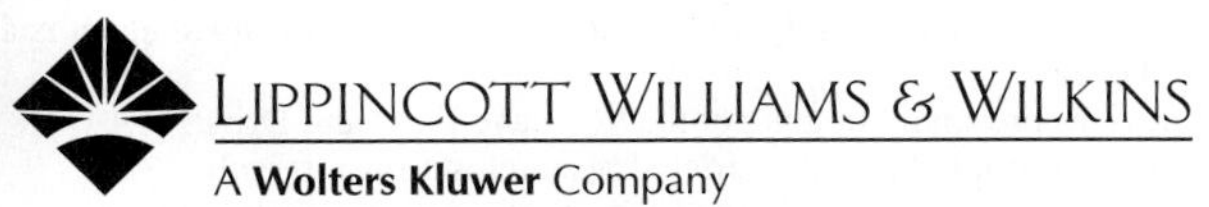

Philadelphia • Baltimore • New York • London
Buenos Aires • Hong Kong • Sydney • Tokyo

Acquisitions Editor: R. Craig Percy
Developmental Editor: Stephanie Harris
Production Editor: Melanie Bennitt
Manufacturing Manager: Kevin Watt
Cover Illustrator: Patricia Gast
Compositor: Circle Graphics
Printer: R. R. Donnelley–Crawfordsville

Published by Lippincott Williams & Wilkins
530 Walnut Street
Philadelphia, PA 19106 USA
LWW.com

Printed in the USA

Library of Congress Cataloging-in-Publication Data

Manual of intensive care medicine : with annotated key references / edited by Richard S. Irwin, James M. Rippe.—3rd ed.
p. ; cm.
Based on: Irwin and Rippe's intensive care medicine / edited by Richard S. Irwin, Frank B. Cerra, and James M. Rippe. 4th ed. c1999.
Includes bibliographical references and index.
ISBN 0-7817-1986-0
1. Critical care medicine—Handbooks, manuals, etc. I. Irwin, Richard S. II. Rippe, James M.
[DNLM: 1. Intensive Care. 2. Intensive Care Units. WX 218 M2945 2000]
RC86.7 .M365 2000
616′.028—dc21

99-087836

---

10 9 8 7 6 5 4 3 2 1

CONTENTS

I. PROCEDURES AND TECHNIQUES

Editor—Stephen O. Heard

II. CARDIOVASCULAR PROBLEMS IN THE INTENSIVE CARE UNIT

Editor—Richard C. Becker

III. CORONARY CARE

Editor—Richard C. Becker

VII. GASTROINTESTINAL AND HEPATOBILIARY PROBLEMS IN THE INTENSIVE CARE UNIT

Editor—Ray E. Clouse

VIII. ENDOCRINE PROBLEMS IN THE INTENSIVE CARE UNIT

Editor—Michael J. Thompson

IX. HEMATOLOGIC PROBLEMS IN THE INTENSIVE CARE UNIT

Editor—F. Marc Stewart

X. PHARMACOLOGY, OVERDOSES, AND POISONINGS

Editor—Christopher H. Linden

XII. SHOCK AND TRAUMA

Editor—Arthur L. Trask

XIII. NEUROLOGIC PROBLEMS IN THE INTENSIVE CARE UNIT

Editors—David A. Drachman and David Paydarfar

XIV. TRANSPLANTATION

Editor—David L. Dunn

XV. RHEUMATOLOGIC AND IMMUNOLOGIC PROBLEMS IN THE INTENSIVE CARE UNIT

Editor—David F. Giansiracusa

XVI. PSYCHIATRIC ISSUES IN THE INTENSIVE CARE UNIT

Editor—Theodore A. Stern

XVII. MORAL, ETHICAL, LEGAL, AND PUBLIC POLICY ISSUES IN THE INTENSIVE CARE UNIT

Editors—James M. Rippe and Richard S. Irwin

APPENDIX

CONTRIBUTING AUTHORS

Syed Adil Ahmed, M.D.
Assistant Professor, Department of Anesthesiology, UMass Memorial Health Care, Worcester, Massachusetts 01655

David H. Ahrenholz, M.D.
Associate Professor, Department of Surgery, University of Minnesota Medical School; Department of Surgery, Regions Hospital, St. Paul, Minnesota 55101

Ahmad-Samer Al-Homsi, M.D.
Assistant Professor of Medicine, Department of Hematology and Medical Oncology, University of Massachusetts Medical Center; Attending Hematologist and Medical Oncologist, Milford-Whitinsville Regional Hospital, UMass Memorial Health Care, Worcester, Massachusetts 01655

Joseph S. Alpert, M.D.
Professor and Head, Department of Medicine, University of Arizona Health Sciences Center, Tucson, Arizona 85724

Neil M. Ampel, M.D.
Associate Professor of Medicine, Department of Infectious Diseases, University of Arizona; Tucson Veterans Affairs Medical Center, Tucson, Arizona 85723

Neil Aronin, M.D.
Professor of Cell Biology and Medicine, University of Massachusetts Medical School, Worcester, Massachusetts 01655

Gerald P. Aurigemma, M.D.
Associate Professor of Medicine and Radiology, Director, Non-Invasive Cardiology, Department of Cardiovascular Medicine, UMass Memorial Health Care, Worcester, Massachusetts 01655

Karen K. Ballen, M.D.
Assistant Professor of Medicine, Department of Medicine, University of Massachusetts School of Medicine; Director, Bone Marrow Transplant Program, UMass Memorial Health Care, Worcester, Massachusetts 01655

Daniel T. Baran, M.D.
Department of Orthopedics and Physical Rehabilitation, University of Massachusetts Medical School, Worcester, Massachusetts 01655

Steven P. Beaudette, M.D.
The Heart Institute, Nashua, New Hampshire 03060

Pamela S. Becker, M.D., Ph.D.
Associate Professor of Medicine, Department of Hematology and Medical Oncology, University of Massachusetts Medical School and UMass Memorial Health Care, Worcester, Massachusetts 01655

Richard C. Becker, M.D.
Professor, Department of Medicine, University of Massachusetts Medical School; Director, Coronary Care Unit, Department of Medicine, UMass Memorial Health Care, Worcester, Massachusetts 01655

Isabelita R. Bella, M.D.
Assistant Professor, Department of Neurology, University of Massachusetts Medical School and UMass Memorial Health Care, Worcester, Massachusetts 01655

Joseph R. Benotti, M.D.
Department of Cardiology, St. Vincent's Hospital, Worcester, Massachusetts 01604

Steven Borzak, M.D.
Assistant Professor, Department of Medicine, Case Western Reserve University; Associate Division Head, Department of Cardiovascular Medicine, Henry Ford Hospital, Detroit, Michigan 48202

Suzanne F. Bradley, M.D.
Associate Professor, Department of Internal Medicine, University of Michigan Medical School; Physician Scientist, Geriatric Research Education and Clinical Center, Veterans Affairs Medical Center, Ann Arbor, Michigan 48105

Kenneth L. Brayman, M.D., Ph.D.
Associate Professor of Surgery, Director of Pancreas Transplant Program, University of Pennsylvania School of Medicine and University of Pennsylvania Hospital, Philadelphia, Pennsylvania 19104

Doreen B. Brettler, M.D.
Professor of Medicine, Department of Hematology and Medical Oncology, University of Massachusetts Medical School, UMass Memorial Health Care, Worcester, Massachusetts 01605

Christopher P. Cannon, M.D.
Assistant Professor of Medicine, Department of Cardiovascular Medicine, Harvard Medical School; Associate Physician, Department of Cardiovascular Medicine, Brigham and Women's Hospital, Boston, Massachusetts 02115

Ronald P. Caputo, M.D.
Assistant Clinical Professor, Department of Medicine, SUNY Health Science Center; Invasive Attending Physician, Department of Cardiology, St. Joseph's Hospital Health Care, Syracuse, New York 13203

Karen C. Carroll, M.D.
Director of Diagnostic Infectious Diseases Laboratory, ARUP Laboratories, Inc.; Associate Professor of Pathology, Adjunct Associate Professor of Infectious Diseases, Department of Pathology, University of Utah Health Sciences Center, Salt Lake City, Utah 84132

David A. Chad, M.D.
Department of Neurology, UMass Memorial Health Care, Worcester, Massachusetts 01655

G. Muqtada Chaudhry, M.D.
Department of Cardiology—Cardiac Electrophysiology and Pacing, St. Elizabeth's Medical Center, Boston, Massachusetts 02135

Sarah H. Cheeseman, M.D.
Professor of Medicine, Pediatrics, Molecular Genetics, and Microbiology, University of Massachusetts Medical School; Infectious Disease Specialist, Department of Medicine, UMass Memorial Health Care, Worcester, Massachusetts 01655

David M. Clive, M.D.
Associate Professor of Medicine, Department of Renal Medicine, UMass Memorial Health Care, Worcester, Massachusetts 01655

Ray E. Clouse, M.D.
Department of Internal Medicine, Washington University School of Medicine, Barnes-Jewish Hospital, St. Louis, Missouri 63110

Christopher A. Clyne, M.D.
Assistant Clinical Professor, Department of Internal Medicine, Yale University School of Medicine; Department of Cardiology, St. Raphael's Hospital, New Haven, Connecticut 06511

Gerald Alexander Colvin, D.O.
Senior Research Fellow, Department of Hematology and Medical Oncology, UMass Memorial Health Care, Worcester, Massachusetts 01655

Ann E. Connolly, R.N., B.S.N.
Department of Pulmonary, Allergy, and Critical Care Medicine, University of Massachusetts Medical School, UMass Memorial Health Cares, Worcester, Massachusetts 01655

Jonathan F. Critchlow, M.D.
Assistant Professor of Surgery, Harvard Medical School; Co-Director, Respiratory—Surgical Intensive Care Unit, Department of Surgery, Beth Israel Hospital, Boston, Massachusetts 02215

Frederick J. Curley, M.D.
Department of Pulmonary and Critical Care Medicine, Milford-Whitinsville Hospital, Milford, Massachusetts 01757

Jennifer S. Daly, M.D.
Associate Professor, Department of Medicine, University of Massachusetts Medical School; Infectious Disease Specialist, Department of Infectious Diseases and Immunology, UMass Memorial Health Care, Worcester, Massachusetts 01655

Raul Davaro, M.D.
Assistant Professor, Department of Medicine, University of Massachusetts Medical School; Infectious Disease Specialist, Department of Infectious Diseases and Immunology, UMass Memorial Health Care, Worcester, Massachusetts 01655

Daniel A. Devereaux, M.D.
UMass Memorial Health Care, Worcester, Massachusetts 01655

David A. Drachman, M.D.
Professor and Chairman, Department of Neurology, UMass Memorial Health Care, Worcester, Massachusetts 01655

David L. Dunn, M.D., Ph.D.
Jay Phillips Professor and Chairman, Department of Surgery, University of Minnesota, Minneapolis, Minnesota 55455

Kevin M. Dwyer, M.D.
Associate Chief, Department of Trauma Services, Inova Fairfax Hospital, Falls Church, Virginia 22042

Charles H. Emerson, M.D.
Professor of Medicine, Department of Endocrinology and Metabolism, University of Massachusetts Medical School, Worcester, Massachusetts 01655

Robert V.B. Emmons, M.D.
Cancer Center, UMass Memorial Health Care, Worcester, Massachusetts 01655

Alan P. Farwell, M.D., F.A.C.P.
Associate Professor of Medicine, Department of Endocrinology and Metabolism, University of Massachusetts Medical School, Worcester, Massachusetts 01655

Kevin J. Felice, D.O.
Department of Neurology, University of Connecticut Health Center, Farmington, Connecticut 06030

Marc Fisher, M.D.
Department of Neurology, UMass Memorial Health Care, Worcester, Massachusetts 01605

Nancy M. Fontneau, M.D.
Department of Neurology, UMass Memorial Health Care, Worcester, Massachusetts 01655

Cynthia T. French, R.N., C.S., A.N.P.
Department of Pulmonary, Allergy, and Critical Care Medicine, UMass Memorial Health Care, Worcester, Massachusetts 01655

Nelson M. Gantz, M.D.
Clinical Professor, Department of Medicine, Hahnemann University School of Medicine; Chairman, Department of Medicine, Chief, Department of Infectious Diseases, Pinnacle Health Hospitals, Harrisburg, Pennsylvania 17110

Leonard I. Ganz, M.D.
Assistant Professor of Medicine, Department of Electrophysiology, Allegheny University of the Health Sciences, Allegheny University Hospitals, Pittsburgh, Pennsylvania 15212

Marie Juliet George, M.D.
Assistant Professor, Department of Medicine, University of Massachusetts Medical School, Worcester, Massachusetts; Medical Director of Infectious Diseases, Department of Medicine, Southwestern Vermont Medical Center, Bennington, Vermont 05201

Edith S. Geringer, M.D.
Instructor in Psychiatry, Harvard Medical School; Co-Director, Department of Psychiatry, Massachusetts General Hospital, Boston, Massachusetts 02114

Edward P. Gerstenfeld, M.D.
Electrophysiology Fellow, Department of Medicine, University of California, San Francisco, California 94143

Reem Ghalib, M.D.
Department of Gastroenterology, Washington University School of Medicine and Barnes-Jewish Hospital, St. Louis, Missouri 63110

David F. Giansiracusa, M.D.
Professor of Medicine, Vice Chair, Department of Medicine, UMass Memorial Health Care, Worcester, Massachusetts 01655

Richard H. Glew, M.D.
Professor, Department of Medicine, Molecular Genetics and Microbiology, University of Massachusetts Medical School; Associate Chair, Department of Medicine and Director, Division of Infectious Diseases and Immunology, UMass Memorial Health Care, Worcester, Massachusetts 01655

Jack L. Gluckman, M.D.
Chairman, Department of Otolaryngology—Head and Neck Surgery, University of Cincinnati Medical Center, Cincinnati, Ohio 45267

Christopher Greene, M.D.
Department of Anesthesiology, UMass Memorial Health Care, Worcester, Massachusetts 01655

Ronald F. Grossman, M.D., F.R.C.P.(C), F.A.C.P.
Professor, Department of Medicine, University of Toronto; Head, Department of Respiratory Medicine, Mount Sinai Hospital, Toronto, Ontario M5G 1X5, Canada

Scott A. Gruber, M.D.
Associate Professor, Departments of Surgery, Immunology, and Organ Transplant, University of Texas at Houston, Houston, Texas 77225

Rainer W.G. Gruessner, M.D., Ph.D.
Department of Surgery, University of Minnesota, Minneapolis, Minnesota 55455

Charles I. Haffajee, M.D.
Professor, Department of Medicine, Tufts University School of Medicine; Director of Cardiac Electrophysiology and Pacing, Department of Medicine, St. Elizabeth's Medical Center, Boston, Massachusetts 02135

Daniel F. Hanley, M.D.
Director, Neurosciences Critical Care Unit, Johns Hopkins Medical Center, Baltimore, Maryland 21287

Robert A. Harrington, M.D.
Assistant Professor, Department of Medicine, Duke University; Director, Cardiovascular Clinical Trials, Duke Clinical Research Institute, Duke University Medical Center, Durham, North Carolina 27705

Leslie R. Harrold, M.D.
Assistant Professor, Department of Medicine, University of Massachusetts Medical School; Rheumatologist, Department of Medicine, UMass Memorial Health Care, Worcester, Massachusetts 01655

Stephen O. Heard, M.D.
Professor, Department of Anesthesiology, University of Massachusetts Medical School; Co-Director, Surgical Intensive Care, Department of Anesthesiology, UMass Memorial Health Care, Worcester, Massachusetts 01655

Stephan Heckers, M.D.
Massachusetts General Hospital, Charlestown, Massachusetts 02129

Robert C. Hendel, M.D.
Associate Professor of Medicine, Northwestern University Medical School; Associate Director, Critical Care Unit, Northwestern Memorial Hospital, Chicago, Illinois 60611

Hashim M. Hesham, M.D.
Assistant Professor, Department of Surgery, Albany Medical College; Attending Surgeon, Department of Surgery, Albany Medical Center, Albany, New York 12110

Robert J. Heyka, M.D.
Department of Hypertension and Nephrology, Cleveland Clinic Foundation, Cleveland, Ohio 44195

Helen Hollingsworth, M.D.
Associate Professor, Department of Medicine, Pulmonary Center, Boston University School of Medicine; Director, Adult Asthma and Allergy Services, Department of Medicine, Boston Medical Center, Boston, Massachusetts 02118

Abhinav Humar, M.D.
Assistant Professor, Department of Surgery, University of Minnesota; Transplant Surgeon, Department of Surgery, Fairview—University Medical Center, Minneapolis, Minnesota 55455

Eric S. Iida, M.D.
Department of Renal Medicine, UMass Memorial Health Care, Worcester, Massachusetts 01655

Richard S. Irwin, M.D.
Professor of Medicine, University of Massachusetts Medical School; Director, Department of Pulmonary, Allergy, and Critical Care Medicine, UMass Memorial Health Care, Worcester, Massachusetts 01655

Teresa E. Jacobs, M.D.
Clinical Instructor, Department of Medicine, University of Washington Medical School, Seattle Pulmonary Associates, Seattle, Washington 98104

Peter J. Jederlinic, M.D.
Associate Professor, College of Physicians and Surgeons, Columbia University; Department of Medicine, Mary Imogene Bassett Hospital, Cooperstown, New York 13326

Paul G. Jodka, M.D.
Assistant Professor, Department of Medicine, Tufts University School of Medicine, Boston, Massachusetts; Attending Physician, Department of Medicine, Critical Care, BayState Medical Center, Springfield, Massachusetts, 01199

Carol A. Kauffman, M.D.
Chief, Department of Infectious Diseases, Veterans Affairs Medical Center; Professor, Department of Medicine, University of Michigan Medical Center, Ann Arbor, Michigan 48109

Shubjeet Kaur, M.D.
Assistant Professor, Department of Anesthesiology, University of Massachusetts Medical School; Vice-Chair, Clinical Affairs, Co-Medical Director, Operative Services, Department of Anesthesiology, UMass Memorial Health Care, Worcester, Massachusetts 01655

Carey D. Kimmelstiel, M.D.
Assistant Professor, Tufts University School of Medicine; Associate Director, Cardiac Catheterization Laboratory; Director, Clinical Cardiology, New England Medical Center, Boston, Massachusetts 02111

John Kitzmiller, M.D.
Associate Professor, Department of Plastic Surgery, University of Cincinnati College of Medicine, Cincinnati, Ohio 45267

Lawrence A. Labbate, M.D.
Ralph H. Johnson Veterans Affairs Medical Center, Charleston, South Carolina 29401

Jean-François Lambert, M.D.
Research Fellow, Department of Hematology and Medical Oncology, UMass Memorial Health Care, Worcester, Massachusetts 01655

Stephen E. Lapinsky, M.D.
Assistant Professor, Department of Medicine, University of Toronto, Toronto, Ontario M65 4E9, Canada

Rhonda L. Larsen
PA-C, MHS, Department of Medicine, Duke University; Director, Cardiology Site Coordination, Duke Clinical Research Institute, Duke University Medical Center, Durham, North Carolina 27710

Poh Hock Leng, M.D.
Department of Pulmonary, Allergy, and Critical Care Medicine, UMass Memorial Health Care, Worcester, Massachusetts 01655

Erica L. Liebelt, M.D.
Assistant Professor, Department of Pediatrics, Johns Hopkins School of Medicine; Medical Toxicologist, Johns Hopkins Hospital, Baltimore, Maryland 21287

Christopher H. Linden, M.D.
Associate Professor, Department of Emergency Medicine—Toxicology, UMass Memorial Health Care, Worcester, Massachusetts 01655

Carol F. Lippa, M.D.
Department of Neurology, Medical College of Pennsylvania, Hahnemann University, Philadelphia, Pennsylvania 19129

N. Scott Litofsky, M.D.
Associate Professor, Department of Neurosurgery, University of Massachusetts Medical School and UMass Memorial Health Care, Worcester, Massachusetts 01655

Nancy Y.N. Liu, M.D.
Department of Rheumatology, UMass Memorial Health Care, Worcester, Massachusetts 01655

Randall R. Long, M.D., Ph.D.
Associate Professor, Department of Neurology, University of Massachusetts Medical School and UMass Memorial Health Care, Worcester, Massachusetts 01655

Christopher Longcope, M.D.
Professor of Obstetrics, Gynecology, and Medicine, University of Massachusetts Medical School, Worcester, Massachusetts 01655

Donald G. Love, M.D.
Instructor, Department of Medicine, Harvard Medical School, Beth Israel Deaconess Medical Center; Director of Cardiology Rehabilitation, Co-director of Electrophysiology, Department of Cardiology, MetroWest Medical Center, Framingham, Massachusetts 01701

Fred A. Luchette, M.D.
Associate Professor of Surgery, University of Cincinnati College of Medicine; Department of Surgery—Trauma and Critical Care, University of Cincinnati Medical Center, Cincinnati, Ohio 45267

J. Mark Madison, M.D.
Associate Professor of Medicine and Physiology, Director, Pulmonary Diagnostic Laboratories; Department of Pulmonary, Allergy, and Critical Care Medicine, UMass Memorial Health Care, Worcester, Massachusetts 01655

Brian J. Mady, M.D.
Assistant Professor of Medicine, Department of Infectious Diseases and Immunology, University of Massachusetts Medical School; Infectious Disease Specialist, Department of Infectious Diseases and Immunology, UMass Memorial Health Care, Worcester, Massachusetts 01655

Paul Ellis Marik, M.D., M.B.B.cH., F.C.P.(S.A.), F.C.C.M.
Director, MICU, Department of Medicine, Washington Hospital Center, Washington, DC 20010

Deborah H. Markowitz, M.D.
Assistant Professor of Medicine, Department of Pulmonary, Allergy, and Critical Care Medicine, University of Massachusetts School of Medicine; Assistant Director, Pulmonary Function Laboratory, UMass Memorial Health Care, Worcester, Massachusetts 01655

Freda D. McCarter, M.D.
Research Fellow, Department of Surgery, University of Cincinnati, Cincinnati, Ohio 45267

Robert M. Mentzer, M.D.
Department of Surgery, University of Cincinnati Medical Center, Cincinnati, Ohio 45267

Ann L. Mitchell, M.D.
Department of Neurology, UMass Memorial Health Care, Worcester, Massachusetts 01655

Robert S. Mittleman, M.D.
Associate Professor of Medicine, Director, Section of Cardiac Electrophysiology and Pacing, Department of Cardiovascular Medicine, UMass Memorial Health Care, Worcester, Massachusetts 01655

M. Ryan Moon, M.D.
Department of Surgery, University of Cincinnati Medical Center, Cincinnati, Ohio 45267

Majaz Moonis, M.D.
Assistant Professor, Department of Anesthesiology and Surgery, UMass Memorial Health Care, Worcester, Massachusetts 01655

John P. Mordes, M.D.
Department of Medicine, University of Massachusetts Medical School and UMass Memorial Health Care, Worcester, Massachusetts 01605

J. Cameron Muir, M.D.
Department of Oncology, Northwestern Memorial Hospital, Chicago, Illinois 60611

Michael S. Niederman, M.D.
Chief, Department of Pulmonary and Critical Care Medicine, Winthrop University Hospital, Mineola, New York 11501

Dominic J. Nompleggi, M.D., Ph.D.
Associate Professor of Medicine and Surgery, Director, Adult Nutrition Support Service, UMass Memorial Health Care, Worcester, Massachusetts 01655

Frank M. O'Connell, M.D.
Assistant Professor, Department of Anesthesiology and Surgery, UMass Memorial Health Care, Worcester, Massachusetts 01655

Steven M. Opal, M.D.
Professor of Medicine, Department of Infectious Diseases, Brown University School of Medicine; Memorial Hospital of Rhode Island, Pawtucket, Rhode Island 02860

Linda A. Pape, M.D.
Associate Professor of Medicine, Department of Cardiovascular Medicine, UMass Memorial Health Care, Worcester, Massachusetts 01655

Nereida A. Parada, M.D.
Assistant Professor, Department of Medicine, Boston University School of Medicine and Boston Medical Center, Boston, Massachusetts 02118

John A. Paraskos, M.D.
Professor of Medicine, Director, Cardiovascular Center and Ambulatory Cardiology Services; Department of Cardiovascular Medicine, UMass Memorial Health Care, Worcester, Massachusetts 01655

John J. Paris, S.J., Ph.D.
Walsh Professor of Bioethics, Department of Theology, Boston College, Chestnut Hill, Massachusetts 02167

David Paydarfar, M.D.
Department of Neurology, UMass Memorial Health Care, Worcester, Massachusetts 01655

Catherine A. Phillips, M.D.
Associate Professor, Department of Neurology, University of Massachusetts Medical School and UMass Memorial Health Care, Worcester, Massachusetts 01655

Mark H. Pollack, M.D.
Associate Professor, Department of Psychiatry, Massachusetts General Hospital, Boston, Massachusetts 02114

Jahn A. Pothier, M.D.
Department of Pulmonary, Allergy, and Critical Care Medicine, UMass Memorial Health Care, Worcester, Massachusetts 01655

Debra D. Poutsiaka, M.D., Ph.D.
Staff Physician, Department of Medicine, New England Medical Center; Assistant Professor, Department of Medicine, Tufts University School of Medicine, Boston, Massachusetts 02111

Chandra Prakash, M.D., M.R.C.P.
Department of Gastroenterology, Washington University School of Medicine; Department of Gastroenterology, Barnes-Jewish Hospital, St. Louis, Missouri 63110

Melvin R. Pratter, M.D.
Department of Pulmonary and Critical Care Medicine, University of Medicine and Dentistry of New Jersey; Robert Wood Johnson School of Medicine at Camden, Cooper Hospital—University Medical Center, Camden, New Jersey 08103

Juan Carlos Puyana, M.D.
Assistant Professor, Department of Surgery, Harvard Medical School; Director, Surgical Critical Care, Department of Surgery, Brigham and Women's Hospital, Boston, Massachusetts 02115

John Querques, M.D.
Clinical Fellow in Psychiatry, Massachusetts General Hospital, Boston, Massachusetts 02114

Paula D. Ravin, M.D.
Associate Professor, Department of Neurology, University of Massachusetts Medical School; Clinical Faculty, Department of Neurology, UMass Memorial Health Care, Worcester, Massachusetts 01655

Frank E. Reardon, J.D.
Hassan and Reardon, P. C., Boston, Massachusetts 02116

Lawrence D. Recht, M.D.
Department of Neurology, UMass Memorial Health Care, Worcester, Massachusetts 01655

Randall R. Reves, M.D., M.S.C.
Associate Professor, Department of Infectious Diseases, University of Colorado Health Science Center; Denver Public Health, Denver Health and Hospital Authority, Denver, Colorado 80204

Peter E. Rice, M.D.
Clinical Assistant Professor, State University of New York Health Science Center at Brooklyn; Department of Surgery, Brookdale Hospital Medical Center, Brooklyn, New York 11212

James M. Rippe, M.D.
Associate Professor of Medicine (Cardiology), Tufts University School of Medicine, Boston, Massachusetts; Director, The Center for Clinical and Lifestyle Research, Shrewsbury, Massachusetts 01545

Mark J. Rosen, M.D.
Chief, Department of Pulmonary and Critical Care Medicine, Beth Israel Medical Center; Professor of Medicine, Albert Einstein College of Medicine, New York, New York 10003

Marjorie Ross, M.D.
Department of Neurology, Newton Wellesley Hospital, Newton, Massachusetts 02462

Aldo A. Rossini, M.D.
Department of Diabetes, University of Massachusetts Medical School, UMass Memorial Health Care, Worcester, Massachusetts 01605

Alan L. Rothman, M.D.
Associate Professor, Department of Medicine, Molecular Genetics and Microbiology, University of Massachusetts Medical School; Attending Physician, Department of Medicine, UMass Memorial Health Care, Worcester, Massachusetts 01655

Lewis J. Rubin, M.D.
Department of Pulmonary and Critical Care Medicine, University of California at San Diego, San Diego, California 92103

Steven A. Sahn, M.D.
Professor of Medicine, Director, Department of Pulmonary and Critical Care Medicine, Allergy, and Clinical Immunology, Medical University of South Carolina, Charleston, South Carolina 29425

Diane M. F. Savarese, M.D.
Assistant Professor, Department of Medicine, University of Massachusetts Medical School, Department of Hematology and Medical Oncology, UMass Memorial Health Care, Worcester, Massachusetts 01655

Claire A. Scanlon, M.D.
Department of Renal Medicine, UMass Memorial Health Care, Worcester, Massachusetts 01655

Oren P. Schaefer, M.D.
Assistant Professor, Department of Medicine, University of Massachusetts Medical School; Director, Pulmonary Medicine Fellowship, Department of Medicine, Division of Pulmonary, Allergy, and Critical Care Medicine, UMass Memorial Health Care, Worcester, Massachusetts 01655

Mrinal Sharma, M.D.
Clinical Assistant Professor of Medicine, Georgetown Medical School, Washington, DC 20007; Virginia Medical Associates, Springfield, Virginia 22151

Sara J. Shumway, M.D.
Professor of Surgery, University of Minnesota, Minneapolis, Minnesota 55455

Nicholas A. Smyrnios, M.D.
Associate Professor, Department of Medicine, University of Massachusetts Medical School; Director, Medical Intensive Care Unit, Department of Medicine, Division of Pulmonary, Allergy, and Critical Care Medicine, UMass Memorial Health Care, Worcester, Massachusetts 01655

Frederick A. Spencer, M.D.
Assistant Professor, Associate Director of Coronary Care Unit, Medical Director of Cardiac Rehabilitation, UMass Memorial Health Care, Cardiovascular Thrombosis Research Center, Worcester, Massachusetts 01655

David H. Spodick, M.D., D.Sc., F.A.C.C.
Professor, Department of Medicine/Cardiology, University of Massachusetts Medical School; Director, Clinical Cardiology and Cardiovascular Fellowships, Department of Medicine/Cardiology, Worcester Medical Center, Worcester, Massachusetts 01604

Michael L. Steer, M.D.
Professor of Surgery, Beth Israel Deaconess Medical Center, Harvard Medical School, Boston, Massachusetts 02215

Theodore A. Stern, M.D.
Associate Professor of Psychiatry, Harvard Medical School; Chief, The Avery D. Weisman Consultation Service; Department of Psychiatry, Massachusetts General Hospital, Boston, Massachusetts 02114

Donald S. Stevens, M.D.
Department of Anesthesiology, UMass Memorial Health Care, Worcester, Massachusetts 01655

F. Marc Stewart, M.D.
Chief, Department of Hematology and Medical Oncology, University of Massachusetts Medical School, UMass Memorial Health Care, Worcester, Massachusetts 01655

Peter H. Stone, M.D.
Co-Director, Samuel A. Levine Cardiac Unit; Director, Clinical Trials Center, Department of Cardiovascular Medicine, Brigham and Women's Hospital, Boston, Massachusetts 02115

Naveen A. Syed, M.D.
UMass Memorial Health Care, Worcester, Massachusetts 01655

George E. Tesar, M.D.
Chairman, Department of Psychiatry and Psychology, The Cleveland Clinic Foundation, Cleveland, Ohio 44195

Pierre Théroux, M.D.
Research Center, Institut de Cardiologie, University of Montreal—Montreal Heart Institute, Montreal, Quebec H1T 1C8, Canada

Michael J. Thompson, M.D.
Assistant Professor of Medicine, Department of Diabetes, University of Massachusetts Medical School, UMass Memorial Health Care, Worcester, Massachusetts 01655

Arthur L. Trask, M.D., F.A.C.S.
Trauma Services, Fairfax Hospital, Falls Church, Virginia 22046

Christoph Troppmann, M.D.
Department of Surgery, University of Zurich, CH-8091 Zurich, Switzerland

Jeffrey R. Tucker, M.D.
Department of Emergency Medicine, Connecticut Children's Medical Center, Hartford, Connecticut 06106

Joseph Varon, M.D., F.A.C.P., F.C.C.P., F.C.C.M.
Associate Professor, Department of Medicine, Baylor College of Medicine; Research Director, Department of Emergency Services, The Methodist Hospital, Houston, Texas 77030

Michael C. Vredenburg, D.O.
Section Chief, Department of Cardiology, St. Mary's Medical Center, Grand Rapids, Michigan 49503

Michael J. Waligora, M.D.
Northwestern Memorial Hospital, Chicago, Illinois 60611

William V. Walsh, M.D.
Assistant Professor, Department of Medicine, University of Massachusetts Medical School; Physician, Department of Hematology and Medical Oncology, UMass Memorial Health Care, Worcester, Massachusetts 01655

Richard Y. Wang, D.O.
Assistant Professor, Department of Medicine, Brown University School of Medicine; Director, Medical Toxicology, Department of Emergency Medicine, Rhode Island Hospital, Providence, Rhode Island 02903

John P. Weaver, M.D.
Associate Professor, Department of Neurosurgery, University of Massachusetts Medical School; Director, Cerebrovascular Program, Co-Director, Surgical Epilepsy Program, Department of Neurosurgery, UMass Memorial Health Care, Worcester, Massachusetts 01655

John G. Weg, M.D.
Professor of Internal Medicine, Medical Director of Critical Care Support Services, Department of Pulmonary and Critical Care Medicine, University of Michigan Medical Center, Ann Arbor, Michigan 48109

Arthur Williams, M.D.
Senior Resident, Department of General Surgery, University of Cincinnati, Cincinnati, Ohio 45267

Mark M. Wilson, M.D.
Assistant Professor, Department of Medicine, University of Massachusetts Medical School; Associate Director of Medical Intensive Care Unit, Department of Pulmonary, Allergy, and Critical Care Medicine, UMass Memorial Health Care, Worcester, Massachusetts 01655

Dietmar H. Wittmann, M.D., Ph.D.
Professor of Surgery, Medical College of Wisconsin, Milwaukee, Wisconsin 53045

Janice Zaleskas
University of Massachusetts Medical School, Worcester, Massachusetts 01655

PREFACE

We are proud to present the third edition of the *Manual of Intensive Care Medicine*. The first two editions established this *Manual* as a leading source of information in the complex field of critical care. The practical format and user-friendly, portable size of the *Manual* have made it a particularly useful addition to bedside practice in critical and intensive care, and a valuable teaching tool and reference for students, interns, residents, fellows, and others practicing in the intensive care environment.

Since the publication of the second edition of *Manual of Intensive Care Medicine* nearly 10 years ago, dramatic changes have swept the field of critical care. Much of this new knowledge has been summarized in the fourth edition of our large-format textbook, *Irwin and Rippe's Intensive Care Medicine* (Lippincott Williams & Wilkins, 1999). The third edition of the *Manual* is intended to parallel the fourth edition of our textbook. Although this has increased the scope of the *Manual* compared with previous editions, we feel that this approach will be most beneficial to practitioners of intensive care. As in previous editions, chapters are pared down to emphasize essential concepts, and, whenever possible, information is presented in tables and illustrations. Annotated references are provided to guide the interested reader through key articles in the relevant literature.

The *Manual of Intensive Care Medicine* opens with an extensive section on Procedures and Techniques. The next eight sections are divided according to organ systems. In each chapter, discussions of key entities that present in the intensive care or coronary care environment are presented together with targeted discussions focusing on treatment.

Section 10 conveys a thorough review of Pharmacology, Overdoses, and Poisonings, recognizing that these remain important issues in intensive care. The next two sections focus on Surgical Issues in critical care as well as Shock and Trauma. These sections are intended to provide practitioners with a thorough overview of these important aspects of intensive care medicine. Finally, the *Manual* closes with sections on Neurology, Transplantation, Rheumatology and Immunology, Psychiatry, and Moral, Ethical, and Legal Issues in intensive care—all crucial to a comprehensive view of adult intensive care medicine.

The third edition of the *Manual of Intensive Care Medicine* has been totally rewritten to incorporate modern understandings of both medical and surgical intensive care. Although it is intended to stand alone to provide useful information to the bedside practice of intensive care, it also has a direct relationship with *Irwin and Rippe's Intensive Care Medicine*, Fourth Edition, and can be effectively used both as an entrée into the larger book, as well as a study guide and companion.

We acknowledge the contributors to the fourth edition of our textbook, *Irwin and Rippe's Intensive Care Medicine*. Although the *Manual of Intensive Care Medicine* has been edited and revised with the expert guidance of many section editors, the chapters were developed based on the expert knowledge of the original textbook contributors, reorganized and rewritten in a style necessary for the scope of this portable text.

We also acknowledge and thank a number of individuals, without whose able assistance, the third edition of this *Manual* would not have been possible. First and foremost, Dr. Rippe's Editorial Director, Elizabeth Porcaro, has provided expert work organizing and expediting all aspects of manuscript preparation. Without Beth's superb editorial skills, this project would be inconceivable. Karol Lempicki, Dr. Irwin's Administrative Assistant has provided important assistance in managing his complex clinical and academic endeavors. Carol Moreau, Executive Assistant to Dr. Rippe, expertly juggled the diverse aspects of his clinical, research, and travel calendar to allow time for efforts of this magnitude. A special word of thanks to our Editor, Craig Percy, who strongly urged us to generate this third edition and supported the process every step of the way. Stephanie Harris at Lippincott Williams & Wilkins lent expert editorial assistance throughout the process.

We particularly thank the section editors for the *Manual*—each of whom contributed long hours and expert guidance required to ensure that the *Manual* would contain state-of-the-art, yet user-friendly information.

Finally, we thank our families: Diane, Jamie, and Rebecca Irwin; Rachel and Andrew Koh; Sara, John, and Ben DiIorio; and Stephanie, Hart, Jaelin, and Devon Rippe, who continue to love and support us in all of our efforts, both personal and academic.

We hope that what has emerged from the efforts of all of these outstanding people is a practical, user-friendly book that will continue to advance the knowledge and efforts of the many fine clinicians who practice in the intensive care environment.

James M. Rippe, M.D.
Richard S. Irwin, M.D.

I. PROCEDURES AND TECHNIQUES

1. AIRWAY MANAGEMENT AND ENDOTRACHEAL INTUBATION

Shubjeet Kaur and Stephen O. Heard

Management of the airway to ensure optimal ventilation and oxygenation, with or without endotracheal intubation, is a skill every critical care specialist should possess.

I. **Anatomy.** The respiratory passage includes the nose, the nasopharynx, the mouth, the oropharynx, the hypopharynx, the larynx, and the trachea. The tracheal carina is located at the fourth thoracic vertebral level. The right main bronchus takes off at a less acute angle than the left, a configuration making right main bronchial intubation more common if the endotracheal tube is placed too far down the respiratory passage. Abnormal anatomy in any of the foregoing can preclude successful attempts at mask ventilation and endotracheal intubation.

   A. **Airway obstruction.** Upper airway obstruction may occur secondary to the tongue's falling backward or to soft tissue collapse in the oropharynx. In a patient suspected of having a cervical spine injury, the jaw thrust maneuver can be used. In other patients, the head tilt–chin lift maneuver can be used. The head tilt is accomplished by placing one's palm on the patient's forehead and applying pressure to extend the patient's head about the atlantooccipital joint. Alternatively, the chin lift, performed by placing several fingers of the other hand in the patient's submental area to lift the mandible, can be used in conjunction with the head tilt. In a spontaneously breathing patient, establishing this head position may constitute sufficient treatment.

   B. **Airway adjuncts.** An oropharyngeal (Fig. 1-1) or nasopharyngeal airway (Fig. 1-1) can be used to establish an adequate airway when head positioning alone is inadequate. The oropharyngeal airway is semicircular and can be inserted by turning the curved portion toward the palate as it enters the mouth. It is then advanced beyond the posterior portion of the tongue and is rotated 180 degrees into position. An oropharyngeal airway should only be used in unconscious patients because it can cause gagging and vomiting. Alternatively, in the semi-awake patient who does not have extensive facial trauma or cerebrospinal rhinorrhea, a nasopharyngeal airway can be used. This is a soft rubber or plastic tube inserted, after lubrication, through the nostril into the posterior pharynx.

   C. **Use of face mask and bag valve device.** In a patient in respiratory arrest, one may deliver oxygen through a mask and bag valve device. One ensures a tight mask fit over the patient's mouth and nose by using one's left hand and alternately compressing and releasing the bag with the right hand. Rise and fall of the chest indicate good air exchange.

   D. **Other airway adjuncts.** The laryngeal mask airway (Fig. 1-2) can be positioned without direct visualization of the vocal cords and conforms to the shape of the laryngeal inlet.

II. **Indications for intubation.** The following broad categories encompass the majority of indications for endotracheal intubation: (a) acute airway obstruction, (b) secretions, (c) loss of protective reflexes, and (d) respiratory failure.

   Rapid assessment of the patient's airway anatomy can be performed even in the most urgent of situations. Evaluation of mouth opening (normal is 40 mm), dentition, cervical spine mobility (flexion-extension), thyromental distance (normal is three finger breadths), and the function of the temporomandibular joints is key to subsequent success and avoidance of complications. A history of degenerative arthritis (especially rheumatoid arthritis with its risk of atlantooccipital dislocation) should be carefully taken. Removable bridge work and dentures should be taken out before intubation. Mallampati and associates developed a clinical classification based on the size of the posterior aspect of the tongue relative to the oropharynx to predict the ease of intubation. In patients with a class I airway (Fig. 1-3) (faucial pillars, uvular, soft palate, and posterior pharyngeal well visualized),

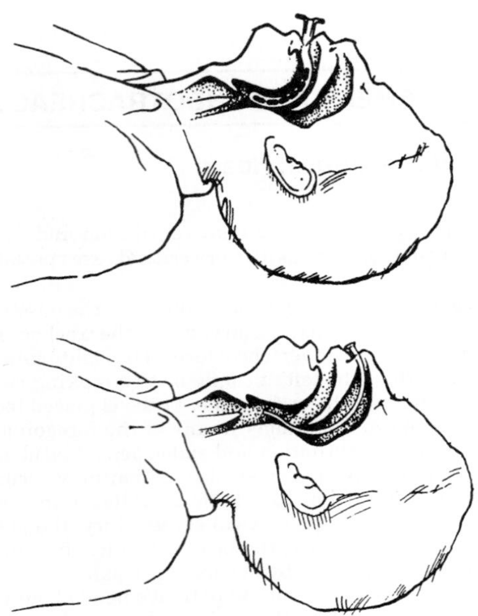

FIG. 1-1. Top: The proper position of the oropharyngeal airway. **Bottom:** The proper position of the nasopharyngeal airway. (Reprinted with permission from *Textbook of advanced cardiac life support.* Dallas, TX: American Heart Association, 1997.)

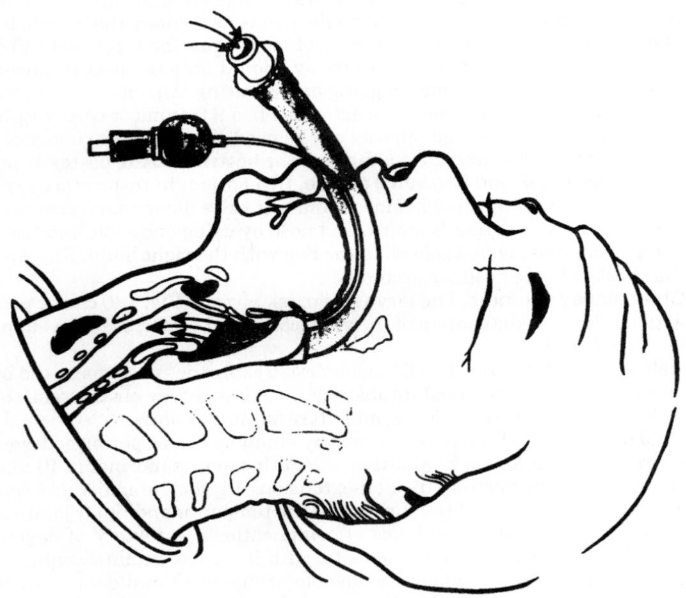

FIG. 1-2. Correct position of the laryngeal mask airway. (From Maltby JR, Loken RG, Watson NC, et al. The laryngeal mask airway: clinical appraisal in 250 patients. *Can J Anaesth* 1990;37:509, with permission.)

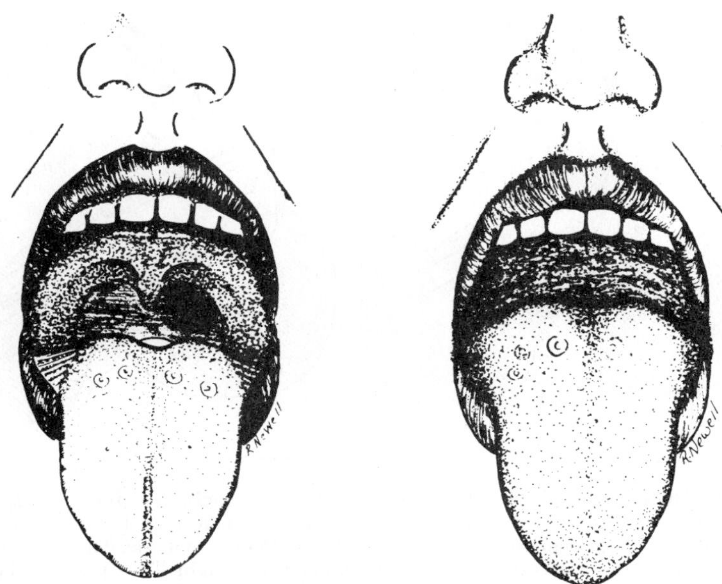

FIG. 1-3. The faucial pillars, soft palate, and uvula are not visible in the patient on the **right.** One should expect difficulty in orotracheal intubation. (From Mallampati SR, Gatt SP, Gugino LD, et al. A clinical sign to predict difficult tracheal intubation: a prospective study. *Can Anaesth Soc J* 1985;32:420, with permission.)

a relatively easy intubation can be anticipated. In those with a class III airway (Fig. 1-3) (only soft palate visualized), it may be extremely difficult to expose the glottic opening by direct laryngoscopy.

III. Equipment. To complete intubation successfully, the following must be readily available: a source of 100% oxygen, suction plus a large-bore tonsil suction tip (Yankauer), and a well-fitting mask with bag valve device. Other necessary supplies include a functional laryngoscope handle and blades (curved and straight), a tongue depressor, endotracheal tubes of different sizes, a stylet, and a syringe for cuff inflation.

A. Laryngoscopes. The choice of laryngoscope blade shape is a matter of personal preference and experience. The curved blade (MacIntosh) is placed in the vallecula, and the handle of the laryngoscope is pulled up and away from the operator (at a 45-degree angle) to lift the epiglottis indirectly and to expose the glottic opening (Fig. 1-4). The tip of the straight blade (Miller) is used to lift the epiglottis directly (Fig. 1-4) and is more useful in patients who have a cephalad and anterior laryngeal inlet.

B. Endotracheal tubes. Selection of proper tube diameter is important because resistance to airflow varies with the fourth power of the radius of the endotracheal tube. Guidelines for appropriate tube selection are summarized (Table 1-1).

IV. Technique of intubation.

A. Orotracheal intubation. This is the most commonly employed route for emergency intubations. Successful orotracheal intubation requires alignment of the oral, pharyngeal, and laryngeal axes (Fig. 1-5). The patient's head should be in the sniffing position (neck flexed and head slightly extended). In the unconscious patient who is considered to have a full stomach, laryngoscopy can

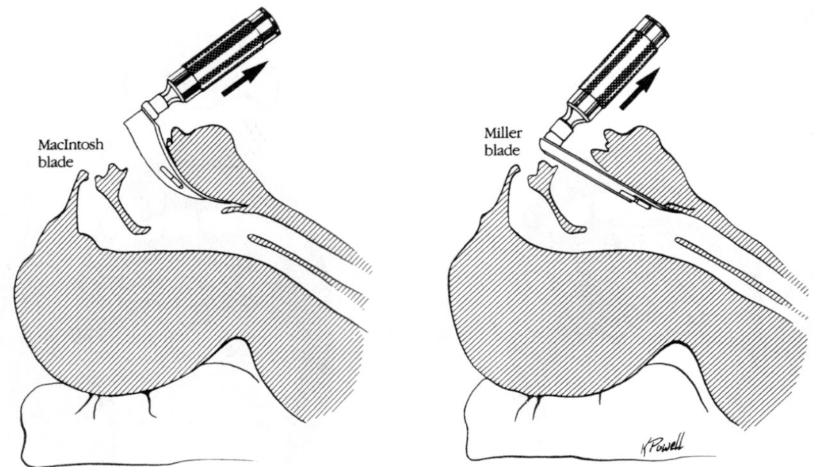

FIG. 1-4. The two basic types of laryngoscope blades, MacIntosh **(left)** and Miller **(right).** The MacIntosh blade is curved. The blade tip is placed in the vallecula, and the handle of the laryngoscope pulled forward at a 45-degree angle. This maneuver allows visualization of the epiglottis. The Miller blade is straight. The tip is placed posterior to the epiglottis, thus pinning the epiglottis between the base of the tongue and the straight laryngoscope blade. The motion on the laryngoscope handle is the same as that used with the MacIntosh.

be performed with cricoid pressure (Sellick maneuver). The Sellick maneuver is applied by compressing the cricoid cartilage posteriorly against the vertebral body to occlude the esophagus. This maneuver can prevent passive regurgitation of stomach contents into the trachea during intubation.

The laryngoscope handle is grasped in the left hand while the patient's mouth is opened with the gloved right hand. Often in the sniffing position, the

TABLE 1-1. Dimensions of endotracheal tubes based on patient age

Age	Internal Diameter (mm)	French Unit	Distance inserted from Lips for Tip Placement in Mid-trachea* (cm)
Premature	2.5	10	10
Full term	3.0	12	11
1–6 mo	3.5	14	11
6–12 mo	4.0	16	12
2 yr	4.5	18	13
4 yr	5.0	20	14
6 yr	5.5	22	15–16
8 yr	6.0	24	16–17
10 yr	6.5	26	17–18
12 yr	7.0	28–30	18–22
≥14 yr	7.0 (females)	28–30	20–24
	8.0 (males)	32–34	

*Add 2 to 3 cm for nasal tubes.

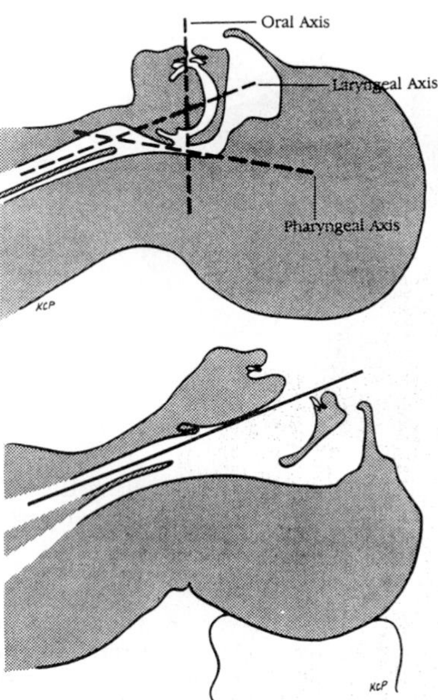

FIG. 1-5. Top: In the supine patient, the axes of the mouth, pharynx, and the larynx lie in divergent directions. To facilitate intubation, the axes of these three regions must be brought into close approximation. **Bottom:** With the patient's head in the proper position and with the use of the laryngoscope, the axes of the mouth, pharynx, and larynx can be brought into approximation, thus allowing easy visualization of the opening to the larynx.

unconscious patient's mouth will open; if not, the thumb and index finger of the operator's right hand are placed on the patient's lower and upper incisors, respectively, and are moved past each other in a scissorlike motion. The laryngoscope blade is inserted on the right side of the patient's mouth, is advanced to the base of the tongue, and pushes it toward the left.

With the blade in place, the operator should lift it forward in a plane 45 degrees from the horizontal to expose the vocal cords (Figs. 1-4 and 1-6). It is essential to keep the left wrist stiff and to do all lifting from the arm and shoulder, to avoid turning the patient's teeth into a fulcrum. The endotracheal tube is then held in the right hand and is inserted at the right corner of the patient's mouth in a plane that intersects with the laryngoscope blade at the level of the glottis. This technique prevents the endotracheal tube from obscuring the operator's view of the vocal cords. The endotracheal tube is advanced through the vocal cords until the cuff just disappears from sight. The cuff is then inflated with enough air to prevent a leak during positive-pressure ventilation with a bag valve device.

Proper depth of tube placement is clinically ascertained by observing symmetric expansion of both sides of the chest and auscultating equal breath sounds in both lungs. A useful rule of thumb for tube placement in adults of average size is that the incisors should be at the 23-cm mark in men and at the 21-cm mark in women. The stomach should also be auscultated to ensure that the esophagus has not been entered.

In the awake patient, the tongue and posterior pharynx may be anesthetized using a combination of lidocaine spray (1% to 9%) or a viscous lidocaine gel (20%).

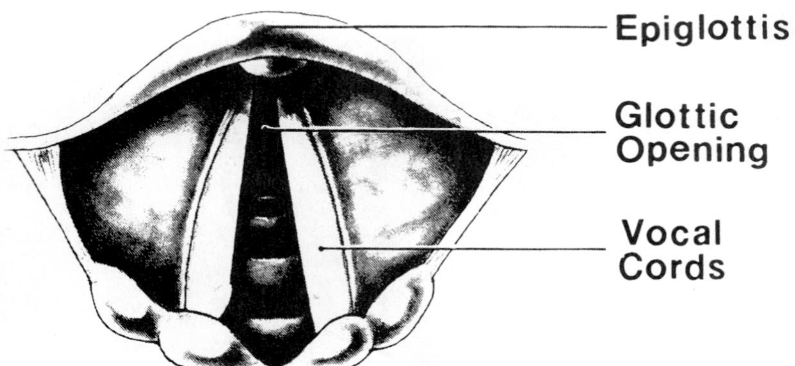

FIG. 1-6. Superior view of the larynx. (From Stoelting RK, Miller RD. *Basics of anesthesia.* New York: Churchill Livingstone, 1989, with permission.)

Anesthesia below the vocal cord is obtained by performing a transtracheal block with 4% lidocaine administered by cricothyroid membrane puncture with a small needle. Blind nasotracheal intubation and fiberoptic (oral or nasal) intubation are other viable options. Alternatively, general anesthesia may need to be administered by an anesthesiologist to intubate the patient.

B. Fiberoptic bronchoscope intubation. This is an extremely useful technique in patients with distorted airway anatomy or suspected cervical spine injury. After obtaining adequate topical anesthesia and with the endotracheal tube positioned over the bronchoscope, the operator introduces the fiberoptic bronchoscope into the patient's mouth or nose and advances it through the vocal cords into the trachea. The endotracheal tube is then advanced over the bronchoscope.

C. Cricothyrotomy. When intubation is unsuccessful and the situation is emergent, a cricothyrotomy may be required. A needle cricothyrotomy can be done by introducing a large-bore (i.e., 14-gauge) catheter attached to a syringe into the airway through the cricothyroid membrane while applying constant aspiration. Aspiration of air confirms tracheal placement. The catheter can be threaded in and then attached to a 3 cc syringe which can be connected to the endotracheal tube adapter from a size 7-mm ID endotracheal tube. A bag valve device and a high frequency jet ventilator can then be used to maintain oxygenation. Techniques of performing a standard cricothyrotomy are outlined in Chapter 12.

V. Airway management in the intubated patient. Once the endotracheal tube is in place and proper placement has been assessed by auscultation, the tube should be securely taped. A chest radiograph should be obtained to confirm optimal position and to rule out right main bronchus intubation. In patients requiring prolonged ventilatory support, intracuff pressures should be monitored daily and should be maintained between 17 and 23 mm Hg, thereby reducing the risk of tracheal mucosal ischemia.

If an *endotracheal tube change* is required because of an air leak or obstruction, one must approach the problem with the utmost caution. Review of the history to assess ease or difficulty of previous intubation and mask ventilation should be done. Any change in the patient's condition (e.g., fluid overload, facial or upper airway swelling) should be carefully evaluated. It is preferable that the tube be changed under direct vision by doing a laryngoscopy. If visualization is difficult, a tube changer (Eschmann stylet) can be used as a stent over which the old endotracheal tube is pulled out and the new one is threaded. Equipment (fiberoptic bronchoscope or a laryngeal mask airway) to deal with unanticipated airway problems should be readily available.

VI. Complications of endotracheal intubation. Complications may occur during intubation and include aspiration, damage to teeth, perforation of the oropharynx or larynx, epistaxis, hypoxemia, myocardial ischemia, and noncariogenic pulmonary edema.

Long-term intubation may result in tracheal mucosal ulceration or blockage or kinking of tube. Postextubation sore throat, hoarseness, or even stridor (in the pediatric population) may occur secondary to some degree of vocal cord or subglottic edema. Tracheal stenosis is a feared late complication of long-term endotracheal intubation.

VII. Extubation. Criteria for safe extubation are based on appropriate weaning from mechanical ventilation, a fully awake patient who is able to protect his or her airway, and sufficient resolution of the initial indication for intubation.

Emergency airway equipment to manage postextubation problems (e.g., laryngospasm) should be available. With the head of the bed at a 45-degree angle, the patient's oropharynx should be suctioned and the endotracheal tube removed under positive pressure after cuff deflation. Supplemental oxygen is then provided, and the patient is observed in a monitored setting until the physician rules out the need for reintubation.

Selected Readings

Bishop MJ, Weymuller EA, Fink BR. Laryngeal effects of prolonged intubation. *Anesth Analg* 1984;63:335.

Good review article describing the complications of long-term endotracheal intubation.

Holinger P, Johnson K. Factors responsible for laryngeal obstruction in infants. *JAMA* 1950;143:1229.

Good article about laryngeal obstruction in infants.

Koch E, Benumof JL. Percutaneous transtracheal jet ventilation: an important airway adjunct. *AANA J* 1990;58:337.

Description of the use of transtracheal jet ventilation to gain airway control in an emergency obstructed upper airway situation.

Mallampati SR, Gatt SP, Gugino LD, et al. A clinical sign to predict difficult tracheal intubation: a prospective study. *Can Anaesth Soc J* 1985;32:420.

Landmark article describing the Mallampati grading of airway to predict the degree of difficulty in laryngeal exposure during intubation.

Messeter KH, Pettersson KI. Endotracheal intubation with the fiberoptic bronchoscope. *Anaesthesia* 1980;35:294.

Basic description of endotracheal intubation with a fiberoptic bronchoscope.

Owen RI, Cheney FW. Endobronchial intubation: a preventable complication. *Anesthesiology* 1987;67:255.

Assessment of the correct depth of endotracheal tube placement to prevent mainstem intubation.

Rosenbaum SH, Rosenbaum LM, Cole RP, et al. Use of the flexible fiberoptic bronchoscope to change endotracheal tubes in the critically ill patient. *Anesthesiology* 1981;54:169.

Case report of use of fiberoptic bronchoscope to change the endotracheal tube.

Sellick BA. Cricoid pressure to control regurgitation of stomach contents during induction of anaesthesia. *Lancet* 1961;2:404.

Initial article describing the use of cricoid pressure to prevent regurgitation and aspiration of stomach contents.

Taylor PA, Towey RM. The broncho-fiberscope as an aid to endotracheal intubation. *Br J Anaesth* 1972;44:611.

Basic review of the use of the fiberoptic bronchoscope for endotracheal intubation.

Tintinall JE, Claffey J. Complications of nasotracheal intubation. *Ann Emerg Med* 1981;10:142.

Good review of the complications and difficulties associated with blind nasotracheal intubation.

Willms D, Shure D. Pulmonary edema due to upper airway obstruction in adults. *Chest* 1988;94:1090.

Case report describing pulmonary edema after acute airway obstruction.

2. CENTRAL VENOUS CATHETER

Shubjeet Kaur and Stephen O. Heard

I. Indications. Major indications for central venous catheter (CVC) placement include (a) monitoring of fluid status, (b) administration of irritant medications or vasoactive substances, (c) total parenteral nutrition, (d) hemodialysis, (e) placement of a temporary transvenous pacing wire, (f) procurement of venous access when peripheral vein cannulation is not possible, and (g) management of aspiration of air in surgical procedures considered high risk for venous air embolism (e.g., posterior fossa craniotomy with the patient in the sitting position).

II. Site selection. The major sites for CVC placement include (a) the internal jugular vein (IJV), (b) the subclavian vein (SCV), (c) the external jugular (ELV), (d) the femoral vein, and (e) the antecubital vein (peripherally inserted central catheters).

III. General Considerations and Complications

A. Catheter tip location. The ideal location for the catheter tip is the distal innominate or proximal superior vena cava, 3 to 5 cm proximal to the caval atrial junction. Positioning of the catheter tip within the right atrium or right ventricle may result in perforation of the cardiac wall and tamponade. Arrhythmias from mechanical irritation may also result from catheter tip malposition. The caval atrial junction is approximately 13 to 17 cm from the right-sided SCV or IJV insertion sites and 15 to 20 cm for left-sided insertions. Although an intracardiac electrogram can be used to position the catheter tip accurately, a chest radiograph to confirm appropriate placement and to rule out other complications (e.g., pneumothorax) is mandatory.

B. Vascular erosions. Large vessel erosion may occur 1 to 7 days after catheter insertion and is more common with left-sided insertions. Ideally, the catheter should be positioned parallel to the vessel wall to avoid this complication.

C. Air and catheter embolism. Air embolism during central line insertion may prove fatal and can be prevented by increasing venous pressure (Trendelenburg position) during catheter placement. Unexplained hypoxemia or cardiovascular collapse may occur. Immediate treatment entails placing the patient in the left lateral decubitus position and using the catheter to aspirate air from the right ventricle.

When a catheter-through or over-needle technique is used, catheter tip embolism can be prevented by not withdrawing the catheter over the needle during the insertion.

D. Coagulopathy. In patients with underlying coagulopathy (prothrombin time greater than 15 seconds, platelet count less than 50,000, or bleeding time greater than 10 minutes), CVC insertion may result in serious hemorrhagic complications, and EJV cannulation may be the safest approach. Alternatively, the IJV site is a safe alternative because it can be compressed.

E. Thrombosis. The incidence of thrombosis probably increases with the duration of catheterization, but it does not appear to be related to the site of insertion. All catheter materials currently used are thrombogenic; however, polyurethane coated with hydromer appears to be the best available material for bedside catheterization.

F. Antecubital approach

1. Anatomy. The basilic vein, found in the medial part of the antecubital fossa, is formed in the ulnar part of the dorsal venous network of the hand (Fig. 2-1). It joins the brachial vein in the upper arm to form the axillary vein, which provides an unimpeded path to the central venous circulation.

The cephalic vein is found in the lateral part of the antecubital fossa and, because of considerable interpatient anatomic variability, is a less reliable route to access the central circulation.

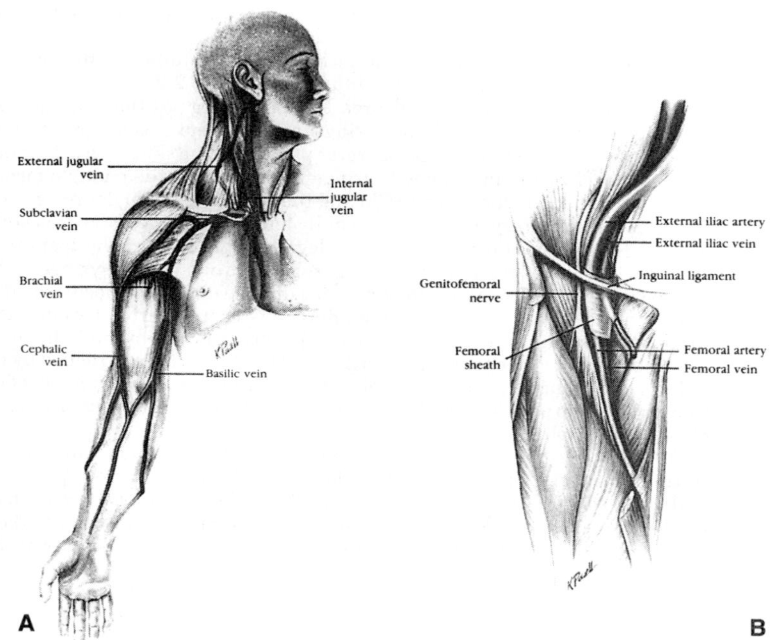

FIG. 2-1. A: Venous anatomy of the upper extremity. The internal jugular, external jugular, and subclavian veins are also shown. **B:** Anatomy of the femoral vein.

2. **Technique.** With the patient's arm at his or her side, the antecubital fossa (preferably the right) is prepared and draped with strict aseptic technique. A tourniquet is placed proximally to distend the vein, which is entered at a 45-degree angle with the needle level pointing upward and cephalad. To avoid catheter breakage and embolism secondary to bending at the patient's elbow, the point of insertion should be proximal to the antecubital crease if possible. When free backflow of blood is confirmed, the tourniquet is released, and the catheter is advanced over the guidewire using the Seldinger technique. The length of insertion is estimated by measuring the distance from the venipuncture site to the manubriosternal junction. The appropriate position is subsequently confirmed using a chest radiograph. The first-pass success rate is 70% with the basilic vein approach and 40% to 50% with the cephalic vein using this technique.
3. **Complications.** Complications associated with antecubital CVC include sterile phlebitis, thrombosis, infection, and pericardial tamponade.

G. Internal jugular approach

1. **Anatomy.** The IJV emerges from the base of the skull and enters the carotid sheath dorsally with the internal carotid artery (Fig. 2-1). It courses posterolateral to the artery beneath the sternocleidomastoid muscle (SCM) and lies medial to the anterior portion of the SCM in its upper part and beneath the triangle formed by the two heads of the muscle in the lower part, to enter the superior vena cava near the medial border of the anterior scalene muscle, beneath the sternal border of the clavicle. The straight path provided to the central venous circulation results in a high success rate of cannulation. The close anatomic relation of the IJV to the carotid artery, the stellate ganglion and cervical sympathetic trunk, the dome of the pleura (left higher

than right), and the thoracic duct on the right can result in complications from a misdirected needle.

2. **Technique.** The three general approaches to IJV cannulation are the anterior, central, and posterior and are illustrated in Fig. 2-2.

The patient is placed in a 15-degree Trendelenburg position and the head is turned to the contralateral side. Using standard aseptic technique, after infiltration of local anesthetic, the operator punctures the skin with a 22-gauge "finder" needle with an attached syringe at the apex of the triangle formed by the two muscle bellies of the SCM and the clavicle (central approach). The internal carotid artery pulsation is usually felt 1 to 2 cm medial to this point. The finder needle is directed at a 45-degree angle toward the ipsilateral nipple while the operator applies constant aspiration on the syringe. After successful venipuncture with the finder needle, the large-bore needle is introduced in the identical plane. The guidewire is then inserted through this large needle while one takes care to avoid ventricular arrhythmia by limiting insertion to no deeper than 15 to 20 cm. The CVC is then threaded by the Seldinger technique, using a scalpel to make a larger skin incision if needed. The catheter tip position should be confirmed by an immediate postprocedure chest radiograph.

The anterior approach (Fig. 2-2) is a viable alternative to IJV cannulation. Initial needle insertion is 0.5 to 1 cm lateral to the carotid artery pulsation at the midpoint of the sternal head of the SCM. The posterior approach uses the EJV as a landmark. The needle is inserted 1 cm dorsal to point where the EJV crosses the posterior border of the SCM or 5 cm cephalad from the

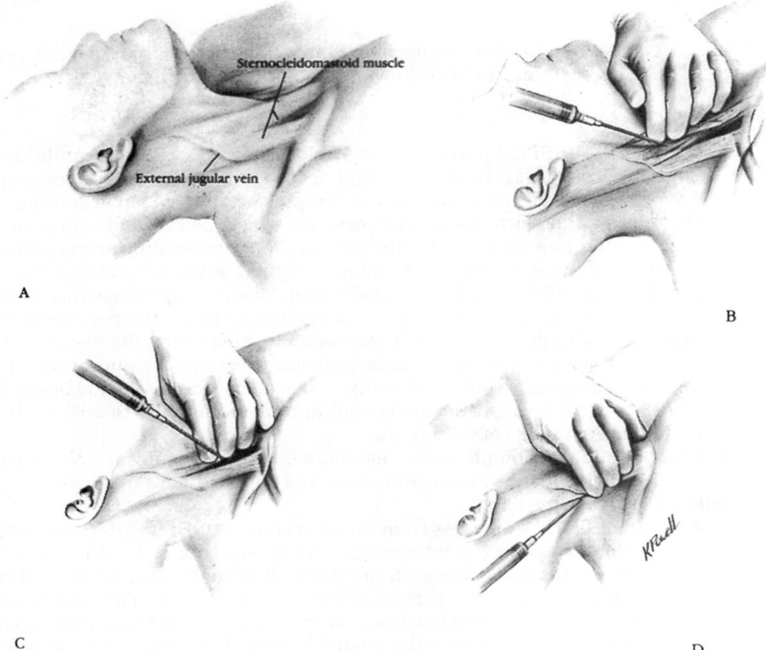

FIG. 2-2. Surface anatomy and various approaches to cannulation of the internal jugular vein. **A:** Surface anatomy. **B:** Anterior approach. **C:** Central approach. **D:** Posterior approach.

clavicle along the clavicular head of the SCM and is directed caudally and ventrally toward the suprasternal notch at an angle of 45 degrees from the sagittal plane and a 15-degree upward angulation.

3. **Complications.** The overall incidence of complications with the IJV approach ranges from 0.1% to 4.2% and includes carotid artery puncture, pneumothorax, vessel erosion, thrombosis and infection. Carotid artery puncture with a finder or larger needle, in the absence of a coagulopathy, can be managed by applying firm pressure to prevent hematoma formation. Accidental cannulation of the carotid artery with a 7-Fr catheter may require surgical exploration.

H. External jugular vein approach

1. **Anatomy.** The EJV is formed by the union of the posterior auricular and retromandibular veins, anterior and caudal to the ear, and courses obliquely across the anterior surface of the SCM (Fig. 2-1). It pierces the deep fascia posterior to the SCM and joins the SCV at a sharp acute angle behind the medial third of the clavicle.
2. **Technique.** The patient is placed in a slight Trendelenburg position, with arms by the side and face turned to the contralateral side. After sterile preparation, the venipuncture is performed with the 16-gauge catheter over the needle, using the operator's left index finger and thumb to distend and anchor the vein. The needle is advanced in the axis of the vein at 20 degrees to the frontal plane. When free backflow of blood is established, the needle is advanced a few millimeters further, and the catheter is threaded into the vein over the needle. A guidewire can be introduced through this catheter, and a CVC can be placed using the Seldinger technique. Abduction of the ipsilateral arm and anteroposterior pressure exerted on the clavicle may help the guidewire to negotiate the angle formed at the junction of the EJV with the SCV.

   The EJV can be successfully cannulated in 80% of patients, and serious associated complications are rare.

I. Femoral vein approach

1. **Anatomy.** The femoral vein (Fig. 2-1) is a direct continuation of the popliteal vein and becomes the external iliac vein at the inguinal ligament. At the ligament, it lies in the femoral sheath medial to the femoral artery and nerve.
2. **Technique.** Femoral vein cannulation can be performed with relative ease and a high success rate. The patient is placed supine, the groin is prepared and draped, and the venipuncture is made 1 to 1.5 cm medial to the femoral arterial pulsation. The femoral arterial pulsation is usually found at the junction of the medial and middle third of a line joining the anterior superior iliac spine and the pubic tubercle. An 18-gauge thin-walled needle attached to a syringe and is inserted at a 45-degree angle pointing cephalad, 2 to 3 cm inferior to the inguinal ligament, to minimize the risk of a retroperitoneal hematoma in the event of an arterial puncture. Once venous blood return is established, the syringe is depressed to skin level, and free aspiration of blood is reconfirmed. A guidewire and subsequently a dilator are advanced, and the catheter is finally threaded using the Seldinger technique.

   Arterial puncture, infection, and thromboembolic events are the most common complications of this approach.

J. Subclavian vein approach

1. **Anatomy.** The SCV is a direct continuation of the axillary vein, beginning at the lateral border of the first rib and extending 3 to 4 cm along the undersurface of the clavicle to join the ipsilateral IJV behind the sternoclavicular articulation to become the brachiocephalic vein (Fig. 2-1). Fibrous attachment to the clavicle prevents collapse of the vein even with significant hypovolemia. The SCV is bordered by muscles anteriorly, the subclavian artery and brachial plexus posteriorly, and the first rib inferiorly.
2. **Technique.** The infraclavicular or supraclavicular technique may be used to cannulate the SCV (Fig. 2-3). The patient is placed in a 15- to 30-degree Trendelenburg position, with a small bedroll between the scapulae. The head

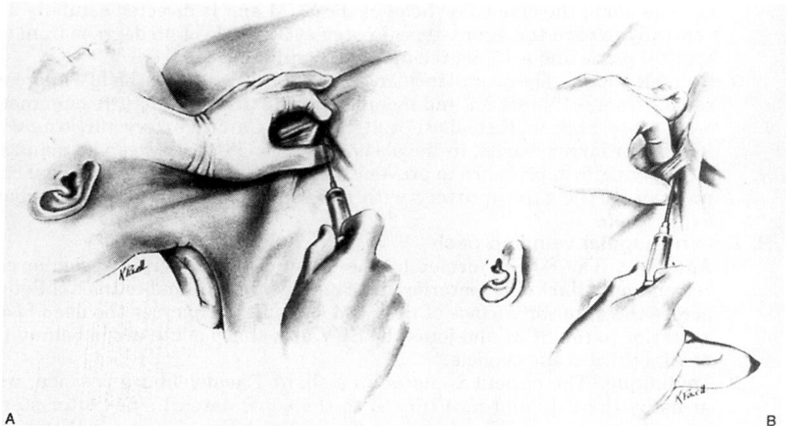

FIG. 2-3. A: Patient positioning for subclavian cannulation. **B:** Cannulation technique for the supraclavicular approach.

is turned to the contralateral site, and arms are by the side. For the infraclavicular approach (Fig. 2-3), skin puncture is made with an 18-gauge thin-wall needle attached to a syringe, 2 to 3 cm caudal to the midpoint of the clavicle and directed toward the suprasternal notch until it abuts the clavicle. The needle is then "walked" down the clavicle until the inferior edge is cleared. As the needle is advanced, it is kept as close to the inferior edge of the clavicle as possible to avoid puncturing the dome of the pleura. When blood return is established, the needle bevel (initially facing upward) is turned 90 degrees toward the heart, the syringe is removed, the guidewire is inserted, the needle is removed, and the CVC is advanced over the guidewire to the appropriate depth.

For the supraclavicular approach (Fig. 2-3), skin puncture is just above the clavicle and is lateral to the insertion of the clavicular head of the SCM. The needle is advanced toward the contralateral nipple, just under the clavicle, and it should enter the jugular subclavian at a depth of 1 to 4 cm. Depending on the operator's experience, a 90% to 95% success rate can be achieved with this approach. Major complications include pneumothorax, arterial puncture, and thromboembolism.

3. **Infection.** Infection is a dreaded risk of central venous cannulation. Methods to reduce risk include the use of sterile technique including maximum barrier precautions, chlorhexidine preparation, use of the SCV site for catheter insertion, and use of catheters impregnated with antiseptics or antibiotics.

Selected Readings

Ahmed N, Payne RF. Thrombosis after central venous cannulation. *Med J Aust* 1976; 1:217.

Good prospective analysis of the incidence of thrombosis after central venous cannulation.

Blitt CD, Wright WA, Petty WC, et al. Central venous catheterization via the external jugular vein: a technique employing the J-wire. *JAMA* 1974;229:817.

Basic description of CVC insertion using a J-wire through the EJV.

Bridges BB, Camden E, Takacs IA. Introduction of central venous pressure catheters through arm veins with a high success rate. *Can Anaesth Soc J* 1979;26:128.

Good description of how to optimize the success rate of CVC using the arm vein approach.

Czepiak CA, O'Callaghan JM, Venus B. Evaluation of formulas for optimal positioning of central venous catheters. *Chest* 1995;107:1662.

Good article validating the use of formulas to predict accurately the required length of CVC for optimal positioning.

Defalque RJ. Percutaneous catheterization of the internal jugular vein. *Anesth Analg* 1974;53:1.

Good basic review of the technique of CVC insertion using the IJV.

Doering RB, Stemmer EA, Connolly JE. Complications of indwelling venous catheters with particular reference to catheter embolism. *Am J Surg* 1967;114:259.

Good review of complications related to indwelling venous catheters.

Dripps RD, Eckenhoff JE, Vandam LD. *Introduction to anesthesia: the principles of safe practice,* 6th ed. Philadelphia: WB Saunders, 1982.

Excellent basic anesthesia textbook.

Lumley J, Russell WJ. Insertion of central venous catheters through arm veins. *Anaesth Intensive Care* 1975;3:101.

Review of a procedure to insert a CVC through the arm veins.

McGee WT, Mallory DL, Johans TG, et al. Safe placement of central venous catheters is facilitated using right atrial electrocardiography. *Crit Care Med* 1988;4:S434.

Abstract describing the use of right atrial electrocardiography to optimize placement of a CVC.

Morgan RNW, Morrell DF. Internal jugular catheterization: a review of a potentially lethal hazard. *Anaesthesia* 1981;36:512.

Case report describing a near-fatal hemorrhage resulting from vertebral artery laceration during IJV cannulation.

Seneff MG. Central venous catheterization: a comprehensive review: part 1. *J Intensive Care Med* 1987;2:163.

Excellent review of CVC insertion.

Wanscher M, Frifelt JJ, Smith-Sivertsen C, et al. Thrombosis caused by polyurethane double-lumen subclavian superior vena cava catheter and hemodialysis. *Crit Care Med* 1988;16:624.

Good article describing the incidence of thrombosis in patients with double-lumen catheters used for hemodialysis.

3. ARTERIAL LINE PLACEMENT AND CARE

Syed Adil Ahmed

I. Indications. Indications for arterial catheter insertion include hemodynamic monitoring, frequent arterial blood gas sampling, arterial administration of drugs such as thrombolytics, and use of an intraaortic balloon pump.

II. Equipment and sources of error. The equipment necessary to display and measure arterial waveform includes the following: (a) an appropriate intravascular catheter; (b) fluid-filled noncompliant tubing with stopcocks; (c) a transducer; (d) a constant flush device; and (e) electronic monitoring equipment, consisting of a connecting cable, a monitor with amplifier, an oscilloscope display screen, and a recorder.

Improper zeroing of the system is the single most important source of error. Calibration of the system is usually not necessary, because of standardization of the current disposable transducer. If the zero referencing and calibration are correct, a fast-flush test (Fig. 3-1) will assess the system's dynamic response. Overdamped tracings are usually caused by air bubbles, kinks, clot formation, compliant tubing, loose connections, a deflated pressure bag, or anatomic factors. All these problems are usually correctable.

III. Methods of cannulation

A. Insertion sites. The most commonly used sites for arterial cannulation in the adult are the radial, femoral, axillary, dorsalis pedis, and brachial arteries. Radial artery cannulation is attempted initially unless the patient is in shock or pulses are not palpable. If this technique fails, femoral artery cannulation should be performed.

B. Radial artery cannulation. Anatomy of the radial artery is shown in Fig. 3-2. The anastomoses between radial and ulnar arteries provide excellent collateral flow to the hand. A competent superficial or deep arch must be present to ensure adequate collateral flow. At least one of these arches may be absent in up to 20% of individuals.

1. **Modified Allen test.** The modified Allen test is sometimes used to assess the degree of collateral flow. To perform this test, the examiner compresses both radial and ulnar arteries and asks the patient to clinch and unclinch the fist repeatedly until pallor of the palm is produced. Hyperextension of the hand is avoided, because it may cause a false-negative result. One artery is then released, and the time to blushing of the palm is noted. The procedure is repeated with the other artery. Normal palmar blushing is complete before 7 seconds (positive test); 8 to 14 seconds is considered equivocal; and a result of 15 or more seconds is abnormal (negative test). The modified Allen test does not necessarily predict the presence of collateral circulation, and some centers have abandoned its use as a routine screening procedure.

2. **Percutaneous insertion.** The hand is placed in 30 to 60 degrees of dorsiflexion. The volar aspect of the wrist is prepared and draped using the sterile technique, and approximately 0.5 mL of lidocaine is infiltrated on the both sides of the artery through a 25-gauge needle. A 20-gauge, nontapered, Teflon 1.5- to 2-inch catheter-over-needle apparatus is used for the puncture. Entry is made at a 30- to 60-degree angle to the skin approximately 5 to 8 cm proximal to the distal wrist crease. The needle and cannula are advanced until blood return is noted in the hub, signifying intraarterial placement of the tip of the needle (Fig. 3-3). A small amount of further advancement is necessary for the cannula to enter the artery as well. With this accomplished, needle and cannula are brought flat to the skin, and the cannula is advanced to its hub with a firm, steady rotary action. Correct positioning is confirmed by pulsatile blood return on removal of the needle.

   Catheters with self-contained guidewires to facilitate passage of cannula into the artery are available. Percutaneous puncture is made in the same

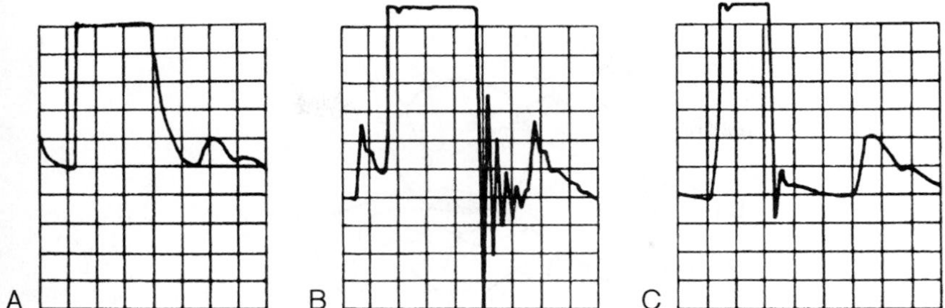

FIG. 3-1. Fast-flush test. **A:** Overdamped system. **B:** Underdamped system. **C:** Optimal damping.

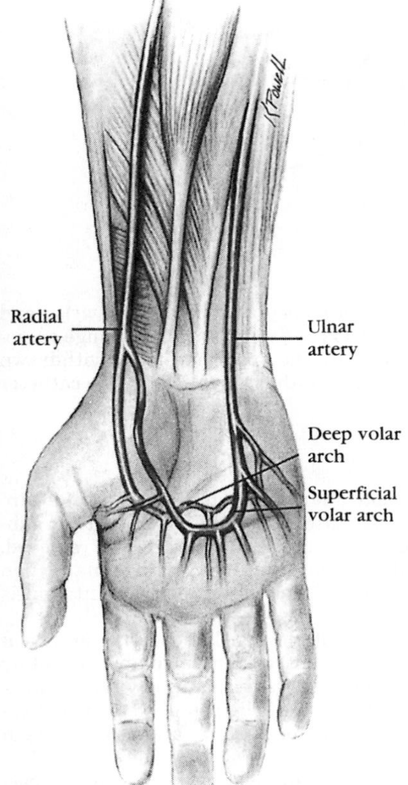

FIG. 3-2. Anatomy of the radial nerve. Note the collateral circulation to the ulnar artery through the deep volar arterial arch and dorsal arch.

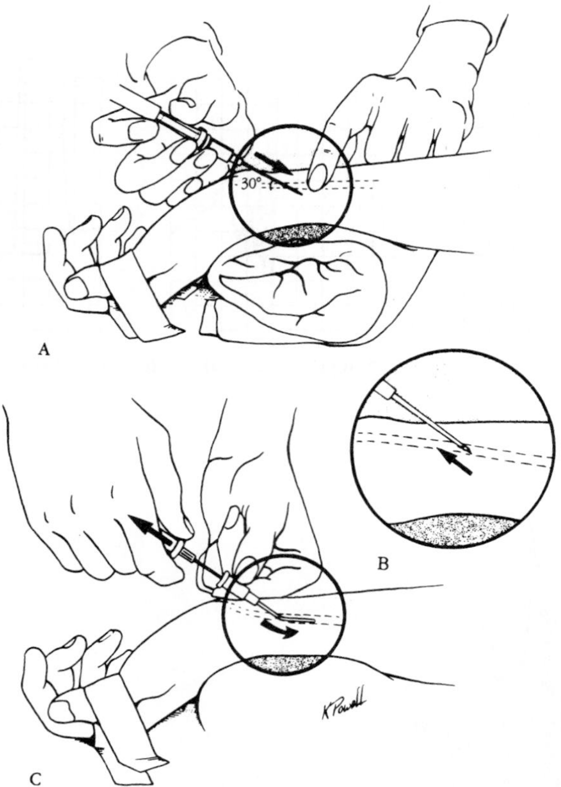

FIG. 3-3. Cannulation of the radial artery. **A:** A towel is placed behind the wrist, and the hand is immobilized with tape. The radial artery is fixated with a 20-gauge angiocatheter connected to a 5-mL syringe (optional). **B:** The angiocatheter is withdrawn until pulsatile blood return is noted. **C:** The trocar is withdrawn as the Teflon catheter is simultaneously advanced.

manner, but when blood return is noted in the catheter hub, the guidewire is passed through the needle into the artery to serve as a stent for subsequent catheter advancement. The guidewire and needle are then removed, and placement is confirmed by pulsatile blood return. The cannula is then secured firmly, it is attached to the transducer tubing, aseptic ointment is applied, and the site is bandaged.

C. Dorsalis pedis artery cannulation. The patient's foot is placed in plantar flexion and is prepared in the usual fashion. Vessel entry is obtained approximately halfway up the dorsum of the foot; advancement is the same as with cannulation of the radial artery. Systolic pressure readings are usually 5 to 20 mm Hg higher with dorsalis pedis catheters than with radial artery catheters, but mean pressure values are generally unchanged.

D. Brachial artery cannulation. Brachial artery cannulation is infrequently performed because of concern regarding the lack of effective collateral circulation. The median nerve lies in close proximity to the brachial artery in the antecubital fossa and may be punctured in 1% to 2% of cases. Cannulation of the brachial artery can be performed with a 2-inch catheter over-the-needle apparatus as described for radial artery catheterization.

E. **Femoral artery cannulation.** Anatomy of the femoral artery is shown in Fig. 3-4. The artery is cannulated using the Seldinger technique and any one of several available prepackaged kits. The patient lies supine with the leg extended and slightly abducted. Skin puncture should be made a few centimeters caudal to the inguinal ligament, to minimize the risk of retroperitoneal hematoma or bowel perforation. The thin-walled needle is directed, bevel up, cephalad at a 45-degree angle. When arterial blood return is confirmed, the needle and syringe are brought down against the skin to facilitate guidewire passage. The guidewire is inserted, the needle is withdrawn, and a stab incision is made with a scalpel at the skin puncture site. The catheter is threaded over the guidewire to its hub, and the guidewire is withdrawn. The catheter is then sutured securely to the skin and is connected to the transducer tubing.

F. **Axillary artery cannulation.** The patient's arm is abducted, externally rotated, and flexed at the elbow by having the patient place the hand under his or her head. The artery is palpated at the lower border of the pectoralis major muscle. The remainder of the catheterization proceeds as described for femoral artery cannulation.

IV. **Complications.** The complications associated with arterial catheterization are listed in Table 3-1.

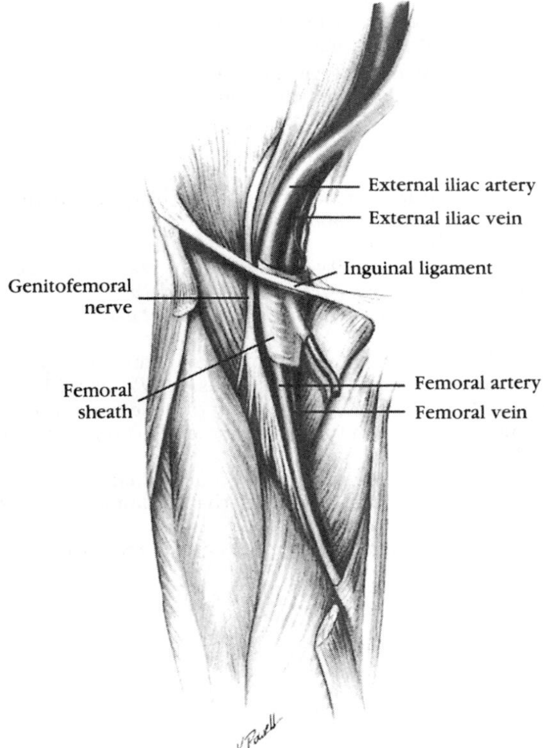

FIG. 3-4. Anatomy of the femoral artery and adjacent structures. The artery is cannulated below the inguinal ligament.

TABLE 3-1. Complications associated with arterial cannulation

Site	Complication
All sites	Pain and swelling
	Thrombosis
	Asymptomatic
	Symptomatic
	Embolization
	Hematoma
	Hemorrhage
	Limb ischemia
	Catheter-related infection
	Local
	Systemic
	Diagnostic blood loss
	Pseudoaneurysm
	Heparin-associated thrombocytopenia
Radial artery	Cerebral embolization
	Peripheral neuropathy
Femoral artery	Retroperitoneal hemorrhage
	Bowel perforation
	Arteriovenous fistula
Axillary artery	Cerebral embolization
	Brachial plexopathy
Brachial artery	Median nerve damage
	Cerebral embolization

Selected Readings

Ejrup B, Fischer B, Wright IS. Clinical evaluation of blood flow to the hand: the false-positive Allen test. *Circulation* 1966;33:778.
More detail about the Allen test.

Gardner RM. Accuracy and reliability of disposable pressure transducer coupled with modern pressure monitors. *Crit Care Med* 1996;24:879.
Good material to read for understanding of equipment used to monitor arterial pressure invasively.

Mann S, Jones RI, Miller-Craig MW, et al. The safety of ambulatory intraarterial pressure monitoring: a clinical audit of 1000 studies. *Int J Cardiol* 1984;5:585.
Details about complications related to brachial artery cannulation.

Slogoff S, Keats AS, Arlund C. On the safety of radial artery cannulation. *Anesthesiology* 1983;59:42.
Good review about the safety of radial artery cannulation.

Wilkins RG. Radial artery cannulation and ischemic damage: a review. *Anesthesia* 1985;40:896.
This article provides more detail about safety of this procedure.

4. PULMONARY ARTERY CATHETERS

Christopher Greene

I. General principles. Pulmonary artery (PA) catheterization and monitoring has four central objectives: (a) to assess left ventricular (LV) or right ventricular (RV) function, (b) to monitor hemodynamic status, (c) to guide treatment, and (d) to provide prognostic information.

The catheter is constructed from polyvinylchloride and has a pliable shaft that softens at body temperature. Because polyvinylchloride has a high thrombogenicity, the catheters are generally coated with heparin. The standard catheter length is 110 cm, and the most commonly used external diameter is 5 or 7 French. A balloon is fastened 1 to 2 mm from the tip; when it is inflated, it guides the catheter from the greater intrathoracic veins through the right heart chambers into the PA. Progression of the catheter is stopped when it makes impact in a PA slightly smaller in diameter than the fully inflated balloon. From this position, the PA wedge pressure (PAWP) is obtained. Balloon capacity varies. The balloon is usually inflated with air or filtered carbon dioxide but never liquids.

The most commonly employed PA catheter in the intensive care setting is a quadruple-lumen catheter, which has a lumen containing electrical leads for a thermistor positioned at the catheter surface 4 cm proximal to its tip. The thermistor measures PA blood temperature and allows thermodilution cardiac output measurements.

Several special-purpose PA catheter designs are available. Pacing PA catheters incorporate two groups of electrodes on the catheter surface, enabling intracardiac electrocardiographic (ECG) recording or temporary cardiac pacing. These catheters are used for emergency cardiac pacing, although it is often difficult to position the catheter for reliable simultaneous cardiac pacing and PA pressure measurements. A five-lumen catheter (Paceport RV catheter, CR Bard, Billerica, MA) allows passage of a specially designed 2.4-Fr bipolar pacing electrode probe through the additional lumen. This allows emergency temporary intracardiac pacing without the need for a separate central venous puncture. Continuous mixed venous oxygen saturation measurement is clinically available using a fiberoptic five-lumen PA catheter. Catheters equipped with fast-response (95 milliseconds) thermistors allow determination of RV ejection fraction (RVEF) and RV systolic time intervals.

II. Catheter insertion procedure. Techniques for insertion of Swan-Ganz catheters and handling of the monitoring equipment are described in many sources. Manufacturers' recommendations should be carefully followed, as should the individual institution's uniform procedure techniques and equipment preferences. Central venous access using the appropriate size of introducer sheath must first be obtained using sterile technique. Continuous monitoring of the ECG and pressure waveforms of the catheter is required as well as equipment and supplies for cardiopulmonary resuscitation.

Pass the catheter through the introducer sheath into the vein. Advance it, using the marks on the catheter shaft indicating 10-cm distances from the tip, until the tip is in the right atrium. This maneuver requires advancement of approximately 35 to 40 cm from the left antecubital fossa, 10 to 15 cm from the internal jugular vein, 10 cm from the subclavian vein, and 35 to 40 cm from the femoral vein. A right atrial waveform on the monitor with appropriate fluctuations accompanying respiratory changes or cough confirms proper intrathoracic location.

With the catheter tip in the right atrium, inflate the balloon with the recommended amount of air or carbon dioxide. Inflation of the balloon should be associated with a slight feeling of resistance—if it is not, suspect balloon rupture, and do not attempt further inflation or advancement of the catheter until balloon integrity has been properly reevaluated. If significant resistance to balloon inflation is encountered, suspect malposition of the catheter in a small vessel; withdraw the catheter and readvance it to a new position. Do not use liquids to inflate the balloon because they may be irretrievable and could prevent balloon deflation.

With the balloon inflated, advance the catheter until an RV pressure tracing is seen. Continue advancing the catheter until the diastolic pressure tracing rises above that observed in the RV center, thus indicating PA placement. Advancement beyond the PA position results in a fall on the pressure tracing from the levels of systolic pressure noted in the RV and PA. When this is noted, record the PAWP and deflate the balloon. Phasic PA pressure should reappear on the pressure tracing when the balloon is deflated. If it does not, pull back the catheter with the deflated balloon until the PA tracing appears.

Carefully record the balloon inflation volume needed to change the PA pressure tracing to the PAWP tracing. If the inflation volume is significantly lower than the manufacturer's recommended volume, or if subsequent PAWP determinations require decreasing balloon inflation volumes as compared with an initial appropriate volume, the catheter tip has migrated too far peripherally and should be pulled back immediately.

Secure the catheter in the correct PA position by suturing or taping it to the skin to prevent unintentional advancement. Apply a germicidal agent and dress the skin appropriately.

Order a chest radiograph to confirm the catheter's position; the catheter tip should appear no more than 3 to 5 cm from the midline.

III. Paceport catheter insertion procedure. The Paceport catheter has an additional lumen 19 cm from the catheter tip (the RV port), which allows passage of a specially designed 2.4-Fr pacemaker wire (probe). These catheters are used in patients who require hemodynamic monitoring and temporary ventricular pacing. When the probe is not in use, the RV port may be used to infuse fluid or medication. The catheter is inserted as described for a standard PA catheter. The pacemaker is introduced as follows:

Connect the RV port to a pressure transducer to verify the location of the orifice in the RV. Ideally, the RV orifice is positioned 1 to 2 cm distal to the tricuspid valve. To achieve this after initial placement, pull the catheter back until a right atrial pressure tracing is recorded from the RV port. Advance the catheter (with balloon inflated) until an RV pressure tracing is first obtained. At this point, the opening of the RV port is at the level of the tricuspid valve; simply advancing the catheter an additional 1 to 2 cm will place the opening in the desired position. The pacemaker probe can be introduced now or later.

A special package enables sterile introduction of the pacemaker probe. Mark the external part of the RV lumen to indicate how far the probe extends from the RV lumen opening into the RV. Attach the tip of the pacemaker probe introducer package to the hub of the RV port. Advance the 2.4-Fr pacing probe gently through the Paceport lumen. Passage of the probe is facilitated by keeping the extravascular portion of the PA catheter as straight as possible and by keeping the probe on its packaging spool during insertion. Allow the spool to spin slowly as the probe is advanced. When the marker on the probe reaches the 0 marking on the external part of the RV lumen, the tip of the probe is at the lumen opening.

Connect the distal electrode of the probe to the V lead of an ECG and advance it until ST-segment elevation occurs, thereby indicating contact with the endocardium. Connect the probe to a pacemaker generator and check the thresholds. Obtain a chest radiograph to ensure proper probe placement at the RV apex.

IV. Pressure and waveform interpretation

A. Right atrium. Normal resting right atrial pressure is 0 to 6 mm Hg. Three major positive-pressure waves, the A, C, and V waves, can usually be recorded (Fig. 4-1). The A wave is due to atrial contraction and follows the P wave of the ECG by approximately 80 msec. The C wave is due to the sudden motion of the atrioventricular valve ring toward the right atrium at the onset of ventricular systole. The C wave follows the A wave by a time period equal to the PR interval. The V wave represents the pressure generated by venous filling

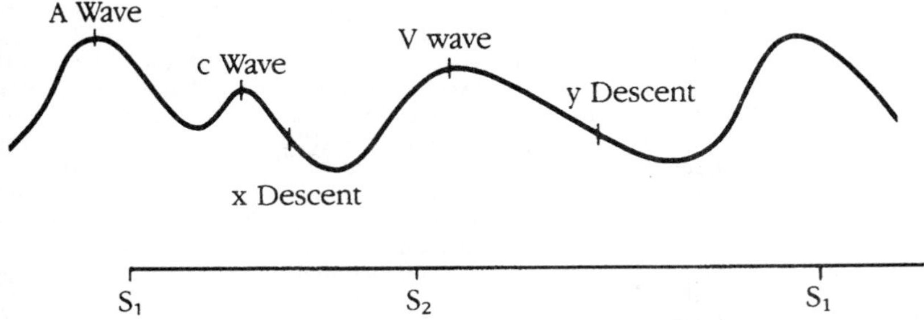

FIG. 4-1. Stylized representation of a right atrial waveform in relation to heart sounds. See text for discussion of A, C and V waves and *x* and *y* descents. (Adapted from Gore JM, Zwerner PL. Hemodynamic monitoring of acute myocardial infarction. In: Alpert JS, Francis GS, eds. *Modern coronary care.* Boston: Little, Brown, 1990, with permission.)

of the right atrium while the tricuspid valve is closed. The peak of the V wave occurs at the end of ventricular systole when the atrium is maximally filled and occurs near the end T wave. The *x* descent follows the c wave and reflects atrial relaxation. The *y* descent is due to rapid emptying of the atrium after opening of the tricuspid valve. The mean right atrial pressure decreases during inspiration (secondary to a decrease in intrathoracic pressure), whereas the A and V waves and the *x* and *y* descents become more prominent.

B. Right ventricle. The normal resting RV pressure is 17 to 30/0 to 6 mm Hg recorded when the PA catheter crosses the tricuspid valve. The RV systolic pressure should equal the PA systolic pressure (except in cases of pulmonic stenosis or RV outflow tract obstruction). The RV pressure should equal the mean right atrial pressure during diastole when the tricuspid valve is open.

C. Pulmonary artery. With the catheter in proper position and the balloon deflated, the distal lumen transmits PA pressure. Normal resting PA pressure is 15 to 30/5 to 13 mm Hg with a normal mean pressure of 10 to 18 mm Hg. The PA waveform is characterized by a systolic peak and diastolic trough with a dicrotic notch resulting from closure of the pulmonic valve. The peak PA systolic pressure occurs in the T wave of a simultaneously recorded ECG. Because the pulmonary vasculature is normally a low-resistance circuit, PA diastolic pressure is closely related to mean PAWP (usually 1 to 3 mm Hg higher than mean PAWP) and thus can be used as an index of LV filling pressure. However, if pulmonary vascular resistance is increased, PA diastolic pressure may markedly exceed mean PAWP.

D. Pulmonary artery wedge pressure. The PAWP is a phase-delayed, amplitude-dampened version of the left atrial pressure. The normal resting PAWP is 2 to 12 mm Hg and averages 2 to 7 mm Hg below the mean PA pressure. The PAWP waveform is similar to that of the right atrium with A, C, and V waves and *x* and *y* descents. Because of the time required for left atrial mechanical events to be transmitted through the pulmonary vasculature, PAWP waveforms are further delayed when they are recorded with a simultaneous EGG. The peak of the A wave follows the P wave by approximately 240 msec, and the peak of the V wave occurs after the T wave has been inscribed. Wedge position may be confirmed by measuring an oxygen saturation of 95% or more from blood withdrawn from the distal lumen. A valid PAWP measurement requires a patent vascular channel between the left atrium and the catheter tip. Thus, the PAWP approximates pulmonary venous pressure (and therefore left atrial pressure) only if the catheter tip lies in zone 3 of the lungs. A catheter wedged outside zone 3 shows marked respiratory variation, an unnaturally smooth vascular waveform, and misleadingly high pressures. Mean

PAWP correlates well with LV end-diastolic pressure (LVEDP), provided the patient has a normal mitral valve and normal LV function. The LVEDP may be significantly higher than mean left atrial pressure or PAWP in patients with decreased LV compliance. PAWP should be measured at end expiration because pleural pressure returns to baseline at the end of passive deflation. How much positive end-expiratory pressure (PEEP) is transmitted to the pleural space depends on lung compliance and other factors. Although it is difficult to estimate precisely the true transmural vascular pressure in a patient on PEEP, PCWP may still correspond closely with LVEDP even at high levels of PEEP. Temporarily disconnecting PEEP to measure PAWP is not recommended. Any measurements will be of questionable value because removing PEEP destabilizes the existing hemodynamics.

V. Cardiac output:thermodilution technique. Most PA catheters are equipped with a thermistor 4 cm from the tip that allows calculation of cardiac output using the thermodilution principle. In practice, a known amount of cold solution (typically 10 mL of 5% dextrose in water in adults and 5 mL of 5% dextrose in water in children) is injected into the right atrium through the catheter's proximal port. The thermistor allows recording of the baseline PA blood temperature and subsequent temperature change. Cardiac output is inversely proportional to the integral of the time-versus-temperature curve. Thermodilution cardiac output is inaccurate in low-output states, tricuspid regurgitation, and atrial or ventricular septal defects.

VI. Hemodynamic patterns in common clinical situations. Table 4-1 summarizes specific hemodynamic patterns for various disease entities. Preexisting hypertension or abnormal myocardial compliance can markedly alter these idealized values.

VII. Complications

A. Balloon rupture. Balloon rupture occurred more frequently in the early 1970s and was generally related to exceeding of recommended inflation volumes. The main problems posed by balloon rupture are air or balloon fragment emboli with attendant endocardial damage and thrombotic and arrhythmic complications.

B. Knotting. Knotting of a catheter around itself is most likely to occur when loops form in the cardiac chambers and the catheter is repeatedly withdrawn and readvanced. Knotting is avoided if care is taken not to advance the catheter significantly beyond the distances at which entrance to the ventricle or PA would ordinarily be anticipated.

C. Pulmonary infarction. Peripheral migration of the catheter tip (caused by catheter softening and loop tightening with time) with persistent, undetected wedging in small branches of the PA is the most common mechanism underlying pulmonary ischemic lesions attributable to PA catheters. These lesions are usually small and asymptomatic and are often diagnosed solely on the basis of changes in the chest radiograph demonstrating a wedge-shaped pleural-based density with a convex proximal contour. Severe infarctions are produced if the balloon is left inflated in the wedge position for an extended period. Boyd and colleagues found a 1.3% incidence of pulmonary infarction in a prospective study of 528 PA catheterizations done before the introduction of heparin-bonded catheters.

D. Pulmonary artery perforation. PA rupture or perforation has been reported in approximately 0.1% to 0.2% of patients, although recent pathologic data suggest that the true incidence of PA perforation is higher. Patient risk factors for PA perforation include pulmonary hypertension, mitral valve disease, advanced age, hypothermia, and anticoagulant therapy. Another infrequent but life-threatening complication is false aneurysm formation associated with rupture or dissection of the PA. Technical factors related to PA hemorrhage are distal placement or migration of the catheter, failure to remove large catheter loops placed in the cardiac chambers during insertion, excessive catheter manipulation, use of stiffer catheter designs, and multiple overzealous or prolonged balloon inflations. PA perforation typically presents with massive

TABLE 4-1. Hemodynamic parameters in commonly encountered clinical situations (idealized)

	RA	RV	PA	PAWP	AO	CI	SVR	PVR
Normal	0–6	25/0–6	25/6–12	6–12	130/80	≥2.5	1,500	≤250
Hypovolemic shock	0–2	15–20/0–2	15–20/2–6	2–6	≤90/60	<2.0	>1,500	≤250
Cardiogenic Shock	8	50/8	50/35	35	≤90/60	<2.0	>1,500	≤250
Septic Shock								
Early	0–2	20–25/0–2	20–25/0–6	0–6	≤90/60	≥2.5	<1,500	<250
Late[a]	0–4	25/4–10	25/4–10	4–10	≤90/60	<2.0	>1,500	>250
Acute massive pulmonary embolism	8–12	50/12	50/12–15	≤12	≤90/60	<2.0	>1,500	>450
Cardiac tamponade	12–18	25/12–18	25/12–18	12–18	≤90/60	<2.0	>1,500	≤250
AMI without LVF	0–6	25/0–6	25/12–18	≤18	140/90	≤2.5	1,500	≤250
AMI with LVF	0–6	30–40/0–6	30–40/18–25	>18	140/90	>2.0	>1,500	>250
Biventricular failure secondary to LVF	>6	50–60/>6	50–60/25	18–25	120/80	~2.0	>1,500	>250
RVF secondary to RVI	12–20	30/12–20	30/12	<12	≤90/60	<2.0	>1,500	>250
Cor pulmonale	>6	80/>6	80/35	<12	120/80	~2.0	>1,500	>400
Idiopathic pulmonary hypertension	0–6	80–100/0–6	80–100/40	<12	100/60	<2.0	>1,500	>500
Acute VSR[b]	6	60/6–8	60/35	30	≤90/60	<2.0	>1,500	>250

RA, right atrium; RV, right ventricle; PA, pulmonary artery; PAWP, pulmonary artery wedge pressure; AO, aortic; CI, cardiac index; SVR, systemic vascular resistance; PVR, pulmonary vascular resistance; AMI, acute myocardial infarction; LVF, left ventricular failure; RVF, right ventricular failure; RVI, right ventricular infarction; VSR, ventricular septal rupture.

[a]Hemodymanic profile seen in approximately one-third of patients in late septic shock.

[b]Confirmed by appropriate RA-PA oxygen saturation step-up.

Adapted from Gore JM, Albert JS, Benotti JR, et al. *Handbook of hemodynamic monitoring*. Boston: Little, Brown, 1984.

hemoptysis. Emergency management includes immediate wedge arteriography and bronchoscopy, intubation of the unaffected lung, and consideration of emergency lobectomy or pneumonectomy. PA catheter balloon tamponade resulted in rapid control of bleeding in one case report. Application of PEEP to intubated patients may also produce tamponade of hemorrhage caused by a PA catheter.

E. **Thromboembolic complications.** PA catheters are associated with an increased incidence of thrombosis. Thrombi encasing the catheter tip and aseptic thrombotic vegetations forming at endocardial sites in contact with the catheter have been reported. Heparin-bonded catheters reduce thrombogenicity and have become the most commonly employed PA catheters. An important complication of heparin-bonded catheters is heparin-induced thrombocytopenia. Routine platelet counts are recommended for patients with heparin-bonded catheters in place.

F. **Rhythm disturbances.** Atrial and ventricular arrhythmias occur commonly during insertion of PA catheters. Studies have reported advanced ventricular arrhythmias (three or more consecutive ventricular premature beats) in approximately 30% to 60% of patients undergoing right heart catheterization. Most arrhythmias are self-limited and do not require treatment, but sustained ventricular arrhythmias requiring treatment occur in 0% to 3% of patients. Risk factors associated with increased incidence of advanced ventricular arrhythmias are acute myocardial ischemia or infarction, hypoxia, acidosis, hypocalcemia, and hypokalemia. Patients with preexisting left bundle branch block are at risk of developing complete heart block during catheter insertion, although the frequency of catheter-induced right bundle branch block may be low.

G. **Intracardiac damage.** Damage to the right heart chambers, tricuspid valve, pulmonic valve, and their supporting structures as a consequence of PA catheterization has been reported. The incidence of catheter-induced endocardial disruption detected by pathologic examination varies from 3.4% to 75%, but most studies suggest a range of 20% to 30%. These lesions consist of hemorrhage, sterile thrombus, intimal fibrin deposition, and nonbacterial thrombotic endocarditis. The clinical significance is not clear, but there is concern that these lesions may serve as a nidus for infectious endocarditis. The incidence of intracardiac and valvular damage discovered on postmortem examination is considerably higher than that of clinically significant valvular dysfunction.

H. **Infections.** Several studies have suggested a rate of catheter-related septicemia of 0% to 1%. *In situ* time of more than 72 to 96 hours significantly increases the risk of catheter-related sepsis. The incidence of catheter colonization or contamination varies from 5% to 20%, depending on the duration of catheter placement and criteria used to define colonization.

VIII. **Appropriate use of pulmonary artery catheters.** A prospective, cohort study by Connors and colleagues reported an association between the use of PA catheterization and an increased risk of death, costs, length of stay, and intensity of care. Two previous retrospective studies had reported similar results. Until the results of future studies are available, clinicians employing hemodynamic monitoring should carefully assess the risk-to-benefit ratio on an individual basis.

Selected Readings

Becker RC, Martin RG, Underwood DA. Right sided endocardial lesions and flow directed pulmonary artery catheters. *Cleve Clin J Med* 1987;54:384.

Autopsy study with a 36% incidence of hemorrhagic or thrombotic lesions.

Boyd KD, Thomas SJ, Gold J, et al. A prospective study of complications of pulmonary artery catheterizations in 500 consecutive patients. *Chest* 1983;84:245.

"Serious" complications in 4.4% of patients, but no deaths attributable to the use of a PA catheter.

Connors, AF, Speroff T, Dawson NV, et al. The effectiveness of right heart catheterization in the initial care of critically ill patients. *JAMA* 1996;276:889.

Prospective cohort study of 5,735 patients in an intensive care unit illustrating the need for a randomized control trial of PA catheters.

Fraser RS. Catheter-induced pulmonary artery perforation: pathologic and pathogenic features. *Hum Pathol* 1987;18:1246.

Case report of four patients with PA perforation at autopsy.

Gore JM, Goldberg RJ, Spodick DH, et al. A community-wide assessment of the use of pulmonary artery catheters in patients with acute myocardial infarction. *Chest* 1987;92:721.

Retrospective study of 3,263 patients showing increased mortality in those receiving a PA catheter.

Laster JL, Nichols K, Silver D. Thrombocytopenia associated with heparin-coated catheters in patients with heparin-associated antiplatelet antibodies. *Arch Intern Med* 1989;149:2285.

Report of 12 cases.

Mark JB. *Atlas of cardiovascular monitoring.* New York: Churchill Livingstone, 1998.

Clear, concise manual for expert interpretation of hemodynamic waveforms.

O'Quin R, Marini JJ. Pulmonary artery occlusion pressure: clinical physiology, measurement, and interpretation. *Am Rev Respir Dis* 1983;128:319.

Nice discussion of possible errors made in the measurement of PAWP.

Patel C, Laboy V, Venus B, et al. Acute complications of pulmonary artery catheter insertion in critically ill patients. *Crit Care Med* 1985;14:195.

Forty-five percent incidence of transient, benign ventricular arrhythmias.

Pinilla JC, Ross DF, Martin T, et al. Study of the incidence of intravascular catheter infection and associated septicemia in critically ill patients. *Crit Care Med* 1983; 11:21.

Prospective study of 250 patients with a 16% and 2.7% respective incidence of PA catheter infection and septicemia.

Teboul JL, Zapol WM, Brun-Bruisson C, et al. A comparison of pulmonary artery occlusion pressure and left ventricular end-diastolic pressure during mechanical ventilation with PEEP in patients with severe ARDS. *Anesthesiology* 1989;70:261.

PAWP as a reliable indicator of LVEDP in adult respiratory distress syndrome with up to 20 PEEP.

Walston A, Kendall ME. Comparison of pulmonary wedge and left atrial pressure in man. *Am Heart J* 1973;86:159.

Retrospective review of 700 patients showing excellent correlation between PAWP and left atrial pressure over a wide range of cardiac diseases.

Zion, MM, Balkin J, Rosenmann D, et al. Use of pulmonary artery catheters in patients with acute myocardial infarction: analysis of experience in 5841 patients in the SPRINT registry. *Chest* 1990;98:1331.

Higher in-hospital mortality with the use of a PA catheter, but the authors conclude that "it is unlikely that PAC increases mortality."

5. TEMPORARY CARDIAC PACING

Paul G. Jodka

I. Indications. Temporary cardiac pacing is a potentially lifesaving treatment modality for the management of symptomatic, medically refractory rhythm and conduction disturbances. Indications for temporary pacing (both for treatment and diagnosis) are summarized in Table 5-1.

A. Diagnosis. The recording of an intraatrial electrocardiogram (ECG) through a temporary atrial pacing electrode can be helpful in the differential diagnosis of narrow- or wide-complex tachycardias whose mechanism is not readily apparent from the surface ECG. This technique can help define sites of origin of cardiac impulses as well as their path of conduction. For example, the conduction pattern between atria and ventricles may be shown to be antegrade, simultaneous, retrograde, or dissociated by comparison of limb lead tracings with simultaneous intraatrial recordings.

B. Treatment

1. Bradyarrhythmias. Sinus bradycardia, high-grade atrioventricular (A-V) block, and bradycardia-dependent ventricular tachycardia are examples of rhythm disturbances that typically respond to temporary pacing. In these disorders, etiologic factors may include myocardial ischemia or infarction, electrolyte disturbances, drug intoxications, and certain other processes that may influence cardiac impulse generation or propagation. Such precipitants should be sought, and corrected, concurrent with temporary pacing therapy.

2. Tachyarrhythmias. Temporary cardiac pacing has been used for both prevention and termination of some supraventricular and ventricular tachycardias.

Atrial pacing can be effective in the termination of atrial flutter and paroxysmal supraventricular tachycardia. Classic atrial flutter nearly always responds to electrical stimulation that provides a critical pacing rate (typically 125% to 135% of the flutter rate) lasting approximately 10 seconds. Pacing termination of atrial flutter is the preferred treatment in patients with epicardial wires in place after cardiac surgery, and it may also be attempted for conversion of atrial flutter in patients taking digoxin and those with sick sinus syndrome.

Rapid atrial pacing to induce atrial fibrillation has been used to prevent cases of recurrent supraventricular tachycardia with persistently rapid ventricular rate refractory to other interventions.

With atrial pacing, care must be exercised to avoid rapid ventricular stimulation and possible unstable ventricular rhythms.

Temporary pacing can be lifesaving in the prevention of paroxysmal ventricular tachycardia related to a prolonged QT interval (torsades de pointes), especially when this condition is secondary to drugs. When pacing is used for this indication, the aim is to achieve a mild tachycardia, thereby effectively shortening the QT interval.

The success of pacing for the treatment of tachyarrhythmias depends on a close familiarity with the available pacing modes and the clinical context in which the arrhythmias occur. This pacing application should be approached with extreme caution, because further ventricular rate acceleration or rhythm deterioration may occur.

3. Acute myocardial infarction. After acute myocardial infarction, numerous rhythm and conduction disturbances may be seen. Symptomatic bradyarrhythmias refractory to medical therapy require urgent treatment. A task force of the American College of Cardiology and the American Heart Association provided guidelines for temporary cardiac pacing in this setting (Table 5-2). Temporary cardiac pacing may be accomplished either transcutaneously or transvenously.

TABLE 5-1. Indications for acute (temporary) cardiac pacing

A. Conduction disturbances
  1. Symptomatic persistent complete heart block with inferior myocardial infarction
  2. Complete heart block, Mobitz type II AV block, new bifascicular block (e.g., right bundle branch block and left anterior hemiblock, left bundle branch block, first-degree heart block), or alternating left and right bundle branch block complicating acute anterior myocardial infarction
  3. Symptomatic idiopathic complete heart block, or high-degree AV block

B. Rate disturbances
  1. Hemodynamically significant or symptomatic sinus bradycardia
  2. Bradycardia-dependent ventricular tachycardia
  3. AV dissociation with inadequate cardiac output
  4. Polymorphic ventricular tachycardia with long QT interval (torsades de pointes)
  5. Recurrent ventricular tachycardia unresponsive to medical therapy
  6. Evaluation and treatment of supraventricular arrhythmias, including atrial flutter, AV nodal tachycardia, and Wolff-Parkinson-White syndrome

C. During electrophysiologic studies
  1. Evaluation of sinus node, AV node, and His bundle function
  2. Evaluation of wide QRS tachycardias
  3. Evaluation of therapeutic modalities for inducible ventricular and supraventricular tachycardia

AV, atrioventricular.

II. Equipment. Temporary cardiac pacing may be achieved by transvenous, transcutaneous, intraesophageal, or epicardial routes.

A. Transvenous pacing catheters. Transvenous pacing is the most commonly used technique for temporary pacing, and numerous pacing catheter designs and sizes are available. After central venous access has been obtained, standard stiff pacing catheters as well as flexible J-shaped catheters can be placed under fluoroscopic guidance. Flexible, balloon-tipped, flow-directed catheters are available for emergency use or in the absence of fluoroscopic capabilities.

TABLE 5-2. Recommendations for temporary pacemaker in acute myocardial infarction

A. Class I (indicated)
  1. Asystole
  2. Complete heart block
  3. Right bundle branch with left anterior or posterior hemiblock developing in acute myocardial infarction
  4. Type II second-degree atrioventricular block
  5. Symptomatic bradycardia unresponsive to atropine

B. Class IIa (probably indicated)
  1. Type I second-degree heart block with hypotension unresponsive to atropine
  2. Sinus bradycardia with hypotension unresponsive to atropine
  3. Recurrent sinus pauses unresponsive to atropine
  4. Atrial or ventricular overdrive pacing for incessant ventricular tachycardia

C. Class IIb (possibly indicated)
  1. Left bundle branch block with first-degree heart block of unknown duration
  2. Bifascicular block of unknown duration

From Gunnar RM, Passamani ER, Bourdillon PD, et al. Guidelines for the early management of patients with acute myocardial infarction: a report of the American College of Cardiology/American Heart Association Task Force on Assessment of Diagnostic and Therapeutic Cardiovascular Procedures. *J Am Coll Cardiol* 1990; 16:249, with permission.

Also available is a pulmonary artery catheter with a designated port that accommodates a pacing wire designed to allow right ventricular pacing.

B. Esophageal electrodes. Electrode designs include gelatin-coated bipolar "pill" electrodes that can be swallowed, as well as dedicated flexible transesophageal pacing catheters that do not require the patient's cooperation. Such devices can aid in the diagnosis of tachyarrhythmias and can be used to terminate supraventricular tachycardia and atrial flutter.

C. Transcutaneous external pacemakers. Transcutaneous external pacing has been used as an initial pacing mode in the treatment of bradyarrhythmia–asystolic arrest situations, medically refractory symptomatic bradyarrhythmias, overdrive pacing of tachyarrhythmias, and prophylactic pacing applications. Ease and rapidity of application, as well as its noninvasive nature, make transcutaneous pacing attractive, especially for emergency and prehospital use. Principal disadvantages of this form of pacing include a variable incidence of failure to capture and patient intolerance of the obligatory skeletal muscle stimulation.

D. Epicardial pacing. This pacing modality is primarily confined to the postoperative cardiac surgery setting. Placement of epicardial electrodes requires a thoracotomy or sternotomy.

E. Pulse generators for temporary pacing. Modern temporary pulse generators are capable of ventricular, atrial, and A-V–sequential pacing as well as allowing for synchronous or asynchronous pacing at variable rates, current outputs, sensing thresholds, and A-V pacing intervals or delays.

III. Choice of pacing mode. Common cardiac pacing modes are outlined in Table 5-3.

In emergencies, ventricular pacing should be established before attempting A-V–sequential pacing. Ventricular pacing treats bradycardia, but it does not restore the more ideal physiology of synchronized, sequential atrial and ventricular contractions. Possible consequences of A-V asynchrony are delineated in Table 5-4.

IV. Procedure. Once central venous access has been obtained, the pacing catheter is advanced under fluoroscopic guidance. In the absence of fluoroscopy, a flexible balloon-tipped pacing catheter can be placed using ECG guidance; here, the distal electrode of the catheter becomes a unipolar intracardiac lead by being attached to lead V_1 of an ECG machine while the patient is attached to standard limb leads. The catheter is advanced to the right ventricular apex. When the catheter contacts the ventricular endocardium, the ST segment of the intracardiac ECG is elevated ("current of injury") (Fig. 5-1).

Once the pacing catheter tip is positioned in the right ventricular apex, the pacer is put on asynchronous mode and is set at 10 to 20 beats per minute faster than the patient's intrinsic ventricular rate. The threshold current is set at 5 to 10 mA. Ventricular capture is evidenced by a pacemaker spike followed by a wide QRS complex. By gradually decreasing the current output of the pacemaker, the pacing threshold can be defined, ideally a value of less than 0.5 to 1.0 mA. The ventricular

TABLE 5-3. Common pacemaker modes for temporary cardiac pacing

Mode	Description
AOO	Atrial pacing: pacing is asynchronous
AAI	Atrial pacing, atrial sensing: pacing is on demand to provide a minimum programmed rate
VOO	Ventricular pacing: pacing is asynchronous
VVI	Ventricular pacing, ventricular sensing: pacing is on demand to provide a minimum programmed rate
DVI	Dual-chamber pacing, ventricular sensing: atrial pacing is asynchronous, ventricular pacing is on demand following a programmed atrioventricular delay
DDD	Dual-chamber pacing and sensing: atrial and ventricular pacing is on demand to provide a minimum rate, ventricular pacing follows a programmed atrioventricular delay, and upper-rate pacing limit should be programmed

TABLE 5-4. Adverse effects of ventricular pacing

Loss of atrial "kick"
Decreased left ventricular stroke volume
Increased left and right atrial pressure, Cannon A waves
Intermittent mitral and tricuspid regurgitation
Vasodepressor reflexes with hypotension, especially orthostatic
Potential arrhythmia induction (AF, SVT)
Ventriculoatrial conduction in some patients

AF, atrial fibrillation; SVT, supraventricular tachycardia.

output is then set to exceed the threshold current at least threefold. To convert the pacemaker from this VOO mode to the more desirable VVI mode, the pacing rate is set at 10 beats per minute less than the intrinsic rate, and the sensitivity control is changed from asynchronous to the minimum sensitivity level. Increasing the sensitivity until pacing spikes appear defines the sensing threshold. The pacing rate is then reset to the desired rate, with the sensitivity set at a level just below the sensing threshold.

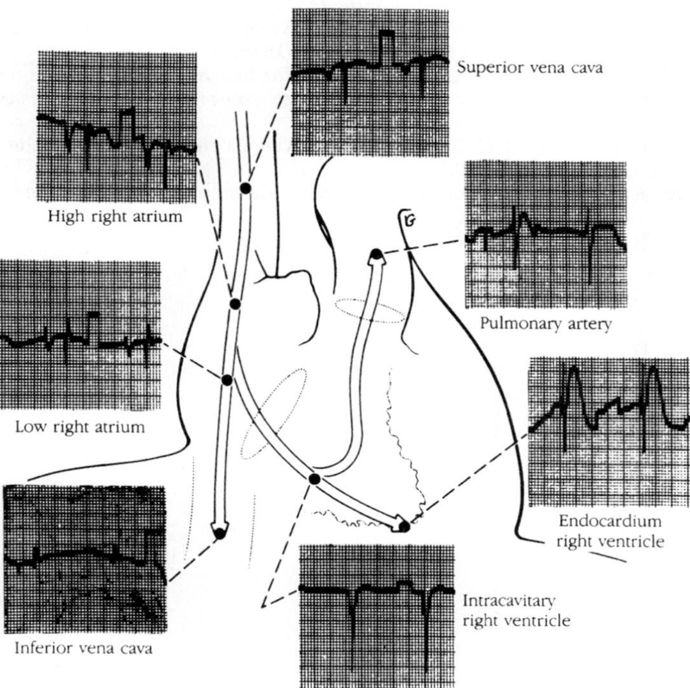

FIG. 5-1. Pattern of recorded electrogram at various locations in the venous circulation. (From Hawthorne JW, Eisenhauer AC, et al. Cardiac pacing. In: Eagle KA, Haber E, De Sanctis RW, eds. *The practice of cardiology: the medical and surgical cardiac units at the Massachusetts General Hospital.* Boston: Little, Brown, 1989, with permission.)

A-V sequential pacing requires catheter placement in the right atrial appendage under fluoroscopy. Atrial current is set to 20 mA at a rate exceeding the intrinsic atrial rate, and the A-V interval is set at 100 to 200 milliseconds. Atrial capture is manifested as atrial depolarization immediately after the pacing spike. A-V synchrony can be demonstrated by turning off the ventricular portion of the pacemaker.

V. Complications. Complications of temporary pacing from any venipuncture site include arrhythmias, pericardial friction rub, right ventricular perforation, cardiac tamponade, infection, pneumothorax, and diaphragmatic stimulation in addition to complications associated with venipuncture itself. Vascular access through the internal jugular or subclavian vein is generally preferred, and the incidence of complications is low in skilled hands. Insertion through the brachial vein is preferred in the patient receiving thrombolytic therapy or full-dose anticoagulation, although the risk of catheter-tip dislodgment from arm movement is increased relative to other access sites. The femoral venous approach is less desirable given an increased risk of deep venous thrombosis formation around the catheter.

Selected Readings

Das G, Anand K, Ankinfedu K, et al. Atrial pacing for cardioversion of atrial flutter in digitalized patients. *Am J Cardiol* 1978;41:308.

An early study demonstrating efficacy of atrial pacing for rhythm conversion in digitalized patients with atrial flutter.

Gunnar RM, Bourdillon PDV, Dixon DW, et al. Guidelines for the early management of patients with acute myocardial infarction: ACC/AHA Task Force Report. *J Am Coll Cardiol* 1990;16:249.

Guidelines for early management of patients with acute myocardial infarction.

Scarovsky S, Strasberg B, Lewin RF, et al. Polymorphous ventricular tachycardia: clinical features and treatment. *Am J Cardiol* 1979;44:339.

An early description of polymorphous ventricular tachycardia in patients with prolonged QT interval; 50% of patients had no recurrence of ventricular tachycardia with rapid ventricular pacing.

Silver MD, Goldschlager NG. Temporary transvenous cardiac pacing in the critical care setting. *Chest* 1988;93:607.

An overview of pacing applications with a brief discussion of complications.

6. CARDIOVERSION AND DEFIBRILLATION

Poh Hock Leng and Deborah H. Markowitz

I. General principles. The process of cardioversion and defibrillation involves delivering a quantity of electrical energy to depolarize the myocardium to terminate a tachyarrhythmia. Cardioversion delivers the shock at a specific point in the electromechanical cycle, before the termination of ventricular systole. The energy pulse is therefore *synchronized* to coincide with the R or S waves of the electrocardiographic (ECG) tracing. There is a significant risk of inducing ventricular fibrillation (VF) should the countershock fall on the "vulnerable" period of late ventricular systole. Thus, under most circumstances, emergency and elective treatment of various tachyarrhythmias requires *synchronized* cardioversion. Alternatively, defibrillation delivers electrical energy to terminate any fibrillating rhythm, including VF and atrial fibrillation (AF). Because VF is immediately life-threatening, and because there is no well-defined QRS complex, random delivery of an electrical pulse in VF is necessary for *unsynchronized* countershocks. Converting AF with electrical shocks is *technically defibrillation,* but the shocks are synchronized to the well-formed QRS complexes, as described earlier, to prevent degeneration into VF. Because the shocks are synchronized, many clinicians refer to the process as *cardioverting* AF.

II. Cardioversion procedure. Elective cardioversion should preferably only be performed in areas fully equipped for cardiopulmonary resuscitation. The patient's electrolytes should be normalized, and acidosis and hypoxemia should be corrected for greater success in maintaining normal sinus rhythm after cardioversion. The digoxin level should be within normal limits to prevent proarrhythmic side effects. Ideally, the patient should fast for at least 8 hours to prevent aspiration. A 12-lead ECG should be obtained before and after the procedure, and an intravenous catheter should be placed in case antiarrhythmic medications or pressors need to be infused on an emergency basis. The patient's blood pressure, heart rate and rhythm, and respiratory status should be monitored throughout the procedure. Short-acting sedatives, such as the benzodiazepine midazolam or propofol, are effective in providing anesthesia, carefully titrated to avoid respiratory depression and the need for mechanical ventilation.

The efficacy of the countershock depends on the size of the paddles, the skin-electrode interface, and the location of the paddles on the thorax. Hand-held paddles are traditional, but self-adhesive pads are available. The advantage of the self-adhesive pads is that the operator does not come into contact with the bed and thus avoids the risk of receiving an electrical shock. Moreover, if the defibrillator is equipped with pacing capabilities, the pads may be used for external pacing should unanticipated bradycardia or asystole occur after countershocking. Alternatively, hand-held paddles allow the operator to apply firm pressure during the procedure. Both electrode types need uniform application to the skin. Hand-held electrodes require a layer of conductive gel over their entire surface to prevent skin burns.

The electrodes may be placed in either the anterolateral or the anteroposterior location. Incorrect placement of the electrodes is the most common cause of unsuccessful cardioversion or defibrillation. When using the anterolateral position, one should place the anterior paddle just to the right of the patient's sternum and below the manubriosternal joint and the lateral paddle over the cardiac apex. If the anteroposterior position is selected, one should place the anterior paddle over the left precordium and the posterior paddle just below the tip of the left scapula. The monitor should be checked to ensure synchronization before discharge, when indicated. Discharge should occur, ideally, during patient exhalation to minimize the distance between the electrode and the heart, thereby decreasing transthoracic impedance. The electrical current is discharged only after the operator has ensured that no assisting personnel are in contact with the patient or the bed, because the electrical energy may be transmitted to other persons. It is important to recheck that synchronization is reestablished after each countershock with repeated attempts.

III. Cardioversion for specific arrhythmias

A. Atrial fibrillation. Cardioversion in AF should be performed in the hemodynamically unstable patient or under elective circumstances to attempt reversion to normal sinus rhythm. Before the procedure, the operator should consider the duration of AF, the embolic risk, and the likelihood of maintaining sinus rhythm after countershocking. In general, large atrial size (larger than 45 mm), long-standing arrhythmia (more than 1 year's duration), previous unsuccessful attempts, and intolerance to antiarrhythmic medications are believed to predict unsuccessful cardioversion. For elective cardioversion in patients with AF of undetermined onset or AF lasting longer than than 48 hours, anticoagulation is recommended for 3 weeks before and 4 weeks after cardioversion to minimize the risk of subsequent embolic events. A randomized trial is currently being conducted to determine whether a transesophageal echocardiogram allows for safe and immediate cardioversion without prior anticoagulation. Anticoagulation after the cardioversion is still indicated because residual electromechanical instability persists, despite the emergence of normal conduction. The starting dose for cardioverting AF is usually 100 J. If conversion does not occur, then each successive dose should be increased by 100 J to a maximum dose of 360 J.

B. Atrial flutter. Atrial flutter is a rhythm that responds to electrical cardioversion. Recommended starting doses are 25 to 50 J. The role of anticoagulation in atrial flutter to prevent thromboembolic events is controversial. However, because this rhythm may also represent an unstable atrial electromechanical process, most clinicians recommend anticoagulation, particularly when cardioversion is anticipated.

C. Supraventricular tachycardia. The success rate for cardioverting supraventricular tachycardia is high, approximately 75% to 80%. However, medications, especially adenosine, can also be used effectively. Increasing ventricular ectopy after low-dose shocks suggests the presence of digoxin toxicity, and further attempts at cardioversion should be abandoned.

D. Wolff-Parkinson-White syndrome. In Wolff-Parkinson-White (WPW) syndrome, patients have an accessory pathway that bypasses the atrioventricular node. Conduction down this pathway results in the familiar "delta" wave seen on the surface ECG, representing myocardial depolarization. Occasionally, supraventricular tachycardia reentrant circuits develop involving the atrioventricular node and the accessory pathway. Cardioversion may be beneficial for supraventricular tachycardias in WPW syndrome because countershocking breaks the reentrant circuit. Cardioversion is the treatment of choice for unstable AF in WPW syndrome. Most medications used to control ventricular rate in AF slow the atrioventricular node. However, blocking the atrioventricular node directs all the depolarizing atrial waves down the accessory path, which has a shorter refractory property than the atrioventricular node. Consequently, conduction proceeds down the accessory pathway and bombards the ventricle with depolarizations, risking VF. For hemodynamically stable patients, procainamide may also be used that stabilizes the myocardium and prolongs refractoriness of the accessory pathway.

E. Ventricular tachycardia. Cardioversion is one of the leading therapeutic options for monomorphic ventricular tachycardia. The starting energy dose required to convert ventricular tachycardia is typically 100 J, and the success rate is approximately 95% to 100%. It is preferable to employ cardioversion in the synchronized mode, except in an extreme emergency with rapid hemodynamic compromise that leaves insufficient time for synchronization and in ventricular flutter in which the presence of tall T waves may be mistaken for QRS complexes. Delivering an electrical current on a T wave risks degeneration to VF. Under these special circumstances, *unsynchronized* countershocking is warranted.

IV. Defibrillation. Rapid defibrillation is the major determinant of survival in cardiac arrest resulting from VF. The advanced cardiac life support guidelines for treating VF recommends three sequential shocks, beginning with 200 J. If VF persists, one should deliver a second shock at a dose of 300 J. The dose of the third and all subsequent shocks should be 360 J. The three shocks should be delivered sequentially before other therapies are initiated because the transthoracic impedance decreases immediately after the initial countershock. Consequently, subsequent shocks may be effective even when the initial shock had been unsuccessful. If the third shock fails to restore the rhythm, then one should continue cardiopulmonary resuscitation and follow the advanced cardiac life support protocol.

V. Cardioversion and defibrillation under special circumstances

A. Pediatric population. In general, the energy level needed to revert any arrhythmia should be reduced for the pediatric patient. The recommended starting dose for defibrillation is 2 J/kg, which should be doubled on the second countershock. VF is uncommon in pediatric patients and should prompt vigorous correction of acidosis and hypoxia.

B. Pacemakers. Permanent pacemakers are susceptible to dysfunction after exposure to countershocks. Potential complications include lead dislodgment, especially for newly implanted devices, acute or chronic impairment of pacing and sensing capabilities, reprogramming of pacing modes, and general damage to the electrical circuitry. For patients with pacemakers, one should use the lowest possible defibrillation energy dose and place the electrodes as far away from the device as possible (more than 10 cm), angling them perpendicular to the ventricular pacing leads. A backup pacing system should always be available in case a malfunction of pacing capabilities develops after a delivered countershock.

C. Implantable cardioverter-defibrillators. Implantable cardioverter-defibrillators (ICDs) are increasingly used to prevent sudden cardiac death. As with pacemakers, ICDs are susceptible to the same types of damage after exposure to a countershock. If elective cardioversion is planned, one should inactivate the device before the procedure. In patients with epicardial ICD patches, higher energies may be necessary because of increased transthoracic impedance. The electrodes should be placed perpendicular to the orientation of the epicardial patches. Urgent defibrillation should not be withheld because the tachyarrhythmia may be due to ICD malfunction, and the ICD should always be rechecked after countershocking.

VI. Automatic external defibrillators. These devices analyze cardiac rhythms. Two types are available, one that requires the operator to discharge the electrical shock with prompting by the device and another that is entirely automated and analyzes and discharges a countershock according to a preprogrammed algorithm. Inappropriate shocks may be initiated as a consequence of improper sensing, such as misinterpreting patient movement as VF. Thus, patients should be in full cardiac arrest before the clinician applies this device, to prevent unnecessary countershocks. Pulse checks are delayed while the automatic external defibrillator is analyzing the rhythm, to minimize movement and to reduce the risk of electrical countershock to the operator.

VII. Complications. Complications of countershocking include thermal burns to the chest and the risk of thromboembolic events, particularly when cardioverting AF or atrial flutter. Countershocks can induce tachyarrhythmias different from the original rhythm, bradycardias, or asystole, which require prompt recognition and treatment, either with another shock or with medications, as necessary. Defibrillation in asystole should always be avoided because excessive vagal response may suppress intrinsic nodal activity. Moreover, depolarizing the myocardium may inhibit the recovery of ventricular escape beats. Yet, one should always consider the possibility that VF with small-amplitude waves ("fine VF") may mimic asystole; a useful cautionary step would be to check more than one lead before assuming a diagnosis of asystole. Finally, applying countershocks to patients with digoxin toxicity may be proarrhythmogenic and could induce serious ventricular dysrhythmias such as VF.

Selected Readings

Cummins RO, ed. *Advanced cardiac life support.* Dallas, TX: American Heart Association, 1997.

An updated and comprehensive manual on cardiopulmonary resuscitation.

Cummins RO, Eisenberg MS, Stults KR. Automatic external defibrillators: clinical issues for cardiology. *Circulation* 1986;73:381.

An article that provides a broad perspective on the clinical issues involved in the use of automatic external defibrillators.

Dick M, Curwin J, Tepper D. Digitalis intoxication recognition and management. *J Clin Pharmacol* 1991;31:444.

An article describing the pharmacologic basis for the treatment of digitalis toxicity.

Emergency cardiac care committee and subcommittees: pediatric advanced life support. *JAMA* 1992;268:2262.

A comprehensive guide to pediatric resuscitation.

Eysmann SB, Marchlinski FE, Buxton AE, et al. Electrocardiographic changes after cardioversion of ventricular arrhythmias. *Circulation* 1986;73:73.

An article describing the ECG changes seen after cardioversion of ventricular arrhythmias.

Golzari H, Cebul RD, Bahler RC. Atrial fibrillation: restoration and maintenance of sinus rhythm and indications for anticoagulation therapy. *Ann Intern Med* 1996; 125:311.

A comprehensive review of the clinical trials pertaining to the management of AF.

Kerber RE, Grayzel J, Hoyt R, et al. Transthoracic resistance in human defibrillation. *Circulation* 1981;63:676.

A study of the factors contributing to transthoracic resistance during defibrillation.

Klein GJ, Bashore TM, Sellers TD, et al. Ventricular fibrillation in the Wolff-Parkinson-White syndrome. *N Engl J Med* 1997;301:1080.

An electrophysiologic study on the risk factors for the development of VF in the WPW syndrome.

Laupacis A, Albers G, Dalen J, et al. Antithrombotic therapy in atrial fibrillation. *Chest* 1998;114:579S.

An updated approach to anticoagulation in patients with AF.

Munter DW, DeLacey WA. Automatic implantable cardioverter-defibrillators. *Emerg Med Clin North Am* 1994;12:579.

A practical review of automatic implantable cardioverter-defibrillators and the management of potential complications in the emergency department setting.

Sellers TD, Campbell RWF, Bashore TM, et al. Effects of procainamide and quinidine sulfate in the Wolff-Parkinson-White syndrome. *Circulation* 1977;55:15.

A discussion on the electrophysiologic effects of procainamide and quinidine in patients with the WPW syndrome.

7. PERICARDIOCENTESIS

Jahn A. Pothier and Deborah H. Markowitz

I. General principles. Pericardiocentesis is a procedure whereby a needle is inserted into the space between the visceral and parietal pericardium for the purpose of sampling or draining pericardial fluid. Normally, there is only 10 to 15 mL of clear fluid in that space, and its composition is similar to that of plasma ultrafiltrate. Several disease states lead to inflammation of the pericardium and subsequent fluid accumulation, including infections, malignancy, diffuse rheumatologic disorders, myocardial infarction, and even myocardial rupture. The composition of the fluid therefore may be exudative, purulent, or frank blood, depending on the underlying cause.

Diagnostic pericardiocentesis is performed to obtain small amounts of pericardial fluid for culture, cytologic study, or other fluid analyses. A therapeutic pericardiocentesis is intended to drain fluid from the pericardial space and to relieve pressure that limits diastolic filling. Diagnostic and therapeutic pericardiocenteses are best performed electively, under controlled circumstances, with echocardiographic or fluoroscopic support. Occasionally, pericardiocentesis needs to be performed on an emergency basis to treat cardiac tamponade, and, as a consequence, the risk of complications such as pneumothorax and myocardial puncture increases.

The visceral pericardium is composed of a single layer of mesothelial cells covering the myocardium and is loosely adherent to the underlying muscle by a network of blood vessels, lymphatics, and connective tissue. In contrast, the parietal pericardium is composed of a thick layer of fibrous connective tissue surrounding another mesothelial monolayer. This fibrous capsule is relatively nondistensible. Effusions that develop rapidly, over minutes to hours, are limited by this noncompliant fibrous parietal pleura, thus placing the fluid under tension. Abrupt accumulation of only 250 mL or less may lead to the clinical signs and symptoms of tamponade, with equalization of pressures in all four cardiac chambers. However, if the effusion develops slowly, the parietal pericardium is allowed to stretch, and significantly larger amounts of fluid (more than 2 L) may accumulate without hemodynamic compromise.

II. Procedure. The materials required for bedside pericardiocentesis are listed in Table 7-1. If time allows, a coagulation profile (prothrombin time, partial thromboplastin time, and platelets) should be checked and corrected. If the procedure is performed on an emergency basis, then hemodynamic compromise is implied. Aggressive resuscitation measures should be ongoing, with infusion of fluids, blood products, or vasopressors, as indicated.

The pericardial space may be entered at various points along the anterior thorax, as demonstrated in Fig. 7-1. The subxiphoid approach (locations 1–3) is preferred in an emergency situation, and is described as follows:

A. Patient preparation. The patient should be placed in a comfortable supine position with the head of the bed elevated to approximately 45 degrees or more. A fully upright position may be necessary for extremely dyspneic patients. This position allows free-flowing effusions to collect inferiorly and anteriorly where they are easiest to access through the subxiphoid approach. A right-handed operator should stand to the patient's right for best entry position, and a left-handed person should stand to the patient's left. The bed should be adjusted to a comfortable height for the person performing the procedure.

B. Pericardiocentesis needle preparation. Some operators prefer to attach an electrocardiographic (ECG) lead to the pericardiocentesis needle to help prevent advancing the needle through the myocardium. This lead substitutes for a precordial V lead on the ECG recording and allows for continuous monitoring throughout the procedure. ST-segment elevation will occur if the needle comes in contact with cardiac muscle or the epicardium. Sterile leads are preferable

TABLE 7-1. Materials for pericardiocentesis

1. *Site preparation:* providone-iodine solution; sterile drapes, gowns, gloves; 1% lidocaine (without epinephrine), atropine, and code cart to bedside
2. *Procedure:* a pericardiocentesis kit or an 18-gauge, 8-cm thin-walled needle with blunt tip; no.11 blade; multiple syringes (20–60 ML); ECG machine; hemostat; sterile alligator clip; and specimen collection tubes
3. *Postprocedure:* sterile gauze, dressings, and sutures

and are available in some pericardiocentesis kits or from the cardiac catheterization laboratory. The alligator clamp should be attached close to the hub of the needle to allow maximum penetration of the needle. The distance between the skin and the parietal pericardium is typically between 6.0 and 7.5 cm, but it may be more in obese patients or in those with a protuberant abdomen. The clinician should attach the needle to a 10-mg syringe, approximately half filled with 1% lidocaine. This technique permits one to anesthetize the subcutaneous tissues and pericardium during needle entry while still allowing sufficient space in the syringe for withdrawal of pericardial fluid.

C. Needle entry site selection. The xiphoid process and the border of the left costal margin are located by inspection and careful palpation. The needle entry site should be 0.5 cm to the left of the xiphoid process and 1.0 cm inferior to the costal margin.

D. Site preparation. Strict sterile technique should be followed at all times. A wide area of the skin in the xiphoid region is prepared with a 10% povidone-iodine solution, and the area is draped with sterile towels while leaving the subxiphoid area exposed. The patient's skin is anesthetized with 1% lidocaine without epinephrine. A small skin incision is made at the needle entry site with a scalpel to

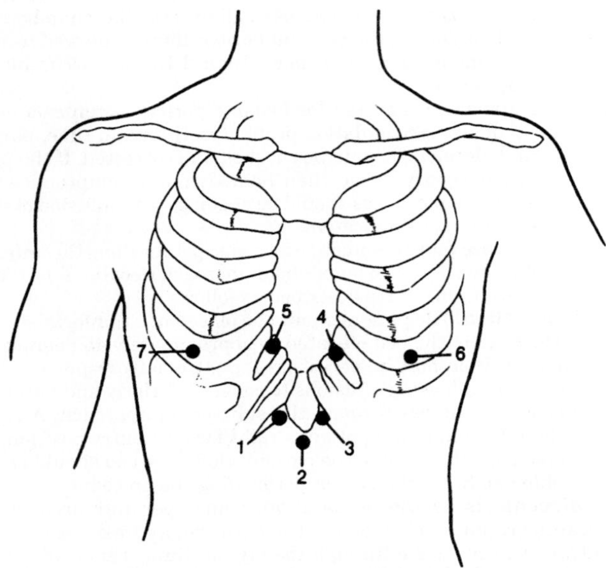

FIG. 7-1. Selected locations for pericardiocentesis. (From Spodick DH. *Acute pericardiocentesis.* New York: Grune & Stratton, 1959, with permission.)

facilitate inserting the blunt needle through the skin; the pericardiocentesis needle does not have a beveled edge, to minimize the risk of myocardial puncture.

E. Needle insertion. The needle is inserted into the subxiphoid incision. Initially, when passing through the skin, the angle of entry should be 45 degrees. The needle is directed superiorly and to the left, aiming for the patient's left shoulder (Fig. 7-2). One should always remember to draw back on the plunger of the syringe while advancing the needle and before injecting the lidocaine. If the bony thorax is hit during needle entry, one should reposition the needle so it may be advanced under the costal margin. The posterior edge of the bony thorax is usually between 1.0 and 2.5 cm below the skin, but it may be more in obese patients. Once the needle has passed beyond the posterior border of the bony thorax, one should reduce the angle that the needle makes with the skin to 15 degrees (Fig. 7-2). This angle is maintained while the needle is still directed at the patient's left shoulder.

F. Needle advancement. The needle should only be moved in a straight trajectory from front to back. Moving the needle from side to side may injure epicardial blood vessels and lymphatics. One should remember to aspirate whenever advancing the needle, then pause to inject the subcutaneous tissue with lidocaine at periodic intervals. The needle is advanced until a "give" is felt and fluid is aspirated from the pericardial space. Some patients may experience a vasovagal response when the pericardium is breached and may need intravenous atropine or saline infusion to reverse bradycardia and hypotension. Should the ECG tracing from the precordial needle lead demonstrate new ST-segment elevations or premature ventricular contractions, one should immediately and carefully withdraw the needle. One continues to aspirate on the syringe while withdrawing the needle. Rapid entry may have caused the needle to go through the pericardial space unknowingly, and correct positioning may be identified with slow extraction of the needle. If one is unsuccessful in isolating the pericardial space, one should completely withdraw the needle, reposition, and try again.

If the procedure was performed to relieve tamponade, the patient's hemodynamic status should improve promptly. Such improvement may be observed after the evacuation of only 50 to 100 mL of fluid. Clinical signs that tamponade has been alleviated include an increase in systemic blood pressure and cardiac output with a fall in right atrial pressure and resolution of pulsus paradoxus.

A large-volume pericardial effusion may be evacuated by attaching a 50-mL syringe onto the pericardiocentesis needle with repeated aspiration attempts. Alternatively, a pericardial drain may be placed by passing a catheter over a guidewire,

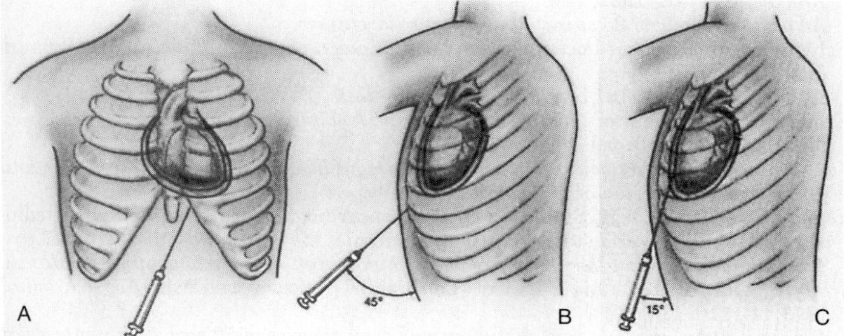

FIG. 7-2. A: Needle direction aiming toward the left shoulder throughout procedure. **B:** Needle angle during skin entry for the first 1.0 to 2.5 cm. **C:** Needle angle after passing the posterior wall of the bony thorax for entry into the pericardial space.

TABLE 7-2. Diagnostic studies to perform for pericardial fluid

1. White count with differential, hematocrit
2. Glucose, total protein, lactate dehydrogenase
3. Gram stain and culture for bacteria, fungi, and acid-fast bacilli
4. Cytology
5. Other studies as indicated: amylase, cholesterol, antinuclear antibody, rheumatoid factor, total complement, C3, viral or parasite studies

as in the Seldinger technique. Samples of the collected pericardial fluid should be sent for the studies listed in Table 7-2.

III. Postprocedure considerations. After pericardiocentesis, close monitoring is required to gauge the rate of pericardial effusion reaccumulation and the potential return of tamponade. All patients should have an end-expiratory chest radiograph immediately after the procedure to detect the presence of a pneumothorax. If not available during the procedure, a transthoracic echocardiogram should be obtained within several hours of the pericardiocentesis to confirm the adequacy of pericardial drainage. Potential complications include cardiac puncture with or without hemopericardium or myocardial infarction, pneumothorax, ventricular tachycardia; bradycardia, trauma to abdominal organs, cardiac arrest, coronary artery laceration, infection, fistula formation, and pulmonary edema. Complications are most likely when the effusion is small (less than 250 mL), is located posteriorly, is loculated, or if the maximum anterior pericardial space is less than 10 mm as determined by echocardiography, because the margin for error is greater. Unguided pericardiocenteses, performed under emergency conditions, are also associated with higher complication rates.

Selected Readings

Kirkland LL, Taylor RW. Pericardiocentesis. *Crit Care Clin* 1992;8:699.
A review of the pathophysiology of pericardial effusions and the pericardiocentesis procedure.

Lovell BH, Braunwald E. Pericardiocentesis. In: Braunwald E, ed. *Heart disease: a textbook of cardiovascular medicine.* Philadelphia: WB Saunders, 1992:1479.
A comprehensive guide to pericardiocentesis.

Meyers DG, Meyers RE, Prendergast TW. The usefulness of diagnostic tests on pericardial fluid. *Chest* 1997;111:1213.
A comprehensive treatises on the prognostic value of various biochemical tests for pericardial fluid analysis; probably the definitive article at this time.

Prager RL, Wilson CH, Bender HW. The subxiphoid approach to pericardial disease. *Ann Thorac Surg* 1982;34:6.
An earlier review of 25 subxiphoid pericardiocenteses.

Scheinman MM. Pericardiocentesis. In: *Cardiac emergencies.* Philadelphia: WB Saunders, 1984:264.
A practical guide to performing pericardiocentesis.

Spodick DH. Technique of pericardiocentesis, in *The pericardium: a comprehensive textbook.* New York: Marcel Dekker, 1997:145.
A practical guide to the diagnostic and treatment benefits of pericardiocentesis and the relevant discussion of pericardial anatomy.

Tsang TS, Freeman WK, Sinak LJ, et al. Echocardiographically guided pericardiocentesis: evolution and state-of-the-art technique. *Mayo Clin Proc* 1998;73:647.
An extensive review of the procedure with emphasis on echocardiographic guidance.

Wong B, Murphy J, Chang CJ, et al. The risk of pericardiocentesis. *Am J Cardiol* 1979;44:1110.
A review of the outcomes and complications from a series of 52 pericardiocenteses at one institution.

8. THE INTRAAORTIC BALLOON AND COUNTERPULSATION

Paul G. Jodka

I. General principles. The intraaortic balloon (IAB) pump is designed to assist an ischemic ventricle through improvement in coronary artery perfusion and reduction in systemic afterload by counterpulsation.

II. Equipment. The balloon is made from a thin film of polyurethane because of its strength and antithrombotic properties. IABs are available in variable sizes, with different balloon volumes and catheter diameters. The catheter itself has two concentric lumina. The central lumen is used to pass a guidewire during insertion and to monitor central aortic pressure. The outer lumen is the passageway for gas exchange and is connected to a console that controls balloon operation as well as having a monitoring function. Helium is used as the driving gas.

III. Physiology. Counterpulsation increases myocardial oxygen supply by diastolic augmentation of coronary perfusion, and it decreases myocardial oxygen requirements through afterload reduction. Counterpulsation causes an increase in cerebral and peripheral blood flow but no significant alteration of renal perfusion.

IV. Indications

A. Cardiogenic shock. The IAB was developed with the hope of reversing cardiogenic shock after myocardial infarction. Counterpulsation should be initiated as soon as it is determined that the shock state is not responsive to intravascular volume manipulation and drug therapy. The ideal candidate for IAB placement should have a reversible anatomic or functional derangement responsible for the shock state.

B. Reversible mechanical defects. Counterpulsation is effective in the initial stabilization of patients with mechanical intracardiac defects complicating myocardial infarction, such as acute mitral regurgitation and ventricular septal perforation, while preparations for definitive intervention are underway.

C. Unstable angina. Counterpulsation is indicated for ongoing myocardial ischemia in the face of maximal medical therapy.

D. Weaning from cardiopulmonary bypass. One of the most useful indications for IAB is to aid in weaning patients from cardiopulmonary bypass who have suffered perioperative myocardial injury.

E. Preoperative use. Most centers use preoperative counterpulsation selectively, rather than routinely, for high-risk patients such as those with critically stenosed coronary arteries or severely depressed left ventricular function.

F. Bridge to transplantation. Counterpulsation has been used to provide mechanical support for patients in congestive heart failure who are awaiting cardiac transplantation.

G. Other indications. Many centers now use counterpulsation to control unstable angina before and during coronary angioplasty and atherectomy. Counterpulsation may be lifesaving after a failed angioplasty, to support the myocardium until emergency aortocoronary revascularization can be performed. The IAB has also been used during interhospital transfers of unstable patients, for treatment of heart failure after myocardial trauma, and for perioperative support for high-risk noncardiac surgery.

V. Contraindications. Aortic valvular insufficiency, aortic dissection, and severe aortoiliac disease are absolute contraindications to counterpulsation. Because of the need for anticoagulation during use of the IAB, gastrointestinal bleeding, thrombocytopenia, and other bleeding diatheses are relative contraindications to counterpulsation.

VI. Insertion technique. The technique of IAB insertion described here is generally applicable to all guidewire-directed IABs and is covered in greater detail in Irwin and Rippe's Intensive Care Medicine, fourth edition textbook.

The following equipment is needed: a manufacturer-supplied sterile insertion kit, a portable fluoroscope, items required for preparation of a sterile field, a no. 11 scalpel, a dilute heparin solution, suturing equipment, 5,000 units of heparin, and a 10-mL syringe.

After careful assessment of the patient, the side with the best circulation is chosen for IAB insertion. The procedure should be performed with the patient supine on a bed or table that permits the use of fluoroscopy. Both inguinal areas are prepared and draped in sterile fashion. The instructions for preparing the IAB should be followed closely, because the technique varies with the manufacturer. Lidocaine (1%) is instilled subcutaneously and subdermally over the femoral artery pulse. The puncture site should be 1 cm below the inguinal crease directly over the femoral pulsation (Fig. 8-1). After cannulation of the artery, a J-guidewire is passed and advanced under fluoroscopy until the tip is in the thoracic aorta (Fig. 8-2). At this point, the patient should be intravenously anticoagulated with 5,000 units of heparin. A small incision is made at the puncture site to allow passage of dilators and the sheath (Fig. 8-3). The IAB is advanced over the guidewire so that its radiopaque tip is positioned 2 cm distal to the ostium of the left subclavian artery (Fig. 8-4).

When the IAB is properly positioned, the central lumen is aspirated and then is flushed with heparinized saline and used to monitor intraaortic pressure and to time counterpulsation. The IAB and sheath are secured with sutures.

Alternatively, the IAB may be inserted without the use of the sheath, a technique that reduces the intraluminal arterial obstruction and may decrease the risk of ischemic complications to the lower limb.

Anticoagulation with a heparin infusion is recommended to reduce the risk of thromboembolic complications related to the IAB. When anticoagulation is contraindicated, an infusion of low-molecular-weight dextran may be used. Prophylactic antibiotics effective against skin flora are recommended.

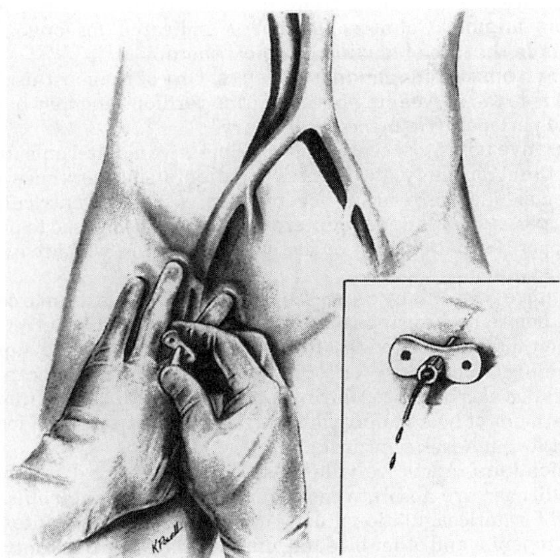

FIG. 8-1. The Potts-Cournand needle is inserted at a 45-degree angle into the common femoral artery. **Inset:** Pulsatile jet of blood indicates that the needle is properly located in the center of the arterial lumen.

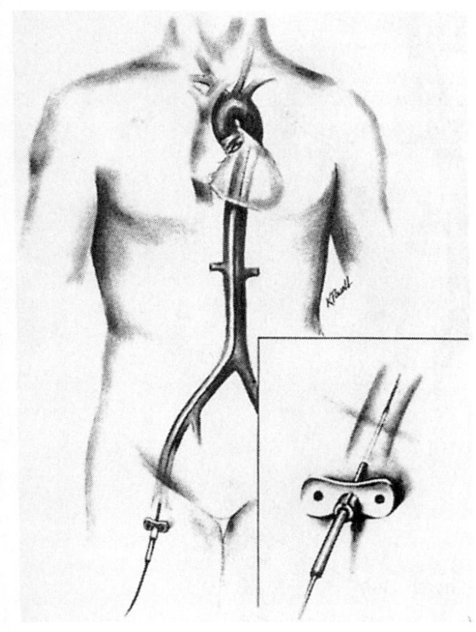

FIG. 8-2. When the Potts-Cournand needle is properly placed in the artery, the guidewire is advanced under fluoroscopic control until the tip is in the thoracic aorta **(inset).**

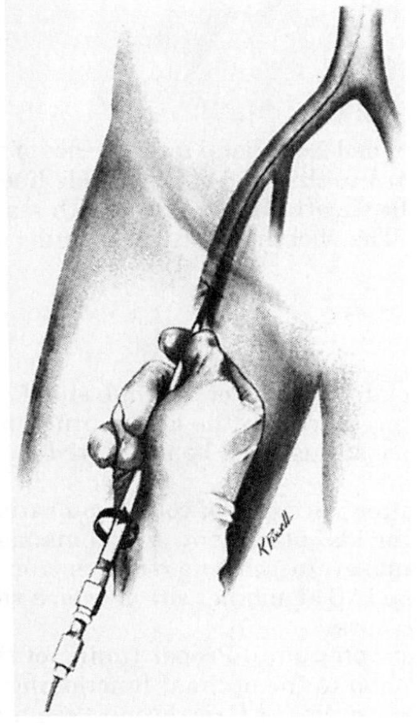

FIG. 8-3. A 9.5-Fr dilator with overlying Teflon sheath is passed over the guidewire. A rotary motion and firm pressure are necessary to enter the lumen of the femoral artery.

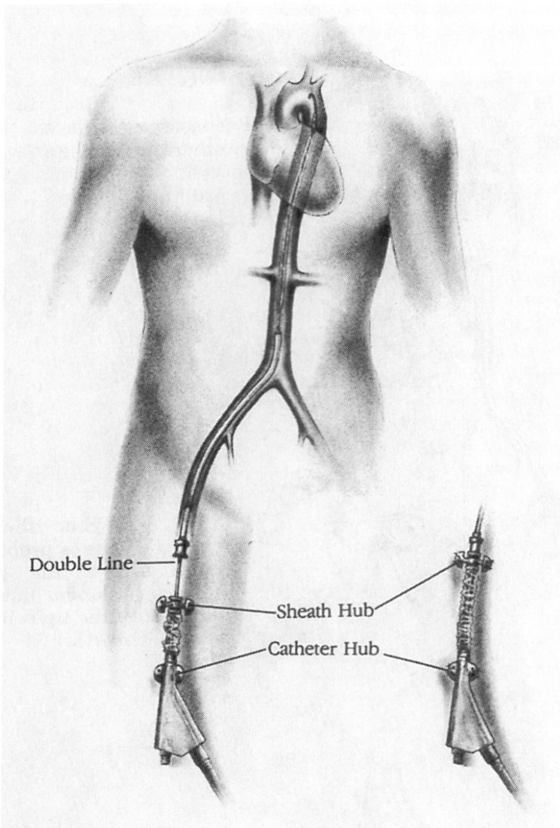

FIG. 8-4. The tip of the intraaortic balloon is positioned 2 cm distal to the orifice of the left subclavian artery. The balloon must be inserted to the level of the double line to be sure the entire membrane had emerged from the sheath. **Inset:** The sheath seal is pushed over the sheath hub to control bleeding. The sheath and catheter hubs are sutured in place.

As soon as the IAB is in position, the circulatory status of the limb should be checked by assessing pulses, Doppler ankle pressures, or the ankle-arm index. While the device is in position, the circulatory status must be monitored every 2 to 4 hours.

Acute limb ischemia may occur anytime after initiation of counterpulsation, but it is most likely to occur immediately after IAB placement. Initial management is conservative if the ischemia is mild, but severe ischemia requires prompt treatment, which may involve placement of the IAB at another site or even a vascular bypass procedure in IAB-dependent patients.

VII. Triggering and timing of the intraaortic balloon pump. Proper timing of the inflation-deflation cycle of the balloon is crucial to the optimal functioning of the IAB. The R wave of the patient's electrocardiogram (ECG) is the most common means of triggering balloon deflation. The IAB is initially set so inflation occurs at the peak of the T wave, which corresponds approximately with closure of the aortic valve. Deflation is then timed to occur just before the next QRS complex, which correlates with ventricular systole. It is important to select the lead with the most pronounced R wave to minimize the likelihood of triggering problems (Fig. 8-5). The IAB may also be triggered by the arterial waveform, or, in an emergency, by an external pacemaker if triggering cannot be effected by ECG or arterial waveform.

When counterpulsation is initiated, the console should be set to a 1:2 assist ratio so the effects of augmentation on every other beat can be analyzed. The IAB should be inflated initially to one-half the operating volume until proper timing is effected. Ideally, IAB inflation should occur just after closure of the aortic valve, which corresponds with the dicrotic notch of the aortic root pulse when it is measured through the lumen of the IAB (Fig. 8-5). Deflation should occur just before systole and thus should be timed so the intraaortic pressure is at a minimum when the aortic valve opens. Improperly timed inflation or deflation negates the potential benefit of the IAB and may even be detrimental to the patient.

When triggering and timing are satisfactory, the IAB may be fully inflated and set to a 1:1 ratio to assist each cardiac cycle. IAB inflation results in a diastolic pressure that exceeds the systolic pressure. Conversely, deflation of the balloon reduces end-diastolic pressure by 15 to 20 mm Hg and systolic pressure by 5 to 10 mm Hg. Timing should be rechecked every 1 to 2 hours or when there is a change in triggering mode or in the patient's clinical status.

Some of the functions monitored by the IAB console include the volume and pressure in the IAB, the presence of gas leaks, the loss of ECG or arterial trigger signal, and improper deflation of the IAB.

VIII. Weaning from counterpulsation. Cessation of counterpulsation involves two steps: weaning and IAB removal. The patient may be weaned by progressively reducing the assist ratio or IAB volume. Usually, a period of 1 to 2 hours is required to

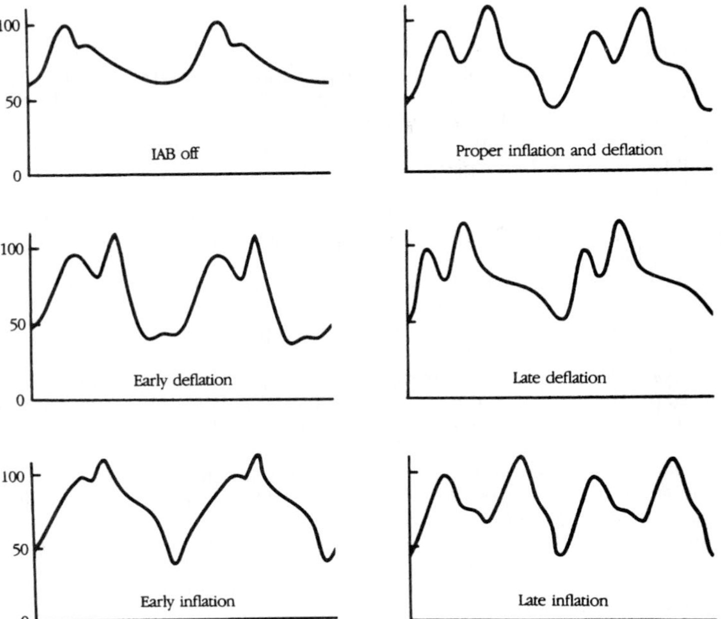

FIG. 8-5. Slide switches on the intraaortic balloon console permit proper timing of inflation and deflation during the cardiac cycle.

establish stability at each new assist level. When the patient has been weaned to 1:3 and has been stable, the IAB may be removed.

The heparin infusion should be stopped 2 hours before IAB removal. The operator should not attempt to withdraw the balloon into the sheath. The IAB and sheath are removed as a unit, and prolonged pressure is applied to the puncture site. The use of sandbags is not recommended. Rarely, surgical management is required to control ongoing bleeding from the insertion site.

IX. Complications of counterpulsation. The overall complication rate for percutaneous IAB is about 15%.

A. Complications during insertion. The most common complication related to insertion is failure of the IAB to pass the iliofemoral system because of atherosclerotic occlusive disease. The reported failure rate ranges from 5% to 7%. Other complications of IAB insertion include aortic dissection and arterial perforation, with a reported incidence of 1% to 2%. Arterial perforation is an acute emergency requiring surgical intervention.

B. Complications while the intraaortic balloon is in place. Limb ischemia is the most common complication of counterpulsation and is sufficiently severe to require removal of the IAB in 11% to 27% of patients. Several large reviews suggest that the most important risk factors for limb ischemia are the female gender, insulin-dependent diabetes, and significant peripheral vascular occlusive disease.

Infection, thrombocytopenia, and embolization of platelet aggregates or atherosclerotic debris have been reported. Rupture of the IAB occurs in 2% to 4% of patients and may cause gas embolization. Blood in the connecting tubing is a hallmark of rupture, and its presence requires immediate cessation of counterpulsation and IAB removal.

C. Complications during or after removal. Arterial perfusion of the limb should be checked soon after removal of the IAB by palpation of pulses and measurement of the ankle-arm index. The puncture site should be examined for hematoma, false aneurysm formation, and arteriovenous fistula.

Selected Readings

Eltchaninoff H, Dimas AP, Whitlow PL. Complications associated with percutaneous placement and use of intraaortic balloon counterpulsation. *Am J Cardiol* 1993;71:328.
A report of 231 cases of IAB use that suggests predictors of limb ischemia.

Irwin RS, Cerra FB, Rippe JM (eds). Irwin and Rippe's Intensive Care Medicine, 4th ed. Philadelphia, PA: Lippincott–Raven, 1999.
A good intensive care medicine textbook.

Isner JM, Cohen SR, Virmani R, et al. Complications of the intraaortic balloon counterpulsation device: clinical and morphologic observations in 54 necropsy patients. *Am J Cardiol* 1980;45:260.
This study suggests that most complications are consequences of insertion of the device, not consequences of its being in place.

Jacobs JP, Horowitz MD, Ladden DA, et al. Case report: intra-aortic balloon counterpulsation in penetrating cardiac trauma. *J Cardiovasc Surg* 1992;33:38.
A case report that describes the management of a patient with a cardiac stab wound.

Kantrowitz A, Wasfie T, Freed PS, et al. Intraaortic balloon pumping 1967 through 1982: analysis of complications in 733 patients. *Am J Cardiol* 1986;57:976.
A good review of complications of IAB.

Katz ES, Tunick PA, Kronzon I. Observations of coronary flow augmentation and balloon function during intraaortic balloon counterpulsation using transesophageal echocardiography. *Am J Cardiol* 1992;69:1635.
A report of six patients studied with transesophageal echocardiography while assisted with IAB; it suggests that transesophageal echocardiography can be used to evaluate IAB positioning and to monitor coronary artery flow augmentation during counterpulsation.

O'Murchu B, Foreman RD, Shaw RE, et al. Role of intraaortic balloon pump counterpulsation in high risk coronary rotational atherectomy. *J Am Coll Cardiol* 1995;26:1270.

A retrospective review of elective use of IAB in high-risk patients before coronary rotational atherectomy.

Scheidt S, Wilner G, Mueller H, et al. Intra-aortic balloon counterpulsation in cardiogenic shock: report of a cooperative clinical trial. *N Engl J Med* 1973;288:979.

A report involving 87 patients with cardiogenic shock. Precise indications for initiation or termination of balloon counterpulsation in this study were elusive.

Siu SC, Kowalchuk GJ, Welty FK, et al. Intra-aortic balloon counterpulsation support in the high-risk cardiac patient undergoing urgent noncardiac surgery. *Chest* 1991;99:1342.

A report of perioperative use of IAB in eight patients with unstable coronary syndromes or severe coronary artery disease who underwent urgent noncardiac surgery.

9. CHEST TUBE INSERTION AND CARE

Hashim M. Hesham

I. General principles. Chest tube insertion (tube thoracostomy) involves placement of a sterile tube into the pleural space for evacuation of air or fluid. Although tube thoracostomy is not complex in the scope of all surgical procedures, it may result in serious and life-threatening complications if it is performed without proper preparation.

II. Indications

- **A. Pneumothorax**
- **B. Hemothorax**
- **C. Empyema**
- **D. Chylothorax**
- **E. Pleural effusion**

III. Contraindication. The most obvious contraindication to chest tube insertion is lack of a pneumothorax or fluid collection in the pleural space. Yet this distinction is not always clear. If one is in doubt, checking x-ray films with a radiologist or a chest computed tomographic (CT) scan may confirm the diagnosis. Past history of a process such as sclerosing procedure, pleurodesis, or thoracotomy on the affected side should raise caution and should prompt evaluation with CT scanning. This is important to avoid placement of the tube in areas of disease or where the lung is adherent to the chest wall. In addition, coagulopathies should be corrected before tube insertion in a nonemergency setting.

IV. Preparation. Chest tube insertion requires not only knowledge of the anatomy of the chest wall and the intrathoracic and abdominal structures but also general aseptic technique. The procedure should be performed or supervised by experienced personnel. The patient must be evaluated by physical examination and chest radiography, to avoid insertion of the tube into the abdomen or into the wrong side. Particular care must be taken before and during the procedure to avoid intubation of the pulmonary parenchyma.

Sterile technique is mandatory whether the procedure is performed in the operating room, the intensive care unit, the emergency room, or on the ward. Obtaining a detailed informed consent contributes to reducing patient anxiety during the procedure. Administration of parenteral narcotics or benzodiazepines provides a relatively painless procedure. Drainage tubes or chest tubes are made from either Silastic or rubber, are either angled or straight, have multiple drainage holes, and contain a radiopaque strip. Chest tubes are available in various sizes ranging from 6 to 40 Fr, with size selection depending on the patient population (6 to 24 Fr for infants and children) and the collection being drained (24 to 28 Fr for air, 32 to 36 Fr for pleural effusions, and 36 to 40 Fr for blood or pus). Before performing the procedure, one should review all the steps that will be taken and make sure that all necessary equipment is available (Table 9-1).

V. Technique

1. The patient should be placed in supine position, and the head of the bed should be adjusted for comfort by having the involved side elevated slightly with the patient's ipsilateral arm brought up over the head (Fig. 9-1).
2. In most instances, the tube is inserted into the fourth or fifth intercostal space in the anterior axillary line, occasionally in the second intercostal space for pneumothorax only.
3. The area is prepared under sterile conditions with 10% povidone-iodine solution. The area is draped to include the ipsilateral nipple, which serves as a landmark. Lidocaine (1%) is infiltrated in the anterior axillary line two finger breadths below the intercostal space to be penetrated.
4. To confirm location of air or fluid, a thoracentesis is performed. If air or fluid is not aspirated, one should reassess the chest radiograph or chest CT scan.

TABLE 9-1. Chest tube insertion equipment

1. Povidone-iodine solution
2. Sterile towels and drapes
3. Sterile sponges
4. 40 mL of 1% lidocaine without epinephrine
5. 10-mL syringe
6. 18–21- and 25-gauge needles
7. Two large Kelly clamps
8. Mayo scissors
9. Standard tissue forceps
10. Needle holder
11. 0 silk suture with cutting needles
12. Scalpel no. 10 blade
13. Chest tubes (24, 28, 32, and 36 Fr)
14. Chest tube drainage system (filled appropriately)
15. Petrolatum (Vaseline) gauze
16. 2-in. adhesive tape
17. Sterile gowns, gloves, masks, and caps

5. A 2-cm transverse incision is made, and additional lidocaine is administered to infiltrate the tissues through which the tube will pass as well as a generous area in the intercostal space including the periosteum of the ribs above and below the insertion site. Care should be taken to anesthetize the parietal pleura fully, because it contains pain fibers. In this case, 30 to 40 mL of lidocaine may be needed to achieve adequate local anesthesia.
6. A short tunnel is created in the chosen intercostal space using Kelly clamps. The closed Kelly clamp is carefully inserted through the parietal pleura into the pleural cavity, hugging the superior portion of the lower rib to prevent injury to intercostal nerves and vessels of the above rib. The clamp is placed to a depth of less than 1 cm in the pleural cavity and is spread open about 2 cm.
7. A finger is inserted into the pleural space to confirm proper location. Only easily disrupted adhesions should be broken.
8. The chest tube is inserted into the pleural space and is positioned appropriately (apically for pneumothorax and dependently for fluid removal). All holes of the chest tube must be within the pleural space.
9. The location of the tube should be confirmed by flow of air or fluid from the tube. The tube is sutured to the skin securely to prevent slippage. A horizontal mattress suture of 0 silk may be used to allow the hole to be tied closed when the tube is removed. Petrolatum gauze can be applied, and the tube can be connected to a drainage apparatus. The tube and connectors should be securely taped.

VI. Complications. Chest tube insertion may be accompanied by significant complications. Unintentional placement of the tube through the intercostal vessels or into the lung, heart, liver, or spleen can result in considerable morbidity and possible mortality. In addition, secondary infection of the pleural space may occur after chest tube insertion and may result in empyema. Prophylactic antibiotics directed against *Staphylococcus aureus* may be of benefit in patients undergoing tube thoracostomy in the trauma setting.

VII. Chest tube management and care. While a chest tube is in place, the tube and drainage system must be checked daily for adequate functioning. In the past, drainage systems employed one to three bottles, closed to the environment, serving as a one-way valve to allow egress of air and fluid while preventing their return back into the pleural space. Today, most institutions use a one-piece thru-chambered system. Suction is routinely established at 15 to 20 cm H_2O.

Connection between the chest tube and the drainage system should be tightly fitted and securely taped. Dressing changes should be preformed every 2 to 3 days

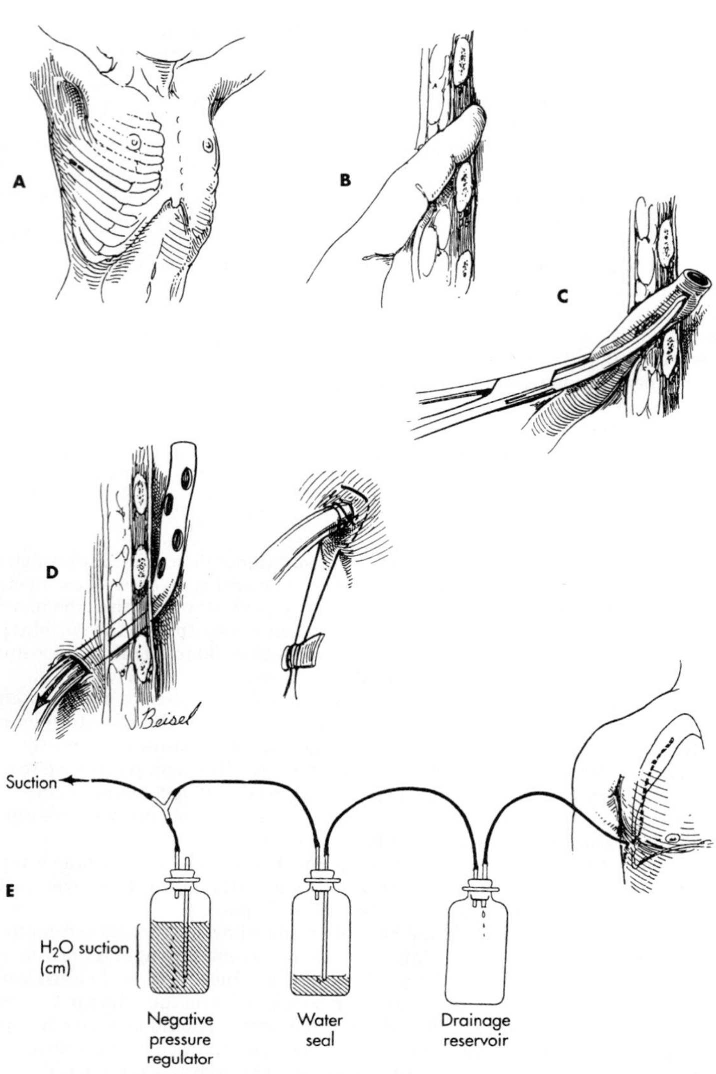

FIG. 9-1. A: Incision in the fourth of fifth intercostal space. **B:** Confirmation of proper location by inserting a finger in the pleural cavity. **C:** Introduction of the chest tube to the chest cavity. **D:** Securing of the chest tube with stitches. **E:** Connection of the chest tube to the bottles and suction (Pleurovac). (From Waldenhausen JA, Pierce WS, Campbell DB (eds.). *Surgery of the chest,* 6th ed. St. Louis: Mosby–Year Book, 1996, with permission.)

or as needed. Serial chest radiographs should be obtained to evaluate the result of drainage and to ensure that the most proximal hole has not migrated from the pleural space. A tube should not be readvanced into the pleural space, and if a tube is to be replaced, it should always be at a different site rather than the same hole.

VIII. Chest tube removal. Indications for removal of chest tubes include resolution of the pneumothorax or fluid accumulation in the pleural space. For pneumothorax, the drainage system is left on suction until the air leak stops. If an air leak persists, brief clamping of the chest tube is performed to be sure that the leak is indeed from the patient and not from the system itself. If after several days an air leak persists, placement of an additional tube may be indicated. When the leak has ceased for more than 24 to 48 hours, the drainage system is placed on water seal by disconnecting the suction, and a chest radiograph is obtained several hours later. If no reaccumulation of air is identified and no air leak appears in the system when the patient coughs and with reestablishment of suction, the tube may be removed. For fluid collection, the tube may also be removed when the drainage is minimal.

Tube removal is often preceded by oral or parenteral analgesia. With a petrolatum gauze dressing, suture removal kit, and tape ready, the physician instructs the patient to take maximal deep breaths slowly. The suture that is holding the tube with the skin is cut and is removed while the hole is simultaneously dressed with petrolatum gauze at the peak of inspiration. If a horizontal mattress suture is in place, it should be tied to close the skin. Chest radiography should then be performed several hours later.

Selected Readings

Advanced trauma life support instructor manual. Chicago: American College of Surgeons, 1989:105.

Tube thoracostomy and sustained sterile technique in emergency situations.

Cameron EW, Mirvis SE, Shamnuganathan K, et al. Computed tomography of malpositioned thoracostomy drains: a pictorial essay. *Clin Radiol* 1997;52:187.

Evaluation of chest drain placement by portable chest radiography is essential for patient management, but in some cases, a chest CT scan reveals unexpected placement of chest tube.

Daly RC, Mucha P, Pairolero PC, et al. The risk of percutaneous chest tube thoracostomy for blunt thoracic trauma. *Ann Emerg Med* 1985;14:865.

Complications of percutaneous tube thoracostomy in victims of blunt trauma.

Evans JT, Green JD, Carlin PE, et al. Meta-analysis of antibiotics in tube thoracostomy. *Am Surg* 1995;61:215.

This study's results suggest that antibiotics should be used in patients undergoing tube thoracostomy.

Millikan JS, Moore EE, Steiner E, et al. Complications of tube thoracostomy for acute trauma. *Am J Surg* 1980;140:738.

Tube thoracostomy is both diagnostic and therapeutic in trauma patients. There is a 4% technical complication rate in tube thoracostomy in the emergency room.

10. BRONCHOSCOPY

Oren P. Schaefer and Richard S. Irwin

I. **General principles.** Bronchoscopy is the endoscopic examination of the bronchial tree. Flexible bronchoscopy is easily performed and is associated with few complications. Compared with rigid bronchoscopy, flexible bronchoscopy is more comfortable, safer for the patient, allows for greater visualization of the entire tracheobronchial tree, and does not require general anesthesia or the use of an operating room. Rigid bronchoscopy remains the procedure of choice for massive hemoptysis, the extraction of foreign bodies, endobronchial resection of tumor or granulation tissue, endoscopic laser surgery, and the dilation of endobronchial strictures and placement of airway stents.

II. **Diagnostic indications**

A. **Hemoptysis.** The evaluation of hemoptysis, whether just blood streaking or massive (more than 600 mL in 24 to 48 hours) is easily done with bronchoscopy. The goal is twofold: localization of the bleeding and diagnosis of its cause. The former is critical if definitive therapy, surgery or embolization, becomes necessary. When bronchoscopy is performed before bleeding ceases, the site and origin are disclosed in approximately 90% of cases. The yield drops to 50% after bleeding has ceased.

B. **Atelectasis.** In the critically ill patient, atelectasis is most often caused by mucus plugging. Flexible bronchoscopy helps to rule out endobronchial obstruction by malignancy or foreign body.

C. **Diffuse parenchymal disease.** Transbronchoscopic lung biopsy and bronchoalveolar lavage (BAL) can offer information about parenchymal processes. BAL is particularly useful in diagnosing opportunistic infections in the immunocompromised host. Transbronchial lung biopsy is done under fluoroscopic guidance to improve localization and to minimize pneumothorax.

D. **Acute inhalation injury.** Upper airway obstruction may develop during the initial 24 hours after an inhalation injury. Acute respiratory failure is more likely in patients with mucosal changes seen at segmental or lower levels. Fiberoptic bronchoscopy is indicated to identify the anatomic level and severity of injury after smoke inhalation.

E. **Blunt chest trauma.** Airway fracture after blunt chest trauma is suggested by hemoptysis, lobar atelectasis, pneumomediastinum, or pneumothorax. Because this condition requires surgical intervention, flexible bronchoscopy should be performed immediately.

F. **Assessment of intubation damage.** Flexible bronchoscopy is easily performed to assess laryngeal or tracheal damage from endotracheal tubes. It can be of value in the decision to perform tracheostomy in the ventilated patient and in the evaluation of a possible tracheoesophageal fistula.

G. **Cultures.** Aspirates obtained from the bronchoscope in a nonintubated patient are no more predictive than cultures obtained by expectorated sputum. Both are associated with high false-positive and false-negative rates. Bronchoscopic aspirates are useful in identifying organisms that do not colonize the respiratory tract when a patient is unable to expectorate adequate amounts of sputum. A protected specimen brush improves on the accuracy of routine bronchoscopic culture when specimens are cultured quantitatively.

H. **Diagnosing ventilator-associated pneumonia.** This condition can be difficult to diagnose. Flexible bronchoscopy can be helpful by providing a specimen for culture. The visualization of distal purulent secretions seen surging from distal bronchi during exhalation may be predictive of ventilator-associated pneumonia.

III. Therapeutic indications

A. Excessive secretions and atelectasis. Lobar atelectasis that does not respond to chest physical therapy, incentive spirometry, and cough is an indication for flexible bronchoscopy. Direct instillation of *N*-acetylcysteine (NAC) through the bronchoscope may help to liquify thick, tenacious, inspissated mucus. NAC may induce bronchospasm in asthmatic patients; pretreatment with a bronchodilator is recommended.

B. Foreign bodies. Rigid bronchoscopy is considered the procedure of choice in removing aspirated foreign bodies. However, devices, such as the basket, are available to help the clinician remove such objects with the flexible scope.

C. Endotracheal intubation. In certain patients with mechanical problems of the neck, the flexible bronchoscope may be used as an obturator for endotracheal intubation. The bronchoscope, with an endotracheal tube passed over it, can be placed transnasally or orally through the vocal cords into the trachea. The tube is then placed under direct vision by passing it over the scope.

D. Hemoptysis. When bleeding threatens to asphyxiate the patient, endobronchial tamponade may stabilize the patient and may allow for more definitive therapy. Tamponade can be achieved with the use of a Fogarty balloon catheter inflated and wedged in the bleeding lobar orifice. Massive hemoptysis can also be controlled with the technique of iced saline lavage. Once stabilized, the patient can then be taken to surgery or for bronchial artery angiography and embolization.

E. Central obstructing airway lesions. Cancer or benign lesions can obstruct the larynx, trachea, and major bronchi and can be treated with photoresection using a laser or airway stenting through the bronchoscope.

F. Closure of bronchopleural fistula. Bronchoscopy can be used to visualize a proximal bronchopleural fistula. A more distal bronchopleural fistula can be localized as well by segmental occlusion with a balloon catheter. Various materials injected through the bronchoscope may successfully seal the fistula.

IV. Complications. When performed by a trained specialist, routine flexible bronchoscopy is extremely safe. Mortality clearly should not exceed 0.1%, and the overall complication rate is no greater than 8.0%. The rare deaths have come from excessive premedication or topical anesthesia, respiratory arrest from hemorrhage, laryngospasm or bronchospasm, and cardiac arrest from acute myocardial infarction. Nonfatal complications include fever, pneumonia, vasovagal reactions, laryngospasm and bronchospasm, hypotension, cardiac arrhythmia, pneumothorax, anesthesia-related problems, and aphonia. These complications usually occur within 24 hours of the procedure.

V. Contraindications. Bronchoscopy should not be performed without a properly experienced physician, in an uncooperative patient, when adequate oxygen tension cannot be maintained during and after the procedure, when coagulation studies cannot be normalized in patients in whom biopsy specimens (brush or forceps) will be taken, in unstable cardiac patients, and in untreated symptomatic asthmatic patients. In patients with severe chronic obstructive pulmonary disease and associated hypercapnea, premedication, sedation, and supplemental oxygen must be used with caution. Patients with elevated intracranial pressure should be anesthetized using a combination of medications for cerebral protection, pharmacologically paralyzed to prevent cough, and monitored to ensure adequate cerebral perfusion pressure.

VI. Procedural considerations

A. Preprocedural. The following must be considered: Does the patient have asthma, cardiovascular disease, or uremia? Does the patient have any drug allergies? Has the patient had a chest radiograph, electrocardiogram, and assessment of oxygenation? Does the patient have a bleeding diathesis, or is the patient receiving any medication that may interfere with coagulation? Has the patient fasted before the procedure? Has an informed consent form been signed? Has premedication been ordered? Does the patient have intravenous access?

B. Procedural. In nonintubated patients, flexible bronchoscopy can be performed by the transnasal or transoral route. Most physicians prefer the former. Adequate local anesthesia is achieved by nebulized lidocaine and topical lidocaine jelly. Lidocaine is absorbed through the mucous membranes, and significant, even toxic, blood levels can be reached after topical administration. Levels in the low therapeutic range are achieved if a total of less than 200 mg is used. A sudden change in mental status, hallucinations, increased sedation, or hypotension should suggest lidocaine toxicity.

In intubated, mechanically ventilated patients, the flexible bronchoscope is easily passed through a swivel adapter with a rubber diaphragm that prevents loss of the delivered respiratory gases. The following should be considered before and during bronchoscopy: (a) an endotracheal tube should be at least 8 mm internal diameter to ensure the delivery of an adequate tidal volume; (b) positive end-expiratory pressure (PEEP) of 20 cm H_2O may develop with standard bronchoscopes, with the attendant risk of barotrauma; (c) PEEP already being delivered should be discontinued; (d) inspired oxygen concentration must be increased to 100%; (e) expired volumes should be constantly measured by a respiratory therapist to ensure that they are adequate (tidal volumes usually have to be increased by 40% to 50%); and (f) suctioning that decreases delivered tidal volume should be minimized. During bronchoscopy, continuous oxygen therapy, oximetry, electrocardiography, and blood pressure monitoring are necessary.

C. Postprocedural. A chest radiograph should be obtained after transbronchoscopic biopsy in the nonintubated patient and after routine bronchoscopy in the intubated mechanically ventilated patient to rule out pneumothorax. The ventilated patient should be returned to preprocedure ventilator settings, and in the nonintubated patient, supplemental oxygen should be continued for 4 hours after the procedure. Frequent vital signs are taken until the patient has been stable for at least 2 hours. Patients must not eat or drink until local anesthesia has worn off, in approximately 1 to 2 hours. Fever after the procedure is not uncommon; if it lasts more than 24 hours, one should evaluate the patient for postbronchoscopy pneumonia.

Selected Readings

Cavaliere S, Foccoli P, Farina PL. Nd: YAG laser bronchoscopy: a five-year experience with 1,396 applications in 1,000 patients. *Chest* 1988;94:15.

Laser bronchoscopy was found to be a safe and effective method in the treatment of obstructive lesions of the tracheobronchial tree.

Conlan AA, Hurwitz SS. Management of massive hemoptysis with the rigid bronchoscope and cold saline lavage. *Thorax* 1980;35:901.

The authors describe the technique of iced saline lavage to control hemorrhage.

Dellinger RP. Fiberoptic bronchoscopy in adult airway management. *Crit Care Med* 1990;18:882.

The author provides an in-depth review of the use of the flexible bronchoscope in management of the airway: intubation with single- and double-lumen endotracheal tubes, tube changes and extubation, and other aspects of airway management.

Imgrund SP, Goldberg SK, Walkenstein MD, et al. Clinical diagnosis of massive hemoptysis using the fiberoptic bronchoscope. *Crit Care Med* 1985;13:438.

Illustrative cases are presented with a review of the use of the flexible bronchoscope in the evaluation and treatment of massive hemoptysis.

Jolliet PH, Chevrolet JC. Bronchoscopy in the intensive care unit. *Intensive Care Med* 1992;18:160.

Brochoscopy in the intensive care unit, including its effects on respiratory mechanics, gas exchange, and hemodynamics and performing the procedure in high-risk patients, is reviewed.

Pisani RJ, Wright AJ. Clinical utility of bronchoalveolar lavage in immunocompromised hosts. *Mayo Clin Proc* 1992;67:221.

The sensitivity and specificity of BAL were found to be 82% and 53%, respectively. The strengths and weaknesses of BAL in this patient population are discussed.

Timsit J-F, Misset B, Azoulay E, et al. Usefulness of airway visualization in the diagnosis of nosocomial pneumonia in ventilated patients. *Chest* 1996;110:172.

Direct visualization of the bronchial tree by bronchoscopy was found to predict nosocomial pneumonia accurately in ventilated patients.

Torres A, Bellacasa JP, Xauber A, et al. Diagnostic value of quantitative cultures of bronchoalveolar lavage and telescoping plugged catheters in mechanically ventilated patients with bacterial pneumonia. *Am Rev Respir Dis* 1989;140:306.
The diagnostic value of quantitative cultures of BAL and telescoping plugged catheter samples in 34 immunocompetent patients suspected of having bacterial pneumonia was studied. Both techniques were found to diagnose pneumonia with similar accuracy.

11. THORACENTESIS

Mark M. Wilson and Richard S. Irwin

I. General principles. Thoracentesis is an invasive procedure, first described in 1852, that involves the introduction of a needle, cannula, or trocar into the pleural space to remove accumulated fluid or air. Although history (cough, dyspnea, or pleuritic chest pain) and physical findings (dullness to percussion, decreased breath sounds, and decreased tactile fremitus) suggest that an effusion is present, a chest radiograph or ultrasonic examination is essential to confirm the clinical suspicion. Analysis of pleural fluid has been shown to yield clinically useful information in more than 90% of cases. Thoracentesis may be performed for diagnostic (generally 50 to 100 mL) or therapeutic (evacuation of air or more than 100 mL fluid) reasons. The four most common causes of pleural effusions are congestive heart failure, parapneumonic, malignancy, and postoperative sympathetic effusions.

II. Contraindications and complications. Relative contraindications to thoracenteses include those settings in which a complication from the procedure may prove catastrophic for the patient (i.e., known underlying bullous disease, the presence of positive end-expiratory pressure, a patient with only one functional lung). Absolute contraindications to thoracenteses include an uncooperative patient, the inability to identify the top of the rib at the planned puncture site clearly, operator inexperience with the procedure, and coagulopathy that cannot be corrected. The overall complication rate from thoracentesis has been reported to be as high as 50% to 78%. Major, possibly life-threatening, complications occur in 15% to 19% and include pneumothorax, hemorrhage, hypotension, reexpansion pulmonary edema, venous or cerebral air embolism (rare), and sheared catheter fragments left in the pleural space (rare). The risk of pneumothorax varies depending on baseline patient characteristics (e.g., presence or absence of chronic obstructive pulmonary disease), operator experience, and the method used to perform the procedure. Minor complications also depend on the method used and occur in 16% to 63%, including dry tap, anxiety, dyspnea, cough, pain, and subcutaneous hematoma or seroma.

III. Procedures

A. Technique for diagnostic (needle only) thoracentesis

1. Obtain a lateral decubitus chest radiograph to confirm a free-flowing pleural effusion.
2. Obtain informed written consent for the procedure.
3. With the patient sitting, arms at side, mark the inferior tip of the scapula on the side to be tapped. This approximates the eighth intercostal space, the lowest interspace punctured unless previous sonography determined that a lower interspace can safely be entered.
4. Position the patient sitting at the edge of the bed, comfortably leaning forward over a pillow-draped, height-adjusted, bedside table. The patient's arms should be crossed in front to elevate and spread the scapulae. An assistant should stand in front of the table to prevent any unexpected movements.
5. Percuss the patient's posterior chest to determine the highest point of the effusion. The interspace below this point should be entered in the posterior axillary line, unless it is below the eighth intercostal space (see no. 3 above). Mark the superior aspect of the rib with your fingernail (the inferior border of each rib contains an intercostal artery and should be avoided).
6. Cleanse the area with iodophor and allow it to dry. Using sterile technique, drape the area surrounding the puncture site.
7. Anesthetize the superficial skin with 2% lidocaine using a 25-gauge needle. Change to a 18-to 22-gauge needle and generously anesthetize the deeper soft tissues, aiming for the top of the rib. Always aspirate as the needle is advanced and before instilling lidocaine to ensure that the needle is not in

a vessel or the pleural space. After passing the rib (1 to 2 cm thick), fluid enters the syringe on reaching the pleural space. The patient may experience discomfort as the needle penetrates the well-innervated parietal pleura. Be careful not to instill anesthetic into the pleural space; it is bactericidal for most organisms, including *Mycobacterium tuberculosis.* Place a gloved finger at the point on the needle where it exits the skin (to estimate the required depth of insertion) and remove the needle.

8. Attach a three-way stopcock to a 20-gauge, 1.5-inch needle and to a 50-mL syringe. The valve on the stopcock should be open to the needle to allow aspiration of fluid during needle insertion.
9. Insert the 20-gauge needle along the anesthetic tract, always aspirating through the syringe as the needle is slowly advanced. When pleural fluid is obtained, stabilize the needle by attaching a clamp to the needle where it exits the skin, to prevent further advancement of the needle into the pleural space.
10. Once pleural fluid is obtained, fill a heparinized blood gas syringe from the side port of the three-way stopcock. Express all air from the sample, cap it, and place in a bag containing iced slush for immediate transport to the laboratory.
11. Fill the 50-mL syringe and transfer its contents into appropriate collection tubes and containers. Always maintain a closed system during the procedure to prevent room air from entering the pleural space. When changing syringes, be sure to place the three-way stopcock with the valve closed to the needle. One hundred milliliters should be ample fluid for most diagnostic studies.
12. When the thoracentesis is complete, remove the needle from the patient's chest. Apply pressure to the wound for several minutes, and apply a sterile bandage.
13. Obtain a postprocedure upright end-expiratory chest radiograph if a pneumothorax is suspected.
14. Immediately after the procedure, draw venous blood for total protein and lactate dehydrogenase determinations. These studies are necessary to interpret pleural fluid values.

B. Technique for therapeutic thoracentesis

1. Follow steps 1 to 7 as described previously.
2. Removal of more than 100 mL of pleural fluid generally involves placement of a catheter into the pleural space to minimize the risk of pneumothorax from a needle during this longer procedure. Commercially available kits use either catheter-over-needle or catheter-through-needle procedures. Each may have a specific set of instructions for performing this procedure. Operators should be thoroughly familiar with the recommended procedure for the catheter system they will use and should receive appropriate supervision from an experienced operator before performing therapeutic thoracentesis on their own.

C. Technique for removal of freely moving pneumothorax

1. Position the patient supine with the head of the bed elevated 30 to 45 degrees.
2. Prepare the anterior second or third intercostal space in the midclavicular line (to avoid the more medial internal mammary artery) for the needle and catheter insertion.
3. Have the bevel of the needle facing upward, and direct the needle superiorly so the catheter can be guided to the superior aspect of the hemithorax.
4. Air may be actively withdrawn by syringe or pushed out when intrapleural pressure is supraatmospheric (e.g., during a cough), as long as the catheter is intermittently open to the atmosphere. In the latter setting, air can leave but not reenter if the catheter is attached to a one-way valve apparatus (Heimlich valve) or if it is put to underwater seal.
5. If a tension pneumothorax is known or suspected to be present and a chest tube is not readily available, quickly insert a 14-gauge angiocatheter into

the second intercostal space according to the foregoing technique. If a tension pneumothorax is present, air will escape under pressure. When the situation has been stabilized, replace the catheter with a sterile chest tube.

IV. Interpretation of pleural fluid analysis. The initial diagnostic determination of a pleural effusion is to classify it as a transudate or an exudate. A transudate is biochemically defined by meeting *all* the following criteria: pleural fluid-to-serum ratio for total protein less than 0.5, pleural fluid-to-serum ratio for lactate dehydrogenase less than 0.6, and an absolute pleural fluid lactate dehydrogenase less than 200 IU. If a transudate is present, then generally no further tests on pleural fluid are indicated. An exudate is present when any of the foregoing criteria for transudate are not met. Further laboratory evaluation is warranted in the setting of an exudative pleural effusion.

A. pH. Pleural fluid pH may have diagnostic and therapeutic implications. With a pleural fluid pH less than 7.2, the differential diagnosis can be narrowed to include systemic acidemia, empyema or parapneumonic effusion, malignancy, rheumatoid or lupus effusion, extrapulmonary tuberculosis, ruptured esophagus, or urinothorax. Effusions with a fluid pH less than 7.2 are potentially sclerotic and require consideration for chest tube drainage to aid resolution.

B. Amylase. Pleural fluid amylase levels twice the serum level or with absolute values greater than 160 Somogyi units may be seen in patients with pancreatitis (acute or chronic), ruptured pancreatic pseudocyst, malignancy, or esophageal rupture.

C. Glucose. Pleural fluid glucose levels less than 50% of the serum level may be found in patients with empyema effusion, malignancy, rheumatoid or lupus effusion, extrapulmonary tuberculosis, or ruptured esophagus.

D. Cell counts and differential. Although not diagnostic, pleural fluid white blood cell counts exceeding 50,000/mm^3 strongly suggest an associated bacterial pneumonia or empyema. Pleural fluid lymphocytosis is nonspecific, but when severe (>80% of cells) it suggests tuberculosis or malignancy. Red blood cell counts of 5,000 to 10,000 cells/mm^3 are needed to make pleural fluid appear pinkish and are nonspecific. Grossly bloody effusions contain more than 100,000 cells/mm^3 and are seen in patients with trauma, malignancy, or pulmonary infarction. A hemothorax is defined by a pleural fluid hematocrit 50% or greater of the serum hematocrit.

E. Cultures and stains. To maximize the yield from pleural fluid cultures, anaerobic and aerobic cultures should be obtained. Fungal and mycobacterial cultures and smears should also be considered in the appropriate clinical setting. Because acid-fast stains may be positive in 20% of tuberculous effusions, they should always be performed in addition to Gram smears. The addition of a pleural biopsy increases the yield for *M. tuberculosis* even further to 80% to 90%.

F. Cytology. Malignant diseases (most commonly lung or breast cancers or lymphoma) can produce pleural effusions by implantation of malignant cells on the pleura or by impairment of lymphatic drainage resulting from tumor obstruction. If initial cytologic results are negative and a strong clinical suspicion exists, additional pleural fluid samples can increase the chance of a positive result. The addition of a pleural biopsy increases the yield even further. Heparin should be added to the container to prevent clotting of the fluid. In addition to malignancy, cytologic examination can definitively diagnose rheumatoid pleuritis.

Selected Readings

Bowditch HI. Paracentesis thoracis. *Am J Med Sci* 23:105, 1852.
The first description of thoracentesis.

Collins TR, Sahn SA. Thoracentesis: clinical value, complications, technical problems, and patient experience. *Chest* 1987;91:817.

Grogan D, Irwin RS, Channick R, et al. Complications associated with thoracentesis: a prospective randomized study comparing three different methods. *Arch Intern Med* 1990;150:873.
The foregoing two articles provide an excellent overview of the complications and pitfalls associated with thoracentesis.

Good JT, Taryle DA, Maulitz RM, et al. The diagnostic value of pleural fluid pH. *Chest* 1980;78:55.
Light RW, Ball WC. Glucose and amylase in pleural effusions. *JAMA* 1973;225:257.
Sahn SA. The differential diagnosis of pleural effusions. *West J Med* 1982;137:99.
The last three readings provide a good review of the use of biochemical testing in the evaluation of pleural effusions.

Light RW, MacGregor MI, Luchsinger PC, et al. Pleural effusions: the diagnostic separation of transudates and exudates. *Ann Intern Med* 1972;77:507.
A must-read classic article!

12. TRACHEOTOMY

Hashim M. Hesham

I. **General principles.** The term tracheotomy derives from the Greek words *trachea arteria* (rough artery) and *tome* (incision) and refers either to the operation that opens the trachea and results in the formation of a tracheostomy or to the opening itself. The procedure was not performed regularly until the 1800s, when it was used for management of diphtheria. Tracheotomy and emergency surgical airways are occasionally required in critically ill patients; thus, the indications, contraindications, complications, and techniques should be familiar to all physicians involved in intensive care.

II. **Indications.** The indication of tracheotomy is divided into three general categories, as discussed in the following sections.

A. **Tracheotomy to bypass airway obstruction**

1. Laryngeal dysfunction from vocal cord paralysis after surgery, recurrent laryngeal nerve injury, or upper respiratory infection can result in stridor or even complete obstruction.
2. In trauma, tracheotomy may be indicated when oral or nasotracheal intubation is impossible for any reason (hemorrhage, edema, direct crush, transection).
3. Inhalation of hot smoke or corrosives may result in significant upper airway edema immediately after burn or later in the hospital.
4. Foreign bodies are most commonly seen in the pediatric age group.
5. In patients with congenital anomalies, significant stenosis of glottic and subglottic structures are indications for emergency tracheotomy.
6. Neglected malignancies of the larynx may present with progressive upper airway obstruction.
7. Certain surgical procedures such as surgery of the base of the tongue or hypopharynx may require prophylactic tracheotomy in anticipation of postoperative edema of the upper airway.
8. In obstructive sleep apnea, tracheotomy is curative because it bypasses the upper airway obstruction.

B. **Tracheotomy for tracheal toilet.** Because of age, weakness, or neuromuscular disease, many patients are unable to clear respiratory tract secretions effectively and therefore require frequent suctioning. Tracheotomy provides an easy access to the lower airway.

C. **Tracheotomy for ventilatory support.** Although endotracheal intubation is usually the initial method of providing ventilatory support, tracheotomy is generally preferred for long-term management. Tracheotomy in patients with chronic lung disease reduces dead-space ventilation. (Although some physicians perform tracheotomy to prevent aspiration, it may actually cause aspiration. In general, tracheotomy to prevent aspiration is not recommended.)

III. **Contraindications.** There are no absolute contraindications to tracheotomy, but certain conditions such as coagulopathies and significant medical problems warrant special attention before anesthesia and surgery.

IV. **Timing.** When to convert from endotracheal tube to tracheotomy has been a matter of great controversy, and a range of 2 to 3 weeks has been advised. The decision should be based on the expected duration of intubation.

V. **Emergency tracheotomy.** Emergency tracheotomy is a moderately difficult procedure. When time is short, the patient's anatomy is distorted, and assistance is inadequate, tracheotomy can be hazardous. Emergency tracheotomy can pose significant risk to nearby neurovascular structures, particularly in children, in whom the trachea is small and not well defined. The incidence of complications of emergency tracheotomy is two to five times higher than for elective tracheotomy. Nonetheless, there are occasional indications for emergency tracheotomy, including a transected trachea, anterior neck trauma, and pediatric (younger than 12 years) patients requiring an emergency surgical airway in whom cricothyrotomy is generally not advised.

VI. Tracheotomy in the intensive care unit. Although tracheotomy is best performed in the operating room, bedside tracheotomy can be performed safely as well. The incidence of complications is low (5% to 6%) when the procedure is performed by an experienced surgeon with proper assistance, lighting, and equipment. The exact technique is described in standard surgical texts.

VII. Postoperative care. The care of a tracheotomy tube after surgery is important. Until the first tracheotomy tube is changed, the tapes should not be changed! Ideally, the first tube change should not be attempted until the tract has matured, a process that requires at least 7 to 10 days.

If the tube has been sutured into position, the suture should be left in place until the first tube change. The inner cannula of the tube should be removed regularly for inspection and cleaning. Humidification is important in preventing obstruction. Before discharge from the hospital, the family of the patient with a permanent tracheotomy must be fully instructed in the care and cleaning of the tube and in techniques for replacing it if it becomes dislodged.

VIII. Complications. Various complications are associated with tracheotomy at a variable rate of 6% to 50% and a mortality rate from 0.9% to 4.5%. Tracheotomy is more hazardous in children than in adults. Occasionally, a tube becomes obstructed with clotted blood or inspissated secretions. In that case, the inner tube should be removed, and suctioning should be performed on the patient. Obstruction may also result from angulation of the distal tube against the anterior tracheal wall.

A. Tube displacement or dislodgment. Dislodgment of a tracheotomy tube that has been in place for 2 weeks or longer can be managed by replacing the tube. If the tube cannot be replaced immediately and the patient cannot be ventilated (indicating that the tube is not in the trachea), orotracheal intubation should be performed. Immediate postoperative displacement can be fatal if the tube cannot be promptly replaced or if the patient cannot be orally intubated.

B. Hemorrhage

1. **Early.** Minor hemorrhage in postoperative fresh tracheotomy occurs in up to 37% of cases. Elevating the head of the bed and packing the wound usually control minor bleeding. Major bleeding occurs in 5% of tracheotomies and is due to bleeding from the thyroid isthmus or from the anterior jugular veins. Persistent bleeding may require a return to the operating room.
2. **Delayed.** Late bleeding after tracheotomy is from granulation tissue or other relatively minor causes. Another more serious cause of bleeding is rupture of the innominate artery caused by erosion through the trachea into the artery resulting from tracheotomy tube angulation or excessive cuff pressures. Pulsation of the tracheotomy tube is an indication of potentially fatal positioning.

C. Bronchorrhea. The tracheotomy tube virtually always irritates the trachea early on and results in an increase in normal secretions.

D. Stomal infection. An 8% to 12% incidence of cellulitis or purulent exudate is reported. Other complications include pneumothorax, pneumomediastinum, tracheoesophageal fistula, subglottic edema and stenosis, dysphagia, and aspiration.

IX. Percutaneous tracheotomy. The concept of tracheotomy by percutaneous dilatation was described by Toye and Weinstein in 1969 and again in 1986. Percutaneous methods of creating a surgical airway can be used whenever elective or emergency tracheotomy is indicated.

A. Advantages

1. Percutaneous tracheotomy can be preformed in 10 to 15 minutes compared with the more than 20 minutes that is required for standard operative tracheotomy.
2. Immediate bleeding is less severe because of less dissection and because the tube fits snugly in the hole that is created.

3. The risk of perforation of the posterior trachea and esophagus is low.
4. The scar is more cosmetically acceptable.
5. The rates of infection and stenosis are low.
6. The procedure can be performed by nonsurgeons.
7. The procedure can be performed at the patient's bedside.

B. Techniques and instruments. Several percutaneous tracheotomy and cricothyrotomy techniques and instruments have been developed over the last 15 years. All use some form of the Seldinger cannulation technique, with various adaptations for cutting (using a tracheostome) or dilating the pretracheal tissues and trachea. In a study using percutaneous dilatational tracheotomy from 1985 to 1992, Ciaglia and Graniero reported significant success rates and fewer complications. The techniques of percutaneous tracheotomy procedure are as follows (Fig. 12-1):

1. Intubate the trachea and monitor oxygen saturation.
2. Loosen the tape fixing the endotracheal tube in place and secure the tube by hand throughout the procedure.
3. Identify neck landmarks.
4. After preparation with 10% povidone-iodine solution and drapes, intravenous sedation and local anesthesia with 1% lidocaine, insert the needle between the first and second tracheal rings.
5. Access the trachea by the Seldinger technique. Use of a bronchoscope is helpful to ensure proper placement of the guidewire.
6. With a guidewire in place, advance a guiding catheter to the trachea (keep the guidewire in the patient's trachea until the end of procedure).
7. Perform serial dilations of the trachea to establish an adequate stoma for insertion of the tracheostomy tube.

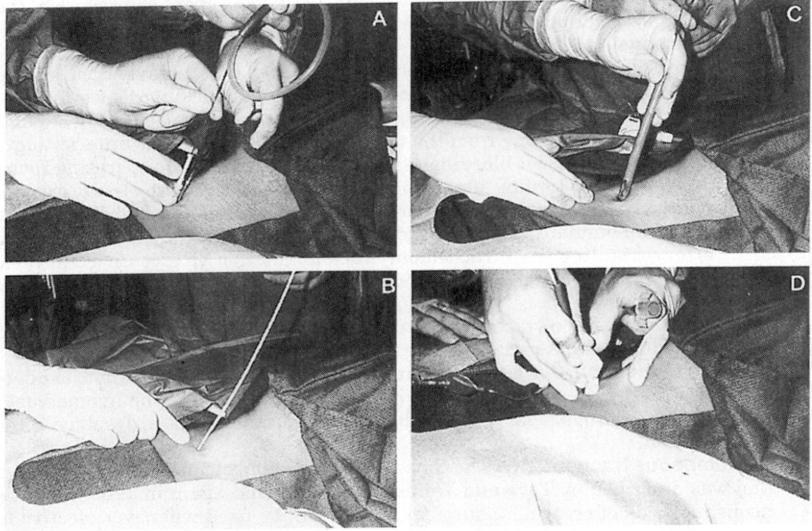

FIG. 12-1. **A:** Access to the trachea is obtained by the Seldinger technique. **B:** With a guidewire in place, a guiding catheter is advanced into the trachea. **C:** Serial dilations of the trachea are then performed to establish an adequate stoma for insertion of the tracheostomy tube. **D:** The tracheostomy tube is introduced; the guidewire and dilators are removed. (From *Cook Critical Care brochure on percutaneous dilatational tracheostomy,* Bloomington, IN, with permission.)

8. Insert the tracheotomy tube and remove the guidewire and dilators. The tracheotomy tube should be secured with stitches and tape, followed by the removal of the endotracheal tube and connection of the ventilation system to the tracheotomy tube. Reported complications include many of the same for standard tracheotomy. However, early and late complications have been fewer than with standard tracheotomy.

Selected Readings

American College of Surgeons Committee on Trauma. *Advanced trauma life support course for physicians: instructor manual.* Chicago: American College of Surgeons, 1985:159.

Emergency tracheotomy is rarely necessary in trauma cases.

Astrachan DI, Kirchner JC, Goodwin JW Jr. Prolonged intubation vs. tracheostomy: complications, practical and psychological considerations. *Laryngoscope* 1988;98:1165.

There is significant practical and psychological benefit in tracheotomy versus prolonged intubation.

Ciaglia P, Graniero KD. Percutaneous dilatational tracheostomy: results and long-term follow-up. *Chest* 1992;101:464.

Good review of success rates and complication of percutaneous dilatational tracheotomy.

D'Amelio LF, Hammond JS, Spain DA, et al. Tracheostomy and percutaneous endoscopic gastrostomy in the management of the head-injured trauma patient. *Am Surg* 1994;60:180.

Early tracheotomy and percutaneous endoscopic gastrostomy within the first 7 days of injury in patients with head trauma are the procedures of choice.

Dunham CM, LaMonica C. Prolonged tracheal intubation in the trauma patient. *J Trauma* 1984;24:120.

There was no difference in complications in intubation versus tracheotomy in the first 2 weeks of administration.

Kline SN. Maxillofacial trauma. In: Kreis DJ, Gomez GA, eds. *Trauma management.* Boston: Little, Brown, 1989.

Carefully performed tracheotomy in critically ill patients is safe and should be considered.

Rodriques JL, Steinberg SM, Luchetti FA, et al. Early tracheostomy for primary airway management in the surgical critical care setting. *Surgery* 1990;108:655.

Early tracheotomy in critically ill patients has significantly decreased the duration of mechanical ventilation as well as the length of hospital stays.

Toye FJ, Weinstein JD. Clinical experience with percutaneous tracheostomy and cricothyroidotomy in 100 patients. *J Trauma* 1986;26:1034.

Good description of tracheotomy performed by percutaneous dilatation.

Wease GL, Frikker M, Villalba M, et al. Bedside tracheostomy in the intensive care unit. *Arch Surg* 1996;131:552.

Bedside tracheotomy is safe and cost effective and should be done with bronchoscopic assistance.

13. GASTROINTESTINAL ENDOSCOPY

Daniel A. Devereaux

I. General principles. This chapter reviews the indications, contraindications, techniques, and complications of gastrointestinal endoscopy in critically ill patients.

Charged couple device chip technology and video monitors have replaced fiberoptic bundles on newer instruments, although fiberoptic and rigid endoscopes are still in use. Wheels and buttons on the handle of the flexible instrument control tip deflection, suction, and air and water insufflation.

II. Indications. Although cardiopulmonary complications of gastrointestinal endoscopy are infrequent, the procedure should be performed only when the tangible benefits clearly outweigh the risks. Gastrointestinal endoscopy in patients with clinically insignificant bleeding or minimally troublesome gastrointestinal complaints should be postponed until the medical-surgical illnesses improve. All endoscopists performing diagnostic gastrointestinal procedures should be competent in endoscopic therapy.

A. Upper gastrointestinal endoscopy. The indications for upper gastrointestinal endoscopy include upper gastrointestinal bleeding, caustic ingestion, and foreign body ingestion.

Patients with upper gastrointestinal bleeding, evidence of hemodynamic instability, and continuing need for transfusions should undergo urgent upper endoscopy with plans for appropriate endoscopic therapy. Percutaneous endoscopic gastrostomy tubes can be inserted at the bedside with the patient under intravenous and local sedation. Life-threatening complications are rarely associated with percutaneous endoscopic gastrostomy placement.

B. Endoscopic retrograde cholangiopancreatography. Endoscopic retrograde cholangiopancreatography (ERCP) is used only occasionally in the intensive care unit (ICU). It is indicated in patients in the ICU who have cholangitis unresponsive to medical therapy and acute gallstone pancreatitis complicated by cholangitis or jaundice. ERCP, combined with a sphincterotomy and stone extraction, reduces complications in patients with cholangitis. In acute gallstone pancreatitis, early ERCP does not lessen mortality, and its effect on complications is controversial.

C. Lower gastrointestinal endoscopy. Lower gastrointestinal endoscopy can be performed for acute lower gastrointestinal bleeding, but this procedure is technically difficult. Colonoscopy appears to have the highest yield in diagnosing and sometimes treating lower gastrointestinal bleeding. It is safe when appropriate resuscitation has been performed. Technetium-labeled erythrocyte scanning and angiography are other methods commonly used for localizing a bleeding site.

Endoscopic colonic decompression has been advised in critically ill patients with acute adynamic ileus when the diameter of the right colon exceeds 12 cm. Other studies suggest that the colonic dilation may not progress to life-threatening complications and decompression is unnecessary.

III. Contraindications. Endoscopy (and the associated air insufflation) should be avoided in patients with known or suspected gastrointestinal perforation and those known to be at high risk of perforation. Hemodynamic instability is a relative contraindication for endoscopy, but the benefit of therapeutic endoscopy may outweigh the risks in critically ill patients. The risk of a bleeding complication of endoscopic sphincterotomy is higher in patients with gross coagulopathy, and ERCP may be delayed while the coagulopathy is corrected. Endotracheal intubation and heavy sedation or general anesthesia may be necessary to facilitate the procedure. Patients with acute upper gastrointestinal bleeding who are confused or stuporous should have their airway protected with an endotracheal tube before endoscopy is performed.

IV. Complications. The principal risks of any endoscopic procedure are bleeding and perforation. Most bleeding is minimal and self-limited, but repeat endoscopy and surgery may be necessary to control recurrent bleeding. Angiography can assist in localizing the bleeding source in postendoscopy bleeding. Perforation of the bowel may result, and antibiotics and intravenous fluids should be given; surgery may be required. If duodenal perforation is encountered after endoscopic sphincterotomy, early medical therapy and stabilization of the patient may preclude the need for surgery. Aspiration of stomach contents and blood in acute upper gastrointestinal bleeding can be minimized by protecting the airway with endotracheal intubation in patients with severe bleeding or an altered mental state.

Sedative medications have their own complications, usually as a consequence of medication-induced hypoxemia (2 to 5/1,000 cases). Other complications can occur, including apnea, hypotension, and, rarely, death (0.3 to 0.5/1,000 cases).

V. Techniques

A. Upper gastrointestinal endoscopy. Fluid resuscitation and optimal treatment of hypoxemia should precede all endoscopic examinations. Endotracheal intubation should be considered in obtunded patients with severe bleeding and those undergoing foreign body removal. Nasogastric or orogastric lavage with a large-bore tube (greater than 40 Fr) should be performed to evacuate blood and clots from the stomach before endoscopy is performed in a patient with acute gastrointestinal bleeding.

Upper gastrointestinal bleeding is the most common indication for upper endoscopy in the ICU. Patients with continued or recurrent upper gastrointestinal bleeding should have urgent upper endoscopy as early as possible, certainly within 6 to 8 hours after presentation. In patients with massive hemorrhage, endoscopy may be performed in the operating room in anticipation of surgical therapy.

The team consists of an experienced endoscopist, a specially trained endoscopy assistant, and a nurse skilled in monitoring patients undergoing endoscopy.

A topical anesthetic is applied to the patient's pharynx to reduce the gag reflex. Intravenous anxiolytics or narcotics are used. I prefer midazolam and fentanyl because of their amnestic effect and short half-life, respectively. Proper patient monitoring is needed, with frequent (every 5 minutes) blood pressure and pulse measurements and continuous measurement of oxygen saturation by pulse oximetry.

Endoscopy is performed with a "therapeutic" instrument, equipped with a large operating channel to allow suctioning of blood, and hemostatic therapy. The endoscope is passed, and the upper gastrointestinal tract is rapidly surveyed to locate the site of bleeding to facilitate surgical therapy if endoscopic therapy fails. If an active bleeding site is found, hemostatic therapy may be attempted immediately.

In patients with significant recent bleeding and endoscopic evidence of recent hemorrhage (a visible vessel or adherent clot on an ulcer), hemostatic therapy to prevent recurrent bleeding should be strongly considered.

Actively bleeding lesions in the upper gastrointestinal tract can be treated with laser photocoagulation, heater probe therapy, monopolar and bipolar electrocoagulation, or injection therapy. Injection therapy is simple and inexpensive, requiring only a needle catheter and various liquid media to effect hemostasis, including absolute ethanol, sclerosants (sodium morrhuate), or vasoconstrictors (epinephrine). Injection therapy may be less effective in briskly bleeding ulcers or in bleeding esophageal varices. A newer method of banding esophageal varices is superior to sclerotherapy in terms of overall complications, recurrent bleeding, and mortality. Heater probes generate heat using electrical current delivered to the tip of the catheter, whereas bipolar electrocautery delivers electrical currently directly to the tissue and causes coagulation necrosis.

Because hemostatic therapy with the heater probe or bicap equipment requires an *en face* view, lesions seen tangentially may be difficult to treat with these methods. Injection therapy using epinephrine, absolute alcohol, or sclerosants (sodium morruhate, ethanolamine) allows treatment of lesions even when seen tangentially. Injection therapy generally begins on the periphery of the lesion, with injections in all four quadrants. Variceal sclerotherapy involves a direct or paravariceal injection of 1 to 4 mL of sclerosant. Banding of varices is performed with an endoscopic adaptor that allows placement of small rubber bands directly on to a varix.

B. Lower gastrointestinal endoscopy. Lower gastrointestinal endoscopy can be extremely difficult to perform in critically ill patients with colonic hemorrhage. Instruments available for the examination of the lower gastrointestinal tract include the following: the anoscope, which is useful mainly to evaluate for hemorrhoids or fissures; the sigmoidoscope; and the colonoscope. Colonoscopes are generally 140 to 180 cm long and are necessary to reach colonic lesions situated proximal to the splenic flexure.

Patient preparation for colonoscopy usually consists of a gallon of nonabsorbed polyethylene glycol given by mouth over 4 to 6 hours or by nasogastric tube 12 hours before examination. Magnesium citrate may be used over 24 to 48 hours in patients who have been taking clear liquids. Abdominal pressure that is applied by an assistant during colonoscopy may assist in advancing the colonoscope.

Colonoscopy has been reported as therapy for pseudoobstruction. Decompression by colonoscopy should not be first-line therapy for pseudoobstruction. Nasogastric and rectal tube placement, discontinuation of offending medications (narcotics and phenothiazines), treatment of underlying illness, and frequent repositioning (every 2 hours) of debilitated patients in the ICU often allows resolution of pseudoobstruction. In patients who have not had a response to conservative therapy, treatment with neostigmine should be tried.

Selected Readings

Fan S, Lai E, Mok F, et al. Early treatment of acute biliary pancreatitis by endoscopic papillotomy. *N Engl J Med* 1993;328:228.

A controversial article that ERCP is indicated in the early treatment of patients with acute pancreatitis.

Freeman ML, Cass OW, Peine CJ, et al. The non-bleeding visible vessel versus the sentinel clot: natural history and risk of rebleeding. *Gastrointest Endosc* 1993;39:3.

An evaluation of the stigmata of ulcers and the need for early surgical intervention.

Hirschowitz BI. Development and application of endoscopy. *Gastroenterology* 1993; 104:337.

An excellent review of the development of GI endoscopy from the use of rigid tubes and candlelight to the charge couple device chip and sophisticated flexible instruments.

Laine L. Refining the prognostic value of endoscopy in patients with bleeding ulcers. *Gastrointest Endosc* 1993;39:436.

A good review supporting of the efficacy of early endoscopy of ICU GI bleeders.

Lin HJ, Perng CL, Lee FY, et al. Endoscopic injection for the arrest of peptic ulcer hemorrhage: final results of a prospective, randomized comparative trial. *Gastrointest Endosc* 1993;39:1.

A review of the two various treatment options of UGI bleed and their efficacy.

Ponec RJ, Saunders MD, Kimmey MB. Neostigmine for the treatment of acute colonic pseudoobstruction. *N Engl J Med* 1999;341:137.

The usefulness of neostigmine was shown in the randomized, placebo controlled study.

Sloyer AF, Panella VS, Demas BE, et al. Olgivie's syndrome: successful management without colonoscopy. *Dig Dis Sci* 1988;33:1391.

An outline of the noninvasive management of pseudoobstruction.

14. PARACENTESIS AND DIAGNOSTIC PERITONEAL LAVAGE

Syed Adil Ahmed and Naveen A. Syed

I. Abdominal paracentesis

A. Indications. Diagnostic abdominal paracentesis is usually performed in any clinical situation in which the analysis of a sample of peritoneal fluid may be useful in ascertaining a diagnosis and in guiding therapy.

As a therapeutic intervention, abdominal paracentesis is usually performed to drain large volumes of abdominal ascites. When tense or refractory ascites is present, large-volume paracentesis is safe and effective. One study documented that large-volume paracentesis decreases esophageal variceal pressure, size, and wall tension in cirrhotics and may be an effective adjunct in the treatment of esophageal variceal bleeding.

B. Techniques. Before abdominal paracentesis is initiated, a catheter must be inserted to drain the urinary bladder, and any underlying coagulopathy or thrombocytopenia must be corrected. If the patient is critically ill, the procedure is performed while the patient is in the supine position. Clinically stable patients can be placed in the sitting position.

The site for paracentesis on the anterior abdominal wall is then chosen (Fig.14-1). The preferred site is in the lower abdomen, just lateral to the rectus abdominis muscle, in the midclavicular line, and inferior to the umbilicus. It is important to stay lateral to the rectus abdominal muscle to avoid injury to the inferior epigastric artery and vein.

Abdominal paracentesis can be performed by the needle technique, the catheter technique, or with ultrasound guidance.

1. **Needle technique.** The patient's abdomen is prepared with 10% povidone-iodine solution, and sterile drapes are applied. Local anesthesia, using 1% or 2% lidocaine with 1:200,000 epinephrine, is infiltrated into the site. Before infiltrating the anterior abdominal wall and peritoneum, the skin is pulled taut inferiorly, a maneuver that allows the peritoneal cavity to be entered at a different location than the skin entrance site, thereby decreasing the chance of ascitic leak. This is known as the Z-track technique. While tension is maintained inferiorly on the abdominal skin, the needle is advanced through the abdominal wall fascia and peritoneum, and local anesthetic is injected. Intermittent aspiration identifies when the peritoneal cavity is entered, with return of ascitic fluid into the syringe. The needle is held securely in this position with the operator's left hand, and the right hand is used to withdraw approximately 20 to 50 mL of ascitic fluid into the syringe for diagnostic paracentesis. Once adequate fluid is withdrawn, the needle and syringe are withdrawn from the anterior abdominal wall, and the paracentesis site is covered with a sterile dressing. A small amount of peritoneal fluid is sent in a sterile container for Gram stain and culture and sensitivity testing. The remainder of the fluid is sent for appropriate studies.
2. **Catheter technique.** The peritoneal cavity is entered in the same manner as for the needle technique. The catheter-over-needle assembly is inserted perpendicular to the anterior abdominal wall using the Z-track technique; once peritoneal fluid returns into the syringe barrel, the catheter is advanced over the needle, the needle is removed, and a 20- or 50-mL syringe is connected to the catheter. The tip of the catheter is now in the peritoneal cavity and can be left in place until the appropriate amount of peritoneal fluid is removed.
3. **Ultrasound guidance technique.** This technique is used in patients who have had previous abdominal surgery or peritonitis. These patients are predisposed to abdominal adhesions.

C. Complications. The most common complications related to abdominal paracentesis are bleeding and persistent ascitic leak. Other complications include

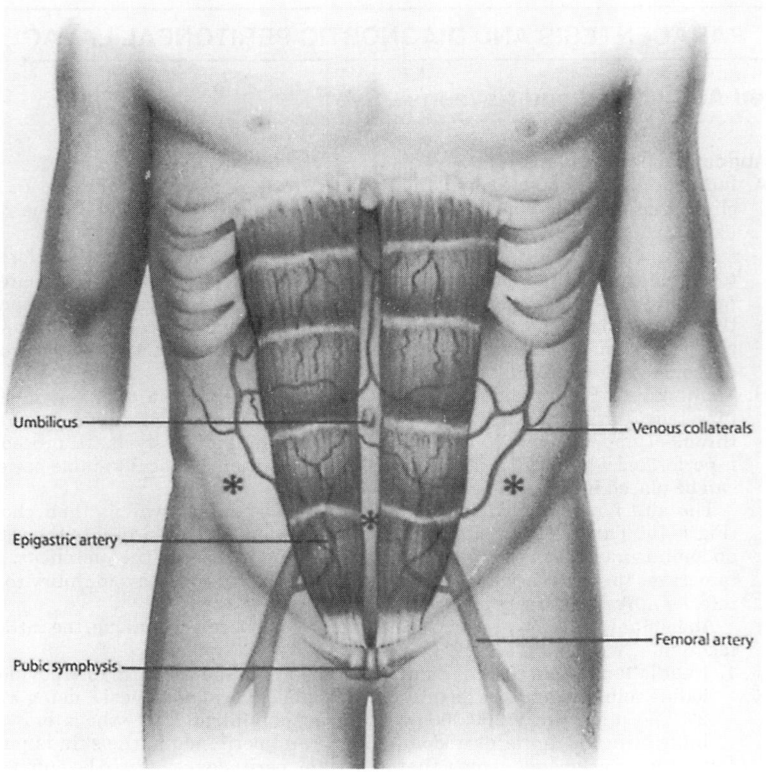

FIG. 14-1. Suggested sites for paracentesis.

intestinal or urinary bladder perforation, with associated peritonitis and infection. Transient hypotension may develop when a considerable amount of ascitic fluid is removed during therapeutic abdominal paracentesis.

II. Diagnostic peritoneal lavage. Since its introduction in 1965, diagnostic peritoneal lavage (DPL) has become a cornerstone in the evaluation of blunt and penetrating abdominal injuries. More recent advances have led to the use of ultrasound and rapid helical computed tomography in the emergency evaluation of abdominal trauma and may decrease the use of DPL in the future.

A. Indications. The primary indication for DPL is evaluation of blunt abdominal trauma in patients with associated hypotension or altered level of consciousness. Patients with associated thoracic or pelvic injuries should also have definitive evaluation for abdominal trauma, and DPL can be used in these patients.

DPL can be used to evaluate penetrating abdominal trauma. It is not recommended in patients with gunshot wounds to the thorax or abdomen, and mandatory exploratory laparotomy or thoracotomy is indicated in these patients.

DPL may prove useful in evaluation for possible peritonitis or ruptured viscus in patients with an altered level of consciousness but no evidence of traumatic injury. DPL can be considered in critically ill patients with sepsis to determine whether intraabdominal infection is the underlying source. DPL is also effective in rewarming patients with significant hypothermia.

B. Contraindications. DPL should not be performed in patients with clear signs of significant abdominal trauma and hemoperitoneum associated with hemodynamic instability. Pregnancy and multiple previous abdominal surgeries are relative contraindications to DPL.

C. Techniques. The three techniques of DPL are the closed percutaneous technique, the semiclosed technique, and the open technique.

The patient must be placed in the supine position for all three techniques. A catheter is placed into the urinary bladder, and a nasogastric tube is inserted into the stomach to prevent iatrogenic bladder or gastric injury. The skin of the anterior abdominal wall is prepared and anesthetized as described for paracentesis. The infraumbilical site is used unless there is clinical concern of possible pelvic fracture and retroperitoneal or pelvic hematoma, in which case the supraumbilical site is optimal.

1. **Closed percutaneous technique.** A 5-mm skin incision is made just at the inferior umbilical edge (Fig. 14-2). An 18-gauge needle is inserted through

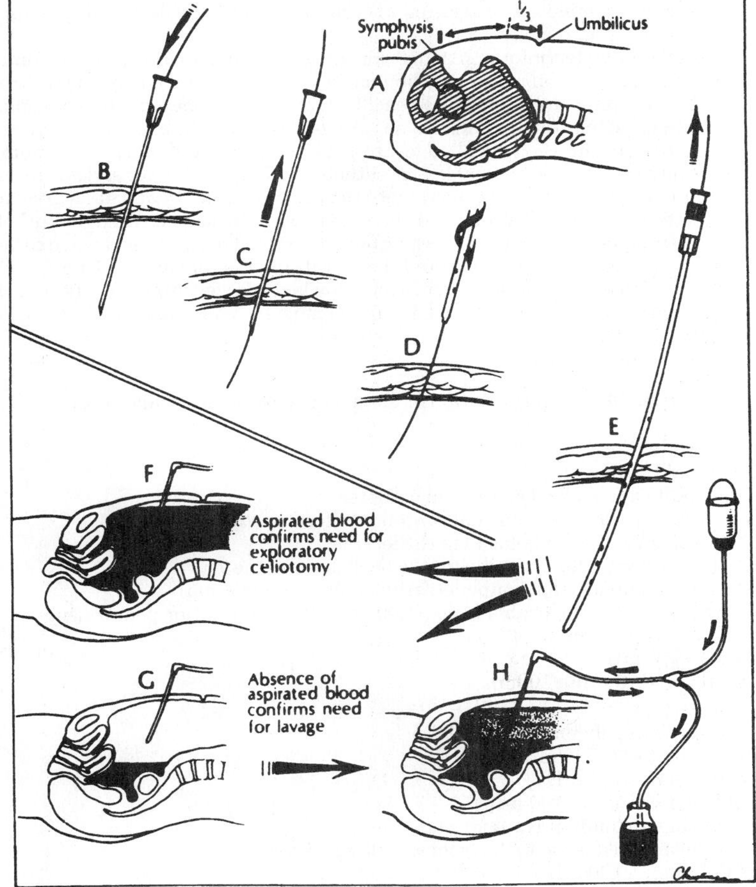

FIG. 14-2. The closed percutaneous technique for diagnostic peritoneal lavage, using a Seldinger guidewire method.

this incision and into the peritoneal cavity, angled toward the pelvis at approximately a 45-degree angle with the skin. The penetration through the linea alba and then through the peritoneum is felt as two separate "pops." A J-tipped guidewire is passed through the needle and into the peritoneal cavity. The 18-gauge needle is then removed, and the peritoneal lavage catheter is inserted over the guidewire into the peritoneal cavity, by using a twisting motion and guiding it inferiorly toward the pelvis. The guidewire is then removed, and a 10-mL syringe is attached to the catheter for aspiration. If free blood returns from the peritoneal catheter before the syringe is attached or if gross blood returns in the syringe barrel, then hemoperitoneum has been documented; the catheter is removed, and the patient is transported quickly to the operating room for emergency celiotomy. If no gross blood returns on aspiration through the catheter, then peritoneal lavage is performed using 1 L of Ringer's lactate solution or normal saline previously warmed to prevent hypothermia. A minimum of 250 mL of lavage fluid is considered a representative sample of the peritoneal fluid. A sample is sent to the laboratory for determination of red blood cell count, white blood cell count, amylase concentration, and the presence of bile, bacteria, or particulate matter. When the lavage is completed, the catheter is removed, and a sterile dressing is applied over the site.

2. **Semiclosed technique.** A 2- to 3-cm vertical incision made in the infraumbilical or supraumbilical area. The incision is continued sharply down through the subcutaneous tissue and linea alba, and the peritoneum is then visualized. Forceps, hemostats, or Allis clamps are used to grasp the edges of the linea alba and to elevate the fascial edges, to prevent injury to underlying abdominal structures. The peritoneal lavage catheter with a metal inner stylet is inserted through the closed peritoneum into the peritoneal cavity at a 45-degree angle to the anterior abdominal wall, directed toward the pelvis. When the catheter–metal stylet assembly is in the peritoneal cavity, the peritoneal lavage catheter is advanced into the pelvis, and the metal stylet is removed. A 10-mL syringe is attached to the catheter, and aspiration is conducted as previously described. When the lavage is completed, the fascia must be reapproximated with sutures, the skin closed, and a sterile dressing applied.

TABLE 14-1. Interpretation of diagnostic peritoneal lavage results

- Positive results
  - Abdominal trauma
    - Immediate gross blood return via catheter
    - Immediate return of intestinal contents or food particles
    - Aspiration of 10 mL of blood via catheter
    - Return of lavage fluid via chest tube or urinary catheter
    - RBC >100,000/mL (for nonpenetrating abdominal trauma)
    - RBC count used is variable from >1,000 to >100,000/mL (for penetrating abdominal trauma)
    - WBC >500/mL
    - Amylase >175 units/100mL
- Negative results
  - Nonpenetrating abdominal trauma
    - RBC count <50,000/mL
    - WBC count <100/mL
    - Amylase <75 units/100 mL
  - Penetrating abdominal trauma
    - RBC count used is variable, from <1,000 to <50,000/mL
    - WBC count <100/mL
    - Amylase <75 units/100 mL

RBC, red blood cell; WBC, white blood cell.

3. **Open technique.** A vertical midline incision approximately 3 to 5 cm long is made. The vertical midline incision is carried down through the skin, subcutaneous tissue, and linea alba, under direct vision. The peritoneum is identified, and a small vertical peritoneal incision is made to gain entrance into the peritoneal cavity. The peritoneal lavage catheter is then inserted into the peritoneal cavity under direct visualization and is advanced inferiorly toward the pelvis. It is inserted without the stylet or metal trocar. Peritoneal lavage is performed as described earlier.

D. **Interpretation of results.** The current guidelines for interpretation of positive and negative results of DPL are listed in Table 14-1.

E. **Complications.** Complications of DPL by any of the techniques described here include malposition of the lavage catheter, injury to the intraabdominal organs or vessels, iatrogenic hemoperitoneum, wound infection or dehiscence, evisceration, and possible unnecessary laparotomy.

Selected Readings

Branney SW, Moore EE, Cantrill SV, et al. Ultrasound based key clinical pathway reduces the use of hospital resources for the evaluation of blunt abdominal trauma. *J Trauma* 1997;42:1086.

An article about ultrasound as a diagnostic tool.

Catre MG. Diagnostic peritoneal lavage versus abdominal computed tomography in blunt abdominal trauma: a review of prospective studies. *Can J Surg* 1995;38:117.

Good article to review to compare DPL and computed tomography to evaluate victims of blunt abdominal trauma.

Gerber DR, Bekes CE. Peritoneal catheterization. *Crit Care Clin* 1992;8:727.

Good reference for indications for abdominal paracentesis.

Inturri P, Graziotto A, Roxxaro L. Treatment of ascites: old and new remedies. *Dig Dis* 1996;14:145.

Description of the role of paracentesis for the treatment of ascites.

Kravetz D, Romero G, Argonz J, et al. Total volume paracentesis decreases variceal pressure, size, and variceal wall tension in cirrhotic patients. *Hepatology* 1997;25:59.

More detail about decrease in esophageal variceal pressure after abdominal paracentesis.

McKenney MG, Martin L, Lentz K, et al. 1,000 consecutive ultrasounds for blunt abdominal trauma. *J Trauma* 1996;40:607.

More details about sonography as a diagnostic tool for patients with blunt abdominal trauma.

Sweeney JF, Albrink MH, Bischof E, et al. Diagnostic peritoneal lavage: volume of lavage effluent needed for accurate determination of a negative lavage. *Injury* 1994; 25:659.

More material about DPL and its interpretation.

Wherrett LJ, Boulanger BR, McLellan BA, et al. Hypotension after blunt abdominal trauma: the role of emergent abdominal sonography in surgical triage. *J Trauma* 1996;41:815.

Discusses the reliability of sonography to rule out intraperitoneal bleeding in trauma victims.

15. MANAGEMENT OF ACUTE ESOPHAGEAL VARICEAL HEMORRHAGE WITH GASTROESOPHAGEAL BALLOON TAMPONADE

Juan Carlos Puyana

I. General principles. Esophageal variceal hemorrhage is an acute, severe, dramatic complication of the patient with portal hypertension that carries a high mortality and significant incidence of recurrence. Until recently, balloon tamponade of the esophagus was considered the first line of treatment to control variceal hemorrhage; however, management of this entity has changed during the last decade, mainly because of the results obtained with urgent diagnostic and therapeutic endoscopy and sclerotherapy. This chapter describes the use of devices designed for gastric and esophageal balloon tamponade, summarizes the experience with these tubes, and describes the current role of balloon tamponade in the overall management of bleeding esophageal varices (Fig. 15-1).

II. Indications and contraindications. A Sengstaken-Blakemore tube is indicated in patients with a diagnosis of esophageal variceal hemorrhage and in whom sclerotherapy is not technically possible or readily available or has failed. An adequate anatomic diagnosis is imperative before any of these balloon tubes are inserted. Severe upper gastrointestinal bleeding attributed to esophageal varices in patients with clinical evidence of chronic liver disease results from other causes in 40% of cases. Use of the tube is contraindicated in patients with recent esophageal surgery or esophageal stricture. Some authors do not recommend balloon tamponade when a hiatal hernia is present, but there are reports of successful hemorrhage control in some of these patients.

III. Technical and practical considerations

A. Airway control. Endotracheal intubation is imperative in patients with hemodynamic compromise or encephalopathy. The incidence of aspiration pneumonia is directly related to the presence of encephalopathy or impaired mental status. Suctioning of pulmonary secretions and blood accumulated in the hypopharynx is facilitated in patients with endotracheal intubation. Sedatives and analgesics are more readily administered in intubated patients and may be required often, because these tubes are poorly tolerated in most patients. Sedatives must be used cautiously, however, because some of these patients have impaired liver metabolism. The incidence of pulmonary complications is significantly lower when endotracheal intubation is routinely used.

B. Hypovolemia, shock, and coagulopathy. Adequate intravenous access should be obtained with large-bore venous catheters, and aggressive fluid resuscitation should be undertaken with crystalloids and colloids. A central venous catheter or pulmonary artery catheter may be required to monitor intravascular filling pressures, especially in patients with severe cirrhosis, advanced age, or underlying cardiac and pulmonary disease. The hematocrit should be maintained at levels higher than 28%, and coagulopathy should be treated with fresh frozen plasma and platelets. Four to 6 units of packed red cells should always be available in case of severe recurrent bleeding, which commonly occurs in these patients.

C. Clots and gastric decompression. Placement of a Ewald tube and aggressive lavage and suctioning of the stomach and duodenum facilitate endoscopy and diminish the risk of aspiration and may help to control hemorrhage from causes other than esophageal varices.

The diagnostic endoscopic procedure should be done as soon as the patient is stabilized after basic resuscitation. Endoscopy is performed in the intensive care unit or operating room under controlled monitoring and with adequate equipment and personnel. An endoscope with a large suction channel should be used.

D. Tubes, ports, and balloons. Minnesota (Fig. 15-2) and Sengstaken-Blakemore (Fig. 15-3) tubes are most commonly used. Other tubes have been described for

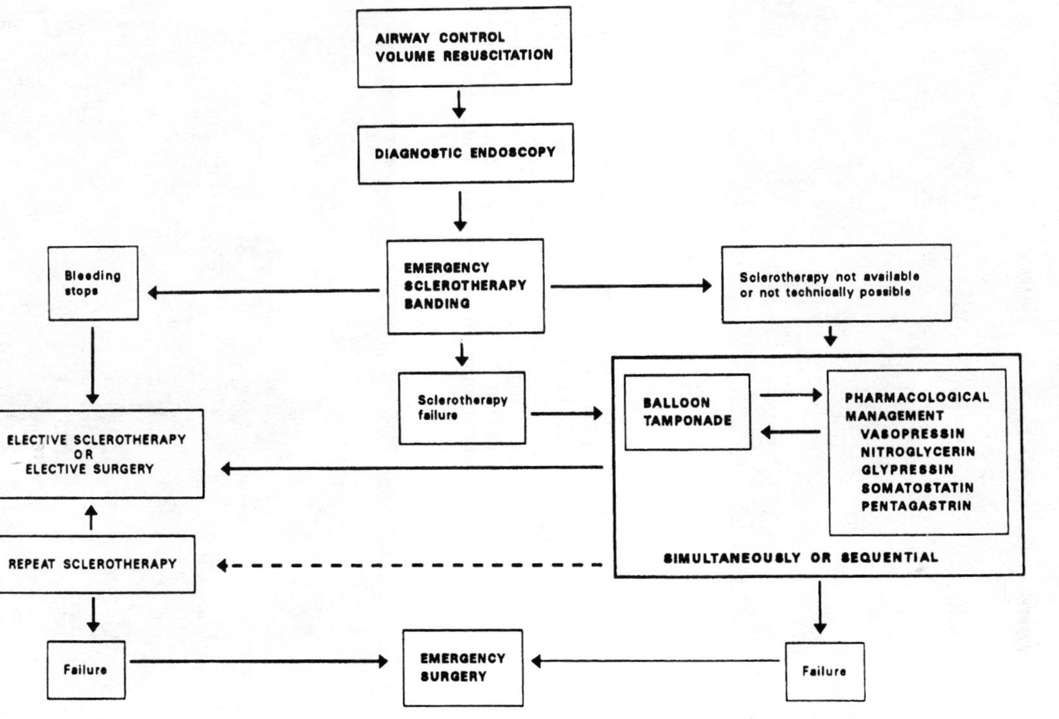

FIG. 15-1. Management of esophageal variceal hemorrhage.

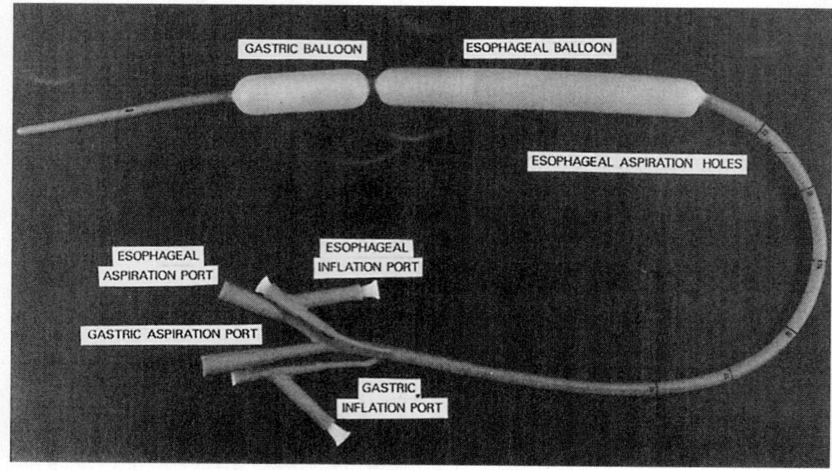

FIG. 15-2. Minnesota tube.

balloon tamponade (Table 15-1). The techniques described here are limited to the use of the Minnesota and Sengstaken-Blakemore tubes. All lumina should be patent, and balloons should be inflated and checked for leaks. The Minnesota tube has a fourth lumen that allows intermittent suctioning above the esophageal balloon, thus facilitating suctioning of saliva, blood, and pulmonary secretions in the hypopharynx (Fig. 15-4). When using a standard Sengstaken-Blakemore tube, a no. 18 Salem sump with surgical ties is attached above the

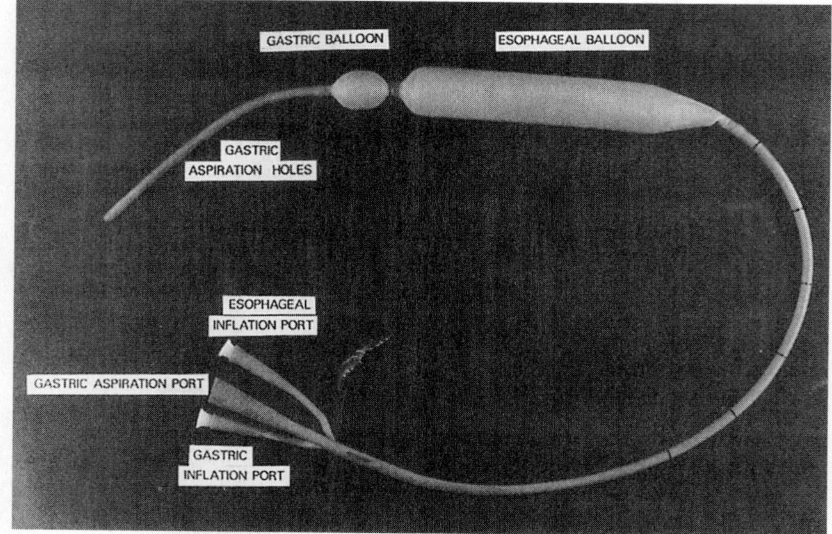

FIG. 15-3. Sengstaken-Blakemore tube.

TABLE 15-1. Tubes available for balloon tamponade

Tube	Manufacturer	Description
Minnesota four-lumen tube	Davol	18-Fr, 42-in.-long tube, 1.5-in. gastric balloon, 8-in. esophageal balloon; rubber, nonsterile, single use
Blakemore tube	Davol, Rush	12-, 16-, and 20-Fr, child, medium and adult sizes (adult, 39 in. long); rubber, nonsterile, single use
Nachlas gastrointestinal tube	Davol	20-Fr, 52-in., triple-lumen, gastric balloon only; two suction ports (above and below balloon); rubber, nonsterile, single use
Linton esophageal tube	Davol	20-Fr, 42-in., 3.5-in. gastric balloon, 800-mL air; two suction ports (above and below balloon); rubber, nonsterile, single use
Idezuki tube	See Idezuki, et al. *Am J Surg* 1990; 160:98.	Gastric and esophageal balloon; transparent tube with significantly larger inner diameter that allows passage of bronchoscope for direct visualization of bleeding varices, permitting "titration" of balloon pressure; polyurethane and polyvinyl chloride

esophageal balloon and is inserted through the patient's mouth. Suctioning above the esophageal balloon and hypopharynx diminishes but does not eliminate the risk of aspiration pneumonia.

E. Tube insertion and placement. The tube should be generously lubricated with lidocaine jelly. It can be inserted through the patient's nose or mouth, but the nasal route is not recommended in patients with coagulopathy. The tube is passed into the stomach. Auscultation in the epigastrium while a flush of air is injected through the gastric lumen verifies the position of the tube, but the position of the gastric balloon must be confirmed radiologically at this time. The gastric balloon is inflated with no more than 80 mL of air, and a (portable) radiograph is obtained that includes the upper abdomen and lower chest (Fig. 15-5). When it is documented that the gastric balloon is below the diaphragm, the balloon should be further inflated with air, slowly, to a volume of 250 to 300 mL. The gastric balloon of the Minnesota tube can be inflated to 450 mL. Tube balloon inlets should be clamped with rubber shod hemostats after insufflation. Hemorrhage is frequently controlled with insufflation of the gastric balloon alone without applying traction, but in patients with torrential hemorrhage it is necessary to apply traction, as described later. If the bleeding continues, the esophageal balloon should be inflated with a bedside manometer to about 45 mm Hg, and this pressure should be monitored and maintained. Some authors inflate the esophageal balloon in all patients immediately after it is inserted.

F. Fixation and traction techniques. Fixation and traction on the tube depend on the route of insertion. When the nasal route is used, traction should not be applied against the nostril, because this can easily cause skin and cartilage

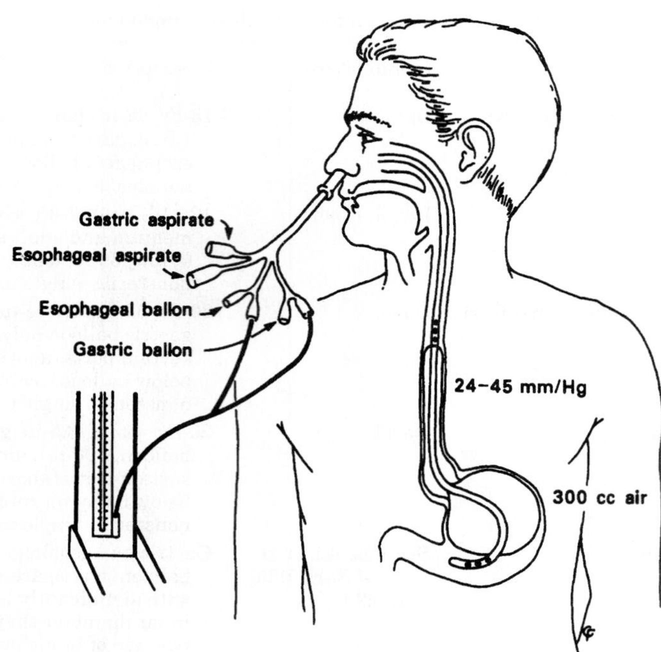

FIG. 15-4. Proper positioning of the Minnesota tube.

necrosis. When traction is required, the tube should be attached to a cord that is passed over a pulley in a bed with an overhead orthopedic frame and aligned directly as it comes out of the nose to avoid contact with the nostril. This system allows maintenance of traction with a known weight (500 to 1500 g) that is easily measured and constant. When the tube is inserted through the mouth, traction is better applied by placing a football helmet on the patient and attaching the tube to the bar of the helmet after a similar weight is applied for tension. Pressure sores can occur in the head and forehead when the helmet does not fit properly or when it is used for a prolonged period. Several authors recommend overhead traction for both oral and nasal insertion.

G. Maintenance and monitoring. The gastric lumen is placed to intermittent suction. The Minnesota tube has an esophageal lumen that can also be placed to low intermittent suction. If the Salem sump has been used as previously described, then continuous suction can be used on the sump tube. The tautness and inflation of balloons should be checked an hour after insertion and periodically by experienced personnel. The tube should be left in place a minimum of 24 hours. The gastric balloon tamponade can be maintained continuously up to 48 hours. The esophageal balloon, however, must be deflated for 30 minutes every 8 hours. The position of the tube should be monitored radiologically every 24 hours or sooner if there is any indication of tube displacement. A pair of scissors should be at the bedside in case the balloon ports need to be cut for rapid decompression, because the balloon can migrate and acutely obstruct the airway.

H. Tube removal. Once hemorrhage is controlled, the esophageal balloon is deflated first; the gastric balloon is left inflated for an additional 24 to 48 hours.

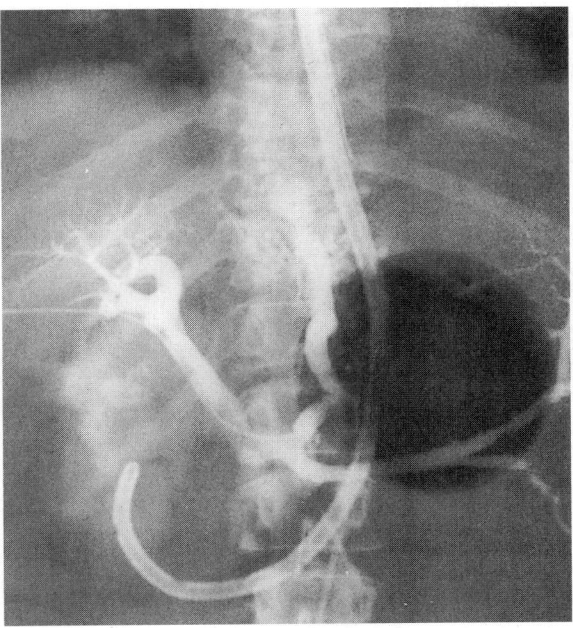

FIG. 15-5. Radiograph showing correct position of the tube; the gastric balloon is seen below the diaphragm. Note the Salem sump above the gastric balloon and adjacent to the tube. (Courtesy of Ashley Davidoff, M.D.)

If there is no evidence of bleeding, the gastric balloon is deflated, and the tube is left in place 24 hours longer. If bleeding recurs, the appropriate balloon is reinflated. The tube is removed if no further bleeding occurs.

IV. Complications. Aspiration pneumonia is the most common complication of balloon tamponade. The severity and fatality rate are related to the presence of impaired mental status and encephalopathy in patients with poor control of the airway. The incidence ranges from 0% to 12%. Acute laryngeal obstruction is the most severe of all complications and the worst example of tube migration. Migration of the tube occurs when the gastric balloon is not inflated properly after adequate positioning in the stomach or when excessive traction (more than 1.5 kg) is used. Aspiration pneumonia and esophageal perforation can both occur when the balloon migrates into the esophagus or hypopharynx. Mucosal ulceration of the gastroesophageal junction is common and is directly related to prolonged traction time (longer than 36 hours). Perforation of the esophagus is reported as a result of misplacing the gastric balloon above the diaphragm (Fig. 15-6). The position must be confirmed radiologically immediately after passing the tube and before the gastric balloon is inflated with more than 80 mL of air. Rupture of the esophagus carries a high mortality, especially in patients with severe hemorrhage who already have serious physiologic impairment. The incidence of complications that are a direct cause of death ranges from 0% to 20%. Unusual complications, such as impaction, result from obstruction of the balloon ports that makes it impossible to deflate the balloon. Occasionally, surgery is required to remove the tube. Other complications include necrosis of the nostrils and nasopharyngeal bleeding.

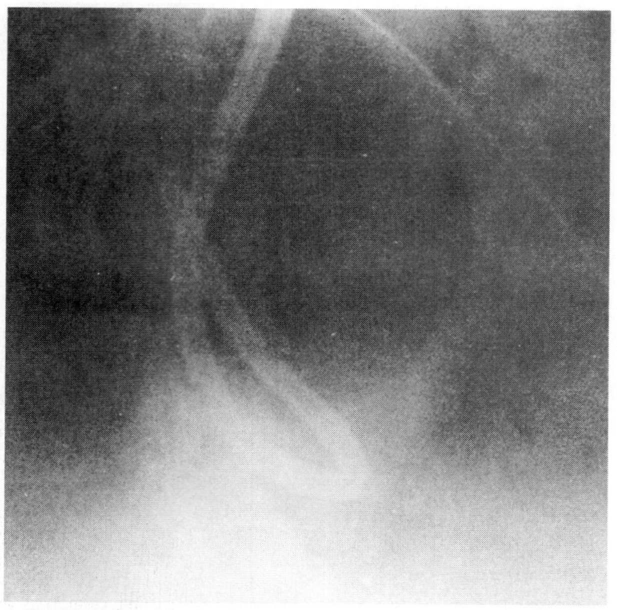

FIG. 15-6. Chest radiograph, showing distal segment of the tube coiled in the chest and the gastric balloon inflated above the diaphragm in the esophagus. (Courtesy of Ashley Davidoff, M.D.)

Selected Readings

Cello JP, Crass RA, Grendell JH, et al. Management of the patient with hemorrhaging esophageal varices. *JAMA* 1986;256:1480.

A review of the management for esophageal varices.

Duarte B. Technique for the placement of the Sengstaken-Blakemore tube. *Surg Gynecol Obstet* 1989;168:449.

Description of a technique for Sengstaken-Blakemore tube placement.

Fleisher D. Etiology and prevalence of severe persistent upper gastrointestinal bleeding. *Gastroenterology* 1983;80:800.

A prospective study documenting the etiology and prevalence of episodes of upper gastrointestinal bleeding over a 12-month period.

Lee H, Hawker FH, Selby W, et al. Intensive care treatment of patients with bleeding esophageal varices: results, predictors of mortality, and predictors of the adult respiratory distress syndrome. *Crit Care Med* 1992;20:1555.

Independent predictors of mortality were total volume of sclerotherapy injectate, multiple blood transfusions, Glasgow Coma Score, International Normalized Ratio (INR), and the presence of shock on admission to the intensive care unit.

Terblanche J, Krige JE, Bornman PC. The treatment of esophageal varices. *Annu Rev Med* 1992;43:69.

Good review of the therapeutic options for the management of esophageal varices.

Westaby D, MacDougall BRD, Williams R. Improved survival following injection sclerotherapy for esophageal varices: final analysis of a controlled trial. *Hepatology* 1985; 5:827.

Survival was better and cumulative proportion of patients with recurrent bleeding was less when patients received sclerotherapy.

16. ENDOSCOPIC PLACEMENT OF FEEDING TUBES

Stephen O. Heard

I. Indications for enteral feeding. Nutritional support is an essential component of intensive care medicine. Provision of nutrition through the enteral route aids in prevention of gastrointestinal mucosal atrophy, thereby maintaining the integrity of the gastrointestinal mucosal barrier. Advantages of enteral nutrition are preservation of immunologic gut function and normal gut flora, improved use of nutrients, and reduced cost and infectious complications.

Enteral feeding at a site proximal to the pylorus may be absolutely or relatively contraindicated in patients with increased risk of pulmonary aspiration, but feeding more distally (particularly distal to the ligament of Treitz) decreases the likelihood of aspiration. Other relative or absolute contraindications to enteral feeding include fistulas, intestinal obstruction, upper gastrointestinal hemorrhage, and severe inflammatory bowel disease. Enteral feeding is not recommended in patients with severe malabsorption or early in the course of severe short gut syndrome.

II. Access to the gastrointestinal tract. Gastric feeding provides the most normal route for enteral nutrition, but it is commonly poorly tolerated in the critically ill patient because of gastric dysmotility with delayed emptying. Enteral nutrition infusion into the duodenum or jejunum may decrease the incidence of aspiration because of the protection afforded by a competent pyloric sphincter; however, the risk of aspiration is not completely eliminated by feeding distal to the pylorus. Infusion into the jejunum is associated with the lowest risk of pulmonary aspiration. An advantage of this site of administration is that enteral feeding can be initiated early in the postoperative period, because postoperative ileus primarily affects the colon and stomach and only rarely involves the small intestine.

III. Techniques. Enteral feeding tubes can be placed by the transnasal, transoral, or percutaneous transgastric routes. If these procedures are contraindicated or unsuccessful, the tube may be placed using endoscopic and laparoscopic techniques or surgically through a laparotomy.

A. Nasoenteric route. Nasoenteric tubes are the most commonly used means of providing enteral nutritional support in critically ill patients. This route is preferred for short- to intermediate-term enteral support when eventual resumption of oral feeding is anticipated. It is possible to infuse enteral formulas into the stomach using a conventional 16- or 18-Fr polyvinylchloride nasogastric tube, but patients are usually much more comfortable if a small-diameter silicone or polyurethane feeding tube is used. Nasoenteric tubes vary in luminal diameter (6 to 14 Fr) and length, depending on the desired location of the distal orifice: stomach, 30 to 36 in.; duodenum, 43 in.; jejunum, at least 48 in. Some tubes have tungsten-weighted tips designed to facilitate passage into the duodenum by normal peristalsis; others have a stylet. Most are radiopaque. Newer tubes permit gastric decompression while delivering formula into the jejunum.

Nasoenteric feeding tubes should be placed with the patient in a semi-Fowler or sitting position. The tip of the tube should be lubricated, placed in the patient's nose, and advanced to the posterior pharynx. If possible, the patient should be permitted to sip water as the tube is slowly advanced into the stomach. Once the tube is in position, air should be insufflated through the tube while the physician auscults over the patient's stomach with a stethoscope. The presence of a gurgling sound suggests, but does not prove, that the tube is in the gastric lumen. *A chest radiograph should be obtained to confirm the position of the tube before feeding is initiated.* The tube should be securely taped to the patient's forehead or cheek without tension. If the tube is placed for duodenal or jejunal feeding, a loop 6 to 8 in. long may be left extending from the nose, and the tube may be advanced 1 to 2 in. every hour. Placing the patient in a right lateral decubitus position may facilitate passage of the tube through the pylorus.

Spontaneous transpyloric passage of enteral feeding tubes in critically ill patients is commonly unsuccessful secondary to the preponderance of gastric atony in these patients. The addition of a tungsten weight to the end of enteral feeding tubes and the development of wire or metal stylets in enteral feeding tubes are aimed at improving the success rate for spontaneous transpyloric passage. The administration of intravenous metoclopramide and erythromycin has been recommended to improve spontaneous transpyloric placement of enteral feeding tubes.

If the tube does not migrate into the duodenum over several hours, tube placement can be attempted under endoscopic assistance or fluoroscopic guidance. The patient is sedated appropriately, and topical anesthetic is applied to the posterior pharynx with lidocaine or benzocaine spray. A nasoenteric feeding tube 43 to 48 in. long with an inner wire stylet is passed transnasally into the stomach. The endoscope is inserted and is advanced through the esophagus into the gastric lumen. Endoscopy forceps are passed through the biopsy channel of the endoscope and are used to grasp the tip of the enteral feeding tube. The endoscope, along with the enteral feeding tube, is advanced distally into the duodenum as far as possible (Fig. 16-1**A**). The endoscopy forceps and feeding tube remain in position in the distal duodenum as the endoscope is withdrawn back into the gastric lumen. The endoscopy forceps are opened, the feeding tube is released, and the endoscopy forceps are withdrawn carefully back into the stomach. On first pass, the feeding tube is usually lodged in the second portion of the duodenum. The portion of the feeding tube that is redundant in the stomach is advanced slowly into the duodenum with the endoscopy forceps; the aim is to achieve a final position distal to the ligament of Treitz (Fig. 16-1**B**). An abdominal radiograph is obtained at the completion of the procedure to document the final position of the nasoenteral feeding tube.

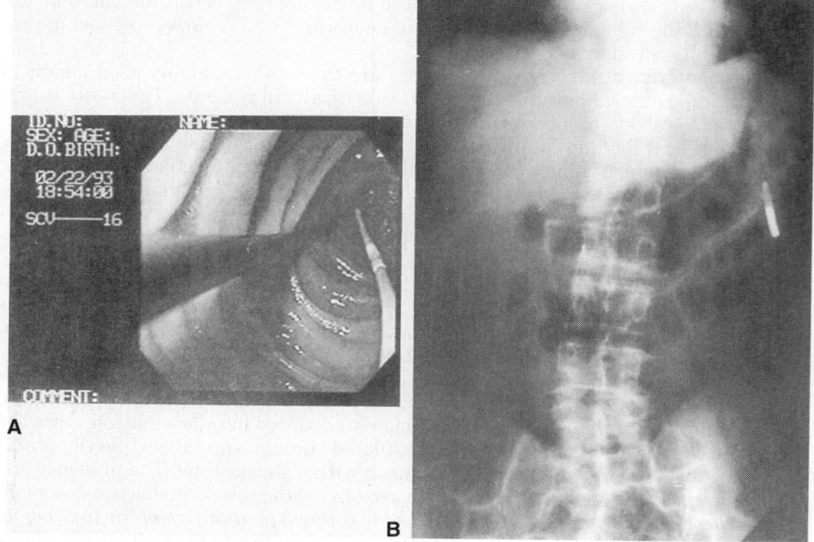

FIG. 16-1. **A:** Endoscopic placement of nasoenteral feeding tube. Endoscopy forceps and gastroscope advancing the feeding tube in the duodenum. **B:** Abdominal radiograph, documenting the optimal position of an endoscopically placed nasoenteral feeding tube, past the ligament of Treitz.

B. Percutaneous route. Percutaneous endoscopic gastrostomy (PEG) tube placement has become the procedure of choice for patients requiring prolonged enteral nutritional support and can be performed in the operating room, in an endoscopy unit, or at the patient's bedside in the intensive care unit with portable endoscopy equipment. Tubes range in size from 20 to 28 Fr. PEG should not be performed in patients with near or total obstruction of the pharynx or esophagus, in the presence of coagulopathy, or when transillumination is inadequate. Relative contraindications are ascites, gastric cancer, and gastric ulcer. Previous abdominal surgery is not a contraindication.

1. **Pull technique.** The procedure is performed with the patient in the supine position. The abdomen is prepared and draped. The posterior pharynx is anesthetized with a topical spray or solution (e.g., benzocaine spray or viscous lidocaine), and intravenous sedation (e.g., 1 to 2 mg midazolam) is administered. A prophylactic antibiotic, usually a first-generation cephalosporin, is administered before the procedure. The fiberoptic gastroscope is inserted into the stomach, which is then insufflated with air. The lights are dimmed, and the assistant applies digital pressure to the patient's anterior abdominal wall in the left subcostal area approximately 2 cm below the costal margin, to look for the brightest transillumination. The endoscopist should be able to identify clearly the indentation in the stomach created by the assistant's digital pressure on the anterior abdominal wall; otherwise, another site should be chosen. When the correct spot has been identified, the assistant anesthetizes the anterior abdominal wall. The endoscopist then introduces a polypectomy snare through the endoscope. A small incision is made in the skin, and the assistant introduces a large-bore catheter-needle-stylet assembly into the stomach and through the snare. The snare is then tightened securely around the catheter. The inner stylet is removed, and a looped insertion wire is introduced through the catheter and into the stomach. The cannula is slowly withdrawn so the snare grasps the wire. The gastroscope is then pulled out of the patient's mouth with the wire firmly grasped by the snare. The end of the transgastric wire exiting the patient's mouth is then tied to a prepared gastrostomy tube. The assistant pulls on the end of the wire exiting from the abdominal wall while the endoscopist guides the lubricated gastrostomy tube into the posterior pharynx and the esophagus. With continued traction, the gastrostomy tube is pulled into the stomach so it exits on the anterior abdominal wall. The gastroscope is reinserted into the stomach to confirm adequate placement of the gastrostomy tube against the gastric mucosa and to document that no bleeding has occurred. The intraluminal portion of the tube should contact the mucosa, but excessive tension on the tube should be avoided, because this can lead to ischemic necrosis of the gastric wall. The tube is secured to the abdominal wall using sutures. Feedings may be initiated immediately after the procedure or 24 hours later (Fig. 16-2).
2. **Push technique.** This method is similar to the pull technique. The gastroscope is inserted, and a point on the anterior abdominal wall is localized as for the pull technique. Rather than introducing a looped insertion wire, however, a straight guidewire is snared and is brought out through the patient's mouth by withdrawing the endoscope and snare together. A commercially developed gastrostomy tube (Sachs-Vine, Bard Guidewire PEG System, Bard, Inc. Billerica, MA 01821) with a tapered end is then passed in an aboral direction over the wire, which is held taut. The tube is grasped and is pulled the rest of the way outward. The gastroscope is reinserted to check the position and tension on the tube.
3. **Introducer technique.** This method uses a peel-away introducer technique originally developed for the placement of cardiac pacemakers and central venous catheters. The gastroscope is inserted into the stomach, and an appropriate position for placement of the tube is identified. After infiltration of the skin with local anesthetic, a 16- or 18-gauge needle is introduced into the stomach. A J-tipped guidewire is inserted through the needle into the stomach, and the needle is withdrawn. Using a twisting motion, a 16-Fr introducer with a peel-away sheath is passed over the guidewire into the

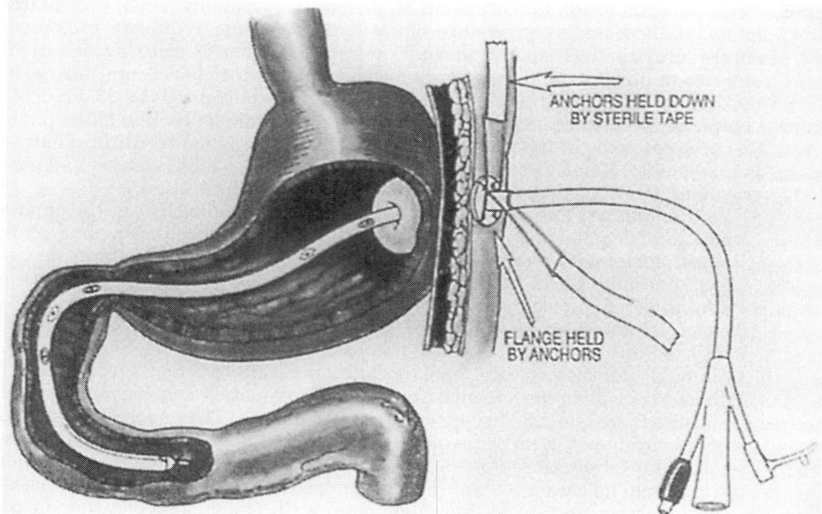

FIG. 16-2. Transgastric duodenal feeding tube, which allows simultaneous gastric decompression and duodenal feeding, can be placed percutaneously (with endoscopic or fluoroscopic assistance) or surgically.

gastric lumen. The guidewire and introducer are removed, leaving in place the sheath that allows placement of a 14-Fr Foley catheter. The sheath is peeled away after the balloon is inflated with 10 mL of normal saline.

4. **Percutaneous endoscopic jejunostomy.** If postpyloric feeding is desired (especially in patients at high risk of pulmonary aspiration), a percutaneous endoscopic jejunostomy (PEJ) may be performed. The PEJ tube allows for simultaneous gastric decompression and duodenal or jejunal enteral feeding. A second smaller feeding tube can be attached and passed through the gastrostomy tube and advanced endoscopically into the duodenum or jejunum. When the PEG is in position, a guidewire is passed through the PEG and is grasped using endoscopy forceps. The guidewire and endoscope are passed into the duodenum as distally as possible. The jejunal tube is then passed over the guidewire through the PEG into the distal duodenum and is advanced into the jejunum, and the endoscope is withdrawn. An alternative method is to grasp a suture at the tip of the feeding tube or the distal tip of the tube itself and pass the tube into the duodenum by using forceps advanced through the biopsy channel of the endoscope. This obviates the need to pass the gastroscope into the duodenum, a maneuver that may result in dislodgment of the tube when the endoscope is withdrawn.
5. **Complications.** The most common complication of percutaneous placement of enteral feeding tubes is infection, usually involving the cutaneous exit site and surrounding tissue. Other complications include gastrointestinal hemorrhage, gastrocolic fistula, peritonitis, and persistent pneumoperitoneum.

IV. **Delivering the tube feeding formula.** The enteral formula can be delivered by intermittent bolus feeding, gravity infusion, or continuous pump infusion. Continuous pump infusion is the preferred method for the delivery of enteral nutrition in the critically ill patient because problems with distention, diarrhea, and elevated gastric residuals are decreased.

V. **Medications.** When medications are administered through an enteric feeding tube, it is important to be certain that the drugs are compatible with each other and with the enteral formula. In general, medications should be delivered separately, rather than as a combined bolus. For medications that are better absorbed in an empty stomach, tube feedings should be suspended for 30 to 60 minutes before administration of the drug. Medications should be administered in an elixir formulation through enteral feeding tubes whenever possible to prevent occlusion of the tube. Enteral tubes should always be flushed with 20 mL of saline after medications are administered.

VI. Complications. Enteral tube placement is associated with few complications, if physicians adhere to appropriate protocols and pay close attention to the details of the procedures. However, nasopulmonary intubation, aspiration, gastrointestinal intolerance to enteral nutrition, prerenal azotemia, hypernatremia, deficiencies of essential fatty acids and fat-soluble vitamins, bacterial contamination of enteral formulas, and occluded feeding tubes are potential complications. Occluded tubes can be cleared by irrigation with warm saline, a carbonated liquid, cranberry juice, and digestive enzymes (Viokase and Pancrease, dissolved in a sodium bicarbonate solution).

Selected Readings

Baskin WN. Advances in enteral nutrition techniques: clinical review. *Am J Gastroenterol* 1992;87:1547.
Nice review of PEG and PEJ techniques.

Bower RH, Cerra FB, Bershadsky B, et al. Early enteral administration of a formula supplemented with arginine, nucleotides, and fish oil in intensive care unit patients: results of a multicenter, prospective, randomized, clinical trial. *Crit Care Med* 1995;23:436.
Patients fed a formula supplemented with arginine, nucleotides, and fish oil had a significant reduction in nosocomial infections and hospital length of stay.

Kalliafas S, Choban PS, Ziegler D, et al. Erythromycin facilitates postpyloric placement of nasoduodenal feeding tubes in intensive care unit patients: randomized, double-blinded, placebo-controlled trial. *JPEN J Parenter Enteral Nutr* 1996;20:385.
Erythromycin increased the success of nasoduodenal intubation from 35% to 61%.

Lord LM, Weiser-Maimone A, Pulhamus M, et al. Comparison of weighted vs unweighted enteral feeding tubes for efficacy of transpyloric intubation. *JPEN J Parenter Enteral Nutr* 1993;17:271.
The unweighted feeding tubes had a higher rate of passing through the pylorus into the small bowel: 84% within 4 hours.

Marcuard SP, Perkins AM. Clogging of feeding tubes. *JPEN J Parenter Enteral Nutr* 1988;12:403.
This study evaluated the potential for various formulas to clog feeding tubes and suggested several procedures to minimize the risk of occlusion.

Montecalvo MA, Steger KA, Farber HW, et al. Nutritional outcome and pneumonia in critical care patients randomized to gastric versus jejunal tube feedings: the Critical Care Research Team. *Crit Care Med* 1992;20:1377.
Feeding through a jejunal tube translated into a higher proportion of patients' receiving their daily caloric goal, higher prealbumin concentrations, and lower incidence of nosocomial pneumonia compared with continuous gastric tube feeding.

Moore FA, Feliciano DV, Andrassy RJ, et al. Early enteral feeding, compared with parenteral, reduces postoperative septic complications: the results of a meta-analysis. *Ann Surg* 1992;216;172.
This meta-analysis of eight prospective, randomized studies showed that septic complications were reduced in high-risk surgical patients who received early enteral nutritional support.

Paz HL, Weinar M, Sherman MS. Motility agents for the placement of weighted and unweighted feeding tubes in critically ill patients. *Intensive Care Med* 1996;22:301.
This study supported the use of weighted tubes but found no utility with motility agents.

Zaloga GP. Bedside method for placing small bowel feeding tubes in critically ill patients: a prospective study. *Chest* 1991;100:1643.
A detailed description of a method for the placement of feeding tubes in the small bowel.

17. CEREBROSPINAL FLUID ASPIRATION

Christopher Greene

I. Cerebrospinal fluid access for diagnostic purposes. A basic cerebrospinal (CSF) test profile includes glucose and protein values, a cell count, a Gram stain, cultures, and a pressure reading. CSF glucose is usually equivalent to two-thirds of serum glucose and lags behind blood levels by about 2 hours. Increased CSF glucose is nonspecific and usually reflects hyperglycemia. Hypoglycorrhachia can be the result of any inflammatory or neoplastic meningeal disorder.

CSF protein content is usually less than 0.5% of that in plasma. Although it is nonspecific, an elevated protein level in the CSF is a reliable indicator of CNS disease. Total protein content in the CSF exhibits a gradient with its highest level normally found in the lumbar subarachnoid space at 20 to 50 mg/dL, followed by the cisterna magna at 15 to 25 mg/dL and the ventricles at 6 to 12 mg/dL. A value exceeding 500 mg/dL is compatible with an intraspinal tumor with a complete subarachnoid block, meningitis, or bloody CSF. Low protein levels are seen in healthy children younger than 2 years of age and in patients with pseudotumor cerebri, acute water intoxication, and leukemia.

Normal CSF cell counts include no erythrocytes and a maximum of 5 leukocytes/mL. Greater numbers of cells are normally found in children (up to 10/mL, mostly lymphocytes). CSF cytologic studies can be helpful in identifying cells from CNS primary or metastatic tumors and differentiation from inflammatory disorders.

A. Hemorrhage. Lumbar puncture (LP) is indicated after subarachnoid hemorrhage (SAH) if the head computed tomographic (CT) scan is not diagnostic and if the clinical history and presentation are atypical. An LP should not be performed without prior CT if the patient has any focal neurologic deficits because transtentorial herniation may occur.

A traumatic LP presents a diagnostic dilemma in the context of a possible SAH. Consistent with a traumatic LP are a decreasing red blood cell count in serially collected tubes, the presence of a fibrinous clot, and a ratio of 1 white blood cell per 700 red blood cells. Xanthochromia is more indicative of SAH. Associated findings of SAH include a slightly depressed glucose concentration, increased protein, and an elevated opening pressure. The mean corpuscular volume (MCV) of erythrocytes in the CSF is lower than that in venous blood in SAH, but it is similar if the hemorrhage was induced by the LP.

B. Infection. CSF evaluation is the most important aspect of the laboratory diagnosis of meningitis. It includes a Gram stain, cell count with differential, protein and glucose levels, and aerobic and anaerobic cultures with antibiotic sensitivities. If tuberculosis or fungal infection is suspected, the fluid is analyzed by acid-fast stain, India ink preparation, and cryptococcal antigen and then is cultured in appropriate media. More extensive cultures are performed in the immunocompromised patient.

Immunoprecipitation tests identify bacterial antigens for *Streptococcus pneumoniae, Streptococcus* group B, *Haemophilus influenzae,* and *Neisseria meningitidis* (meningococcus). Viral cultures or polymerase chain reaction tests can rapidly identify herpes, varicella zoster, cytomegalovirus, and Epstein-Barr virus as well as *Toxoplasma* and *Mycobacterium tuberculosis.*

C. Shunt system failure. A ventriculoperitoneal shunt most commonly consists of a ventricular catheter connected to a reservoir and valve complex at the skull and a catheter that continues subcutaneously into the peritoneum, jugular vein, pleura, or urinary bladder. Shunt failure is often due to obstruction, disconnection, or infection of the shunt system. If shunt failure is suspected, a CT scan should be performed immediately. Aspiration from the reservoir or valve system of a shunt can be performed to determine patency and to collect CSF to rule out an infectious process.

D. Benign intracranial hypertension (pseudotumor cerebri). Benign intracranial hypertension occurs in young persons, often obese women. The patients have an elevation in intracranial pressure (ICP) without focal deficits in the absence of ventriculomegaly and mass lesions. Symptoms develop over several months: headache (most common), dizziness, blurred vision, diplopia, transient visual obscurations, and abnormal facial sensations. Objective signs include visual impairment, papilledema, and sixth nerve palsy. An LP demonstrates elevated ICP (up to 40 cm H_2O). Serial daily punctures can be therapeutic, with CSF aspirated until closing pressure is within normal limits (less than 20 cm H_20).

E. Neoplasms. The subarachnoid space can be infiltrated by various primary or secondary tumors, giving rise to symptoms of meningeal irritation. A CSF cytologic study can determine the presence of neoplastic cells, although complete identification is not always possible. Individual proliferating T and B lymphocytes can also be detected in the CSF and may aid in the differentiation of an opportunistic infection from a leukemic infiltration. CSF analysis for autoantibodies could play a role in the diagnosis of some paraneoplastic syndromes, such as anti-Yo titers in paraneoplastic cerebellar degeneration. A cisternal puncture may enhance the diagnosis if the lumbar CSF is nondiagnostic.

F. Other neurologic disorders. Typical LP findings in multiple sclerosis are normal ICP, normal glucose, mononuclear pleocytosis, and elevated protein levels. Immunoelectrophoresis reveals elevated immunoglobulin G and oligoclonal bands. Antibodies against CSL, a lectin protein involved in the structural stabilization of myelin, have been detected in the CSF of patients with multiple sclerosis, and they may constitute a sensitive and specific diagnostic test. CSF findings described in other disease states include elevated tau protein and decreased beta-amyloid precursor protein in Alzheimer's disease and the presence of anti-GM1 antibodies and cytoalbumin dissociation in Guillain-Barré syndrome.

II. Cerebrospinal fluid access for therapeutic intervention

A. Fistulas. CSF leaks occur for a variety of reasons, including nontraumatic and traumatic causes. Postoperative CSF leaks commonly occur after resection of tumors of the skull base as a result of dural or bony defects despite intraoperative attempts at a watertight dural closure. Leaks after lumbar surgery are unusual but may result from recent myelography, dural tear, or inadequate dural closure. In the pediatric population, repairs of meningoceles or other spina bifida defects are more likely to present with a CSF leak, because of dural or fascial defects. Basilar skull fractures and fractures along the long axis of the petrous bone can lead to CSF rhinorrhea.

The diagnosis of a leak is often easily made clinically. If laboratory characterization is necessary, identification of beta$_2$-transferrin is diagnostic for CSF. This protein is produced by neuraminidase in the brain and is uniquely found in the spinal fluid and perilymph.

First-line treatment of a leak consists of postural drainage by keeping the patient's head elevated for several days. Placement of a lumbar drainage catheter or daily LPs can be useful nonoperative approaches should conservative therapy fail. To help prevent intracranial contamination from the sinuses with lowered ICP, the lumbar drain collection bag should be maintained no lower than the patient's shoulder level, and the duration of drainage should not exceed 5 days.

B. Intracranial hypertension. A ventriculostomy is used to measure ICP and to treat intracranial hypertension by CSF drainage. Indications for ventriculostomy include head trauma, ischemic cerebral insults, obstructive hydrocephalus, aneurysmal SAH, spontaneous cerebral hematoma, and intraventricular hemorrhage. An elevated ICP secondary to cerebral edema may occur in the setting of inflammatory and infectious disorders such as Reye's syndrome or meningitis or as a result of hyperthermia, carbon dioxide retention, or intravascular congestion.

C. Drug therapy. Treatment of lymphoma and leukemia often involves lumbar intrathecal injections of various agents or an intraventricular injection through an Ommaya reservoir. The treatment of meningitis and ventriculitis may require intrathecal antibiotics in addition to systemic therapy. Careful dosage and administration are recommended, especially if the ventricular route is used, because many antibiotics can cause seizures or an inflammatory ventriculitis when they are given intrathecally.

III. Lumbar puncture. LP is a common procedure that is readily performed by the general practitioner and rarely requiring radiologic or other assistance. Contraindications to LP include skin infection at the entry site, anticoagulation or blood dyscrasias, known spinal subarachnoid block or known spinal cord arteriovenous malformations, papilledema in the presence of supratentorial masses, and posterior fossa lesions.

Figures 17-1 and 17-2 depict some of the steps for LP. The patient is placed in the lateral knee-chest position or is sitting while leaning forward over a table at the bedside. Local anesthetic is injected subcutaneously using a 25- or 27-gauge needle. A 1.5-in. needle is then inserted through the skin wheal, and additional local anesthetic is injected along the midline, thus anesthetizing the interspinous ligaments and muscles.

The point of skin entry is midline between the spinous processes of L3-4, at the level of the superior iliac crests. Lower needle placement at L4-5 or L5-S1 is required in children and neonates to avoid injury to the conus medullaris, which lies more caudal than in adults. The needle is advanced with the stylet or obturator in place to maintain needle patency and to prevent iatrogenic intraspinal epidermoid tumors. The bevel of the needle should be parallel to the longitudinal fibers of the dura or to the spinal column. The needle should be oriented rostrally at an angle of about 30 degrees to the skin and virtually aiming toward the umbilicus. When properly oriented, the needle passes through the following structures before entering the subarachnoid space: skin, superficial fascia, supraspinous ligament, interspinous ligament, ligamentum flavum, epidural space with its fatty areolar tissue and internal vertebral plexus, dura, and arachnoid membrane. The total depth varies from less than 1 in. in the extremely young patient to as much as 4 in. in the obese adult. An 18- to 20-gauge spinal needle should be used for pressure measurement. The opening pressure is best measured with the patient's legs relaxed and extended partly from the knee-chest position. Pressure measurements may be

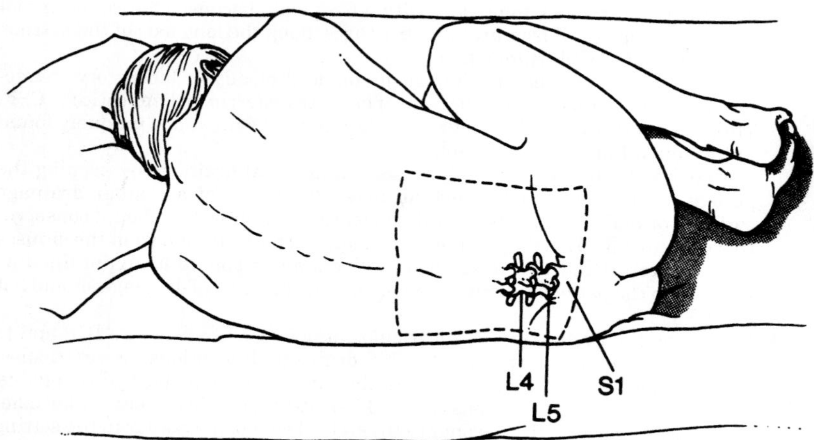

FIG. 17-1. The patient is in the lateral decubitis position with the back at the edge of the bed and the knees, hips, back, and neck flexed. (From Vander Salm TJ, Cutler BS, Wheeler HB, eds. *Atlas of bedside procedures,* 2nd ed. Boston: Little, Brown, 1988, with permission.)

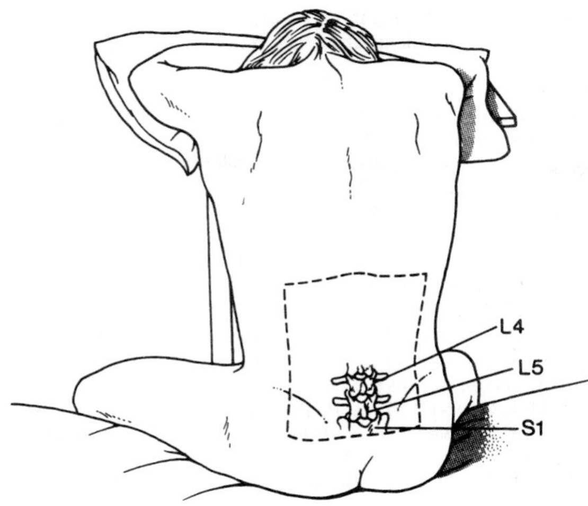

FIG. 17-2. The patient is sitting on the edge of the bed and is leaning on the bedside stand. (From Vander Salm TJ, Cutler BS, Wheeler HB, eds. *Atlas of bedside procedures,* 2nd ed. Boston: Little, Brown, 1988, with permission.)

difficult in children and may be estimated using CSF flow rate. Once CSF is collected, the closing pressure is measured before needle withdrawal. It is best to replace the stylet in the needle before exiting the subarachnoid space. CSF pressure measurements are not accurate if they are performed while the patient is sitting because of the hydrostatic pressure of the CSF column above the entry point; a significant amount of CSF could be lost when the stylet is first withdrawn. Hemorrhage is uncommon but can be seen in association with bleeding disorders and anticoagulation. Spinal SAH can result in blockage of CSF outflow with subsequent back and radicular pain with sphincter disturbances and even paraparesis. Spinal subdural hematoma is similarly infrequent, but it is associated with significant morbidity. Surgical intervention for clot evacuation must be prompt. Infection by introduction of skin flora in the subarachnoid spaces causing meningitis is uncommon and preventable if aseptic techniques are used.

Postdural puncture headache is the most common post LP complication. Its reported frequency varies from 1% to 70%. A smaller needle size, parallel orientation to the dural fibers, and a paramedian approach are associated with a decreased risk of this complication. The reinsertion of the stylet prior to withdrawal of the spinal needle has also been reported to decrease the risk of post-LP headache. Atraumatic (pencil point) needles are associated with a lower risk of postdural puncture headache. CSF flow rate is slow in the smaller size atraumatic needle, and a 20-gauge needle is probably required for large-volume drainage or pressure measurements.

Postdural puncture headaches typically develop within 72 hours and last 3 to 5 days. Conservative treatment consisting of bed rest, hydration, and analgesics should be the first line of treatment. Nonphenothiazine antiemetics are administered if the headache is associated with nausea. If the symptoms are more severe, methylxanthines (caffeine or theophylline) may be successful in up to 85% of patients. If the headache persists or is unaffected, an epidural blood patch is then recommended, because it is one of the most effective treatments for this condition.

Uncommon sequelae of LP are hearing loss and transient sixth nerve palsy.

IV. Aspiration from other sites. CSF may be aspirated from C1-2 (lateral cervical puncture) and cisternal punctures as well as from Ommaya reservoirs, ventriculostomies, ventriculoperitoneal shunts, lumboperitoneal shunts, and lumbar catheters. Consultation with a radiologist or neurosurgeon is recommended.

Selected Readings

Agrillo U, Simonetti G, Martino V. Postoperative CSF problems after spinal and lumbar surgery: general review. *J Neurosurg Sci* 1991;35:93.
Good review of postoperative CSF complications.

Bigner SH. Cerebrospinal fluid cytology: current status and diagnostic applications. *J Neuropathol Exp Neurol* 1992;51:235.
Review of CSF cytology.

Davidson RI. Lumbar puncture. In: Vander Salm TJ, Cutler BS, Wheeler HB, eds. *Atlas of bedside procedures,* 2nd ed. Boston: Little Brown, 1988.
Good description and illustrations of bedside procedures.

Ellis RW III, Strauss LC, Wiley JM, et al. A simple method of estimating cerebrospinal fluid pressure during lumbar puncture. *Pediatrics* 1992;89:895.
On-site calibration recommended.

Leibold RA, Yealy DM, Coppola M, et al. Post-dural puncture headache: characteristics, management and prevention. *Ann Emerg Med* 1993;22:1863.
Short review of postdural puncture headache.

Nandapalan V, Watson ID, Swift AC. Beta$_2$-Transferrin and CSF rhinorrhea. *Clin Otolaryngol* 1996;21:259.
A first-line test if not limited by availability.

Wood J. Cerebrospinal fluid: techniques of access and analytical interpretation. In: Wilkins R, Rengachary S, eds. *Neurosurgery,* 2nd ed. New York: McGraw-Hill, 1996:165.
Comprehensive textbook of neurosurgery.

Yurdakok M, Kocabas CN. CSF erythrocyte volume analysis: a simple method for the diagnosis of traumatic tap in newborn infants. *Pediatr Neurosurg* 1991–1992;17:199.
CSF MCV approximately equal to 20% venous MCV.

Zanetta JP, Tranchant C, Kuchler-Bopp S, et al. Presence of anti-CSL antibodies in the cerebrospinal fluid of patients: a sensitive and specific test in the diagnosis of multiple sclerosis. *J Neuroimmuol* 1994;52:175.
Study of 1,388 patients: 95% sensitivity and 68% to 80% specificity.

18. NEUROLOGIC AND INTRACRANIAL PRESSURE MONITORING

Christopher Greene

I. General principles. Neurologic monitoring falls into two distinct categories. The first category, which includes electroencephalography (EEG) and evoked potentials (EPs), defines a qualitative threshold consistent with the onset of cerebral ischemia. The second category, which includes monitors of intracranial pressure (ICP), cerebral blood flow (CBF), and cerebral metabolism, provides quantitative physiologic information. Cerebral ischemia, defined as cerebral oxygen delivery (C_{DO_2}) insufficient to meet metabolic needs, can result from a critical reduction of any of the components of C_{DO_2}, including CBF, hemoglobin concentration, and arterial hemoglobin saturation (S_aO_2).

II. Techniques

A. Systemic monitoring. Pulse oximetry and blood pressure monitoring provide important clues about the adequacy of global brain oxygenation. Changes in cerebral perfusion pressure (CPP = mean arterial pressure [MAP] – ICP) do not alter CBF over a range of pressures of about 50 to 130 mm Hg. Normally, P_aCO_2 regulates cerebral vascular resistance over a range of P_aCO_2 of 20 to 80 mm Hg. CBF is acutely halved if P_aCO_2 is halved, and it is doubled if P_aCO_2 is doubled. A decreasing C_aO_2, resulting from a decrease in hemoglobin or in S_aO_2, normally causes CBF to increase. Injured brain has impaired ability to increase CBF.

B. Neurologic examination. Frequent, accurately recorded neurologic examinations are an essential aspect of neurologic monitoring. Neurologic examination quantifies three key characteristics: level of consciousness, focal brain dysfunction, and trends in neurologic function. The Glasgow Coma Scale (GCS), originally developed as a prognostic tool, has become popular as a quick, reproducible estimate of level of consciousness (Table 18-1). The GCS should be supplemented by recording pupillary size and reactivity and the status of focal neurologic findings.

C. Neuroimaging. Cerebral computed tomographic (CT) and magnetic resonance imaging scans are indicated if a new or progressive anatomic lesion is suspected (e.g., new or expanded subdural hematomas) and if confirmation of that change is likely to alter treatment. However, CT scanning provides static, infrequent information about brain structure, not function.

CT scans obtained at the time of the patient's admission to the hospital can provide valuable prognostic information about ultimate neurologic outcome and about the risk of subsequent intracranial hypertension. A normal CT scan at admission in patients with GCS scores higher than 8 is associated with a 10% to 15% incidence of ICP elevation; however, the risk of ICP elevation increases in patients who are more than 40 years old, in those with unilateral or bilateral motor posturing, or in those with systolic blood pressure higher than 90 mm Hg.

D. Cerebral blood flow monitoring

1. **Xenon-133 clearance and computed tomography.** Intracarotid, intravenous, or inhaled administration of xenon-133 uses gamma detectors to generate washout curves for the tracer, the rate of clearance being inversely proportional to CBF. Clinical use is limited because of cumbersome regulations governing the administration of radionuclides, the technically demanding nature of the measurements, and the sustained stable conditions (5 to 15 minutes) required to perform a single measurement.
2. **Transcranial Doppler flow velocity.** In most patients, arterial flow velocity (but not actual CBF) can be readily measured in intracranial vessels, especially the middle cerebral artery, using transcranial Doppler equipment. Velocity is a function not only of blood flow rate but also of vessel diameter. If the diameter of the middle cerebral artery remains constant, changes in velocity are proportional to changes in CBF. Transcranial Doppler flow velocity measurements have been used to identify vasospasm after traumatic and nontraumatic subarachnoid hemorrhage.

TABLE 18-1. Glasgow coma score

Component	Response	Score
Eye opening	Spontaneously	4
	To verbal command	3
	To pain	2
	None	1
		Subtotal: 1–4
Motor response (best extremity)	Obeys verbal command	6
	Localizes pain	5
	Exhibits flexion-withdrawal	4
	Exhibits flexor response (decorticate posturing)	3
	Exhibits extensor response (decerebrate posturing)	2
	Shows no response (flaccid)	1
		Subtotal: 1–6
Best verbal response	Oriented and converses	5
	Disoriented and converses	4
	Uses inappropriate words	3
	Makes incomprehensible sounds	2
	Has no verbal response	1
		Subtotal: 1–5
		Total: 3–15

3. **Thermal diffusion.** If the brain surface adjacent to a thermal detector is slightly heated, the rate at which the added thermal energy is dissipated can be used to calculate local blood flow. Because the device determines CBF in one small region of cortex, the technique could be a useful monitor of global CBF or of a specific region at risk of ischemia. The necessity of surgical placement and of maintenance of an invasive intracranial device carries a risk of infection.
4. **Intracranial pressure monitoring.** ICP functions as the outflow pressure for the cerebral circulation (assuming jugular venous pressure is lower than ICP), according to the equation: CPP = MAP – ICP. Although CBF cannot be directly inferred from MAP and ICP, severe increases in ICP reduce both CPP and CBF. Although intracranial hypertension contributes to morbidity and mortality in such diverse diseases as traumatic brain injury, subarachnoid hemorrhage, stroke, and postischemic encephalopathy, the use of ICP monitoring is best established in patients with traumatic brain injury.

   Unlike the modalities previously discussed, ICP monitoring has been used for surveillance and goal-directed therapy. The Brain Trauma Foundation and the American Association of Neurologic Surgeons have published guidelines for the management of traumatic brain injury, including standards, guidelines, and options for the use of ICP monitoring. ICP monitoring is

   1. Appropriate in patients with an abnormal admission CT scan and severe head injury (GCS score of 3 to 8) after cardiopulmonary resuscitation.
   2. Appropriate in patients with severe head injury and a normal CT scan if two or more of the following are noted at admission: age greater than 40 years, unilateral or bilateral motor posturing, and systolic blood pressure less than 90 mm Hg.
   3. Not indicated in patients with mild or moderate head injury. However, a physician may choose to monitor ICP in certain conscious patients with traumatic mass lesions.

   The consensus committee also provided a guideline for treatment of ICP at a threshold of 20 to 25 mm Hg and suggested as an option that treatment of ICP should be corroborated by frequent clinical examination and CPP data. They ranked devices based on their accuracy, stability, and ability to drain CSF in the following order: (a) intraventricular monitors; (b) parenchymal catheter-tip transducers; (c) subdural, including catheter-tip transducers and fluid-coupled catheters; (d) subarachnoid fluid-coupled devices; and (e) epidural devices.

In addition to intracranial hypertension, other data that may prompt concern include widening of the pulse ICP (indicating diminishing intracranial compliance) and plateau waves (cyclic increases in ICP, often 50 mm Hg or greater and lasting as long as 15 to 30 minutes). The pressure volume index (PVI) assesses intracranial compliance by adding or withdrawing CSF through a ventricular cannula, then substituting measured values in the equation: $PVI = V/\log P0/P_{m\ or\ p}$. V is the volume withdrawn or injected, P0 is the pressure before withdrawing or injecting fluid, P_m is the minimum pressure after fluid withdrawal, and P_p is the peak pressure after volume addition. Treatment of ICP is likely to be necessary if PVI is less than 13 mL and is nearly always required if PVI is less than 10 mL. Complications of ICP monitoring include aggravation of cerebral edema, intracranial hemorrhage, cortical damage, and infection, as well as device-related malfunction and injuries.

E. Cerebral oxygen extraction

1. **Jugular venous saturation.** Jugular venous bulb oxygenation reflects the balance between CDO_2 and $CMRO_2$. Experience with tissue oxygen pressure (PO_2) monitoring in traumatic brain injury suggests a correlation between poor outcome and tissue hypoxia. Mortality doubles with a single episode of jugular venous desaturation. Jugular venous bulb monitoring can detect excessive hyperventilation and may also distinguish between vasospasm or hyperemia. Retrograde cannulation of the jugular bulb is a low-risk, technically simple procedure. Fiberoptic catheters are commercially available. The catheter is most accurate if it is placed in the dominant jugular vein, defined as the jugular vein, which, when compressed, produces the greatest increase in ICP or the side with the larger jugular foramen as detected by CT.

   CBF, $CMRO_2$, C_aO_2, and jugular venous oxygen content ($C_{jv}O_2$) are related according to the following equation: $C_{jv}O_2 = C_aO_2 \times CMRO_2/CBF$. By inference, $S_{jv}O_2$, a major determinant of $C_{jv}O_2$, represents a monitor of the ability of CBF to support $CMRO_2$. However, mixed cerebral venous blood may not reflect regional hypoperfusion.

2. **Near-infrared spectroscopy.** Near-infrared spectroscopy may eventually offer the opportunity to assess the adequacy of brain oxygenation continuously and noninvasively by determining the relative concentrations of oxygenated and deoxygenated hemoglobin in brain tissue. Extensive preclinical and clinical data demonstrate the sensitivity of the technique for the detection of qualitative changes in brain oxygenation. Technical challenges remain.

F. Neurochemical monitoring. Microdialysis is a promising new technique in which fluid is infused and withdrawn through a catheter inserted into the brain parenchyma. The recovered dialysate can be analyzed for neurotransmitters or metabolic intermediates such as lactate, pyruvate, and adenosine. Microdialysis may be useful in guiding therapy or establishing prognosis.

G. Electrophysiologic monitoring. EEG monitoring can be used to detect potentially damaging cerebral hypoperfusion, isolated seizures, and status epilepticus and to define the depth or type of coma. Whereas the EEG may document focal or lateral intracranial abnormalities, it has limited value as a precise diagnostic tool. Quantitative EEG monitoring has been used to identify delayed ischemic deficits after subarachnoid hemorrhage, occasionally before clinical deterioration. Sensory EPs, which include somatosensory evoked potentials (SSEPs), brainstem auditory evoked potentials (BAEPs), and visual evoked potentials (VEPs), can be used as qualitative threshold monitors to detect severe neural ischemia by evaluating characteristic waveforms to specific stimuli. Signal averaging and high-quality amplifiers are necessary because the evoked response is approximately one-tenth the amplitude of the EEG. Because obliteration of

EPs occurs only under conditions of profound cerebral ischemia or mechanical trauma, EP monitoring is one of the most specific ways in which to assess neurologic integrity. However, EPs are insensitive to less severe deterioration of cerebral or spinal cord oxygen availability and are modified by sedatives, narcotics, and anesthetics.

Selected Readings

Bouma GJ, Muizelaar JP, Stringer WA, et al. Ultra-early evaluation of regional cerebral blood flow in severely head-injured patients using xenon-enhanced computerized tomography. *J Neurosurg* 1992;77:360.
Thirty-one percent incidence of ischemia; xenon CT is useful as an initial diagnostic study.

Brain Trauma Foundation, American Association of Neurological Surgeons, Joint Section on Neurotrauma and Critical Care. Guidelines for the management of severe head injury. *J Neurotrauma* 1996;13:641.
Guidelines for the management of severe head injury.

Goetting MG, Preston G. Jugular bulb catheterization: experience with 123 patients. *Crit Care Med* 1990;18:1220.
Description of technique.

Gopinath SP, Robertson CS, Contant CF, et al. Jugular venous desaturation and outcome after head injury. *J Neurol Neurosurg Psychiatry* 1994;57:717.
Poor outcome in 74% of patients with a single episode of $S_{jv}O_2$ *less than 50%.*

Jones TH, Morawetz RB, Crowell RM, et al. Thresholds of focal cerebral ischemia in awake monkeys. *J Neurosurg* 1981;54:773.
Critical values of CBF determined.

Marshall LF, Marshall SB, Klauber MR, et al. A new classification of head injury based on computerized tomography. *J Neurosurg* 1991;75:S14.
Initial CT predictive of outcome.

Martin NA, Doberstein C, Zane C, et al. Posttraumatic cerebral arterial spasm: transcranial Doppler ultrasound, cerebral blood flow, and angiographic findings. *J Neurosurg* 1992;77:575.
Twenty-seven percent incidence of vasospasm in 30 patients with closed head injury.

Maset AL, Marmarou A, Ward JD, et al. Pressure-volume index in head injury. *J Neurosurg* 1987;67:832.
Low PVI predictive of high ICP and poor outcome.

Smith DS, Levy W, Maris M, et al. Reperfusion hyperoxia in brain after circulatory arrest in humans. *Anesthesiology* 1990;73:12.
There was an increase in the hemoglobin saturation signal from the brain vasculature to above baseline in patients who were having their automatic internal cardioverter-defibrillator checked.

Strandgaard S, Paulson OB. Cerebral autoregulation. *Stroke* 1984;15:413.
Short review.

Tasker RC, Boyd S, Harden A. Monitoring in non-traumatic coma. II: electroencephalography. *Arch Dis Child* 1988;63:895.
The EEG was found to be useful in predicting a poor outcome in 48 children in non-traumatic coma.

Teasdale G, Jennett B. Assessment of coma and impaired consciousness: a practical scale. *Lancet* 1974;2:81.
Classic article.

19. PERCUTANEOUS CYSTOSTOMY

Paul G. Jodka

I. General principles. Percutaneous suprapubic cystostomy is a proven method of treatment of acute urinary retention when standard bladder catheterization is impossible or contraindicated. This procedure is generally safe and is readily accomplished at the bedside.

II. Indications. The indications for percutaneous suprapubic cystostomy in the intensive care unit are shown in Table 19-1. The most common indication is the inability to place a urethral catheter in the setting of acute urinary retention. Occasionally, the need for suprapubic cystostomy can be averted by proper technique of urethral catheterization.

III. Urethral catheterization. A thorough history and physical examination with particular attention to the patient's genitourinary system are important, along with knowledge of the specific indication for catheterization, because this can influence the type and size of catheter used. For instance, men with a history of prostatism might be difficult to catheterize and may require placement of a well-lubricated larger-bore catheter. A history of previous open, radical, or transurethral prostate resection may also make catheterization difficult. The use of a Coudé-tip catheter with an upper deflected tip may help to negotiate a high bladder neck as a result of contracture after surgery. Urethral catheterization should not be performed in the setting of suspected traumatic urethral disruption until urethral integrity has been demonstrated by retrograde urethrography.

The indication for catheter insertion dictates the type and size of catheter to be placed. Gross hematuria requires a 22- or 24-Fr catheter for irrigation and clot removal. Occasionally, a three-way urethral catheter is needed for continuous bladder irrigation to prevent recurrent clotting. Because prolonged use of large indwelling catheters can lead to urethritis and epididymitis in men, a 16- or 18-Fr Foley catheter should be placed unless otherwise indicated.

After the patient is prepared and draped, 10 mL of local anesthetic in lubricant (2% lidocaine hydrochloride jelly) may be injected into the urethra in male patients. For adequate topical anesthesia, 5 to 10 minutes of dwell time is required, which is facilitated by occlusion of the urethral meatus. After the balloon of the catheter has been tested and the catheter has been lubricated, the physician inserts the catheter into the patient's external meatus with one hand while the other hand stretches the patient's penis perpendicular to his body. If no urine return occurs after catheter advancement, the balloon should not be inflated because this may cause urethral disruption. Instead, irrigation with normal saline should be attempted. In male patients, the involuntary contraction of the external urinary sphincter may cause resistance that can be overcome by gentle, constant pressure to the catheter. Any other form of resistance may represent a stricture requiring urologic consultation. In patients with a history of prostatic surgery, digital transrectal pressure by an assistant may elevate the urethra and may allow passage of the catheter.

In female patients, short, straight catheters are preferred. Because of the shorter urethra, less local anesthetic and less lubricant are needed. Rarely, the urethral meatus is not visible for anatomic reasons, requiring blind catheter placement at the palpated site of the meatus.

IV. Contraindications to suprapubic cystostomy. The contraindications to percutaneous suprapubic cystostomy are listed in Table 19-2.

The bladder may not be palpable in the setting of renal failure with oliguria or anuria, a contracted neurogenic bladder, or incontinence. In male patients with a nonpalpable bladder, saline instillation through a urethral catheter may allow for palpation of the bladder and subsequent suprapubic tube placement. Bladder distention using this method may be impossible in the patient with a small, contracted neurogenic bladder. Ultrasound guidance can be used to direct a 22-gauge spinal

TABLE 19-1. Indications for percutaneous cystostomy

1. Unsuccessful urethral catheterization in the setting of
   - Acute urinary retention
   - Need for accurate urinary output monitoring
   - Prostatic hyperplasia, cancer, or prior prostatic surgery
2. Urethral disruption from pelvic trauma
3. Bladder drainage required in the presence of severe urethral, prostatic, or epididymal infection

needle into the bladder to allow saline infusion, bladder distention, and suprapubic tube placement.

In patients with prior lower abdominal surgery, ultrasound evaluation may be necessary before cystostomy catheter placement to avoid possible injury to a loop of bowel confined to the insertion area by adhesions. Coagulopathy is a relative contraindication to this procedure. In patients with a known bladder tumor, this form of bladder access should be avoided. Percutaneous suprapubic catheters are generally ineffective for bladder drainage in patients with retained clots. Open surgical placement of a large-caliber tube is necessary if urethral catheterization is impossible in this setting.

V. Technique. Several kits are available for percutaneous suprapubic cystostomy, one of which is the Stamey unit (Cook Urological, Spencer, IN), which uses a trocar for placement. The patient is placed in the supine position. The suprapubic area is shaved, prepared, and draped in sterile fashion. Local anesthetic is used to anesthetize the skin and deeper tissues at a location about 4 cm above the pubis (Fig. 19-1).

A 22-gauge spinal needle is used to find the bladder (Fig. 19-1). Bladder puncture is confirmed by aspirating urine with a syringe. The angle and depth of puncture can be noted by placing the fingers on the spinal needle at the junction of the skin and withdrawing the needle. The fingers are placed at an equivalent position on the cystostomy trocar to determine appropriate depth of insertion. A 2-mm stab wound is made at the site of spinal needle puncture. The catheter, mounted on the trocar, is then inserted with one hand placed on the trocar shaft and the other hand on the site marking the depth of the bladder. The trocar is advanced at the same angle and depth as marked by the spinal needle. Urine is aspirated to confirm placement in the bladder, and the trocar is removed, leaving the suprapubic tube in the bladder.

VI. Complications. The complications of percutaneous suprapubic cystostomy are listed in Table 19-3.

Bladder spasms are the most common complication and can be avoided by pulling the cystostomy tube against the bladder wall immediately after placement and then advancing the tube 2 cm into the bladder to allow for movement. Severe bladder spasms can be treated with oxybutynin. This medication must be withdrawn before suprapubic tube removal because its anticholinergic activity may aggravate urinary retention in patients with underlying obstructive uropathy.

Hematuria is also common, but it is rarely severe enough to require open cystostomy for placement of a large-bore catheter for irrigation.

TABLE 19-2. Contraindications to percutaneous cystostomy

1. Nonpalpable bladder
2. Previous lower abdominal surgery
3. Coagulopathy
4. Known bladder tumor
5. Clot retention

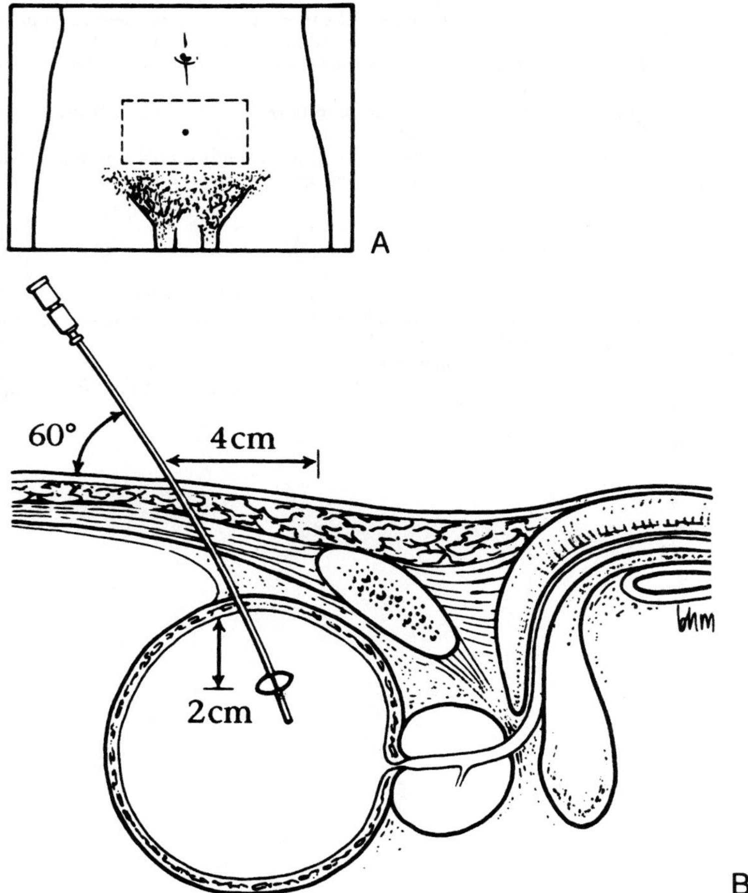

FIG. 19-1. Technique of suprapubic trochar placement. **A:** The area to be shaved, prepared, and draped before trochar placement. **B:** Position of the Stamey trochar in the bladder. The angle, distance from the pubis, and position of the catheter in relation to the bladder wall are demonstrated.

TABLE 19-3. Complications of percutaneous cystostomy

1. Bladder spasms
2. Hematuria
3. Bowel perforation
4. Hypotension
5. Postobstructive diuresis
6. Loss of a portion of the catheter in the bladder

Bowel perforation can be avoided by attempting the procedure only on well-distended bladders and by taking a midline approach no more than 4 cm above the pubis. An ultrasound study should be performed before the procedure in patients with prior abdominal or pelvic surgery, to rule out entrapped bowel.

Hypotension rarely occurs after suprapubic cystostomy and generally is easily treated with intravenous fluids.

Postobstructive diuresis after suprapubic tube placement has been described and may require fluid replacement for its management.

Other rare but possible complications include through-and-through perforation of the bladder and loss of a portion of the catheter in the bladder.

Selected Readings

Morehouse DD. Emergency management of urethral trauma. *Urol Clin North Am* 1982;9:251.

An article describing the management of traumatic urethral injuries.

Vaughn ED, Gillenwater JY. Diagnosis, characterization and management of post-obstructive diuresis. *J Urol* 1973;110:537.

An early descriptive study of 22 patients with postobstructive diuresis.

Walsh PC, Retik AB, Stamey TA, et al, eds. *Campbell's urology,* 6th ed. Philadelphia: WB Saunders, 1992.

A standard textbook of urology.

20. ASPIRATION OF JOINTS

Paul G. Jodka

I. General principles. Arthrocentesis involves the introduction of a needle into a joint space to remove synovial fluid. The presentation of various conditions, such as septic arthritis and crystalline arthritis, may be similar, yet treatment may be different. Thus, arthrocentesis and synovial fluid analysis are important for accurate diagnosis.

II. Indications. Arthrocentesis is performed for both diagnostic and therapeutic reasons. The evaluation of arthritis of unknown cause is the main indication for this procedure. In the intensive care unit, arthrocentesis is most commonly performed to rule out septic arthritis in a patient with acute monoarthritis or oligoarthritis. Table 20-1 lists types of inflammatory arthritides that can mimic septic arthritis and can be differentiated from it by synovial fluid analysis.

Before performing arthrocentesis, one must be certain that a true joint space inflammation with effusion is present rather than a periarticular inflammatory process, such as bursitis, tendinitis, or cellulitis. In the knee, the presence of an effusion may be confirmed by the bulge test (Fig. 20-1) or patellar tap. Examples of diagnostic maneuvers used in the evaluation of joints are described in detail elsewhere.

Arthrocentesis may also be used therapeutically, as in the serial aspiration of a septic joint for drainage and monitoring of the response to treatment. Furthermore, arthrocentesis allows for injection of corticosteroid preparations into the joint space, a form of therapy useful for various forms of inflammatory and noninflammatory arthritis.

III. Contraindications. Absolute contraindications to arthrocentesis include infection of the overlying skin or periarticular structures and severe coagulopathy. If septic arthritis is suspected in the presence of severe coagulopathy, efforts to correct the bleeding diathesis should be made before joint aspiration is performed. Therapeutic anticoagulation is not an absolute contraindication. Although known bacteremia is a contraindication to arthrocentesis given the potential for joint space seeding, joint aspiration is nonetheless indicated if septic arthritis is the presumed source of the bacteremia. Articular damage and instability constitute relative contraindications to arthrocentesis.

IV. Complications. The major complications of arthrocentesis are bleeding and iatrogenically induced infection. These complications occur exceedingly rarely with strict adherence to aseptic technique and with correction of significant coagulopathy before joint aspiration. Direct cartilaginous damage by the needle is difficult to quantitate and likely is minimized by avoidance of excessive needle movement or complete drainage of the joint, as well as avoiding advancement of the needle any deeper than needed to obtain fluid.

V. Technique. Joint aspiration requires knowledge of the relevant joint and periarticular anatomy and strict adherence to aseptic technique. Joints other than the knee should probably be aspirated by an appropriate specialist, such as a rheumatologist or an orthopedic surgeon. Aspiration of some joints, such as the hip or sacroiliac joints, may require fluoroscopic or computed tomographic guidance. Details of the aspiration technique of other joints are presented elsewhere. The technique for knee aspiration is as follows (Fig. 20-2):

1. Confirm the presence of an effusion with the patient supine and the knee extended.
2. Obtain written informed consent from the patient or legal guardian.
3. Collect the items required for the procedure (Table 20-2).
4. The superior and inferior borders of the patella are landmarks for needle placement. Entry should be halfway between these borders just inferior to the undersurface of the patella, either from a medial or lateral approach, the former being

TABLE 20-1. Common causes of inflammatory arthritis

Rheumatoid arthritis
Spondyloarthropathies
Psoriatic arthritis
Reiter's syndrome/reactive arthritis
Ankylosing spondylitis
Ulcerative colitis/regional enteritis
Crystal-induced arthritis
Monosodium urate (gout)
Calcium pyrophosphate dehydrate (pseudogout)
Hydroxyapatite
Infectious arthritis
Bacterial
Mycobacterial
Fungal
Connective tissue diseases
Systemic lupus erythematosus
Vasculitis
Scleroderma
Polymyositis
Hypersensitivity
Serum sickness

more commonly used and preferable with small effusions. Cleanse the area with an iodine-based antiseptic solution. Allow the area to dry, then wipe once with an alcohol swab. Universal precautions apply, as with any procedure.

5. Local anesthesia can be achieved either with sterile ethyl chloride spray or infiltration of local anesthetic solution (e.g. 1% lidocaine) into the subcutaneous and deeper tissues.
6. To enter the knee joint, use an 18-gauge, 1.5-in. needle with a sterile 20- to 60-mL syringe. Use a quick thrust through skin and capsule. Avoid periosteal bone to minimize pain. Aspirate fluid to fill the syringe. If the fluid appears purulent or hemorrhagic, try to tap the joint dry. Drainage of large effusions may require additional syringes, which may be exchanged for the original one while leaving the needle in place.

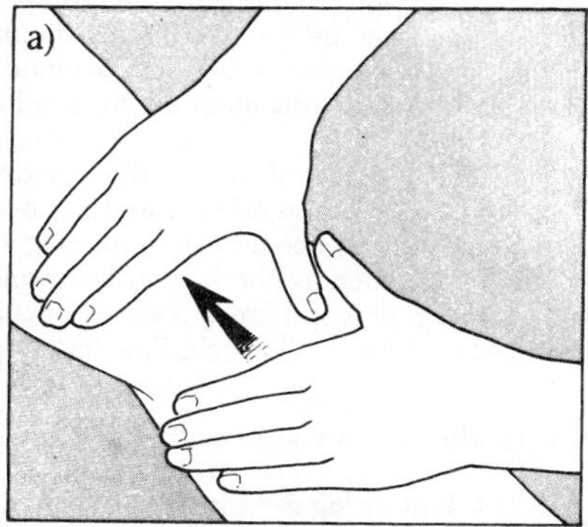

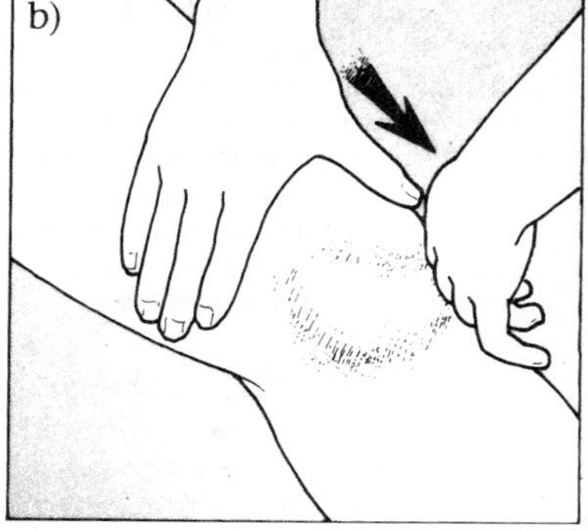

FIG. 20-1. The bulge test. **A:** Milk fluid from the suprapatellar pouch into the joint. **B:** Slide the hand down the lateral aspect of the joint line and watch for a bulge medial to the joint.

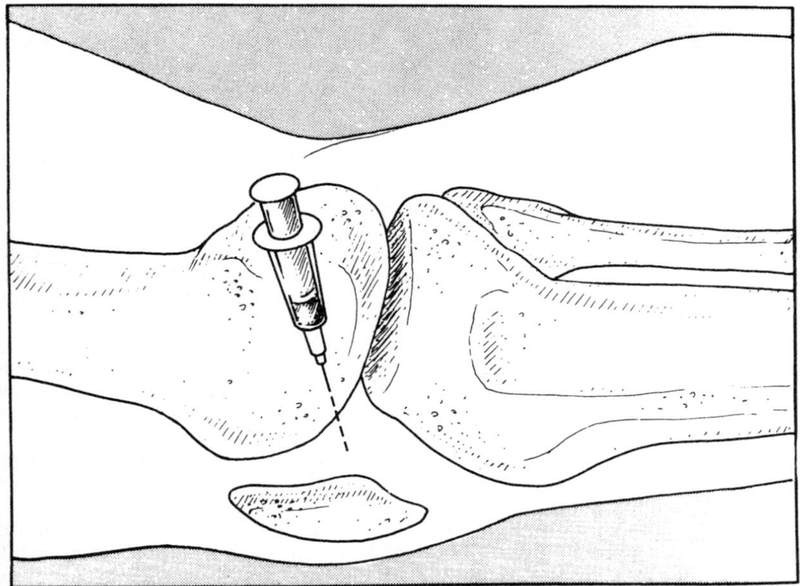

FIG. 20-2. Technique of aspirating the knee joint. The needle enters halfway between the superior and inferior borders of the patella and is directed just inferior to the patella.

TABLE 20-2. Arthrocentesis equipment

Skin preparation and local anesthesia	Iodophor solution Alcohol swab Ethyl chloride spray For local anesthesia: 1% lidocaine, 25-gauge, 1-in. needle, 22-gauge, 1.5-in. needle, 5-mL syringe Sterile sponge/cloth
Arthrocentesis	Gloves 10–60-mL syringe (depending on size of effusion) 18–20-gauge, 1.5-in. needle Sterile sponge/cloth Sterile clamp Adhesive bandage (Band-Aid)
Collection	15-mL anticoagulated tube (with sodium heparin or EDTA) Sterile tubes for routine cultures Slide, cover slip

7. When the fluid has been obtained, the needle is removed, and pressure is applied to the puncture site with sterile gauze. Apply an adhesive bandage after cleaning the area with alcohol. Apply prolonged pressure if the patient has a bleeding diathesis of any type.
8. Document the amount, color, clarity, and viscosity (see string sign, later) of the fluid. Send the fluid for cell count with differential, Gram stain, routine culture, cultures for gonococcus, mycobacteria, and fungi, if indicated, and polarized microscopic examination for crystal analysis. Other tests, including glucose and complement levels, are generally not helpful. Anticoagulated tubes are needed for accurate assessment of fluid for cell count and crystal analysis. Sodium heparin and ethylenediamine tetraacetic acid (EDTA) are appropriate anticoagulants. Fluid may be sent for Gram stain and culture in the syringe or in a sterile red-top tube.

VI. Synovial fluid analysis. Synovial fluid is divided into noninflammatory versus inflammatory types based on the total nucleated cell count. A white blood cell count of 2,000/mm^3 defines an inflammatory fluid. Table 20-3 shows how joint fluid can be categorized based on its characteristics.

A. Color. Color and clarity can be assessed using a clear glass tube. Normal synovial fluid is colorless. Noninflammatory and inflammatory joint fluid have a yellow hue. Septic effusions often appear whitish to frankly purulent. Hemorrhagic effusions appear red or brown. A repeated aspiration from an alternate site may be required if there is a question of a traumatic tap. In case of continued doubt, the hematocrit of the aspirate can be compared with that of peripheral blood. The hematocrit in a hemorrhagic effusion is typically lower than that of a peripheral sample and is equal to it in the case of traumatic tap.

B. Clarity. The clarity of the synovial fluid depends on the amount of cellular or particulate matter within it. Based on how well, if at all, black print on a white background can be read through a glass tube filled with synovial fluid, the fluid is categorized as being transparent, translucent, or opaque (Table 20-3).

C. Viscosity. The viscosity of synovial fluid is a measure of the hyaluronic acid content. Degradative enzymes such as hyaluronidase are produced in inflammatory conditions resulting in a thinner, less viscous fluid. The string sign is a bedside measure of viscosity. Normal synovial fluid forms at least a 6 cm continuous string when a drop of fluid is allowed to fall from the needle or syringe. Inflammatory fluid drips like water and will not form a string. The mucin clot, another measure of viscosity, is a test performed by mixing several drops of synovial fluid in 5% acetic acid. A good, tenacious mucin clot forms only with normal, noninflammatory fluid, but not with an inflammatory sample.

TABLE 20-3. Joint fluid characteristics

	Normal	Group I (noninflammatory)	Group II (inflammatory)	Group III (septic)
Color	Clear	Yellow	Yellow or opalescent	Variable, may be purulent
Clarity	Transparent	Transparent	Translucent	Opaque
Viscosity	Very high	High	Low	Typically low
Mucin clot	Firm	Firm	Friable	Friable
WBC/mm^3	200	200–2,000	2,000–100,000	>50,000, usually >100,000
PMN (%)	<25	<25	>50	>75
Culture	Negative	Negative	Negative	Usually positive

PMN, polymorphonuclear cells; WBC, white blood cell count.

D. Cell count and differential. The cell count should be obtained as soon as possible after arthrocentesis to avoid a falsely low white blood cell count caused by delayed analysis. In general, the technique for the cell count is identical to that used with blood samples. Viscous fluid with much debris may give erroneous results with automated counters, thus making a manual count more accurate in these circumstances. The differential white blood cell count is based on direct visualization. In general, the total white blood cell count and polymorphonuclear cell count increase with infection and inflammation. Septic fluid typically has a differential of greater than 75% polymorphonuclear cells (Table 20-3).

E. Crystals. As with the cell count, crystal analysis should be performed as soon as possible after arthrocentesis for optimal diagnostic yield. Fluid is examined for crystals using a compensated polarized light microscope. The presence of intracellular monosodium urate or calcium pyrophosphate dihydrate (CPPD) crystals confirms the diagnosis of gout or pseudogout, respectively. Monosodium urate crystals are usually needle shaped, are negatively birefringent, and appear yellow when oriented parallel to the compensator axis. CPPD crystals typically are smaller and rhomboid, are weakly positively birefringent, and appear blue when parallel to the plan of reference. If the fluid cannot be examined immediately, it should be refrigerated to preserve the crystals. Even when crystals are found in a sample, infection must be considered, because crystals can occur concomitantly with a septic joint.

F. Gram stain and culture. The Gram stain is performed as with other body fluids. Synovial fluid should routinely be cultured for aerobic and anaerobic organisms. Additional cultures for fungi and mycobacteria should be sent in some circumstances, such as in chronic monoarticular arthritis. Special growth media are required when disseminated gonorrhea is suspected. A positive culture confirms septic arthritis.

Selected Readings

Gottlieb NL, Riskin WG. Complications of local corticosteroid injections. *JAMA* 1980; 243:1547.

Four case reports of less common complications associated with steroid injections.

Kelley WN, Harris ED, Ruddy S, et al. *Textbook of rheumatology,* 2nd ed. Philadelphia: WB Saunders, 1985.

A standard, comprehensive text of rheumatology.

21. ANESTHESIA FOR BEDSIDE PROCEDURES

Frank M. O'Connell

I. General principles. Specialists in intensive care are much better equipped to deal with issues of sedation and analgesia for procedures in the intensive care unit (ICU) than in previous decades primarily because of the numerous pharmacologic agents that are now available. Despite the many intravenous treatment alternatives from which to choose, pain continues to be undertreated. Inadequate treatment of pain may have significant physiologic consequences including pulmonary compromise, thrombotic diathesis, exacerbation of negative nitrogen balance, and an increased stress response.

II. Common pain management problems in the intensive care unit. Titrating the appropriate level of analgesia in critically ill patients is complicated by difficulties in patient assessment, altered pharmacokinetics, and the altered physiology of aging. Because of delirium, the presence of an endotracheal tube, or other causes of altered mental status, patients in the ICU may be unable to communicate their level of pain and anxiety. Clinicians are left to monitor vital signs (e.g., tachycardia and hypertension) that may also result from the patient's severity of illness. The pharmacokinetic profile of an agent has been expressed by the term elimination half-life ($t_{1/2}$), that is, the concentration of drug remaining in the circulation after intravenous administration. The elimination $t_{1/2}$ is related to the volume of distribution at steady state (V_dSS, the volume of the various body compartments over which the drug is distributed), divided by its rate of elimination from the body (clearance, Cl): $t_{1/2} = V_dSS/Cl$.

Factors such as hypoalbuminemia with decreased tissue binding or increased capillary permeability tend to increase V_dSS compared with healthy persons and thereby alter the pharmacokinetic profile in critically ill patients. More recent clinical observations such as the rapid recovery from propofol infusion have suggested that redistribution from the intravascular compartment may be more important than $t_{1/2}$. Older patients exhibit an altered pharmacokinetic profile because of a decrease in lean body mass and an increase in body fat, which may augment V_dSS for lipid-soluble drugs. In addition, aging is associated with a reduction in renal and hepatic drug clearance and an increased sensitivity to the central nervous system depressant effects of opioids and benzodiazepines. Finally, a wide spectrum of bedside procedures of differing length and pain intensity is commonly performed in the ICU. These procedures require careful titration of sedation and analgesia based on the anticipated duration of the procedure and the level of discomfort. Despite these challenges, providing sedation and analgesia at the bedside offers the opportunity for significant cost savings by eliminating operating room time and by preventing complications that may arise during transportation of an unstable patient.

III. Advantages and disadvantages of specific drugs

A. Opioids. Morphine and its analogues (fentanyl, sufentanil, alfentanil, and remifentanil) blunt pain by their effects on various opioid receptors located in the spinal cord, brainstem, thalamus, limbic system, and cerebral cortex (Table 21-1). Analgesia is achieved through inhibition of the nociceptive pathways of the spinal cord and activation of the inhibitory pathways of the brainstem as well as modulation of the emotional response to pain by the limbic system. Differences in lipid solubility influence the ability of an agent to cross the blood-brain barrier and hence its onset of action (e.g., morphine enters the central nervous system slowly and has a 15-minute latency until its peak effect whereas alfentanil or remifentanil are highly lipid soluble and have a rapid onset of action). Gastrointestinal side effects of these agents include reduced intestinal motility, delayed gastric emptying, ileus, nausea, and vomiting. Cardiovascular side effects include hypotension with rapid administration. This effect may be due to histamine release in the case of morphine or vasomotor medullary

TABLE 21-1. Characteristics of intravenous anesthetics (bolus)

Properties	Etomidate	Midazolam	Ketamine	Propofol
Dose (mg/kg)	0.5	0.05–0.1	1–2	1–2
Onset	Rapid	**Intermediate**	Rapid	Rapid
Duration (min)	5–10	10–15	5–10	5–10
Cardiovascular effects	None	Minimal	8	9
Respiratory effects	Minimal	9	Minimal	9
Analgesia	None	None	**Potent**	None
Amnesia	None	**Potent**	**Potent**	None

Dose indicated should be reduced 50% in elderly patients. Entries in bold type indicate noticeable differences among the drugs.

center depression in the case of fentanyl. Respiratory depression, manifested by a blunting of the ventilatory response to hypercarbia and hypoxia, occurs with all opioids and in some cases may result in apnea. Selection of an opioid should be based on the duration of action desired. Agents such as alfentanil or remifentanil are used for procedures of short duration (e.g., cardioversion) or for patients in whom a rapid return to baseline mental status is desired (e.g., head trauma). Morphine may be appropriate for procedures of longer duration or in situations in which a longer duration of analgesia is required (e.g., multiple orthopedic injuries). Because opioids only provide analgesia and are not amnestic or anxiolytic agents, the simultaneous administration of other medications for this purpose may be dictated by the clinical circumstance.

B. Etomidate. Etomidate causes rapid onset of unconsciousness with recovery in 5 to 10 minutes. This agent decreases cerebral metabolic rate in a manner similar to barbiturates, but it does not depress myocardial contractility or reduce baseline sympathetic output. Being the most hemodynamically stable intravenous anesthetic agent known, etomidate is frequently used to induce unconsciousness in patients with tenuous cardiovascular status, including patients with severe aortic stenosis, hypovolemia, left main coronary artery occlusion, and cardiomyopathy. A known pitfall of this drug is its ability to produce adrenal cortical suppression even with a single dose. This may require the concurrent administration of exogenous steroids in physiologic doses.

C. Benzodiazepines. Diazepam, lorazepam, and midazolam are included in this class of compounds whose sedative properties are mediated by the potentiation of gamma-amino butyric acid (GABA), a powerful inhibitory neurotransmitter in the brain. Because of their ability to induce anxiolysis and amnesia, these agents are useful adjuncts to analgesics. Midazolam has a much shorter duration of activity than either diazepam or lorazepam and causes less pain on injection as a result of its water solubility. Because midazolam is highly protein bound, conventional doses may have an exaggerated effect on patients with hypoalbuminemia in the ICU. The conjugated active metabolites of midazolam may accumulate in patients with diminished renal function, and recovery from sedation may also be prolonged in obese or elderly individuals. Recovery of cognitive function after benzodiazepine administration may be delayed for up to 24 hours and may thus interfere with neurologic assessment. Respiratory depression with a diminished ventilatory response to hypercarbia is an effect common to all benzodiazepines and may be more pronounced in patients with chronic obstructive pulmonary disease. Flumazenil may be used to reverse the sedative effects of benzodiazepines, but its duration of action is limited (15 to 20 minutes). Furthermore, it may induce seizure activity, especially in patients receiving prolonged benzodiazepine administration.

D. Ketamine. This intravenous anesthetic is unique in its ability to induce a dissociative state characterized by sedation, amnesia, and significant analgesia. Ketamine has many beneficial respiratory effects such as decreasing airway resistance, preserving airway reflexes, and only mildly depressing the ventilatory response to hypercarbia. Because of these properties, ketamine is considered the intravenous anesthetic of choice in patients with bronchospasm. Because of ketamine's ability to stimulate salivary and tracheobronchial secretions, an antisialagogue such as glycopyrrolate should be administered before ketamine injection. Ketamine also causes cardiovascular stimulation through its ability to augment sympathetic tone and to decrease norepinephrine reuptake. However, ketamine has been reported to cause hypotension in patients with chronic catecholamine depletion secondary to marginal cardiovascular reserve. Drawbacks to the use of this drug include emergence dysphoria, which may be profound, and increased myocardial oxygen consumption resulting from sympathetic stimulation. The second concern is particularly germane to patients at risk of coronary artery disease. Both these pitfalls may be minimized by the concomitant administration of benzodiazepines or propofol.

E. Propofol. Propofol is a sedative-hypnotic agent devoid of amnestic properties that has gained wide popularity as a substitute for barbiturates (e.g., thiopental) in many operating rooms because of the rapid emergence associated with its use. Extensive tissue distribution and a high rate of clearance are responsible for the rapid recovery of consciousness without residual sedation. This characteristic of propofol makes administration by continuous infusion an attractive option for patients in whom a rapid recovery of neurologic status is desirable. Recovery times after termination of infusion in elderly patients and in those with liver dysfunction are similar to recovery times in physiologically normal persons. The soybean emulsion that functions as the vehicle for propofol supports bacterial growth, a feature that has led to episodes of septic shock after iatrogenic contamination. This complication has been reduced by the addition of ethylenediamine tetraacetic acid (EDTA) to the formulation. Nevertheless, strict aseptic technique should be used when handling this drug. Propofol may cause respiratory depression in a manner similar to other sedative agents. Pain on injection is common with propofol, but the use of small doses of lidocaine (20 mg) or opioids before propofol infusion may minimize this effect. Propofol depresses myocardial function and causes afterload reduction resulting from vasodilatation. Because of these circulatory effects, bolus dosing may be unsuitable for elderly or hemodynamically unstable patients.

Selected Readings

Boukoms AJ. Pain relief in the intensive care unit. *J Intensive Care Med* 1988;3:32.
Excellent review article on the different types of opioid receptors.

Bourke DL, Malit LA, Smith TC. Respiratory interactions of ketamine and morphine. *Anesthesiology* 1987;66:153.
This study highlights the minimal amount of respiratory depression observed with the use of ketamine compared with other anesthetic drugs.

Brandt MR, Fernandes A, Mordhurst R, et al. Epidural analgesia improves postoperative nitrogen balance. *BMJ* 1978;1:1106.
This article describes how attenuation of the stress response improves nitrogen balance.

Chang KSK, Davis RF. Propofol produces endothelium-independent vasodilation and may act as a Ca^{2+} channel blocker. *Anesth Analg* 1993;76:24.
This study elucidates mechanisms of propofol-induced hypotension.

Dundee JW, Collier PS, Carlisle RJT, et al. Prolonged midazolam elimination half-life. *Br J Clin Pharmacol* 1986;21:425.
This study describes patient groups for whom midazolam clearance is decreased.

Ebert TJ, Muzi M, Berens R, et al. Sympathetic responses to induction of anesthesia in humans with propofol or etomidate. *Anesthesiology* 1992;76:725.
This article describes the hemodynamic stability with etomidate and the mechanisms involved.

Forster A, Gardaz JP, Suter PM, et al. Respiratory depression by midazolam and diazepam. *Anesthesiology* 1980;53:494.

This study describes the enhanced respiratory depression by benzodiazepines seen in patients with chronic obstructive pulmonary disease.

Fragen RJ, Shanks CA, Molteni A, et al. Effects of etomidate on hormonal responses to surgical stress. *Anesthesiology* 1984;61:652.

This study documents the time course of adrenal suppression with etomidate.

Greenblatt DJ, Locniskar AA, Shader RI. Lorazepam kinetics in the elderly. *Clin Pharmacol Ther* 1979;26:103.

This article documents the increased central nervous system depression seen in the elderly compared with younger patients given an identical dose of a benzodiazepine.

Koch-Weser J, Sellers EM. Binding of drugs to serum albumin. *N Engl J Med* 1976; 294:311.

This is a good review of protein binding of drugs.

Modig J, Borg T, Karistrom G, et al. Thromboembolism after total hip replacement: role of epidural and general anesthesia. *Anesth Analg* 1983;62:174.

This classic article describes how reduction of stress response postoperatively by improved analgesia decreases thromboembolic risk.

Scott JC, Stanski DR. Decreased fentanyl and alfentanil dose requirements with age: a simultaneous pharmacokinetic and pharmacodynamic evaluation. *J Pharmacol Exp Ther* 1987;240:160.

This article describes the augmented effect of synthetic opioids in elderly patients.

Waxman K, Shoemaker WC, Lippmann M. Cardiovascular effects of anesthetic induction with ketamine. *Anesth Analg* 1980;59:335.

This article emphasizes the negative inotropic effects of ketamine and the reasons to use this agent with caution in catecholamine-depleted patients in the ICU.

Winters WD, Ferrer-Allado T, Guzman-Flores C. The cataleptic state induced by ketamine: a review of the neuropharmacology of anesthesia. *Neuropharmacology* 1972; 11:303.

This is a nice review giving a detailed description of the myriad central nervous system effects of ketamine.

22. MONITORING IN THE INTENSIVE CARE UNIT

Nicholas A. Smyrnios, Frederick J. Curley, and Richard S. Irwin

I. **General principles.** This chapter deals with the routine, predominantly noninvasive monitoring that is done for most patients in the intensive care unit (ICU).

II. **Temperature monitoring.** Critically ill patients are at high risk of temperature disorders resulting from debility, impaired voluntary control of temperature, sedative drugs, and predisposition to infection. All critically ill patients should have core temperature measured at least every 4 hours. Patients with temperatures higher than 39°C or lower than 36°C and patients who are undergoing interventions to alter temperature such as breathing heated air or using a cooling-warming blanket should have their temperature monitored continuously. The types of thermometers and sites of temperature used commonly in the ICU are listed in Table 22-1.

Continuous temperature monitoring is best accomplished by measurement of great vessel, rectal, or bladder temperature. Patients with a thermistor-tipped pulmonary artery catheter already in place require no additional monitoring. Rectal probes are often extruded and may be refused by patients. Bladder temperature can be measured at a low cost with a thermistor-equipped catheter. Intermittent measurements should probably be rectal.

III. **Arterial pressure monitoring**

A. **Indirect blood pressure measurement.** Cuffs of inadequate width and length provide falsely elevated readings. Bladder width should equal 40%, and length should be at least 60% of the circumference of the extremity.

Auscultatory pressures are the traditional method of blood pressure measurement using a sphygmomanometer cuff. Sounds from the vibrations of the artery under pressure (Korotkoff sounds) indicate systolic and diastolic pressures. The level at which the sound first becomes audible is the systolic pressure. The point at which there is an abrupt diminution or disappearance of sounds indicates the diastolic pressure.

Palpatory systolic pressure is obtained by detecting a pulse in the radial artery as the cuff is deflated.

Automated indirect blood pressure devices provide measurements of arterial blood pressure without manual inflation and deflation of the cuff. Although many different techniques of measurement have been used, only four of these methods (infrasound, oscillometry, Doppler flow, and volume clamp) have had significant clinical experience. Infrasound devices are rarely used in critical care. Oscillometric methods correlate well with group average values, but they correlate poorly with intraarterial pressures in individual patients. Doppler sensing devices are slightly better but still vary enough to be clinically suspect. Volume clamp devices respond rapidly to changes in blood pressure, give excellent correlation in group averages, and may be appropriate for use in critical care in the future.

B. **Direct invasive blood pressure measurement.** Direct arterial pressure measurement offers several advantages. Arterial catheters can (a) measure the end-on pressure propagated by the arterial pulse, (b) detect pressures at which Korotkoff sounds are either absent or inaccurate, (c) provide beat-to-beat changes in blood pressure, and (d) eliminate the need for multiple percutaneous punctures when frequent blood drawing is necessary. Technical problems affecting invasive arterial pressure measurement are listed in Table 22-2.

IV. **Electrocardiographic monitoring**

A. **Arrhythmia monitoring.** Continuous electrocardiographic (ECG) monitoring is performed routinely in almost all ICUs in the United States. Skin electrodes detect cardiac impulses and transform them into an electrical signal, which is transmitted over wires directly to the signal converter and display unit.

TABLE 22-1. Temperature measurement

Types of thermometers	Sites of measurement
Mercury in glass	Sublingual, Rectal
Liquid crystal display	Forehead
Thermocouples	Axillary, Rectal
Thermistors	Pulmonary artery
Tympanic infrared emission detection devices	Tympanic

In coronary care, arrhythmia monitoring is necessary for the following reasons: (a) up to 95% of patients with acute myocardial infarction (AMI) have some disturbance of their rate or rhythm within 48 hours of admission; (b) ventricular tachycardia occurs in approximately one-third of patients with AMI; monitoring enables the rapid detection of ventricular fibrillation or ventricular tachycardia and increases the likelihood of successful resuscitation; (c) arrhythmia monitoring has been shown to improve prognosis in the postinfarction period when it is combined with an aggressive, formalized approach to the treatment of arrhythmias; (d) thrombolytic therapy for AMI leads to a slight increase in arrhythmias within 8 to 12 hours after successful reperfusion; this result may be used as one indicator of successful reperfusion; and (e) arrhythmia monitoring also allows the measurement of heart rate variability, which may be useful in postinfarction risk stratification.

B. Ischemia monitoring. Significant episodes of myocardial ischemia often go undetected. Automated ST-segment monitoring may be useful in the ICU for the following reasons: (a) early detection of ischemic episodes could lead to early interventions; (b) continuous ST-segment monitoring can lead to the treatment of an expanded group of patients with thrombolytic therapy, including patients whose initial 12-lead ECGs were not diagnostic of AMI; (c) the degree of ST-segment resolution after thrombolysis may be a marker for prognosis after AMI; and d) ST-segment elevation may indicate ischemia acting as a barrier to weaning from mechanical ventilation. In most ST-segment monitoring systems, the computer initially creates a template of the patient's "normal" QRS complexes. It then recognizes the QRS complexes and the J points of subsequent beats and compares an isoelectric point just before the QRS complex with a portion of the ST segment 60 to 80 milliseconds after the J point. It compares this relationship to that of the same points in the QRS complex template. In most systems, 3 leads are monitored simultaneously. These leads are usually chosen to represent the 3 major axes (anteroposterior, left-right, and craniocaudal). They can be displayed individually, or ST-segment deviations can be summed up and displayed in a graph over time. Table 22-3 lists several technical and personnel issues that may impede our ability to generate and interpret high-quality ECG monitoring information in the ICU.

V. Respiratory monitoring. The respiratory parameters that must be monitored in critically ill patients include respiratory rate (f), tidal volume (V_T) or minute ventilation (V_E), and oxygenation. In mechanically ventilated patients, f, V_T, and V_E can be monitored continuously by the ventilator.

TABLE 22-2. Technical problems in direct blood pressure measurement.

Transducers not calibrated to zero at the level of the heart
Thrombus occluding the catheter tip
Movement of the limb possibly interrupting the column of fluid
Natural frequency of system less than five times greater than the fundamental frequency (i.e., the range of expected heart rates)
Tubing longer than 60 cm
Air in the measurement system
Comparison between different measurement sites (e.g., femoral vs. dorsalis pedis)

TABLE 22-3. Technical and personnel issues

1. Patient safety requirements
   a. All equipment in contact with patient at the same ground potential as the power ground line
   b. Insulation of exposed lead connections
   c. Use of appropriately wired three-prong plugs (32ECG,33ECG)
2. Adequate signal size
   a. Matching of skin electrode and preamplifier impedance
   b. Good skin preparation
   c. Site selection
   d. Conducting gels
   e. High preamplifier input impedance
   f. Use of buffer amplifiers
   g. Appropriate signal "damping"
   h. Correct frquency response
   i. Unwanted ambient voltages
3. Personnel issues
   a. Initial formal training for all staff responsible for interpreting ECG monitoring
   b. Formal hospital interpretation and response protocols
   c. Physician backup available in house

ECG, Electrocardiogram.

A. Respiratory rate, tidal volume, and minute ventilation

1. **Impedance monitors.** Impedance monitors employ ECG leads to measure changes in impedance generated by the change in distance between leads during breathing. To obtain a high-quality signal, leads must be placed at points of maximal change in thoracoabdominal contour. Impedance monitors are inexpensive when ECG monitoring is already in use, but they lack the accuracy to make precise measurements.
2. **Respiratory inductive plethysmography.** Respiratory inductive plethysmography measures the changes in the cross-sectional area of the chest and abdomen that occur with respiration and processes these values into respiratory rate and tidal volume. Two bands consisting of elastic fabric containing a wire sewn in a zigzag fashion are placed around the patient's upper chest and around the abdomen below the ribs. As the length of the bands changes with respiration, the coils generate an electric signal that is translated into a volume measurement. This technique can accurately measure f and the percentage of change in V_T, can provide continuous measurement of asynchronous and paradoxic breathing, and can detect obstructive apnea.

B. Pulse oximetry. Oximeters should be used continuously in most critically ill patients because of the frequency of hypoxemia in these patients, the need to adjust oxygen flow to avoid toxicity and insufficiency, and the unreliability of visual inspection to detect mild hypoxemia.

Pulse oximeters measure the saturation of hemoglobin in the tissue during the arterial and venous phases of pulsation and mathematically derive arterial saturation. Oximeters distinguish between oxyhemoglobin and reduced hemoglobin on the basis of their different absorption of light. When red light and infrared light are directed from light-emitting diodes to a photodetector across a pulsatile tissue bed, the absorption of each wavelength by the tissue bed varies with the pulse. The difference between absorption in systole and diastole is due to arterialized blood. The change in the ratio of red to infrared spectrum absorption between systole and diastole can then be used to calculate arterial saturation (SaO_2). Most pulse oximeters measure the saturation to within 2% of actual SaO_2. Table 22-4 lists conditions that adversely affect the results of pulse oximetry.

C. Transcutaneous measurement of oxygen and carbon dioxide. Transcutaneous systems measure partial pressures of oxygen ($P_{tc}O_2$) and carbon dioxide

TABLE 22-4. Conditions that adversely affect the results of pulse oximetry

Poor signal detection
Probe malposition
Motion
Hypothermia
No pulse
Vasoconstriction
Hypotension
Falsely low S_pO_2
Nail polish
Dark skin
Ambient light
Elevated serum lipids
Methylene blue
Indigo carmine
Indocyanine green
Falsely elevated S_pO_2
Elevated carboxyhemoglobin
Elevated methemoglobin
Ambient light
Hypothermia

($P_{tc}CO_2$) that diffuse out of the vasculature and through the skin. An electrode heats the skin, promotes arterialization of capillaries, and improves diffusion of gases through the skin's lipid layers. The measured transcutaneous values of oxygen and carbon dioxide are typically 10 mm Hg lower and 5 to 23 mm Hg higher than arterial values, respectively. Factors that may cause $P_{tc}O_2$ and $P_{tc}CO_2$ to differ from partial pressures of arterial oxygen and carbon dioxide include a shift in the oxyhemoglobin dissociation curve caused by the heating of the skin, fever, hypoperfusion of the area being monitored, the variable effects of local cellular metabolism, edema, burns, abrasions, and scleroderma.

Transcutaneous monitoring is useful in patients for whom changes in either perfusion or gas exchange are likely, but not both. When perfusion is stable, values reflect gas exchange. When gas exchange is stable, values reflect perfusion. When both are unstable, results cannot be interpreted without additional information.

D. Capnography. Capnography involves the measurement and display of expired concentrations of carbon dioxide partial pressure (PCO_2). It is used most often to determine the presence or absence of respiration by detecting cyclic variation of end-tidal PCO_2. Capnography is a useful adjunct for detecting unintentional extubation, malposition of the endotracheal tube, or absence of perfusion.

E. Arterial blood gas analysis. Clinical evaluation is not sensitive enough to detect hypoxemia and hypercapnia. Arterial blood gas (ABG) analysis furnishes rapid and accurate information on these parameters. Therefore, the clinician should have a high index of suspicion that a respiratory or metabolic disorder is present in patients with a variety of central nervous system or cardiovascular signs and should use ABG analysis as part of the evaluation of these abnormalities.

Table 22-5 describes potential sources of error in ABG measurement. Entry should be made at a location where the artery has good collaferal circulation and is just beneath the skin. In most cases, the radial artery fulfills both these criteria. If the radial arteries are not accessible, the dorsalis pedis, posterior tibial, superficial temporal (in infants), brachial, and femoral arteries are alternatives. Brachial and femoral punctures are discouraged in patients with abnormal hemostatic mechanisms. A vessel that has been reconstructed should not be punctured.

The method (radial artery) is as follows:

1. Put on protective gloves and seat yourself in a comfortable position facing the patient.

TABLE 22-5. Potential sources of error in arterial blood gas measurement

Plastic syringes allow oxygen to leak out: lowers Po_2
Suction applied to the plunger pulls gas bubbles out of solution: lowers Po_2, Pco_2
Excess heparin: lowers measured Pco_2 and calculated HCO^{3-}
Failure to analyze or cool the specimen immediately: lowers Po_2, pH; raises Pco_2
Sampling a vein instead of an artery: lowers Po_2

2. Turn the patient's palm up and slightly hyperextend the wrist. The radial artery should be palpable.
3. Cleanse the skin with an alcohol swab.
4. With a 25-gauge needle, inject 1% lidocaine to raise a small wheal at the point where the skin puncture will be made.
5. Attach a needle no smaller than a 22-gauge to a glass syringe that will accept 5 mL of blood.
6. Wet the needle and the syringe with a sodium heparin solution (1,000 units/mL). Express all excess solution.
7. Insert the needle into the artery at an angle of approximately 30 degrees to the long axis of the vessel. This insertion angle minimizes pain from unintentional scraping of the periosteum below the artery.
8. As soon as the artery is entered, blood will appear in the syringe. Allow the arterial pressure to fill the syringe with at least 3 mL of blood. Do not apply suction by pulling on the syringe plunger.
9. Squirt out any tiny air bubbles. Cap the syringe by removing the needle and plugging the syringe with an appropriate rubber stopper. Dispose of the needle in an appropriately designated location.
10. Roll the syringe between both palms for 5 to 15 seconds to mix the heparin and blood. Apply pressure to the puncture site for 5 minutes. If a brachial artery site was used, the vessel should be compressed so the radial artery pulse cannot be palpated.
11. Immerse the capped syringe in a bag of ice and water and immediately transport it to the blood gas laboratory.
12. Write on the ABG slip the time of day, ventilator settings, fraction of inspired oxygen (FiO_2), and position of the patient.

Selected Readings

Carrol GC. Blood pressure monitoring. *Crit Care Clin* 1988;4:411.
A general review of the topic of blood pressure measurement.

Clements FM, Bruijn NP. Noninvasive cardiac monitoring. *Crit Care Clin* 1988;4:435.
A more in-depth explanation of the procedure of ischemia monitoring is described.

Kimball JT, Killip T. Aggresive treatment of arrhythmias in acute myocardial infarction: procedures and results. *Prog Cardiovasc Dis* 1968;10:483.
A classic article validating the treatment of arrhythmias in the post-AMI period.

New W. Pulse oximetry. *J Clin Monit* 1985;1:126.
General review of the technique of pulse oximetry.

Nystrom E, Reid KH, Bennett R, et al. A comparison of two automated indirect arterial blood pressure meters: with recordings from a radial arterial catheter in anesthetized surgical patients. *Anesthesiology* 1985;62:526.
Indicates lack of correlation between indirect and invasive blood pressure measurements.

Stock MC. Noninvasive carbon dioxide monitoring. *Crit Care Clin* 1988;4:511.
A more in-depth description of the technique of capnography.

Tobin MJ, Jenouri G, Lind B, et al. Validation of respiratory inductive plethysmography in patients with pulmonary disease. *Chest* 1983;83:615.
Study demonstrating the accuracy of plethysmography measurements in patients with respiratory disease.

II. CARDIOVASCULAR PROBLEMS IN THE INTENSIVE CARE UNIT

23. CARDIOPULMONARY RESUSCITATION

John A. Paraskos and Richard C. Becker

I. **History.** Since the introduction of cardiopulmonary resuscitation (CPR), we have been forced to rethink our definitions of life and death. Although sporadic accounts of attempted resuscitations are recorded from antiquity, until recently no rational quarrel could be found with the sixth century B.C. poetic fragment of Ibycus, "You cannot find a medicine for life once a man is dead."

II. **Efficacy.** CPR does not seem to go beyond the short-term sustaining of viability until definitive therapy can be administered. Data from prehospital care systems in Seattle show that 43% of patients found in ventricular fibrillation are discharged from the hospital if CPR (i.e., basic life support [BLS]) is applied within 4 minutes and defibrillation (i.e., advanced cardiac life support [ACLS]) is administered within 8 minutes. Survival rates for patients in asystole or with pulseless electrical activity (PEA) are much lower. Even though patients experiencing cardiac arrest in the hospital can be expected to receive CPR and definitive therapy well within the 4- and 8-minute time frames, their chances of being discharged alive are in general worse than for out-of-hospital victims.

III. **Mechanisms of blood flow during resuscitation**

A. **Cardiac compression theory.** According to this theory, during sternal compression the intraventricular pressures would be expected to rise higher than the pressures elsewhere in the chest. With each sternal compression, the semilunar valves would be expected to fall and the atrioventricular values to open, allowing the heart to fill from the lungs and systemic veins.

B. **Thoracic pump theory.** According to this theory, during CPR the heart serves only as a conduit. Forward flow is generated by a pressure gradient between intrathoracic and extrathoracic vascular structures. Interposed abdominal compression CPR (IAC-CPR) is now advised for in-hospital CPR, Active Compression-Decompression CPR (ACD-CPR), and Vest CPR are optional techniques for rescuers adequately trained in these techniques.

C. **Open chest cardiopulmonary resuscitation.** Mechanistically, open chest CPR involves direct cardiac compression without the use of a thoracic gradient. Patients with penetrating chest trauma are unlikely to respond to chest compression and are candidates for open chest CPR. If open chest CPR is to be used, it should be used early. Patients with blunt chest and abdominal trauma may also be considered candidates for open chest CPR. This technique should not be attempted unless adequate facilities and trained personnel are available.

D. **Cardiopulmonary bypass for unresponsive cardiac arrest.** Cardiopulmonary bypass is not a form of routine life support; however, it represents a possible adjunct to artificial circulation. It is an indispensable adjunct to cardiac surgery and is being used more frequently for invasive procedures as a standby for sudden cardiac collapse.

IV. **Infectious diseases and implications for health care professionals.** The fear provoked by the spread of human immunodeficiency virus (HIV) may lead to excessive caution when dealing with strangers; it has clearly decreased the willingness of the lay public as well as health professionals to learn and perform CPR.

Bag-valve mask devices should be available as initial ventilation equipment, and early endotracheal intubation should be encouraged when equipment and trained professionals are available. Masks with one-way valves and plastic mouth and nose covers with filtered openings provide some protection from transfer of oral fluids and aerosols. S-shaped mouthpieces, masks without one-way valves, and handkerchiefs provide little if any barrier protection and should not be considered for routine use.

V. **Advanced cardiac life support in adults.** The use of adjunctive equipment, more specialized techniques, and pharmacologic and electrical therapy in the treatment of cardiac or respiratory arrest victims is generally referred to as ACLS. These techniques and their interface with BLS and the emergency medical services system are considered in the American Heart Association's ACLS teaching program.

A. Airway and ventilatory support. Oxygenation and optimal ventilation are prerequisites of successful resuscitation. Ventilation with the rescuer's exhaled breath, which provides 16% to 17% oxygen, may produce an alveolar partial pressure of oxygen (PAO_2) of 80 mm Hg. Arterial hypoxemia is inevitable because of diminished cardiac output (including pulmonary blood flow), intrapulmonary shunting, and ventilation-perfusion (V/Q) mismatch). Therefore, supplemental oxygen should be administered as soon as it becomes available, beginning with 100%.

Endotracheal intubation is required if the patient cannot be rapidly resuscitated or when adequate spontaneous ventilation does not resume quickly. Experienced personnel should attempt intubation.

B. Circulatory support. Chest compression should not be unduly interrupted while adjunctive procedures are instituted. The rescuer coordinating the resuscitative effort must ensure that adequate pulses are generated by the compressor. The carotid or femoral pulse should be evaluated every few minutes.

Electrocardiographic (ECG) monitoring is necessary during resuscitation to guide appropriate electrical and pharmacologic therapy. Until ECG monitoring allows diagnosis of the rhythm, the patient should be assumed to be in ventricular fibrillation (see later). Most defibrillators currently marketed have built-in monitoring circuitry in the paddles ("quick-look" paddles). On application of the defibrillator paddles, the patient's ECG tracing is displayed on the monitor screen. This facilitates appropriate initial therapy.

Defibrillation is the definitive treatment for most cardiac arrests. It should be delivered as early as possible and repeated frequently until ventricular fibrillation or pulseless ventricular tachycardia has been terminated. If an electrical defibrillator is not immediately available, a precordial thump may be used.

Proper use of the defibrillator requires special attention to the following:

1. **Selection of proper energy levels.** This lessens myocardial damage and arrhythmias occasioned by unnecessarily high energies. Inadequate energies do not terminate the arrhythmia. An initial energy of 200 joules appears to be safer than higher energies and equally effective.
2. **Proper asynchronous mode.** The proper mode must be selected if the rhythm is ventricular fibrillation. The synchronizing must be deactivated or the defibrillator will dutifully await the nonforthcoming R wave. For rapid pulseless ventricular tachycardia (approximately 150 to 200 beats per minute), it is best not to attempt synchronization with the R wave because this increases the likelihood of delivering the shock on the T wave.
3. **Proper position of the paddles.** The anterolateral position requires that one paddle be placed on the right of the upper sternum, just below the clavicle. The other paddle is positioned to the left of the nipple in the left midaxillary line. In the anteroposterior position, one paddle is positioned under the left scapula with the patient lying on it. The anterior paddle is positioned just to the left of the lower sternal border.
4. **Adequate contact between paddles and skin.** The rescuer should hold the paddles with firm (approximately 25 pounds) pressure.
5. **No contact with anyone other than the victim.** The rescuer must be sturdily balanced on both feet and not standing on a wet floor. CPR must be discontinued with no one remaining in contact with the patient.
6. **Rechecking of equipment.** If no skeletal muscle twitch or spasm has occurred, the equipment, contacts, and synchronizer switch used for elective cardioversions should be rechecked.
7. **Rhythm assessment.** The rhythm should be assessed after each countershock, and the patient should be checked for a pulse at appropriate times. *This must be done before proceeding with therapeutic interventions.*

Venous access with a reliable intravenous route must be established early in the course of the resuscitative effort to allow administration of necessary drugs and fluids. Drugs such as epinephrine, atropine, and lidocaine can be administered by the endotracheal tube if there is delay in achieving venous access.

However, this route requires a higher dose to achieve an equivalent blood level, and a sustained duration of action (a "depot effect") can be expected if a return in spontaneous circulation occurs.

VI. Drug therapy

A. Correction of hypoxia. Hypoxemia should be corrected early during CPR with administration of the highest possible oxygen concentration.

B. Correction of acidosis. Correction of acidosis must be considered when the cardiac arrest has lasted more than several minutes. *Metabolic acidosis* develops because of tissue hypoxia and conversion to anaerobic metabolism. *Respiratory acidosis* occurs because of the apnea or hypoventilation with intrapulmonary ventilation-perfusion abnormalities; the marked decrease in pulmonary blood flow that exists even with well performed CPR also contributes. The American Heart Association guidelines suggest that sodium bicarbonate be avoided until successful resuscitation has reestablished a perfusing rhythm. An exception is the patient who has known preexisting hyperkalemia, in whom the administration of bicarbonate is recommended.

C. Volume replacement. Increased central volume is often required during CPR, especially if the initial attempts at defibrillation have failed. Simple crystalloids, such as 5% dextrose in water, are inappropriate for rapid expansion of the circulatory blood volume. Isotonic crystalloids (0.9% saline, Ringer's lactate), colloids, or blood are necessary for satisfactory volume expansion.

D. Sympathomimetic drugs and vasopressors. Sympathomimetic drugs either act directly on adrenergic receptors or act indirectly by releasing catecholamines from nerve endings.

1. **Epinephrine.** This is the pressor agent used most frequently during CPR. Epinephrine is a naturally occurring catecholamine with both alpha and beta activity.

   Indications for the use of epinephrine include all forms of cardiac arrest. The beta action of epinephrine is useful in asystole and bradycardic arrests. The beta effect has also been touted to convert asystole to ventricular fibrillation or to convert "fine" ventricular fibrillation to "coarse."
2. **Norepinephrine.** This is a potent alpha-agonist with beta activity. Its salutary alpha effects during CPR are similar to those of epinephrine. Indications for the use of norepinephrine during cardiac arrest are similar to those for epinephrine, although there does not appear to be any reason to prefer it to epinephrine. Norepinephrine appears to be most useful in the treatment of septic shock and neurogenic shock.
3. **Isoproterenol.** This synthetic catecholamine has almost pure beta-adrenergic activity. Its cardiac activity includes potent inotropic and chronotropic effects. Indications for isoproterenol are primarily in the setting of atropine-resistant, hemodynamically significant bradyarrhythmias, including profound sinus and junctional bradycardia, as well as various forms of high-degree atrioventricular block. *Under no circumstances should isoproterenol be used during cardiac arrest.*
4. **Dopamine hydrochloride.** This naturally occurring precursor of norepinephrine has alpha-, beta-, and dopamine-receptor stimulating activity. Indications for the use of dopamine are primarily significant hypotension and cardiogenic shock.
5. **Dobutamine.** This potent synthetic beta-adrenergic agent differs from isoproterenol in that tachycardia is less problematic. Dobutamine is indicated primarily for the short-term enhancement of ventricular contractility in the patient with heart failure.
6. **Vasopressin.** During cardiac arrest, vasopressin has been used in experimental protocols as an adjunct or alternative to epinephrine.

E. Antiarrhythmic agents. Antiarrhythmics play an important role in stabilizing rhythm in many resuscitation situations.

1. **Lidocaine.** Lidocaine is indicated primarily to suppress ventricular arrhythmias in patients with myocardial ischemia and recent myocardial infarction.
2. **Amiodarone.** Amiodarone given intravenously has been found successful in terminating a variety of reentrant and non-reentrant supraventricular and

ventricular arrhythmias. It may be used during VT/VF arrest, especially if lidocaine has failed or if defribrillation attempts have failed. Some suggest its use as a first antiarrhythmic in VT/VF arrest if defibrillation attempts have failed and should take the place of Bretylium tosilate in the appended algorithms.

3. **Procainamide hydrochloride.** Procainamide, an antiarrhythmic agent with quinidine-like activity, is indicated for the suppression of ventricular arrhythmias refractory to lidocaine or both lidocaine and bretylium. It may also be used in patients with supraventricular arrhythmias.
4. **Adenosine.** Adenosine is an endogenous purine nucleoside that depresses atrioventricular nodal conduction and sinoatrial nodal activity. Adenosine is effective in terminating arrhythmias that involve the atrioventricular node in a reentrant circuit (e.g., paroxysmal supraventricular tachycardia [PSVT]). In supraventricular tachycardias such as atrial flutter, atrial fibrillation, or atrial or ventricular tachycardias that do not use the atrioventricular node in a reentrant circuit, blocking transmission through the atrioventricular node may prove helpful in clarifying the diagnosis.
5. **Verapamil and diltiazem.** Unlike other calcium channel blocking agents, verapamil and diltiazem increase refractoriness in the atrioventricular node and significantly slow condution. This action may terminate reentrant tachycardias that use the atrioventricular node in the reentrant circuit (e.g., PSVT). These drugs may also slow the ventricular response in patients with atrial flutter or fibrillation and in patients with multifocal atrial tachycardia.
6. **Magnesium.** Magnesium is administered intravenously. For rapid administration during ventricular tachycardia (torsades de pointes) or ventricular fibrillation with suspected or documented hypomagnesemia, 1 to 2 g may be diluted in 100 mL of 5% dextrose in water and given over 1 to 2 minutes.
7. **Atropine sulfate.** Atropine is a vagolytic drug of use in increasing heart rate by stimulating pacers and facilitating atrioventricular conduction suppressed by excessive vagal tone. Atropine is indicated primarily in bradycardias causing hemodynamic difficulty or associated with ventricular arrhythmias. It is also used in asystole and bradycardic arrests.
8. **Calcium.** Calcium is indicated *only* in calcium channel blocker toxicity, severe hyperkalemia, severe hypocalcemia, cardiac arrest after multiple transfusions with citrated blood, and fluoride toxicity, as well as in patients who are being removed from heart-lung bypass after cardioplegic arrest.

VII. Clinical setting. The procedures involved in resuscitation of a victim of cardiovascular or respiratory collapse are part of a continuum progressing from initial recognition of the problem and institution of CPR to intervention with defibrillators, drugs, pacemakers, transport, and postresuscitative evaluation and care. The following sections focus on the pharmacologic and electrical interventions appropriate to various clinical settings common in cardiac arrest.

A. Ventricular fibrillation. Ventricular fibrillation is the initial rhythm encountered in 50% to 70% of prehospital cardiac arrests and 30% to 40% of hospital cardiac arrests. In a significant percentage of hospital cardiac arrests and in a smaller number of prehospital arrests, pulseless ventricular tachycardia is the first rhythm encountered by rescue personnel. Electrical defibrillation is the most important intervention in treating these arrhythmias (Fig. 23-1). The sooner it is administered, the more likely it is to succeed.

B. Asystole. Asystole (Fig. 23-2) is the first rhythm encountered in 30% to 40% of prehospital as well as hospital cardiac arrests. Asystole is obviously the end result of any pulseless rhythm, and as such, when it is the presenting rhythm it is often the termination of untreated ventricular fibrillation.

C. Pulseless electrical activity. PEA is present when an arrest victim is found to have organized ECG ventricular complexes (QRS) unassociated with a palpable pulse. Electromechanical dissociation is a form of PEA in which the QRS complex is unaccompanied by any evidence of ventricular contraction and the emergency response is the same (Fig. 23-3).

D. Other clinical situations

1. **Bradycardia with a pulse (Fig. 23-4)**
2. **Sustained ventricular tachycardia (Fig. 23-5)**

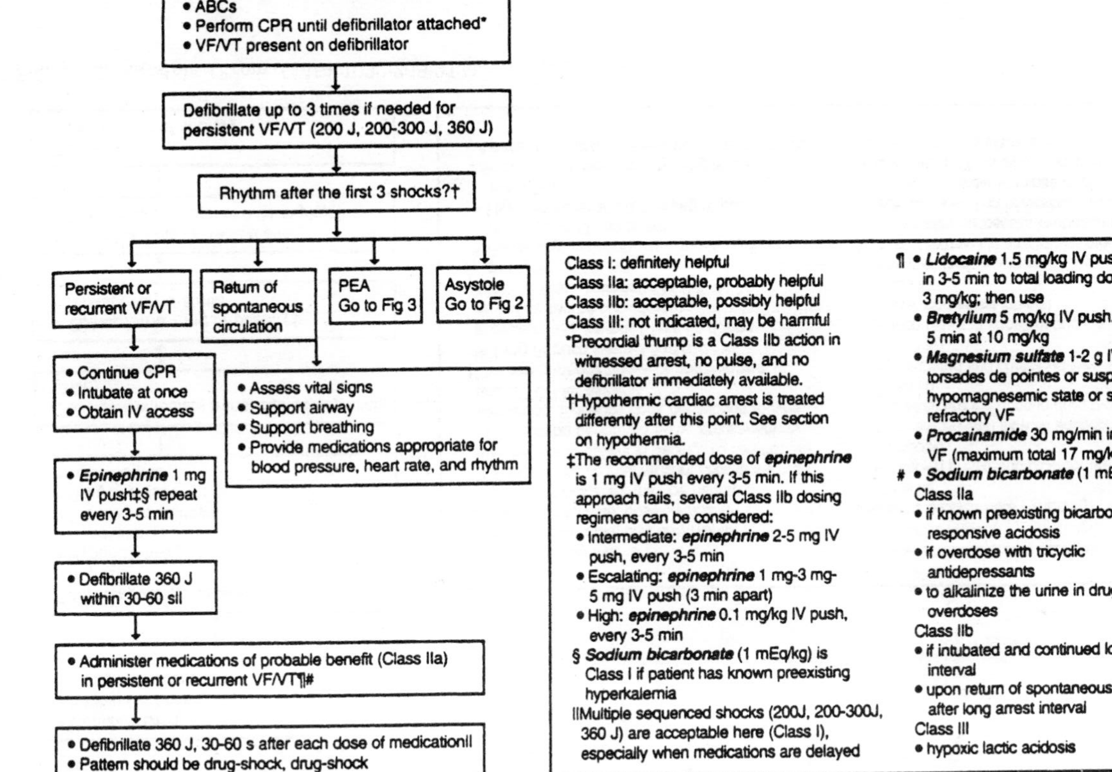

FIG. 23-1. Ventricular fibrillation and pulseless ventricular tachycardia (VF/VT). (From *JAMA* 1992;268:2171, with permission.)

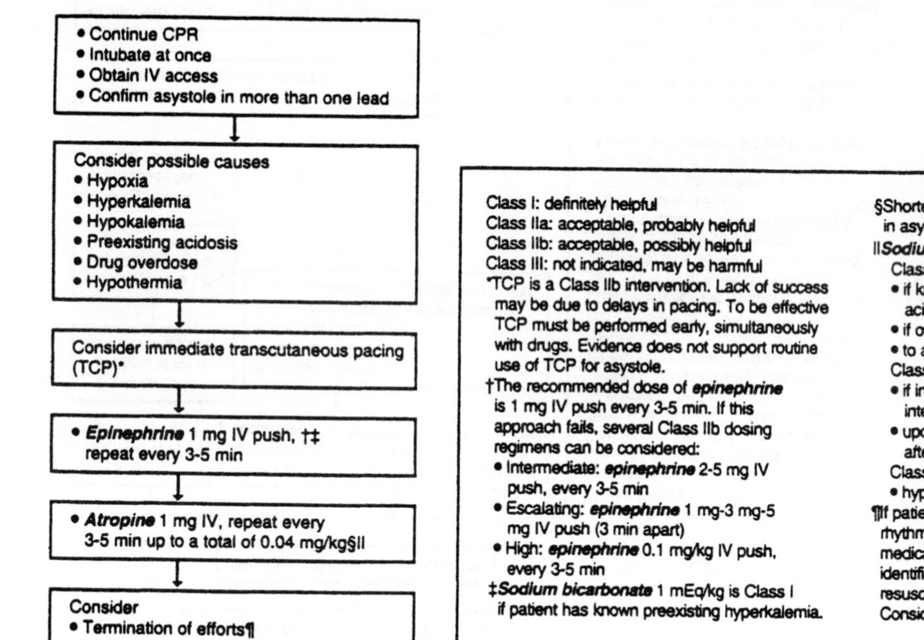

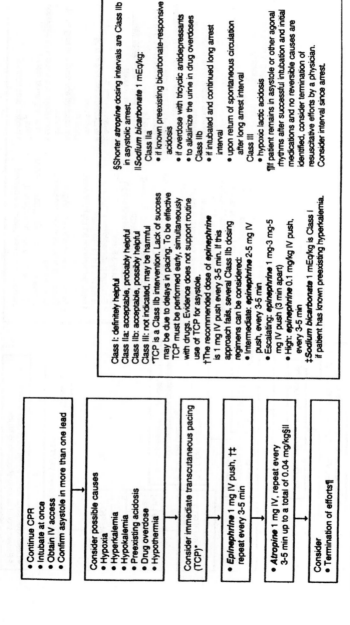

FIG. 23-2. Asystole. (From *JAMA* 1992;268:2171, with permission.)

PEA includes
- Electromechanical dissociation (EMD)
- Pseudo-EMD
- Idioventricular rhythms
- Ventricular escape rhythms
- Bradyasystolic rhythms
- Postdefibrillation idioventricular rhythms

- Continue CPR
- Intubate at once
- Obtain IV access
- Assess blood flow using Doppler ultrasound

↓

Consider possible causes
(Parentheses=possible therapies and treatments)
- Hypovolemia (volume infusion)
- Hypoxia (ventilation)
- Cardiac tamponade (pericardiocentesis)
- Tension pneumothorax (needle decompression)
- Hypothermia (see hypothermia algorithm, Section IV)
- Massive pulmonary embolism (surgery, ***thrombolytics***)
- Drug overdoses such as tricyclics, digitalis, β-blockers, calcium channel blockers
- Hyperkalemia*
- Acidosis†
- Massive acute myocardial infarction (go to Fig 9)

↓

- ***Epinephrine*** 1 mg IV push, *‡ repeat every 3-5 min

↓

- If absolute bradycardia (<60 beats/min) or relative bradycardia, give ***atropine*** 1 mg IV
- Repeat every 3-5 min up to a total of 0.04 mg/kg§

Class I: definitely helpful
Class IIa: acceptable, probably helpful
Class IIb: acceptable, possibly helpful
Class III: not indicated, may be harmful

****Sodium bicarbonate*** 1 mEq/kg is Class I if patient has known preexisting hyperkalemia.

†***Sodium bicarbonate*** 1 mEq/kg:
Class IIa
- if known preexisting bicarbonate-responsive acidosis
- if overdose with tricyclic antidepressants
- to alkalinize the urine in drug overdoses

Class IIb
- if intubated and long arrest interval
- upon return of spontaneous circulation after long arrest interval

Class III
- hypoxic lactic acidosis

‡The recommended dose of ***epinephrine*** is 1 mg IV push every 3-5 min. If this approach fails, several Class IIb dosing regimens can be considered.
- Intermediate: ***epinephrine*** 2-5 mg IV push, every 3-5 min
- Escalating: ***epinephrine*** 1 mg-3 mg-5 mg IV push (3 min apart)
- High: ***epinephrine*** 0.1 mg/kg IV push, every 3-5 min

§ Shorter ***atropine*** dosing intervals are possibly helpful in cardiac arrest (Class IIb).

FIG. 23-3. Pulseless electrical activity (PEA) and electromechanical dissociation (EMD).(From *JAMA* 1992;268:2171, with permission.)

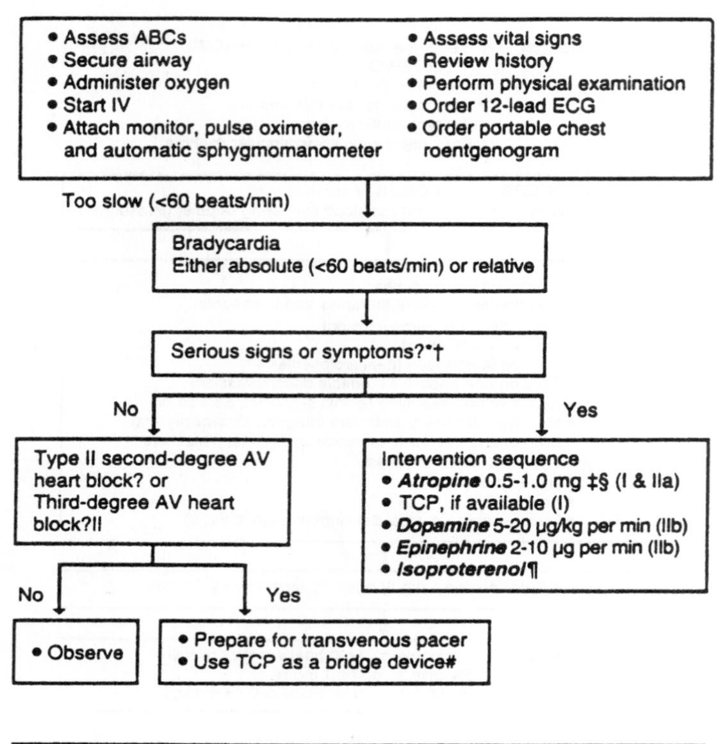

• Assess ABCs
• Secure airway
• Administer oxygen
• Start IV
• Attach monitor, pulse oximeter, and automatic sphygmomanometer
• Assess vital signs
• Review history
• Perform physical examination
• Order 12-lead ECG
• Order portable chest roentgenogram
Too slow (<60 beats/min)
Bradycardia
Either absolute (<60 beats/min) or relative
Serious signs or symptoms?*†
No
Yes
Type II second-degree AV heart block? or Third-degree AV heart block?||
Intervention sequence
• *Atropine* 0.5-1.0 mg ‡§ (I & IIa)
• TCP, if available (I)
• *Dopamine* 5-20 μg/kg per min (IIb)
• *Epinephrine* 2-10 μg per min (IIb)
• *Isoproterenol*¶
No
Yes
• Observe
• Prepare for transvenous pacer
• Use TCP as a bridge device#

*Serious signs or symptoms must be related to the slow rate. Clinical manifestations include:
symptoms (chest pain, shortness of breath, decreased level of conciousness) and
signs (low BP, shock, pulmonary congestion, CHF, acute MI).

†Do not delay TCP while awating IV access or for ***atropine*** to take effect if patient is symptomatic.

‡Denervated transplanted hearts will not respond to ***atropine***. Go at once to pacing, ***catecholamine*** infusion, or both.

§***Atropine*** should be given in repeat doses in 3-5 min up to total of 0.04 mg/kg. Consider shorter dosing intervals in severe clinical conditions. It has been suggested that atropine should be used with caution in atrioventricular (AV) block at the His-Purkinje level (type II AV block and new third-degree block with wide QRS complexes) (Class IIb).

||Never treat third-degree heart block plus ventricular escape beats with ***lidocaine***.

¶***Isoproterenol*** should be used, if at all, with exteme caution. At low doses it is Class IIb (possibly helpful); at higher doses it is Class III (harmful).

#Verify patient tolerance and mechanical capture. Use analgesia and sedation as needed.

FIG. 23-4. Bradycardia with a pulse.(From *JAMA* 1992;268:2171, with permission.)

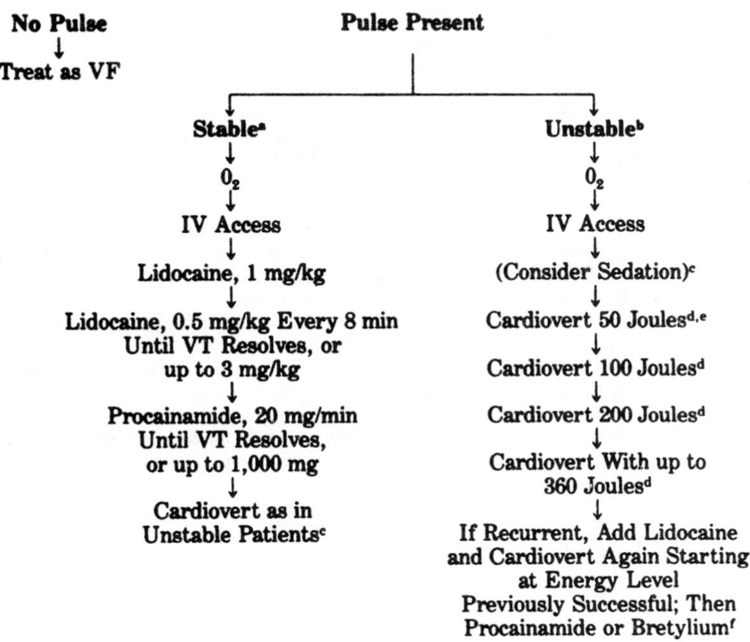

FIG. 23-5. Sustained ventricular tachycardia. This sequence was developed to assist in teaching how to respond to a broad range of patients with sustained ventricular tachycardia. Some patients may require therapy not specified herein. This algorithm should not be construed as prohibiting such flexibility. **a.** If a patient becomes unstable (see **b**) at any time, move to "unstable" arm of the algorithm. **b.**"Unstable" indicates symptoms (e.g., chest pain, dyspnea), hypotension, congestive heart failure, ischemia, or infarction. **c.** Sedation should be considered for all patients except those who are unconscious or who cannot wait because of severe hemodynamic instability. **d.** For patients in shock or marked pulmonary edema, unsynchronized cardioversion should be performed if synchronization would cause a delay; for patients with rapid ventricular tachycardia greater than 150 beats per minute, unsynchronized cardioversion is preferable to avoid synchronizing on the T wave. If ventricular fibrillation appears to result on the monitor and the patient is pulseless, countershock should be given immediately without synchronization. **e.** A precordial thump may be used before cardioversion. **f.** If ventricular tachycardia resolves, one should begin intravenous infusion of the antiarrhythmic drug that aided resolution; if cardioversion is unsuccessful, one should use intravenous lidocaine, followed by bretylium. Procainamide may also be considered. (From *JAMA* 1985;255:2843, with permission.)

Selected Readings

Babbs CF, Sack JB, Kern KB. Interposed abdominal compression as an adjunct to cardiopulmonary resuscitation. *Am Heart J* 1994;127:412.

Randomized trials show that survival of patients resuscitated in the hospital with IAC CPR was improved over standard CPR.

Guidelines for the determination of death. Report of the medical consultants on the diagnosis of death to the President's Commission for the Study of Ethical Problems in Medicine and Biomedical and Behavioral Research. *JAMA* 1981;246:2184.

Guidelines for determining and defining clinical death and biologic death.

Kudenchuk PJ, Cobb LA, Copass MK, et al. Amiodarone for resuscitation after out-of-hospital cardiac arrest due to ventricular fibrillation. *New Engl J Med* 1999;341:871.
In patients with out-of-hospital refractory VT/VF, amiodarone resulted in higher rate of survival to hospital admission, but not to hospital discharge.

Lindner KH, Dirks B, Strohmenger HU, et al. Randomised comparison of epinephrine and vasopressin in patients with out-of-hospital ventricular fibrillation. *Lancet* 1997;349:535.
Vasopressin led to more frequent resuscitation than epinephrine in a preliminary study.

Plaisance P, Lurie KG, Vicaut E, et al. A comparison of standard cardiopulmonary resuscitation and active compression-decompression resuscitation for out-of-hospital cardiac arrest. French Active Compression-Decompression Cardiopulmonary Resuscitation Study Group. *N Engl Med* 1999;341:569.
ACD-CPR performed during ACLS significantly improved long-term survival rates among patients with out-of-hospital cardiac arrests.

Waxman HL, Groh WC, Marchlinski FE, et al. Amiodarone for control of sustained ventricular tachyarrhythmias: clinical and electrophysiologic effects in 51 patients. *Am J Cardiol* 1982;50:1066.
The use of intravenous amiodarone among patients with sustained ventricular arrhythmias is highlighted and is gaining more widespread acceptance.

24. CRITICAL AORTIC STENOSIS AND HYPERTROPHIC CARDIOMYOPATHY

Gerard P. Aurigemma, John A. Paraskos, and Richard C. Becker

I. General principles. Obstruction to the left ventricular outflow, resulting either from valvular aortic stenosis or from hypertrophic obstructive cardiomyopathy, may lead to syncope, congestive heart failure, or sudden cardiac death. In addition, supraventricular tachyarrhythmias in patients with marked ventricular hypertrophy may be met with dire hemodynamic consequences (Table 24-1).

II. Aortic stenosis

A. Pathophysiology. In valvular aortic stenosis, increased impedance to left ventricular ejection is the primary hemodynamic disturbance; the severity of the obstruction determines the hemodynamic consequences for the left ventricle. In fixed valvular stenoses, a cross-sectional area as small as 1.0 cm^2 (compared with the normal 3.0 to 3.5 cm^2) causes a significant rise in left ventricular outflow impedance and results in a pressure gradient across the valve, even at rest; with further reduction of the orifice size to 0.6 to 0.8 cm^2, outflow impedance increases.

Both myocardial hypertrophy and ischemia may lead to increased left ventricular chamber stiffness or reduced diastolic compliance.

The rate of progression of valvular aortic stenosis is highly variable, but it may be more rapid in patients with degenerative calcific than congenital or rheumatic disease. The peak systolic gradient across the valve has been observed to proceed at rates of 0.8 to 1.3 mm Hg per month; however, an individual patient with initially mild stenosis may develop severe stenosis as quickly as in 2 years.

B. History. The cardinal symptoms associated with outflow obstruction include angina pectoris, dizziness, syncope, and dyspnea (Table 24-2). Angina pectoris is the most commonly encountered symptom, occurring in more than half of patients with symptomatic aortic stenosis. Syncope occurring with or immediately after physical exertion is the next most common symptom, elicited from approximately one-third of symptomatic patients. More frequently, however, patients complain of effort-induced dizziness or lightheadedness.

Patients presenting with left ventricular systolic failure resulting from unrelieved aortic stenosis may complain of progressive dyspnea on exertion, paroxysmal nocturnal dyspnea, orthopnea, cough, or generalized fatigue. Rarely, an adult with unrecognized aortic valvular stenosis may suffer sudden death without premonitory symptoms.

Once the symptoms of angina pectoris, syncope, or dyspnea develop, mean life expectancy is several years, and prompt measures should be taken to define the severity of the lesion and to determine the need for surgical intervention. An analysis of survival curves of unoperated patients with aortic stenosis indicates that median survival after onset of heart failure is 2 years; for syncope, it is 3 years, and for, it is angina 5 years.

C. Physical examination. In patients with aortic stenosis, blood pressure is usually normal, although pulse pressure tends to be restricted; significant hypertension is not rare, especially in the elderly. Systolic vibrations or "shudders" of the carotid pulse correlate with the presence of a transmitted murmur but not with the severity of the stenosis. Careful palpation of the carotid artery may reveal a delayed upstroke, following the slow rise in the aortic pressure curve (pulsus parvus et tardus), a finding that identifies hemodynamically severe aortic stenosis with great specificity.

An aortic ejection click may be audible at the onset of the murmur (Table 24-3). In severe aortic stenosis, the second heart sound is expected to be paradoxically split because of the prolongation of left ventricular ejection time. However,

TABLE 24-1. Causes of left ventricular outflow obstruction

A. Congenital lesions
  1. Valvular
    a. Unicuspid
    b. Bicuspid with degeneration
    c. Deformed three- or four-cusped valves with degeneration (rare)
  2. Subvalvular
    a. Discrete fibromembranous
    b. Tunnel lesion (diffuse fibromuscular)
    c. Hypertrophic cardiomyopathy
  3. Supravalvular
    a. Hourglass deformity
    b. Hypoplastic
    c. Membranous
B. Acquired lesions
  1. Degenerative changes (fibrocalcific deformity)
    a. Of congenitally abnormal valve
    b. Of normal three-cusped valve
  2. Rheumatic heart disease

in adult patients with critical aortic stenosis, the aortic closure sound is diminished in intensity, precluding the auscultation of paradoxic splitting. A fourth heart sound should be audible in all forms of severe left ventricular outflow obstruction (unless atrial fibrillation has supervened).

An ausculatory finding common to all forms of left ventricular outflow obstruction is a systolic ejection (crescendo-decrescendo) murmur. The intensity of the murmur is related poorly to the severity of stenosis; the duration of the murmur is a better index of the severity of obstruction. A late-peaking, prolonged murmur suggests severe stenosis.

An aortic regurgitation murmur is common in valvular as well as discrete subvalvular aortic stenosis (Table 24-4).

D. Laboratory studies

1. Electrocardiography. In severe aortic stenosis, evidence of left ventricular hypertrophy is present in the majority of patients. Increased R-wave voltage over left precordial leads is expected with associated ST-segment sagging and T-wave inversion (strain pattern), typical of pressure overload left ventricular hypertrophy. Left bundle branch block may also be appreciated.

2. Chest radiography. In most patients, the heart is not dilated, and the cardiothoracic ratio is normal on a posteroanterior chest radiograph. However, the left lower border of the heart shadow is often rounded or convex as a result of left ventricular hypertrophy. With systolic failure of the left ventricle, the chest radiograph reveals cardiac enlargement, as well as evidence

TABLE 24-2. Features common to all forms of severe left ventricular outflow obstruction

Angina, syncope, dyspnea
Systolic ejection murmur
Paradoxically split-second sound
Fourth sound
Sustained apical impulse
Left ventricular hypertrophy

TABLE 24-3. Differentiating features among causes of left ventricular outflow obstruction

Age at onset of symptoms
Years symptoms have been present
Maximal location of systolic murmur
Systolic ejection click
Dilatation of ascending aorta
Differential carotid delay and brachial pressures
Presence of aortic regurgitation
Presence of mitral disease
Decreased aortic closure sound

of pulmonary venous engorgement or congestion. Calcification of the aortic valve is expected in adults with valvular aortic stenosis.

3. **Echocardiography.** In patients with critical aortic stenosis, the echocardiogram is expected to demonstrate concentric left ventricular hypertrophy, as well as thickened aortic valve cusps with diminished mobility (Fig. 24-1).
4. **Doppler echocardiography.** Echocardiographic investigation of the aortic valve for stenosis requires careful Doppler analysis and a skilled and meticulous ultrasonographer. The velocity of the jet of blood traversing the stenotic valve correlates with the transvalvular gradient (Fig. 24-2).

E. Cardiac catheterization. Cardiac catheterization is warranted in any patient with suspected severe symptomatic aortic stenosis. With a normal cardiac output, a mean systolic gradient of 50 mm Hg or more is usually found with severe aortic stenosis. In such severe cases, the calculated valve area is usually less than 0.8 cm^2; however, as cardiac output decreases because of systolic pump failure, mean systolic gradients less than 50 mm Hg are often recorded. The calculated valve area, however, should accurately estimate the severity of stenosis in these cases.

F. Management. In general, asymptomatic persons with aortic stenosis do not require surgical intervention. Valve replacement is recommended if the valve area is found to be less than 0.8 cm^2 in the symptomatic patient. Once angina, syncope, or left ventricular failure occurs, urgent cardiac catheterization is necessary, and early surgical correction is warranted if catheterization corroborates the presence of severe stenosis.

G. Intensive care unit management. Medical therapy of symptomatic aortic stenosis in the intensive care unit is at best a temporizing measure until definitive diagnosis and surgical correction can be undertaken.

While awaiting surgical correction, the patient with both fixed aortic stenosis and myocardial ischemia may be treated with judicious use of nitrates. Both systolic and diastolic aortic pressures tend to drop, so overall wall stress and myocardial oxygen requirements may be lessened dramatically. Excessive nitrate effect, however, is potentially deleterious, because preload reduction may drop the stroke volume and precipitously lower the blood pressure.

Patients with left ventricular failure and pulmonary congestion may be cautiously treated with diuretics. Careful monitoring of the pulmonary capillary wedge pressure is recommended to prevent excessive reduction in preload and subsequent hypotension.

H. Surgical therapy. A symptomatic patient with valvular stenosis and a valve area of less than 0.8 cm^2 should be offered aortic valve replacement. If left ventricular systolic function is preserved, the mean gradient usually exceeds 50 mm Hg in these patients.

The presence of a mean transvalvular gradient of less than 30 mm Hg and a critically narrowed aortic valve identifies a subgroup of patients in whom valve replacement is associated with poor outcome. Preoperative ejection fraction

TABLE 24-4. Aortic stenosis: physical findings

Lesion	Murmur	Ejection Click	Aortic Closure Sound	Aortic Regurgitation	Carotid Pulse
Congenital					
Unicuspid valvular	Aortic area to neck and apex	Common	Normal or loud in children	Uncommon in children	Delayed
Bicuspid valvular	Aortic area to neck and apex	Common in young adults	Decreased in adults	Common	Delayed
Discrete subvalvular	Left sternal border	Rare	Normal or decreased	Very common	Delayed
Hypertrophic	Left sternal border and apex	Rare	Normal or decreased	Uncommon	Brisk
Supravalvular	Aortic area to neck	Rare	Normal or decreased	Uncommon	Rapid right; delayed left
Acquired					
Degenerative	Aortic area to neck and apex	Uncommon	Decreased	Common	Delayed
Rheumatic	Aortic area to neck and apex with mitral murmurs	Uncommon	Decreased	Very common	Delayed

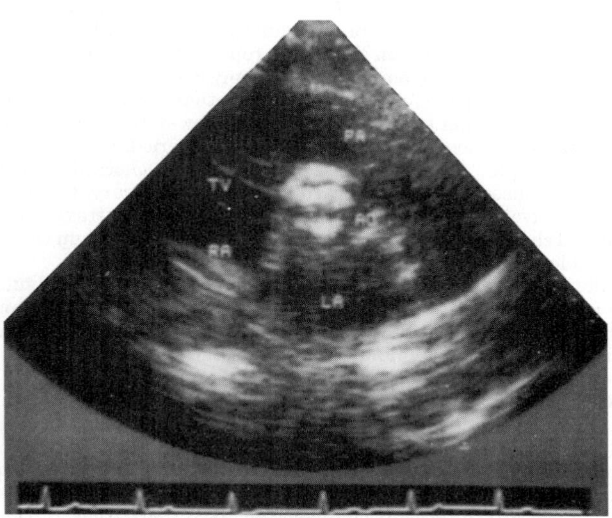

FIG. 24-1. Echocardiogram in calcific valvular aortic stenosis. Thickened immobile valve cusps are seen to fill the aortic valve area in the cross-sectional view in diastole. Systolic views failed to demonstrate significant opening. *AO,* aortic valve; *LA,* left atrium; *RA,* right atrium; *TV,* tricuspid valve.

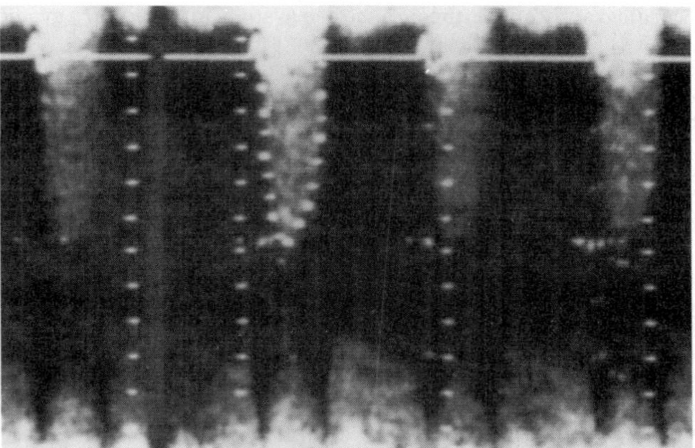

FIG. 24-2. Continuous-wave Doppler recording across the left ventricular outflow tract and aortic valve. The maximum velocity is almost 7 m per second, giving a peak gradient of 189 mm Hg and a mean gradient of 188 mm Hg. The mean gradient at catheterization was 100 mm Hg.

alone does not correlate well with surgical risk or postoperative morbidity; in fact, ejection fraction may improve dramatically after valvular replacement.

I. **Postoperative hypotension.** Numerous reports have described the coexistence of aortic stenosis and hypertrophic cardiomyopathy. The coexistence of these lesions is likely to come to attention in the patient who undergoes initially successful aortic valvular surgery but develops a low-output state, with or without pulmonary congestion, in the early postoperative period. Treatment of this potentially catastrophic situation is best dictated by the echocardiographic findings, including transesophageal echocardiography if necessary. Optimal treatment usually involves fluid administration, discontinuation of intravenous positive inotropic and chronotropic support, and administration of calcium channel blockers or beta-blockers.

J. **Percutaneous valvuloplasty.** Percutaneous balloon aortic valvuloplasty has been used to increase the orifice size of a stenotic aortic valve. This technique has been applied successfully in children and young patients to cure the stenosis or to improve hemodynamics enough to allow for valve replacement.

III. Hypertrophic cardiomyopathy

A. **Etiology.** Hypertrophic cardiomyopathy comprises a wide spectrum of structural abnormalities resulting in a variety of clinical syndromes. Marked degrees of hypertrophy may accompany hypertension and aortic stenosis (secondary hypertrophy); however, hypertrophic cardiomyopathy refers to a disorder whose structural features include marked left ventricular wall thickness, asymmetric hypertrophy of the interventricular septum, narrowed outflow tract, and systolic anterior motion of the mitral valve.

B. **Pathophysiology.** The left ventricle of patients with hypertrophic obstructive cardiomyopathy is found to be massively hypertrophied in an asymmetric fashion, with disordered histologic architecture. Most often, the interventricular septum is both disproportionately hypertrophied and hypokinetic. In some patients, the hypertrophied ventricle displays evidence of an apparent obstruction to outflow, denoted by associated systolic apposition of the mitral valve apparatus and the interventricular septum on M-mode or two-dimensional echocardiography or the appearance of a systolic intracavitary gradient in association with systolic anterior motion.

C. **History.** Most patients with hypertrophic cardiomyopathy have only mild symptoms. The diagnosis is often made in adulthood, with patients usually in their fourth or fifth decade of life. Clinical manifestations vary widely; many patients are asymptomatic, whereas the first presentation in some affected individuals may be sudden cardiac death. There appears to be a male preponderance.

Common symptoms include dyspnea, which is the result of abnormal diastolic filling, angina, and syncope. As in aortic stenosis, it is common for typical angina pectoris (and even myocardial infarction) to occur despite the presence of normal epicardial coronary arteries. Near syncope and syncope are also common symptoms and may indicate a predisposition to serious ventricular arrhythmias.

D. **Physical examination.** The apical impulse may be laterally displaced, and a presystolic impulse may be palpable. In hypertrophic cardiomyopathy with obstruction, the carotid pulse has a "bisfieriens" quality, characterized by an abrupt decline in midsystole.

The murmur of hypertrophic obstructive cardiomyopathy is usually best heard between the apex and the left sternal border and is usually made louder by the Valsalva maneuver and by standing. This murmur is therefore distinguished from all other outflow murmurs, which tend to decrease in intensity with these maneuvers.

E. **Laboratory studies**

1. **Electrocardiogram.** In hypertrophic cardiomyopathy, the asymmetric nature of the septal hypertrophy may cause deep Q waves in inferior and lateral leads, mimicking a prior infarction (Fig. 24-3).
2. **Chest radiograph.** Enlargement of the cardiac silhouette is seen in approximately one-half of patients with hypertrophic cardiomyopathy.

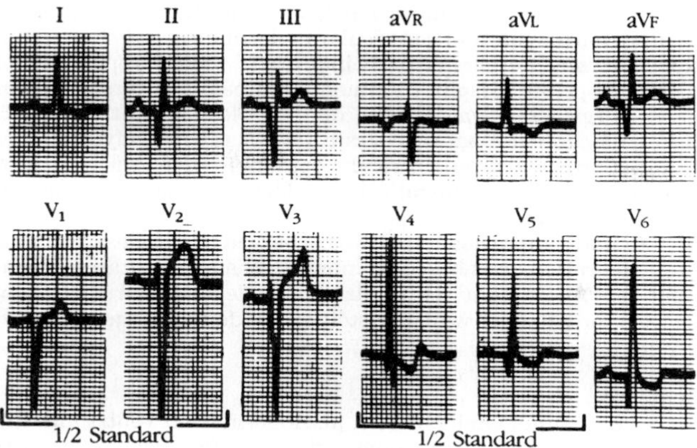

FIG. 24-3. Electrocardiogram of a patient with asymmetric septal hypertrophy. Q waves in leads II, III, aVF, V_5, and V_6. Precordial leads exhibit voltage criteria for left ventricular hypertrophy with ST-segment and T-wave abnormalities suggestive of strain. (From *Circulation* 1964;29 [Suppl IV]: 1, with permission.)

3. **Echocardiogram.** A universal echocardiographic feature of hypertrophic cardiomyopathy is marked left ventricular hypertrophy, which often predominantly involves the interventricular septum. The left ventricular cavity is diminished in both systole and diastole. Patients with systolic gradients have systolic anterior motion of the mitral valve apparatus, prolonged contact of the anterior mitral leaflet with the septum, and early closure of the aortic valve.
4. **Doppler echocardiogram.** Doppler echocardiography has also been successfully used to record the subaortic gradient of hypertrophic obstructive cardiomyopathy.

F. Cardiac catheterization. In nonvalvular obstructions, cardiac catheterization allows localization of the site of obstruction by recording, on careful retrograde pullback of the catheter, the pressure gradient either above or below the aortic valve. Hypertrophic obstructive cardiomyopathy is characterized by a variable gradient below the aortic valve. This gradient is dynamic in that it is markedly affected by physiologic or pharmacologic interventions. Any decrease in left ventricular size or increase in contractility raises the gradient.

G. Medical therapy. The medical treatment of hypertrophic cardiomyopathy is aimed at providing symptomatic relief and preventing sudden death. Diuretics may be used cautiously in patients with pulmonary congestion; *care must be taken not to reduce preload excessively.*

Beta-blockers have salutary effects for patients with hypertrophic cardiomyopathy and symptoms: they decrease both contractility and heart rate and therefore lessen myocardial oxygen demand. Calcium channel blockers may also have salutary effects on left ventricular diastolic function by relieving ischemia, lowering blood pressure, or reducing asynchrony of relaxation.

Nitrates have proved helpful in treating angina in patients with hypertrophic cardiomyopathy and coronary artery disease, but, as in valvular stenosis, these agents must be used with caution because of the potentially deleterious effects of preload reduction.

Patients with hypertrophic cardiomyopathy may experience incapacitating or life-threatening arrhythmias. Recurrent syncope and symptomatic palpitations require investigation into possible arrhythmias and may require antiarrhythmic therapy. Amiodarone appears to be efficacious in the treatment of both supraventricular and ventricular arrhythmias.

H. Surgical therapy. Surgery is rarely indicated for hypertrophic cardiomyopathy. If symptoms persist despite treatment with beta-blockers or calcium channel blockers, surgical removal of ventricular muscle may be attempted. Surgery for hypertrophic cardiomyopathy generally involves a septal myomectomy to remove a portion of proximal interventricular septum to widen the left ventricular outflow tract. Occasionally, mitral valve replacement may be performed to relieve mitral regurgitation.

Symptomatic improvement may be observed in response to a dual-chamber pacing. The rationale is based on knowing that preexcitation of the interventricular septum by right ventricular pacing leads to paradoxic septal motion away from the posterior wall in systole and widening of the left ventricular outflow tract.

Selected Readings

Aurigemma GP, Battista S, Orsinelli D, et al. Abnormal left ventricular intracavitary flow acceleration in patients undergoing aortic valve replacement for aortic stenosis: a marker for high post-operative morbidity and mortality. *Circulation* 1992;86:926.

Patients with aortic stenosis and increased ventricular wall thickness may exhibit features of outflow tract obstruction after valve replacement. Hemodynamic deterioration may accompany the use of inotropic agents.

Bonow RO, Udelson JE. LV diastolic dysfunction as a cause of congestive heart failure. *Ann Intern Med* 1992;117:502.

An important concept for hypertrophic states, including aortic stenosis, is left ventricular diastolic dysfunction and the steep pressure-volume relationship that can lead to congestive heart failure.

Dexter L, Harken DE, Cobb LA Jr, et al. Aortic stenosis. *Arch Intern Med* 1958;101:754.

The father of cardiovascular hemodynamics, Louis Dexter, describes the key physiologic features of aortic stenosis.

Maron BJ, Bonow RO, Cannon RO III, et al. Hypertrophic cardiomyopathy: interrelations of clinical manifestations, pathophysiology, and therapy. 1. *N Engl J Med* 1987;316:780.

A comprehensive review of hypertrophic cardiomyopathy including its clinical presentation, diagnosis, and management.

25. CRITICAL CARE OF PERICARDIAL DISEASE

David H. Spodick and Richard C. Becker

I. General principles. Pericardial diseases cover a wide etiopathogenetic spectrum, including every kind of medical and surgical disease. For practical purposes, there are three pericardial conditions to be considered: (a) acute pericarditis with or without pericardial effusion; (b) cardiac tamponade; and (c) constrictive pericarditis, including effusive-constrictive pericarditis.

II. Acute pericarditis. Acute pericarditis most often is a strictly inflammatory fibrinous lesion without clinically recognizable pericardial fluid.

A. Etiology. A burgeoning list of diseases, syndromes, and agents has been shown to produce pericarditis. The cause in any given case can be found in nine major categories (Table 25-1).

B. Symptoms. Acute pericarditis may be asymptomatic, but more often the patient has central chest pain, usually sharp with a pleuritic component but sometimes with only vague precordial distress. Precordial distress may closely mimic angina, including a predominant pressure sensation. The onset is frequently perceived as sudden, particularly when it interrupts sleep; the pain is frequently reduced by sitting up. It may radiate in an anginal distribution, remain precordial, or migrate to one side of the chest. A quasispecific feature is its frequent radiation to the trapezius ridge; pain may also be confined to one or both trapezius ridges. Patients describe breathing difficulty, but not true dyspnea. Odynophagia (pain on swallowing) occasionally occurs and can be the only symptom. Patients with myopericarditis may also have considerable skeletal muscle pain. Fever varies, depending on the cause. Anorexia and anxiety are common. Etiologic or associated diseases (e.g., acute myocardial infarction, tuberculosis, and rheumatic fever) may produce signs that can coexist or may even dominate the clinical tableau.

C. Signs. The pericardial rub (friction sound) is pathognomonic of pericarditis and remains common in pericardial effusions. Rubs are sometimes faint and nearly always wax and wane, even to the point of disappearing and reappearing within the same hour. A fully developed rub has three components, usually distinguishable by careful auscultation even at rapid heart rates: a ventricular systolic rub, preceded by an atrial rub, and followed by an early diastolic rub.

D. Laboratory studies. Except in the presence of significant accompanying myocarditis or other heart disease, true cardiomegaly does not occur with pure pericarditis. About 250 mL of pericardial fluid is needed to begin to enlarge the roentgenographic cardiac silhouette. The white blood cell count, sedimentation rate, and other acute-phase reactants vary according to the etiologic agent or primary illness.

Electrocardiographic (ECG) changes (Fig. 25-1) are of three types: typical, typical variants, and atypical (the last including no change). Of four potential ECG stages, an entirely typical stage I ECG is virtually diagnostic. Stage I produces concave ST-segment elevation in most ECG leads, particularly those of left ventricular epicardial deviation (i.e., mainly leads I, II, aVL, aVF, and V_3 to V_6). Lead aVR consistently shows ST-segment depression. V_1 usually shows ST-segment depression; less often it shows an isolectric ST segment, and occasionally it shows ST-segment elevation.

During the evolutionary phase (stage II), all ST junctions return to baseline more or less "in phase," with little change in T waves. The T waves progressively flatten and invert in all or most of the leads that showed ST-segment elevations. In stage III, T-wave inversions appear and are not distinguishable from those of diffuse myocardial injury, myocarditis, or biventricular injury. In stage IV, the T waves return to their prepericarditic condition. The entire ECG evolution occurs in a matter of days or weeks.

TABLE 25-1. Major etiologic categories of acute pericarditis and myopericarditis overlapping pathogenesis

1. Idiopathic pericarditis (syndrome)
2. Pericarditis due to living agents
3. Pericarditis in the vasculitis—connective tissue disease group
4. Immunopathic pericarditis; pericarditis in "hypersensitivity" states
5. Pericarditis in diseases of contiguous structures
6. Pericarditis in disorders of metabolism
7. Neoplastic pericarditis
8. Traumatic pericarditis
9. Pericarditis of uncertain origin or in association with syndromes of uncertain cause

E. Management. The treatment of clinically noneffusive pericarditis or pericarditis without overly compressing effusion is symptomatic (i.e., aimed at pain, malaise, and fever). The optimal treatment is to begin with ibuprofen (Motrin) 600 mg every 6 hours, which sometimes relieves pain within 15 minutes to 2 hours of the first dose. Should this approach fail, aspirin, up to 900 mg four times per day, may be given. In patients with myocardial infarction and peri-

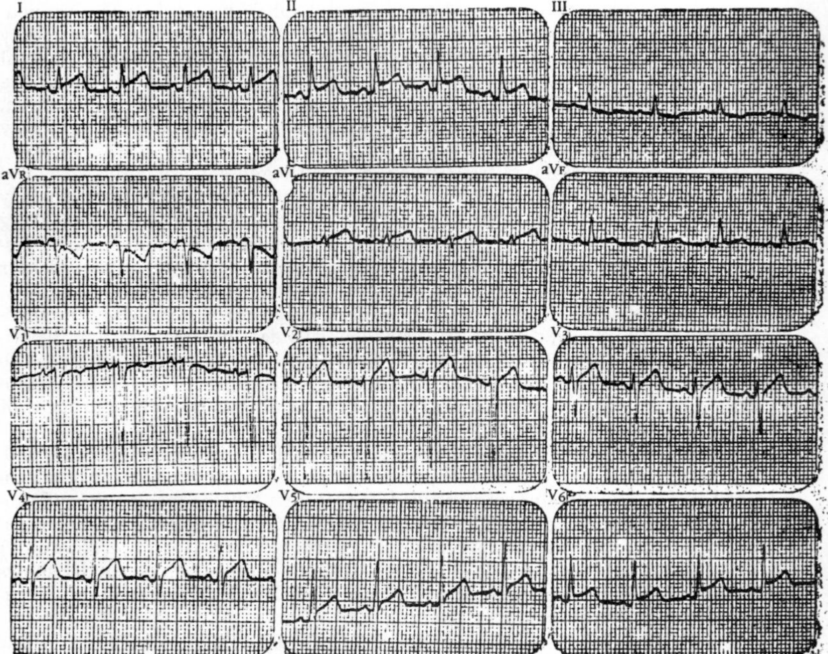

FIG. 25-1. Acute pericarditis. Typical stage I electrocardiogram showing J-ST elevations in most leads (I, II, aVL, aVF, and V_3 to V_6) and J-ST depressions in leads aVF and V_1. PR segments are depressed below the TP baseline in leads I, II, aVL, aVF, and V_3 to V_6. PR-segment depression is the earliest change, occurring sooner after onset of symptoms. ST (J) elevation follows.

carditis, indomethacin perhaps should not be used because of experimental work showing that it reduces coronary flow, increases experimental infarction size, and raises blood pressure.

Intractably symptomatic pericarditis occasionally calls for an alternative, even more drastic treatment, such as phenylbutazone over 2 or 3 days beginning with extremely small doses and with constant vigilance for side effects. Corticosteroid therapy may be employed at the lowest effective dose with appropriate tapering, but it should be avoided if at all possible because patients may become addicted, with consequent extreme difficulty in weaning.

III. Noncompressing (lax) pericardial effusion. Most cases of acute pericarditis *without* tamponade probably involve some excess fluid resulting from intrapericardial exudation, with those amounting to 250 mL or more becoming clinically obvious either on physical examination or (more likely) chest radiograph. Yet even large effusions may not clinically embarrass the heart as long as the rate of exudation is slow enough to permit the pericardium to stretch.

A. Clinical features. Noncompressing effusions may produce no clinical manifestations and may be the only sign of pericardial disease, so any symptoms or signs are those of pericarditis itself, either occurring with or preceding the effusion. If a systemic or extrapericardial disease is responsible for the pericarditis, signs and symptoms of that condition may dominate the picture. Extremely large, although noncompressing, effusions may produce precordial discomfort and symptoms resulting from pressure on adjacent structures, such as dyspnea (from reduced lung capacity), cough, hoarseness, dysphagia, and hiccups. Heart sounds may be reduced with massive effusions.

B. Laboratory studies. Radiography shows an increased cardiac silhouette and, in the absence of cardiac and pulmonary disease, clear lung fields and often left pleural effusion. The ECG may show low-voltage QRS complex and T waves (nearly always with normal P-wave voltage). Low voltage is nonspecific and not sensitive. Echocardiography at first reveals a small amount of fluid posteriorly at the left ventricular level in systole only (Table 25-2).

Swinging on alternate beats may produce electrical alternation, owing to repetitive change of the heart position with respect to the fixed positions of the ECG electrodes (more typical of tamponade).

IV. Cardiac tamponade. Cardiac tamponade is defined as hemodynamically significant cardiac compression resulting from accumulating pericardial contents that evoke and defeat compensatory mechanisms (Fig. 25-2). A wide range of severity of cardiac compression may be encountered. The pericardial contents may be effusion fluid, blood, pus, or gas (including air), singly or in combination, occasionally with underlying constrictive epicarditis. Tamponade must be considered in any patient with cardiogenic shock and systemic congestion.

A. Physiology. For significant cardiac compression, the pericardial contents must increase at a rate exceeding the rate of stretch of the parietal pericardium and, to some degree, the rate at which venous blood volume expands to maintain the small filling gradient to the right heart. Relentlessly increasing intrapericardial pressure progressively reduces ventricular volume, producing rising diastolic pressures that resist filling to the point that even a high ejection fraction cannot avert critical reduction of stroke volume at any heart rate.

B. Compensation. Beyond pericardial stretch, compensatory mechanisms for tamponade are mainly adrenergically mediated, including tachycardia, peripheral vasoconstriction, and maintained ejection fraction (in pure tamponade without heart disease, the ejection fraction is normal or increased).

C. Pulsus paradoxus. Excessive fluid in the pericardium increases the normal pericardial effect on ventricular interaction and exaggerates the normal inspiratory decrease in systemic blood pressure, thus leading to pulsus paradoxus. Although pulsus paradoxus is the hallmark of tamponade, at the bedside it must be borne in mind that pulsus is common to other disorders: obstructive lung disease (including severe asthma), pulmonary embolism, tense ascites, obesity, mitral stenosis with right heart failure, right ventricular infarction, and hypovolemic and cardiogenic shock.

TABLE 25-2. Echo Doppler in pericardial effusion and cardiac tamponade[a]

I. Pericardial effusion: M-mode and 2-D
  A. Echo-free space
    1. Posterior to LV (small to moderate effusions)
    2. Posterior and anterior (moderate to large effusions)
    3. Behind left atrium in some large to very large effusions
  B. Decreased movement of posterior pericardium-lung interface
  C. RV pulsations brisk (with anterior fluid)
  D. Aortic root movement abnormal or attenuated
  E. "Swinging heart" (large effusions)
    1. Periodicity 1:1 or 2:1 (rarely 3:1)
    2. RV and LV walls move synchronously
    3. Mitral-tricuspid pseudoprolapse (pansystolic at HR > 120 beats/min)
  F. 2-D only
    1. Loculated fluid
    2. Adhesions (fibrinous and fibrous)

II. Cardiac tamponade: M-mode and 2-D evidence of effusion plus
  A. Cardiac compression
    1. Decreased total transverse dimension (RV epicardium to LV epicardium at end diastole: may be apparent only after tap)
    2. RV diameters decreased (may be apparent only after tap), unless previous RV enlargement
    3. Early diastolic collapse of RV outflow tract with continued diastolic inward wall motion (≥ 50 msec after mitral D point)
  B. Inspiratory effects (with pulsus paradoxus)
    1. RV expands from greatly reduced expiratory end-diastolic size
    2. IV septum shifted to left
    3. LV compressed
    4. Mitral excursion-D/E amplitude and open valve area decreased
      a. E/F slope decreased or rounded
      b. Open time[b] decreased
    5. Aortic valve[b] opening decreased; premature closure
    6. Reduced increase in inferior vena cava diameter (<25%)
    7. Echocardiographic stroke volume decreased
    8. Decreased fractional shortening (short axis)
    9. Doppler: Right-sided transvalvular flows greatly exaggerated; left-sided flows greatly reduced (reversed during expiration)
  C. Notch in RV epicardium during isovolumic contraction (M-mode)
  D. Coarse oscillations of LV posterior wall (2-D echocardiography only)
  E. RA free wall indentation (buckling) during late diastole or isovolumic contraction
  F. RV indentation (buckling) during early diastole
  G. LA free wall indentation (cases with fluid behind LA)
  H. SVC and IVC dilation (unless volume depletion) and relatively fixed diameter during respiration
  I. Presystolic reflux or contrast media into IVC

[a] Sensitivities and specificities vary for each item.
[b] Often difficult to define during pericardial effusion; mitral valve may open with atrial systole only during inspiration.
HR, heart rate; IV, interventricular; IVC, inferior vena cava; LA, left atrium; LV, left ventricle; RA, right atrium; RV, right ventricle; SVC, superior vena cava; 2-D, two-dimensional.

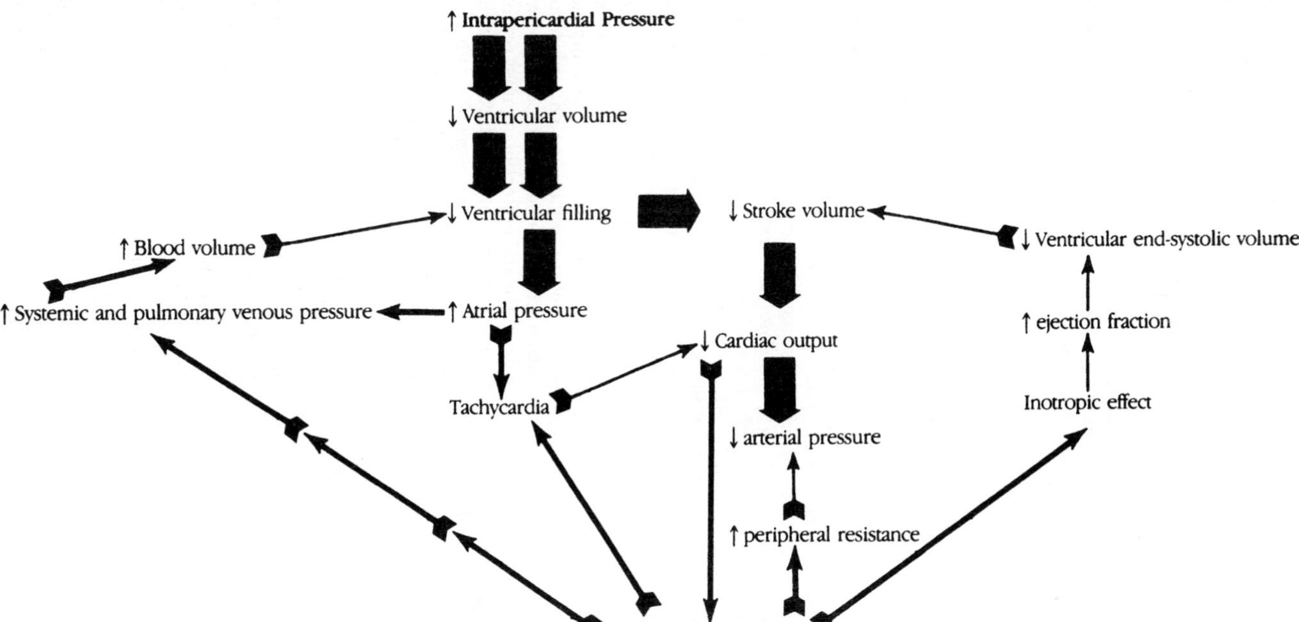

FIG. 25-2. Cardiac tamponade *(heavy arrows without tails)* and compensatroy mechanisms *(arrows with tail). Thin-tailed arrows* represent immediate mechanisms directed against tamponade changes; intermediate mechanisms are represented by *heavier tailed arrows.* For example, decreased ventricular filling resulting from decreased ventricular volume is immediately supported by increased blood volume. Development of the latter is stimulated by the intermediate mechanism, increased venous pressures (see text).

D. Clinical features. Tamponade may appear insidiously as the first sign of pericardial injury or intrapericardial bleeding, especially in conditions such as neoplasia, trauma, and connective tissue disorders. Commonly, however, it follows clinical acute pericarditis. The symptoms of tamponade are not specific, and patients may have symptoms and signs of an associated disease. Usually, these patients are dyspneic and progressively feel "sicker," and with advanced cardiac compression they have pallor, tachycardia, cyanosis, impaired cerebral function, sweating, and cold acral points. Most patients (clearly not all until late) are relatively or absolutely hypotensive.

In patients with rapid tamponade resulting from hemorrhage, as in wounds and cardiac or aortic rupture, the dominant picture is one of shock. If unchecked, this leads to electromechanical dissociation.

E. Physical examination. When tamponade results from inflammatory or neoplastic lesions, pericardial rubs frequently are present and can be loud, although the heart sounds themselves may be distant because of insulation by the surrounding fluid and feeble heart action. Heart sounds are usually better heard over the base of the heart, sometimes with relative accentuation of the pulmonic second sound (P_2). Neck veins are usually engorged, even with the patient sitting at 90 degrees, and sometimes there are prominent forehead, scalp, and retinal veins. If the venous level can be accurately discerned, the single negative systolic phase in midsystole (*x* trough) is a valuable finding that may be timed while listening to the heart sounds as one watches a rapid inward darting of the neck veins between S_1 and S_2.

Pulsus paradoxus occurs when respiratory changes alternatively favor right and left heart filling. *It is absent or minimal with any significant degree of constriction.* On the other hand, advanced left ventricular hypertrophy or severe left heart failure (i. e., greatly reduced ventricular chamber compliance) complicating tamponade may maintain pressures higher than right or opposite ventricular and pericardial pressures. Finally, severe tamponade with extreme hypotension may not show measurable respiratory changes.

F. Critical care. Removal of pericardial fluid as soon as possible by paracentesis or surgical drainage is the definitive treatment, indeed the only rational treatment. Surgical drainage is optimal, especially for either traumatic tamponade or tamponade from pericarditis caused by pyogenic organisms. Otherwise, needle aspiration can be used with the introduction of a pericardial catheter with minimal trauma to permit continued drainage and protection against refilling. The pericardium can be tapped from almost any reasonable place on the chest wall, and it is desirable to use two-dimensional echocardiography as a guide. The subxiphoiod approach is preferred for the usual blind pericardiocentesis.

V. Pericarditis versus myocardial infarction. Special consideration must be given to differentiating acute pericarditis, with or without effusion or tamponade, from both acute myocardial infarction and acute pericarditis in the setting of (and presumably resulting from) myocardial infarction. Because pericarditic pain may occasionally masquerade as ischemic pain, it sometimes becomes critical, particularly in older patients, to distinguish between the two (Table 25-3).

VI. Constrictive pericarditis. Constrictive pericarditis is seen less in its traditional chronic form and more often in subacute and acute forms, soon after a detectable bout of acute pericarditis with or without effusion. Today most cases are idiopathic or follow cardiopericardial surgery. The causes are essentially the same as for acute pericarditis (Table 25-1), although acute rheumatic fever with pericarditis, even when severe, does not produce constriction. Certain etiologic factors, however, are especially likely to lead to constriction, sometimes without evidence of antecedent acute pericarditis. These include tuberculosis, therapeutic irradiation of the chest, trauma, and a new form during uremia under dialysis.

Like tamponade, constriction severely limits ventricular filling, with equalization of left and right heart diastolic pressures. Systolic right ventricular pressure rises, but usually to less than 50 mm Hg, and the ratio of right ventricular end-diastolic pressure to systolic pressure is usually greater than 0.3. Respiratory changes in cardiac pressures are minimal, and jugular venous pressure increases

TABLE 25-3. Differential diagnosis of acute pericarditis

Finding	Acute Pericarditis	Acute Ischemia
Pain		
Onset	More often sudden	Usually gradual, crescendo
Main location	Substernal or left precordial	Same or confined to zones of radiation
Radiation	May be same as ischemic, also trapezius ridges	Shoulders, arms, neck back; not trapezius ridges
Quality	Usually sharp; stabbing, "background" ache	Usually "heavy" or "burning"
Inspiration	Worse	No effect unless with infarct in pericarditis
Duration	Persistent; may wax and wane	Usually intermittent
Electrocardiogram		
J-ST	Diffuse elevation usually concave, without reciprocal depressions	Localized deviation usually convex (with reciprocal infarction)
PR segment depressions	Frequent	Rarely
Abnormal Q waves	None unless with infarction	Common with infarction ("Q wave" infarcts)
T waves	Inverted after J points return to baseline	Inverted while ST still elevated (infarct)
Myocardial enzymes	Normal or elevated	Elevated (infarct)
Pericardial friction	Rub (most cases)	Rub only if with pericarditis
Abnormal S_3	Absent unless preexisting	May be present
Abnormal S_4	Absent unless preexisting	Nearly always present
S_4	Intact	Often dull, mushy after first day
Pulmonary congestion	Absent	May be present
Arrhythmia	None (in absence of heart disease)	Frequent
Conduction abnormalities (AV and IV)	None (in absence of heart disease)	Frequent

AV, atrioventricular; IV, interventricular.

during inspiration (Kussmaul's sign, also seen in right ventricular infarction, acute cor pulmonale, and tricuspid stenosis). Inspiratory decrease in arterial pressure in pure constriction is slight, nearly always less than 10 mm Hg.

Unlike in cardiac tamponade, the heart is not compressed in early diastole and relaxes normally or abruptly (rubber bulb effect) as filling proceeds until it reaches its pericardial limit. There is, therefore, a "square-root" configuration to the diastolic pressure (not seen in tamponade, particularly when measured by manometer tip catheters). Unlike the situation in tamponade, venous and atrial pressures show prominent *y* as well as *x* troughs. The *y* descent tends to be deeper and precipitous as it corresponds to the ventricular pressure dip when the atrioventricular valves are open (Fig. 25-3).

The clinical picture of constrictive pericarditis depends on the tempo of onset. Patients have mainly the following signs and symptoms of systemic congestion, usually with clear lung fields and a normal or slightly enlarged (rarely small) cardiac size: easy fatigability; dyspnea on exertion, usually without orthopnea; pedal edema, ascites, or both; hepatomegaly (and, in some chronic cases, splenomegaly); and, above all, distention of the neck veins in which the *x* and *y* descent both collapse, departing from a high standing level of pressure.

The echocardiographic diagnosis of constrictive pericarditis is not specific, although the echocardiogram may be helpful in conjunction with the clinical picture. Echocardiographic findings in constriction are summarized in Table 25-4.

A. Management. Medical management of constrictive pericarditis resembles that of congestive heart failure, because most signs and symptoms are related to systemic congestion. Digitalis therefore has been used, although its effect in the absence of complicating heart disease is uncertain. It is, however, useful in the presence of certain arrhythmias. Antiarrhythmic agents other than digitalis can also be used for particular arrhythmias; however, in the usual subacute or acute constriction, they are generally not needed (acute pericarditis, in the absence of heart disease, does not produce arrhythmias). Diuretics have long been a mainstay to relieve systemic congestion and its symptoms. The definitive treatment of constrictive pericarditis is always surgical removal of as much of the pericardium as possible.

B. Cardiac compression after cardiac surgery. The rapidly increasing number of patients undergoing cardiac surgery is producing significant increased in postsurgical cardiac compression from four major causes: bleeding, pericardial effusion, postpericardiotomy syndrome, and constrictive pericarditis.

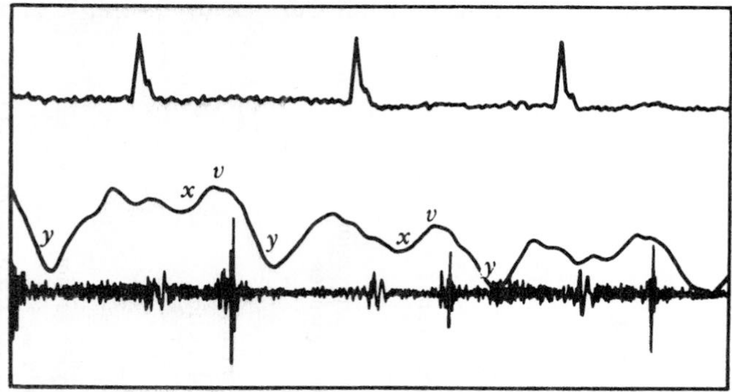

FIG. 25-3. Constrictive pericarditis. Jugular venous pulse tracing taken 2.5 months after successful coronary bypass surgery. The patient developed systemic congestion and distention of neck veins with prominent *x* and *y* descents. The *x* trough falls between the first and second heart sounds, and the *y* trough follows the second heart sound on the phonocardiogram.

TABLE 25-4. Echocardiography of pericardial scarring and constriction[a]

A. Pericardial thickening
  1. Condensed parietal pericardial echo
  2. Doubled parietal pericardial echo
B. Adhesions (fibrous or fibrinous)
  1. Adhesive strands seen (2-D) between LVPW and parietal pericardial echo (fluid present)
  2. Parietal pericardium moves with LVPW
    a. Without intervening space
    b. With intervening space = residual pericardial fluid ("halo sign")
C. Constrictive pericarditis
  1. Reduced ventricular size
  2. Atrial dilated
  3. Flat LVPW motion in mid- to late diastole
  4. Usually no posterior "depression" after atrial systole (post-P wave endocardial echo moves <1 mm posteriorly)
  5. Mitral E/F slope sharp
  6. Early atrioventricular valve closure
  7. IVS notchings: sharp posterior, men anterior motion (septal "flip-flop")
    a. During atrial systole
    b. During early diastole
  8. Inspiratory effects
    a. Interatrial and interventricular septa bulge to left
    b. Premature (pre-P wave) pulmonary valve opening (at very high RVDP)
    c. Marked inspiratory post-P wave deepening of pulmonary valve A wave
    d. Mitral and aortic Doppler flow velocities reduced from first inspiratory beat[b]
    e. Tricuspid and pulmonic transvascular velocities increased from first inspiratory beat[b]
D. 2-D only (most of A, B, and C on both M-mode and 2-D)
  1. Pericardium forms immobile single or double "shell"
  2. Ventricular expansion ends abruptly
  3. Atrioventricular valves hyperactive
  4. SVC, IVC, and hepatic veins dilated and lack normal inspiratory narrowing

[a] Most signs are relatively nonspecific.
[b] Distinguish constriction from restrictive cardiomyopathy.
IVC, inferior vena cava; IVS, interventricular septum; LVPW, left ventricular posterior wall; RVDP, right ventricular diastolic pressure; SVC, superior vena cava; 2-D, two-dimensional.

Selected Readings

Shabetai R, Fowler NO, Fenton JC, et al. Pulsus paradoxus. *J Clin Invest* 1965;44:1882.
The physiology of pulsus paradoxus, an important finding among patients with pericardial effusions with tamponade, is outlined in a landmark study.

Spodick DH. Acute pericardial disease: pericarditis, effusion, and tamponade. *JCE Cardiol* 1979;14:9.
A comprehensive review of pericardial diseases by the world's leading authority.

Spodick DH. Arrhythmias during acute pericarditis: a prospective study of one hundred consecutive cases. *JAMA* 1976;235:39.
Arrhythmias, mostly supraventricular in origin, can occur in patients with acute pericarditis.

Spodick DH. *The Pericarditis: a comprehensive textbook.* New York: Marcel Dekker, 1997.

26. SUDDEN CARDIAC DEATH

Charles I. Haffajee, G. Muqtada Chaudhry, and Richard C. Becker

I. General principles. Sudden cardiac death (SCD) occurs in approximately 400,000 patients per year in the United States and accounts for almost half of all cardiovascular mortality. SCD is generally defined as loss of consciousness resulting from a cardiac cause within 1 hour of the onset of symptoms in an individual with or without known preexisting heart disease. It does not spare any age, gender, or socioeconomic group and is much more common in patients with underlying coronary artery disease (CAD).

Each year, 1.5 million Americans experience myocardial infarction (MI), of which about 40% die. Of these patients, roughly two-thirds die before they reach a hospital or receive medical attention. Of the remaining one-third, about half die after reaching the hospital, and most of the remaining deaths occur in the first year after discharge.

Most advances in treatment and a better understanding of the mechanisms leading to SCD have resulted from monitoring during the process of cardiac arrest and evaluation of the survivors. Substudies have suggested that most patients die either of primary ventricular fibrillation (VF) (40%) or rapid ventricular tachycardia (VT) leading to VF (60%) (Table 26-1 and Fig. 26-1).

CAD is the major cause of SCD. Acute MI causes only about 20% of these deaths, and global ischemia (left main triple-vessel atherosclerotic CAD or coronary artery spasm) accounts for another 15% to 20%. The remaining 50% to 60% of SCDs appear to result from VT or VF, most often associated with prior MI. This is particularly true in patients with either left ventricular (LV) aneurysms or markedly lowered ejection fractions (EFs).

A smaller percentage of SCD is due to cardiac diseases other than CAD, such as cardiomyopathies (dilated, hypertrophic, infiltrative, and right ventricular dysplasia), primary electrical disease (primary VF, long QT syndrome, and Wolff-Parkinson-White syndrome), end-stage valvular heart disease, congenital heart disease, acute massive pulmonary embolism, high-risk behavior (cocaine use, bulimia, anorexia nervosa), and rupture or dissection of the aorta. Blunt impact to the chest, probably delivered at an electrically vulnerable phase of ventricular excitability, has been implicated in SCD during sports activities. Bradyarrhythmia leading to cardiac standstill occasionally causes SCD, more often in the setting of end-stage congestive heart failure (CHF).

II. Diagnosis of arrhythmias leading to sudden cardiac death. Arrhythmias observed in the immediate postresuscitation period are frequently different from those responsible for the VT/VF initiating death in SCD victims. After resuscitation, once hemodynamic stability has been achieved, only a few patients exhibit spontaneous arrhythmias that may have resulted in SCD.

The arrhythmias leading to SCD may be identified by extensive Holter monitoring or exercise testing or, more reliably, by electrophysiologic (EP) testing. Approximately 25% of patients resuscitated from SCD do not exhibit ambient significant arrhythmias during Holter monitoring or exercise testing even though their SCD resulted from VT/VF. On the other hand, EP testing using programmed electrical stimulation in these patients has a higher probability of exposing arrhythmia leading to SCD. Unfortunately, a significant percentage of patients can have polymorphic VT or VF as the only inducible arrhythmia during EP study, and this may be the only arrhythmia recorded during resuscitation.

About 30% to 40% of survivors of SCD may have no identifiable arrhythmia on the aforementioned tests, and additional diagnostic evaluation may not yield any significant underlying cardiac abnormality. Subtle abnormalities, such as long QT syndrome, may be sought in these patients, and that may involve repetitive monitoring or exercise testing.

TABLE 26-1. Cardiac causes of ventricular tachycardia and fibrillation in the absence of acute myocardial infarction

1. Prior myocardial infarction
2. Cardiomyopathies
   - Idiopathic dilated
   - Valvular heart disease
   - Hypertrophic myopathies
   - Arrhythmogenic right ventricular dysplasia
   - Congenital heart disease
   - Infiltrative disease (sarcoid, collagen, vascular, malignancy)
3. Electrical disorders
   - Long QT syndrome
   - Preexcitation syndromes (e.g., Wolff-Parkinson-White syndrome)
   - Conduction disorders
   - Primary idiopathic ventricular fibrillation

III. Management. Prevention rather than treatment has been the goal for the management of SCD. However, prevention can fail only once! Therefore, recent years have noticed increasing emphasis on treatment (i.e., implantable cardiovertor-defibrillators [ICDs]) of arrhythmic sudden death. However, because of the magnitude of the problem and the cost involved with this strategy, primary prevention of the conditions predisposing to SCD remains the cornerstone of management. Determining the most effective treatment for SCD prevention and identifying high-risk subgroups continue to pose a challenge (Table 26-2).

A. Primary prevention. Because CAD remains the most common condition associated with SCD, its prevention will have the most significant impact. CAD risk

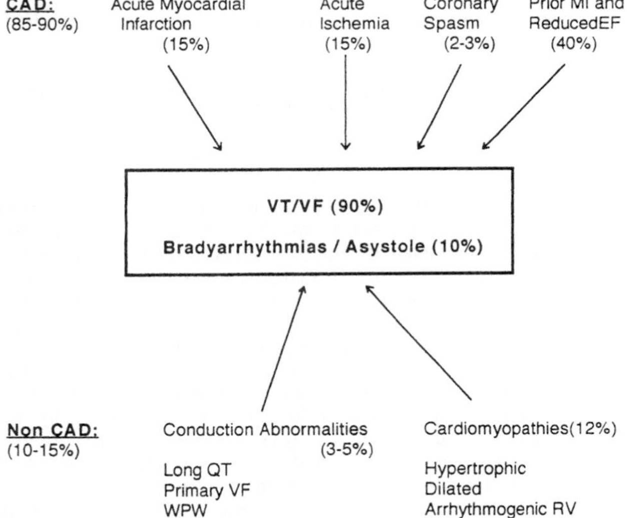

FIG. 26-1. Mechanisms of sudden cardiac death. *CAD,* coronary artery disease; *EF,* ejection fraction; *MI,* myocardial infarction; *RV,* right ventricle; *VF,* ventricular fibrillation; *VT,* ventricular tachycardia; *WPW,* Wolff-Parkinson-White syndrome.

TABLE 26-2. Approach to management of sudden cardiac death

- Primary prevention
  - Coronary risk factor modification
    - Management of hypertension, diabetes, hypercholesterolemia, smoking cessation, lifestyle modification
  - Treatment of at-risk patients
    - Aspirin and beta-blockers in patients after myocardial infarction, surgical or percutaneous revascularization, "prophylactic" ICD, or amiodarone in high-risk subsets
- Secondary prevention
  - SCD Survivor
  - ↓
  - Stabilize
    - Treat complications of resuscitation
    - Assess neurologic status
    - Extubate
  - ↓
  - Identify reversible causes
    - Acute myocardial infarction
    - Electrolyte imbalance
    - Drug-induced torsades des pointes
  - ↓
  - Define coronary anatomy and cardiac status
    - Echocardiography (LVEF, chamber size, valvular status)
    - Exercise/pharmacologic stress test with imaging modality
    - Cardiac catheterization
  - ↓
  - Define conduction abnormalities, tachyarrhythmias
    - Holter monitoring
    - Exercise testing
    - Signal averaged electrocardiogram
    - Electrophysiologic testing
  - ↓
  - Select therapy
    - Implantable cardiovertor defibrillator
    - Guided/empiric antiarrhythmic drug therapy
    - CABG ± implantable defibrillator

CABG, coronary artery bypass graft; ICD, implantable cardiovertor defibrillator; LVEF, left ventricular ejection fraction: SCD, sudden cardiac death.

factors have been recognized for years, but not until recently did conclusive cumulative evidence demonstrate the benefits of aggressive interventions. Management of hypertension is important, especially in patients with LV hypertrophy. Intensive diabetes control has also been shown to be vital in preventing cardiac events. Cholesterol-lowering therapy with hydroxymethylglutaryl coenzyme A (HMG-CoA) reductase inhibitors assumed increasing significance after the 4S and West of Scotland coronary prevention trials, which established the role of these agents in patients with and without prior CAD. Smoking cessation and lifestyle modification remain valuable aspects of CAD prevention. In relatives of patients with premature CAD, risk factors should be assessed and treadmill testing considered when they reach the age of 40 to 45 years.

Patients with known CAD and previous MI should be assessed for risk of SCD. Patients with multivessel disease and angina with reduced LVEF should be revascularized percutaneously or surgically (coronary artery bypass graft), because revascularization has been shown to decrease myocardial reinfarction and SCD. The role of aspirin is now established in prevention of recurrent cardiac events in patients who have had an MI. Numerous trials have shown the efficacy of beta-blockers in reducing mortality, primarily by reduction of SCD, after MI. Although the reduction of myocardial ischemia and cardiac sympathetic activation appears to be the basis of their cardioprotective effect, more recent animal data revealed that attenuation of stress-induced vagal withdrawal, which is probably mediated at the level of the central nervous system, is an important determinant in increasing the threshold of arrhythmia induction. This is of interest when noting that the long-term reduction of SCD has only been clearly shown with lipophilic (e.g., metoprolol, propranolol) and not with hydrophilic (e.g., atenolol, sotalol) beta-blockers.

The enthusiasm of assessing the efficacy of antiarrhythmic agents after MI has considerably waned in the post-Cardiac Arrhythmia Suppression Trial (CAST) era. The use of *d*-sotalol in the Survival With Oral *d*-Sotalol (SWORD) trial met with a similar fate in patients with LV dysfunction after MI. Amiodarone was evaluated in two recently completed studies. The European Myocardial Infarct Amiodarone Trial (EMIAT) enrolled survivors of MI with LVEF of at least 40%, and after a mean follow-up of 21 months failed to show any significant difference in total mortality compared with placebo. The Canadian Amiodarone Myocardial Infarction Arrhythmia Trial (CAMIAT) study evaluated post-MI patients with frequent or repetitive ventricular ectopy. There was no difference in all-cause mortality between those receiving amiodarone or placebo after a mean of 21 months. Although the routine use of amiodarone in such patients is not supported by these trials, the demonstration of lack of increased mortality in the treatment group and of a reduction in SCD fills the balance in favor of amiodarone in post-MI patients in whom antiarrhythmic therapy is indicated.

In post-MI patients in whom at least 3 weeks have passed since their most recent MI with nonsustained VT, LVEF less than or equal to 0.35, and inducible-nonsuppressible VT, the Multicenter Automatic Defibrillator Implantation Trial (MADIT) showed significant benefit with prophylactic ICD implant in contrast to conventional therapy.

Asymptomatic ventricular arrhythmias in patients with CHF are associated with increased incidence of SCD. Use of amiodarone was evaluated in such patients. In the Grupo de la Sobrevida en la Insuficiencia Cardiaca en Argentina (GESICA) trial, significant reduction in mortality was achieved in the treatment group among patients with CHF and nonsustained VT on Holter monitor. In the Congestive Heart Failure Survival Trial of Antiarrhythmic Therapy (CHF-STAT) study, patients with frequent repetitive ventricular ectopy did not show any difference in mortality with amiodarone; however, the trend was toward reduced mortality among those with nonischemic cardiomyopathy. Again, these trials attest to the safety of amiodarone in patients with CHF and make it the preferred agent when antiarrhythmic therapy is indicated.

High-risk patients with hypertrophic cardiomyopathy should be considered for prophylactic amiodarone therapy. Beta-blockers are recommended for patients with congenital long QT syndrome, and those at high risk may benefit from left cardiac sympathetic denervation. Nearly one-third of patients who die suddenly of an anomalous origin of the left coronary artery had prior exertional syncope or angina. Identification of such high-risk individuals and surgical correction of their anomaly are imperative. The aforementioned disorders are frequently encountered in young persons. It is important to counsel them to avoid participation in competitive sports until the disorder is corrected.

B. Secondary prevention. Patients who have experienced a life-threatening arrhythmia or who have been resuscitated from arrhythmic SCD should be considered for aggressive individualized therapy for the prevention of SCD recurrence. If VT/VF occurred in these patients in the setting of a reversible factor, such as electrolyte imbalance, drug-induced torsades de pointes, or global ischemia, corrective steps should be taken to prevent their recurrence.

Resuscitated victims of SCD in whom VT/VF occurred in the absence of a reversible factor or acute MI should be stabilized. Once neurologic status returns to baseline, cardiac catheterization and EP evaluation should be considered (Fig. 26-2).

1. Sudden cardiac death survivor

↓

2. Stabilize
   —Treat complications of resuscitation
   —Assess neurological status
   —Extubate

↓

3. Identify reversible causes
   —Acute myocardial infarction
   —Hypokalemia
   —Drug-induced torsades de pointes

↓

4. Define cardiac status and anatomy
   —Exercise/persantine thallium scan
   —Echocardiography (LVEF, valvular status, four chamber size)
   —Nuclear (MUGA) scan
   —Cardiac catheterization

↓

5. Define VT/VF; conduction abnormalities
   —EP study
   —Holter
   —Exercise testing

↓

6. Select therapy
   —Implantable defibrillator
   —CABG ± defibrillator
   —Empiric amiodarone
   —Possibly sotalol

FIG. 26-2. Management of patients with sudden cardiac death.

Cardiac catheterization allows assessment of the extent of CAD and the degree of LV dysfunction. Revascularization should be performed, if indicated, not only to eliminate ischemia as a trigger for future events but also to improve LV function in patients with possible hibernating myocardium. EP studies should be performed after normalization of electrolytes and elimination of all antiarrhythmic agents.

Antiarrhythmic therapy alone, whether empiric or EP guided, has not been unequivocally shown to prevent recurrent arrhythmic events. Because of the inherent lethal nature of arrhythmia recurrence, the increasing emphasis is on treating these arrhythmias with ICD, especially in high-risk subgroups. Adjuvant antiarrhythmic drug therapy after the implantation of ICD is also an option for patients who have frequent recurrences and whose arrhythmia can either be prevented or modified by such agents.

Several uncontrolled, nonrandomized studies appear to demonstrate that the ICD can decrease the recurrence of sudden cardiac death to 1% or less per year. However, in follow-up studies of patients who have received the ICD, the total mortality in 3 to 5 years after ICD implantation remains high (20% to 35%) and may be more dependent on LV dysfunction or CAD.

An organized approach should be made for the management of survivors of SCD. Individualized therapy has been shown to decrease the recurrence of death from 30% per year to less than 10% per year. In particular, use of the ICD for survivors of arrhythmic SCD appears to reduce the incidence of recurrent sudden death to 1% to 2% per year.

More problematic is the appropriate preventive therapy for survivors of SCD who have CAD and LV dysfunction and no inducible arrhythmias by programmed ventricular stimulation, exercise testing, or prolonged Holter monitoring and for patients with other types of structural heart disease and no inducible or documented arrhythmias. The incidence of recurrent arrhythmic sudden death appears to be high in these patients. Unless some obvious, correctable, reversible factor for SCD can be identified in these patients, ICD implantation is recommended.

Selected Readings

Cairns JA, Connolly SJ, Roberts R, et al for the Canadian Amiodarone Myocardial Infarction Arrhythmia Trial Investigators. Randomised trial of outcome after myocardial infarction in patients with frequent or repetitive ventricular premature depolarisations: CAMIAT. *Lancet* 1997;349:675.

The importance of amiodarone as a pharmacologic means to prevent postinfarction arrhythmic death was highlighted in the CAMIAT study.

Cardiac Arrhythmia Suppression Trial (CAST) Investigators. Preliminary report: effect of encanide and flecainide on mortality in a randomized trial of arrhythmia suppression after myocardial infarction. *N Engl J Med* 1989;321:406.

The CAST trial provided a vital understanding of the association between antiarrhythmic agents and their potential "proarrhythmic" properties in selected patients.

Greene HL. Sudden arrhythmic cardiac death: mechanisms, resuscitation and classification. The Seattle perspective. *Am J Cardiol* 1990;65:4B.

A comprehensive review of the mechanisms, epidemiology, and outcomes among patients with sudden arrhythmic cardiac death.

Moss AJ, Hall J, Cannon DS, et al for the Multicenter Automatic Defibrillator Implantation Trial Investigators. Improved survival with an implanted defibrillator in patients with coronary disease at high risk for ventricular arrhythmia. *N Engl J Med* 1996;335:1933.

The MADIT Study was among the first to identify the benefit of cardioverter-defibrillator implantation in patients at risk of sudden cardiac death.

27. DISSECTION OF THE AORTA

Linda A. Pape and Richard C. Becker

I. General principles. Aortic dissection occurs when a hematoma develops within the wall of the aorta and advances, sometimes along the entire length of the aorta. The clinical presentation is varied, and the condition is life-threatening. The hematoma may rupture into the pericardial sac or the pleural space, thus causing cardiac tamponade or massive hemothorax. It often disrupts the aortic valve and causes acute aortic insufficiency and left ventricular failure. Compromise of branch vessels may lead to stroke or limb ischemia.

Over the past 20 years, faster and more accurate diagnosis, advances in surgical technique, and more rapidly instituted medical and surgical treatment have transformed aortic dissection from an almost uniformly fatal process to one with a 5-year survival rate of up to 75%.

II. Etiology

A. Anatomy. The thoracic aorta includes the aortic valve and sinuses of Valsalva, from which originate the coronary arteries, the ascending aorta, the aortic arch, and the descending aorta. Two-thirds of all dissections originate in the ascending aorta, the 5-cm segment above the aortic valve.

B. Histology. Aortic dissection appears to begin when an intimal tear permits blood to enter the aortic media and to advance along a plane within the outer third of the aortic wall. The transversely oriented intimal tear most commonly occurs in the proximal ascending aorta (61%). The next most common sites are the proximal descending aorta between the origin of the left subclavian artery and the ligamentum arteriosum (16%), the remainder of the descending aorta (10%), the aortic arch (9%), and the abdominal aorta (3%).

The cause of the break in the intima that allows dissection to occur is unknown. Atherosclerosis does not seem to be an etiologic factor; intimal tears were found to originate in an atherosclerotic plaque in only 5% of cases in two series. Because penetrating atherosclerotic ulcers of the aorta may lead to localized hematoma formation and aortic rupture, clinical distinction from typical aortic dissection may be difficult.

The histologic finding of cystic medionecrosis is associated with defects in elastic tissue and collagen organization, and the term has become almost synonymous with Marfan syndrome.

C. Etiologic factors. Hypertension is by far the most important disease associated with the development of aortic dissection. After hypertension, congenitally malformed aortic valves are the most common factor predisposing to aortic dissection. Other conditions associated with aortic dissection include Marfan syndrome, Ehlers-Danlos syndrome, coarctation of the aorta, Turner syndrome, relapsing polychondritis, pregnancy (usually in the third trimester), giant cell aortitis, syphilitic aoritis, and cocaine use. Iatrogenic causes include cardiac catheterization, femoral artery insertion of an intraaortic balloon catheter, and balloon angioplasty of aortic coarctation. Cardiovascular surgery is a rare cause of acute aortic dissection (Table 27-1).

III. Classification. The original classification of DeBakey divides aortic dissection into three types. Type I dissection begins in the ascending aorta and extends distally to the arch and descending aorta. Type II dissection begins in and is limited to the ascending aorta. Type II is more likely in patients with the Marfan syndrome. Type III begins in and is limited to the descending aorta. Recognizing the distinct difference in clinical course and prognosis, Daily and associates in 1970 divided dissection patients into two groups: those with involvement of the ascending aorta (type A) and those in whom the dissection was limited to the descending aorta (type B).

TABLE 27-1. Causes and associations of aortic dissection

1. Hypertension
2. Congenital aortic valve disease
   - Bicuspid
   - Unicuspid
3. Coarctation of aorta
4. Marfan syndrome
5. Ehlers-Danlos syndrome
6. Turner syndrome
7. Relapsing polychondritis
8. Pregnancy
9. Giant cell arteritis
10. Syphilitic aortitis
11. Cocaine use
12. Iatrogenic
    - Cardiac catheterization
    - Intraaortic balloon insertion
    - Cardiac surgery

IV. Pathophysiology. Most intimal tears occur in those portions of the aorta that seem to be subject to the greatest mechanical stress: the ascending aorta immediately above the aortic valve and the proximal descending aorta just beyond the origin of the left subclavian artery. As blood enters the intima and media, it usually tracks along in a plane between the inner two-thirds and outer one-third of the media, creating a double-lumened aorta. There is often more than one communication between true and false lumina.

The most important factors influencing the progression of aortic dissection, aside from the tissue characteristics of the aorta itself, are left ventricular contracility, aortic compliance, and stroke volume. *Left ventricular contractility determines the rate of rise of the aortic pressure pulse and is thought to be the most important single factor.*

The consequences of aortic dissection may be divided into three main groups: arterial compromise, aortic insufficiency, and external rupture.

External rupture constitutes the most frequent cause of death. External rupture through the thoracic aortic adventitia most frequently causes hemorrhage into the pericardium or left pleural space. Dissection of the descending thoracic aorta and abdominal aorta (the latter is rare) may also rupture into the retroperitoneum (Table 27-2).

V. Diagnosis

A. History. The predominant symptom in patients with acute aortic dissection is the abrupt onset of severe chest pain often described as "ripping" or "tearing." Anterior chest pain is most common, radiating to the interscapular region of the back. If pain is limited to the anterior chest, ascending aortic dissection is

TABLE 27-2. Site of external rupture in relation to site of intimal tear

Site	Ascending Aortic (%) ($n = 227$)	Aortic Arch (%) ($n = 37$)	Descending Aorta (%) ($n = 97$)
Pericardium	70	35	12
Left pleural space	6	32	44
Mediastinum	6	8	15
Esophagus	—	8	1

n, number of patients studied.

more likely. The same is true for pain in the neck, throat, or jaw. If pain is limited to the back, the dissection is more likely due to dissection of the descending aorta; however, pain in both the anterior chest and back is common enough in either type of dissection that pain location alone, although suggestive, is not specific to the site of dissection.

Other presenting symptoms include the following: syncope, usually resulting from cardiac tamponade; congestive heart failure, resulting from acute aortic insufficiency; stroke or limb ischemia, caused by arterial compression; abdominal pain; restlessness; acute myocardial infarction, resulting from involvement of a coronary artery; fever; anterior spinal artery ischemia with motor and sensory deficits; disseminated intravascular coagulation; renal failure; and renovascular hypertension.

B. Physical examination. Hypertension (systolic blood pressure higher than 160 mm Hg) is present in more than half of patients who present with dissection of the descending aorta (Table 27-3). Primarily because of the complication of cardiac tamponade, 20% to 25% of patients with acute ascending aortic dissection present with hypotension (systolic blood pressure higher than 100 mm Hg).

Absent or markedly diminished arterial pulses are the hallmark of ascending aortic dissection. Only 10% to 15% of patients with descending aortic dissection have demonstrable pulse deficits at the time of presentation. In most cases, the pulse deficit is asymptomatic, although stroke, limb ischemia, and neurologic syndromes of spinal artery involvement may be seen. *Pulses must be routinely carefully examined in all patients with suspected myocardial infarction, and the presence of a pulse deficit should alert the physician to the possible presence of aortic dissection.*

Aortic regurgitation is found in the majority of patients with ascending aortic dissection. If acute severe aortic regurgitation results in left ventricular failure, the wide pulse pressure typically associated with aortic regurgitation will *not* be present.

Cardiac tamponade from rupture of ascending aortic dissection into the pericardial sac causes syncope and hypotension. Distended neck veins, elevated central venous pressure, tachycardia, pulsus paradoxus, and hypotension are typical features of tamponade. External rupture of descending aortic dissection may occur into the left pleural space and may cause dullness to percussion at the left base. Neurologic deficits may be due to carotid compromise resulting in hemiplegia or to spinal artery occlusion leading to paraplegia. In major limb ischemia, loss of deep tendon reflexes, anesthesia, and paralysis may result.

C. Laboratory findings. Tables 27-4 and 27-5 list the typical laboratory findings in aortic dissection.

TABLE 27-3. Physical findings in aortic dissection

Finding	Ascending	Descending
Hypertension	+	++
Absent or changing pulses	++	±
Aortic regurgitation murmur	++	±
Left ventricular failure	+	±
Stroke	+	–
Shock	++	±
Elevated central venous pressure with pulsus paradoxus	++	±
Dullness at left lung base	–	+
Pericardial friction rub	±	–
Arterial compromise	++	±

++, often present; +, occasionally present; ±, rarely present; –, not present.

TABLE 27-4. Laboratory findings in acute aortic dissection

A. Electrocardiogram
  1. Nonspecific
    a. LVH
    b. ST-T abnormalities
  2. Absence of ST elevations (usual)
  3. If coronary ostium involved, MI or ischemia may be seen
B. Chest radiograph
  1. Widened superior mediastinum
  2. Haziness or enlargement of aortic knob
  3. Irregular aortic contour
  4. Double density of descending aorta
  5. Separation (>5 mm) of intimal calcium from outer aortic contour
  6. Rightward displacement of trachea
  7. Enlargement of cardiac silhouette from pericardial effusion
  8. Left pleural effusion

LVH, left ventricular hypertrophy; MI, myocardial infarction.

1. **Electrocardiography.** No electrocardiographic findings are specific to aortic dissection. Left ventricular hypertrophy with pressure overload resulting from hypertension or left ventricular diastolic overload from prior chronic aortic regurgitation may be present. With cardiac tamponade, electrical alternans may be seen. In the case of dissection involving a coronary artery, typical electrocardiographic changes of ischemia or infarction are present.
2. **Chest radiography.** The most common finding on plain chest radiography, seen in more than 80% of patients with aortic dissection, is widening of the superior mediastinum resulting from the increased diameter of the aorta (Fig. 27-1).

   Enlargement or haziness of the aorta knob, irregularity of the aortic shadow, and double density of the descending aorta are seen. A less common but nearly diagnostic finding is the separation of intimal calcification from the outer contour of the descending aorta by more than 5 mm (calcium sign). Dilation of the aorta with intimal calcification less than 5 mm from the outer contour is more suggestive of atherosclerotic aneurysmal dilation of the aorta. Other chest radiographic findings include rightward displacement of the trachea, enlargement of cardiac silhouette by hemopericardium, and left pleural effusion.

TABLE 27-5. Laboratory findings in acute aortic dissection

	Echo/ Doppler TEE	Angiography	Contrast CT	MRI
Anatomic findings				
Two lumens	+	+	+	+
Intimal flap	+	+	+	+
Intramural hematoma	+	–	+	+
Aortic valve involvement	+	+	–	+
Pericardial effusion	+	–	+	+
Physiologic findings				
Site (flow through) intimal tear	+	+cine	–	+cine
Aortic insufficiency	+	+	–	+cine

CT, computed tomography; MRI, magnetic resonance imaging; +, present; –, not present; TEE, transesophageal echocardiography.

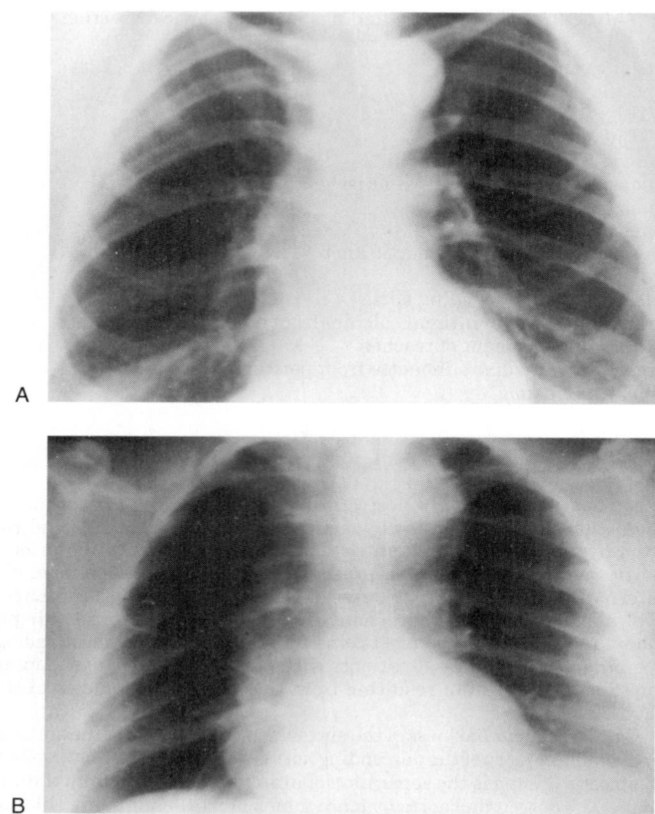

FIG. 27-1. Chest radiographs taken in a 57-year-old woman. When a radiograph taken 3 years previously **(A)** is compared with that taken at presentation with acute dissection of the ascending aorta **(B),** widening of the mediastinum is noted.

3. **Echocardiography.** Multiplane transesophageal echocardiography (TEE) represents a major advance in diagnosing aortic dissection by allowing visualization of the ascending aorta, aortic arch, and descending aorta. After a screening transthoracic echocardiogram to assess the proximal ascending aorta, the presence of wall motion abnormalities, pericardial effusion, and aortic insufficiency, a TEE can be performed rapidly in the emergency room or at the patient's bedside. With TEE, one can demonstrate the intimal flap, false lumen, and the communications between lumina and intramural hematomas, as well as the mechanism for aortic regurgitation and more complex anatomy.
4. **Intravascular ultrasound.** Initial reports of intravascular ultrasound suggest that it, too, can accurately diagnose aortic dissection and may have greater sensitivity than TEE in certain cases.
5. **Computed tomography.** The computed tomographic findings in aortic dissection include identification of two lumina, detection of an intimal flap, compression of the true due to clotted blood in the false lumen, pleural, or pericardial fluid, quantification of lumen diameter, and displacement of intimal calcium. Differentiation from an atherosclerotic aneurysm is not always

possible, especially if the false lumen is thrombosed. Contrast enhancement has resulted in improved diagnostic accuracy.

6. **Magnetic resonance imaging.** Magnetic resonance imaging provides superb anatomic detail of the aorta, intimal tear, and false channel. Sensitivity and specificity are as high as 98%.
7. **Angiography.** Aortography has historically been the definitive diagnostic procedure in the evaluation of suspected aortic dissection. Angiographic diagnosis depends on demonstration of both true and false lumina within the aorta. Deformity of the true lumen by the false lumen is also seen in nearly all cases and may be the only angiographic finding suggestive of dissection when the false lumen is not opacified. Visualization of the intimal flap, aortic valvular incompetence, and involvement of aortic major branches as well as the coronary arteries may likewise be demonstrated. Additional injections and use of biplane technique increase the likelihood of demonstrating the intimal tear. Ulcerlike projections of contrast from the lumen help to identify penetrating atherosclerotic ulcers, which may have a clinical presentation similar to that of aortic dissection.

D. Comparison of imaging techniques. The right diagnostic strategy for suspected aortic dissection depends on the availability of imaging techniques and experienced personnel at each institution. Although the sensitivity and specificity of magnetic resonance imaging may be slightly superior, TEE is rapidly becoming the diagnostic test of choice because it is extremely accurate and can be performed more readily in the emergency setting.

VI. Treatment. In few medical conditions is survival as dependent on rapid diagnosis and institution of treatment as in acute aortic dissection. Untreated, acute dissection has an extremely rapid, usually fatal clinical course.

One of the main goals in surgical treatment of ascending aortic dissection is to repair or replace the ascending aorta. Aortic valve resuspension or reconstruction is preferred to replacement, except in cases of Marfan syndrome or aortic root dilatation in which composite grafts should be used. The operative mortality rate for acute ascending dissection is approximately 25%.

With medical therapy, the short-term survival rate for acute dissection of the descending aorta is reported to be as high as 80%; however, as many as 30% to 50% of patients have progression of dissection despite intensive drug therapy and require either emergency or elective surgery. Definite indications for surgical treatment include failure to control pain, progressive dissection, expansion, and rupture or arterial compromise (Table 27-6). Patients with failed medical treatment of acute descending aortic dissection have a predicted surgical mortality of 75%.

TABLE 27-6. Indications for surgery

1. Ascending aorta involvement
2. Contraindications to myocardial depressants
   a. Aortic insufficiency
   b. Left ventricular failure
3. External rupture
   a. Hemopericardium
   b. Hemothorax
   c. Other
4. Arterial compromise
   a. Limb ischemia
   b. Renal failure
   c. Cerebral ischemia or infarction
5. Progression
   a. Continued pain
   b. Expansion of dissecting hematoma as seen on chest radiograph, computed tomography, or magnetic resonance imaging

TABLE 27-7. Initial medical therapy for acute aortic dissection

Drug	Dosage
One of	
Propranolol hydrochloride	0.5 mg i.v. test dose; 1.0 mg q5 min until HR <60/min; repeat as need q2–3h
Esmolol	0.5 mg/kg i.v. for 1 min followed by 50 μg/kg/min for 4 min; titrate upward by repeat of same loading dose with 50 μg/kg/min incremental increases in maintenance dose
Labetalol	0.20 mg i.v. over 2 min; 40–80 mg q10 min up to 300 mg; continuous infusion 2 mg/min according to BP
In combination with	
Sodium nitroprusside	25 μg/min i.v.; titrate by 25 μg/min increments q3–5 min to achieve systolic BP 100–120 mm Hg (Caution: urine output and mental status must be monitored)

BP, blood pressure; HR, heart rate.

In all patients except those who are hypotensive, initial management of acute aortic dissection is directed at lowering both myocardial contractility and systemic arterial pressure, the two factors most important in the progression of dissection. Intensive medical treatment should be instituted as soon as the clinical diagnosis of acute dissection is made and should not be delayed for definitive testing (Table 27-7). Vasodilators should always be used in combination with beta-blockers.

Patients who present with hypotension are likely to have hemopericardium with tamponade or rupture into the left pleural space. In these patients, intravenous volume should be expanded with saline, colloid, or lactated Ringer's solution. The presence of cardiac tamponade indicates the need for emergency surgery.

The goals of medical therapy are to stop the spread of the intramural hematoma and to prevent rupture. Control of pain is one of the best indications that these goals have been attained. Continued pain may suggest progressive dissection. Other indications of ongoing dissection and failure of medical therapy are increasing mediastinal dimension on chest radiograph, loss of a pulse, development of a stroke, renal failure, aortic insufficiency, and congestive heart failure.

Selected Readings

DeBakey ME, Henly WS, Cooley DA, et al. Surgical management of dissecting aneurysms of the aorta. *J Thorac Cardiovasc Surg* 1965;49:130.

The surgical approach to aortic dissection was pioneered by DeBakey and Cooley.

Goldstein SA, Mintz GS, Lindsay J, et al. Aorta: comprehensive evaluation by echocardiography and transesophageal echocardiography. *J Am Soc Echocardiogr* 1993; 6:634.

TEE has become a mainstay in the diagnosis of aortic dissection and, at many institutions, is the diagnostic modality of choice.

McCloy RM, Spittell JA Jr, McGoon DC. The prognosis in aortic dissection (dissecting aortic hematoma or aneurysm). *Circulation* 1965;31:665.

Aortic dissection has been recognized as a vascular emergency for decades with considerable morbidity and mortality if the diagnosis is not made promptly, followed by appropriate treatment.

Spittell PC, Spittell JA, Joyce JW, et al. Clincal features and differential diagnosis of aortic dissection experience with 236 cases (1980 through 1990). *Mayo Clin Proc* 1993;68:642.

The Mayo experience as elegantly outlined by Spittell provides a comprehensive review for clinicians.

28. ACUTE AORTIC INSUFFICIENCY

Joseph S. Alpert, Joseph R. Benotti, and Richard C. Becker

I. General principles. Aortic insufficiency (AI) manifests itself in a variety of ways (Fig. 28-1). At one end of the spectrum are patients with chronic hemodynamically significant AI who may be asymptomatic, with only a heart murmur or evidence of progressive cardiac enlargement. At the opposite end of the spectrum are patients who present with acute, severe AI and cardiogenic shock resulting from acute destruction or disruption of a previously normal aortic valve.

II. Definition and etiology. Acute, severe AI is defined as hemodynamically significant AI of sudden onset, occurring across a previously competent aortic valve into a left ventricle not previously subjected to volume overload. The causes of acute AI are summarized in Table 28-1.

A. Infective endocarditis. Acute bacterial endocarditis is commonly the result of *Staphylococcus aureus.* This organism often produces necrosis and perforation or detachment of one or more aortic valve leaflets. An annular abscess may distort the annulus and may cause one or more aortic commissures to fail to coapt or to prolapse into the left ventricular outflow tract during diastole. One or more large valvular vegetations may prevent proper diastolic coaptation of the aortic valve commissures. Although present on occasion in staphylococcal endocarditis, such bulky vegetations are more characteristic of fungal endocarditis caused by *Aspergillus, Candida albicans, Histoplasma capsulatum,* or other such species.

Acute endocarditis with an organism of sufficient virulence to cause valve destruction or perforation can infect a previously normal valve. Although common in narcotic addicts as a result of intravenous injections, acute endocarditis may also occur secondary to abscess formation complicating subcutaneous drug use (skin popping). More commonly, infection involves an anatomically bicuspid aortic valve.

Annular abscess, nearly always associated with hemodynamically severe AI, may result in gradual or sudden onset of first- or second-degree atrioventricular block, left bundle branch block, or complete heart block secondary to inflammation and necrosis of the atrioventricular node and proximal His-Purkinje region of the conduction system. Infection may erode into the pericardium, resulting in purulent pericarditis, hemopericardium, and cardiac tamponade. Annular abscess extending into the membranous intraventricular septum may cause septal rupture and a left-to-right shunt. Extension of infection into the muscular septum can cause ventricular irritability in conjunction with a variety of infranodal heart block patterns. Infection may extend from the aortic valve and annulus into the contiguous right ventricle or anterolaterally situated right atrium, resulting in the development of an aortic–right ventricular or right atrial fistula. These complications are associated with the development of a continuous murmur (related to the substantial left-to-right shunt) and severe congestive heart failure. Superior extension of infection can cause a mycotic aneurysm involving the sinus of Valsalva or proximal ascending aorta. The development of any of these complications in the setting of acute endocarditis mandates urgent aortic valve replacement.

B. Dissection. Dissection of the ascending aorta with medial hematoma may involve the aortic valve. The hematoma can displace the attachments of the aortic valve cusps downward and medially, such that one or more cusps prolapse or evert into the outflow tract of the left ventricle during diastole, thereby leading to incompetence of the valve. AI occurs in approximately 65% of patients with dissection of the ascending aorta.

C. Connective tissue diseases. There are reports of acute, severe AI complicating systemic lupus erythematosus. Aortitis, with inflammation and furling of

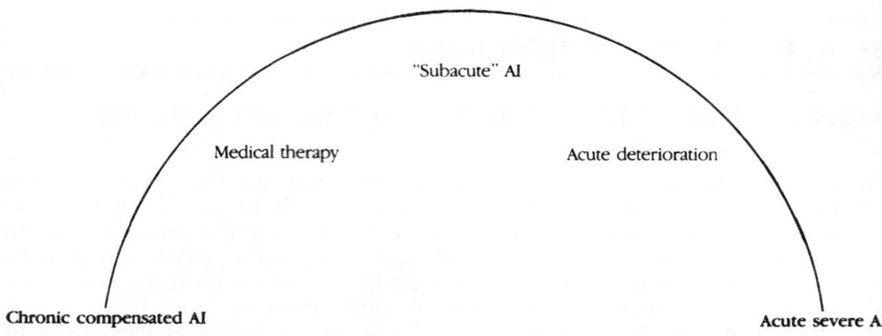

FIG. 28-1. Clinical spectrum of aortic insufficiency (AI). A patient with chronic compensated AI is hemodynamically stable, has an enlarged left ventricle and widened pulse pressure, and is asymptomatic. A patient with acute, severe AI is hemodynamically unstable, has a normal-sized left ventricle and normal pulse pressure, and presents with acute pulmonary edema and cardiogenic shock.

the aortic valve leaflet, extraarticular manifestations of ankylosing spondylitis, or Whipple disease can also result in progressive severe AI. In idiopathic giant cell aortitis and Takayasu arteritis, the inflammatory process can result in severe AI. It is likely that some cases of spontaneous acute, severe AI are related to noninfectious inflammatory processes involving the aortic valve.

D. Trauma. Acute disruption of the aortic valve may result from closed chest or abdominal trauma, such as that caused by automobile accidents, crush injuries, or falls. Sudden compression of the thoracoabdominal aorta during diastole when the aortic valve is closed can elevate intravascular pressure and may cause aortic cuspal tearing, perforation, or detachment. Trauma can damage a previously normal aortic valve; however, it is likely that myxomatous valves are more susceptible to physical injury.

E. Spontaneous aortic insufficiency. Sudden eversion of an aortic cusp may result in spontaneous acute, severe AI. This may occur with a myxomatous valve or, occasionally, with a previously normal aortic valve.

F. Prosthetic valve aortic insufficiency. Sudden, partial dehiscence of the sewn ring of a prosthetic valve from the aortic annulus causes acute AI. This is an occasional complication of emergency aortic valve replacement for bacterial endocarditis with the valve implanted into an infected annulus. Pannus ingrowth, thrombus formation, or a vegetation may impede proper seating of the ball or poppet during diastole and may result in severe AI. Homograft valves and porcine bioprostheses fixed in formaldehyde undergo progressive degeneration that frequently culminates in severe AI. Glutaraldehyde-fixed porcine valves can also spontaneously degenerate after a number of years of flawless performance; however, this complication fortunately occurs much less frequently than is the case with formaldehyde-fixed valves.

TABLE 28-1. Causes of acute aortic insufficiency

1. Infective endocarditis
2. Dissection of the ascending aorta
3. Connective tissue diseases
4. Trauma
5. "Spontaneous" or idiopathic aortic insufficiency
6. Prosthetic or bioprosthetic valve aortic insufficiency

III. Pathophysiology. The left ventricular response elicited by the volume-overload state characteristic of AI is conditioned by the severity of the hemodynamic insult and the rapidity with which it develops.

In chronic, severe AI, the volume of blood regurgitating back into the left ventricle during diastole increases slowly over time. To accommodate this regurgitant volume, the left ventricle slowly dilates, its walls undergo minimal thickening, and its compliance increase. As long as systolic function is preserved, the ventricle is capable of ejecting the abnormally large total volume (stroke volume and regurgitant stroke volume), so organ perfusion is maintained and ejection fraction is preserved, left ventricular diastolic pressure does not rise, and symptoms of cardiac decompensation do not ensue. Ejection of the large total stroke volume results in a widened arterial pulse pressure.

The clinical situation seen with acute AI is different. If the acute AI is severe, end-diastolic left ventricular pressure may approach aortic diastolic pressure. The normal ventricle, neither hypertrophied nor dilated, cannot acutely increase its total left ventricular stroke volume sufficiently to maintain forward stroke volume.

The patient with acute, severe AI and reduced cardiac output has impaired regional arterial flow, oliguria, pallor and coolness of the skin, deranged temperature regulation secondary to reduced cutaneous blood flow, and gastrointestinal and hepatic dysfunction. With extreme reduction in tissue perfusion, patients may have cardiogenic shock and lactic acidosis. Table 28-2 compares and contrasts the hemodynamic features of chronic, severe and acute, severe AI.

IV. Clinical presentation

A. History. The patient with acute, severe AI presents with acute symptoms resulting from the precipitous rise in left atrial pressure (pulmonary congestion) and an abrupt reduction in forward cardiac output. Symptoms attributable to chronic AI are those of progressive, severe pulmonary congestion and include the following:

1. Dyspnea with exertion.
2. Orthopnea and a dry or minimally productive cough aggravated by recumbency.
3. Paroxysmal nocturnal dyspnea.
4. Dyspnea at rest even while sitting upright.

TABLE 28-2. Comparison of major hemodynamic features of acute and chronic aortic regurgitation

Hemodynamic Feature	Acute	Chronic[a]
Left ventricular compliance	Not increased	Increased
Regurgitant volume	Increased	Increased
Left ventricular end-diastolic pressure	Markedly increased	May be normal
Left ventricular ejection velocity (dp/dt)	Not significantly increased	Markedly increased
Aortic systolic pressure	Not increased	Increased
Aortic diastolic pressure	Normal to decreased	Markedly decreased
Systemic arterial pulse pressure	Slightly to moderately increased	Markedly increased
Ejection fraction	Not increased	Normal to increased
Effective stroke volume	Decreased	Normal
Effective cardiac output	Decreased	Normal
Heart rate	Increased	Normal
Peripheral vascular resistance	Increased	Not increased

[a] Without left ventricular failure.

Adapted from Morganroth J, Perloff JK, Zeldis SM, et al. Acute, severe aortic regurgitation. *Ann Intern Med* 1977;87:223, with permission.

Symptoms reflecting the reduction in cardiac output are more subtle and are often overshadowed by those resulting from pulmonary congestion. There may be fatigue on exertion, apathy, agitation, and a deterioration in intellectual function reflecting impaired skeletal muscle and cerebral perfusion.

Severe chest or back pain, abrupt in onset, characterizes aortic dissection. Fever, chills, malaise, and evidence of peripheral arterial emboli implicate infective endocarditis. A history of recent chest or abdominal trauma raises the likelihood of traumatic disruption of the aortic valve. The abrupt onset of cardiac decompensation in the absence of ancillary symptoms or known heart disease suggests sudden disruption or perforation of an aortic valve intrinsically weakened by myxomatous degeneration.

B. Physical examination. Physical findings in the patient with acute, severe AI relate to the severity of pulmonary congestion and impairment in forward cardiac output and tissue perfusion. The clinical findings in acute AI and the important differences between chronic and acute AI with respect to the overall presentation are presented in Table 28-3.

Fever, petechiae, purpura, and small or large arterial embolic events implicate infective endocarditis. Excruciating chest or back discomfort and an inequality of pulses in the neck, upper, or lower extremities suggest aortic dissection. AI in a tall, thin patient with a long arm span, hyperextensile joints, and ectopia lentis points to the diagnosis of annuloaortic ectasia or aortic dissection complicating Marfan syndrome. Figure 28-2 is an algorithm that directs the clinician to the origin of AI as a function of associated ancillary clinical information.

V. Laboratory studies

A. Chest radiography. The chest radiograph usually reveals bilateral patchy interstitial infiltrates that progress to confluent alveolar infiltrates emanating from the hilar regions as pulmonary congestion progresses to fulminant pulmonary edema. The cardiac silhouette is not enlarged unless the patient has preexisting chronic valvular, myocardial, or pericardial dysfunction. The absence of cardiomegaly essentially rules out the presence of chronic AI of hemodynamic consequence.

B. Electrocardiography. The initial echocardiogram and Doppler study provide information concerning the hemodynamic severity of the AI, the involvement of other valves, and the presence of preexisting heart disease. The echocardiogram may also provide information regarding the cause of AI (e.g., infective endocarditis and aortic dissection) (Table 28-4).

C. Cardiac catheterization. If there is clear-cut echocardiographic evidence of aortic valve leaflet destruction, severe AI, and premature closure of the mitral valve in a patient previously free of cardiac disease and presenting with shock or pulmonary edema refractory to inotropic afterload reduction therapy, urgent aortic valve replacement may be lifesaving. The inherent delay and hemodynamic stress associated with cardiac catheterization and angiography put the patient at added risk and may reduce the likelihood of a successful surgical outcome. However, cardiac catheterization, left ventricular angiography, and coronary arteriography are usually required in patients with clinical or echocardiographic evidence of preexisting heart disease.

In patients with AI and suspected aortic dissection, further assessment of the ascending thoracic aorta is required to confirm (a) the presence and extent of dissection, and (b) the presence and severity of AI. This can be accomplished by magnetic resonance imaging, computed tomography, transesophogeal echocardiography, or angiography.

VI. Treatment. The treatment of patients with acute, severe AI may be categorized as follows:

1. General supportive cardiovascular measures.
2. Pharmacologic (medical) management.
3. Surgical management.

TABLE 28-3. Comparison of clinical findings in acute and chronic aortic insufficiency

Clinical Finding	Acute	Chronic[a]
Congestive heart failure	Early and sudden	Late and insidious
Arterial pulse		
Rate per minute	Increased	Normal
Rate of rise	Not increased	Increased
Systolic pressure	Normal to decreased	Increased
Diastolic pressure	Normal to mildly increased	Decreased
Pulse pressure	Near normal	Increased
Contour of peak	Single	Bisferiens
Pulsus alternans	Common	Uncommon
Left ventricular impulse	Near normal to laterally displaced, not hyperdynamic	Laterally displaced, hyperdynamic
Auscultation		
First heart sound	Soft to absent	Normal
Aortic component of second heart sound	Soft	Normal or decreased
Pulmonic component of second heart sound	Normal or increased	Normal
Fourth heart sound	Consistently absent	Usually absent
Third heart sound	Common	Uncommon
Aortic systolic murmur	Grade 3 or less	Grade 3 or more
Aortic regurgitant murmur	Short, medium-pitched	Long, high-pitched
Austin Flint murmur	Mid-diastolic	Presystolic, mid-diastolic, or both
Peripheral arterial auscultatory signs	Absent	Present
Electrocardiogram	Normal left ventricular voltage with minor repolarization abnormalities	Increased left ventricular voltage with major repolarization abnormalities
Chest radiograph		
Left ventricle	Normal to slightly increased	Markedly increased
Aortic root and arch	Usually normal	Prominent
Pulmonary venous pattern	Redistributed to upper lobes	Normal
Interstitial and alveolar fluid	Usually present	Usually absent, unless terminally decompensated

[a] Without left ventricular failure.

Adapted from Benotti JR. Acute aortic insufficiency. In: Alpert JS, Dalen JE, eds. *Valvular heart disease,* 2nd ed. Boston: Little, Brown, 1987, with permission.

General supportive cardiovascular measures include supplementary inspired oxygen to maintain the arterial oxygen pressure (P_aO_2) in excess of 65 mm Hg or arterial oxygen saturation (S_aO_2) in excess of 95%. Pulmonary edema is managed by the intravenous administration of a potent loop diuretic as well as with morphine sulfate and positioning the patient with the head and thorax elevated at least 45 degrees above the horizontal plane.

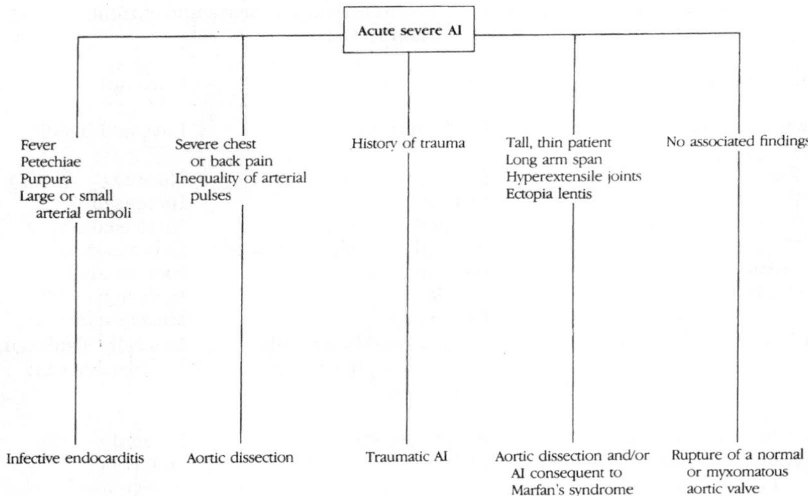

FIG. 28-2. Etiology of acute, severe aortic insufficiency as determined by ancillary clinical findings.

Evidence of peripheral organ hypoperfusion in the setting of acute AI mandates pulmonary artery catheterization and intraarterial cannulation so right and left heart filling pressures, cardiac output, and arterial blood pressure can be monitored continuously. A cardiac index less than 2.0 L/min/m^2, mean pulmonary artery pressure greater than 20 mm Hg, arterial systolic pressure less than 90 mm Hg, oliguria (urine output less than 30 mL per hour), and other indirect evidence of impaired tissue perfusion (e.g., decreased mental acuity, cool moist skin, pallor) substantiate the presence of cardiogenic shock.

TABLE 28-4. Comparison of echocardiographic manifestations of acute and chronic aortic regurgitation

Echocardiographic Variable	Acute	Chronic[a]
Mitral valve		
Closure	Early	Normal
Opening	Late	Normal
Anterior leaflet E/F slope	Reduced	Normal
Diastolic fluttering	Yes	Yes
Aortic valve presystolic opening	Yes	No
Septal wall motion	Normal	Hyperkinetic
Posterior wall motion	Normal	Hyperkinetic
End-diastolic dimension	Normal	Increased
End-systolic dimension	Normal	Normal
Shortening fraction	Normal	Increased

[a] Without left ventricular failure.

Adapted from Alpert JS. Acute aortic insufficiency. In: Alpert JS, Dalen JE, Rahimtoola SH, eds. *Valvular heart disease,* 3rd ed. Philadelphia: Lippincott Williams & Wilkins, 2000, with permission.

Vasodilator therapy may stabilize and may improve the patient's tenuous clinical and hemodynamic status. Nitroprusside can produce a 30% to 50% increase in cardiac output. Should the cardiac index not rise above 2.0 to 2.2 L/min/m^2 in response to nitroprusside infusion despite a dose sufficient to lower systolic blood to 90 mm Hg or to reduce mean blood pressure by at least 15 mm Hg, an inotropic agent should be added. Dobutamine, a relatively pure beta$_1$-myocardial stimulant, selectively augments myocardial contractility, thereby raising cardiac index with little or no increase in heart rate.

Definitive management of acute AI resulting from infective endocarditis often requires early aortic valve replacement. Patients with severe heart failure from aortic valve endocarditis have a higher mortality rate than patients with heart failure from mitral valve endocarditis. Although it is desirable to delay aortic valve replacement until antibiotic therapy is completed, this luxury may, at any moment, be precluded by a precipitous deterioration in the patient's condition. Nevertheless, valve replacement can be performed on an emergency basis or after only a few days of antibiotic therapy with an acceptably low risk of reinfection (usually less than 10%). If the patient presents with cardiogenic shock from acute AI, aortic valve replacement should be undertaken immediately even though there is little or no time for antibiotic administration. All patients should receive 4 to 6 weeks of parenteral antibiotic therapy after aortic valve replacement.

Other indications for surgery in acute AI complicating infective endocarditis include infection of a prosthetic valve, infection with an organism refractory to antibiotic therapy, continued sepsis despite appropriate antimicrobial therapy, recurrent large vessel emboli, fungal endocarditis, and myocardial abscess as manifested by the development of high-grade atrioventricular block or the inability to sterilize the blood with appropriate antibiotics.

Selected Readings

Alpert JS. Acute aortic regurgitation. In: Alpert JS, Dalen JE, Rahimtoola SH, eds. *Valvular heart disease,* 3rd ed. Philadelphia: Lippincott Williams & Wilkins, 2000:269.
An extensive overview of acute AI by one of the leading authorities in the field.

Miller RR, Vismara LA, DeMara AN, et al. Afterload reduction therapy with nitroprusside in severe aortic regurgitation: improved cardiac performance and reduced regurgitant volume. *Am J Cardiol* 1976;38:564.
Afterload reduction therapy with nitroprusside can improve stroke volume and overall cardiac performance.

Wigle ED, Labrosse CJ. Sudden, severe aortic insufficiency. *Circulation* 1965;32:708.
Acute AI, unlike chronic AI, can present with sudden hemodynamic decompensation and cardiogenic shock.

29. ACUTE MITRAL REGURGITATION

Robert A. Harrington, Rhonda L. Larsen, James M. Rippe, and Richard C. Becker

I. General principles. Acute mitral regurgitation (MR) may result from sudden disruption of any portion of the mitral valve apparatus: valve leaflets, chordae tendineae, papillary muscle, or attachments of the papillary muscles to the left ventricular wall. Acute MR may occur in a variety of situations commonly treated in the intensive care unit.

II. Etiology. The mitral valve apparatus consists of the valve leaflets, annulus, chordae tendineae, and papillary muscles. Normal function of the mitral valve depends on coordinated interplay of all structures (Table 29-1 and Fig. 29-1).

A. Mitral valve leaflets. Disruption of the mitral valve leaflets, although a common cause of chronic MR (in rheumatic valvular disease), is a rare cause of acute MR. Acute MR may occur after infective endocarditis, when vegetations may inhibit normal leaflet closure; actual leaflet destruction may occur. Leaflet disruption has also been reported after trauma and with left atrial myxoma, in which the impact of the swinging mass on the leaflets may prevent proper closure. Connective tissue disorders involving the leaflets, such as the severe myxomatous degeneration occasionally seen in floppy valve syndrome or Marfan syndrome, may result in acute MR, although other portions of the mitral valve apparatus, such as the annulus or chordae tendineae, are also typically involved.

B. Annulus. Chronic MR can result from dilatation of the valve annulus, particularly in conditions causing left ventricular failure and dilatation. Acute MR is rarely caused by annular dilatation, except in the setting of a connective tissue disorder involving the heart's fibrous skeleton (floppy valve syndrome, Marfan syndrome). There is a subgroup of patients with ischemic MR on the basis of generalized ventricular and annular dilatation caused by diffuse left ventricular ischemic dysfunction. Calcification of the annulus may cause MR, but it does not lead to acute decompensation.

C. Chordae tendineae. Ruptured chordae tendineae is a common cause of acute MR and may complicate infective endocarditis (either active or healed) or rheumatic valvulitis. Other causes of ruptured chordae include trauma, myxomatous degeneration, Marfan syndrome, systemic lupus erythematosus, congenital aortic valve disease with aortic regurgitation, Libman-Sacks endocarditis, acute rheumatic fever, and pregnancy. In most cases of ruptured chordae, no underlying origin can be determined, and it is termed *spontaneous.*

D. Papillary muscles. Acute MR due to papillary muscle dysfunction may be caused by ischemia and may be transient or permanent, by altered geometry of a dilated ventricle that inhibits normal leaflet coaptation or by blunt chest trauma with subsequent myocardial contusion causing papillary muscle dysfunction. Because the papillary muscles are supplied by the most distal portions of the coronary arterial tree, these muscles are vulnerable to transient ischemia or infarction; hence, during episodes of angina, temporary ischemia may result in acute MR. Intense ischemia during myocardial infarction may lead to papillary muscle necrosis and permanent MR or the catastrophic complication of papillary muscle rupture (Fig. 29-2). Because its entire blood supply comes from branches of the posterior descending artery, the posteromedial papillary muscle is more vulnerable to ischemia than is the anterolateral.

Dilatation of the left ventricle may lead to acute MR by altering the geometric relation of the papillary muscles to the leaflets. This may occur in left ventricular failure of any cause, in dilated cardiomyopathies, or in left ventricular

TABLE 29-1. Causes of acute mitral regurgitation

A. Disorders of the mitral valve leaflets
   1. Infective endocarditis
   2. Trauma
   3. Left atrial myxoma
   4. Methysergide (Sansert) therapy
   5. Ankylosing spondylitis
   6. Severe myxomatous degeneration
   7. Trauma of mitral vulvuloplasty
B. Disorders of the mitral valve annulus
   1. Connective tissue disorders
   2. Severe calcification
C. Disorders of the chordae tendineae
   1. Infective endocarditis
   2. Rheumatic valvulitis
   3. Trauma
   4. Myxomatous degeneration
   5. Marfan syndrome
   6. Systemic lupus erythematosus
   7. Congenital aortic valve disease
   8. Libman-Sacks endocarditis
   9. Acute rheumatic fever
   10. Pregnancy
   11. "Spontaneous"
D. Disorders of the papillary muscles
   1. Dysfunction
      a. Ischemia
      b. Myocardial infarction
      c. Left ventricular dilatation
      d. Left ventricular aneurysm
      e. Amyloidosis
      f. Sarcoidosis
      g. Other infiltrative cardiomyopathies
      h. Trauma and myocardial contusion
      i. Papillary muscle cryoablation
   2. Rupture
      a. Trauma
      b. Acute myocardial infarct
      c. Myocardial abscess
      d. Syphilis
      e. Periateritis nodosa
E. Prosthetic valve malfunction
   1. Deterioration of Silastic disc
   2. Lodging of the ball or disc in the open position
   3. Dislodgment of the ball or disc
   4. Ring or strut fracture
   5. Paravalvular leak
   6. Suture or pledger dislodgment
   7. Deterioration of leaflets of tissue valve
   8. Prosthetic valve endocarditis
   9. Porcine valve cuspal tear

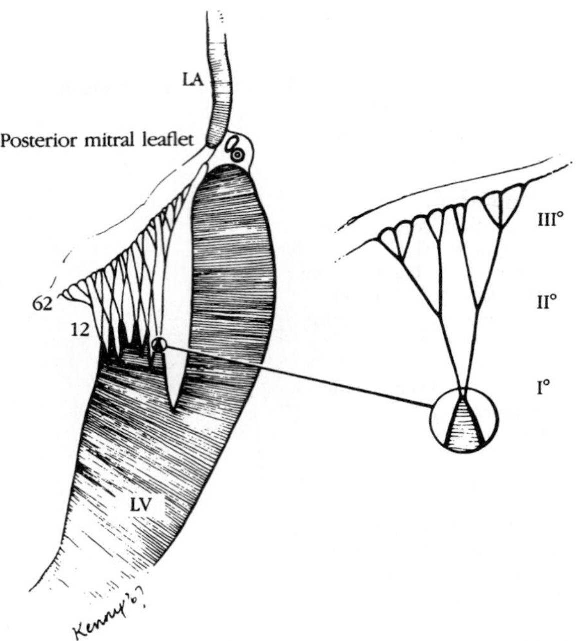

FIG. 29-1. The average number of chordae tendineae normally originating from each left ventricular papillary muscle. Although greater variation exists, each left ventricular papillary muscle contains about 6 heads, each of which contains 2 primary or first-order chordae tendineae. Each primary cord subdivides into 2 secondary chordae, each of which divides into 2 or 3 tertiary or third-order chordae. The number of chordae attached to each left ventricular papillary muscle thus averages 12, and the number of chordae inserting directly into the mitral leaflets from a single papillary muscle averages 62. (These numbers were found by counting chordae and papillary muscle heads in 12 normal hearts.) *LA,* left atrium; *LV,* left ventricle. (From Perloff JK, Roberts WC. The mitral apparatus. Functional anatomy of mitral regurgitation. *Circulation* 1972;46:227, with permission.)

aneurysm. Occasionally, infiltrative diseases (amyloidosis, sarcoidosis) may cause sufficient papillary muscle dysfunction to result in acute MR.

E. Prosthetic valve. Deterioration of Silastic discs can produce acute MR. The discs may lodge in the supporting cage in the open position, intermittently stick in the open position, occasionally break free, and lodge elsewhere in the arterial circulation. Deterioration of the outer margins of the disc has also been described. Pledgets from the sewing ring may erode, particularly in patients with connective tissue disease. Paravalvular leaks have been reported in up to 10% of patients receiving mitral valve prostheses and may be severe enough to cause acute MR. Prosthetic valve endocarditis occurs in approximately 2% of patients with a mitral valve prosthesis and may lead to acute MR. Porcine valves have reduced the incidence of thromboembolic phenomena but have shown a tendency to degenerate, with studies reporting up to a 16% incidence of degenerative failure at 7 years, particularly in patients younger than 35 years.

III. Pathophysiology. The hemodynamic effect is that of sudden, dramatic afterload reduction, allowing the left ventricle to eject blood into the relatively low-pressure

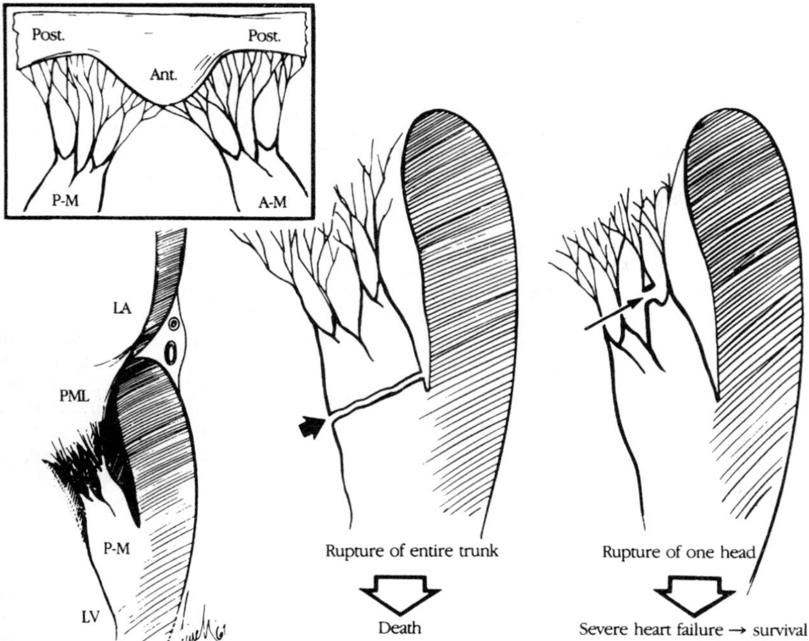

FIG. 29-2. Syndromes arising from rupture of various portions of the papillary muscle. Both the posterior (*P-M*) and anterior (*A-M*) papillary muscles give rise to branching chordae tendineae that attach to both anterior and posterior leaflets **(inset)**. Rupture of the entire central body (trunk) of the papillary muscle **(center)** leads to overwhelming mitral regurgitation (*MR*), shock, and death, whereas rupture of one head **(right)** leads to pulmonary edema and survival if it is promptly treated. *LA,* left atrium; *LV,* left ventricle; *PML,* papillary muscle leaflet. (From Roberts WC, Perloff JK. Mitral valve disease. A clinicopathologic survey of the conditions causing the mitral valve to function abnormally. *Ann Intern Med* 1972;77:939, with permission.)

left atrium during both isometric contraction and early ejection. Approximately 50% of the regurgitant volume is ejected into the left atrium before opening of the aortic valve.

Two factors determine the volume of regurgitant flow: the regurgitant orifice size and the pressure gradient between the left ventricle and the left atrium. Interventions that decrease left ventricular systolic pressure, such as arterial dilators (nitroprusside, hydralazine, or angiotensin-converting enzyme [ACE] inhibitors) or the intraaortic balloon pump, decrease regurgitant volume by reducing the left ventricular to left atrial pressure gradient.

IV. Diagnosis

A. History. In contrast to patients with chronic MR, who become symptomatic slowly as left ventricular failure develops, patients with acute MR can generally pinpoint a date when symptoms began.

Patients with ruptured chordae may give a history of previous rheumatic fever or long-standing asymptomatic murmur complicated by a sudden exacerbation of symptoms. A history of mitral valve prolapse also should suggest ruptured chordae as a cause of acute decompensation. The patient may give a history of infective endocarditis or trauma. In contrast, rupture of a papillary muscle is a catastrophic event, generally occurring during acute myocardial infarction and resulting in pulmonary edema and shock. Without prompt surgical repair, mortality approaches 100%.

The symptoms of acute MR are those of pulmonary edema and pulmonary hypertension. Depending on the volume of regurgitation, the patient may experience symptoms ranging from dyspnea on exertion to acute pulmonary edema. Abrupt elevation of pulmonary vascular pressures may cause acute right heart failure, with its attendant signs and symptoms (e.g., hepatomegaly, ascites, peripheral edema) and evidence of low-output congestive heart failure.

B. Physical examination. A summary of the physical examination findings in acute MR is found in Table 29-2. It is a spectrum of findings, ranging from the presence of a new systolic murmur with hemodynamic stability to cardiogenic shock. Fever and occasionally Roth spots, Janeway lesions, or splinter hemorrhages may be present in infective endocarditis. Skeletal, ophthalmologic, or dermatologic abnormalities suggestive of connective tissue disease may be present.

Patients with chronic MR are typically in atrial fibrillation, a finding suggesting a chronically dilated left atrium. S_1 is often soft and blowing; a high-pitched murmur heard best at the apex and radiating to the axilla is present. The murmur begins with S_1 and extends throughout systole, often obscuring A_2 (reflecting the persistence of a gradient between the left ventricle and left atrium throughout systole). The murmur changes little in response to changes in left ventricular volume typical of atrial fibrillation, and the intensity of the murmur correlates poorly with the severity of regurgitation if the intensity of the murmur is graded III/VI or lower; however, when the murmur intensity is IV/VI or greater, there is good correlation with severity of regurgitation as measured by echocardiography.

In acute MR, the underlying rhythm is typically sinus tachycardia. A prominent, often palpable presystolic gallop is frequently present as the hypertrophied left atrium forcefully ejects blood into the left ventricle. S_2 may be widely split (reflecting early closure of the aortic valve), and if pulmonary hypertension is present, P_2 may be accentuated. The murmur of acute MR often suggests dysfunction of a specific portion of the valvular apparatus. The resultant murmur, best heard at the base of the heart, may be confused with that of aortic stenosis. Overwhelming MR may present *without* an audible murmur. No murmur is audible in 50% of patients with acute papillary muscle rupture, probably because of left ventricular failure.

C. Laboratory studies. A summary of laboratory findings pertinent to acute MR is found in Table 29-3.

1. **Electrocardiography.** Sinus tachycardia is typical in acute MR, whereas atrial fibrillation suggests a chronic condition. Occasionally, a biphasic P wave with large terminal forces in lead V_1 suggests left atrial volume overload. Acute papillary muscle infarction may be accompanied by electrocardiographic changes typical of acute myocardial infarction.

TABLE 29-2. Physical examination findings in acute mitral regurgitation

1. Evidence of systemic manifestations of any disorder listed in Table 29-1
   a. Fever, Roth spots, Janeway lesions
   b. Evidence of blunt chest trauma
2. Cardiovascular findings
   a. Prominent (often palpable) S_4
   b. Sinus tachycardia
   c. Widely split S_2
   d. Systolic murmur (may mimic murmur of aortic stenosis)
3. Other findings
   a. Evidence of pulmonary congestion
   b. Evidence of shock

TABLE 29-3. Laboratory findings in acute mitral regurgitation

1. Electrocardiogram
   a. Sinus tachycardia
   b. Large terminal forces in P wave in V_1
   c. Acute ischemic changes
2. Chest radiograph
   a. Pulmonary congestion without cardiomegaly
   b. Left atrial enlargement (rare)
3. Echocardiogram
   a. Systolic expansion of left atrium (two-dimensional echocardiogram)
   b. Flail leaflet
   c. Vegetation
   d. Flattened septal or posterior wall motion (infarction)
   e. Hyperdynamic septal and posterior wall motion (acute volume overload)
   f. Increased E/F slope
   g. Demonstration of regurgitant flow by pulse and/or color flow Doppler
   h. Absence of evidence of AS, HOCM, or VSD
4. Gated cardiac blood pool scan
   a. Left-to-right stroke volume index of greater than 1.5–2.0 : 1.0
   b. Elevated left ventricular ejection fraction
5. Cardiac catheterization
   a. Giant CV waves (see text)
   b. Absence of oxygen content step-up between right atrium and right ventricle
   c. Angiographic evidence of regurgitation
   d. Presence or absence of other cardiac abnormalities

AS, aortic stenosis; HOCM, hypertrophic obstructive cardiomyopathy; VSD, ventricular septal defect.

2. **Chest radiography.** The chest radiograph in acute MR typically reveals the striking findings of interstitial or alveolar edema with a normal-sized cardiac silhouette.
3. **Echocardiography.** M-mode and two-dimensional echocardiography techniques, including pulse Doppler and Doppler color flow techniques, make several important contributions to the diagnosis of acute MR. First, these studies help to differentiate the many possible underlying conditions causing acute MR. Second, they can rule out conditions that may mimic acute MR. Recent work has suggested that transesophageal echocardiography is superior to transthoracic echocardiography in quantifying acute MR. Use of intraoperative transesophageal echocardiography may guide decision making in surgical repair of the mitral valve.

D. Cardiac catheterization

1. **Right heart catheterization.** This technique provides important diagnostic information in patients with suspected acute MR and is useful in optimizing vasodilation therapy. The procedure may be performed at the bedside in an unstable patient, by using a balloon-tipped, flow-directed catheter (Fig. 29-3). Bedside right heart catheterization is particularly helpful in distinguishing acute MR from rupture of the interventricular septum. In the latter condition, a step-up in oxygen content of greater than 1% volume between the right atrium and the right ventricle is present with a hemodynamically significant left-to-right shunt. Pulmonary artery pressures are typically elevated in acute MR, although this finding is nonspecific. Oxygen saturation in pulmonary arterial finding is nonspecific. Oxygen saturation in pulmonary arterial blood is often diminished, resulting from low cardiac output.
2. **Left heart catheterization.** Although angiography is still far from ideal in its ability to quantify regurgitation absolutely, left heart catheterization pro-

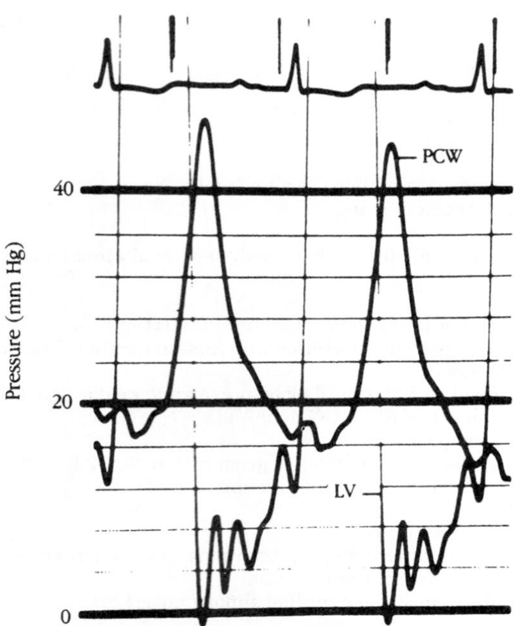

FIG. 29-3. Pressure tracings obtained during cardiac catheterization from a patient with acute MR caused by ruptured chordae tendineae. The top tracing is the patient's electrocardiogram. Large CV waves are present in the pulmonary capillary wedge *(PCW)* pressure tracing. *LV,* left ventricular diastolic pressure. (From Howe JP III, Alpert JS. Acute mitral regurgitation. In: Dalen JE, Alpert JS, eds. *Valvular heart disease.* Boston: Little, Brown, 1981:147, with permission.)

vides useful information about the severity of regurgitation, the degree of coexisting coronary artery disease, left ventricular function, and the presence or absence of any other valvular lesions. Prompt opacification of the entire left atrium (within 1 or 2 systoles) indicates severe MR. The functional status of the left ventricle is important when considering surgical intervention, because patients with diffuse left ventricular dysfunction and poor residual myocardium have an extremely high in-hospital mortality, regardless of the therapy chosen.

V. Treatment

A. Intensive care unit management. Medical therapy in the intensive care unit should focus on hemodynamic stabilization and rapid identification of the mechanical defect and underlying cause. If the acute MR is ischemic in origin with papillary muscle dysfunction, reperfusion therapy, with either thrombolytic agents or percutaneous transluminal coronary angioplasty, may be indicated.

The mainstays of medical therapy are vasodilating drugs and the intraaortic balloon pump. Afterload reducing agents, such as nitroprusside, hydralazine, and ACE inhibitors, improve hemodynamics in acute MR by several mechanisms. First, by lowering systemic vascular resistance and impedance to left ventricular ejection, forward cardiac output is increased and regurgitant volume is diminished. Second, by decreasing left ventricular volume, these agents decrease the size of the regurgitant orifice. Although ACE inhibitors, hydralazine, or vasodilating calcium channel blockers are often sufficient for long-term management of patients with chronic MR, nitroprusside is the agent of choice for acute MR. Patients with low systemic arterial pressures (systolic pressure less than 90 mm Hg, diastolic pressure less than 60 mm Hg) may benefit from judicious use of inotropic agents such as dopamine or dobutamine. Such patients are probably best managed with a combination of vasodilator drugs and intraaortic balloon pump therapy. Patients with low arterial pressures or in whom systemic pressures fall before a decrease in pulmonary artery pressures are candidates for prompt insertion of the intraaortic balloon pump.

B. Surgical therapy. Various techniques for repair of specific portions of the valve apparatus may be employed, including leaflet or annulus plication, Carpentier ring annuloplasty, placement of artificial chordae, and direct suture repair of chordae tendineae or papillary muscle head; however, repair of the valve, when technically possible, is the surgical therapy of choice.

The results of surgical intervention depend on the following: age of the patient; the cause of acute regurgitation; the existence of other cardiac lesions (e.g., coronary artery disease and ventricular aneurysm); the functional capacity of the left ventricle; the presence of pulmonary hypertension; the presence of cardiogenic shock; the coexistence of hepatic, renal, or pulmonary disease; the need for intraaortic balloon pump therapy; and the urgency of surgery.

Selected Readings

Burch GE, DePasquale NP, Phillips JH. Clinical manifestations of papillary muscle dysfunction. *Arch Intern Med* 1963;112:158.

Papillary muscle dysfunction as a cause of mitral insufficiency is common among patients with myocardial ischemia and infarction. "Dynamic" mitral insufficiency can be severe and may lead to congestive heart failure.

Silverman B, Kozma G, Silverman M, et al. Echocardiographic manifestations of postinfarction ventricular septal rupture. *Chest* 1975;68:778.

Ventricular septal rupture after myocardial infarction can lead to cardiogenic shock and death. The echocardiographic manifestations of acute ventricular septal rupture are described.

Smith MD, Cassidy JM, Gurley JC, et al. Echo doppler evaluation of patients with acute mitral regurgitation: superiority of transesophageal echocardiography with color flow imaging. *Am Heart J* 1995;129:967.

Transesophageal echocardiography is an important diagnostic tool for evaluating patients with suspected mitral insufficiency.

III. CORONARY CARE

30. ACUTE HEART FAILURE

Ronald P. Caputo and Richard C. Becker

I. Epidemiology. Heart failure is a major health problem in Western society. Despite advances made in the diagnosis and treatment of congestive heart failure, the incidence and prevalence of this devastating syndrome continue to increase.

II. Pathophysiology. The heart may fail by several mechanisms (Table 30-1), which may be classified according to three etiologic categories (Table 30-2).

A. Systolic and diastolic dysfunction. Systolic and diastolic dysfunction are terms frequently used to describe the abnormal function of the left ventricle in patients presenting with heart failure. Systolic dysfunction refers to heart failure occurring as a result of poor contractility, whereas diastolic dysfunction generally refers to heart failure that occurs despite normal or supernormal contractility, presumably on the basis of impaired ventricular filling.

B. Forward and backward heart failure. Forward heart failure and backward heart failure are terms used in regard to patients with symptomatic heart failure. Forward failure describes the clinical symptoms resulting from decreased forward cardiac output and tissue perfusion, including fatigue, exercise intolerance, and decreased mental status. Backward failure describes the syndrome of tissue congestion resulting from, at least in the acute setting, increased venous hydrostatic pressure. The most notable symptom of backward failure is pulmonary edema.

Similarly, the terms *right* and *left heart failure* are used to describe signs and symptoms of either right or left ventricular dysfunction. Classically, signs of right ventricular dysfunction include ascites, edema, and hepatic congestion, whereas signs of left ventricular dysfunction include pulmonary congestion and decreased tissue perfusion.

III. Compensatory mechanisms. The Frank-Starling mechanism is a well-described phenomenon in which an increase in end-diastolic volume results in increased cardiac wall stretch, increased myofibril stretch, and a more optimal alignment of myofibrils for cross-bridge cycling. This results in an increased force of contraction; it occurs in both acute and chronic situations.

IV. Diagnostic tools

A. Pulmonary artery catheterization. There has been some discussion regarding the utility of the balloon-tipped pulmonary artery catheter. Although debate continues, we believe that hemodynamic monitoring is useful in the following circumstances:

1. When the diagnosis of cardiogenic versus noncardiogenic pulmonary edema is unclear from data obtained from history, physical examination, or radiography.
2. When knowledge of the patient's intravascular volume status is critical but not discernible by noninvasive means.
3. For diagnostic purposes in certain cases of acute cardiac failure (i.e., tamponade or left-to-right shunt).
4. To assess the therapeutic efficacy of cardiotonics, vasopressors, or vasodilators by means of cardiac output and intracardiac pressures.

B. Indwelling arterial catheter. The indwelling arterial catheter has a low diagnostic yield and should mainly be used for blood pressure monitoring or frequent blood gas sampling. Situations in which close observation of blood pressure is indicated include hypertensive crisis, vasodilator therapy, and severe hemodynamic derangement (shock).

C. Echocardiography. A transthoracic echocardiogram provides information regarding atrial and ventricular size and function, valvular structure and function, intracardiac blood flow, anatomy of the ascending and transverse aorta, pericardium, intracardiac masses, and right-sided cardiac pressures.

TABLE 30-1. Common causes of acute heart failure

Pressure overload	Systemic hypertension Aortic stenosis Hypertrophic cardiomyopathy Pulmonary embolism Cessation of afterload therapy Dysfunctional prosthetic aortic valve
Volume overload	Aortic insufficiency (trauma, dissection, ABE) High-output failure (thyrotoxicosis, beriberi, severe anemia) Cessation of diuretic therapy
Impaired ventricular filling	Mitral stenosis (RHD, MAC, myxoma) Tamponade (neoplasm, viral, uremia) Constriction (post-XRT, postsurgery) Restriction (amyloid, hemochromatosis)
Myocardial diseases	Myocarditis (viral, etc.) Dilated cardiomyopathy (ischemic, ETOH, idiopathic) Metabolic diseases (hypocalcemia, hypophosphatemia) Toxic insult (cocaine, lead, antineoplastic therapy)
Dysrhythmias	Ischemia Bradyarrhythmias (heart block, sick sinus, iatrogenic) Tachyarrhythmias (VT, SVT)

ABE, acute bacterial endocarditis; ETOH, ethanol induced; MAC, mitral annular calcification; RHD, rheumatic heart disease; SVT, supraventricular tachycardia; VT, ventricular tachycardia; XRT, external beam radiation therapy.

D. Transesophageal echocardiography. Transesophageal echocardiography provides similar information to that provided by transthoracic studies but is a more technically involved procedure. Although transesophageal echocardiography provides superior visualization of the aortic root, all heart valves, intraatrial structures, and the atrial-basal ventricular septum, the apical portion of the heart and the upper portion of the ascending aorta are not well seen.

E. Cardiac catheterization. By using intracardiac pressure measurements, oxygen saturation data, ventriculography, aortography, and angiography, cardiac

TABLE 30-2. Etiologic categories of cardiac failure

Impediments to cardiac filling and emptying
- Valvular disease
- Pericardial disease
- Restrictive disease
- Pulmonary embolism
- Extreme hypertension

Primary myocyte dysfunction
- Myocarditis
- Cardiomyopathies
- Toxic injury
- Metabolic disturbances
- Ischemic disease

Abnormal organization or signaling of cardiac contraction
- Tachyarrhythmias
- Bradyarrhythmias
- Asystole

catheterization provides information regarding right and left ventricular function, valvular function, pulmonary-systemic-intracardiac hemodynamics, intracardiac shunting, aortic disease, and coronary anatomy.

V. Treatment

A. Nonspecific therapy. All patients presenting with acute congestive heart failure should be considered for admission to a critical care unit. This opinion has been reinforced by a study demonstrating that physicians display a poor predictive ability for survival in such patients both at 90 days and 1 year. Several simple therapeutic maneuvers are beneficial in most cases of acute heart failure (Table 30-3).

B. Principles of pharmacologic therapy. The concept of using single or combined pharmacologic agents to improve the hemodynamic status of patients with uncompensated heart failure is straightforward (Table 30-4). One strategy is to improve the pumping function of the heart directly using inotropic agents; another strategy is to optimize or normalize hemodynamic status by altering other components of the circulatory system, that is, reducing preload (diuretics, nitrates) and afterload (nitroprusside, hydralazine, angiotensin-converting enzyme inhibitors).

C. Circulatory support with vasopressors. In patients whose mean arterial pressure is less than 70 mm Hg, norepinephrine or high-dose dopamine should be used promptly to restore blood pressure and perfusion to the vital organs and the coronary circulation.

D. Intraaortic balloons counterpulsation. Intraaortic balloon pumping reduces ST-segment abnormalities in patients with acute myocardial infarction or unstable angina and is effective in the treatment of angina unresponsive to medical therapy. Intraaortic balloon pumping may be useful in rescue angioplasty after failed thrombolysis. Other indications include the following: cardiogenic shock; mechanical complications of acute myocardial infarction, such as acute ventricular septal defect and mitral regurgitation; the inability to wean the patient from cardiopulmonary bypass support; and prophylactic applications, including patients with clinically unstable left main coronary stenosis who are awaiting surgery.

E. Left ventricular assist devices. External pulsatile assist devices have been used successfully both as a bridge to cardiac transplantation and in patients in postcardiotomy cardiogenic shock.

VI. Diagnosis and management in specific situations

A. Pressure overload

1. **Hypertension.** The magnitude of hypertension required to precipitate acute heart failure depends on a patient's baseline cardiac function. In the case of malignant hypertension-hypertensive crisis (defined as a diastolic pressure greater than 130 mm Hg and evidence of end-organ compromise), left ventricular dysfunction and acute heart failure may occur in patients with normal baseline function.
2. **Aortic stenosis.** Aortic stenosis does not develop acutely, except in the case of prosthetic valve dysfunction. Patients with aortic stenosis can, however,

TABLE 30-3. Nonspecific therapy of acute heart failure

1. Place patient in proper position
2. Ensure adequate oxygenation
3. Obtain sufficient venous access
4. Optimize blood pressure
5. Rapidly determine heart rhythm (antiarrhythmic, cardioversion, pacemaker)
6. Sedate patient
7. Consider fluid restriction/diuresis
8. Rapidly diagnose cardiac disease

TABLE 30-4. Pharmacologic therapies

Diuretics	Thiazide (metolazone, chlorothiazide) Loop (furosemide, bumetanide)
Nitrates	
Inotropic agents and vasopressors	Sympathomimetic amines (dopamine, etc.) Phosphodiesterase inhibitors (amrinone) Cardiac glycosides (digitalis) Miscellaneous inotropic agents
Afterload reducers	ACE inhibitors Hydralazine Nitroprusside

ACE, angiotensin-converting enzyme.

present with acute heart failure. This occurs when a sudden alteration occurs in the compensatory balance on which these patients depend.

Acute heart failure associated with aortic stenosis is best managed by treating the precipitating event. By correcting heart rate, rhythm, contractility, and blood pressure toward normal, the pressure-wall stress mismatch is also normalized, and left ventricular function is consequently improved. In the case of atrial fibrillation, for example, cardioversion can restore sinus rhythm, decrease heart rate, and eventually restore atrial systole. All these changes have a favorable effect on left ventricular function and systemic hemodynamics. Rarely, symptoms persist despite treatment of the acute precipitants. In these cases, emergency balloon aortic valvuloplasty or aortic valve replacement must be considered.

3. **Hypertrophic cardiomyopathy.** Therapy for acute heart failure that occurs in the setting of hypertrophic cardiomyopathy centers on improving diastolic left ventricular function and reducing the ventricular gradient if present. This is best accomplished using medications that slow heart rate, enhance ventricular relaxation, and decrease the force of contraction. Beta-blockers and calcium channel blockers, particularly verapamil, have been shown to be effective. A critical mistake is the use of inotropic agents in these patients. These drugs speed the heart rate, impair diastolic relaxation, and exacerbate the intraventricular gradient. Diuretics must be used cautiously.
4. **Pulmonary embolism.** Pulmonary embolism is not an uncommon medical problem and is underdiagnosed. Acute pulmonary embolism results in decreased flow across the pulmonary bed, decreased left ventricular filling, and diminished cardiac output.

   If life-threatening pulmonary embolism is suspected, definitive therapy must be initiated immediately (thrombolytics, surgical or mechanical embolectomy), even without the benefit of pulmonary angiography in extreme cases. Supportive care should include volume administration and supplemental oxygen as needed.
5. **High-output heart failure.** In certain circumstances, heart failure can occur in the setting of a supernormal cardiac output, termed *high-output failure.* Increased cardiac output is due mainly to either increased circulatory volume (preload) or decreased peripheral resistance (afterload), although heart rate and contactility are also mildly increased. Specific causes of high-output failure include anemia, thyrotoxicosis, beriberi, arteriovenous fistulas, Paget's disease, polyostotic fibrous dysplasia (Albright syndrome), cirrhosis, and carcinoid syndrome. Pathophysiologically, pulmonary or systemic congestion occurs secondary to a sustained rise in left ventricular diastolic pressure. This is due to increased end-systolic volume and a shortened diastolic filling period that is a consequence of tachycardia.

   Although the development of high-output failure is not an acute process, the congestive symptoms may appear abruptly. Typically, symptoms appear when cardiac output, although remaining at supernormal levels, begins to decline slightly. The time frame in which this happens depends partially on baseline ventricular function. Initial therapy includes reduction of circulatory volume with diuretics and, in some instances (thyrotoxicosis), controlling heart rate with beta-blockers. Long-term therapy is focused on treating the underlying pathologic process, for example, thyroid ablation, correction of anemia, and thiamin supplementation.

B. Myocardial diseases

1. Myocarditis. Myocarditis is an inflammatory process that involves the myocardium; it may be an acute or a chronic process and may occur in the peripartum period. Acute heart failure can occur with acute fulminant myocarditis. In North America, viruses are presumed to be the most common agents producing myocarditis, whereas in South America, Chagas disease (caused by *Trypanosoma cruzi*) is far more common. Among viruses, Coxsackie B virus is the most frequent cause of myocarditis.

Therapy is usually supportive, with prolonged bed rest, digitalis, diuretics, and afterload reduction with angiotensin-converting enzyme inhibitors. The use of corticosteroids is controversial. Antimicrobial agents may be used in patients with susceptible infections.

2. Cardiomyopathies

a. Idiopathic dilated cardiomyopathy. Dilated cardiomyopathy is a syndrome characterized by cardiac enlargement and impaired systolic function of one or both ventricles. This condition most probably represents the result of a variety of disease processes involving the myocardium. The disease is most common in middle age and is more frequent in men. The course of dilated cardiomyopathy is usually one of progressive deterioration.

b. Alcoholic cardiomyopathy. Chronic excessive alcohol consumption can be associated with dilated cardiomyopathy, which may lead to congestive heart failure. Possible mechanisms include a direct toxic effect of alcohol or its metabolites, nutritional deficiencies (thiamine), and a toxic effect of additives (cobalt).

3. Metabolic disturbances. Severe hypophosphatemia may result in a reversible left ventricular dysfunction that resolves with restoration of serum phosphate to normal levels. Severe chronic hypocalcemia may rarely cause congestive heart failure, which resolves when the serum calcium is raised. Severe hypomagnesema may result in focal myocardial necrosis. Thiamine deficiency can cause a reversible myocardial dysfunction (beriberi). Carnitine and selenium deficiencies may also lead to dilated cardiomyopathy.

4. Toxic injury. Many different substances may act on the heart and damage the myocardium. Cocaine increases myocardial oxygen demand by increasing heart rate and blood pressure, causes coronary vasoconstriction, may accelerate atherosclerosis, and can lead to thrombotic occlusion of the coronary arteries, with resultant acute myocardial infarction. Lead poisoning may lead to overt congestive heart failure secondary to left ventricular dysfunction that is reversible with chelation therapy. The venom of the scorpion may lead to severe left ventricular dysfunction and resultant acute congestive heart failure. Treatment includes adrenergic blocking agents and specific antivenom. Arsenicals can lead to a dilated cardiomyopathy that is reversible with chelation therapy.

Antineoplastic agents can have a deleterious effect on the heart. Interferon-alpha treatment has been reported to cause a dilated cardiomyopathy that resolves with discontinuation of therapy. High doses of cyclophosphamide have been associated with heart failure secondary to a hemorrhagic myocarditis. Anthracycline cardiotoxicity may be early or late. The early cardiotoxicity is not dose dependent and includes electrocardiographic abnormalities, left ventricular dysfunction, and myopericarditis. The late cardiotoxicity is related to the development of dose-dependent degenerative cardiomyopathy.

Selected Readings

Braunwald E, ed. *Heart disease,* 4th ed. Philadelphia: WB Saunders, 1992:397.
A description of the Frank-Starling mechanism, an important compensatory response in disease states and disorders characterized by impaired ventricular systolic function.

Konstam MA. Heart failure: evaluation and care of patients with left ventricular systolic dysfunction. Rockville, MD: Agency for Healthcare Policy and Research, Dept. of Health and Human Services AHCPR publication No. 94-0612, 1994.
An excellent overview of pathophysiologic mechanisms, epidemiology, and management of congestive heart failure.

Poawa BM, Smith WR, McClish DK, et al. Physicians' survival predictions for patients with acute congestive heart failure. *Arch Intern Med* 1997;157:1001.
The management of patients with congestive heart failure is complex, and the severity of disease is frequently underestimated by physicians.

31. UNSTABLE ANGINA

Pierre Théroux and Richard C. Becker

I. **General principles.** Unstable angina is a well-defined clinical entity with specific causes, pathophysiologic mechanisms, clinical manifestations, laboratory findings, and treatment.

II. **Pathogenic mechanisms.** Pathophysiologic processes involved in acute ischemic syndromes are shown in Fig. 31-1.

A. **Myocardial ischemia.** Myocardial ischemia is the consequence of an imbalance between myocardial oxygen demand and supply. In stable angina, the ischemia is induced by excess demand relative to the capability of supply. In acute coronary syndromes, ischemia is caused by a primary decrease in coronary artery blood flow and, typically, by an occluding thrombus. The ischemia can be more or less severe and may cause transmural or subendocardial ischemia, and it may be more or less sustained, possibly to result in myocardial necrosis.

B. **Plaque rupture.** Plaque rupture triggers thrombus formation. The plaque that ruptures is histologically young (causing less than 50% stenosis), is rich in cholesterol and cholesterol esters, and has a thin, fibrous cap infiltrated by monocytes-macrophages and other inflammatory cells secreting matrix-degrading enzymes.

C. **Plaque inflammation.** A toxic or immune reaction can drive the response-to-injury reaction, leading to atherosclerosis, inflammation, matrix degradation, and plaque erosion. Candidate offenders are modified low-density lipoprotein cholesterol, free radicals, or antigens derived from intracellular pathogens such as cytomegalovirus and *Chlamydia pneumoniae.*

D. **Platelet activation.** Platelets interact with adhesive proteins from the subendothelium (and disrupted plaque) exposed to circulation, leading to platelet adhesion, activation, and secretion.

E. **Thrombin generation.** Tissue factor, present in a variety of tissues and in the atherosclerotic plaque, and also expressed by monocytes-macrophages, forms a complex with factor VII to activate factor X and lead to thrombin generation. Thrombin converts fibrinogen to fibrin, activates platelet, and self-amplifies its reaction by feedback stimulation of factors V, VIII, and XI.

III. **Diagnosis.** The diagnosis of unstable angina is based on recognition of symptoms and implies an evaluation of the risk associated with the disease. Practical guidelines have been published for early management, incorporating clinical elements and electrocardiographic (ECG) findings (Table 31-1).

A. **Symptom recognition.** Symptom recognition is fundamental in the diagnosis of unstable angina. The key diagnostic feature of unstable angina is the presence of more severe (or new) symptoms, departing from the usual pattern of angina for a given patient. Unstable angina is routinely classified as follows: (a) new-onset or crescendo angina, with chest pain occurring at rest or at a progressively lower threshold of exercise; (b) prolonged chest pain, poorly relieved with nitroglycerin; and (c) recurrence of angina pain after myocardial infarction. The Braunwald classification is now most frequently used (Table 31-2).

B. **Differential diagnosis.** When cardiac pain is the likely diagnosis, the diagnosis of secondary unstable angina must be excluded. The causes of an excess in myocardial oxygen demand are as follows: (a) inappropriate tachycardia (anemia, fever, hypoxia, tachyarrhythmias, thyrotoxicosis); (b) high afterload (aortic valve stenosis, hypertrophic cardiomyopathy, hypertension with left ventricular hypertrophy); (c) high preload (cardiac chamber dilation and congestive heart failure); (d) high cardiac output conditions (arteriovenous fistula, beriberi heart disease, Paget's disease); and (e) hyperdynamic states (sympathomimetic drugs, cocaine intoxication).

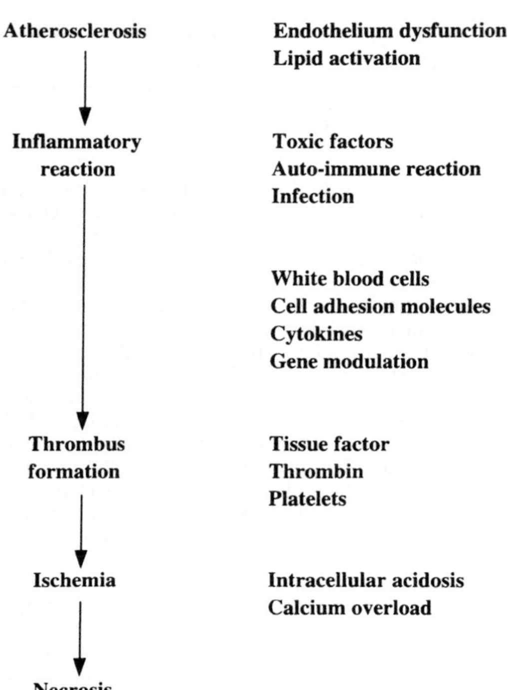

FIG. 31-1. Pathophysiologic processes involved in acute ischemic syndromes. Unstable angina is a buildup of various pathophysiologic mechanisms within the atherosclerotic plaque leading to plaque activation, rapid progression of lumen obstruction, myocardial ischemia, and, eventually, cell necrosis.

IV. Specific presentations

A. Unstable angina after coronary angioplasty. Restenosis after balloon angioplasty occurs within the first 6 months in 30% to 50% of patients and is frequently evident as pain at rest.

B. Unstable angina after bypass surgery. Unstable angina occurring in the first few years after coronary artery bypass surgery may be related to a single active lesion; later, it is frequently associated with more extensive graft disease.

C. Non–Q-wave myocardial infarction. Non–Q-wave myocardial infarction is recognized by an elevation of cardiac enzymes in serial plasma samples obtained in the first 12 hours after the onset of an episode of chest pain, usually prolonged (lasting 30 minutes or longer), and accompanied by ST-T–segment changes. Non–Q-wave myocardial infarction is managed as unstable angina, because the pathophysiologic features are similar.

D. Prinzmetal's variant angina. Prinzmetal's variant angina represents the extreme manifestation of coronary artery vasomotion. The primary spasm is usually focal, at the site of a significant or nonsignificant coronary artery stenosis. The pain in variant angina typically occurs at rest, often at night and more frequently in the early morning hours.

V. Diagnosis

A. Twelve-lead electrocardiography. The presence of ST-T–segment changes on the presenting ECG is a useful diagnostic aid in unstable angina. The absence

TABLE 31-1. Risk stratification in unstable angina

Gradient in Risk	High	Intermediate[a]	Low[a]
EARLY RISK EVALUATION (HOSPITAL ADMISSION)			
Clinical features			
Clinical presentation	Prolonged chest pain: hemodynamic compromise during pain; transient S_3	Chest pain at rest	New-onset exertional, more severe exertional
ECG			
T wave ST segment	Deep T wave in anterior leads ST elevation, pseudo-normalization, ST depression ≥1 mV	T-wave changes ST depression <1 mV	
Biochemical tests			
CK	Elevated		
Troponin T	Elevated		
Troponin I	Elevated		
IN-HOSPITAL RISK STRATIFICATION			
Evolution	Recurrent ischemia	Inducible ischemia, silent ischemia	No pain, no inducible ischemia

[a] Mainly determined by the absence of high-risk features. Other determinants of risk are older age, previous bypass surgery, previous myocardial infarction, and comorbid conditions such as diabetes mellitus, renal failure, and obstructive coronary disease. S_3, third heart sound, CK, creatine kinase; ECG, electrocardiogram.

of these changes, however, does not rule out the disease. The ECG obtained during an episode of chest pain can add information.

B. Creatine kinase and creatine kinase containing M and B enzymes. Cardiac enzyme activity and more specifically, activity of creatine kinase (CK) and of its MB isoform are determined in all patients with unstable angina and more particularly when the acute chest pain is prolonged. An elevation in values is associated with a less favorable prognosis.

C. Troponin T and troponin I. These markers are highly sensitive and specific to myocardial cell damage. Many studies have not documented elevated levels in 30% to 40% of patients with unstable angina, often when plasma CK and MB-CK values are normal. Elevated values are also associated with impaired prognosis during the hospital stay and during follow-up (independently of CK values).

D. Imaging techniques. Myocardial imaging obtained during an episode of chest pain can detect transient myocardial ischemia with high sensitivity; thallium-201 has been used for this purpose, but technetium-99m offers distinct advantages, because it can be injected during an episode of chest pain and imaging obtained several hours later, when the patient is in a stable condition.

E. Continuous ST-segment monitoring. Holter monitor recordings allow detection of silent ischemia in approximately 20% of patients with unstable angina. Its presence suggests more severe coronary artery disease and has prognostic implications.

TABLE 31-2. Braunwald classification of unstable angina

	Category		
	A	B	C
Clinical circumstances	Develops with extracardiac condition that intensifies myocardial ischemia (secondary UA)	Develops in absence of extracardiac condition (primary UA)	Develops within 2 after AMI (postinfraction UA)
Severity			
I. New onset of severe angina or accelerated angina; no rest pain	IA	IB	IC
II. Angina at rest within past month but not within preceding 48 h (angina at rest, subacute)	IIA	IIB	IIC
III. Angina at rest within 48 h (angina at rest, acute)	IIIA	IIIB	IIIC

Patients with UA may also be classified into the following groups: (a) absence of treatment for chronic stable angina; (b) treatment for chronic stable angina; or (c) maximal antiischemic therapy. They may also be divided into those with transient ST-T wave changes during pain. AMI, acute myocardial infarction; UA, unstable angina.
Reprinted with permission of the American Heart Association from Braunwald E. Unstable angina: a classification. *Circulation* 1989;80:410.

F. Provocative testing. Provocative testing by exercise treadmill or a pharmacologic agent such as dipyridamole or dobutamine allows detection of ischemia in the presence of a significant coronary narrowing. Provocative testing performed when the patient is stable or past the acute phase or in low-risk patients helps to evaluate the severity of the underlying coronary artery disease.

VI. Coronary angiography. Coronary angiography is a useful diagnostic procedure in unstable angina. As many as 15% of patients with symptoms of unstable angina may not have coronary artery disease, whereas 10% have left main coronary artery disease, and 30% have three-vessel disease. Coronary angiography is performed in patients at high risk, in patients with recurrent or refractory angina, and in patients with a low tolerance for exercise, to evaluate the feasibility of revascularization.

VII. Antithrombotic therapy. Antithrombotic therapy with aspirin and heparin is now recognized effective therapy of unstable angina. The use of fibrinolytic therapy has been deceptive, with a trend to an increase in the number of ischemic events. Antianginal therapy with nitroglycerin, beta-blockers and calcium antagonists is also routinely used.

A. Platelet inhibitors. Antiplatelet therapy is highly effective in unstable angina. Drugs that have been evaluated are aspirin, ticlopidine, and glycoprotein IIb/IIIa receptor antagonists. Aspirin has been tested during the acute and subacute phases of the disease and also in secondary prevention. A starting dose of 160 to 325 mg is recommended to achieve rapidly full inhibition of thromboxane A_2 generation by platelets, followed by a maintenance dose of 160 mg per day. Ticlopidine and clopidogrel are acceptable alternatives in patients with poor tolerance to aspirin. Tirofiban (Aggrastat) was evaluated in the Platelet Receptor Inhibition for Ischemic Syndrome Management (PRISM) and the Platelet Receptor Inhibition for Ischemic Symptoms (PRISM-PLUS) trials. The drug, directly compared with heparin in the former trial, reduced the risk of recurrent ischemic events by 36% after 48 hours of treatment. The PRISM-PLUS trial documented a significant gain with tirofiban added to intravenous heparin, with a reduction in the risk of death, myocardial infarction, and refractory ischemia, and in the risk of death and myocardial infarction at 7 days. The gain appeared early and was sustained after 6 months. The Platelet Glycoprotein GPIIb/IIIa in Unstable Angina: Receptor Suppression Using Integelin Therapy (PURSUIT) trial involving 9,375 patients documented significant reduction in the rate of death and myocardial infarction with eptifibatide compared with placebo. Benefits have also been observed with abciximab (ReoPro) in patients with refractory ischemia selected on the basis of a culprit coronary artery lesion suitable for coronary angioplasty.

B. Heparin. Intravenous heparin reduces the risk of death, myocardial infarction, refractory ischemia, and silent ST-segment depression during the acute phase of the disease. A weight-adjusted bolus dose of 5,000 U, followed by an infusion of 1,000 U per hour titrated to an activated partial thromboplastin time 2 to 2.5 times control is recommended. The optimal duration of treatment should be

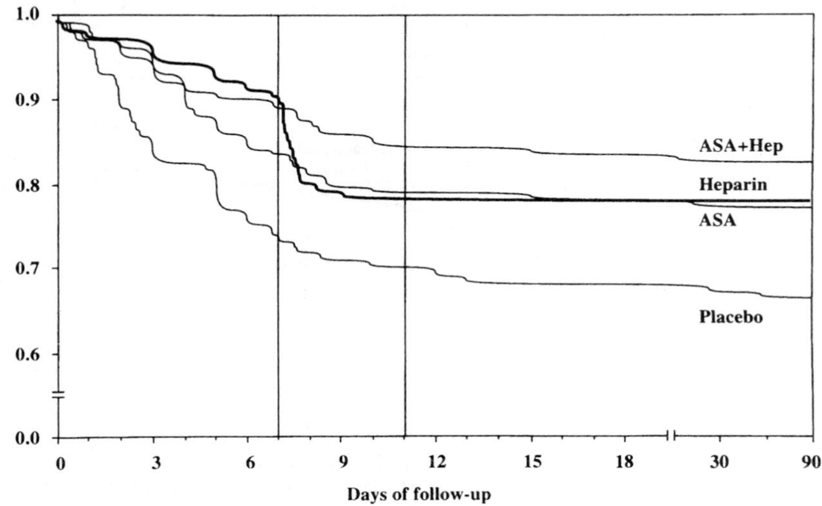

FIG. 31-2. Reactivation of unstable angina after the discontinuation of heparin. The part of the survival curves to the right shows the event rates in patients randomized to placebo, aspirin, heparin, or the combination of aspirin plus heparin. Within the rectangle are the event rates following the discontinuation of study drugs, illustrating a high event rate in the heparin groups. (From *Lancet* 1990;335:615, with permission.)

individualized, from 48 hours in patients with no recurrent angina until after an intervention procedure in patients with persisting symptoms (Fig. 31-2).

C. Direct thrombin inhibitors. Clinical trials have shown excess bleeding with higher doses and lack of efficacy with low doses. The GUSTO-2B trial has shown a benefit of hirudin during drug administration, but the benefits were not sustained long term. Further studies are in progress.

D. Low-molecular-weight heparins. Low-molecular-weight heparins (Fig. 31-3) present distinct advantages over fractionated heparins. These advantages have been well demonstrated in venous disease and are now clearly emerging in unstable angina (Fig. 31.3).

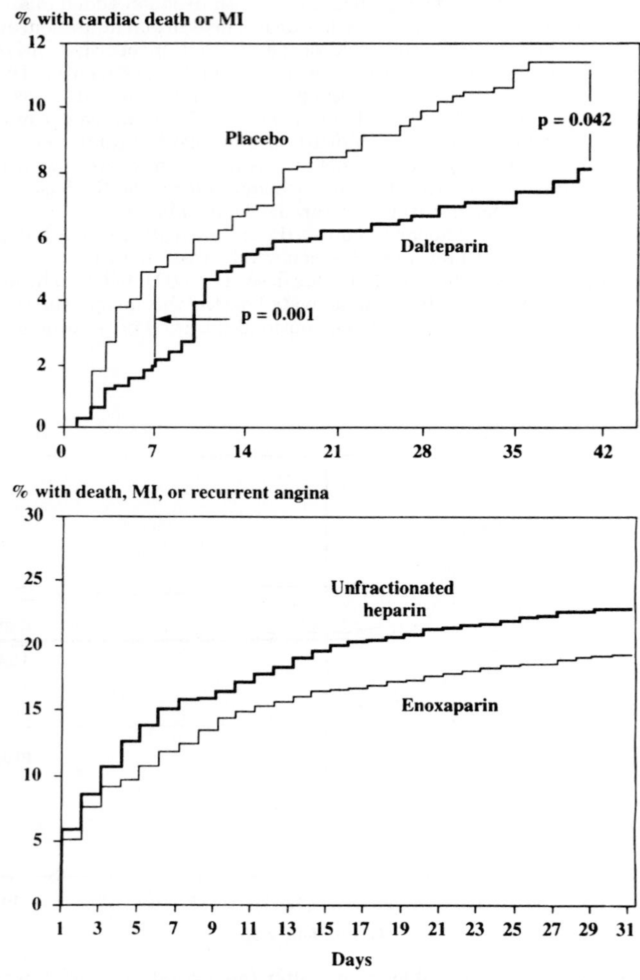

FIG. 31-3. Low-molecular-weight heparins in unstable angina. **Top:** Survival curves of patients randomized to dalteparine or placebo, showing the efficacy of the low-molecular-weight heparin. (From ref. 13, with permission.) **Bottom:** Direct comparison of enoxaparin and unfractionated heparin. (From ref. 14, with permission.)

VIII. Antiischemic therapy

A. Nitroglycerin. Nitroglycerin is widely used in unstable angina, based on a consensus that the drug is effective to prevent recurrent chest pain. It is generally initiated as an intravenous infusion in higher-risk patients. Transdermal or oral administration is adequate in lower-risk patients.

B. Beta-blockers. Beta-blockers preserve myocardial oxygen needs by reducing heart rate, blood pressure, and myocardial contractility and are useful antianginal agents.

C. Calcium antagonists. Calcium antagonists are the treatment of choice, along with nitrates, for the management of Prinzmetal's variant angina. They are also recommended for patients with refractory chest pain and those with contraindications to beta-blockers. Nifedipine should not be used without a beta-blocker.

IX. Medical versus invasive treatment. The two most important randomized trials that have compared surgical versus medical therapy for unstable angina are the National Cooperative Study, published in 1978, and the Veterans Administration Cooperative study, published in 1987. The TIMI-3B study has compared an early invasive strategy to an early conservative strategy. None of the three studies documented that routine surgery (or angioplasty) reduces the rate of fatal and nonfatal myocardial infarction. All three, however, document an important crossover from medical to surgical therapy.

Important subsets of patients in the Veterans Administration Study benefited in the long term from surgery. The 5-year survival in patients with three-vessel disease was 89%, compared with 75% with medical treatment ($p = .02$). Mortality in patients with an ejection fraction between 30% and 49% was reduced from 27% to 14% with surgical intervention. Patients with an ejection fraction of 50% or more did better with medical therapy. On the other hand, a recent study from Scandinavia performed in 2,457 patients has shown a significant reduction in the risk of death and myocardial infarction with routine invasive management per-

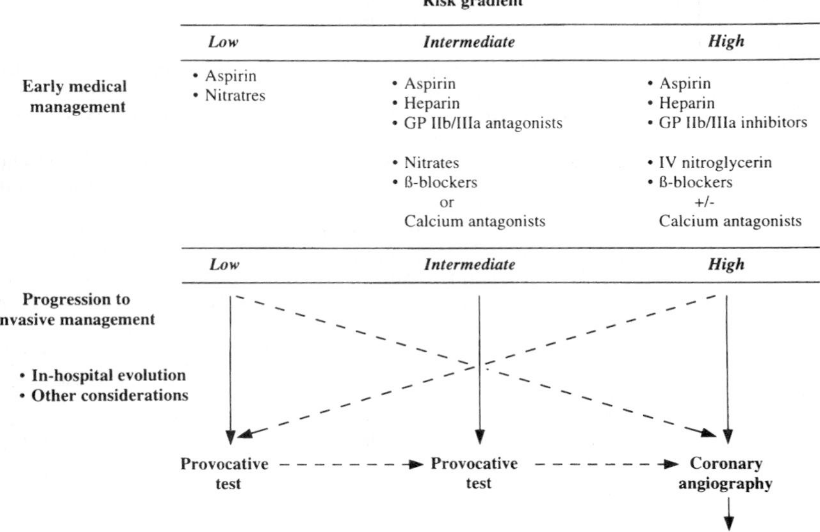

FIG. 31-4. General approach to management of unstable angina, with rapid progression from medical to invasive treatment, by risk, in-hospital evolution, results of provocative testing, and various considerations. The benefits of medical and invasive treatment are often additive.

formed after a minimum of five days of medical therapy including aspirin and dalteparine, a low molecular-weight heparin. Therefore, the best strategy may be individualized to patients' risk and among low-risk patients, the ones in whom risk stratification suggests significant ischemia.

Selected Readings

Braunwald E. Unstable angina: a classification. *Circulation* 1989;80:410.

The Braunwald classification of unstable angina is used widely in clinical practice and provides prognostic and management insights.

CAPTURE Investigators. Randomized placebo-controlled trial of abciximab before and during coronary intervention in refractory unstable angina: the CAPTURE trial. *Lancet* 1997;349:1429.

Abciximab, a platelet glycoprotein IIb/IIIa antagonist, was beneficial among patients with refractory unstable angina when coronary angioplasty was carried out within 12 to 24 hours.

Cohen M, Demers C, Gurfinkel EP, et al for the Efficacy and Safety of Subcutaneous Enoxaparin in Non–Q-Wave Coronary Events Study Group. Low molecular weight heparin versus unfractionated heparin for unstable angina and non–Q-wave myocardial infarction. *N Engl J Med* 1997;337:447.

A large comparative trial of enoxaparin, a low-molecular-weight heparin, and unfractionated heparin showed superiority for the former, reducing the composite outcome of death, myocardia infarction, and refractory angina.

Davies MJ, Thomas AC. Plaque fissuring:the cause of acute myocardial infarction, sudden ischemic death, and crescendo angina. *Br Heart J* 1985;53:363.

The pathophysiology of unstable angina and non–Q-wave myocardial infarction was first described by Davies in a series of elegant studies.

Fragmin and Fast Revascularization during Instability in Coronary Artery Disease (FRISC-2) Investigators. Invasive compared with non-invasive treatment in unstable coronary-artery disease: FRISC II prospective randomized multicenter study. *Lancet* 1999;354:708.

The study has documented a reduction in the risk of death or myocardial infarction in high-risk patients with routine invasive management performed after 5 days of intensive medical therapy.

Hamm CW, Ravkilde J, Gerhardt W, et al. The prognostic value of troponin T in unstable angina. *N Engl J Med* 1992;327:146.

Troponin T is a useful prognostic marker that identifies patients at risk for myocardial infarction and cardiovascular death.

PRISM (Platelet Receptor Inhibition for Ischemic Syndrome Management) Investigators. A comparison of aspirin plus tirofiban with aspirin plus heparin for unstable angina. *N Engl J Med* 1998;338:1498.

The PRISM Trial showed the benefit of tirofiban, a potent platelet antagonist, in the treatment of patients with unstable angina and non–Q-wave myocardial infarction.

PURSUIT (Platelet IIb/IIIa in Unstable Angina: Receptor Suppression Using Integrilin) Investigators. Inhibition of platelet glycoprotein IIb/IIIa with eptifibatide in patients with acute coronary syndromes. *N Engl J Med* 1998;339:436.

The PURSUIT Trial, a global study of patients with acute coronary syndromes, identified benefit when eptifibatide was added to a background of antiischemic and antithrombotic therapy.

TIMI IIIB Investigators. Effects of tissue plasminogen activator and a comparison of early and conservative strategies in unstable angina and non–Q-wave myocardial infarction: results of the TIMI IIIB trial. *Circulation* 1994;89:1545.

A "watchful waiting" approach to patients with unstable angina and non–Q-wave myocardial infarction effectively identifies those at high-risk for recurrent cardiovascular and thrombotic events.

32. COMPLICATED MYOCARDIAL INFARCTION

Christopher P. Cannon, Leonard I. Ganz, Peter H. Stone, and Richard C. Becker

I. General principles. Patient care after acute myocardial infarction (MI) initially focuses on limiting myocardial injury but then turns to preventing, identifying, and treating complications. Most complications and the highest mortality occur in the first months after the acute event (Fig. 32-1); thus, prompt identification and treatment of any established or potential complications are necessary. It has been well established that the proximate cause of acute MI in the most patients is acute coronary occlusion resulting from thrombosis. The sequelae of coronary occlusion are depicted in Fig. 32-2. After a period of prolonged ischemia, myocardial necrosis occurs, leading to myocardial dysfunction and, in some cases, death. Major processes play a significant role in determining the prognosis following acute MI: (a) persistent ischemic jeopardy with the potential for recurrent infarction and further loss of myocardial function; (b) left ventricular (LV) dysfunction occurring either in the acute setting or as part of a more insidious process of LV remodeling; and (c) electrical disturbances that can lead to significant arrhythmias or conduction disorders.

The categories of complications that may follow acute MI are shown in Table 32-1.

II. Recurrent ischemia or infarction. Recurrent ischemic events after acute MI are a major cause of subsequent mortality; therefore, prompt identification and therapy are needed.

A. Incidence and clinical consequences. Recurrent infarction may occur in patients whose initial MI was treated with thrombolytic agents and in those whose MI evolved without such therapy. Reinfarction occurs in 4% to 10% of patients after thrombolytic therapy.

The consequences of reinfarction with regard to short- and long-term mortality are great. In the Multicenter Investigation of Limitation of Infarct Size (MILIS) study, patients who had an infarct extension had an in-hospital mortality more than fourfold higher than patients without an extension (30% versus 7%, $p < .01$). In the TIMI trials, patients who had reinfarction had an approximately 2.5 times higher mortality at 1- to 3-year follow-up compared with those who did not.

B. Prevention. The management of recurrent ischemic events falls into two categories: prevention and treatment of the acute event.

1. Antithrombotic therapy. The first component of antithrombotic therapy is aspirin, which has been shown to be of benefit across the spectrum of ischemic heart disease.

The second component of antithrombotic therapy for prevention of recurrent infarction after MI is heparin. After thrombolytic therapy with tissue-type plasminogen activator (tPA), intravenous unfractionated heparin has been clearly shown to improve infarct-related artery patency. The effect of heparin is greatest when anticoagulation is effective, with a therapeutic activated partial thromboplastin (at least twice times control). Its role after streptokinase administration is less clear.

2. Beta-adrenergic blockade. Beta-blockade in the setting of acute MI and after MI has been studied extensively and has been found almost uniformly to be beneficial.

3. Platelet receptor glycoprotein IIb/IIIa inhibition. In non–ST-segment elevation MI and unstable angina, platelet receptor glycoprotein IIb/IIIa inhibition has been shown to be beneficial.

C. Treatment. After preventive antithrombotic and antiischemic medical therapy, the treatment of an acute ischemic event depends on whether acute reocclusion

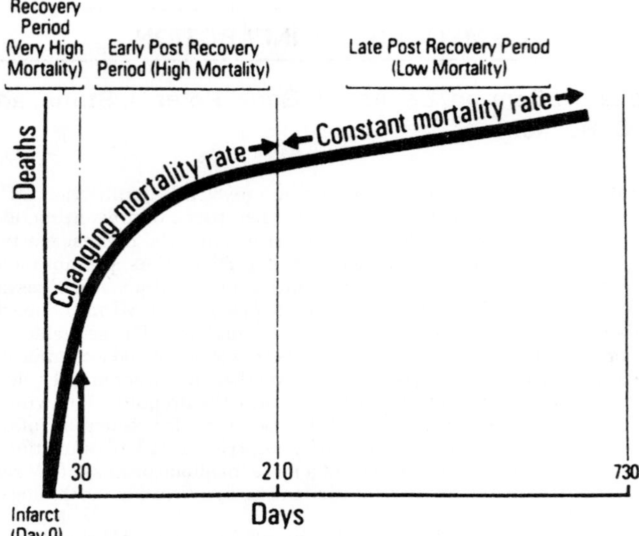

FIG. 32-1. Cumulative mortality after an acute myocardial infarction. (From Sherry S. The Anturane Reinfarction Trial. *Circulation* 1908;62[Suppl 5]:73, with permission. Copyright 1980, American Heart Association.)

is occurring. Figure 32-3 outlines an approach to the acute evaluation and treatment of a recurrent ischemic event.

III. Right ventricular infarction. Right ventricular infarction occurs in 35% to 50% of patients with inferior MI (themselves accounting for over half of all MIs) and therefore requires special diagnostic evaluation and therapy.

A. Identification. The simplest test by which to identify right ventricular infarction uses right precordial electrocardiographic leads placed in the usual positions except beginning in the left second intercoastal space and moving over to the right side of the chest. The acute presence of ST-segment elevation in lead V_{4R} has a sensitivity and specificity of 85% to 90% for the diagnosis of right ventricular infarction. The differential diagnosis for right ventricular

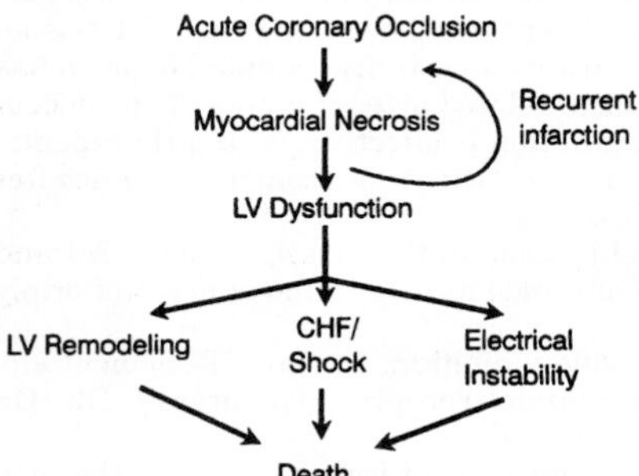

FIG. 32-2. Sequelae of acute myocardial infarction. *CHF,* congestive heart failure; *LV,* left ventricular.

TABLE 32-1. Complications following acute myocardial infarction

1. Recurrent infarction or ischemia
   a. Q wave or non-Q wave
   b. Right ventricular infarction
2. Left ventricular dysfunction
   a. Diastolic dysfunction
   b. Systolic dysfunction
   c. Left ventricular dilation and remodeling
   d. Left ventricular aneurysm
3. Disruption of cardiac structures
   a. Rupture of left ventricular free wall
   b. Rupture of intraventricular septum
   c. Rupture of papillary muscle
4. Miscellaneous
   a. Thromboembolism
   b. Pericarditis
5. Electrical disturbances and conduction disorders
   a. Ventricular arrhythmias
   b. Supraventricular arrhythmias
   c. Conduction disorders and bradyarrhythmias

infarction includes hypotension resulting from LV infarction, pericardial tamponade, constrictive pericarditis, and pulmonary embolism.

B. Clinical manifestations. Initial descriptions of right ventricular infarction focused on hemodynamic complications, namely, decreased performance of the right ventricle with consequent increased filling pressures and isolated right-sided congestion. Jugular venous distention and clear lungs distinguish right ventricular infarction from combined right-and left-sided congestion resulting from LV dysfunction. Systemic hypotension is a frequent complication of right ventricular infarction, in which poor right ventricular output leads to decreased LV filling.

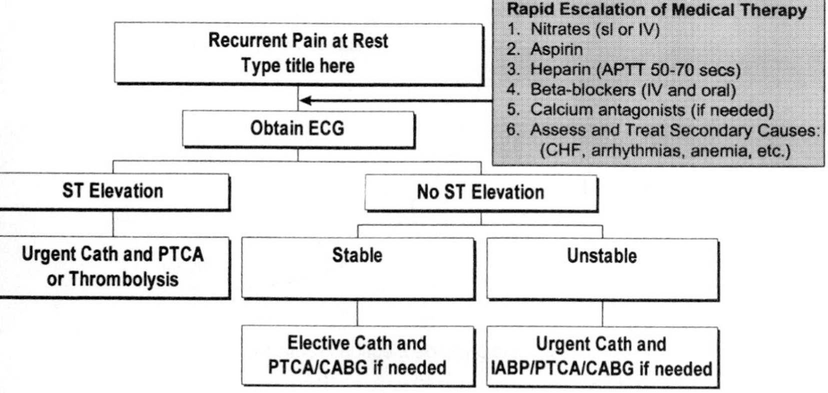

FIG. 32-3. Treatment of recurrent ischemic events.

Atrioventricular or sinoatrial nodal block occurs in 10% to 15% of patients with inferior MI but is particularly prevalent in those with right ventricular infarction; nearly 25% of patients with inferior MI with right ventricular infarction exhibit atrioventricular block, compared with 4% of those without right ventricular infarction.

C. Management. Initial treatment of right ventricular infarction involves early reperfusion therapy directed at limiting infarct size. If hemodynamic compromise is present, measures should be used to increase forward output of the right ventricle. Volume expansion is the mainstay of therapy, with the aim of a right atrial or central venous pressure as high as necessary to fill the LV adequately. A pulmonary artery catheter is essential for optimal management of these patients with combined ventricular failure.

If volume expansion alone does not restore systemic blood pressure to greater than 90 mm Hg, dobutamine or dopamine should be used to increase right ventricular output. In contrast to left-sided heart failure, in right-sided heart failure, venous vasodilators, such as nitrates, should be avoided, because they decrease right ventricular filling pressures and hence output. If hemodynamically significant sinus bradycardia or atrioventricular block develops, temporary ventricular pacing may be necessary.

IV. Left ventricular dysfunction. The most important determinant of prognosis after MI is the degree of LV dysfunction (Fig. 32-4), even when reperfusion with thrombolysis is achieved. The following factors influence residual ventricular function: (a) LV function before the acute MI, (b) infarct size, and (c) location of the MI.

A. Congestive heart failure. The clinical consequence of LV dysfunction is congestive heart failure. There may be systolic dysfunction, manifested by reduced systemic perfusion and evidence of pulmonary congestion, or diastolic dysfunction, manifested by increases in LV filling pressures and pulmonary congestion, but no evidence of reduced systemic perfusion.

1. Diastolic dysfunction. Diastolic dysfunction occurs almost uniformly in patients with acute MI, although it becomes clinically significant in only

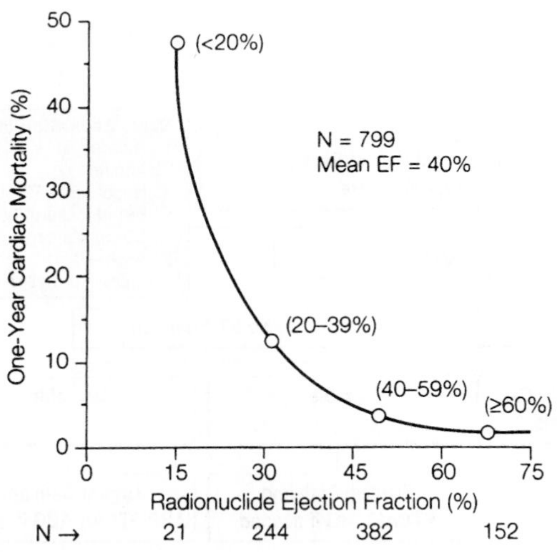

FIG. 32-4. Relationship between left ventricular ejection fraction *(EF)* determined before discharge and 1-year mortality. (From *N Engl J Med* 1983;309:331, with permission.)

one-fourth to one-third of such patients. It is the most common cause of early mild congestive heart failure in the setting of acute MI and can be responsible for acute or flash pulmonary edema.

2. **Treatment.** The treatment goals in patients with diastolic dysfunction include treatment of the pulmonary congestion, which involves diuresis, and treatment of the ischemia.

   Intravenous nitroglycerin has been used widely because it can be rapidly titrated in response to blood pressure. Beta-blockers may be invaluable in patients whose pulmonary congestion is due to isolated diastolic dysfunction. These agents reduce ischemia and thereby improve LV compliance and reduce LV filling pressures.

B. **Systolic dysfunction.** Congestive heart failure resulting from systolic dysfunction is the most serious complication of acute MI. The cause of systolic dysfunction is usually impaired LV contractility from a large MI. Systolic dysfunction, even severe pump failure, may be due to myocardial stunning, not necessarily to frank infarction. Myocardial stunning is a reversible process of myocardial dysfunction resulting from an episode of ischemia (often in border zones surrounding a central zone of infarction). Although necrosis in this ischemic zone does not occur, the dysfunction may persist for days before more normal function is restored.

C. **Cardiogenic shock.** The most malignant end of the spectrum of congestive heart failure is cardiogenic shock, in which congestive heart failure is manifested by frank systemic hypotension and pulmonary congestion. Patients with cardiogenic shock have the highest risk of acute MI.

   The initial treatment goal for patients with severe congestive heart failure is to ensure adequate oxygenation with supplemental oxygen (and endotracheal intubation, if necessary) and to maintain systolic blood pressure at 90 mm Hg or greater, to provide adequate perfusion of vital organs.

   Inotropic agents such as digitalis increase cardiac output associated with a slight decrease in ventricular end-diastolic pressure (preload). Diuretics and nitrates diminish pulmonary congestion, but the patient will have no major improvement in cardiac output. A balanced vasodilator such as nitroprusside reduces both preload and afterload, thereby increasing cardiac output, reducing LV end-diastolic pressure, and alleviating pulmonary congestion. Most effective is administration of both inotropic and vasodilator therapies, with nitroprusside to reduce afterload and dopamine or dobutamine to act as inotropic cardiac stimulants.

   High-risk patients with cardiogenic shock may require insertion of an intraaortic balloon counterpulsation pump as an adjunct in the treatment of severe systolic dysfunction.

   More important in the treatment of patients with cardiogenic shock is reperfusion of the infarct-related artery. Thus, early angiography and mechanical revascularization should be considered.

V. **Disruption of cardiac structures.** Rupture of the myocardial wall is one of the most serious complications of acute MI. Rupture can occur in the free wall, in the intraventricular septum, or in a papillary muscle (Table 32-2). Free wall rupture occurs in approximately 10% of patients who die of acute MI; those at highest risk are women, acutely hypertensive patients, and those with large infarctions. Rupture usually occurs 3 to 5 days after MI but occurs earlier in patients treated with thrombolytic therapy.

VI. **Thromboembolism.** Thromboembolism is a recognized complication of acute MI, occurring in 5% to 10% of patients. Both arterial and venous emboli can occur, with LV mural thrombi accounting for most arterial emboli and right ventricular of deep venous thrombi leading to pulmonary emboli.

VII. **Pericarditis.** Pericardial irritation occurs in approximately one-fourth of patients with acute MI and usually begins 2 to 4 days after MI. It may present as an asymptomatic pericardial effusion, early symptomatic pericarditis with or without effusion, or late pericarditis. Aspirin is given to relieve pain and to decrease

TABLE 32-2. Clinical profile of mechanical complications of acute myocardial infarction

Variable	Ventricular Septal Defect	Free Wall Rupture	Papillary Muscle Rupture
Age (mean, yr)	63	69	65
Days post-MI	3–5	3–5	3–5
Anterior MI	66%	50%	25%
New murmur	90%	25%	50%
Palpable thrill	Yes	No	Rare
Previous MI	25%	25%	30%
Echocardiographic findings 2-D	Visualize defect may have pericardial effusion	—	Flail or prolapsing leaflet
Doppler	Detect shunt	—	Regurgitant jet in LA
PA catheterization	Oxygen stepup in RV	Equalization of diastolic	Prominent V wave in PCW pressure tracing
Incidence	2%–4%	≤10%	1%
Mortality			
Medical	90%	90%	90%
Surgical	50%	Case reports	40%–90%

LA, left atrium; MI, myocardial infarction; PA, pulmonary artery; PCW, pulmonary capillary wedge, RV, right ventricle; 2-D, two dimensional. From Pasternak RC, Braunwald E, Sobel BE. Acute myocardial infarction. In: Braunwald E, ed. *Heart disease,* 4th ed. Philadelphia: WB Saunders, 1992;1257; and Labovitz AJ, et al. Mechanical complications of acute myocardial infarction. *Cardiovasc Rev Rep* 1984; 5:948, with permission.

inflammation; up to 650 mg every 4 hours may be required. Other nonsteroidal antiinflammatory medications relieve pain but may lead to infarct thinning.

VIII. Electrical disturbances

A. Arrhythmias complicating myocardial infarction. Cardiac arrhythmias are an important complication during acute MI. In the prehospital phase, ventricular tachycardia and fibrillation probably account for the majority of sudden deaths. Tachyarrhythmias and bradyarrhythmias are frequently seen in the in-hospital phase of acute MI. Arrhythmias in the setting of acute MI may be due to reentry, abnormal automaticity, or conduction block; these mechanisms are modulated by ischemia, LV failure, and variations in autonomic tone (Tables 32-3 and 32-4).

B. Indications for pacemaker placement during myocardial infarction. Whether a temporary pacemaker is necessary during acute MI is a function of the particular conduction disturbance and its hemodynamic sequelae, as well as the site of infarction (Table 32-5).

Patients who manifest continued symptomatic bradycardia, atrioventricular block, or permanent complete (third-degree) heart block after acute MI should generally receive a permanent pacemaker before hospital discharge. Patients with permanent bundle branch block and transient Mobitz II second-degree or third-degree atrioventricular block should also undergo permanent pacemaker implantation. When the need for permanent pacing is less clear, and the level of atrioventricular block is uncertain (i.e., intranodal versus infranodal), a limited electrophysiology study may be undertaken, with permanent pacemaker implantation if infranodal block is demonstrated.

TABLE 32-3. Arrhythmias during acute myocardial infarction

Category	Arrhythmia	Objective of Therapy	Therapeutic Options
Ventricular tachyarrhythmias	Ventricular fibrillation	Urgent reversion to sinus rhythm	Defibrillation; lidocaine; amiodarone; bretylium
	Ventricular tachycardia	Restoration of hemodynamic stability	Cardioversion/defibrillation; lidocaine; procainamide; amiodarone
	Accelerated idioventricular rhythm	Observation unless hemodynamic compromise	Atropine; atrial pacing
	Ventricular premature beats	None	Observation
Supraventricular tachyarrhythmias	Sinus tachycardia	Reduction of heart rate to diminish myocardial work/oxygen demand	Identify and treat underlying cause; beta-blockers
	Atrial fibrillation/flutter	Reduction of ventricular rate; restoration of sinus rhythm	Cardioversion if unstable; beta-blockers, calcium blockers; digoxin; rapid atrial pacing (for flutter); consider antiarrhythmic therapy
	Paroxysmal supraventricular tachycardia	Reduction of ventricular rate; restoration of sinus rhythm	Vagal maneuvers; adenosine; beta-blockers, calcium blockers; cardioversion if unstable
	Nonparoxysmal junctional tachycardia	Search for precipitating cause (e.g., digitalis toxicity); observation unless hemodynamic compromise	Consider overdrive atrial pacing; consider suppressive antiarrhythmic therapy
Bradyarrhythmias and conduction disturbances	Sinus bradycardia	Increased heart rate only if hemodynamic compromise	Atropine; temporary pacing
	Junctional escape rhythm	Increased heart rate only if hemodynamic compromise	Atropine; temporary pacing
	Atrioventricular block or intraventricular conduction block	Increased heart rate; prophylax against progression to high-grade atrioventricular block	Atropine; aminophylline; ventricular pacing

From Ganz LI, Antman EM. Cardiac arrhythmias during acute myocardial infarction, in: Antman EM, Rutherford JD, eds. *Coronary care medicine: a practical approach,* 2nd ed. Boston: Martinus Nijhoff, in press. Reprinted with permission by Kluwer Academic Publishers.

TABLE 32-4. Intravenous antiarrhythmic drug dosing during acute myocardial infarction

Drug	Bolus	Infusion
Lidocaine	1.0–1.5 mg/kg initially; additional boluses (0.5–0.75 mg/kg every 5–10 min) as necessary to control VT/VF to maximum total load (3.0 mg/kg)	1–4 mg/min
Procainamide	17 mg/kg (maximum 1000 mg) over 15–30 min, monitoring blood pressure	1–4 mg/min
Amiodarone	150 mg over 10 min, monitoring blood pressure	1 mg/min for 6h, then 0.5 mg/min
Bretylium	5 mg/kg initially; additional boluses (10 mg/kg every 5–10 min) as necessary to control VT/VF to maximum total load (35 mg/kg)	1–2 mg/min

VT/VF, ventricular tachycardia/ventricular fibrillation.

TABLE 32-5. Intraventricular block during acute myocardial infarction

	Incidence	Progression to CHB	Management
LAHB	3%–5%	Low	Observe
LPHB	1%–2%	Low	Observe
RBBB	2%–5%	Low	Observe
LBBB	4%–5%	Moderate	Consider temporary pacemaker
RBBB with 1° AVB		Moderate	Consider temporary pacemaker
LBBB with 1° AVB		Moderate–high	Temporary pacemaker
RBBB/LAHB	4.0%	High	Temporary pacemaker
RBBB/LPHB	0.8%	High	Temporary pacemaker
Trifascicular block		High	Temporary pacemaker
Alternating BBB		High	Temporary pacemaker

AVB, atrioventricular block; BBB, bundle branch block; CHB, complete heart block; LAHB, left anterior hemiblock; LBBB, left bundle branch block; LPHB, left posterior hemiblock; RBBB, right bundle branch block.

Selected Readings

Becker RC, Gore JM, Lambrew C, et al. A composite view of cardiac rupture in the United States National Registry of Myocardial Infarction. *J Am Coll Cardiol* 1996;27:1321.

Cardiac rupture, although relatively rare, is responsible for 10% to 15% of all deaths after MI. Thrombolytic therapy accelerates the occurrence of rupture, at times within 24 hours of treatment.

Cannon CP. Optimizing the treatment of unstable angina. *J Thromb Thrombolysis* 1995;2:205.

The treatment of unstable angina includes a full complement of antiischemic and antithrombotic therapies.

Cannon CP, Sharis PJ, Schweiger MJ, et al. Prospective validation of a composite end point in thrombolytic trial of acute myocardial infarction (TIMI 4 and 5). *Am J Cardiol* 1997;80:696.

In the TIMI-4 and TIMI-5 trials, the validation of a composite end point was established and was used to determine the predictors of an adverse outcome after MI.

Loh E, Sutton MS, Wun CC, et al. Ventricular dysfunction and the risk of stroke after myocardial infarction. *N Engl J Med* 1997;336:251.

The risk of thromboembolism following MI is influenced by ventricular performance. An LV ejection fraction of less than 35% increases the risk of stroke, and, therefore, long-term anticoagulant therapy should be considered.

Muller JE, Rude RE, Braunwald E, et al. Myocardial infarct extension: occurrence, outcome, and risk factors in the Multi-center Investigation of Limitation of Infarct Size. *Ann Intern Med* 1988;108:1.

MILIS, a landmark study, provided pivotal insights that paved the way for trials of thrombolytic therapy.

TIMI Study Group. Comparison of invasive and conservative strategies after treatment with intravenous tissue plasminogen activator in acute myocardial infarction: results of the Thrombolysis in Myocardial Infarction (TIMI) phase II trial. *N Engl J Med* 1989;320:618.

The rate and clinical relevance of reinfarction after MI was determined in the TIMI phase II trial.

33. REPERFUSION THERAPY FOR ACUTE MYOCARDIAL INFARCTION: DECISIONS, INDICATIONS, AND MANAGEMENT

Richard C. Becker, Mrinal Sharma, and Frederick A. Spencer

I. General principles. According to the World Health Organization definition, the diagnosis of myocardial infarction (MI) is based on at least two of the following three criteria: (a) a clinical history of ischemic-type chest discomfort, (b) changes on one or more surface electrocardiograms (ECGs), and (c) a characteristic rise and fall in serum cardiac markers that reflect myocardial cell damage.

A. Progress in the management of ST-segment elevation infarction. Most patients with ST-segment elevation MI have occlusive coronary arterial thrombosis that develops at a site of atherosclerotic plaque erosion or rupture. There is little question that prompt restoration of coronary blood flow and of myocardial perfusion limits infarct size, preserves ventricular function, and reduces mortality.

B. Prognostic importance of ventricular performance in myocardial infarction. Left ventricular dysfunction, determined clinically (S_3 gallop, rales, elevated jugular venous pressure), radiographically (pulmonary edema), or with contrast ventriculography, radionuclide ventriculography, or by ECG (increased end-systolic volume, reduced ejection fraction), has been demonstrated to be among the most accurate predictors of cardiac events in both the prereperfusion and reperfusion eras.

The Thrombolysis in Myocardial Infarction (TIMI) investigators established a risk score that predicted the occurrence of in-hospital adverse outcomes. Predictors of early (30-day) mortality were also established by the Global Utilization of Streptokinase and TPA for Occluded Coronary Arteries (GUSTO-1) Investigators. Increasing Killip class (i.e., worsening ventricular performance) was strongly associated with early death (Table 33-1). Similar observations were made in the National Registry of Myocardial Infarction (NRMI-2) that included over 250,000 patients (Table 33-2).

C. Open vessel hypothesis. The open vessel hypothesis states that early reperfusion results in myocardial salvage, which preserves ventricular performance and ultimately is responsible for improved patient survival.

II. Ventricular performance in trials of coronary thrombosis

A. Thrombolytic therapy versus placebo. Several trials performed in the early thrombolytic era determined the impact of reperfusion therapy on left ventricular performance (Table 33-3).

B. Comparative trials of tissue-type plasminogen activator and streptokinase. The most recent (and perhaps the final) comparative trial of tissue-type plasminogen activator (tPA) (accelerated or front-loaded dosing) and streptokinase was performed by the GUSTO Investigators. The major finding of GUSTO was that accelerated tPA resulted in 10 additional lives saved per 1,000 patients treated. This corresponds to a 1% absolute or 14% relative reduction in 30-day mortality. The reduction in mortality is highly statistically significant, whether compared with the streptokinase arms combined ($p = .001$) or separately ($p = .009$ for subcutaneous heparin, $p = .003$ for intravenous heparin) (Table 33-4).

III. Coronary arterial patency and patient outcome

A. Importance of time to treatment. Because achievement of early infarct-related artery (IRA) patency has been shown to be the most important goal in early acute MI management, treatment must be initiated without delay. The TIMI-II trial found that for each hour earlier that a patient was treated, there was a 1% absolute decrease in mortality, translating into an additional 10 lives saved per 1,000 patients treated.

TABLE 33-1. Demographic and clinical predictors of 30-day mortality: GUSTO-1 trial

Subgroups	30-day Mortality (%)
Sex	
Male	5.7
Female	11.1
Age	
<60 yr	2.4
60–75 yr	8.3
>75 yr	20.5
Infarct location	
Anterior	10.0
Inferior	5.0
Killip class	
I	5.1
II	13.9
III	32.7
IV	57.8

GUSTO, Global Utilization of Streptokinase and tPA for Occluded Coronary Arteries: phase I trial. (Adapted from Lee KL, Woodlief LH, Topol EJ, et al for the GUSTO-1 Investigators. Predictors of 30-day mortality in the era of reperfusion for acute myocardial infarction: results from an International trial of 41,021 patients. *Circulation* 1995;91:1659, with permission.)

B. Speeding the door-to-reperfusion time. Initial reports indicated that the use of MI protocols or pathways markedly reduced door-to-reperfusion times. To aid hospitals in their efforts to improve, the NHAAP Coordinating Committee coined the term *the 4 Ds: Door, Data, Decision,* and *Drug* times (Fig. 33-1). These are the four critical time points in evaluating the patient for reperfusion therapy: the time between hospital arrival (door), ECG acquisition (data), assessment of eligibility for thrombolysis (decision), and administration of thrombolytic therapy (drug). Using the 4 Ds has been extremely useful in reducing in-hospital treatment delays, as evidenced by several reports.

TABLE 33-2. National Registry of Myocardial Infarction (NRMI-2) risk assessment assignment: predictors of a poor in-hospital clinical outcome

Risk Characteristic	Odds ratio (95% CI) for adverse outcome[a]
Killip IV	4.46 (3.70–5.39)
Systolic blood pressure <100 mm Hg and heart rate >100 BPM	2.0 (1.61–2.47)
Killip III	1.59 (1.41–1.78)
Age >70 yr	1.42 (1.02–1.97)
Killip II	1.41 (1.32–1.52)
ST segment elevation (first ECG)	1.32 (1.23–1.42)
Anterior site of infarction	1.23 (1.10–1.30)
Prior myocardial infarction	1.10 (1.03–1.17)

[a]Risk of recurrent ischemia, recurrent MI, myocardial infarction, total stroke, major bleeding, death. BPM, beats per minute; CI, confidence interval; ECG, electrocardiogram. (From Bedson RC, Burns SM, Gore JM. Early identification and in-hospital management of patients with acute myocardial infarction at risk for adverse outcomes: a nationwide perspective of routine clinical practice. *Am Heart J* 1998;135:786, with permission.)

TABLE 33-3. Left ventricular performance in early thrombolytic therapy trials

Trial	n	Time to Treatment (hours)	End Point	Assessment Method	Time Assessed	Ejection fraction (%)		
						tPA	Placebo	p value
Guerci et al.	138	<4	LVEF	Gated blood pool scan, rest/exercise	Day 10	53.2	46.4	<.03
National Australian	144	≤4	Global EF	Contrast ventriculogram	Day 5–7	57.7	51.7	.04
TICO	145	<2.4	Global EF	Contrast ventriculogram	Day 21	61	54	.006
ECSG	721	<5	Global EF	Contrast ventriculogram	Day 10–22	50.7	48.5	.04
TPAT	115	≤3.75	Global EF	Radionuclide ventriculogram	Early	49.1	45.4	
					Day 9	53.6	47.8	.017
			Regional wall motion		Early	33.9	32.2	
					Day 9	43.0	36.0	

ECSG, European Cooperative Study Group; EF, ejection fraction; LVEF, left ventricular ejection fraction; TICO, Thrombolysis in Acute Coronary Occlusion; tPA, tissue-type plasminogen activator; TPAT, Tissue Plasminogen Activator-Toronto.

TABLE 33-4. Major clinical outcomes by treatment group: GUSTO-1 trial

	Streptokinase + Subcutaneous heparin (n = 9,796)	Streptokinase + Intravenous heparin (n = 10,377)	Accel. tPA + Intravenous heparin (n = 10,344)	tPA + Streptokinase + Intravenous heparin (n = 10,328)	p
24-h mortality	2.8%	2.9%	2.3%	2.8%	.0005
30-d mortality	7.2%	7.4%	6.3%	7.0%	.001
30-d death or nonfatal disabling stroke	7.7%	7.9%	6.9%	7.6%	.0006

Accel, accelerated; tPA, tissue-type plasminogen activator. p values are for comparisons of accelerated tPA versus both streptokinase groups combined. (Adapted from GUSTO Investigators. An international randomized trial comparing four thrombolytic strategies for acute myocardial infarction. *N Engl J Med* 1993;329:673–682.

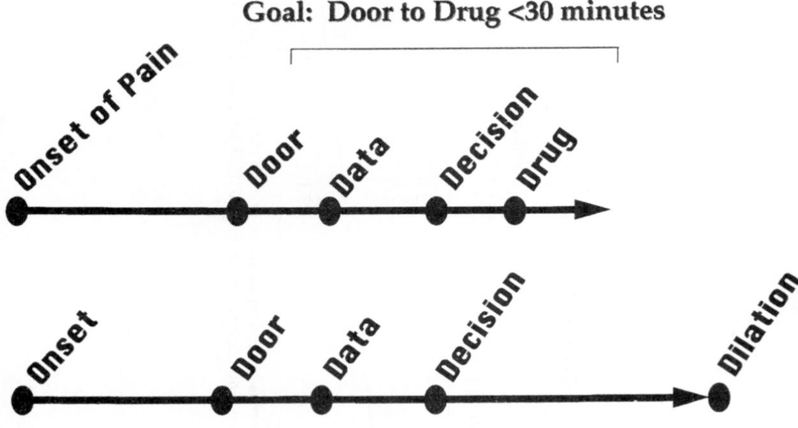

FIG. 33-1. The National Heart Attack Alert Program's (NHAAP) Four D's, designed to reduce time to myocardial perfusion, can be applied on a nationwide basis to treatment algorithms for thrombolytic therapy as well as primary angioplasty.

The University of Massachusetts—Memorial Medical Center, like many other institutions, has endorsed the Time-to-Treatment Continuous Quality Improvement Flowsheet (Fig. 33-2) that can be used to track individual hospital performance and to reduce treatment delays.

C. Time-independent benefit of coronary arterial patency. The open vessel hypothesis can be viewed from two unique perspectives. The first is a time-dependent benefit derived from early coronary arterial reperfusion and myocardial salvage. The second is "time independent" of myocardial salvage and reflects the importance of vessel patency on the detrimental process of ventricular remodeling after infarction (Table 33-5).

D. Thrombolysis in clinical practice. Thrombolytic therapy has been used in the clinical arena to treat a wide variety of venous and arterial thromboembolic disorders.

1. **Streptokinase.** Streptokinase is a nonenzymatic protein produced by beta-hemolytic streptococci. It activates the fibrinolytic system indirectly by forming a 1:1 stoichiometric complex with plasminogen, which then activates plasminogen, converting it to the active enzyme plasmin.
2. **Urokinase.** Urokinase is a trypsinlike serine protease composed of two polypeptide chains, connected by a disulfide bridge. It activates plasminogen directly and converts it to the active enzyme plasmin.
3. **APSAC.** Streptokinase and the plasminogen-streptokinase activator complex are cleared rapidly from the circulation, with half-lives of 15 and 3 minutes, respectively. By temporarily blocking the active center of plasminogen, the plasma half-life can be prolonged substantially.
4. **scu-PA (single-chain urokinaselike plasminogen activator).** scu-PA is a single-chain glycoprotein containing 411 amino acids, which can be converted to urokinase by hydrolysis of the Lys148-149 peptide bond.
5. **Tissue-type plasminogen activator.** Native tPA is a serine protease composed of one polypeptide chain containing 527 amino acids. On limited plasmic action, the molecule is converted to a double-chain activator linked by

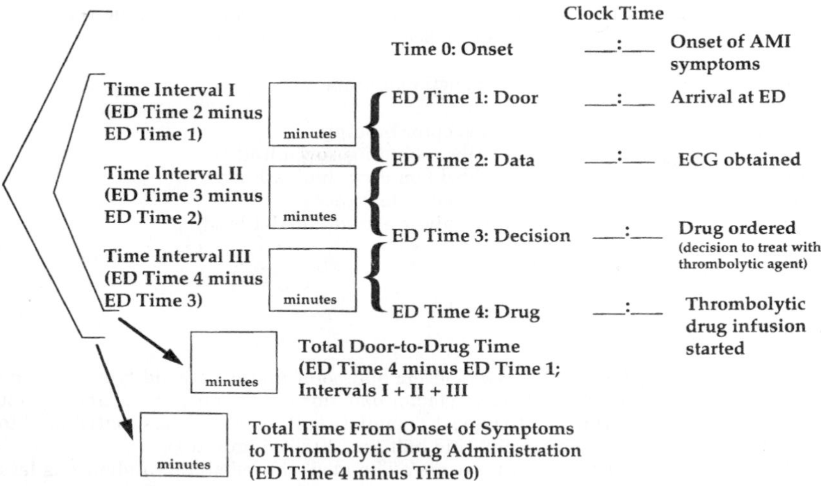

FIG. 33-2. Time-to-treatment flow sheets provide a means to document on-site performance and to reduce treatment delays.

one disulfide bond. This occurs by cleavage of the Arg 275-Ile 276 peptide bond yielding a heavy chain (M_r 31,000) derived from the amino terminal part of the molecule and a light chain (M_r 28,000) comprising the carboxy terminal region. The high affinity of tPA for plasminogen in the presence of fibrin thus allows efficient activation on the fibrin clot, whereas no efficient plasminogen activation by tPA occurs in plasma (Table 33-6).

6. **New-generation thrombolytic agents.** Several mutants, hybrids, and variants of existing thrombolytic agents have been developed and are currently undergoing evaluation (Table 33-7).

   Reteplase (r-PA) is a deletion mutant that contains the Kringle-2 and protease domains of the parent tPA molecule. It has a prolonged half-life (18 minutes) and is given in two abbreviated intravenous infusions (2 minutes) 30 minutes apart. Reteplase is a thrombolytic approved by the United States Food and Drug Administration for the treatment of acute MI and is marketed under the name Retevase.

   Tenecteplase (TNK-tPA) is a multiple point mutation of the parent tPA molecule. In its mutant form, T103N, N117Q, KHRR (296–299), AAAA, threonine 103 has been changed to asparagine 103, creating a new glycosylation site (and a longer half-life). It is administered as a single intravenous bolus.

TABLE 33-5. Proposed mechanisms supporting the open-artery hypothesis: "time independent"

Effect on post-MI LV remodeling
Effect on infarct healing
Electrophysiologic effect
Perfusion of hibernating myocardium
Collateral blood supply to distant ischemic myocardium

LV, left ventricle; MI, myocardial infarction.

TABLE 33-6. Structure-function relationship of the wild-type tissue-type plasminogen activator molecule

Domain/region	Functional property
Kringle-1	Receptor binding
Kringle-2	Fibrin binding (low affinity)
Fibronectin finger	Fibrin binding (high affinity)
Epidermal growth factor	Hepatic clearance
Protease	Catalytic activity; PAI-1 binding

PAI-1, plasminogen activator inhibitor-1.

Lanoteplase (n-PA) is a deletion and point mutant of wild-type tPA. The finger and epidermal growth factor domains have been deleted, and a point mutation within the Kringle-1 domain ($Asn^{117} \rightarrow Gln^{117}$) has contributed to the molecule's long circulating half-life (30 to 45 minutes).

E. Thrombolysis or no thrombolysis? The ideal thrombolytic candidate is less than 75 years of age, is within 6 hours of chest pain onset, has ST-segment elevation in two or more anatomically contiguous ECG leads (or a new left bundle branch block) (Fig. 33-3), and has no absolute contraindications to treatment (Table 33-8).

IV. Noninvasive assessment of coronary arterial reperfusion. Rapid and effective assessment of coronary arterial patency is vital to the treatment of MI. Although coronary angiography is the current standard, cardiac catheterization laboratories are not widely available, and routine coronary angiography has not been shown to be vital component of early management strategies (Table 33-9).

TABLE 33-7. New thrombolytics being investigated for the treatment of acute myocardial infarction

r-PA
- Deletion mutant tPA (K_2 and protease domains preserved)
- Prolonged half-life (18 minutes): bolus dosing
- Reduced fibrin affinity
- Produced in *Escherichia coli*

TNK-tPA
- Multiple point mutation tPA
- Prolonged half-life (18 minutes): bolus dosing
- High fibrin specificity
- Resistant to PAI-1
- Produced in Chinese hamster ovary cells

n-PA
- Deletion and point mutation tPA (K_1, K_2, protease domains preserved; $Asn^{117} \rightarrow Gln^{117}$
- Prolonged half-life (30–45 min): bolus dosing
- Reduced fibrin affinity
- Produced in Chinese hamster ovary cells

n-PA, novel plasminogen activator.
r-PA, recombinant plasminogen activator.
tNK-tPA, TNK tissue plasminogen activator.

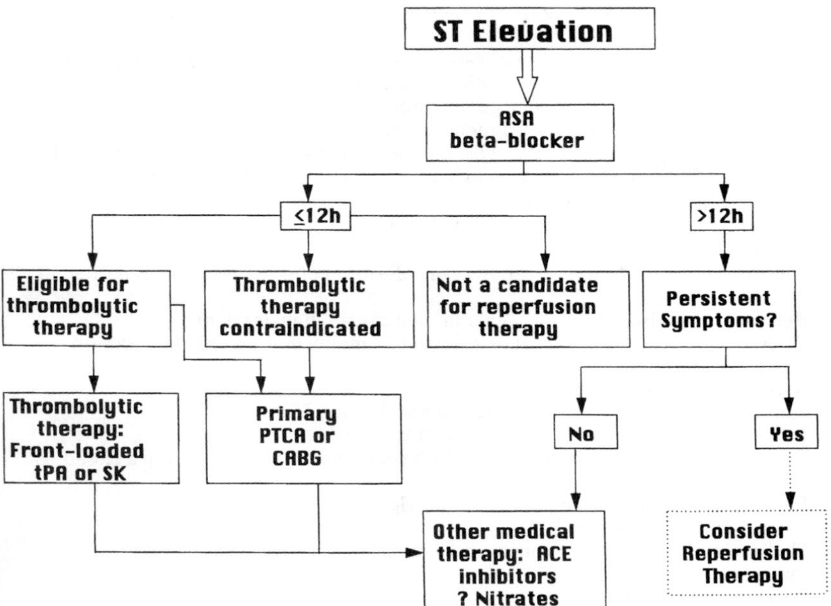

FIG. 33-3. Recommended management algorithm for patients with ST-segment elevation myocardial infarction. This approach can also be applied to patients with new (or presumably new) left bundle branch block. *ACE,* angiotensin-converting enzyme; *ASA,* aspirin; *CABG,* coronary artery bypass grafting; *PTCA,* percutaneous transluminal coronary angioplasty; *SK,* streptokinase; *tPA,* tissue-type plasminogen activator.

A. Symptoms. Rapid relief of chest pain is the earliest symptom-related marker suggesting that reperfusion has occurred. Although relief of chest pain is still considered a *sine qua non* of coronary reperfusion, few patients with angiographically confirmed patency can be identified by symptom relief alone.

B. Electrocardiography

1. **ST-segment elevation.** The magnitude of ST-segment elevation (and reciprocal ST-segment depression) on the admission ECG is a marker of infarct size and in-hospital mortality. The overall ST-segment area is also a predictor of early clinical outcome. Accordingly, the degree of ST-segment resolution on a routine 12-lead ECG may be a readily available tool for assessing coronary arterial reperfusion. A substudy of the International Joint Efficacy Comparison of Thrombolytics (INJECT) trial supports the strong predictive value of ST-segment resolution (Fig. 33-4). Patients without resolution had a high 35-day mortality (17.5%) compared with those with partial (4.3%) and complete resolution (2.5%).
2. **T-wave evolution.** Successful reperfusion accelerates the ECG evolution of infarction. Early (within 24 hours) inversion of T waves is predictive of angiographic patency, preserved ventricular function, and a lower incidence of in-hospital adverse events.

C. Arrhythmias associated with reperfusion. Accelerated idioventricular rhythms and late diastolic ventricular systoles are common reperfusion-related arrhythmias, occurring in 60% to 80% of patients. However, they lack specificity and

TABLE 33-8. Patient selection criteria for thrombolytic therapy

Eligibility criteria; chest pain or chest-pain–equivalent syndrome consistent with AMI ≤12 h from symptom onset with ECG showing:
- ≥1-mm ST elevation in ≥2 contiguous limb leads
- ≥2-mm ST elevation in ≥2 contiguous precordial leads
- New LBBB (or presumed new) with ST elevation (>5 mm) discordant with QRS complex, ≥1 mm ST depression in V_1, V_2, V_3, and/or ST-segment elevation ≥1 mm concordant with QRS complex
- New or preexisting RBBB with ST elevation

Contraindications
- Absolute contraindications: require consideration of an alternative reperfusion strategy
- Active internal bleeding (e.g., melena, hematuria, hemoptysis)
- Known spinal cord or cerebral arteriovenous malformation or tumor, recent lumbar puncture
- Recent head trauma (2 mo)
- Known previous hemorrhagic cerebrovascular accident
- Intracranial or intraspinal surgery within 6 mo
- Trauma or surgery within 2 weeks (which could result in bleeding into a closed space)
- Persistent blood pressure >180/110 mm Hg
- Known bleeding disorder
- Mediastinal lymphoma or cancer metastatic to pericardium
- Pregnancy
- Suspected aortic dissection
- Previous allergy to a streptokinase product (not a contraindication to the use of other thrombolytic agents)

Relative contraindications
- Mitral valve disease with chronic atrial fibrillation (risk of partial lysis and embolization of atrial thrombus)
- Within 1 yr of ischemic or embolic cerebrovascular accident (CVA); however, if moderate or severe residual neurologic deficit, alternative reperfusion strategies should be considered
- Major trauma or surgery within 2 mo
- History of chronic, uncontrolled hypertension (diastolic ≥110 mm Hg), treated or untreated
- Subclavian or internal jugular venous cannulation
- Recent (within 7 d) major organ biopsy
- Menstruation not a contraindication

AMI, acute myocardial infarction; LBBB, left bundle branch block; RBBB, right bundle branch block.

should not be used independently to assess coronary patency. On the other hand, bradyarrhythmias, particularly when accompanied by systemic hypotension (Bezold-Jarisch reflex), may be a useful marker of reperfusion involving the right coronary artery.

V. Coronary angiography:timing and clinical indications. Because investigators have established that early reperfusion limits infarct size and preserves myocardial function, and optimal patient outcome is influenced strongly by the ability of existing therapies to establish physiologic myocardial perfusion, coronary angiography remains an important tool for practicing clinicians (Table 33-10).

VI. Coronary angioplasty: primary and adjunctive use

A. Primary coronary angioplasty. Over the past decade, coronary angioplasty has been increasingly used in the treatment of patients with acute MI. Because

TABLE 33-9. Biochemical markers of coronary arterial reperfusion: creatine kinase and its isoforms

Biochemical Marker	Rate of Rise or Peak Level[a]	Assay	Procedure Time (minutes)
Creatine kinase	<4 h	Radioimmunoassay	>60
MB-creatine kinase	90 mins; >2.4-fold increase above baseline	Radioimmunoassay	>60
		Immunofunctional assay	<15
MB isoform	120 mins; MB_2/MB_1 ratio >3.8 above baseline	High-voltage electrophoresis	25
MM isoform	120 mins; MM_3 (total) MM_3/MM_1, ratio	Minicolumn chromatofocusing	<60

[a]From treatment initiation.

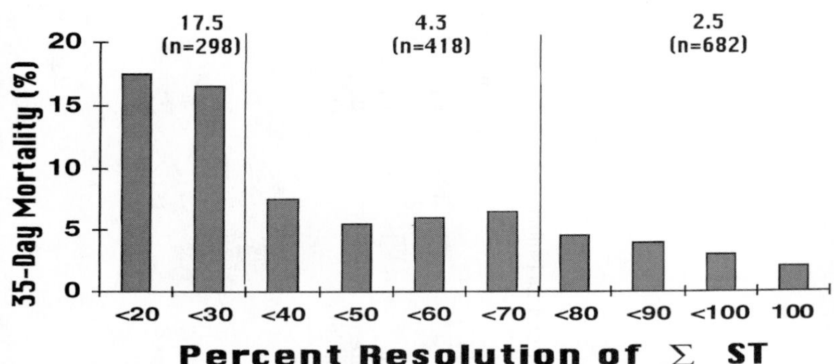

FIG. 33-4. Coronary arterial reperfusion after thrombolytic administration can be determined by noninvasive means. Resolution of ST-segment elevation (70% or greater) within 180 minutes of treatment initiation is associated with a low mortality. (Adapted from International Joint Efficacy Comparison of Thrombolytics. Randomized, double-blind comparison of Reteplase double bolus administration with streptokinase in acute myocardial infarction [INJECT]. *Lancet* 346:329, 1995, with permission.)

interventional capabilities are *not* immediately available in most hospitals, it is important to review the indications as determined by the results of randomized clinical trials and the experience gained from large-scale registries. Rather than being viewed as adversaries, coronary angioplasty and thrombolysis should be considered treatment alternatives to be used as indicated to optimize patient care (Fig. 33-5).

B. Delayed coronary angioplasty. Several clinical trials have addressed the role of routine predischarge coronary angioplasty. In clinical practice, particularly within centers that routinely perform predischarge coronary angiography, the tendency to dilate vessels with more than 70% stenosis is commonplace. Although recurrent episodes of myocardial ischemia may be reduced after this practice, no evidence indicates that the incidence of either death or nonfatal reinfarction is lessened.

TABLE 33-10. Coronary angiography in myocardial infarction

Timing	Potential Indications
Immediate	Diagnosis of MI in question Contraindication to thrombolytics Hemodynamic compromise
Early	Failed thrombolysis Recurrent symptoms, ST-segment elevation (threatened reinfarction) Hemodynamic compromise
Urgent	Recurrent myocardial ischemia, spontaneous or provoked
Deferred	Recurrent myocardial ischemia, spontaneous or provoked
Routine	Risk stratification Early discharge protocol ? Reduce cost

MI, myocardial infarction.

Patient with Suspected Acute Myocardial Infarction

Coronary Thrombolysis

Benefits

•Widescale availability
•Ease of administration
•Proven benefit in large-sclae clinical trials
•Short door to drug time

Limitations

•Suboptimal TIMI 3 flow rates
•Procoagulant state
•Hemorrhage rates relatively high

Primary Angioplasty

Benefits

•High TIMI 3 flow rates
•Define coronary anatomy
•Reduced mortality in cardiogenic shock
•Low intracerebral
•hemorrhage rate

Limitations

•Not widely available
•Repeat procedures common
•Prolonged "door to balloon time" in many centers

FIG. 33-5. The potential benefits and limitations of coronary thrombolysis and primary angioplasty in the treatment of patients with suspected acute myocardial infarction.

Selected Readings

Becker RC, Burns M, Gore JM for the National Registry of Myocardial Infarction Investigators. Early identification and in-hospital management of patients with acute myocardial infarction at risk for adverse outcomes: a nation-wide perspective of routine clinical practice. *Am Heart J* 1998; 135:786.
The NRMI-2 Database was used to identify patients at risk for adverse outcomes as well as routine management strategies.

DeWood MA, Spores J, Notske R, et al. Prevalence of total coronary occlusion during the early hours of transmural myocardial infarction. *N Engl J Med* 1980;303:897.
A landmark study documenting the occurrence of coronary occlusion in patients with acute MI.

GUSTO Investigators. An international randomized trial comparing four thrombolytic strategies for acute myocardial infarction. *N Engl J Med* 1993; 329:673.
In GUSTO-1, accelerated tPA was found to be superior to streptokinase in the management of patients with ST-segment elevation MI.

International Joint Efficacy Comparison of Thrombolytics. Randomized, double-blind comparison of Reteplase double bolus administration with streptokinase in acute myocardial infarction (INJECT). *Lancet* 1995; 346:329.
New-generation fibrinolytics, including rPA, can be administered as a bolus and have shown promise in the treatment of ST-segment elevation MI.

ISIS-2 (Second International Study of Infarct Survival). Randomized trial of intravenous streptokinase, oral aspirin, both, or neither among 17,187 cases of suspected acute myocardial infarction: ISIS-2. *Lancet* 1988; 2:349.
ISIS-2 confirmed the importance of aspirin therapy in acute MI.

Lee KL, Woodlief LH, Topol EJ, et al for the GUSTO-1 Investigators. Predictors of 30-day mortality in the era of reperfusion for acute myocardial infarction: results from an International trial of 41,021 patients. *Circulation* 1995; 91:1659.
The GUSTO investigators identified several patient characteristics and clinical predictors of early mortality.

Sharkey SW, Burnette DD, Ruiz E, et al. An analysis of time delays preceeding thrombolysis for acute myocardial infarction. *JAMA* 1989;262:3171.

"Time to treatment" is a key determinant of patient outcome in MI.

TIMI Study Group. Comparison of invasive and conservative strategies after treatment with intravenous tissue plasminogen activator in acute myocardial infarction: results of the Thrombolysis in Myocardial Infarction (TIMI) phase II trial. *N Engl J Med* 1989;320:618.

Routine early coronary angiography and angioplasty do not save lives after acute MI.

Velury VS, Ma Y, Hurley T, et al. Clinical utility of electrocardiographic ST segment area for predicting unsatisfactory outcomes following thrombolytic therapy. *J Thromb Thrombolysis* 1995;2:51.

The ECG "ST area" can be used to predict outcome, including congestive heart failure and death.

34. SECONDARY PREVENTION AFTER ACUTE MYOCARDIAL INFARCTION: A CORONARY CARE UNIT PERSPECTIVE

Steven Borzak, Michael C. Vredenburg, and Richard C. Becker

I. General principles. Management of the patient with acute myocardial infarction (MI) has undergone radical transformation over the past three decades. Once guided by "the tincture of time" coupled with rest and relaxation, therapy is now based on mortality data from large-scale clinical trials in thousands of patients, whose outcomes may be joined by metaanalysis.

II. Secondary prevention as a treatment strategy. The modern paradigm of acute MI management typically involves several stages. First, acute management focuses on the early and sustained restoration of coronary patency, combined with efforts to limit infarct size and to treat early ventricular arrhythmias. This stage begins with the patient's decision to seek medical attention, continues in the ambulance and emergency department, and may extend to the coronary care unit (CCU) or catheterization laboratory. The next stage, which may begin in the emergency department or CCU, involves early risk stratification, monitoring and treatment of complications, and consideration of adjunctive therapy designed to reduce the risk of death and morbidity during hospitalization and in early recovery.

The final stage involves efforts to restore the patient to the highest possible functional capacity and to modify cardiac risk through prevention strategies.

A diverse array of drugs and other interventions is currently available for the patient experiencing an acute MI. The selection of treatment depends on an understanding of the physiologic principles governing adverse outcome after MI (Table 34-1). Interventions for the patient after MI are also appropriately guided by the risk factor profile (Table 34-2). Patients at higher risk clearly have the most to gain from a secondary prevention strategy.

III. Antiplatelet agents. The most convincing evidence for the routine use of aspirin during and after MI comes from the results of the Second International Study of Infarct Survival (ISIS-2), in which 17,187 patients with suspected MI were randomized to placebo, aspirin 160 mg per day for 30 days, streptokinase 1.5 million units, or aspirin plus streptokinase. This trial demonstrated a 23% reduction in 5-week vascular mortality with aspirin, 25% with streptokinase, and 42% with the combination of aspirin and streptokinase. The beneficial effect on survival persisted in follow-up analysis (mean 15 months).

It is therefore currently recommended that patients with MI receive 160 to 325 mg of aspirin on hospital admission and 160 to 325 mg daily thereafter.

Ticlopidine (Ticlid) was shown to decrease the incidence of MI in an open study of patients with unstable angina and to decrease the incidence of death or recurrent stroke in patients with stroke or transient ischemic attacks. Ticlopidine or clopidogrel (Plavix) are indicated in combination with aspirin for 2 to 4 weeks after intracoronary stenting. One study demonstrated that clopidogrel, which also inhibits adenosine diphosphate–mediated platelet aggregation, has activity in reducing events in patients with vascular disease.

One series of trials evaluated the role of glycoprotein IIb/IIIa antagonists in the setting of non–Q-wave MI or unstable angina. Collectively, preliminary reports are available in more than 15,000 patients who received tirofiban (Aggrastat) or eptifibatide (Integrelin) versus placebo for 2 to 4 days either alone or in conjunction with an angioplasty intervention. The preliminary findings suggest reductions in death or reinfarction at 30 days not offset by an increase in serious hemorrhage.

IV. Early beta-adrenergic blockade. The role of long-term oral administration of beta-adrenergic blocking agents (beta-blockers) for secondary prevention after MI is well established from individual trials and from pooled results revealing a 20% to 25% reduction in long-term mortality.

TABLE 34-1. Mechanistic strategies linking acute treatment and secondary prevention in acute myocardial infarction

Physiologic Variable	Presumed Mechanism	Potentially Applicable Intervention
Interruption of triggering mechanism of infarction	Plaque rupture, platelet aggregation, coronary thrombosis	Antiplatelet agents, antihypertensives, beta-blockers, smoking cessation, anticoagulants
Achievement of coronary patency	Mechanical revascularization, spontaneous or thrombolysis-induced recanalization	Thrombolytic agents, antiplatelet agents, anticoagulants, acute revascularization
Reinfarction	Increase in myocardial oxygen demand or reduction in supply, reocclusion of infarct artery or new site of occlusion	Beta-blockers, calcium channel blockers, cholesterol-lowering drugs, nitrates, antihypertensives, revascularization, antiplatelet agents, anticoagulants, ACE inhibitors
Sudden death	Ventricular arrhythmia	Beta-blockers, antiarrhythmic agents, implantable cardioverter-defibrillator
Progression of coronary artery disease	Atherosclerosis	Cholesterol-lowering strategies, antihypertensives, smoking cessation, calcium channel blockers, ACE inhibitors, exercise training
Development of congestive heart failure	Ventricular expansion or remodeling	ACE inhibitors, nitrates, antihypertensives, revascularization
Comorbid events, e.g., stroke	Cardiogenic embolus	Anticoagulants, antiplatelet agents

ACE, angiotensin-converting enzyme.

TABLE 34-2. Features of myocardial infarction associated with increased 1-year mortality

	Approximate Odds Ratio
Left-ventricular dysfunction	
Ejection fraction <40%	4.2
Congestion on chest radiograph	3.0
Increased ventricular volume	6.0
Previous infarction	1.8
Residual myocardial ischemia	
Angina before discharge	1.3
Angina on exercise test	2.5
Persistent ST-segment depression on ECG	2.5
Electrical instability, autonomic dysfunction	
More than 10 VPB/hr	2.7
Abnormal signal-averaged ECG	8.0
Diminished heart rate variability	3.8
Occluded infarct artery	2.5

ECG, electrocardiogram; VPB, ventricular premature beat.

The combination of thrombolytic therapy and intravenous beta-blockade is a safe and well-tolerated regimen among patients presenting early with signs and symptoms of MI. Insufficient data are available, however, to determine whether the combination lowers mortality beyond that for either agent given alone. Despite this limitation, early beta-blockade should be considered in all eligible patients.

V. Smoking. Approximately 30% of all adults in the United States smoke cigarettes. Many studies have examined the incidence of coronary heart disease events and mortality among smokers who have suffered an MI and subsequently discontinued smoking. These studies have demonstrated a dramatic and consistent reduction in mortality from coronary heart disease of nearly 50% among smokers who have been able to quit. Treatment of nicotine withdrawal is based on the patient's symptom profile, using supportive care and sedation with benzodiazepines. Nicotine replacement therapy may be dangerous in patients with active myocardial ischemia.

VI. Magnesium. The Fourth International Study of Infarct Survival (ISIS-4) randomized 58,000 patients to intravenous magnesium or control. Patients received 8 mmol of magnesium sulfate intravenously over 15 minutes and then 72 mmol intravenously over 24 hours. In contrast to the earlier studies, magnesium administration led to no improvement in 35-day mortality, which was 7.64% in magnesium-treated patients versus 7.24% in control patients, a difference that was not significant.

VII. Angiotensin-converting enzyme inhibition and ventricular remodeling. Pfeffer and colleagues laid the groundwork for clinical studies of angiotensin-converting enzyme (ACE) inhibition. They compared captopril treatment begun 3 to 16 days after MI with placebo in 2,200 patients followed for an average of 42 months. Inclusion criteria included an ejection fraction less than 40% without signs of ischemia or overt congestive heart failure. Captopril treatment resulted in a 19% reduction in total mortality, and significant reductions in congestive heart failure requiring the addition of open-label ACE inhibitor treatment or hospitalization. In addition, captopril demonstrated a 25% reduction in reinfarction. The latter finding is consistent with observations made in the Studies of Left Ventricular Dysfunction (SOLVD) trials and supports the evidence in animal models that ACE inhibition may have an antiatherosclerotic effect.

Long-term secondary prevention studies, beginning at least 3 days after MI, are complemented by a set of trials of earlier intervention begun within 24 hours of MI onset and a shorter course of treatment (Table 34-3). The early-and late-starting trials suggest that overall ACE inhibition started early is a safe but only modestly effective intervention in the unrestricted MI population. The ACE inhibitors are preferred in patients with extensive MI, heart failure, or left ventricular dysfunction and have the most impact when they are continued long term (Table 34-4). A new study demonstrates a reduction in MI and death when patients with coronary and vascular disease, but preserved systolic function, were treated long-term with the ACE inhibitor ramipril.

VIII. Nitrates. Nitrates have been used for more than a century in the treatment of angina. Hemodynamic benefits include a reduction in preload and ventricular filling pressures and coronary vasodilation. Several small clinical trials performed before the widespread use of thrombolytic therapy examined the benefits of nitrate preparations. In the majority of studies, intravenous nitroglycerin was given for 48 hours and was titrated to reduce mean arterial blood pressure by 10%, or up to 30% in hypertensive patients. The available evidence suggests that intravenous nitroglycerin may reduce ischemic pain and may lessen morphine requirements; however, large-scale trials performed in the reperfusion era have not revealed a survival benefit.

Nitrates can be considered for symptom relief of angina or heart failure. Because oral and topical nitrates are safe early in the course of MI, the expense of an intravenous preparation can be obviated by oral administration in those patients who receive treatment. Nitrates should be used with caution if at all, in inferior infarction, and are contraindicated in right ventricular infarction.

IX. Cholesterol-lowering strategies. Elevated total cholesterol, elevated low-density lipoprotein (LDL) cholesterol, and decreased high-density lipoprotein (HDL) cholesterol are associated with an increased risk of coronary heart disease. After MI, elevated cholesterol levels are strongly associated with recurrent cardiac events and cardiovascular mortality. Several studies have demonstrated that lowering cholesterol by behavioral intervention, drug therapy, or a combination can retard and may even reverse the progression of atherosclerotic plaques seen on angiography in both native arteries and bypass grafts. Drug therapy to reduce elevated cholesterol should therefore be considered before patients leave the coronary care unit, and ideally it should be initiated before hospital discharge. For secondary prevention, statin therapy should be begun with a dose expected to reduce LDL cholesterol to 100 mg/dL or less and should be adjusted as necessary in the outpatient setting to achieve this therapeutic goal.

X. Calcium channel blockers. Cellular calcium overload has been identified as a final common pathway of cellular injury in MI. This observation, coupled with several promising animal studies, led to the widespread application of calcium channel blockers to reduce infarction size, to lower mortality, and to reduce reinfarction in patients with MI.

A. Nifedipine and dihydropyridines. Numerous trials examined the effect of nifedipine in patients with acute or threatened MI. A consistent finding was the overall lack of benefit; in fact, several studies revealed evidence of harm.

One leading hypothesis to explain the adverse effects of short-acting dihydropyridines is that their potent peripheral vasodilatory properties simultaneously reduce coronary perfusion pressure and trigger reflex catecholamine release.

B. Calcium blockers and subset analyses. A consistent finding, particularly in studies including rate-slowing calcium channel antagonists (diltiazem, verapamil) has been increased incidence of clinical congestive heart failure. Thus, the benefit of calcium blockers after MI appears to be limited to a lower-risk subset of patients in whom signs or symptoms of congestive heart failure are not present. This observation is in contrast to beta-adrenergic blockers, in which the effect on late mortality, and particularly sudden death, is greater in the setting of heart failure.

XI. Antihypertensive treatment. Hypertension is associated with increased risk of coronary heart disease, cerebrovascular disease, left ventricular hypertrophy, congestive heart failure, and renal failure. There are no trials of antihypertensive therapy for secondary prevention of MI, and most primary prevention trials selectively excluded patients with known coronary disease.

TABLE 34-3. Studies of early angiotensin-converting enzyme inhibitors after myocardial infarction

Trial	Publication Date	Agent	No. of Patients	Inclusion Criteria	Initiation of Treatment	Duration of Treatment	Early Mortality Reduction (4–6 wk)
Consensus II	1992	Enalapril (intravenous)	6,090	Unselected patients	<24 h	6 mo	+10%
ISIS-4	1995	Captopril	58,050	Unselected patients	<24 h	35 d	6.3%
GISSI-3	1994	Lisinopril	18,895	Unselected patients	<24 h	42 d	12%
Chinese Captopril Study	1995	Captopril	11,345	Unselected patients	<36 h	30 d	3.4%
TRACE	1995	Trandolapril	1,749	Echo-defined LV dysfunction	3–7 d	Long-term	21%
SMILE	1995	Zofenopril	1,556	Anterior MI not eligible for thrombolysis	<24 h	42 d	25%

GISSI, Gruppo Italiano per lo Studio della Sopravvivanza nell'Infarto Miocardico; ISIS, International Study of Infarct Survival; SMILE, Survival of Myocardial Infarction Long-Term Evaluation; TRACE, Trandolapril Cardiac Evaluation.

TABLE 34-4. Recommended secondary prevention strategies

Strategy	Patient Selection	Timing	Strength of Evidence
Aspirin	All patients	On presentation and indefinitely	+++
Beta-blockers	All patients without heart block, bronchospastic lung disease, or severe heart failure	Intravenously on presentation and then oral	++
Smoking cessation counseling	All smokers	On admission and repeatedly	+
ACE inhibitors	All nonhypotensive patients without renal dysfunction; greatest benefit with heart failure or LV dysfunction	Initiate within 24 hours; continue beyond 4–6 wks if heart failure or LV dysfunction present	+++
Cholesterol lowering by statin drug	All patients with LDL cholesterol > 100 mg/dL	Measure lipids on admission; initiate treatment before discharge	++
Amiodarone or AICD	Symptomatic sustained and possibly nonsustained ventricular tachycardia	>48 h after presentation	+
Rehabilitation	All patients	In hospital and after discharge	+

ACE, angiotensin-converting enzyme; AICD, automatic implantable cardioverter-defibrillator; LDL, low-density lipoprotein; LV, left ventricular.

The selection of an antihypertensive regimen in patients after MI should be individualized. Beta-blockers and ACE inhibitors, as discussed previously, reduce mortality and should therefore be considered in all patients without contraindications.

XII. Cardiac rehabilitation. Current therapy of patients with MI includes commode privileges on admission, progressing rapidly to ambulation on CCU discharge and performance of tasks simulating those required at home before hospital discharge. If primary angioplasty and risk stratification by angiography are accomplished at hospitalization, one study demonstrated the safety of avoiding a CCU stay altogether and hospital discharge at 72 hours in appropriately selected patients. Cardiac rehabilitation programs have evolved from primary emphasis on exercise training to programs that emphasize reduction in coronary disease risk factors, including smoking cessation, exercise, nutritional counseling, and psychosocial support.

XIII. Estrogen. Estrogen is believed to prevent coronary disease by mediating a favorable change in serum lipids (increased HDL, reduced LDL). It may also reduce vasomotor tone and decrease platelet aggregation. Epidemiologic studies have suggested a 40% to 50% reduction risk of coronary heart disease in general populations with estrogen therapy. In addition to its effect on coronary disease, postmenopausal estrogen replacement therapy reduces the risk of osteoporosis and hip fracture and decreases the symptoms associated with menopause. However, it may also increase the risk of endometrial cancer and possibly breast cancer. The addition of progestin to estrogen may reduce the chance of endometrial cancer, but it could obviate cardiovascular benefit as well, perhaps by having a less favorable change on serum cholesterol fractions or possibly a "prothrombotic" effect. Among women who have had a hysterectomy, the balance would favor a greater benefit. A recently completed prospective trial showed a clinical benefit of estrogen-progestin on manifestations of cardiac disease.

Selected Readings

Antman EM, Lau J, Kupelnick B, et al. A comparison of results of meta-analyses of randomized control trials and recommendations of clinical experts. *JAMA* 1992;268:240.

The "meta" analysis has been used to determine the potential impact of randomized controlled trials on treatment recommendations and practice among physicians.

CAPRIE Steering Committee. A randomized, blinded, trial of dopidogrel versus aspirin in patients at risk of ischaemic events. *Lancet* 1996;348:1329.

Clopidogrel, a novel platelet antagonist, was shown to be superior to aspirin therapy, particularly in patients with peripheral vascular disease and prior MI.

ISIS-2 Collaborative Group. Randomized trial of intravenous streptokinase, oral aspirin, both, or neither among 17,187 cases of suspected acute myocardial infarction: ISIS-2. *Lancet* 1988;2:349.

The ISIS-2 Study, a landmark effort, identified the importance of aspirin therapy either alone or in combination witih a fibrinolytic agent.

ISIS-4 (Fourth International Study of Infarct Survival). A randomized factorial trial assessing early oral captopril, oral mononitrate, and intravenous magnesium sulphate in 58,050 patients with suspected acute myocardial infarction. *Lancet* 1995; 345:669.

The ISIS-4 Study determined that magnesium therapy and nitrate therapy were not beneficial in the routine management of patients with acute MI, but supported early ACE inhibitors.

Krone RJ. The role of risk stratification in the early management of a myocardial infarction. *Ann Intern Med* 1992;116:223.

A comprehensive review of risk stratification strategies in the setting of acute MI.

35. DIAGNOSTIC TESTING IN THE CORONARY CARE UNIT

Michael J. Waligora, Robert C. Hendel, and Richard C. Becker

I. General principles. Myriad diagnostic procedures are available in the coronary care unit. The specialist in intensive care must be familiar with procedures that critically ill patients may require.

II. Electrocardiography. The electrocardiogram (ECG) remains one of the most informative, least expensive, and most rapidly obtainable diagnostic procedures available in the coronary care unit. From this electrical activity, information on chamber size, ischemia, injury, dysthythmias, conduction, and electrolyte disturbances can be obtained.

A. Morphology of the normal electrocardiogram. Atrial depolarization originates in the sinus node and activates the atria from right to left. The normal P wave is less than 0.2 mV (2 mm) in amplitude and less than 0.12 seconds in duration. The PR interval is typically 0.12 to 0.20 second (Fig. 35-1).

Ventricular activation proceeds symmetrically outward from the septum and from endocardium to epicardium. Septal activation produces initial Q waves in leads I, II, III, aVL, V_5, and V_6 and R waves in V_1 to V_4. Right and left ventricular depolarizations next result in R waves in leads I, II, III, aVL, aVF, and V_3 to V_6. Terminal forces produced by the activation of the left ventricular septum result in a terminal S wave in leads I, V_5, and V_6. The ST segment is normally isoelectric. The T wave represents ventricular repolarization, which usually produces upright T waves in all leads except a VR and V_1.

The QT interval reflects the duration of ventricular depolarization and repolarization. Because the duration of the QT interval varies with the heart rate, Bazett proposed the corrected QT interval: QT_c = QT/(square root of RR). Normal valves are less than 0.39 second for men and 0.41 second for women, but many investigators accept a QT_c as long as 0.44 seconds as normal. The causes of QT prolongation include idiopathic long QT interval syndrome, myocardial ischemia, cardiomyopathy, central nervous system disease, autonomic nervous system dysfunction, hypocalcemia, hypokalemia, antiarrhythmic drugs, and psychotropic drugs.

B. Atrial abnormalities. P-wave abnormalities may represent atrial enlargement or hypertrophy or altered intraatrial pressure, volume, or conduction. Right atrial abnormality is manifest by a low P-wave amplitude in lead I and a tall peaked P wave in leads II, III, and aVF (P pulmonale). In adults, the most common cause of right atrial abnormality is chronic obstructive pulmonary disease.

Left atrial abnormality is manifest by prolongation and notching of the P wave with shortening of PR segment (P mitrale). The most frequent cause of P mitrale is left ventricular disease with increased left ventricular end-diastolic pressure. PR-segment depression may be seen in pericarditis, atrial infarction, and atrial injury resulting from penetrating wounds.

C. Ventricular hypertrophy. ECG manifestations of left ventricular hypertrophy include increased voltage, delayed terminal forces, ST-segment and T-wave abnormalities, and left atrial abnormalities. The QRS voltage criteria for left ventricular hypertrophy are listed in Table 35-1.

D. Pulmonary embolus. The most common ECG features of acute pulmonary embolism are sinus tachycardia and nonspecific repolarization abnormalities. The S_1-Q_3-T_3 (Fig. 35-2) pattern, right bundle branch block, right axis deviation, and P pulmonale are seen in only one-fourth of patients.

E. Chronic obstructive pulmonary disease. Chronic obstructive pulmonary disease often results in a peaked P wave in lead II, right axis deviation, and clockwise rotation of the QRS axis. Absence of R waves in the precordial leads may simulate anterior myocardial infarction.

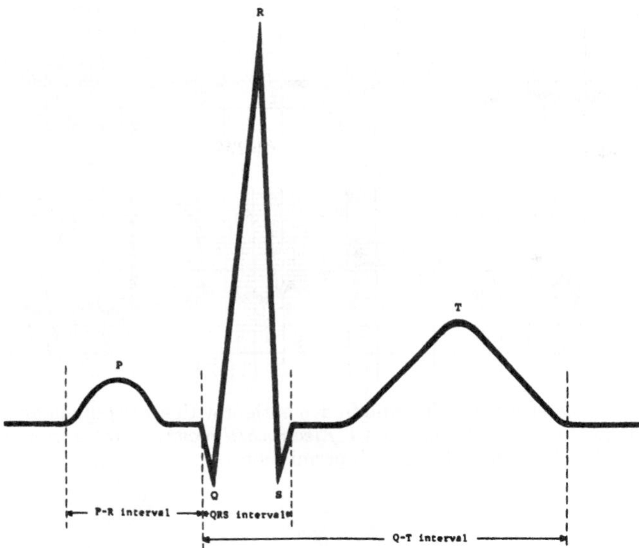

FIG. 35-1. Schematic representation of the surface electrocardiogram. *P,* atrial depolarization; *QRS,* ventricular depolarization; *T,* ventricular repolarization. See the text for further description of intervals and normal values. (From Chung EK, ed. *Principles of cardiac arrhythmias,* 2nd ed. Baltimore: Williams & Wilkins, 1977, with permission.)

F. Myocardial ischemia. Subepicardial ischemia is often manifest by T-wave inversion, but subendocardial ischemia may maintain a positive T wave. ST-segment depression is usually seen with myocardial ischemia, although ST-segment elevation may be seen with coronary arterial spasm. Most important is evidence of changes in the ECG when compared with prior tracings.

G. Myocardial infarction. The ECG changes of myocardial infarction (Fig. 35-3) are caused by ischemia, injury, and cellular death identified by T-wave changes, ST-segment displacement, and the appearance of Q waves. An early tracing in acute myocardial infarction may show increased magnitude of T waves (hyperacute), either upright or inverted. This is followed within minutes by upright displacement of the ST segment in the leads facing the area of injury. Q waves usually occur within hours to days but may be present initially.

TABLE 35-1. Voltage criteria for the diagnosis of left ventricular hypertrophy

One or more of the following:
R wave in lead I + S wave in lead III >25 mm
R wave in aVL >11 mm
R wave in aVF >20 mm
S wave in aVR >14 mm
R wave in V_5 or V_6 >26 mm
R wave in V_5 or V_6 + S wave in V_1 >35 mm
Largest R wave + largest S wave in precordial leads >45 mm

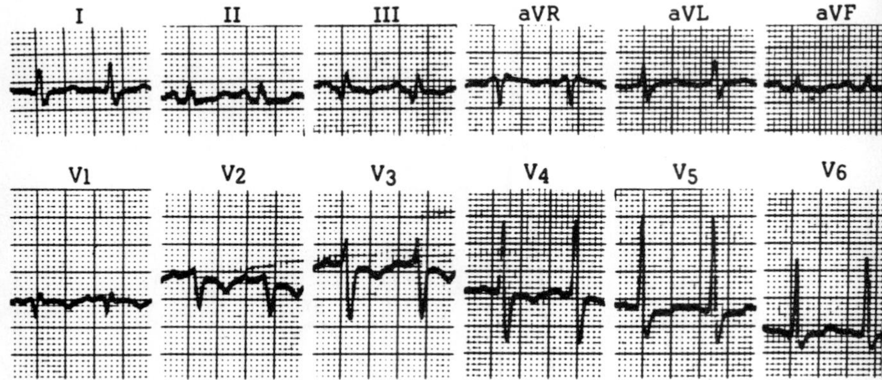

FIG. 35-2. A 12-lead electrocardiogram from a patient with acute pulmonary embolism. Note the S_1-Q_3-T_3 pattern. (From Chou T. *Electrocardiology in clinical practice,* 3rd ed. Philadelphia: WB Saunders, 1991, with permission.)

III. Chest radiography

A. Interpretation of the portable chest film: pulmonary vasculature. In normal pulmonary flow, the pulmonary arteries and veins branch outward from each hilum with gradual peripheral tapering. As pulmonary flow increases to twice normal, the enlarged arteries and veins become apparent on chest radiographs. High-output states, such as anemia, pregnancy, thyrotoxicosis, volume overload, intracardiac shunts, and fever, result in symmetric increases in vascularity. Pulmonary venous hypertension, caused by left ventricular dysfunction, mitral stenosis, or other obstructions to blood flow between the pulmonary capillaries and left ventricle, results in increased flow to the apices, followed by interstitial edema with Kerley lines and finally alveolar edema.

B. Cardiac silhouette. The normal cardiothoracic ratio, which is the ratio of transverse cardiac diameter to the maximum internal diameter of the thorax, is defined as being less than 0.5. Left ventricular enlargement may be secondary to hypertrophy, dilatation, or both.

Left atrial enlargement is easily identified on the chest radiograph as a prominence of the left superior heart border, double density behind the right atrial margin, and splaying of the carina resulting from upward displacement of the left main stem bronchus.

Right atrial enlargement is evidenced by increased fullness and convexity of the right cardiac contour and a filling in of the retrosternal clear space. Right ventricular enlargement displaces the whole heart rotationally to the left. This displacement causes increased convexity of the left upper heart border and elevation of the cardiac apex. Right ventricular enlargement may also obliterate the retrosternal clear space.

IV. Cardiac catheterization and angiography. Although not performed at the bedside, invasive radiographic procedures are often necessary in cardiac patients. The intensive care specialist should be familiar with the applications of such techniques as well as the potential for procedural complications, including cardiac perforation, vascular intimal dissection, myocardial infarction, thromboembolic events, induction of dysrhythmias, and hemodynamic changes.

A. Aortography. The indications for aortography are suspected acute aortic dissection or acute aortic regurgitation.

B. Pulmonary angiography. In suspected pulmonary embolism, the pulmonary angiogram remains the current standard for diagnosis.

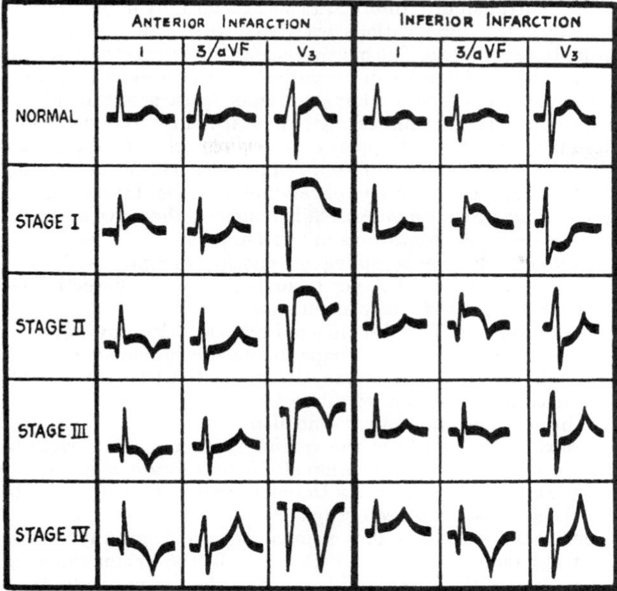

FIG. 35-3. Succession of 12-lead electrocardiograms, demonstrating evolution of an acute anterior wall myocardial infarction *(left)* and inferior wall myocardial infarction *(right)*. Note the progression from isoelectric ST segments to ST-segment elevation in stage I, T-wave inversion in stage II, resolution of ST-segment elevation in stage III, and deep T-wave inversion in stage IV. (From Grossman W, ed. *Cardiac catheterization, angiography and intervention,* 4th ed. Baltimore: Williams & Wilkins, 1991, with permission.)

C. Coronary arteriography. Selective cannulation of the coronary arteries with contrast administration is the standard for determining the presence and extent of critical coronary stenoses.

V. Echocardiography. Echocardiography is a safe, convenient, and efficient method of evaluating cardiac structure and motion, and, in conjunction with Doppler techniques, it may be used to assess ventricular function and blood flow through cardiac structures.

A. Hypertrophic cardiomyopathy. Hypertrophic cardiomyopathy is readily evaluated using echocardiographic techniques. Systolic anterior motion of the mitral valve is associated with left ventricular outflow tract obstruction. Other findings seen in hypertrophic cardiomyopathy are asymmetric or concentric left ventricular hypertrophy and, in the concentric form, left ventricular cavity obliteration during systole.

B. Coronary artery disease: myocardial ischemia. Normally functioning myocardium thickens and contracts during ventricular systole. Echocardiographic findings of ischemic myocardium consist of abnormalities of left ventricular wall thickness, thickening, and motion. Echocardiography may be used to confirm the diagnosis of ischemia and to determine which areas of myocardium are at risk.

C. Myocardial infarction. A strong correlation exists between the extent of echocardiographically determined wall motion abnormalities and the size of a myocardial infarction. Echocardiography may not be sensitive enough to detect small or nontransmural infarcts. Echocardiography may also be used to diagnose many of the complications associated with acute myocardial infarction.

D. Valvular heart disease. The bedside echocardiogram is valuable in confirming suspected valvular disease in the patient in the coronary care unit with severe congestive heart failure or other symptoms. Acute aortic insufficiency or acute mitral regurgitation complicating a myocardial infarction can be quickly recognized using color flow Doppler echocardiography as a turbulent retrograde jet through the valve. In addition, Doppler echocardiography may be used to assess the presence and degree of valvular stenosis. Transesophageal echocardiography may provide a more detailed image of the valve apparatus, function, and the presence of vegetations in endocarditis.

E. Aortic dissection. Transesophageal echocardiography is likely the noninvasive diagnostic method of choice in suspected aortic dissection because of its accuracy, safety, speed, and convenience.

F. Source of embolus. Two-dimensional echocardiography can be used to identify the source of embolus. Perhaps the most common source of embolus in a cardiac patient is an intracavitary thrombus. Patients with atrial fibrillation, left ventricular aneurysm, or dilated cardiomyopathy are prone to develop mural thrombi and subsequent embolism.

Paradoxic embolism from the venous system across a right-to-left shunt may be suggested by identification of a patent foramen ovale or atrial septal defect by Doppler and color flow Doppler examination. This can be confirmed by bubble contrast echocardiography.

G. Pericardial disease. Two-dimensional echocardiography is the method of choice for detecting pericardial effusions. In the hemodynamically compromised patient with clinical evidence of cardiac tamponade, the echocardiogram may be performed quickly and at the bedside with a high sensitivity for pericardial effusion. Echocardiographic findings of a hemodynamically significant pericardial effusion (cardiac tamponade) include a large effusion, right atrial or right ventricular diastolic collapse, and increased respiratory variation in transvalvular flow velocities.

VI. Nulcear cardiology. Imaging with radioisotopes is used to assess a wide variety of cardiac physiologic properties, including myocardial perfusion and ventricular function.

A. Myocardial perfusion imaging. Although the coronary arteriogram is accurate in defining vessel morphology, radionuclide studies to assess myocardial perfusion are superior in determining the physiologic significance of a coronary stenosis. Furthermore, scintigraphy may function as a noninvasive predictor for the presence of and prognosis from such stenoses.

B. Acute imaging. The evaluation of patients with chest pain in the emergency department remains a difficult task. Both the number of patients discharged who subsequently suffer acute MI and the number of coronary care admissions for what eventually is found to be noncardiac chest pain are high. Because little redistribution occurs with sestamibi, it is a promising agent for perfusion imaging during acute ischemic syndromes.

C. Cardiac performance. Right and left ventricular ejection fractions and regional wall motion may be safely and reproducibly determined noninvasively using radionuclide techniques. In addition, ventricular volumes, indices of diastolic dysfunction, indices of valvular regurgitation, and intracardiac shunts may be determined.

VII. Computed tomography. Computed tomography has been successfully employed to detect intracardiac masses, pericardial disease, and aortic dissections.

VIII. Magnetic resonance imaging. Magnetic resonance imaging may be the most accurate procedure for the detection of aortic dissection, with the highest sensitivity and specificity compared with aortography, computed tomography, and transesophageal echocardiography. It is also accurate in determining the site of intimal tear, the presence of thrombus, and the presence of associated pericardial effusion.

Magnetic resonance imaging allows excellent visualization of pericardial effusions and pericardial thickness.

IX. Right heart catheterization. Hemodynamic monitoring via pulmonary artery catheterization allows measurement of pressures in the right-sided cardiac chambers and pulmonary artery, estimates of the left atrial pressure from the pulmonary capillary wedge pressure, and calculation of cardiac output and pulmonary and systemic vascular resistance.

Selected Readings

Bazett HC. An analysis of the time-relations of electrocardiograms. *Heart* 1920; 7:353.

The original work of Bazett shed light on the sequence of events that characterize ventricular depolarization and repolarization. The QT interval is corrected (QTc) for the heart rate.

Cigarroa JE, Isselbacher EM, DeSanctis RW, et al. Diagnostic imaging in the evaluation of suspected aortic dissection: old standards and new directions. *N Engl J Med* 1993; 328:35.

The diagnostic evaluation of patients with suspected aortic dissection includes a variety of modalities including transesophageal echocardiography, computed tomography, and magnetic resonance imaging.

Manning WJ, Silverman DI, Gordon SPF, et al. Cardioversion from atrial fibrillation without prolonged anticoagulation with use of transesophageal echocardiography to exclude the presence of atrial thrombi. *N Engl J Med* 1993; 328:750.

A transesophageal echocardiogram can be used to determine the potential risk for thromboembolism in patients with atrial fibrillation.

36. MECHANISMS OF ACUTE MYOCARDIAL ISCHEMIA AND INFARCTION

Carey D. Kimmelstiel, Christopher A. Clyne, and Richard C. Becker

I. **General principles.** The heart is an aerobic organ that relies almost exclusively on the oxidation of substrates for the generation of energy; therefore it tolerates only a small oxygen debt. Because the heart does not contain oxygen stores, its high rate of energy expenditure, required to meet the needs of actively functioning tissues and organs throughout the body, causes a striking decline in oxygen tension within seconds of coronary arterial occlusion, followed by a loss of myocardial contractility.

II. **Normal coronary anatomy.** Blood and essential substrates are carried to the myocardium through the major epicardial coronary arteries, their branches, intramural and subendocardial extensions, and the collateral circulation.

A. **Right coronary artery.** The right coronary artery, typically 2.5 to 3.0 mm in diameter, originates within the right coronary sinus of Valsalva (Fig. 36-1). In approximately 80% of individuals, this artery reaches the crux cordis and gives rise to posterior descending, atrioventricular node, and left ventricular branches.

B. **Left coronary artery.** The left coronary artery originates in the left coronary sinus of Valsalva. The ostium is typically located at the level of the aortic ring, up to 1.0 cm higher than the ostium of the right coronary artery (Fig. 36-2). The left main coronary artery, which may be up to 4.5 mm in diameter, divides into two major branches—the left anterior descending coronary artery and the left circumflex coronary artery.

The coronary circulation has been divided anatomically into dominant and nondominant, depending on which blood vessel reaches and crosses the crux cordis of the heart. In this instance, the posterior descending artery and often the atrioventricular nodal artery originate from the dominant vessel. Accordingly, the right coronary artery is considered the dominant vessel in approximately 80% of individuals. However, the left coronary artery system provides blood flow to the largest area of myocardium and is therefore the predominant artery in most individuals.

C. **Coronary artery anomalies.** In some cases, anatomic variations (anomalies) preclude normal delivery of essential substrate and compromise myocardial function (Table 36-1).

D. **Coronary ostial abnormalities.** The coronary ostium can be abnormal with respect to its intrinsic anatomy (proper aortic sinus origin), size (ostial hyperplasia, fibrous endoproliferation, atresia), or orientation (tangential orientation, intussusception).

E. **Ectopic coronary artery origination.** One or more of the ectopic coronary arteries may originate from the pulmonic trunk. There may be anomalous origin from an atypical site—a noncoronary cusp, the aortic wall above the coronary sinus, or the descending aorta.

F. **Abnormal connections.** Abnormal connections between a coronary artery and an adjacent vascular structure tend to enlarge with time because of the persistence of a pressure gradient. Examples are a coronary-cameral fistula (right ventricle, left ventricle, right atrium, left atrium), coronary-arteriovenous fistula, and coronary-to-extracardiac artery or vein (coronary-pulmonary, coronary-bronchial, coronary-caval) fistula.

G. **Intramural coursing (muscular bridge).** The main coronary arteries and their branches course on the epicardial surface of the heart. Occasionally, the vessels take a subepicardial course.

H. **Coronary artery size.** The diameter of a coronary artery can be too small (hypoplastic) or too large (ectasic). Either may be a congenital or acquired abnormality.

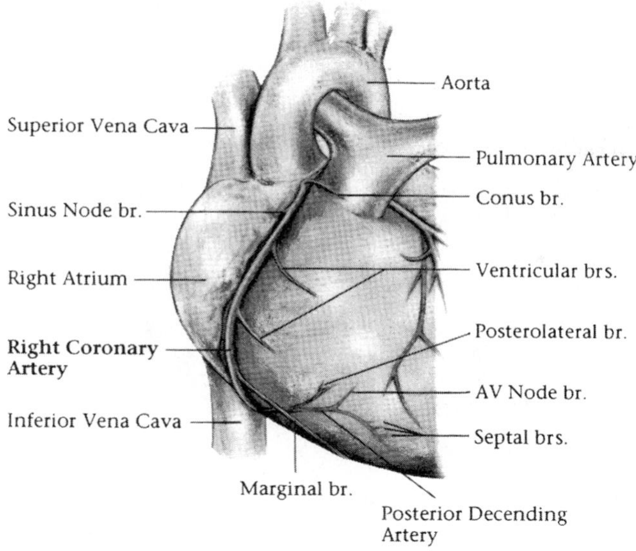

FIG. 36-1. Anatomy of the right coronary artery.

III. Collateral circulation. Vascular connections between two or more coronary arteries that are larger than capillaries are considered collaterals. The presence of a collateral circulation in the human heart is firmly established. Most of these vessels, ranging in size from 50 to 1,500 μm, are located subendocardially; however, epicardial collaterals can be found at the ventricular apex.

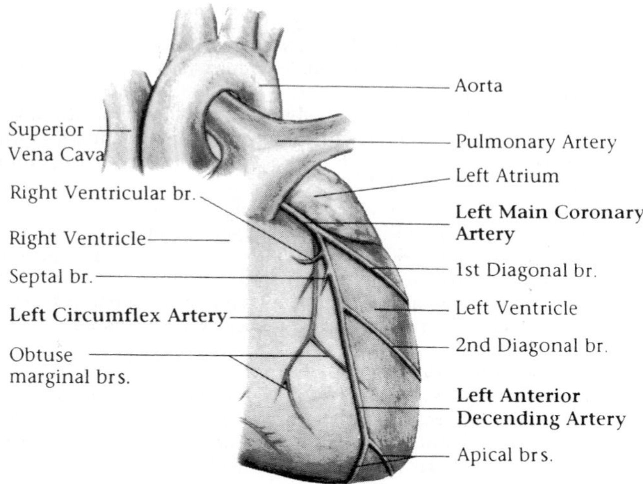

FIG. 36-2. Anatomy of the left coronary artery, including the left main, left anterior descending, and left circumflex coronary arteries.

TABLE 36-1. Classification of anomalous coronary arteries

Ostial abnormality
Origin
Size
Orientation
Ectopic coronary artery origination
Pulmonic trunk
Opposite coronary sinus
Opposite coronary artery
Aortic wall
Extracardial vessels
Cardiac chamber
Abnormal connections
Arteriovenous fistula
Coronary-cameral fistula
Coronary to extracardiac artery or vein
Intramuscular coursing (muscular bridge)
Subepicardial
Subendocardial
Intracavitary
Coronary artery size
Hypoplastic
Elastic

IV. Oxygen carrying capacity of blood. The unique physiologic role of hemoglobin in tissue metabolism is fostered by the sigmoidal shape of its oxygen-binding curve. In reality, hemoglobin has a relatively low oxygen affinity. With decreasing pH and increasing 2,3-diphosphoglyceric acid concentrations or temperature, a further decrease in hemoglobin's affinity for oxygen occurs, causing more oxygen to be released at the tissue level for a given partial pressure of oxygen (PO_2) (Fig. 36-3).

V. Coronary blood flow

A. Oxygen consumption. With increasing myocardial demands, oxygen consumption increases three- to fourfold. Because myocardial oxygen extraction cannot increase substantially, coronary blood flow must increase to meet the demands placed on the heart (Table 36-2).

During diastole, when the aortic valve is in the closed position, aortic diastolic blood pressure is transmitted through the dilated sinuses of Valsalva to the coronary ostia. The coronary sinuses act as reservoirs, thus facilitating uniform blood flow through diastole.

B. Perfusion pressure. Coronary arterial blood flow is determined, to a large extent, by the pressure gradient (driving pressure) between the aorta (in diastole) and the coronary sinus. This relationship is influenced by atherosclerotic narrowings and elevations in left ventricular end-diastolic and right atrial pressure. Coronary blood flow is maintained when the mean arterial pressure exceeds 65 mm Hg. Below this level, myocardial perfusion is significantly reduced.

VI. Disorders of myocardial oxygen supply

A. Coronary atherosclerosis. In most patients with documented myocardial ischemia or infarction, coronary atherosclerosis is the underlying pathologic lesion. Clinical manifestations of coronary atherosclerosis result from chronic as well as acute reductions in myocardial blood flow from epicardial coronary arteries.

A large body of evidence suggests that the conversion from stable to unstable angina is heralded by plaque rupture or fissuring, which exposes the atheroscle-

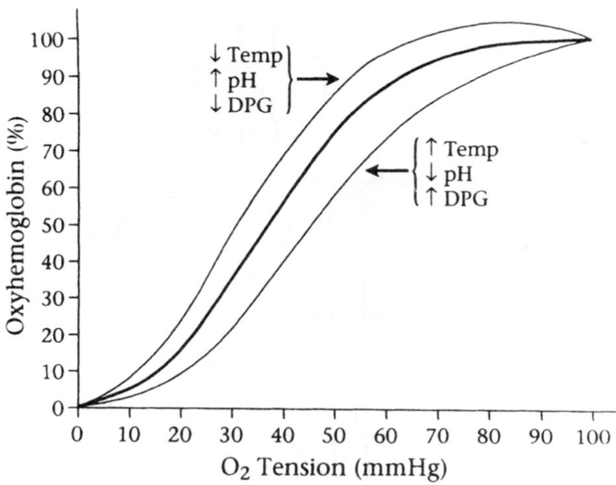

FIG. 36-3. The oxygen binding curve for human hemoglobin under physiologic conditions. The affinity of hemoglobin for oxygen varies with changes in pH, temperature, and 2,3-diphosphoglyceric acid concentrations.

rotic matrix and subendothelium to circulating blood products. Evidence for plaque rupture comes from angiographic studies in unstable angina patients showing a higher prevalence of eccentric, irregular, narrow-necked stenoses with overhanging edges (type II lesion) when compared with patients with stable angina, who are more likely to exhibit concentric, symmetric stenoses or eccentric broad-necked (type I) stenoses (Fig. 36-4).

B. **Coronary vasospasm.** Most ischemic episodes result from an increase in myocardial oxygen demand, but reduction in coronary flow can be associated with ischemic episodes, and in a small percentage of cases vasospasm is the sole cause. Coronary vasospasm most often occurs at the site of arterial segments containing atherosclerotic plaque (Fig. 36-5). In addition, atherosclerosis has been documented to cause endothelial dysfunction.
C. **Nonatherosclerotic coronary artery disease.** Although most patients exhibiting myocardial ischemia and infarction have atherosclerotic disease as the cause of the ischemia, several causes of nonatherosclerotic coronary disease (Table 36-3) may lead to symptoms of angina or precipitation of myocardial necrosis. A comprehensive review is beyond the scope of this chapter, but several are reviewed briefly in the following sections.
D. **Congenital abnormalities.** Isolated congenital anomalies of the coronary arteries are uncovered in fewer than 1% of adults undergoing coronary angiography. Many different anomalies exist.

TABLE 36-2. Factors influencing coronary arterial blood flow

Duration of diastole
Perfusion pressure
Extrinsic coronary arterial compression
Neurohormonal-mediated vasodilation/vasoconstriction
Autoregulation

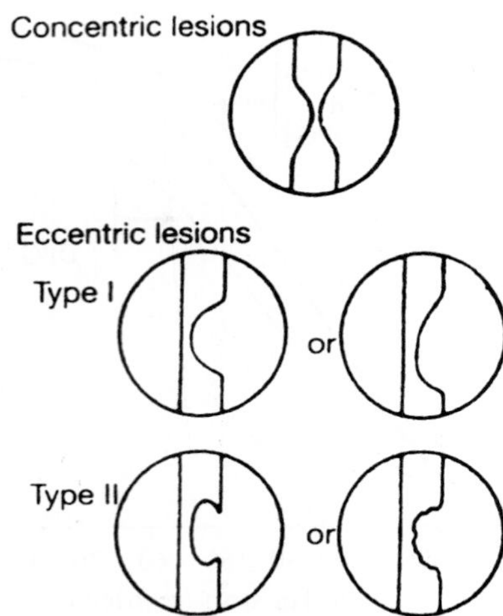

FIG. 36-4. Stenosis morphology in unstable and stable coronary syndromes. (Adapted from Ambrose JA, Winters SL, Stern A, et al. Angiographic morphology in the pathogenesis of unstable angina pectoris. *J Am Coll Cardiol* 1985;5:609, with permission.)

- **E. Trauma.** Penetrating and blunt trauma can cause myocardial infarction. Penetrating trauma such as stab and gunshot wounds can cause coronary laceration, although the primary clinical presentation in this setting is that of pericardial tamponade. Blunt trauma can cause myocardial infarction even in the absence of preexisting atherosclerotic disease.
- **F. Embolism.** Embolism to the coronary arteries can lead to myocardial infarction by acute occlusion of the involved vessel, usually the left anterior descending coronary artery. Potential sources of coronary embolism include left ventricular mural thrombus, endocarditis (either native or prosthetic valve), neoplasia, air and calcium during cardiac surgery or cardiac catheterization, paradoxic embolization across a patent foramen ovale, and atrial septal defect.
- **G. Dissection.** Coronary dissection causes ischemia and infarction when intima separates from media and the resultant flap obstructs blood flow through the vessel lumen. Such obstructive dissections occur most commonly as a complication of coronary intervention and rarely as a result of diagnostic angiography. Aortic dissection also may extend proximally to involve the coronary circulation. Spontaneous coronary dissections occur infrequently. Most cases occur in young women, one-third in the peripartum period.
- **H. Anemia.** Chronic anemia induces a high-output state, resulting in large measure from a reduction in blood viscosity. Ischemia induction is facilitated in this condition primarily in patients with existing coronary artery disease.
- **I. Prothrombotic states.** Ischemia and infarction occasionally occur as a result of one of the so-called prothrombotic or "hypercoagulable" states. Inappropriate thrombosis occurs in these disorders, usually from a breakdown in thromboregulation at the level of the vascular endothelium. These states have been elegantly reviewed.
- **J. Hypotension.** Ischemia, especially of the subendocardium, can manifest during periods of hypotension. In this setting, coronary perfusion is reduced.

VII. Disorders of myocardial oxygen demand

- **A. Aortic stenosis.** Angina pectoris is a common clinical manifestation of acquired aortic stenosis. Even in the absence of coronary disease, myocardial oxygen demand may exceed supply as a result of myocardial hypertrophy, prolongation

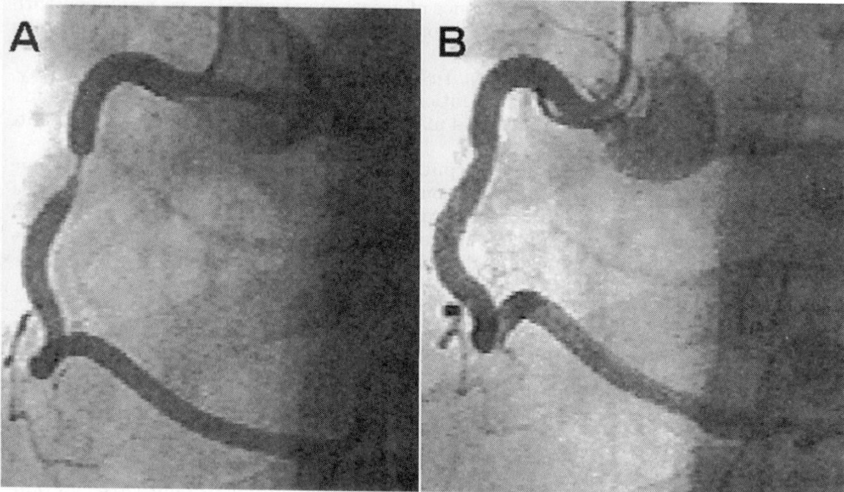

FIG. 36-5. Right coronary angiogram in a patient who presented with clinical and electrocardiographic signs of acute myocardial infarction. **A:** A high-grade stenosis in the midportion of the vessel. **B:** The appearance of the vessel after relief of spasm after the infusion of intracoronary nitroglycerin. Note that spasm occurred at the site of a subcritical stenosis.

of the systolic ejection period, and elevated left ventricular systolic pressure, a triad that in concert greatly augments myocardial oxygen consumption.

B. Aortic insufficiency. Although a less common clinical problem, ischemia can be expressed as a symptom of aortic insufficiency in which increased myocardial oxygen demand and diminished supply coexist.

C. Hypertensive heart disease. Hypertension is well known to be a risk factor for the development of left ventricular hypertrophy as well as coronary artery disease. Left ventricular hypertrophy in the absence of coronary stenoses may pre-

TABLE 36-3. Nonatherosclerotic coronary artery disease: causes

Congenital coronary artery anomalies
Coronary arteriovenous fistulas
Trauma
Coronary embolism
Coronary dissection
Coronary vasculitis
Radiation arteritis
Anemia
Hypercoagulable states
Hypotension
Aortic stenosis and insufficiency
Left ventricular hypertrophy
Hypertrophic cardiomyopathy
High-output states
Dilated cardiomyopathy

cipitate ischemia as a consequence of greater myocardial mass combined with diminished perfusion pressure secondary to elevated ventricular end-diastolic pressure.

D. Hypertrophic cardiomyopathy. In hypertrophic obstructive cardiomyopathy, mechanisms similar to those mentioned earlier may result in ischemia. In addition, myocardial oxygen demand may be especially high in patients with outflow gradients.

E. High-output states. In high-output states such as hyperthyroidism, ischemic symptoms most often occur in patients with underlying coronary artery disease as a consequence of elevated myocardial oxygen demand through augmented contractility and heart rate. Investigators have suggested that the hyperthyroid state predisposes afflicted patients to coronary spasm.

Selected Readings

Bland EF, White PD, Garland J. Congenital anomalies of the coronary arteries: report of an unusual case associated with cardiac hypertrophy. *Am Heart J* 1933;18:787.

One of the most widely cited coronary anomalies is origin of the left anterior descending coronary artery from the pulmonary trunk.

Kurosawa H, Wagenaar SS, Becker AE. Sudden death in a youth: a case of quadricuspid aortic valve with isolation of origin of left coronary artery. *Br Heart J* 1981; 46:211.

Sudden cardiac death in youth may be caused by anomalous coronary arteries that impair myocardial perfusion, thus increasing the risk of malignant arrhythmias.

Nachman RL, Silverstein R. Hypercoagulable states. *Ann Intern Med* 1993;119:819.

A wide variety of primary and secondary hypercoagulable "prothrombotic" states may predispose to coronary arterial events. However, inherited thrombophilias more often lead to venous thromboembolism.

37. NONISCHEMIC CHEST PAIN

Donald G. Love, Richard C. Becker, and John A. Paraskos

I. **General principles.** Chest pain is a common complaint among patients undergoing evaluation in most major medical centers. It may be observed in cardiac, vascular, gastrointestinal, pulmonary, musculoskeletal, psychologic, neurologic, and dermatologic disease entities (Table 37-1). Chest pain accounts for an estimated 2% to 4% of all emergency room visits in the United States. Similarly, more than 1.5 million Americans are admitted to intensive care units for suspected ischemic heart disease yearly.

II. **History.** When the clinician evaluates patients with chest pain, the history should focus on risk factors for atherosclerosis (age, gender, family history, smoking, cholesterol, hypertension, diabetes, peripheral vascular disease, prior coronary artery disease or myocardial infarction [MI], type A personality), precipitating factors, alleviating factors, quality, location, intensity, duration, frequency, radiation, pattern, setting, and associated symptoms.

III. **Ischemic chest pain.** The pain of angina pectoris has a diverse presentation. Some episodes of ischemia or infarction may be painless but may produce "angina equivalents," including profound weakness, diaphoresis, nausea, malaise, dyspnea, and localized discomfort in areas more commonly affected by radiating pain. The incidence of atypical presentation increases with older age, diabetes, history of stroke, spinal cord disease, coronary artery bypass surgery, and cardiac transplant. Up to 25% of infarctions are clinically silent.

A. **Location and radiation.** Ischemic pain is typically located in the lower substernal area. It may radiate to one or both arms, to the shoulders, to the anterior neck, to the lower jaw, and, less often, to the teeth, wrists, and back. The extreme limits of radiation are from the occiput to the epigastrium.

B. **Quality.** Ischemic cardiac pain is typically a deep visceral sensation and is therefore frequently described as follows: choking; constricting; heavy; squeezing; suffocating; strangling; pressure; burning; viselike, bandlike, and discomfort, not pain, as if someone were standing on the patient's chest. The intensity ranges from mild to crushing. Rarely is ischemic chest pain well localized, sharp, stabbing, knifelike, or tearing in quality.

C. **Duration.** In most instances, ischemic chest pain lasts 2 to 20 minutes. Pain lasting longer than 30 minutes should raise the suspicion of acute MI or a nonischemic cause.

D. **Precipitants and alleviants.** Ischemic chest pain is often precipitated by exertion and can be triggered by emotional stress, a large meal, the supine position (angina decubitus), sexual intercourse, cold weather, and use of the upper extremities. The intensity of effort necessary to incite angina often varies from day to day and throughout a given day; often, the threshold is lower in the morning, after large meals, in the cold, and with emotional upset. It may be relieved by rest within 2 to 10 minutes, by nitrates within 2 to 5 minutes, by standing, by carotid sinus massage, by oxygen, or by beta-blockade.

IV. **Diagnosis**

A. **Physical examination.** The examination must include vital signs (temperature, blood pressure in both upper extremities, heart rate, respiratory rate), general appearance (for evidence of diaphoresis, anxiety, cyanosis), gestures (Levine sign), skin examination (for evidence of xanthoma or xanthelasma), chest palpation, lung examination (for evidence of wheezing, consolidation, tympany), heart sounds and murmurs, abdominal examination (for evidence of epigastric tenderness), vascular examination, and special maneuvers (Adson).

The patient's heart rate and blood pressure may be increased, normal, or decreased. A transient regurgitation murmur may be audible in patients with ischemia. In addition, signs of left ventricular dysfunction, such as pallor, cool

TABLE 37-1. Differential diagnosis of chest pain

- Cardiac
  - Ischemic
    - Atherosclerotic
    - Coronary spasm
    - Systemic hypertension
    - Pulmonary hypertension
    - Aortic stenosis
    - Aortic insufficiency
    - Hypertrophic cardiomyopathy
    - Severe anemia
    - Severe hypoxia
    - Polycythemia
    - Nonatherosclerotic epicardial disease
  - Nonischemic
    - Aortic dissection
    - Aortic aneurysm
    - Pericarditis
    - Mitral valve prolapse
    - Myocarditis
    - Cardiomyopathy
- Noncardiac
  - Pulmonary
    - Pulmonary embolism
    - Pneumothorax
    - Pneumonia
    - Pleuritis
    - Bronchospasm
    - Pulmonary hypertension
    - Tracheitis and tracheobronchitis
    - Intrathoracic tumor
  - Gastrointestinal
    - Motility disorders
      - Nutcracker esophagus
      - Diffuse esophageal spasm
      - Lower esophageal sphincter hypertension
      - Nonspecific motility disorder
      - Achalasia
    - Gastroesophageal reflux
    - Esophageal rupture (Boerhaave syndrome)
    - Esophageal tear (Mallory-Weiss syndrome)
    - Esophagitis
      - *Candida*
      - Herpes
      - Irradiation-induced
    - Esophageal foreign body
    - Peptic ulcer disease
    - Pancreatitis
    - Biliary disease-cholecystitis or biliary colic
    - Splenic infarction
    - Gaseous bowel distention
  - Neuromusculoskeletal
    - Thoracic outlet syndrome
      - Anterior scalene hypertrophy
      - Cervical rib
    - Cervical disc disease
    - Costochondritis/Tietze syndrome
    - Chest wall trauma—rib fracture
    - Malignancy
    - Herpes zoster
    - Precordial catch syndrome
    - Sternal wire nerve entrapment
    - Xiphodynia
    - Slipping rib syndrome
    - Ostalgia due to neoplasm, inflammation, or infarction
    - Sternal marrow pain (acute leukemia)
    - Intercostal neuritis
    - Reflex autonomic dysfunction
  - Psychiatric
    - Depression
    - Anxiety
    - Panic attacks
    - Malingering
  - Other
    - Cocaine
    - Lymphoma
    - Diabetes
    - Uremia
    - Renal stones
    - Superficial thrombophlebitis (Mondor syndrome)
    - Mediastinitis
    - Mediastinal emphysema
    - Mediastinal neoplasms

clammy skin, an S_3 gallop, rales, and a dyskinetic point of maximum impulse, may be found. Funduscopic examination may reveal signs of hypertension or diabetes. Peripheral pulses may reveal bruits or diminished pedal pulses consistent with coexisting peripheral vascular disease.

B. Electrocardiography. Emergency room patients with chest pain and both ST-segment elevation and Q waves on the electrocardiogram (ECG) have an 85% chance of having an acute MI. Unfortunately, the sensitivity of ECG for serious disorders is too low to allow reassurance in the absence of abnormalities. Only 13% of patients with acute MI have ST-segment elevation and Q waves on their presenting ECG.

C. Chest radiography. Chest radiographs are routinely obtained in patients admitted to the intensive care unit with a complaint of chest pain. Helpful findings include parenchymal infiltrates, pneumothorax, vascular redistribution, widened mediastinum, cardiomegaly, atelectasis, rib fracture, free air under the diaphragm, hiatal hernia, pleural effusions, cervical ribs, abnormal calcifications, and mass lesions. Pulmonary edema should suggest the possibility of ischemia-mediated left ventricular dysfunction.

D. Other diagnostic tests. Two-dimensional echocardiography may show wall motion abnormalities before chest pain or ECG findings. Echocardiography at the time of presentation with chest pain is sensitive but less specific (53%) for MI. Immediate nuclear imaging may help to identify patients with an ischemic cause of their symptoms.

V. Etiology of nonischemic chest pain. An estimated 10% to 30% of patients with angina in whom coronary angiography is performed have normal-appearing coronary arteries. This results in the diagnosis of more than 100,000 new cases of noncardiac chest pain in the United States each year.

A. Cardiac causes

1. **Abnormal cardiac sensitivity.** Right ventricle catheter manipulation, right atrial pacing, and intracoronary contrast injection are perceived as chest pain more often in patients with chest pain syndromes and normal coronary arteries than in those with angiographically significant coronary disease.
2. **Mitral valve prolapse.** A chest pain syndrome has been described in patients with mitral valve prolapse. It may be substernal but is most often located in the left anterior precordium. It may be precipitated by exertion but not always in a reproducible manner. The duration is variable, lasting from seconds to hours.
3. **Acute pericarditis.** Chest pain associated with pericarditis is most commonly pleuritic, sharp, stabbing, left-sided, and referred to the trapezius ridge and neck if the diaphragmatic surface is involved. At times, it can be relieved by sitting forward and can be aggravated by turning in bed, swallowing, coughing, and twisting. The pain often lasts for hours and is changed little by exertion.

B. Pulmonary causes

1. **Pulmonary hypertension.** The discomfort experienced among patients with pulmonary hypertension may be identical to that described earlier for typical angina. The pain may be caused by right ventricular ischemia or dilation of the pulmonary arteries. Underlying causes include massive pulmonary embolism, primary pulmonary hypertension, severe chronic obstructive lung disease, mitral stenosis, and severe long-standing left ventricular failure.
2. **Pleural disorders.** Inflammation or distention of the pleura causes chest pain that is worsened by deep inspiration and coughing. Movement and palpation have little effect. Physical examination may reveal fever, pleural rub, pleural effusion, and pulmonary consolidation. Pleurodynia is a self-limited disease associated with Coxsackie B infection and causes pleuritic chest pain. Usually, the patient has a viral prodrome.
3. **Pneumonia.** When infectious pneumonia extends from the lung parenchyma to the pleural surface, pleuritic pain may occur. Usually, the accompanying fever, cough, dyspnea, sputum production, elevated white blood count, and radiographic findings eliminate diagnostic confusion.
4. **Pneumothorax.** Spontaneous pneumothorax with attendant lung collapse stretches the pleura, causing pleuritic chest pain and dyspnea. The chest radiograph is usually diagnostic.
5. **Pulmonary embolism.** Chest pain is a common presenting complaint among patients with pulmonary embolism. Pulmonary emboli may cause pleuritic localized pain or deep, vague, visceral, substernal discomfort. Pleuritic pain is associated with smaller emboli, which cause pulmonary infarction and atelectasis. Substernal pain is more common with massive pulmonary emboli producing right ventricular strain.

C. Vascular causes

1. **Aortic dissection.** Aortic dissection may be misdiagnosed as myocardial ischemia or MI. In addition, MI is a possible complication of aortic dissection from proximal extension involving the coronary ostia. Dissection of the aorta is suggested by severe persistent pain radiating to the back or interscapular or lumbar regions. It is often described as sudden, maximal at onset, tearing, ripping, boring, and migratory.
2. **Aortic aneurysm.** Expansion of an aortic aneurysm may cause chest pain by eroding or impinging on nearby structures. Erosion of vertebral bodies may cause boring, aching, throbbing, or localized pain.

D. Musculoskeletal causes

1. **Chest wall pain.** Musculoskeletal thoracic pain is generally of short duration (less than 1 minute), but it can last for days. It may be precipitated by abrupt movement, turning of the head or thorax, or direct palpation. Unlike ischemic pain, which occurs with exercise, musculoskeletal pain often occurs after exercise and subsides over a longer period (hours to days).

   Tietze syndrome, a rare cause of chest pain, is associated with swelling and erythema of the costochondral and costosternal junctions.

   Rib fracture causes a well-localized tenderness usually preceded by a history of trauma, malignancy, or severe osteoporosis.

   Cervical and upper thoracic osteoarthritis and herniated discs may cause chest pain similar to angina pectoris. Distinguishing characteristics of radicular pain include worsening with bending and body movement, accompanying neurologic signs and symptoms (e.g., numbness, weakness, stiffness, vertigo, tingling, paresthesias), radiation to the radial aspect of the arm or fingers, pain with coughing and sneezing, and pain with prolonged bed rest.

   Thoracic outlet syndrome, including anterior scalene muscle and cervical rib syndromes, may be confused with ischemic chest pain. Obliteration of the radial pulse with the chin elevated and rotated toward the affected side (Adson maneuver) is an important clinical finding. Chest radiography may reveal an underlying cervical rib.

   Chest pain may also occur in patients with ankylosing spondylitis, rheumatoid arthritis, psoriatic arthritis, infectious arthritis, xiphoidalgia, precordial catch syndrome, metastatic cancer, chest trauma, osteochondroma, osteosarcoma, multiple myeloma, slipping rib syndrome, and fibromyalgia.

   Precordial catch (Texidor twinge) is believed to result from muscle spasm and causes acute sharp anterior chest pain in young adults that is worse during breathing and is relieved by taking a deep breath or by stretching.

   After open heart surgery, patients may complain of chest discomfort. In addition to concerns about adequate revascularization and technical difficulties, possibilities to consider include nerve entrapment, postpericardiotomy syndrome, mediastinitis, costochondritis, and superficial wound infections.
2. **Herpes zoster.** Herpes zoster (shingles) can affect the anterior chest and can mimic angina pectoris. However, the pain is dermatomal and does not cross the midline. Associated neurologic complaints include hyperesthesia, hypoesthesia, and dysesthesia.

E. Psychiatric causes. Since the Civil War in the United States, chest pain has been recognized as a feature of anxiety (DaCosta syndrome, soldier's heart, neurocirculatory asthenia). The discomfort is more commonly located in the inframammary region, near the cardiac apex. It is variably described as dull and aching or sharp and stabbing. It can last from seconds to hours.

F. Gastrointestinal causes

1. **Esophagus.** Esophageal chest pain is described as a visceral discomfort and may be misdiagnosed as angina pectoris. Among patients with chest pain and angiographically normal-appearing coronary arteries, 20% to 60% have esophageal abnormalities.

   Common descriptors of esophageal pain include heartburn, acid, warmth, fullness, pressure, and gnawing. The symptoms may be provoked by ingestion of food, especially at the extremes of temperature, of large quantity, or immediately before recumbency. Esophageal pain is often substernal, but it may extend to the right or left chest and may radiate to the back.

2. **Gastroesophageal reflux disease.** Recent studies with ambulatory monitoring suggest that the most common esophageal cause of chest pain is gastroesophageal reflux disease. Up to 10% of patients with gastroesophageal reflux disease have chest pain as their only symptom.
3. **Esophageal motility disorders.** Motility disorders have long been recognized as a cause of chest pain. They include "nutcracker" esophagus (high-amplitude, peristaltic contractions of long duration), diffuse esophageal spasm (frequent simultaneous contractions in the distal esophagus), nonspecific abnormalities, lower esophageal sphincter hypertension, and achalasia.

Other esophageal causes of chest pain include esophageal rupture (Boerhaave syndrome), esophageal tear (Mallory-Weiss syndrome), infectious esophagitis (e.g., from herpes, *Candida*), and irradiation-induced esophagitis.

Biliary tract disease, including sphincter of Oddi spasm, cholelithiasis, and cholecystitis, can mimic ischemic chest pain. The discomfort with these diseases may present substernally and may respond to nitroglycerin.

Pancreatitis may mimic myocardial ischemia or infarction. The discomfort associated with pancreatitis is often transmitted to the back.

Peptic ulcer disease may be confused with myocardial ischemic syndromes. The relationship between symptoms and either food intake or relief with antacids is an important clinical feature.

G. Other causes

1. **Myocarditis.** The clinical spectrum of viral myocarditis ranges from asymptomatic ECG abnormalities to fulminant heart failure, cardiogenic shock, and death.
2. **Cocaine.** Cocaine use has been associated with MI. Cocaine increases myocardial oxygen demand and decreases coronary artery blood flow.

Selected Readings

Christie LG, Conti CR. Systematic approach to evaluation of angina-like chest pain: pathophysiology and clinical testing with emphasis on objective documentation of myocardial ischemia. *Am Heart J* 1981;102:897.

A step-wise approach to patients with chest pain and suspected myocardial ischemia.

Kannel WB, Abbott RD. Incidence and prognosis of unrecognized myocardial infarction: an update from the Framingham Study. *N Engl J Med* 1984;311:1144.

The Framingham data provided important information on the incidence and prognosis of unrecognized MI.

Lee TH, Rouan GW, Weisberg MC, et al. Clinical characteristics and natural history of patients with acute myocardial infarction sent home from the emergency room. *Am J Cardiol* 1987;60:219.

One of the most feared situations in clinical medicine is discharging a patient with acute MI from the emergency department. The clinical characteristics and outcomes are reviewed.

38. EVALUATION AND MANAGEMENT OF HYPERTENSION IN THE INTENSIVE CARE UNIT

Robert J. Heyka and Richard C. Becker

I. Hypertensive urgencies and emergencies. Evaluation and management of patients in the intensive care unit (ICU) with elevated blood pressure involve two general situations. Patients may have a hypertensive crisis requiring urgent or emergency therapy, or they may have a transient, more benign elevation in blood pressure that is less critical.

II. Definitions. The term *hypertensive crisis* is loosely defined as a severe elevation in blood pressure. Hypertensive emergencies and urgencies are categories of hypertensive crises that are potentially life-threatening situations that may occur against the background of a sudden worsening of chronic essential hypertension, with secondary forms of hypertension, or *de novo.* Usually, the patient has severe elevation of blood pressure with diastolic blood pressures higher than 120 to 130 mm Hg. However, the level of systolic blood pressure, diastolic blood pressure, or mean arterial pressure itself does not distinguish these two entities. Rather, they are differentiated by the presence or absence of acute and progressive target organ damage (TOD) (Table 38-1).

A hypertensive emergency means that the blood pressure elevation is associated with ongoing central nervous system, myocardial, hematologic, or renal TOD, whereas a hypertensive urgency means that the potential for TOD damage is great and likely if blood pressure is not soon controlled. Accelerated hypertension and malignant hypertension refer to sub-categories of hypertensive crises with exudative retinopathy. They probably represent a continuum of organ damage.

Accelerated hypertension is a hypertensive crisis with grade III Keith-Wagener-Barker retinopathy consisting of constriction and sclerosis (i.e., grades I or II) plus hemorrhages and exudates (making this grade III). The presence of exudate is more worrisome than hemorrhage alone. Accelerated hypertension may be an urgency or an emergency, depending on involvement of other target organs.

Malignant hypertension is a crisis with the presence of Keith-Wagener-Barker grade IV retinopathy involving the foregoing findings plus papilledema. It is frequently associated with diffuse TOD such as hypertensive encephalopathy, left ventricular failure, or fibrinoid necrosis, and it is sometimes associated with microangiopathic hemolytic anemia.

III. Approach to the patient. In the ICU, therapy must often begin before a comprehensive patient evaluation is completed. A systematic approach offers the opportunity to be both expeditious and inclusive (Table 38-2).

A brief history and physical examination should be initiated to assess the degree of TOD and to rule out obvious secondary causes of hypertension. The history should include inquiries about prior hypertension, other significant medical disease, and medication use and compliance. Important symptoms attributable to TOD include neurologic (headache, nausea, and vomiting; visual changes; seizures; focal deficits; mental status changes), cardiac, or renal. This history must sometimes be supplemented by family members. Physical examination should first verify blood pressure readings—in both arms, while the patient is supine and standing, if possible. Intraarterial monitoring may be necessary. Signs of neurologic ischemia, such as altered mental status or focal neurologic deficits, should be sought. Direct ophthalmologic examination, auscultation of the lungs and heart, evaluation of the abdomen and peripheral pulses for bruits, masses, or deficits, and assessment of recent urine output can be quickly accomplished. Ancillary and laboratory evaluation should include electrolytes, blood urea nitrogen and creatinine, complete blood count with differential, assessment of cardiac function, and chest radiography.

IV. Treatment. The intensity of intervention is determined by the clinical situation. Depending on the TOD, interventions such as intubation, control of seizures, hemo-

TABLE 38-1. Examples of hypertensive crises

Generalized	Cardiovascular	Neurologic	Renal
Accelerated and malignant hypertension	Acute left ventricular failure	Hypertensive encephalopathy	Acute renal failure
Microangiopathic hemolytic anemia/ disseminated intravascular coagulation	Unstable angina pectoris	Subarachnoid hemorrhage	Acute glomerulonephritis
Eclampsia	Myocardial infarction	Intracerebral hemorrhage	Scleroderma crisis
Vasculitis	Aortic dissection	Cerebrovascular accident	
Catecholamine excess (drugs, rebound syndrome, pheochromocytoma)	Suture integrity after surgery		

From Vidt DG, Gifford RW. A compendium for the treatment of hypertensive emergencies. *Cleve Clin Q* 1984;51:421, with permission.

dynamic monitoring, and maintenance of urine output can be as important as prompt control of blood pressure. The goal of initial therapy is to terminate ongoing TOD, *not* to return blood pressure to normal levels because cerebral autoregulation determines the initial stop point. In both hypertensive and normotensive patients, this floor is approximately 25% lower than the initial mean arterial pressure or a diastolic blood pressure in the range of 110 to 100 mm Hg. Therefore, a reasonable target for initial therapy is to decrease mean arterial pressure by 20% to 25% with an agent that decreases systemic vascular resistance, taking into consideration the patient's medical history, initiating events, and ongoing TOD. However, patients with acute left ventricular failure, myocardial ischemia, or aortic dissection require more aggressive treatment because both systemic vascular resistance and cardiac output *must* be decreased.

The decision to use oral or parenteral therapy depends on whether the patient is conscious, whether there is TOD, how rapidly the onset of response is needed, how rapidly the pressure must be lowered, and whether the patient is at risk for new complications from overaggressive treatment (Table 38-3). Evidence of cardiac, cerebrovascular, or renovascular disease puts the patient at high risk if therapy overshoots the mark.

TABLE 38-2. Initial evaluation of hypertensive crisis in the intensive care unit

- Continuous blood pressure monitoring
  - Direct (intraarterial) preferred
  - Indirect (cuff)
- Brief initial evaluation—history and physical examination with attention to
  - Neurologic, cardiac, pulmonary, renal symptoms
  - Organ perfusion and function
  - Blood and urine studies: electrolytes, BUN, creatinine, CBC with differential, urinalysis with sediment; if indicated, serum catecholamines, cardiac enzymes
  - ECG
  - Chest radiograph
- Initiation of therapy
- Further evaluation of etiology once stabilized

BUN, blood urea nitrogen; CBC, complete blood count; ECG, electrocardiogram.
From Vidt DG, Gifford RW. A compendium for the treatment of hypertensive emergencies. *Cleve Clin Q* 1984;51:421, with permission.

TABLE 38-3. Parenteral versus oral therapy of hypertension in the intensive care unit

Is this a hypertensive emergency?
Is rapid onset of effect needed?
Is rapid lowering of blood pressure needed?
Is a shorter duration of action important?
Is the patient at risk for overshoot hypotension?
  Atherosclerotic heart disease
  Renovascular hypertension
  Cerebrovascular disease
  Dehydration
  Other recent antihypertensive therapy

The answers to the questions in Table 38-3 guide the decision of parenteral versus oral therapy. Table 38-4 lists recommendations and precautions for therapeutic agents, and Table 38-5 lists proper dosing for each agent.

A. New onset of hypertension. New, unexpected, temporary increases in blood pressure may be seen in the ICU. Secondary causes should be sought. Factors such as pain, anxiety, new onset of angina, hypercarbia or hypoxia, hypothermia, rigors, excessive arousal after sedation, or fluid mobilization with volume overload can all lead to short-term elevations in blood pressure (Table 38-6). If antihypertensive agents are necessary, low doses of short-acting agents should be used to avoid sharp drops in blood pressure in this usually self-limited situation.

B. Perioperative hypertension. Uncontrolled blood pressure can induce new TOD, increase the risk of vascular suture breakdown or bleeding, and worsen overall prognoses.

1. **Preoperative.** Moderate chronic hypertension is not a major risk factor for surgery in otherwise stable patients, but it is a marker for potential coronary artery disease. Routine blood pressure therapy should be continued as regularly scheduled up to the morning of surgery. Pretreatment (up to 2 weeks) before elective surgery with beta-blockers can control blood pressure during anesthesia, intubation, and extubation with decreased risk of ischemia. In patients at risk of or with known coronary artery disease, intravenous atenolol, preoperatively and during hospitalization, can decrease cardiovascular complications and mortality in noncardiac surgery.
2. **Perioperative.** Persistent blood pressure readings higher than 160/100 mm Hg in a previously normotensive patient or an increase of more than 30 mm Hg (systolic or diastolic) above preoperative levels in a known hypertensive patient are worrisome. A useful classification of hypertension associated with cardiovascular surgery considers the clinical situation rather than the specific pathologic mechanism (Table 38-7).
3. **Postoperative.** Once the patient returns to the ICU, the immediate postoperative period (up to 2 hours) represents a time of significant patient instability, and blood pressures can vary widely. There is an increase in pressor reflexes and increased central nervous system activity. Pain, hypothermia with shivering, hypercarbia and hypoxia, or reflex excitement after anesthesia can lead to changes in blood pressure that require minute-to-minute adjustment. The goal is to avoid both overshoot hypotension and inadequate control. Because hypertension in this setting is usually neither severe nor long lasting and is usually sensitive to small doses of antihypertensive medications, intravenous infusion or minibolus therapy allows the most controlled approach to blood pressure regulation. Nitroprusside or labetalol is effective in most situations. In the patient with fixed coronary lesions, nitroglycerin can be used to improve poststenotic collateral flow.

C. Pharmacologic agents. Therapeutic options for treatment of hypertension in the ICU setting are rapidly expanding.

TABLE 38-4. Treatment of hypertensive emergency

Etiology		Recommended drugs	Drugs to avoid
Neurologic	Hypertensive encephalopathy	Nitroprusside, labetalol, diazoxide	M-Dopa, clonidine, beta-blockers
	Intracerebral hemorrhage or subarachnoid hemorrhage	Nitroprusside, labetalol	M-Dopa, clonidine, beta-blockers
	Cerebral infarction	Nitroprusside, labetalol	M-Dopa, clonidine, beta-blockers
	Head injury	Nitroprusside	M-Dopa, clonidine, beta-blockers
Cardiovascular	Myocardial ischemia, infarction	Nitroglycerin, nitroprusside, labetalol, calcium antagonists, beta-blockers	Minoxidil, hydralazine, diazoxide
	Aortic dissection	Nitroprusside, beta-blockers, labetalol, trimethaphan	Minoxidil, hydralazine, diazoxide, nitroglycerin
	Acute left ventricular failure	Nitroprusside, nitroglycerin, loop diuretics, converting enzyme inhibitors	Minoxidil, hydralazine, diazoxide, labetalol, beta-blockers
Renal failure	Acute renal failure	Nitroprusside, labetalol, calcium antagonists	
Other	Microangiopathic hemolytic anemia	Nitroprusside, labetalol, calcium antagonists	
	Malignant hypertension	As with encephalopathy—oral agents may be considered	
	Eclampsia	Hydralazine, diazoxide, labetalol, calcium antagonists	Diuretics, beta-blockers

M-Dopa, methyldopate hydrochloride.
From Vidt DG, Gifford RW. A compendium for the treatment of hypertensive emergencies. *Cleve Clin Q* 1984;51:421, with permission.

TABLE 38-5. Proper dosing for agents to treat hypertensive crisis

Agent	Administration	Onset	Duration
Direct vasodilators			
Nitroprusside	i.v. infusion: 0.25–10.0 mg/kg/min	Immediate	3–5 min
Nitroglycerin	i.v. infusion: 5–100 mg/min	2–5 min	3–5 min
Diazoxide	i.v. bolus: 50–100 mg q10–15 min (total 600 mg)	1–5 min	6–12 h
	i.v. infusion: 10–30 mg/min		
Beta-blockers			
Esmolol	250–500 mg/kg/min for 1 min; then 50–100 mg/kg/min/ for 4 min; may repeat	1–2 min	10–20 min
Labetalol	i.v. bolus: 20–80 mg q10 min	5–10 min	3–6 h
	i.v. infusion: 2mg/min	5–10 min	3–6 h
Calcium antagonists			
Nicardipine	i.v. infusion: 5–15 mg/h	5–10 min	1–4h
Verapamil	i.v. bolus: 5–10 mg over 1–5 min	1–5 min	30–60 min
	i.v. infusion: 3–25 mg/h (maximum 90 mg/h)	1–5 min	30–60 min
Diltiazem	i.v. bolus: 5–20 mg (repeat q15–30 min) up to 20 mg	15–30 min	3 h
	i.v. infusion: 5–10 mg/h ↑ by mg/h, up to 15 mg q30 min	5–10 min	3 h
Nimodipine	60 mg q4h × 21 days; repeat	1 h	2–4 h
Angiotensin-converting enzyme inhibitors			
Captopril	p.o. 6.25–25 mg, repeat q30 min, if necessary	15–50 min	4–6 h
Enalaprilat	i.v. bolus: 1.25–5.0 mg (over 5 min) q6h	15 min	6 h
Central agonists			
Clonidine	p.o. 0.2 mg initially; 0.2 mg/h (total 0.7 mg)	30–120	8–12 h
Methyldopate	i.v. infusion: 250–500 mg	30–60 min	3–6 h
Miscellaneous			
Fenoldopam	i.v. infusion: 0.1 mg/kg/min; ↑ by 0.05–0.2 mg/kg/h at 20-min intervals	20–30 min	1–3 h
Hydralazine	i.v. bolus: 10–20 mg	10–20 min	3–8 h
	i.v. 10–50mg i.m.	20–30 min	
Phentolamine	i.v. bolus: 5–10 mg q5–15 min	1–5 min	3–10 min
Trimethaphan	i.v. infusion: 0.5–5 mg/min	1–5 min	10 min

i.v., intravenous; i.m., intramuscular injection; p.o., oral.
From Vidt DG, Gifford RW. A compendium for the treatment of hypertensive emergencies. *Cleve Clin Q* 1984;51:421, with permission.

TABLE 38-6. New onset of hypertension in the intensive care unit

- Situational
  - Pain
  - Anxiety
  - New-onset angina
  - Hypocarbia
  - Hypoxemia
  - Hypothermia with shivering
  - Rigors
  - Volume overload
- Rebound or discontinuation syndrome
- Prior, undiagnosed, untreated hypertension
  - Fundus, examination
  - Two-dimensional echocardiogram for concentric left ventricular hypertrophy

1. **Direct vasodilators**
   a. **Sodium nitroprusside.** Sodium nitroprusside is the most predictable and effective agent for the treatment of severe hypertension. It dilates both arterioles and venules (reducing both afterload and preload) and lowers myocardial oxygen demands.
   b. **Nitroglycerin.** Nitroglycerin predominantly dilates the venous system.
   c. **Hydralazine.** Parenteral hydralazine was removed from the United States market in 1993 and was returned in 1994. It is a direct arterial vasodilator that increases cardiac output and heart rate.
2. **Beta-blockers.** Several beta-blockers, such as propranolol (nonselective), metoprolol (selective), and the short-acting esmolol (selective), can be given parenterally. Labetalol is the beta-blocker used most commonly for elevated blood pressures in the ICU.

TABLE 38-7. Hypertension with cardiovascular surgery

- Preoperative period
  - Anxiety
  - Pain
  - Angina
  - Discontinuation of antihypertensive or cardiac therapy
  - Rebound hypertension
- Intraoperative period
  - Induction of anesthesia
    - Drug effects—vasodilation, inotropic changes
    - Manipulation of viscera or trachea, urethra, and rectum
    - Stemotomy, chest retraction
  - With initiation of cardiopulmonary bypass
- Postoperative period
  - Early (0–2 h)
    - Hypoxemia, hypercarbia, hypothermia with shivering, postanesthetic excitement or pain
    - After myocardial revascularization, valve replacement, repair of aortic coarctation
  - Intermediate (12–36 h)
    - As above
    - Fluid overload, mobilization
    - Reaction to endotracheal, nasogastric, chest; or bladder tube

From Estafanous FG. Hypertension in the surgical patient: Management of blood pressure and anesthesia. *Cleve Clin J Med* 1989;56:385, with permission.

3. **Calcium antagonists.** Calcium antagonists, particularly the dihydropyridine subclass, have become more widely used in the ICU setting.
   a. **Nifedipine.** Nifedipine is administered orally or sublingually, although an intranasal preparation is being tested in Europe. It decreases peripheral vascular resistance and increases collateral coronary blood flow. There is an uncontrolled and unpredictable reduction in blood pressure after oral or sublingual administration. Serious complications, such as myocardial infarction or ischemia, worsening renal function, and cerebral ischemia, have been reported because of the precipitous reduction in blood pressure to less than autoregulatory limits.
   b. **Nicardipine.** Nicardipine is a dihydropyridine calcium antagonist that is a rapid-acting systemic and coronary artery vasodilator. It has minimal effects on cardiac conductivity or inotropy.
   c. **Nimodipine.** Nimodipine is a dihydropyridine calcium antagonist that crosses the blood-brain barrier and has been used in the ICU. A meta-analysis of its use in subarachnoid hemorrhage showed a statistically significant benefit on risk for severe disability, vegetative state, or death, but its putative effect on preventing vasospasm is less clear. It is currently recommended only for patients with subarachnoid hemorrhage who are on a 21-day oral dosing schedule.
   d. **Verapamil.** Verapamil is a phenylalkylamine calcium antagonist that is an arterial vasodilator. It has a greater effect on atrioventricular conduction than the dihydropyridine subgroup and is useful in the treatment of a variety of tachyarrhythmias. It also has a more pronounced negative inotropic effect and a rapid onset of action with a relatively low incidence of serious side effects. Verapamil can be given as repeated small boluses or a continuous intravenous infusion.
   e. **Diltiazem.** Diltiazem is a benzothiazepine calcium antagonist available as an intravenous preparation. It is a nondihydropyridine calcium antagonist with effects intermediate between those of verapamil and of the dihydropyridine group.
4. **Angiotensin-converting enzyme inhibitors**
   a. **Captopril.** Captopril was the first angiotensin-converting enzyme (ACE) inhibitor available in the United States. It is rapidly absorbed, with peak blood levels reached 30 minutes after administration.

      Captopril has a rapid onset of effect after oral administration. There is no change in cardiac output or reflex tachycardia. ACE inhibitors are particularly effective in patients with congestive heart failure or recent myocardial infarction. There is a risk of acute hypotension or worsening of renal function in patients who are volume depleted, who have bilateral high-grade renal artery stenosis, or who have high-grade stenosis in a solitary functioning kidney. Other acute side effects include bronchospasm, hyperkalemia, cough, angioedema, rash, and dysgeusia. The drug can accumulate in patients with renal failure.
   b. **Enalaprilat.** Enalaprilat is the only ACE inhibitor that can be administered parenterally. It is the active form of the oral agent, enalapril. Enalaprilat is useful when oral therapy is impractical in patients who have been previously treated with an ACE inhibitor, in those with underlying left ventricular dysfunction, or in those with recent myocardial infarction.
5. **Central agonist: clonidine.** Clonidine is an $alpha_2$ central agonist that decreases peripheral vascular resistance. The decrease in venous return and bradycardia can contribute to reduction in cardiac output at rest. Clonidine is available as an oral preparation and a transdermal patch with an effectiveness of approximately 1 week. The patch should not be used to initiate therapy in the ICU because it takes several days to achieve a steady state.
6. **Diuretics.** Diuretics are usually not considered primary agents in managing hypertensive crises because most patients are hypovolemic. However, patients with postoperative hypertension, cardiac dysfunction, or evidence of pulmonary edema may require the use of these drugs. In addition, many par-

enteral antihypertensive agents tend to induce fluid retention that can lead to pseudoresistance to the drug. In these instances, loop diuretics, such as furosemide or bumetanide, can help control intravascular volume, maintain urine output, and prevent resistance to antihypertensive therapy. Loop diuretics can be given intravenously as a bolus or a slow continuous infusion.

Selected Readings

Breslin DJ, Gifford RW, Fairbairn JF, et al. Prognostic importance of ophthalmoscopic findings in essential hypertension. *JAMA* 1966;195:91.

The fundoscopic examination, frequently overlooked in daily clinical practice, provides important prognostic information in patients with hypertension.

Calhoun DA, Oparil S. Treatment of hypertensive crisis. *N Engl J Med* 1990;323:1177.

A review of treatment strategies for use in hypertensive crisis.

Mangano DT, Layug EL, Wallace A, et al. Effect of atenolol on mortality and cardiovascular morbidity after noncardiac surgery. *N Engl J Med* 1996;335:1713.

Beta-blocker therapy has a favorable impact on outcome among patients undergoing noncardiac surgery.

Vidt DG, Gifford RW. A compendium for the treatment of hypertensive emergencies. *Cleve Clin Q* 1984;51:421.

Two of the leaders in hypertension provide an overview of treatment modalities.

39. SUPRAVENTRICULAR TACHYCARDIAS

Edward P. Gerstenfeld, Steven P. Beaudette, Robert S. Mittleman, and Richard C. Becker

I. **General principles.** Supraventricular tachycardias (SVTs) are frequently encountered in the intensive care setting. Since the advent of invasive electrophysiologic studies, insight into the mechanisms responsible for these arrhythmias has dramatically improved.

II. **Definition.** A tachycardia is considered supraventricular in origin if the atrium or atrioventricular (A-V) junction participates in the arrhythmia, either as the origin of the abnormal impulse or as an essential part of a reentrant circuit. The QRS complex is usually narrow; however, at rapid ventricular rates, aberrant ventricular conduction may produce a wide QRS complex.

III. **Pathophysiology.** Two general mechanisms account for the generation of supraventricular arrhythmias, abnormal impulse conduction and abnormal impulse formation. Abnormal impulse conduction occurs in reentry. Abnormal impulse formation includes abnormal or enhanced automaticity and triggered activity. Most clinical arrhythmias are due to reentry.

IV. **Diagnosis.** For a patient who is hemodynamically stable, a 12-lead electrocardiogram (ECG) obtained as rapidly as possible provides essential information. If a 12-lead ECG cannot be obtained, a telemetry recording may be of value. Special attention should be given to identifying the P waves. Usually, leads II and V_1 are the best leads by which to identify atrial activity. After open heart surgery, epicardial recording electrodes are commonly placed; when these electrodes are available, they can be of enormous value in identifying atrial activity (Figs. 39-1 and 39-2).

Vagal maneuvers can provide important insight into the mechanisms of an SVT and can often lead to a diagnosis or termination of the arrhythmia. The carotid arteries should first be auscultated. Firm pressure is then applied for 5 to 10 seconds directly over the carotid pulse near the angle of the mandible. SVTs with reentry circuits involving the sinoatrial (S-A) or A-V nodes may terminate. SVTs caused by reentry circuits that do not involve the S-A or A-V nodes, such as atrial flutter or atrial fibrillation, do not terminate but may be easier to diagnose because the ventricular response slows, thus allowing identification of atrial activity. If the rhythm is sinus tachycardia, there will be gradual slowing, with a return to the former rate once the maneuver is discontinued (Table 39-1).

V. **Treatment.** The treatment of an SVT is geared toward the underlying mechanism (Table 39-2 and Fig. 39-3).

A. **Cardioversion.** Direct current cardioversion is the treatment of choice for patients who are hemodynamically compromised from a reentrant SVT. In addition, synchronized direct current cardioversion can be performed in the hemodynamically stable patient to restore sinus rhythm.

B. **Adenosine.** Adenosine can be effective in both diagnosis and treatment of SVTs. When given by intravenous bolus, the drug produces slowing in sinus and A-V nodal tissues. Therefore, SVTs with reentry circuits that involve these structures can be terminated with immediate return to sinus rhythm.

C. **Drugs for rate control**

1. **Cardiac glycosides.** The cardiac glycosides, primarily digitalis, cause conduction slowing and lengthening of refractoriness in the S-A and A-V nodes. These drugs are useful in acute or chronic treatment for SVTs with a reentry circuit involving the S-A or A-V node or in slowing the ventricular rate in atrial fibrillation or flutter.
2. **Beta-blockers.** Beta-blockers (propranolol, metoprolol, atenolol, esmolol) exert their effect by competitively inhibiting catecholamine binding to beta-adrenergic receptors. They are useful in short-term or long-term treatment

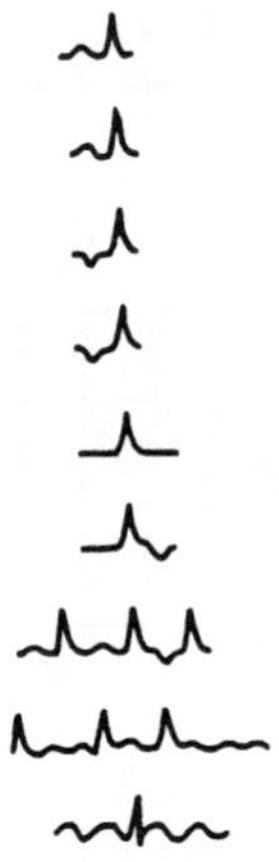

Type	P-Wave Morphology	P-Wave Location	Presumed Mechanism
Sinus Tachycardia	Normal		↑ Automaticity
Sinus Node Re-entry	Normal		Re-entry
Automatic Atrial Tachycardia	Abnormal		↑ Automaticity
Intra-atrial Re-entry	Abnormal		Re-entry
AV Nodal Re-entry	ABN (not seen)		Re-entry
AV-Reciprocating Tachycardia	Abnormal		Re-entry
Multifocal Atrial Tachycardia	Varying		↑ Automaticity
Atrial Fibrillation	Chaotic		Re-entry
Atrial Flutter	Sawtooth		Re-entry

FIG. 39-1. Characteristics of supraventricular tachyarrhythmias.

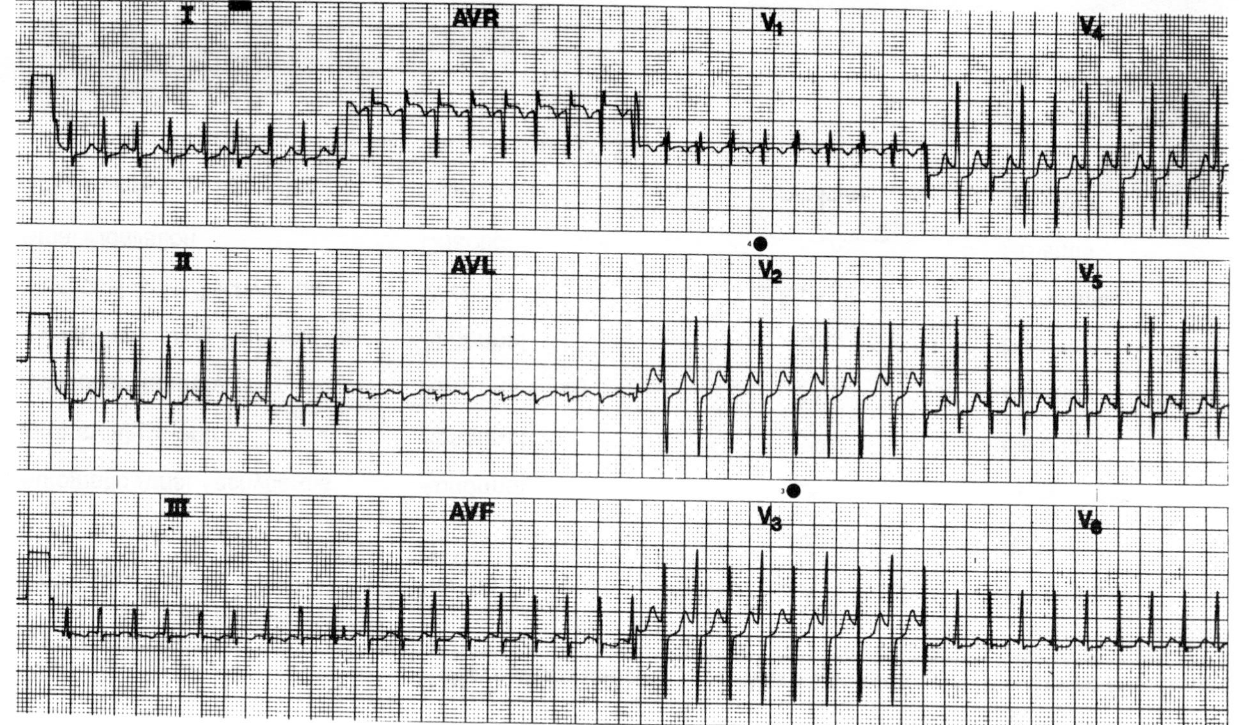

FIG. 39-2. Standard 12-lead electrocardiogram from two young patients with paroxysmal palpitations. **A:** There is a narrow complex rhythm with no visible P waves. By electrophysiologic testing, this patient was found to have an atrioventricular nodal reentry tachycardia. **B:** Patient with an atrioventricular reciprocating tachycardia. Note the P waves, which occur immediately after the QRS complex and are best seen in the inferior leads *(arrows)*.

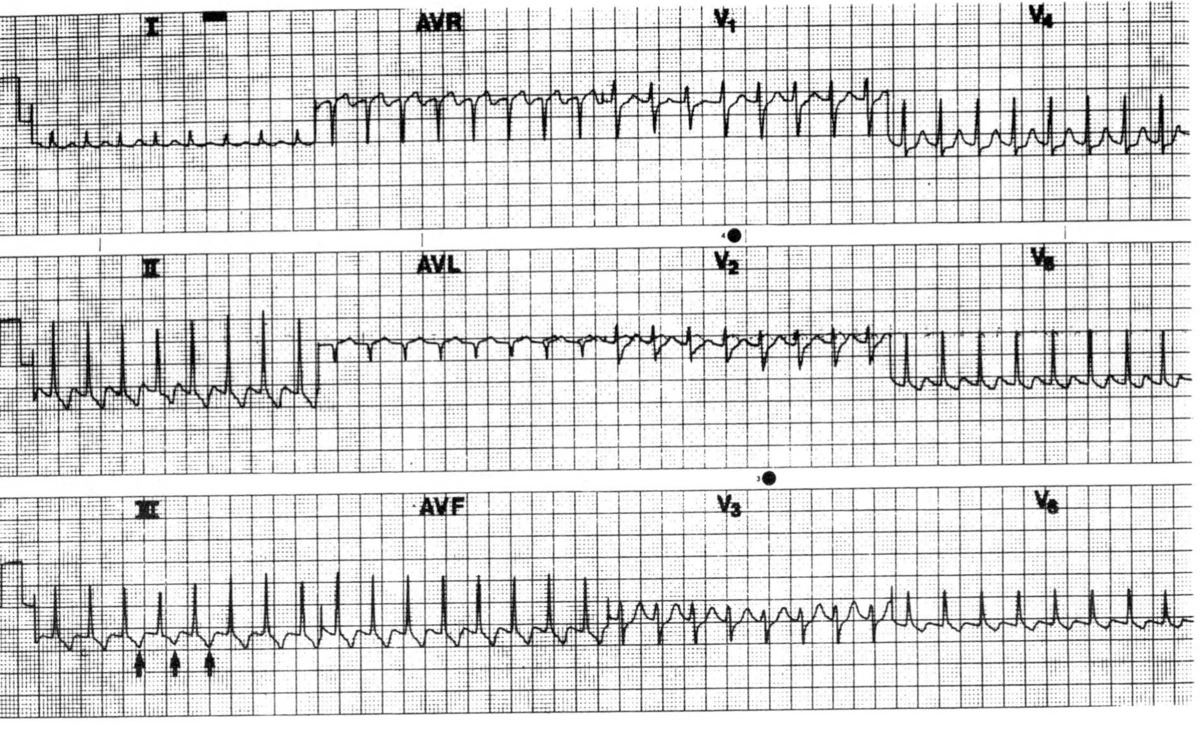

FIG. 39-2. *Continued.*

TABLE 39-1. Effect of vagal maneuvers or adenosine on supraventricular tachycardias

Arrhythmia	Response to Maneuver
A-V nodal reentry tachycardia	No effect or abrupt conversion to NSR
A-V reciprocating tachycardia	No effect or abrupt conversion to NSR
Intraatrial reentry tachycardia	No effect or increase in A-V block
Sinus node reentry tachycardia	No effect or abrupt conversion to NSR
Atrial fibrillation	Increased A-V block, with slowing of the ventricular rate
Atrial flutter	Increased A-V block, with slowing of the ventricular rate
Sinus tachycardia	Gradual slowing, then gradual acceleration
Automatic atrial tachycardia	Increased A-V block, with slowing of the ventricular rate
Multifocal atrial tachycardia	Increased A-V block, with slowing of the ventricular rate

A-V, atrioventricular; NSR, normal sinus rhythm.

of SVTs caused by a reentry circuits and can also be used to slow ventricular response.

3. **Calcium channel blockers.** Verapamil and diltiazem block the slow calcium channels and lead to slowed conduction in the sinus and A-V nodes. These drugs can be used to suppress reentrant arrhythmias that involve the sinus or A-V node. They are also effective in slowing the ventricular response to atrial arrhythmias.

D. Drugs used to convert and maintain normal sinus rhythm

1. **Class I antiarrhythmic agents.** Class IA drugs block fast sodium channels and therefore reduce the maximal rate of rise of the action potential upstroke (V_{max}), slowing conduction velocity in atrial and ventricular myocardium. These effects are manifest as QRS and QT-interval prolongation on the surface ECG. Agents in this class are quinidine and procainamide.

   Class IC drugs markedly decrease V_{max} and lead to a slowing of conduction in atrial and ventricular myocardial tissue. On ECG, this appears as a widening of the QRS complex. Agents currently available in this class are flecainide and propafenone. In general, they are well tolerated but carry a risk of proarrhythmia.

2. **Class III antiarrhythmic agents.** Class III antiarrhythmic agents block potassium channels and prolong repolarization without significantly altering conduction velocity. Each of these drugs, however, has additional electrophysiologic effects. The class III agents currently available to treat SVTs are amiodarone, sotalol, and ibutilide.

E. Electrophysiologic ablation. In patients with recurrent symptomatic episodes of SVT who are refractory to or intolerant of medical therapy, radiofrequency ablation can eliminate many common SVTs (Fig. 39-4).

VI. Individual supraventricular tachycardias

A. Reentrant supraventricular tachycardias

1. Atrial fibrillation

a. **Mechanisms.** Atrial fibrillation is the most common supraventricular arrhythmia. It often occurs in the setting of underlying structural heart or pulmonary disease. It is also associated with valvular heart disease, cardiomyopathies, pericarditis, pulmonary embolism, ethanol excess, and thyrotoxicosis.

b. **Diagnosis.** The symptoms of atrial fibrillation are variable, depending on the ventricular rate and underlying heart disease. Some patients are asymptomatic. Palpitations or irregular pulse are often noted. The increased rate can lead to angina in patients with coronary artery disease. The loss of atrial contraction along with the increased rate can lead to a drop in cardiac output and resultant congestive heart failure. The hemodynamic compromise is often worse in patients with disorders reliant on the atrial component of ventricular filling, such as dilated and hypertrophic cardiomyopathies and aortic stenosis.

On ECG, atrial activity is irregular in both timing and morphology at a rate of 350 to 600 beats per minute. In untreated patients with normal A-V node function, the rate is usually 120 to 180 beats per minute.

c. Management. The management strategy in patients with atrial fibrillation should address three areas: ventricular rate control, anticoagulation, and conversion to or maintenance of sinus rhythm.

Ventricular rate control of patients with acute onset of atrial fibrillation with a rapid ventricular response can be accomplished with any of the A-V nodal blocking drugs, calcium channel blockers, beta-blockers, or digoxin. Critically ill patients in the intensive care unit often have high levels of catecholamines and sympathetic tone, which impairs digoxin's vagally mediated medicated slowing of ventricular rate. Intravenous beta-blockers and calcium channel blockers have a much faster onset and do not require adjustment for renal insufficiency. Once ventricular rate control is achieved with short-acting intravenous medication, therapy should rapidly be changed to the oral route.

The risk of stroke in patients who are more than 65 years old and have nonrheumatic chronic atrial fibrillation but who are not anticoagulated is approximately 4.5% per year and increases with age and risk factors (diabetes, hypertension, pervious thromboembolism, left ventricular dysfunction, and left atrial enlargement). All patients with atrial fibrillation of unknown duration and no contraindications should receive anticoagulant therapy. Patients with new-onset atrial fibrillation while in the hospital may be given 24 hours of observation to convert spontaneously to sinus rhythm but then should be started on heparin therapy if atrial fibrillation persists.

Most patients with new-onset atrial fibrillation who do not convert to sinus rhythm spontaneously should undergo attempts to return them to sinus rhythm. Patients with known atrial fibrillation of less than 48 hours' duration may undergo cardioversion without prior anticoagulation with a low rate of thromboembolism. Patients with atrial fibrillation of longer duration should undergo 3 to 4 weeks of anticoagulation with warfarin before and after cardioversion to sinus rhythm. Patients who do not tolerate atrial fibrillation well or who have contraindications to long-term anticoagulation may undergo cardioversion after a transesophageal echocardiogram to exclude an atrial thrombus. Preliminary evidence indicates that transesophageal echocardiography–guided cardioversion is safe when it is preceded by at least 24 hours of heparin and is followed by 3 weeks of anticoagulation with warfarin.

2. Atrial flutter

a. Mechanisms. Typical atrial flutter is caused by a single reentrant wavefront in the right atrium.

b. Diagnosis. Patients often complain of palpitations and are often more symptomatic than patients with atrial fibrillation.

The ECG of typical atrial flutter is delineated by characteristic sawtooth-shaped flutter waves that are regular in timing and morphology at a rate between 250 and 350 beats per minute. Patients often have 2:1 block in the A-V node, with a resultant ventricular rate of approximately 150 beats per minute.

c. Management. Therapy is similar to that for atrial fibrillation: rate control, anticoagulation, and conversion to sinus rhythm.

TABLE 39-2. Drugs commonly used for treatment of supraventricular tachycardias

Drug	Most Commonly Used Dosage	Half-life	Route of Elimination	Major Adverse Effects	Comments
Adenosine	i.v., bolus: 6–12 mg (3 mg if given centrally)	10 sec	Erythrocytes	Transient dyspnea, flushing, chest pain, S-A and A-V block	Larger dose may be needed in the presence of caffeine and theophylline; reduce dose with concomitant dipyridamole use
Digoxin	i.v. loading: 0.5–1 mg over 24 h p.o.: 0.125–0.5 mg q.d.	36–48 h	Renal	Fatigue, nausea, visual disturbances, arrhythmias	Adjust maintenance dose in renal failure; accelerates accessory bypass tract conduction.
Propranolol	i.v.: 1–3 mg p.o.: 10–80 mg q6h	4–6 h	Hepatic	CHF, bronchospasm. S-A and A-V block, hypotension, masks hypoglycemia, depression	Nonselective beta-receptor blocker
Metoprolol	i.v.: 5 mg q5min (to 15 mg) p.o.: 50–200 mg/qd: 2–4 times/d	3–7 h	Hepatic	See propranolol	$Beta_1$-selective
Esmolol	i.v. loading: 500 μg/kg over 1 min, then 25 μg/kg/min; increase by 25–50 μg/kg/min q4min to desired effect	9 min	Erythrocytes	See propranolol	$Beta_1$-selective; very short half-life
Verapamil	i.v. bolus: 0.10–0.15 mg/kg p.o. 40–120 mg q8h	3–7 h	Hepatic	Hypotension, bradycardia. A-V block. CHF, constipation	Increases digoxin levels; accelerates accessory bypass tract conduction
Diltiazem	i.v. bolus: 0.25 mg/kg: 0.35 mg/kg if ineffective i.v. maintenance: 10–20 mg/h p.o.: 30–120 mg q8h	4–5 h	Hepatic	Hypotension, bradycardia. A-V block. CHF	
Quinidine	p.o.: 300–600 mg q6h	6–7 h	Hepatic	Gastrointestinal distress, diarrhea, thrombocytopenia, anemia, rash, torsades de pointes	Frequent early toxicity causing drug termination

Procainamide	i.v. loading: 15 mg/kg i.v. maintenance: 2–5 mg/min	3–5 h	Hepatic, renal	Lupus-like syndrome, nausea, diarrhea, rash, contusion, myalgias, torsades de pointes	60% develop antinuclear antibodies, with 20–30% developing clinical lupus-like syndrome; NAPA (active metabolite) formed in the liver
Disopyramide	p.o.: 100–200 mg q6h	6–7 h	Renal	Anticholinergic effects: urinary retention, constipation, dry mouth; CHF; torsades de pointes	Greater negative inotropy than other class IA agents
Flecainide	p.o.: 100–200 mg q12h	20 h	Hepatic	Dizziness, visual disturbances, bradycardia, sustained ventricular tachycardia	Increases mortality in patients with depressed ejection fraction and prior myocardial infarction
Propafenone	p.o.: 150–300 mg q8h	5–8 h	Hepatic	Bradycardia, bronchospasm, CHF, sustained ventricular tachycardia	Beta-blocker activity 1/40 that of propranolol, on mg per mg basis
Amiodarone	i.v. loading: 150 mg over 10 min; then 1 mg/min for 6h; then 0.5mg/min p.o. loading: 600–1600 mg/d for 1–3 wk p.o. maintenance: 200–400 mg/d	50 d	Hepatic	Pulmonary fibrosis, hepatitis, hypo- and hyperthyroidism, neuropathy, corneal deposits, photosensitivity	Possesses class, I, II, III, and IV activity; use limited by frequent side effects; most side effects dose related.
Sotolol	p.o.: 80–160 mg q12h	6–18 h	Renal	Bronchospasm, CHF, A-V block, bradycardia, hypotension, torsades de pointes	Potent beta-blocker in addition to class III activity
Ibutilide	i.v. 1 mg over 10 min; repeat in 10 min if ineffective	6 h	Hepatic	Torsades de pointes, 6.7% nonsustained, 1.7% sustained	Correct electrolyte abnormalities before dosing; have i.v. magnesium and a defibrillator available; monitor for 4 h after last dose

A-V, atrioventricular, CHF, congestive heart failure; i.v., intravenous; NAPA, *N*-acetyl procainamide; p.o., oral; S-A, sinoatrial.

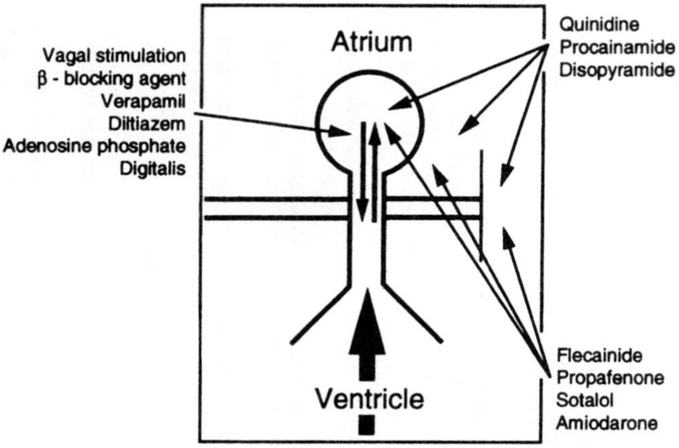

FIG. 39-3. Site of action of antiarrhythmic drugs. The class I and III antiarrhythmic agents affect the atrial and ventricular myocardium and accessory pathway and the atrioventricular node, whereas the class II (beta-blockers) and class IV (calcium channel blockers) agents and digoxin primarily affect the atrioventricular node. (Adapted from Falk PH, Podrid PT. *Atrial fibrillation and management.* New York: Raven Press, 1992, with permission.)

3. **Atrioventricular nodal reentry tachycardia**
   a. **Mechanisms.** A-V nodal reentry tachycardia is the second most common form of SVT. It often presents in young patients without structural heart disease but can present at any age.
   b. **Diagnosis.** The initiation sequence often seen on the surface ECG for typical A-V nodal reentry tachycardia consists of a premature atrial beat followed by a prolonged PR interval, indicating conduction over the slow pathway. This is followed by initiation of a regular, usually narrow-complex tachycardia with a rate generally between 140 and 200 beats per minute (Fig. 39-2A).
   c. **Management.** Vagal maneuvers, which the patient can learn, frequently terminate the tachycardia. Alternatively, agents that prolong A-V refractoriness, such as adenosine, calcium channel antagonists (verapamil and diltiazem), beta-blockers, and digitalis, can be used. If there is hemodynamic compromise, synchronized direct current cardioversion with 25 to 50 J is usually successful.
4. **Atrioventricular reciprocating tachycardia**
   a. **Mechanisms.** A-V reciprocating tachycardia is the third most common form of SVT; like A-V nodal reentry tachycardia, it often occurs in young patients without structural heart disease.
   b. **Diagnosis.** Orthodromic A-V reciprocating tachycardia through a concealed accessory pathway is common. The rate is generally 140 to 240 beats per minute. Because the ventricular activation is over the normal conduction system, the QRS complex is usually narrow. Because atrial activation is retrograde, the P wave is inverted in leads II, III, and aVF (Fig. 39-2B).
   c. **Management.** Acute therapy for A-V reciprocating tachycardia is similar to that for A-V nodal reentry tachycardia. In patients with A-V reciprocating tachycardia who do not respond to A-V nodal blocking agents, intravenous procainamide can be administered. Long-term therapy is necessary if the episodes are frequent or if they cause hemodynamic

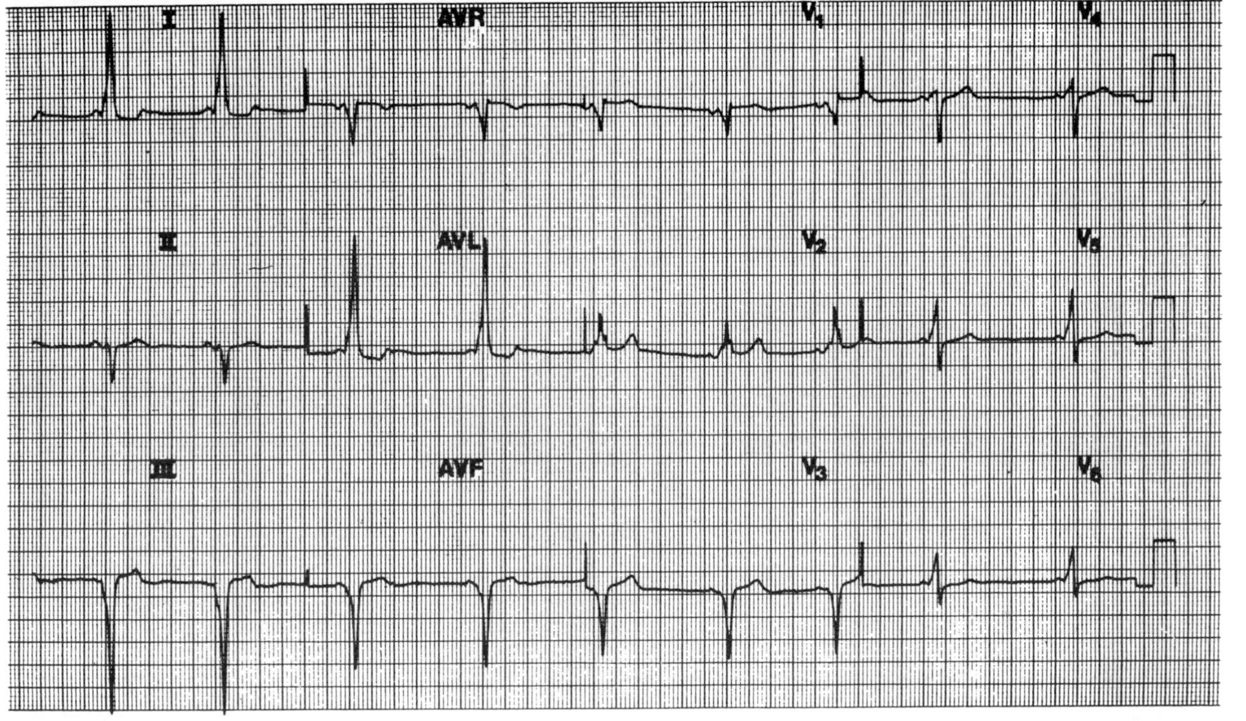

FIG. 39-4. Standard 12-lead electrocardiogram from a young woman before and immediately after radiofrequency catheter ablation of a right-sided accessory pathway producing the Wolff-Parkinson-White syndrome. **A:** The PR interval is short, with a prominent upright delta wave in the lateral leads and a negative delta wave in leads III, aVF, and V_1. **B:** Immediately after ablation, the PR interval and QRS complexes reverted to normal. There are persistent ST–T-wave abnormalities, which also returned to normal within the next few weeks.

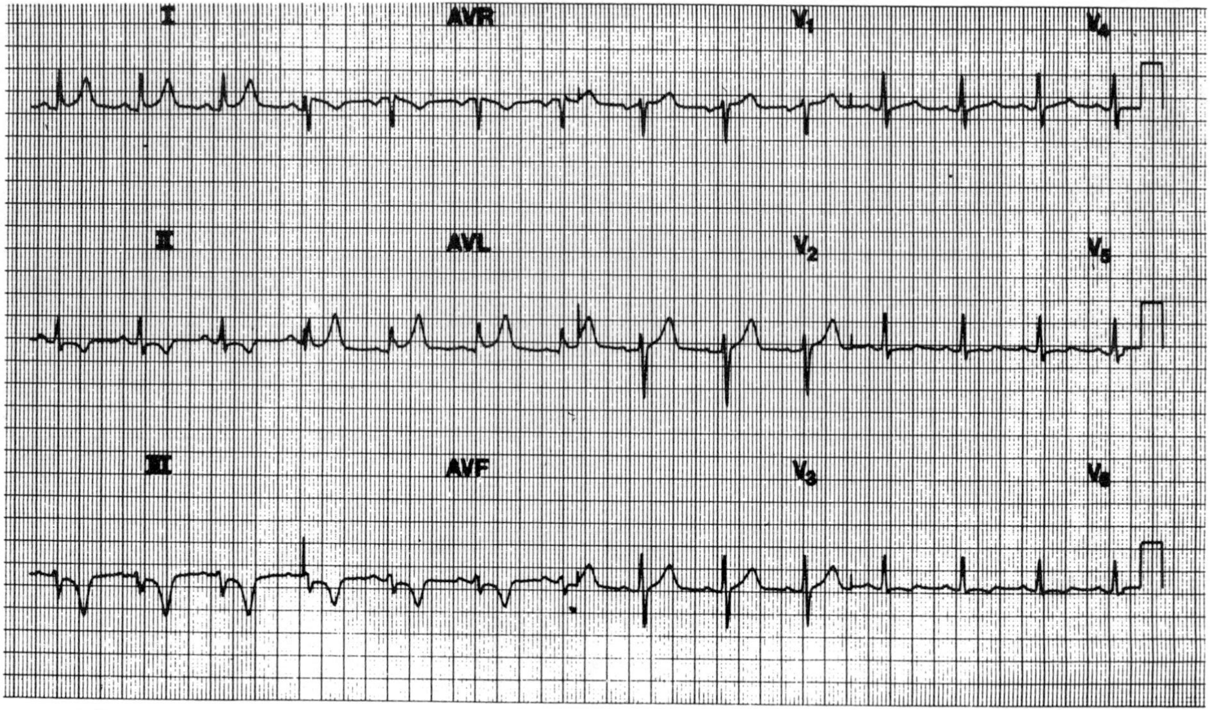

FIG. 39-4. *Continued.*

compromise. Type IC antiarrhythmics (flecainide, propafenone) affect both limbs of the reentrant circuit by increasing conduction time and refractoriness in both the A-V node and accessory bypass tract and are generally the most effective and best tolerated.

Because the effectiveness of radiofrequency catheter ablation is high (greater than 90%) and the complication rate is low, patients with recurrent symptoms should be considered for this procedure.

B. Automatic supraventricular tachycardias

1. Sinus tachycardia

a. Mechanisms. Sinus tachycardia is the most common cause of an atrial tachyarrhythmia and must always be considered in the differential diagnosis. Fever, hypovolemia, hypoxia, anemia, pain, anxiety, exertion, arteriovenous fistulae, and beta-blocker withdrawal all can cause sinus tachycardia. It is commonly seen in myocardial ischemia, left ventricular dysfunction, pulmonary embolism, and thyrotoxicosis. Medications with sympathomimetic activity, including most pressor and inotropic agents, also can be responsible.

b. Diagnosis. The P-wave morphology is normal, with a rate greater than 100 beats per minute. The maximum sinus rate for any patient is normally approximately 220 minus their age, although in high catecholamine states it can be even higher.

c. Management. Treatment is aimed at identifying and correcting the underlying cause.

2. Multifocal atrial tachycardia. Multifocal atrial tachycardia occurs commonly in patients who are acutely ill with chronic obstructive pulmonary disease, congestive heart failure, or theophylline toxicity. At least three ectopic foci compete as the dominant pacemaker. There must, therefore, be at least three different P-wave morphologies on the surface ECG. The atrial rate is greater than 100 beats per minute, and the rhythm is irregularly irregular.

The treatment should first be directed toward the underlying disease. Intravenous verapamil has been shown to be effective in causing a reduction in atrial and ventricular rates.

3. Wolff-Parkinson-White syndrome. Patients with preexcitation may be asymptomatic but are prone to a number of SVTs. Approximately 80% are due to A-V reciprocating tachycardia, 15% to atrial fibrillation and flutter; the accessory bypass facilitates rapid conduction to the ventricle. Some key points common to treatment of all the arrhythmias associated with preexcitation are as follows:

1. Regular narrow complex tachycardias associated with the Wolff-Parkinson-White syndrome can be treated acutely with an agent that lengthens A-V nodal or accessory pathway refractoriness. The drug of choice is adenosine. Verapamil or beta-blocker may be used. Procainamide may work in resistant cases.
2. Patients with an irregular wide complex tachycardia known or suspected to be atrial fibrillation with conduction down an accessory pathway should *not* be treated with A-V nodal blocking agents. This may result in rapid conduction down the accessory pathway to the ventricles and degeneration into ventricular fibrillation. Procainamide is the drug of choice. Synchronized electrical cardioversion should be used if a patient becomes hemodynamically unstable.
3. Long-term prophylactic treatment should not be with A-V blocking agents alone. All adults with Wolff-Parkinson-White syndrome and symptomatic SVT should be strongly considered for electrophysiologic study and possible ablation therapy.

VII. Differential diagnosis. The differential diagnosis of a narrow complex tachycardia is often small when a systematic analysis of the 12-lead ECG is performed. The first helpful decision is whether the ventricular response to the SVT is regular or irregular. The most common irregular SVTs include atrial fibrillation, atrial flutter with variable A-V conduction, and multifocal atrial tachycardia. Any

TABLE 39-3. Supraventricular tachycardias

Regular		Irregular
Short RP (RP < PR)	Long RP (RP > PR)	
Atrioventricular reentrant tachycardia (AVRT)	AVRT with slow bypass tract	Atrial fibrillation
Atrioventricular nodal reentry tachycardia (AVNRT)	Atypical AVNRT	Atrial flutter with variable A-V block
Ectopic atrial tachycardia with A-V conduction delay	Ectopic atrial tachycardia	Multifocal atrial tachycardia
	Sinus tachycardia	
	Intraatrial reentrant tachycardia	
	Sinus node reentrant tachycardia	

A-V, atrioventricular.

atrial tachycardia at a fast enough rate can also occur with variable A-V conduction and an irregular ventricular response. Close scrutiny of atrial activity and use of vagal maneuvers or adenosine often separate these (Table 39-3).

VIII. Wide QRS supraventricular tachycardia. The QRS width during an SVT is occasionally greater than 120 milliseconds. When confronted with a wide QRS tachycardia, an important distinction is whether it is supraventricular or ventricular in origin. Findings suggestive of ventricular tachycardia include A-V dissociation, fusion beats, positive QRS concordance (positive deflections in all precordial leads), QRS duration of greater than 140 milliseconds with a right bundle branch block and 160 milliseconds with a left bundle branch block, left axis deviation greater than minus 90 degrees, and a different QRS morphology during tachycardia compared with a baseline preexisting bundle branch block.

Selected Readings

Akhtar M, Shenasa M, Jazayeri M, et al. Wide QRS complex tachycardia: reappraisal of a common clinical problem. *Ann Intern Med* 1988;109:905.

Keys for differentiating supraventricular and ventricular tachyarrhythmias.

Boston Area Anticoagulation Trial for Atrial Fibrillation Investigators. The effect of low-dose warfarin on the risk of stroke in patients with nonrheumatic atrial fibrillation. *N Engl J Med* 1990;323:1505.

Anticoagulation has been shown to reduce the risk of thromboembolic stroke among patients with nonvalvular atrial fibrillation.

Gilmour RF, Zipes DP. Basic electrophysiologic mechanisms for the development of arrhythmias: clinical applications. *Med Clin North Am* 1984;68:795.

Fundamental mechanisms of atrial arrhythmias that include abnormal impulse formation (enhanced automaticity, triggered activity) and abnormal conduction (reentry).

Haines DE, Dimarco JP. Current therapy for supraventricular tachycardia. *Curr Probl Cardiol* 1992;17:414.

Current therapies for supraventricular arrhythmias and a useful reference for understanding antiarrhythmic agents, dosing, and indications.

Manning WJ, Silverman DI, Gordon SPF, et al. Cardioversion from atrial fibrillation without prolonged anticoagulation with use of transesophageal echocardiography to exclude the presence of atrial thrombi. *N Engl J Med* 1993;328:750.

Transesophageal echocardiography can be used to determine the presence of atrial and atrial appendage thrombi and is an important diagnostic tool for anticoagulation management.

IV. PULMONARY PROBLEMS IN THE INTENSIVE CARE UNIT

40. A PHYSIOLOGIC APPROACH TO MANAGING RESPIRATORY FAILURE

Mark M. Wilson and Melvin R. Pratter

I. Overview. Arterial blood gas analysis is the single most important laboratory test for evaluating respiratory failure and metabolic disorders. Indeed, respiratory failure may be defined by arterial blood gas abnormalities (arterial carbon dioxide tension [P_aCO_2] greater than 50 mm Hg or arterial oxygen tension [P_aO_2] less than 50 to 60 mm Hg]. The proper interpretation of arterial blood gas values requires a working knowledge of the following: (a) the Henderson-Hasselbalch equation, (b) the simplified alveolar air equation, (c) the alveolar O_2 tension (P_AO_2)-arterial O_2 tension gradient concept, (d) the calculation of $\Delta H^+/\Delta P_aCO_2$ ratios and their application in making therapeutic decisions, and (e) the differential diagnosis of various acid-base disorders.

II. Normal gas exchange. The primary function of the respiratory system is gas exchange. This process can be divided into two basic components: (a) the bulk flow of gas between the atmosphere and the terminal airways and (b) the diffusion of gases between terminal lung regions and the pulmonary capillary blood. For routine clinical purposes, the efficiency of these processes may be evaluated by measuring the P_aO_2, the P_aCO_2, and the alveolar-arterial (A-a) PO_2 gradient.

A. P_aO_2. The normal value for P_aO_2 depends on both the position of the patient at the time the sample is obtained and the age of the individual. Formulas predicting normal P_aO_2 are as follows:

In the upright position, $P_aO_2 = 104.2 - 0.27 \times \text{age (yr)}$

In the supine position, $P_aO_2 = 103.5 - 0.47 \times \text{age (yr)}$

B. P_aCO_2. The normal P_aCO_2 is 35 to 45 mm Hg. This value is determined by the level of alveolar ventilation for a given level of CO_2 produced by the body. Unlike P_aO_2, the P_aCO_2 is unaffected by age or body position. Because CO_2 production does not vary widely even in critically ill patients (unless they are on a high-carbohydrate, low-fat diet or have a substantially elevated metabolic rate) it can be generally assumed that P_aCO_2 will vary inversely with alveolar ventilation.

C. P(A-a) O_2 gradient. To interpret a decrease in P_aO_2, one must know the difference between the alveolar and arterial PO_2 values, or the A-a gradient. The alveolar PO_2 (P_AO_2) can be calculated from the simplified alveolar air equation:

$$P_AO_2 = P_IO_2 - P_aCO_2 / R$$

P_IO_2, the partial pressure of inspired O_2, is obtained by multiplying the atmospheric pressure of dry inspired air by the fraction of inspired O_2 being breathed (F_IO_2). At sea level and breathing room air (21% O_2), this value can be assumed to be 150 mm Hg. R is the respiratory exchange ratio and can be assumed to be 0.8, even in critically ill patients with significant lung disease.

The normal A-a gradient is 5 to 10 mm Hg. It is closer to 5 mm Hg in the upright position and closer to 10 mm Hg in the supine position. The A-a gradient is a sensitive indicator of respiratory disease that interferes with gas exchange. It can be helpful in differentiating extrapulmonary from pulmonary causes of hypercapnia and hypoxemia, if it is measured during breathing of room air. At any age, an A-a gradient exceeding 20 mm Hg should be considered abnormal and indicative of pulmonary dysfunction.

III. Abnormal gas exchange

A. Hypoxemia. Five pathophysiologic mechanisms can cause hypoxemia: low P_IO_2, hypoventilation, low ventilation-perfusion (V/Q) mismatch, right-to-left shunting, and diffusion impairment. A low P_{IO_2} is generally seen only at high altitude. Diffusion impairment alone is not the major cause of hypoxemia. In the clinical setting, then, hypoventilation, low V/Q mismatch, and right-to-left shunting are essentially the only important pathophysiologic causes of hypoxemia. In the latter two settings, a decreased cardiac output (resulting in a decreased mixed venous O_2 content) can magnify the resultant arterial hypoxemia. In patients with hypoxemia, calculating the A-a gradient is vital in determining whether the cause is hypoventilation only (a normal A-a gradient) or low V/Q mismatch or right-to-left shunting (both characterized by an elevated A-a gradient).

B. Hypoventilation. Hypoventilation is a decrease in alveolar ventilation for a given level of CO_2 production resulting from a decrease in minute ventilation from extrapulmonary dysfunction. This decreased minute ventilation leads to a proportional decrease in alveolar ventilation, resulting in an increased P_aCO_2. From the simplified alveolar air equation, it is clear that for any constant P_{IO_2} and R values, an increase in P_aCO_2 will cause P_{AO_2} and P_aO_2 to decrease. With no abnormality of distal gas exchange, the A-a gradient remains normal.

C. V/Q mismatch. In areas of inadequate ventilation for a given level of perfusion (low V/Q mismatch), pulmonary venous blood has a relative decrease in both P_{O_2} and O_2 content (decreased percentage of oxyhemoglobin saturation). In areas of lung with excessive ventilation for the amount of perfusion (high V/Q mismatch), pulmonary venous blood has a relatively higher P_{O_2} but only a minimal improvement, if any, in O_2 content (the flat top portion of the sigmoidal shaped oxyhemoglobin dissociation curve). The net result is that P_aO_2 is decreased and the A-a gradient is increased because of the greater effect of low V/Q mismatching.

D. Right-to-left shunting. Right-to-left shunting refers to mixed venous blood going directly into the arterial circulation without having first been exposed to alveolar gas (from cardiac or great vessel, pulmonary vascular, or pulmonary parenchymal sources). When the shunted blood mixes with the rest of the arterial blood, it lowers the average O_2 content, and therefore the average P_aO_2. The A-a gradient is always increased.

E. Differential diagnosis of hypoxemia. To determine the cause of hypoxemia one must evaluate the P_aCO_2, the A-a gradient, and occasionally the patient's response to 100% O_2. During hypoventilation, the P_aCO_2 is always elevated, the A-a gradient is normal (10 mm Hg or less), and the decrease in P_aO_2 is accounted for solely by the low P_{AO_2}. If the patient is given 100% O_2 to breathe (rarely necessary), there will be a dramatic increase in P_aO_2 (to more than 500 mm Hg). During V/Q mismatch and right-to-left shunting, the decreased P_aO_2 is typically accompanied by an elevated A-a gradient. During V/Q mismatch, the P_aCO_2 may or may not be elevated, whereas it is rarely elevated in right-to-left shunt. The P_aO_2 in the patient with V/Q mismatch shows a dramatic rise in response to 100% O_2 (to more than 500 mm Hg). The patient with right-to-left shunting, on the other hand, shows a much smaller response, or, in severe cases, no response at all to 100% O_2. Contrast echocardiography or quantitative nuclear medicine perfusion lung scanning can be obtained to differentiate the right-to-left shunt of cardiac, great vessel, or pulmonary vascular origin from a pulmonary parenchymal cause.

F. Hypercapnia. Three pathophysiologic mechanisms can lead to an elevated P_aCO_2: (a) breathing a gas containing CO_2, (b) hypoventilation, and (c) severe low V/Q mismatch. Clinically, only the last two are important. Hypoventilation has already been discussed. The major mechanism causing arterial hypercapnia in patients with intrinsic lung disease is severe low V/Q mismatch. A substantially greater degree of low V/Q mismatch must be present to cause arterial hypercapnia than to cause hypoxemia (the CO_2 dissociation curve is nearly linear; therefore, high V/Q areas can increase CO_2 elimination much more effectively than they can increase pulmonary capillary O_2 content). Although it is not a primary cause of hypercapnia, respiratory muscle overload (from increased work of breathing and the mechanical disadvantage of the inspiratory muscles associated with severe lung derangement) is commonly a contributing factor. Relative hypoventilation, an inability to increase minute ventilation appropriately in response to increases in CO_2 production, also commonly results from respiratory muscle dysfunction or fatigue.

IV. Respiratory acid-base disorders. Acid-base balance is assessed clinically from the arterial hydrogen ion (H^+) concentration. The ratio of the relative availability of acid versus base determines the H^+ concentration, as shown by the following:

$$H^+ = 24 \times (P_aCO_2 / HCO_3^-) \quad \text{(modified Henderson-Hasselbalch equation)}$$

(Note that a pH of 7.40 corresponds to a H^+ concentration of 40 nM/L and that each change in pH of 0.01 units corresponds to an opposite deviation in H^+ concentration of 1 nM/L when the pH is 7.28 to 7.45. Outside this range, estimated H^+ can be inaccurate by 5% to 11%.) To manage an acid-base abnormality, it should be decided whether it is a respiratory or metabolic disturbance (i.e., a primary change in P_aCO_2 versus a primary change in HCO_3^-, respectively), whether it is a simple or a mixed disturbance (i.e., a primary change in one parameter versus a primary change in both parameters), and whether it is an acute or chronic process (minutes to hours versus days to weeks or longer).

A. Respiratory acidosis. In primary respiratory acidosis, the P_aCO_2 is elevated because of respiratory system dysfunction. Under normal circumstances, an appropriate compensatory change (i.e., increase) will occur in the HCO_3^- level to help minimize the effect on H^+ concentration. To determine how long the P_aCO_2 has been elevated, the ratio of $\Delta H^+/\Delta P_aCO_2$ is computed. In the absence of prior measurements, pH is assumed to have started at 7.40 ($H^+ = 40$) and P_aCO_2 at 40 mm Hg. The changes in H^+ and P_aCO_2 are then calculated by subtracting 40 from the most recently measured values. Acutely, any change in the HCO_3^- level reflects nonrenal body buffering. Chronically, the kidneys gradually increase the HCO_3^- level to bring H^+ concentration back toward, but not to, normal. During the transition from the acute stage of respiratory acidosis to the chronic stage, or when their is an acute increase in P_aCO_2 in the setting of established chronic hypercapnia, an intermediate degree of compensation should be expected. The $\Delta H^+/\Delta P_aCO_2$ ratios for acute, chronic, and acute-on-chronic respiratory acidosis are 0.8, 0.3, and greater than 0.3 but less than 0.8, respectively. The differential diagnosis of respiratory acidosis is the same as that of hypercapnic respiratory failure (Table 40-1). The therapeutic approach is also the same.

B. Respiratory alkalosis. Primary respiratory alkalosis is defined by a decrease in P_aCO_2 with an accompanying compensatory decrease in HCO_3^-. The duration of respiratory alkalosis involves the same determination of $\Delta H^+/\Delta P_aCO_2$ ratios. The values for acute and chronic respiratory alkalosis are 0.8 and 0.17, respectively. The differential diagnosis for respiratory alkalosis is presented in Table 40-2. Note that a primary respiratory alkalosis may have a normal or an elevated A-a gradient. The differential diagnosis of respiratory alkalosis with an elevated A-a gradient is the same as that of nonhypercapnic, hypoxemic respiratory failure. The general approach to a respiratory alkalosis is to direct therapy at the underlying disorder. It is usually not necessary to treat the alkalosis directly unless the serum pH is extremely high (e.g., more than 7.55) and associated with significant cardiac dysrhythmia, evidence of cerebrovascular or cardiovascular vasoconstriction, or manifestations of tetany such as carpopedal spasm. In such a setting, sedation with or without paralysis of skeletal muscles may be useful.

V. Physiologic approach to respiratory failure. Respiratory failure occurs when gas exchange becomes significantly impaired. Because it is impossible to predict P_aO_2 and P_aCO_2 accurately using clinical criteria, the diagnosis of respiratory failure depends on arterial blood gas analysis. With hypercapnic respiratory failure (Table 40-1), the A-a gradient may or may not be increased. In hypoventilation from dysfunction in the extrapulmonary compartment, the A-a gradient is normal. When hypercapnic respiratory failure results from severe V/Q mismatch from abnormalities of the pulmonary compartment, the A-a gradient is typically (but not always) extremely increased (e.g., more than 40 mm Hg). Commonly, a disease process may affect components of both compartments, and the resultant combina-

TABLE 40-1. Causes of hypercapnia and their pathophysiologic mechanisms[a]

Site of Abnormality	Disease	Mechanism
Pulmonary disorders of:		Severe ventilation-perfusion mismatch
Lower airways	Chronic obstructive pulmonary disease, asthma, cystic fibrosis	
Lung parenchyma	Environmental/occupational lung disease	
Pulmonary vasculature	Pulmonary embolism (rarely)	
Extrapulmonary disorders of:		Hypoventilation
Central nervous system	Respiratory center depression due to drug overdose, primary alveolar hypoventilation, myxedema	
Peripheral nervous system	Spinal cord disease, amyotrophic lateral sclerosis, Guillain-Barré syndrome	
Respiratory muscles	Myasthenia gravis, polymyositis, hypophosphatemia	
Chest wall	Ankylosing spondylitis, flail chest, thoracoplasty	
Pleura	Restrictive pleuritis	
Upper airways	Tracheal obstruction, epiglottitis, adenoidal and tonsillar hypertrophy, obstructive sleep apnea	

[a] This table is not an exhaustive listing; it includes the more common causes for each involved compartment of the respiratory system.

TABLE 40-2. Causes of respiratory alkalosis

Normal A-a Gradient	Elevated A-a Gradient
Central nervous system disorder	Sepsis and capillary leak syndrome
Hormones, drugs:	Hepatic failure
Salicylates	Chronic interstitial lung diseases
Catecholamines	Pulmonary edema (cardiogenic, noncardiogenic)
Progesterone	Pulmonary embolism
Analeptic overdose	Pneumonia
Thyroid hormone excess	Asthma
Pregnancy	
High altitude	
Severe anemia	
Psychogenic hyperventilation	
Endotoxemia	
Mechanical hyperventilation with normal lungs	
During menses after ovulation	

tion of mechanisms causes an A-a gradient that is generally only modestly increased (e.g., 15 to 20 mm Hg).

VI. Treatment. Respiratory failure is managed by combined supportive and specific therapies. In nonhypercapnic (hypoxemic) respiratory failure, the major problem is a low P_aO_2. If the mechanism is low V/Q mismatch, supplemental O_2 will prove effective. If the disease process involves a diffuse pulmonary intraparenchymal shunt, as in the acute respiratory distress syndrome, mechanical ventilation with positive end-expiratory pressure may be required in addition to supplemental O_2. If instead the problem is a right-to-left cardiac or pulmonary vascular shunt, supplemental O_2 alone will be of limited benefit; emphasis is on specific therapy (i.e., surgical repair of an atrial septal defect, obliteration of a pulmonary arteriovenous fistula).

The key initial decision in hypercapnic respiratory failure is whether or not the patient requires intubation and mechanical ventilation. In general, intubation should be strongly considered for patients with acute respiratory acidosis that has not rapidly responded to medical therapy. The patient with a $\Delta H^+/\Delta P_aCO_2$ ratio that signifies chronic respiratory acidosis should be followed closely, but these patients rarely need to be intubated. In the acute-on-chronic situation, the trend of the acidosis over time is the crucial factor in deciding on the necessity for intubation.

Specific therapy varies greatly by disease, and therefore no broad generalizations can be made. Examples of potential specific therapy include naloxone to offset respiratory center depression from narcotic overdose, inhaled bronchodilators and systemic corticosteroids for asthma and emphysema, or nasal continuous positive airway pressure for obstructive sleep apnea. Details of therapy for the most common of these diseases are presented in subsequent chapters.

Selected Readings

Demers RR, Irwin RS. Management of hypercapnic respiratory failure: a systematic approach. *Respir Care* 1979;24:328.

Provides a systematic approach to the patient with respiratory acidosis and reviews the concept of the A-a gradient.

Murray JF. *The normal lung: the basis for diagnosis and treatment of lung disease.* Philadelphia: WB Saunders, 1976:171.

This citation reviews the concept of the A-a gradient and the major mechanisms involved in gas exchange impairment.

Narins RG, Emmett M. Simple and mixed acid-base disorders: a practical approach. *Medicine* (Baltimore) 1980;59:161.

Comprehensive and practical review of acid-base physiology and provides an approach to and differential diagnosis for each of the major acid-base disturbances.

Pratter MR, Irwin RS. Extrapulmonary causes of respiratory failure. *J Int Care Med* 1986;1:197.

Reviews how to distinguish extrapulmonary from pulmonary causes of respiratory failure and the mechanisms responsible for arterial hypoxemia and hypercapnia.

Robin ED, Laman PD, Goris ML, et al. A shunt is (not) a shunt is (not) a shunt. *Am Rev Respir Dis* 1977;115:553.

Succinct description of the different right-to-left shunts and how to distinguish them.

West JB. *Pulmonary pathophysiology: the essentials,* 5th ed. Philadelphia: Williams & Wilkins, 1998:17.

This citation reviews the concept of the A-a gradient and the major mechanisms involved in gas exchange impairment.

West JB. Causes of carbon dioxide retention in lung disease. *N Engl J Med* 1971; 284:1232.

Explains how and why V/Q mismatch is the major cause of hypercapnia in lung disease.

41. ACUTE RESPIRATORY DISTRESS SYNDROME

Ann E. Connolly, Mark M. Wilson, and Richard S. Irwin

I. Definition and etiology. Acute respiratory distress syndrome (ARDS) represents a pathophysiologic state of acute, diffuse alveolar damage characterized by pulmonary edema and refractory hypoxemia. The most commonly used definition, proposed by the European-American Consensus Conference on ARDS, includes the following criteria: the ratio of partial pressure of arterial oxygen (P_aO_2) to fraction of inspired oxygen (F_iO_2) less than 200, regardless of the level of positive end-expiratory pressure (PEEP); bilateral pulmonary infiltrates on chest radiograph; and a pulmonary artery occlusion pressure less than or equal to 18 mm Hg or no clinical evidence of elevated left atrial pressure on the basis of chest radiograph or other clinical data.

Conditions associated with ARDS include those that cause lung injury directly (e.g., gastric aspiration, pneumonia or other toxic inhalational injury) and those that cause injury indirectly (e.g., septic shock, trauma, drug ingestion, pancreatitis). Indirect mechanisms are responsible for most cases of ARDS. Up to one-half of all cases of ARDS are associated with the systemic inflammatory response syndrome or sepsis syndrome. The risk of developing ARDS increases as the number of potential causes (risk factors) increases.

II. Pathology and pathogenesis. The initial pathology of ARDS (i.e., diffuse alveolar damage) includes interstitial swelling, proteinaceous intraalveolar edema, alveolar hemorrhage, and fibrin deposition. So-called alveolar flooding characteristically occurs in only some alveoli; others appear to be normal. Degenerative cellular changes occur, and within 1 to 2 days, hyaline membranes are usually seen within the alveoli. The repair from acute lung injury begins quickly after the initial insult. Type II cells (responsible for surfactant production) proliferate several days after the onset of ARDS and eventually differentiate into new type I cells to reline the alveolar walls. Most of the alveolar edema usually resolves after approximately 1 week, and hyaline membranes are much less prominent. Some patients seem to resolve lung injury with little if any fibrosis, whereas others go on to develop severe parenchymal fibrosis. The reason that outcomes are so variable is unknown. The development of diffuse alveolar damage can be categorized into an exudative phase (days 1 to 3), a proliferative phase (days 3 to 7 or more), and a fibrotic phase (after 1 week).

At the time of onset, the clinical hallmarks of ARDS are severe tachypnea and hypoxemia, primarily the result of right-to-left intrapulmonary shunting. The extensive shunt in ARDS (up to 25% to 50% of the cardiac output) results from persistent perfusion of atelectatic and fluid-filled alveoli caused by an ineffective or absent hypoxic pulmonary vasoconstriction response. Because blood flowing through a shunt is not exposed to alveolar gas, supplemental oxygen is of little to no value, thus accounting for the characteristic refractory nature of the hypoxemia. Because alveolar edema resolves during the first week, the amount of shunt and the need for supplemental oxygen and airway pressure therapy decrease and stabilize. Further improvements in oxygenation depend on the fibroproliferative, reparative response to restore normal architecture for gas exchange.

Increased physiologic dead-space ventilation (resulting from hyperventilation and overinflation of still normal or relatively normal alveoli) and intrapulmonary shunt are both responsible for the tachypnea and high minute ventilation required to achieve effective carbon dioxide excretion in ARDS. In severe ARDS, as much as 90% of each tidal volume (V_T) may be "wasted" (i.e., does not participate in gas exchange). If there is relatively rapid improvement (over 10 to 14 days), minute ventilation and dead-space ventilation decrease in tandem with improvements in oxygenation. In patients who develop significant fibrosis, minute ventilatory requirements remain high even as oxygenation improves.

High airway pressures are almost always required to ventilate patients with ARDS with V_T values that otherwise are well tolerated in persons with physiologically normal lungs. Respiratory system (i. e., chest wall and lungs) compliance is dramatically reduced (from normal compliance greater than 100 mL/cm H_2O with V_T values of about 8 mL/kg to less than or equal to 20 mL/cm H_2O). This increase in inflation pressure is a reflection of the amount of edema and atelectasis that is present and is not a measure of the lung injury as such. If fibrosis develops, the elastic properties of the lung parenchyma can change and then can result in true reductions in lung compliance.

Peak airway pressures are also increased during mechanical ventilation of patients with ARDS, sometimes out of proportion to the increase in static inflation pressures, a finding suggesting an increase in airways resistance. This change may be due to secretions, edema, and mediators that cause bronchospasm. This may be amplified by resistance of narrow endotracheal tubes and the mechanical apparatus used to provide ventilatory support.

The work of breathing in ARDS is increased by the pulmonary mechanical properties discussed earlier and may be multiplied by the effect of tachypnea. In ARDS, the work of breathing may be responsible for 25% to 50% of the body's total oxygen consumption. Mechanical ventilatory support in ARDS reduces the work of breathing so oxygen can be redirected to other vital organs.

Given the variety of conditions associated with acute lung injury, it should not be surprising that no characteristic hemodynamic pattern exists. Rather, it is more common for the hemodynamic pattern to reflect the underlying condition itself.

III. Diagnosis. When ARDS presents without preexisting or coexisting conditions, it is easy to recognize. Inhalation of toxic gas or ingestion of certain drugs in toxic doses, severe viral pneumonia, and aspiration of gastric contents during resuscitation from cardiac arrest are examples of well-defined events that can lead to ARDS. If followed by the rapid development of respiratory distress (generally within a few hours to 1 to 3 days) and bilateral alveolar infiltrates on chest radiograph, ARDS is the likely cause.

Respiratory signs and symptoms (dyspnea and tachypnea) often precede the full development of infiltrates on the chest radiograph; however, alveolar infiltrates invariably develop within the next several hours. The most dramatic and consistent findings on physical examination include tachypnea, tachycardia, and increased work of breathing (use of accessory muscles of respiration). The patient may be extremely agitated as well. On examination, dry crackles and scattered rhonchi may be heard throughout the lung fields. Not uncommonly, the chest examination is remarkably normal, despite severe alveolar infiltrates on the chest radiograph. End-expiratory wheezes can often be heard, but frank airway obstruction with prolonged expiratory time is not expected. At the time of presentation, the rest of the physical examination is usually normal, unless other organ systems are involved.

Ideally, the diagnosis of ARDS is made by documenting both diffuse alveolar damage and increased vascular permeability in patients with severe respiratory distress, diffuse radiographic infiltrates consistent with pulmonary edema, and hypoxemia. However, because obtaining lung tissue in these critically ill patients is most often impractical, the diagnosis of ARDS is usually made by inference (see foregoing criteria).

Although severe hypoxemia is generally included as a diagnostic criterion for ARDS, the appropriate threshold for defining the abnormality in P_aO_2 has not been studied systematically. Arbitrarily, a P_aO_2/F_iO_2 ratio less than 300 (normal is greater than 500) has been accepted as the minimum criterion for lung injury, and a level less than 200 indicates ARDS.

Whether noncardiogenic and cardiogenic forms of pulmonary edema can be distinguished radiographically has been controversial, particularly because the radiographic appearance in ARDS can also be strongly influenced by the effects of therapy.

IV. Treatment

A. Specific treatment. No specific therapy exists for ARDS. Identified underlying or complicating conditions (e.g., pneumonia, sepsis) should be treated with specific therapy on an individual basis.

B. Supportive treatment

1. **Mechanical ventilation.** The goals of mechanical ventilation in ARDS are to maintain acceptable gas exchange and to minimize the occurrence of adverse effects associated with its application. The initial ventilator management should include a volume-cycled ventilator in the assist/control mode. Convincing data now favor the use of V_T of 6 mL/kg to keep airway plateau pressures no more than 30 to 35 cm H_2O in an attempt to minimize any alveolar overdistension injury. The use of such low V_T can lead to hypercapnia (not necessarily undesirable, see discussions of permissive hypercapnia or controlled hypoventilation strategies) and atelectasis.

   Attention is being focused on the importance of first recruiting and then maintaining as many alveolar units open as possible. This goal often requires levels of PEEP considerably in excess of those needed simply to lower the F_iO_2 below 0.6 (i.e., to minimize additional lung injury from oxygen toxicity).

   In those patients with ARDS whose oxygenation cannot be maintained with more conventional approaches, growing clinical experience with the use of mechanical ventilation in the inverse-ratio mode or pressure-control mode may be useful strategies for salvaging gas exchange when acceptable P_aO_2 (e.g., greater than or equal to 60 to 80 mm Hg) cannot be achieved with PEEP less than 15 to 20 cm H_2O or when the use of PEEP is associated with excessive plateau pressures. Clinical experience with other nonconventional modes of ventilatory support (e.g., high-frequency ventilation, liquid ventilation, extracorporeal respiratory support, inhaled nitric oxide) is too limited to allow any recommendations on their use.

2. **Patient positioning.** Because of the nonuniform distribution of lung infiltrates in ARDS, repositioning the patient into the prone position can improve oxygenation by relieving atelectasis and by improving the distribution of perfusion relative to ventilation. Improvement occurs in ~66% to 75% of patients, usually within minutes.

3. **Fluid management.** Patients with ARDS should have fluid restriction and should even undergo diuresis when possible, especially during the first few days after onset of the disorder. Any compromise in end-organ function should be carefully monitored and corrected. The benefits of fluid restriction and diuresis after 3 to 4 days remain unclear.

4. **Corticosteroids.** Several prospective, multicenter, placebo-controlled studies have shown no benefit to the use of high-dose corticosteroids early in the course of ARDS. Anecdotal reports and several small trials have suggested, however, that corticosteroids may be beneficial if they are administered during the fibroproliferative phase of ARDS (7 to 10 days after onset). Further studies are needed to establish the role of corticosteroids in the management of ARDS.

5. **Exogenous surfactant.** Because normal surfactant may be dysfunctional in ARDS, the instillation of exogenous surfactant has been proposed as a means to improve airspace stability in ARDS and may have added antibacterial and immunologic properties as well. Although the only prospective trial available showed no benefit on 30-day mortality, duration of mechanical ventilation, or physiologic function, the design of the trial and the efficacy of the inhaled drug have been criticized. Interest in exogenous surfactant remains strong, and additional trials with alternative agents in the future are likely.

6. **Other pharmacologic therapies.** No specific medications have been shown to be of benefit in ARDS. Studies of *N*-acetylcysteine and ibuprofen in patients with sepsis failed to show any significant benefit on patient outcome. Similarly, prospective trials of therapy directed against mediators of sepsis (endotoxin, tumor necrosis factor, interleukin-1) failed to show any significant reduction in overall mortality. Ongoing clinical trials with

antioxidants (procysteine), selective pulmonary vasodilators (inhaled nitric oxide, aerosolized prostacyclin), and antiinflammatory agents (eicosanoid inhibitors, selective prostanoids, lisophylline) are currently under way.

V. Recovery and prognosis. Most patients who die of ARDS do so within the first 2 weeks of the illness. However, for those who survive, recovery often takes 2 weeks or longer. Thus, for most survivors of ARDS, many issues of general supportive care must be addressed.

Many patients with ARDS develop a syndrome of multiorgan dysfunction. Recovery depends on adequate support of vital organ systems. Complications of management are common, and chief among these are barotrauma, nosocomial pneumonia, and so-called stress-related gastrointestinal bleeding.

Outcome for patients is difficult to predict. General scoring systems (e.g., the Acute Physiology and Chronic Health Evaluation) provide an estimate of the probability of mortality after the first 24 hours of intensive care. The number of acquired organ system failures is often the most important prognostic indicator for patients requiring intensive care, including patients with ARDS. Since ARDS was first reported more than 2 decades ago, mortality has remained relatively constant, at 60% to 70%, until recently. Some more recent reports, however, suggest that mortality may be falling to 40% or less. Although the explanation for this is not clear, the decrease could be due to differences in patient populations, less corticosteroid use in early ARDS, more corticosteroid use in late ARDS, greater attention to fluid management, improving hemodynamic or nutritional support, improved antibiotics for nosocomial infection, changes in ventilator support strategies, or the benefits of protocol-driven management in clinical trials.

Selected Readings

Albert RK. Prone position in ARDS: what do we know, and what do we need to know? *Crit Care Med* 1999;27:2574.

This editorial summarizes what we have learned regarding prone positioning.

Anzueto A, Baughman RP, Guntupalli KK, et al. Aerosolized surfactant in adults with sepsis-induced respiratory distress syndrome: Exosurf Acute Respiratory Distress Syndrome Sepsis Study Group. *N Engl J Med* 1996;334:1417.

A prospective, multicenter, double-blind, placebo-control study involving 725 patients with ARDS. Continuous aerosolized surfactant had no effect on mortality.

Bernard GR, Artigas A, Grigham KL, et al. The American-European Consensus conference on ARDS: definitions, mechanisms, relevant outcomes, and clinical trial coordination. *Am J Respir Crit Care Med* 1994;149:818.

Results of a consensus conference, proposing a standard definition for ARDS and a basic framework for studying and comparing groups of patients with ARDS.

Chatte G, Sab JM, Dubois JM, et al. Prone position in mechanically ventilated patients with severe acute respiratory failure. *Am J Respir Crit Care Med* 1997;155:473.

A descriptive study of 32 patients with ARDS. Significant improvement in arterial oxygenation was documented in prone versus supine positioning.

Knaus WA, Wagner DP, Draper EA, et al. The APACHE III prognostic system: risk prediction of hospital mortality for critically ill hospitalized adults. *Chest* 1991;100:1619.

Refining the APACHE methodology in another large database.

Marini JJ. Lung mechanics in the adult respiratory distress syndrome: recent conceptual advances and implications for management. *Clin Chest Med* 1990;11:673.

An excellent review of the pulmonary pathophysiologic effects of ARDS.

Milberg JA, Davis DR, Steinberg KP, et al. Improved survival of patients with acute respiratory distress syndrome (ARDS): 1983–1993. *JAMA* 1995;273:306.

Describes the temporal trends in ARDS mortality in more than 900 patients seen over a decade at one institution.

Schuster DP. What is acute lung injury? What is ARDS? *Chest* 1995;107:1721.

Raises appropriate questions and concerns regarding the use of the consensus conference definition and criteria for ARDS.

Tomashefski JF Jr. Pulmonary pathology of the adult respiratory distress syndrome. *Clin Chest Med* 1990;11:593.

An excellent review of the pathology of ARDS.

42. STATUS ASTHMATICUS

J. Mark Madison and Richard S. Irwin

I. Definition. Asthma is an inflammatory disease of the airways featuring reversible airway obstruction. Typically, intermittent worsening or exacerbation of asthma is triggered by exposure to environmental factors. The term *status asthmaticus* is used to describe moderate to severe exacerbations of asthma that fail to respond rapidly and substantially to intensive bronchodilator therapy.

II. Diagnosis. Patients presenting with an acute asthma exacerbation typically give a history consistent with prior asthma and complain of an acute, progressively worsening shortness of breath, wheezing, cough, or chest tightness that is no longer responding well to inhaled bronchodilators. Usually, one or more factors can be identified as precipitating the exacerbation, and these are commonly inhaled allergens, pollutants, smoke, and viral respiratory tract infections. Congestive heart failure, acute pulmonary thromboembolism, foreign bodies, or obstruction of the upper airway by any cause all produce wheezing that can be confused with asthma. In addition, in the intensive care setting, distinguishing an exacerbation of asthma from an exacerbation of chronic obstructive pulmonary disease sometimes can be difficult when the patient's prior history is unavailable.

III. Assessment. Complaints of severe breathlessness, chest tightness, or difficulty in walking more than 100 feet all suggest severe airway obstruction. Prior endotracheal intubation for asthma, frequent or recent emergency department visits or hospitalizations for asthma, current or recent use of systemic corticosteroids, and a history of syncope or seizures during prior asthma exacerbations are important evidence of a patient's tendency to develop severe airway obstruction.

Physical examination is important for excluding other causes of dyspnea and for assessing the degree of airway obstruction. Tachycardia (more than 120 beats per minute), tachypnea (more than 30 breaths per minute), diaphoresis, bolt upright posture in bed, pulsus paradox (more than 10 mm Hg), and accessory muscle use all should be regarded as signs of severe airway obstruction. However, because the absence of these signs does not rule out severe obstruction, physical examination cannot be relied on exclusively to estimate the severity of airway obstruction. Cyanosis, respiratory muscle alternans, abdominal paradox, and depressed mental status are late and ominous indicators of respiratory failure.

Peak expiratory flow rate (PEFR) and the forced expired volume of air in 1 second (FEV_1) are equally good bedside measures to quantify the degree of airway obstruction, and these objective measures are the essential cornerstone of assessment. In general, a PEFR or FEV_1 less than 50% of baseline (either the predicted value or the patient's best known value) is regarded as severe airway obstruction.

Arterial blood gas analysis should be performed when clinical findings suggest severe airway obstruction. A partial pressure of arterial oxygen (P_aO_2) less than 60 mm Hg on room air should be regarded as additional evidence of severe airway obstruction. Moreover, the partial pressure of arterial carbon dioxide (P_aCO_2) is typically low during an exacerbation of asthma. A normal or high P_aCO_2 (40 mm Hg or more) during a severe exacerbation of asthma mandates careful monitoring and the urgent consideration for mechanical ventilation.

Routine chest radiographs reveal few abnormalities other than hyperinflation. However, chest radiography is useful for identifying other causes of dyspnea and wheezing and for detecting complications of severe airway obstruction (e.g., pneumothorax).

IV. Treatment. Patients with severe airway obstruction who are at high risk of mortality from asthma need close monitoring, often in an intensive care unit. Most patients respond to conventional therapy with inhaled beta-adrenergic agonists, cholinergic antagonists, systemic corticosteroids, supplemental oxygen, and, when necessary, support by mechanical ventilation. For the few patients whose condition deteriorates despite conventional therapy, methylxanthines and intravenous isoproterenol may be started, and consideration may be given to various nonconventional therapies. In general, therapy is not altered in treating asthma exacerbations in the pregnant patient.

A. Bronchodilator therapy

1. **Beta-adrenergic agonists.** Short-acting beta-adrenergic agonists that have relative selectivity for the beta$_2$-adrenergic receptor (e.g., albuterol) are the mainstay of bronchodilator therapy for acute asthma. The major side effects of beta-adrenergic agonists are tremor, cardiac stimulation, and hypokalemia.

   The inhalational route of administration is almost always preferable to systemic delivery. Studies have shown that metered-dose inhalers (MDIs) equipped with spacer devices are as effective as small-volume nebulizers in the treatment of acute asthma. Four puffs of albuterol by MDI have been given at 1-minute intervals and repeated every 20 to 30 minutes for up to six doses.
2. **Cholinergic antagonists.** Inhaled muscarinic cholinergic antagonists are effective bronchodilators, but act more slowly and are less effective than the inhaled beta-adrenergic agonists. Some data suggest that ipratropium may be a useful adjunct to beta-adrenergic agonists in the initial treatment of status asthmaticus, and, therefore, ipratropium has been recommended by some (four to eight puffs by MDI with spacer every 6 hours as needed or 0.5 mg by nebulizer every 6 hours as needed) (see Chapter 53).
3. **Methylxanthines.** Because of toxicity, methylxanthines are mainly reserved for patients in whom conventional therapy fails objectively. For patients not already taking methylxanthines, a loading dose of aminophylline (6 mg/kg lean body weight) is administered over 20 to 30 minutes, followed by an intravenous infusion rate of 0.6 mg/kg per hour. Six hours after initiation of the infusion, the serum theophylline level should be checked, and the infusion rate should adjusted accordingly. The initial infusion rate should be decreased if the patient has conditions that decrease methylxanthine clearance such as congestive heart failure, systemic infections, hepatic cirrhosis, or use of phenobarbital, cimetidine, or macrolide and quinolone antibiotics.
4. **Magnesium sulfate.** Because the bronchodilation is transient, is less than that of beta-adrenergic agonists, and does not augment the response to beta-adrenergic agonists, intravenous magnesium sulfate is not recommended routinely.

B. Antiinflammatory therapy: corticosteroids. Numerous studies have documented the safety and efficacy of short courses of corticosteroids in the treatment of status asthmaticus. Oral administration of corticosteroids is as effective as intravenous therapy. However, because absorption of orally administered drugs may be variable in critically ill patients, many clinicians prefer the intravenous route for initial treatment. The current recommendation is 60 to 80 mg of methylprednisolone every 6 to 8 hours. Inhaled corticosteroids may have a role in non–life-threatening, acute asthma, but further studies are needed.

Once the patient shows evidence of daily improvement, corticosteroids can be administered orally. Usually, prednisone is started at 60 mg per day and gradually is tapered over 7 to 14 days as the patient continues to improve. Notably, the need for gradual tapering is questionable. Whether prednisone is gradually tapered or stopped abruptly, the recovering patient should be started on a corticosteroid aerosol.

C. Other therapy

1. **Oxygen.** Supplemental oxygen therapy should be an initial intervention in the emergency department. In addition to mitigating the complications of hypoxemia, supplemental oxygen minimizes potential episodes of hypoxemia resulting from the acute administration of beta-adrenergic agonists, decreases elevated pulmonary vascular pressures, and improves oxygen delivery to respiratory muscles.
2. **Mechanical ventilation.** For patients in severe distress in whom respiratory arrest has already occurred or is imminent, the need for intubation and

mechanical ventilation is obvious. The possibility of pneumothorax should be promptly addressed in these patients. Patients not *in extremis* should be monitored closely during initial bronchodilator therapy, and the physician should be prepared to perform intubation in case of substantial deterioration. The decision to intubate for status asthmaticus is a clinical judgment based on repeated assessment of whether the patient is responding to therapy, whether hypercapnia is worsening, whether the patient has signs of muscle fatigue as evidenced by paradoxic abdominal wall motion during inspiration, and whether the patient's mental status is deteriorating.

Oral, rather than nasal, intubation is preferred because nasal polyps and sinusitis are common in asthma and because the oral route allows the larger endotracheal tube (internal diameter 8 mm or larger) needed for possible therapeutic bronchoscopy.

Because the risk of barotrauma is related to dynamic hyperinflation of the lungs and high airway pressures, controlled hypoventilation is the ventilatory strategy used to minimize lung volumes and airway pressures. Adequate tissue oxygenation, not a normal P_aCO_2, should be the goal. Physician acceptance of hypercapnia in this setting has been termed *permissive hypercapnia.* Notably, no controlled studies of respiratory acidosis have defined a particular pH value that mandates sodium bicarbonate administration. We prefer to give bicarbonate only when the acidosis appears to be associated with hemodynamic compromise.

To lessen the risk of myopathy associated with the combination of neuromuscular blocking agents and corticosteroids, paralyzing agents should be avoided whenever possible. When paralysis is necessary, muscle function should be allowed to recover partially between repetitive boluses.

3. **Additional and unconventional management measures.** Airway obstruction sometimes may be sufficiently severe to prevent maintenance of adequate gas exchange. Many unconventional measures based on anecdotal experience may be instituted such as inhaled helium-oxygen (heliox), general anesthetics (e.g., halothane), magnesium sulfate, bronchoscopy with therapeutic lavage, hypothermia, and extracorporeal life support.
4. **Therapies with no established role.** There is no established role for fluid administration in excess of euvolemia, mucolytics, or chest physical therapy. Sedatives are contraindicated in the absence of mechanical ventilation. Antibiotics are warranted only when one has a strong suspicion of an active infectious process, particularly pneumonia and bacterial sinusitis.

Selected Readings

Barnes PJ. Pathophysiology of asthma. *Br J Clin Pharmacol* 1996;42:3.

This is an overview of the inflammatory processes underlying asthma.

Darioli R, Perret C. Mechanical controlled hypoventilation in status asthmaticus. *Am Rev Respir Dis* 1984;129:385.

Using low respiratory frequency (6 to 10 cycles / min) and tidal volume (8 to 12 mL / kg), complications of barotrauma were significantly decreased.

Elshami AA, Tino G. Coexistent asthma and functional upper airway obstruction. *Chest* 1996;110:1358.

Case reports of asthma complicated by functional upper airway obstruction are presented.

Fanta CH, Rossing TH, McFadden ER. Glucocorticosteroids in acute asthma: a critical controlled trial. *Am J Med* 1983;74:845.

Parenteral corticosteroids added to standard bronchodilator therapy caused a significant improvement in lung function at 24 hours compared with standard bronchodilator therapy alone.

Fanta CH, Rossing TH, McFadden ER. Treatment of acute asthma: is combination therapy with sympathomimetics and methylxanthines indicated? *Am J Med* 1986;80:5.

Adding methylxanthines to inhaled beta-adrenergic agonists during treatment of acute asthma did not cause significant improvement in lung function compared with beta-adrenergic agonists alone.

Feihl F, Perret C. Permissive hypercapnia. *Am J Respir Crit Care Med* 1994;150:1722.
The consequences of hypercapnia and respiratory acidosis are comprehensively reviewed.

Gluck EH, Onorato DJ, Castriotta R. Helium-oxygen mixtures in intubated patients with status asthmaticus and respiratory acidosis. *Chest* 1990;98:693.
Seven patients with respiratory failure secondary to status asthmaticus had high airway pressures and persistent respiratory acidosis. Patients were mechanically ventilated at lower airway pressures by employing a mixture of helium and oxygen.

Lanes SF, Garrett JE, Wentworth CE III CE, et al. The effect of adding ipratropium bromide to salbutamol in the treatment of acute asthma. *Chest* 1998;114:365.
Based on pooled analysis of three clinical trials for acute asthma, addition of inhaled ipratropium bromide to inhaled beta-adrenergic agonists caused a small improvement in lung function and modestly decreased need for additional treatment, subsequent exacerbations, and hospitalizations.

McFadden ER. Dosages of corticosteroids in asthma. *Am Rev Respir Dis* 1993;147:1306.
This is an excellent review of corticosteroid use in asthma.

Rizk NW, Kalassian KG, Gilligan T, et al. Obstetric complications in pulmonary and critical care medicine. *Chest* 1996;110:791.
This is a review of obstetric issues in critical care medicine, including a section on the treatment of asthma during pregnancy.

Schwartz SH. Treatment of status asthmaticus with halothane. *JAMA* 1984;251:2688.
One general anesthetic used to treat patients with status asthmaticus refractory to conventional therapy is halothane. Two case reports and the possible risks of halothane are discussed.

Shapiro JM, Condos R, Cole RP. Myopathy in status asthmaticus: relation to neuromuscular blockade and corticosteroid administration. *J Intensive Care Med* 1993;8:144.
Case reports of status asthmaticus complicated by myopathy are described. An association exists between the combination of neuromuscular blocking agents plus corticosteroids and the development of myopathy.

Smith DL, Deshazo RD. Bronchoalveolar lavage in asthma. *Am Rev Respir Dis* 1993;148:523.
A review of bronchoalveolar lavage in asthma research and as therapy for status asthmaticus.

Turner, MO, Patel A, Ginsburg S, et al. Bronchodilator delivery in acute airflow obstruction. *Arch Intern Med* 1997;157:1736.
A metaanalysis shows that bronchodilator delivered by MDI or nebulizer is equivalent in the treatment of acute asthma.

US Dept of Health and Human Services, Public Health Service, National Institutes of Health (NIH). *Expert panel report 2: guidelines for the diagnosis and management of asthma.* NIH publication no. 97–4051, 1997.
These are consensus guidelines for the management of asthma.

43. CHRONIC OBSTRUCTIVE PULMONARY DISEASE

Oren P. Schaefer, Stephen E. Lapinsky, and Ronald F. Grossman

I. General principles. Respiratory failure secondary to COPD leads to 75,000 deaths in the United States annually and is the fourth most common cause of death overall and the second most common cause of permanent disability in people older than 40 years of age. Deaths from chronic obstructive pulmonary disease (COPD) over the last 2 decades have increased 71%, the greatest percentage increase among the major causes of death in the United States.

II. Etiology. The major risk factor associated with the development of COPD is cigarette smoking. The total number of pack-years of smoking correlates best, although the total length of time spent smoking likely contributes as well. Only a minority of heavy cigarette smokers develop significant COPD, a finding meaning that additional cofactors are important. Homozygous alpha$_1$-antitrypsin deficiency is a risk factor for the development of COPD even in the absence of cigarette smoking, although nonsmoking patients with alpha$_1$-antitrypsin deficiency may not necessarily develop COPD. Other factors that may increase the risk of COPD, particularly in cigarette smokers, include a history of significant childhood respiratory illnesses, air pollution, and the presence of increased airway reactivity. Occupational exposure to grain and mineral dusts and textile material such as cotton or hemp may be a risk factor even in the absence of cigarette smoking.

III. Physiologic derangements. Expiratory airflow obstruction results from both structural airway narrowing as well as functional narrowing caused by the loss of radial distending forces on the airways. Inflammatory edema, excessive mucus, and glandular hypertrophy are responsible for intrinsic obstruction of airways. Destruction of alveolar walls causes loss of elastic recoil and airflow obstruction that increases in a dynamic fashion with expiratory effort.

The pathophysiologic consequences of severe, chronic airflow obstruction in the lung include the following: reduced flow rates that limit minute ventilation; maldistributed ventilation, resulting in both wasted ventilation (high ventilation-perfusion [V/Q] mismatch) and impaired gas exchange (low V/Q mismatch); increased airway resistance, which causes an increased work of breathing; and air trapping and hyperinflation, which alter the geometry of the respiratory muscles and place them at a mechanical disadvantage. The maximum force they can generate is reduced, and this change predisposes these muscles to fatigue. Some patients with COPD may have a blunted respiratory center drive, which further predisposes them to carbon dioxide retention.

IV. Diagnosis. The diagnosis of COPD is suspected on clinical grounds but confirmed by pulmonary function tests. Arterial blood gases (ABGs) determine the diagnosis of respiratory failure.

A. History. A negative history of cigarette smoking makes the diagnosis of COPD unlikely. Chronic productive cough and dyspnea on exertion are the two symptoms most commonly associated with COPD, but they are associated with a large variety of other causes. Nevertheless, such a history in a heavy cigarette smoker should raise the possibility of COPD.

B. Physical examination. Decreased breath sounds, prolonged expiration, wheezing, and hyperinflation may be present. Examination also aids in the assessment of respiratory distress. A combative, confused, or obtunded patient suggests the possibility of hypercapnia or hypoxia. Respiratory muscle fatigue suggests that mechanical ventilatory support may be required. It is heralded by the onset of paradoxic respiratory motion or respiratory alternans.

C. Radiology. Roentgenographic findings may include hyperinflation with flattened diaphragms and an increased retrosternal and retrocardiac airspace, one of two distinctly different bronchovascular patterns (e.g., vascular attenuation or prominence of lung markings), enlarged hilar pulmonary arteries and right ventricular enlargement, and regional hyperlucency and bullae. Although these findings are common in patients with severe COPD, they lack sensitivity in the diagnosis of mild COPD. In patients with an acute exacerbation, a chest roentgenogram may exclude reversible conditions such as pneumonia, pneumothorax, or pulmonary edema. In the intensive care unit, technical factors limit the quality of the chest films. Although interpretation of a portable film may be difficult, these radiographs nevertheless may provide valuable information, particularly in ventilated patients.

D. Pulmonary function tests. The demonstration of nonreversible expiratory airflow obstruction in the laboratory determines the diagnosis of COPD. A decrease in the ratio of forced expiratory volume in 1 second (FEV_1) to forced vital capacity is the hallmark of obstructive airways disease. However, the FEV_1 correlates with clinical outcome and mortality. Hypercapneic respiratory failure from COPD is usually not observed unless the FEV_1 is less than 1 L. Pulmonary function tests may also reveal an increased total lung capacity and residual volume, as well as a reduction in carbon monoxide diffusing capacity.

ABGs provide the necessary data to diagnose and quantitate the severity of respiratory failure. The patient with severe COPD admitted to the intensive care unit typically presents with an elevated partial pressure of carbon dioxide (P_aCO_2), a decreased partial pressure of oxygen (P_aO_2), and an alveolar-arterial oxygen pressure ($P(A\text{-}a)O_2$) gradient that is substantially increased. The relation between the change in P_aCO_2 and the change in hydrogen ion concentration allows one to determine whether hypercapnia is acute, acute-on-chronic, or chronic (Chapter 40).

V. Differential diagnosis. COPD usually must be distinguished from other conditions that cause expiratory airflow limitation and hypercapnia: asthma, cystic fibrosis, bronchiectasis, and bronchiolitis.

VI. Exacerbations. Many factors may be associated with acute decompensation, the most common being an acute viral upper or lower respiratory tract infection. With an acute exacerbation, the patient describes increased dyspnea and increased cough and sputum production, often accompanied by a change in the color and character. The more severe the symptoms, the more likely there is a bacterial infection. Airflow obstruction is worsened, the work of breathing increases, and mucus production and mucociliary clearance are altered. Pulmonary function tests document worsened expiratory airflow obstruction, whereas the ABGs usually show an additional decrease in the P_aO_2 and, in patients with severe COPD, the development or worsening of arterial hypercapnia. One must also consider the other specific causes of acute decompensation in COPD (Table 43-1).

VII. Treatment. Treatment of the patient with COPD involves long-term management of the stable patient, treatment of acute exacerbations, and treatment of respiratory failure.

A. Long-term management. Management of COPD involves the use of inhaled bronchodilators, and possibly steroids, theophylline, and supplemental oxygen. Smoking cessation, however, clearly remains the first step in management. Long-term management is covered in further depth in *Intensive Care Medicine,* Fourth Edition.

B. Acute exacerbation

1. Supportive therapy

a. Oxygen therapy. Supplemental oxygen should be given to all hypoxemic or hypercapneic patients presenting with an acute exacerbation. P_aCO_2 commonly rises with supplemental oxygen, but carbon dioxide narcosis is uncommon. Patients should not be kept hypoxemic for fear that oxygen therapy will aggravate carbon dioxide retention, but ABGs must be closely monitored.

b. Bronchodilators. Although COPD is characterized by irreversible airflow obstruction, it often has a reversible component, particularly in the setting of an acute exacerbation. Inhaled beta-agonists and ipratropium, administered by nebulizer or by metered-dose inhaler using a spacer

TABLE 43-1. Acute decompensation in chronic obstructive pulmonary disease: differential diagnosis

Air pollution
Aspiration
Bronchiolitis
Cardiac arrhythmia
Chest wall injury (e.g., rib fracture)
Chronic obstructive pulmonary disease
Cigarette smoking
Cystic fibrosis
Lymphangitic carcinomatosis
Metabolic derangements (e.g., hypophosphatemia)
Parasitic infections
Pleural effusion
Pneumonia
Pneumothorax
Pulmonary edema
Pulmonary embolism
Sedation
Surgery
Systemic illness
Tracheobronchial infection
Upper respiratory tract infection

device appear to be equally effective. A metered-dose inhaler with an aerosol holding chamber may also be used to provide bronchodilator therapy effectively to patients receiving mechanical ventilation. Theophylline may offer additional benefit in patients with COPD by increasing central nervous system (CNS) respiratory drive, respiratory muscle contractility, and resistance to respiratory muscle fatigue, although its role in acute exacerbations is not clear.

c. **Antibiotics.** No evidence indicates that antibiotics given routinely are beneficial in all exacerbations of COPD. Clinical benefits are most likely to occur in patients with more serious exacerbations, particularly those with fever and grossly purulent sputum. The organisms usually responsible for bacterial infection in acute exacerbations include *Haemophilus influenzae, Streptococcus pneumoniae,* and *Moraxella catarrhalis.* Antibiotic coverage should be directed against these organisms.

d. **Corticosteroids.** Short-term use of corticosteroids is advocated in acute exacerbations, although not all patients benefit. A dosage of 0.5 mg per kilogram of methylprednisolone intravenously every 6 hours has been shown to be beneficial. The risk of relapse may be reduced if initial treatment includes a course of corticosteroids.

e. **Other interventions.** Nutritional support should be instituted early in the course of hospitalization. Carbon dioxide retention can be made worse if the patient is given too many calories. In the absence of bronchiectasis or bronchorrhea, chest physical therapy is likely of no benefit.

2. **Specific therapy.** Exacerbations of COPD are usually due to upper or lower airway infections (e.g., viral). However, should a specific condition be discovered for which specific treatment exists, therapy should be instituted (Table 43-1).

3. **Respiratory failure**

   a. **Supplemental oxygen.** Supplemental, low-flow oxygen is probably the single most useful treatment in COPD-induced hypercapnic respiratory failure. The use of oxygen leads to (a) a decrease in anaerobic metabolism and lactic acid production, (b) an improvement in brain function,

(c) a decrease in cardiac arrhythmias and ischemia, (d) a decrease in pulmonary hypertension, (e) an improvement in right heart function with improvement in right heart failure, (f) a decrease in the release of antidiuretic hormone and an increase in the ability of the kidneys to clear free water, (g) a decrease in the formation of extravascular lung water, (h) improvement in survival, and (i) a decrease in red blood cell mass and hematocrit.

The administration of oxygen is often associated with a rise in the P_aCO_2. This likely results from a change in dead space or shift of the hemoglobin-oxygen binding curve, rather than decreased respiratory drive. This rise is expected and should not be specifically treated unless it is excessive, resulting in a trend toward acute respiratory acidosis, with CNS or cardiovascular side effects. Should this occur, the supplemental oxygen should not be discontinued abruptly, but rather decreased slowly until the P_aCO_2 returns to a more acceptable level. Because abrupt discontinuation of supplemental oxygen may not be associated with a prompt increase in ventilation, the P_aCO_2 may not fall. The withdrawal of supplemental oxygen then further depresses the already low alveolar PO_2 and causes arterial hypoxemia. Carbon dioxide narcosis may occur with excessive oxygen therapy but is much less likely with low flow-controlled oxygen therapy.

b. Intubation and mechanical ventilation. This decision reflects a continuous reassessment of the patient's status including the trend of ABG values and a determination of whether the patient is strong and alert enough to clear secretions and to protect the airway. Repeat assessment of the relation between the arterial hydrogen ion concentration and P_aCO_2 may be of help in determining whether intubation is required right away (e.g., acute acidosis) or whether it should be prepared for expectantly (e.g., acute-on-chronic) or delayed for the present time (e.g., chronic). The presence of acute respiratory acidosis with a low arterial pH (less than 7.2) and inadequate P_aO_2 (less than 55 mm Hg), or CNS and cardiovascular dysfunction dictates that assisted ventilation is required.

Although it is prudent to avoid intubation in the patient with COPD whenever possible, the development of stupor or coma may necessitate emergency intubation, a potentially disastrous situation. Predictors of which patients will ultimately require mechanical ventilation during the hospitalization include the presence of asynchronous or paradoxic breathing with an initial P_aCO_2 greater than 60 mm Hg and a marked deterioration in ABGs from previous outpatient baseline values. A significant drop in the pH after the administration of low-flow oxygen is also predictive of the ultimate need for mechanical ventilation.

The objectives of ventilation are to support gas exchange and to rest the muscles of respiration, thus enabling the patient to resume spontaneous breathing once the excessive mechanical loads of breathing have been corrected. Adequate nutrition is also essential, as noted previously.

A particular problem in ventilating patients with airflow obstruction is the development of "intrinsic" or "auto" positive end-expiratory pressure (PEEP)—the difference between the alveolar pressure and proximal airway pressure measured by the ventilator at the end of exhalation. Auto-PEEP is the result of "air-trapping" from low expiratory flow through obstructed airways and is aggravated by rapid respiratory rates, slow inspiratory flow rates, and ventilation through narrow endotracheal tubes. The consequences of auto-PEEP include elevation of inspiratory pressures, hypotension, and increased work for spontaneous or triggered breaths. To trigger the ventilator, patients must first develop enough negative intrapleural pressure to reverse the positive auto-PEEP, and then they need further negative intrapleural pressure before inspiratory flow can begin. This effect can be overcome by applying external PEEP equivalent to or slightly less than auto-PEEP. The only effect of this externally applied PEEP is to reduce inspiratory work, and it is therefore of no value in paralyzed patients. Applied PEEP of up to 85% of intrinsic PEEP does not aggravate hyperinflation or compromise hemodynamics.

Ventilatory rate and tidal volume on mechanical ventilation must be regulated to return pH slowly toward normal. Hyperventilation of a patient with chronic carbon dioxide retention can cause marked respiratory alkalosis resulting in seizures or arrhythmias. Attempts to normalize pH and to correct P_aCO_2 too quickly can result in excessive peak airway pressures and elevated auto-PEEP. In this situation, reduction of the ventilator rate and controlled hypoventilation are indicated. Adequate oxygenation must be maintained, but the P_aCO_2 is allowed to rise. Acidosis resulting from this permissive hypercapnia may require treatment with bicarbonate, especially if associated with hemodynamic instability.

4. **Noninvasive ventilation.** Although intubation and mechanical ventilation are lifesaving measures, they carry significant risks. Noninvasive modalities have been successfully used to support gas exchange and to prevent intubation, and, whenever possible, they should be tried before invasive ventilation. Pressure-support ventilation administered by a tight-fitting face or nasal mask may obviate the need for conventional mechanical ventilation. Mask ventilation is generally well tolerated, but it should not be used in patients who are excessively agitated or who are unable to clear secretions or protect their airway.

Selected Readings

Abou-Shala N, Meduri GU. Noninvasive mechanical ventilation in patients with acute respiratory failure. *Crit Care Med* 1996;24:705.

A thorough review that includes the indications for use, technique for application, advantages, and potential complications.

American Thoracic Society. Standards for the diagnosis and care of patients with chronic obstructive pulmonary disease. *Am J Respir Crit Care Med* 1995;152:S77.

A comprehensive review.

Anthonisen NR, Monfreda J, Warren CPW, et al. Antibiotic therapy in exacerbations of chronic obstructive pulmonary disease. *Ann Intern Med* 1987;106:196.

Patients with COPD with increased dyspnea, sputum production, and purulence and treated with antibiotics had overall greater treatment success, and fewer relapses, than those given placebo.

Brochard L, Mancebo J, Wysocki M, et al. Noninvasive ventilation for acute exacerbations of chronic obstructive pulmonary disease. *N Engl J Med* 1995;333:817.

In selected patients, noninvasive ventilation can reduce the need for intubation and can decrease length of stay and in-hospital mortality.

Derenne J-P, Fleury B, Pariente R. Acute respiratory failure of chronic obstructive pulmonary disease. *Am Rev Respir Dis* 1988;138:1006.

A review covering all aspects of this problem, with emphasis on pathophysiology and management.

Gross NJ. Ipratropium bromide. *N Engl J Med* 1988;319:486.

Comprehensive review of this widely used therapy for COPD. It covers its basic and clinical pharmacology and its use in clinical care.

Karpel JP, Pesin J, Greenberg D, et al. A comparison of the effects of ipratropium bromide and metaproterenol sulfate in acute exacerbations of COPD. *Chest* 1990;98:835.

In COPD exacerbations, equivalent bronchodilation was achieved by both drugs. Ipratropium use was not associated with decreased oxygenation, as was seen with metaproterenol.

Leatherman JW. Mechanical ventilation in obstructive lung disease. *Clin Chest Med* 1997;17:577.

A review of topics relevant to the use of mechanical ventilation in patients with severe airflow obstruction including discussions on bedside assessment of respiratory mechanics, dynamic pulmonary hyperinflation, and the role of controlled hypoventilation with permissive hypercapnea.

Ranieri VM, Dambrosio M, Brienza N. Intrinsic PEEP and cardiopulmonary interaction in patients with COPD and acute ventilatory failure. *Eur Respir J* 1996;9:1283.

A review of the concepts of intrinsic PEEP in patients with obstructive airway disease and discussion of the use of extrinsic PEEP in ventilatory strategies.

Sethi S. Infectious exacerbations of chronic bronchitis: diagnosis and management. *J Antimicrob Chemother* 1999;43 [Suppl A]:97.

A review of bacterial acute exacerbations of chronic bronchitis with emphasis on management of the infectious issues.

Weinberger SE, Schwartzstein RM, Weiss JW. Hypercapnia. *N Engl J Med* 1989; 321:1223.

An excellent discussion of the physiology, pathophysiology, and therapeutic implications of hypercapnea.

44. EXTRAPULMONARY CAUSES OF RESPIRATORY FAILURE

Mark M. Wilson and Helen Hollingsworth

I. General principles. This chapter discusses those conditions that cause respiratory failure primarily or exclusively by their effects on structures other than the lungs themselves. The following components make up the extrapulmonary compartment: (a) central nervous system (CNS), (b) peripheral nervous system, (c) respiratory muscles, (d) chest wall, (e) pleura, and (f) upper airway. Because severe impairment of the extrapulmonary compartment produces respiratory failure through the mechanism of hypoventilation, the resultant respiratory failure is always hypercapnic. Extrapulmonary causes can account for up to an estimated 17% of all cases of hypercapnic respiratory failure. Extrapulmonary causes of respiratory failure should also be considered in patients who fail to be weaned from mechanical ventilation despite treatment of the initial pulmonary cause of respiratory failure.

II. Pathogenesis. Arterial hypercapnia in the presence of a normal alveolar-arterial oxygen tension gradient (A-a gradient) on room air is the *sine qua non* of pure extrapulmonary respiratory failure. An A-a gradient less than 20 mm Hg in the presence of an elevated partial pressure of arterial carbon dioxide (P_aCO_2) is, with few exceptions, diagnostic of extrapulmonary respiratory failure.

Functionally, extrapulmonary disorders (Table 44-1) can lead to hypercapnic respiratory failure because of a decrease in normal force generation (e.g., CNS dysfunction, peripheral nervous system abnormalities, or respiratory muscle dysfunction) or an increase in impedance to bulk flow ventilation (e.g., chest wall and pleural disorders or upper airway obstruction).

A. Decrease in normal force generation. Any condition that directly or indirectly impairs respiratory muscle function can result in decreased force generation. If this impairment is severe enough, the level of minute ventilation may be insufficient for the level of (metabolic) production of carbon dioxide, and hypercapnic respiratory failure will result.

A decrease in central drive to breathe may occur from direct central loss of sensitivity to changes in PCO_2 and pH or as a result of a peripheral chemoreceptor loss of sensitivity to hypoxia, such as with CNS depressants, metabolic abnormalities, CNS structural lesions, primary alveolar hypoventilation, and central sleep apnea (Table 44-1).

Disruption of impulse transmission from the respiratory center in the brainstem to the respiratory muscles may result in respiratory failure. The innervation of the inspiratory respiratory muscles may be involved as part of a generalized process, such as in Guillain-Barré syndrome, myasthenia gravis, amyotrophic lateral sclerosis, neuromuscular junction blockade (Table 44-1), or as an isolated abnormality that affects the respiratory system in a variable way that depends on the level of the injury, such as in phrenic nerve palsy and spinal cord trauma (Table 44-1). Peripheral nervous system dysfunction severe enough to produce hypercapnic respiratory failure is always associated with a reduced vital capacity (usually less than 50% of predicted value) and markedly decreased maximal inspiratory and expiratory pressures at the mouth (usually less than 30% of predicted). Clinically, this type of respiratory failure is characterized by an ineffective cough and a high incidence of aspiration, atelectasis and pneumonia.

Certain systemic myopathies feature prominent respiratory muscle involvement, such as muscular dystrophies, myotonic disorders, inflammatory and endocrine myopathies, and electrolyte disturbances (Table 44-1). The clinical presentation generally is one of widespread skeletal muscle weakness. Respiratory muscle involvement and respiratory failure usually develop only as the disease progresses. On occasion, however, respiratory failure may be the presenting manifestation of a generalized myopathy.

TABLE 44-1. Causes of respiratory failure

Central nervous system
- Drug (e.g., narcotics, barbiturates)
- Hypothyroidism
- Starvation
- Metabolic alkalosis
- Brainstem disease (neoplasm, infection, infarction)
- Primary alveolar hypoventilation (Ondine curse)
- Central sleep apnea

Respiratory muscles
- Muscular dystrophies
- Myotonic dystrophies
- Periodic paralyses
- Glycogen storage diseases
- Polymyositis
- Hyper-/Hypothyroidism
- Hyperadrenocorticoism
- Rhabdomyolysis
- Infectious myositis (viral, trichinosis)
- Hypophosphatemia
- Hyper-/Hypomagnesemia
- Hypokalemia
- Hypercalcemia
- Eosinophilia-myalgia syndrome
- Procainamide myopathy
- Drug-induced neuromuscular blockade
- Critical illness myopathy

Chest wall/pleura
- Kyphoscoliosis
- Obesity-hypoventilation syndrome
- Flail chest
- Fibrothorax
- Thoracoplasty
- Ankylosing spondylitis

Peripheral nervous system
- Spinal cord disease (trauma, neoplasm, hemorrhage, infection)
- Tetanus
- Strychnine poisoning
- Amyotrophic Lateral Sclerosis
- Poliomyelitis
- Guillain-Barré syndrome
- Shellfish poisoning ("red tide")
- Ciguatera poisoning (fugu)
- Bilateral phrenic nerve palsy
- Charcot-Marie-Tooth disease
- Diphtheria
- Tick paralysis
- Acute intermittent porphyria
- Beriberi
- Myasthenia gravis
- Eaton-Lambert syndrome
- Critical illness polyneuropathy
- Drug-induced neuromuscular blockade
- Botulism
- Organophosphate poisoning
- Neuralgic amyotrophy

Upper airway
- Acute epiglottitis
- Acute laryngeal edema
- Foreign body aspiration
- Retropharyngeal hemorrhage
- Bilateral vocal cord paralysis
- Laryngeal/tracheal tumors
- Tracheal stenosis
- Tracheomalacia
- Obstructive sleep apnea
- Adenotonsillar hypertrophy
- Obstructive goiter

B. Increased impedance to bulk flow. Any disorder (Table 44-1) that causes a decrease in chest wall or pleural compliance (e.g., kyphoscoliosis, pleural fibrosis) or increases airflow resistance from upper airway obstruction (e.g., tracheal stenosis, laryngeal edema, obstructive sleep apnea) may culminate in hypercapnic respiratory failure if the resultant respiratory muscle force requirements cannot be sustained or overcome.

Lateral curvature of the spine (i.e., scoliosis) is generally a much more important factor in the development of hypercapnic respiratory failure than is dorsal curvature of the spine (i.e., kyphosis). Persons with severe deformity (angle of lateral curvature 120 degrees or more) at a relatively young age are at the greatest risk of eventual development of respiratory failure.

III. Diagnosis. The major differential diagnosis of extrapulmonary respiratory failure is hypercapnic respiratory failure from intrinsic lung disease (e.g., chronic obstructive pulmonary disease or asthma). These latter conditions can be readily distinguished because they are almost always associated with a markedly elevated A-a gradient when calculated on room air, which reflects the severe derangement of distal gas exchange that is present. Pulmonary parenchymal disease can exist concomitantly with extrapulmonary respiratory failure and may be suggested by the combination of hypercapnia and mild to moderate widening of the A-a gradient to 20 to 30 mm Hg. Even when the A-a gradient exceeds 30 mm Hg, some degree of extrapulmonary dysfunction may be present. When primary pulmonary disease is severe enough to cause hypercapnia, the gradient is generally more than 30 mm Hg.

A careful medical history frequently guides the clinician toward a specific cause from among the numerous diagnostic possibilities and should include an assessment of (but not limited to): the presence of muscle weakness and any specific muscle groups involved, duration of symptoms, sleep patterns and daytime somnolence, history of trauma or recent viral illness, dietary habits, and drug ingestions or chemical exposures. A thorough neuromuscular examination may support the initial impression or may suggest additional possibilities for evaluation.

A few laboratory tests may be useful diagnostically. Measurements of maximal inspiratory pressure (MIP) and maximal expiratory pressure (MEP) at the mouth are easy to perform, noninvasive, and highly predictive of the development of hypercapnic respiratory failure when the problem is decreased respiratory muscle force generation. Although normal predicted values vary (primarily on the basis of age and sex), an MIP not as negative as –30 cm H_2O or reduced to up to 30% of normal is likely to be associated with arterial hypercapnia. MEP is also reduced in this setting, and in some neuromuscular disorders the decrease may be even greater than that of the corresponding MIP. An MEP less than 40 cm H_2O is generally associated with a poor cough and difficulty clearing secretions.

Vital capacity measurements may be valuable predictors of the development of arterial hypercapnia and can be performed at the bedside. Although a vital capacity less than or equal to 1 L or less than 15 mL/kg body weight is commonly associated with arterial hypercapnia in patients with neuromuscular weakness, this is a less sensitive predictor than the MIP, particularly in patients with chest wall disorders such as kyphoscoliosis.

Significant upper airway obstruction should be considered in the patient who complains of dyspnea in association with stridor (extrathoracic obstruction) or expiratory wheezing (intrathoracic obstruction), particularly if other symptoms suggest an upper airway process (e.g., dysphagia in epiglottitis). Unless the patient is acutely ill, the presence of upper airway obstruction can usually be confirmed in the pulmonary function laboratory with the results of flow-volume loop analysis or by direct visualization.

Specific laboratory testing (toxicology screens, thyroid function tests, and levels of magnesium, phosphate, potassium, calcium, and creatinine phosphokinase) and other diagnostic studies (computed tomography, lumbar puncture, electromyography, muscle or nerve biopsy, polysomnogram) should be guided by the patient's presentation and physical examination.

IV. Treatment. The treatment of extrapulmonary respiratory failure can be divided into specific and supportive therapy. A description of specific therapies for each of the numerous potential causes of extrapulmonary respiratory failure in Table 44-1 is beyond the scope of this chapter. In the acute life-threatening situation, the first step in treatment is always to establish an adequate airway. Supportive therapy involves the use of mechanical ventilatory assistance (see Chapters 51 and 52), supplemental oxygen, and techniques of airway hygiene.

In the setting of chronic or progressive disease, reversible factors such as pulmonary congestion, infection, retained secretions, and other intercurrent illnesses should be carefully sought and treated. Regardless of the primary cause of respiratory muscle weakness, malnutrition exacerbates muscle weakness, and proper nutritional replacement can be beneficial in increasing respiratory muscle strength and function.

Selected Readings

Braun NMT, Arora NS, Rochester DF. Respiratory muscle and pulmonary function in polymyositis and other proximal myopathies. *Thorax* 1983;38:616.

Fifty-three patients with proximal myopathy were extensively studied to determine at what level of muscle weakness hypercapnic respiratory failure is likely and to sug-

gest which tests of pulmonary function or respiratory muscle strength predict this development.

Brooks BR. Natural history of ALS: symptoms, strength, pulmonary function and disability. *Neurology* 1996;47:S71.

Easy to read general discussion of the changes that occur and the progression expected in amyotrophic lateral sclerosis.

Defusco DJ, O'Dowd P, Hokama Y, et al. Coma due to ciguatera poisoning in Rhode Island. *Am J Med* 1993;95:240.

An interesting case report in a patient from a nonendemic area for this disease.

Hansen-Flaschen J, Cowen J, Raps EC. Neuromuscular blockade in the intensive care unit: more than we bargained for. *Am Rev Respir Dis* 1993;147:234.

A brief, but important, clinical commentary that drew attention to an underappreciated complication of neuromuscular blockade. This article discusses the risk factors and causes of prolonged weakness in this group of patients.

Kelly SM, Rosa A, Field S, et al. Inspiratory muscle strength and body composition in patients receiving total parenteral nutrition therapy. *Am Rev Respir Dis* 1984;130:33.

Small prospective study showing that loss of body mass negatively affects inspiratory muscle strength and contributes to ventilatory failure. Providing nutritional support improves overall nutritional status and inspiratory muscle strength.

NIH Conference. Myositis: immunologic contributions to understanding the cause, pathogenesis and therapy. *Ann Intern Med* 1995;122:715.

A summary of the clinical usefulness of myositis-specific autoantibodies.

Pratter MR, Irwin RS. Extrapulmonary causes of respiratory failure. *J Intensive Care Med* 1986;1:197.

Comprehensive review of the extrapulmonary causes of respiratory failure.

van der Meche FGA, Schmitz PIM, Dutch Guillain-Barré Study Group. A randomized trial comparing intravenous immune globulin and plasma exchange in Guillain-Barré syndrome. *N Engl J Med* 1992;326:1123.

A multicenter trial involving 150 patients treated with either 5 doses of intravenous immunoglobulin or 5 plasma exchanges. At 4 weeks from presentation, 53% of the intravenous immunoglobulin group had improved strength versus 34% in the plasma exchange group.

Williams MH Jr, Shim CS. Ventilatory failure. *Am J Med* 1970;48:477.

Good early review of the clinical conditions associated with ventilatory failure and their evaluation.

Zulueta J, Fanburg B. Respiratory dysfunction in myasthenia gravis. *Clin Chest Med* 1994;15:683.

A general review of the pathophysiology, clinical features, assessment, and management of myasthenia gravis.

45. ACUTE RESPIRATORY FAILURE IN PREGNANCY

Mark M. Wilson and Helen Hollingsworth

I. Overview. Acute respiratory failure remains an important cause of maternal and fetal morbidity and mortality. Thromboembolism, amniotic fluid embolism, and venous air embolism together account for approximately 20% of maternal deaths. Other causes of respiratory failure account for another 10% to 15% of maternal deaths. The physiology of pregnancy, critical to this discussion, can be reviewed in *Intensive Care Medicine,* Fourth Edition.

II. Causes of acute respiratory failure

A. Thromboembolic disease. Pulmonary embolism is the second leading cause of maternal mortality. The increased frequency of venous thromboembolism associated with pregnancy is attributed to an increase in clotting factors VII, VIII, and X, an increased fibrinogen level, and decreased fibrinolytic activity. Additional risks include venous stasis caused by uterine pressure on the inferior vena cava (IVC), cesarean section, increased maternal age, multiparity, obesity, and surgery during pregnancy and the early puerperium.

Symptoms, physical signs, and laboratory, radiographic, and electrocardiographic findings are not specific. Noninvasive tests such as duplex scanning to exclude deep venous thrombosis and perfusion lung scanning should be performed first; pulmonary angiography should be reserved for patients in whom pulmonary embolism cannot be excluded by these studies.

B. Amniotic fluid embolism. Amniotic fluid embolism is rare but usually catastrophic and has a mortality rate of up to 86%. Predisposing factors include older maternal age, multiparity, amniotomy, cesarean section, insertion of intrauterine fetal monitors, and term pregnancy in the presence of an intrauterine device. Ninety percent of cases occur before or during labor. The antemortem diagnosis rests predominantly on the clinical setting and the exclusion of other causes of respiratory failure. Demonstration of fetal elements in the maternal circulation in blood aspirated from central venous and right heart catheters lacks both sensitivity and specificity.

Cardiorespiratory collapse and disseminated intravascular coagulation occur simultaneously or in sequence. Severe dyspnea, tachypnea, and cyanosis during labor or in the early puerperium is the classic presentation. Shock is the first manifestation in 10% to 15% of patients. Excessive bleeding, particularly uterine, may be the first sign. The longer the survival, the greater the likelihood of respiratory failure, cardiovascular collapse, and disseminated intravascular coagulation. Up to 50% of patients who survive the first 60 minutes will have clinical evidence of coagulopathy, and most of the remaining patients will have laboratory evidence of disseminated intravascular coagulation.

C. Venous air embolism. Sudden, profound hypotension, usually followed by respiratory arrest, is the most common presentation of air embolism. Cough, dyspnea, dizziness, tachypnea, tachycardia, and diaphoresis may occur. The classic "mill-wheel" murmur, a drumlike sound, may be heard over the precordium. Electrocardiographic evidence of ischemia, right heart strain, and arrhythmias can be seen. Metabolic acidosis from lactic acid production may be present. Obstruction of the pulmonary circulation can be caused by a bolus of air that forms a block in the apical tract of the right ventricle and by fibrin microemboli that obstruct the pulmonary arterioles and capillaries. Polymorphonuclear leukocytes may be recruited and activated, thus leading to tissue damage.

D. Gastric aspiration. Aspiration into the tracheobronchial tree may be followed by chemical pneumonitis and increased-permeability pulmonary edema. The volume of acid aspiration determines, in part, the rapidity of symptom onset. Massive aspiration leading to immediate asphyxia or pneumonia from aspiration of oropharyngeal bacteria may also occur. The pathogens are usually oropharyngeal anaerobes. Risk factors for aspiration include increased intragastric pressure caused by the gravid uterus, progesterone-induced relaxation of the lower esophageal sphincter, delayed gastric emptying during labor, and analgesia-induced decreased mental status.

E. **Respiratory infections.** The spectrum of organisms found in community-acquired pneumonia in the pregnant woman is similar to that found in the nonpregnant population: *Streptococcus pneumoniae, Mycoplasma pneumoniae,* and *Haemophilus influenzae* are the most common. Primary varicella-zoster infection progresses to pneumonia more commonly in pregnant patients. Coccidioidomycosis is associated with an increased risk of dissemination during pregnancy and is associated with a high mortality rate. In women infected with the human immunodeficiency virus, the spectrum of pathogens includes opportunistic infections. *Listeria monocytogenes* also has a predilection for pregnant women, most commonly resulting in abortion or neonatal sepsis, but it remains rare.

F. **Asthma.** Asthma is the most common respiratory problem during pregnancy. Close monitoring and consistent control of asthma are crucial to maternal and fetal well-being. Assessment of the patient with an exacerbation includes the history, examination, and an objective measure of lung function. Findings that predict hospitalization include diaphoresis, use of accessory muscles, assumption of upright posture, altered level of consciousness, pulse rate greater than 120 beats per minute, respiratory rate greater than 30 breaths per minute, pulsus paradoxus greater than 18 mm Hg, and a peak expiratory flow rate less than 120 L per minute (or less than 50% predicted or personal best). Adequate oxygenation (S_aO_2 greater than 95%) in pregnant women with asthma must be ensured.

During acute attacks, arterial blood gases typically reveal mild hypocapnia and moderate hypoxemia. In pregnancy, the baseline partial pressure of arterial carbon dioxide (P_aCO_2) is often already depressed and likely decreases further with an acute asthma attack. A partial pressure of arterial oxygen (P_aCO_2) of 35 mm Hg therefore may actually represent "pseudonormalization" caused by fatigue and possibly impending respiratory failure. Persistent hypocapnia with associated respiratory alkalosis (pH greater than 7.48) may result in uterine artery vasoconstriction and decreased fetal perfusion.

G. **Beta-adrenergic tocolytic therapy associated with pulmonary edema.** Beta-adrenergic agonists are accepted therapy for inhibition of preterm labor. The use of beta$_2$-selective agents, such as ritodrine and terbutaline, has diminished the frequency of maternal tachycardia, but maternal pulmonary edema remains a serious side effect. Typical symptoms and signs include chest discomfort, dyspnea, tachypnea, rales, and edema on chest roentgenogram. Pulmonary edema may develop after only 24 hours, although usually after 48 hours of tocolytic therapy.

H. **Pneumomediastinum and pneumothorax.** Pneumomediastinum, albeit uncommon, is most often seen in the second stage of labor. Chest or shoulder pain that radiates to the neck and arms, mild dyspnea, and subcutaneous emphysema are common. Prolonged, dysfunctional labor is a predisposing factor.

III. Diagnostic testing

A. **Radiology.** Evaluation of patients with respiratory failure requires radiologic investigation. Concern exists for potential adverse effects on the fetus, but studies do not find an appreciable increased risk of gross congenital abnormalities or intrauterine growth retardation with exposure to less than 5 to 10 rads. Oncogenic risk is similarly small. A posteroanterior chest roentgenogram delivers an estimated fetal radiation exposure of 5 mrads. Careful shielding of the abdomen reduces this further. Pulmonary angiography (with shielding) results in a fetal absorbed dose of less than 50 mrads. Estimates of fetal radiation exposure with a perfusion lung scan are 18 mrads with technetium-labeled albumin. Although all the biologic effects of this type of radiation on the fetus are not known, the risk seems acceptable when compared with the mortality associated with undiagnosed pulmonary embolism.

B. Hemodynamic monitoring. Indications for pulmonary artery catheterization in obstetric patients are similar to those in the nonpregnant patient, but they include monitoring the critically ill patient with severe preeclampsia or eclampsia during labor. Although cardiac output is normally elevated during gestation and parturition, central pressures are not significantly different in pregnant and nonpregnant patients. One should measure the fetal heart rate daily or continuously, depending on the age of the fetus and the clinical situation, to document that the fetus is alive.

C. Tocolytic monitoring. Monitoring for labor contractions may be indicated.

IV. Treatment

A. Supportive therapy

1. Mechanical ventilation. Guidelines for intubation and mechanical ventilation are the same for pregnant as for nonpregnant patients (see Chapter 51). Hyperemia associated with pregnancy can narrow the upper airway. Patients are at increased risk of upper airway trauma during intubation, and small endotracheal tubes may be required. The decreased functional residual capacity may lower the oxygen reserve. At the time of intubation, a short period of apnea may be associated with a precipitous decrease in P_aO_2. Before any attempt at intubation, 100% oxygen should be administered. Hyperventilation to increase the P_aO_2 must be avoided because the associated respiratory alkalosis may decrease uterine blood flow. Cricoid pressure can help to decrease gastric inflation and can prevent regurgitation.

Minute ventilation should be adjusted for a P_aCO_2 of 30 to 32 mm Hg, which is normal in pregnancy. When only small increases in the fraction of inspired oxygen are necessary, one should aim for the usual gestational P_aO_2 of more than 95 mm Hg. Weaning parameters for pregnant patients are not well established. Therefore, one should follow the same guidelines used for nonpregnant patients (Chapter 52). Weaning from the ventilator when the patient is in the lateral decubitus position may be preferable, to avoid compression of the IVC.

2. Reversal of hypotension. The supine position may impair venous return in pregnant patients; the Trendelenburg position is unlikely to help and may further decrease venous return because of IVC compression. One should position the patient with her right hip elevated 10 to 15 cm or in the lateral decubitus position to move the uterus off the IVC. Hypotension not responsive to repositioning or fluid resuscitation requires vasopressors. Predominantly alpha-adrenergic agents, (e.g., norepinephrine) improve maternal blood pressure, but they decrease uterine blood flow because of uterine artery vasoconstriction. Ephedrine, with both alpha- and beta-stimulating effects, tends to preserve uterine blood flow while reversing hypotension. If maternal hypotension persists, drugs with more alpha-adrenergic activity should be tried.

3. Nutrition. Nutritional support is important for both maternal and fetal outcome. Maternal malnutrition may correlate with intrauterine growth retardation and development of preeclampsia. Maternal weight gain correlates with fetal weight gain and a successful outcome. Enteral is preferred over parenteral nutrition, to avoid complications associated with central venous catheters, to reduce expense, and to minimize gastric mucosal atrophy. If delivery occurs while the mother is receiving total parenteral nutrition, the neonate should be observed closely for hypoglycemia.

B. Specific therapy

1. Thromboembolism. The immediate goals of therapy are to provide adequate oxygenation, to treat hypotension and organ hypoperfusion, and to interrupt clot propagation by anticoagulation. Intravenous heparin should be instituted immediately in all patients who do not have contraindications. Heparin does not cross the placenta and is not teratogenic. Pregnancy and the immediate postpartum period are relative contraindications to thrombolysis because of the risk of hemorrhage during labor, delivery, and the first several days postpartum. IVC interruption should be considered in any patient with cardiopulmonary compromise caused by pulmonary embolism who does not receive thrombolytic therapy, who has a contraindication to heparin, or who has recurrent emboli despite heparin anticoagulation.

Heparin by continuous intravenous infusion is given for 7 to 10 days and then is administered subcutaneously in doses adjusted to prolong the activated partial thromboplastin time to 1.5 to 2.5 times control. Anticoagulant therapy is continued throughout pregnancy and for an additional 4 to 6 weeks postpartum. The use of low-molecular-weight heparin in pregnancy appears to be safe and may not be associated with the osteopenia seen with long-term heparin use. Warfarin (Coumadin), a potent teratogen, is not used. When pulmonary embolism occurs late in pregnancy or in the postpartum period, anticoagulant therapy is continued for at least 3 months.

2. **Amniotic fluid embolism.** Treatment is supportive: one should provide adequate ventilation and oxygenation, blood pressure support, and management of bleeding. When bleeding is active, transfusion with fresh frozen plasma, cryoprecipitate, and platelets is indicated. Reduction of uterine bleeding by manual massage, oxytocin infusion, and possibly, methylergonovine maleate, is also important. If bleeding persists, one should consider uterine exploration for tears or retained placenta.
3. **Venous air embolism.** Placing a patient in the left lateral decubitus position may allow the bubble of air to migrate away from the right ventricular outflow tract. Aspiration of air from the right atrium, right ventricle, or pulmonary outflow tract can be attempted with a central venous or pulmonary artery catheter. Emboli that have migrated into the pulmonary vasculature can be decreased in size by providing 100% oxygen. Anticoagulation to treat fibrin microemboli, high-dose corticosteroids to prevent inflammation, and hyperbaric oxygen have all been suggested.
4. **Gastric aspiration.** Prophylactic antibiotics are not beneficial in gastric aspiration. Antibiotics should be prescribed only when infection complicates chemical pneumonitis. Antibiotic choice is guided by the appropriate evaluation of respiratory secretions and other cultures. Current studies do not support a role for corticosteroids.
5. **Respiratory infections.** Selection of antibiotics to treat pneumonia during pregnancy follows the same guidelines used for nonpregnant patients. Drugs with the least risk to the fetus and mother should be chosen. For community-acquired pneumonia in pregnancy, penicillins, cephalosporins, and erythromycin (excluding the estolate that is associated with an increased risk of cholestatic jaundice in pregnancy) are probably safe. Both the American Thoracic Society and the Infectious Disease Society of America have published guidelines on the evaluation and treatment of community-acquired pneumonia. Other infectious agents must be treated according to usual standards, with the safety of drug therapy weighed against the risk of untreated infection.
6. **Asthma.** The prevention or reversal of hypoxemia is paramount. Oxygenation may worsen with bronchodilators, and therefore oxygen should be used in all patients. Pharmacotherapy of severe exacerbations of asthma during pregnancy is similar to that used for the nonpregnant patient (see Chapters 42 and 53). The effects of inhaled bronchodilators are predominantly local, thereby decreasing fetal exposure. The more selective beta$_2$-agonists theoretically do not decrease uterine blood flow unless there is a decrease in maternal systemic vascular resistance. Beta-agonists carry the risk of hypokalemia and pulmonary edema if they are used at high doses for more than 24 to 48 hours. Intravenous theophylline appears safe, but its role in status asthmaticus remains controversial. High-dose intravenous corticosteroids should be given to help reverse airflow obstruction. Prednisone crosses the placenta poorly, and few, if any, untoward fetal effects can be attributed to maternal steroid treatment. Despite therapy, respiratory failure may ensue and may require mechanical ventilation (see Chapter 51). When a pregnant patient has life-threatening refractory asthma, one should consider emergency delivery of the fetus by cesarean section. This difficult decision in part depends on the age and viability of the fetus.

7. **Beta-adrenergic tocolytic pulmonary edema.** Treatment involves the immediate discontinuation of the tocolytic agent, supplemental oxygen, and diuresis. Other respiratory support is given as indicated.
8. **Pneumomediastinum and pneumothorax.** Pneumomediastinum does not often require drainage. Air usually dissects out of the mediastinum into the subcutaneous tissues of the neck. Direct treatment at any underlying cause. A spontaneous pneumothorax occupying less than 20% of the hemithorax in an asymptomatic patient who is not receiving mechanical ventilation can be observed closely. In symptomatic patients, patients receiving mechanical ventilation, or patients with an enlarging pneumothorax, chest tube placement is mandatory.

Selected Readings

Clark SL. New concepts of amniotic fluid embolism: a review. *Obstet Gynecol Surv* 1990;45:360.
A review of pathophysiology, presentation, diagnosis, and treatment.

Clark SL, Hankins GDV, Dudley DA, et al. Amniotic fluid embolism: analysis of the national registry. *Am J Obstet Gynecol* 1995;172:1158.
Forty-six patients were reviewed in this excellent discussion of pathophysiology and similarities among amniotic fluid embolism, anaphylaxis, and septic shock.

Dombrowski MP. Pharmacologic therapy of asthma during pregnancy. *Obstet Gynecol Clin North Am* 1997;24:559.
An in-depth evaluation of prescribing medication for the pregnant asthmatic patient.

Ginsberg JS, Hirsch J, Rainbow AJ, et al. Risks to the fetus of radiologic procedures used in the diagnosis of maternal venous thromboembolic disease. *Thromb Haemost* 1989;61:189.
Fetal absorbed radiation doses with procedures used to diagnose thromboembolic disease. The article includes a literature review.

Lapinsky SE, Kruczynski, Slutsky AS. Critical Care of the pregnant patient. *Am J Respir Crit Care Med* 1995;152:427.
A review of the critically ill obstetric patient.

Mossman KL, Hill LT. Radiation risks in pregnancy. *Obstet Gynecol* 1982;60:237.
Evaluation of radiation exposures in early pregnancy. Procedures to minimize fetal exposure are discussed.

Perry KG, Morrison JC, Rust OA, et al. Incidence of adverse cardiopulmonary effects with low-dose continuous terbutaline infusion. *Am J Obstet Gynecol* 1995;173:1273.
Review of more than 8,700 women given terbutaline as tocolytic therapy for preterm labor. Pulmonary edema developed in 28 (0.32%). Risk of adverse effects appeared much lower than prior literature had suggested.

Schatz M. Asthma during pregnancy: interrelationships and management. *Ann Allergy* 1992;68:123.
A complete review including pathophysiology, management, and pharmacotherapy in pregnancy.

Toglia M, Weg JG. Venous thromboembolism during pregnancy. *N Engl J Med* 1996;335:108.
An outstanding review of venous thromboembolism in the obstetric patient.

Weinberger SE, Weiss ST, Cohen WR, et al. Pregnancy and the lung. *Am Rev Respir Dis* 1980;121:559.
A comprehensive article on the respiratory physiology of pregnancy.

Wilson MW, Curley FJ. Gas embolism. Part I. Venous gas embolism. *J Intensive Care Med* 1996;11:182.
Complete discussion of the problem including diagnosis and treatment.

46. VENOUS THROMBOEMBOLISM: PULMONARY EMBOLISM AND DEEP VENOUS THROMBOSIS

Oren P. Schaefer and John G. Weg

I. General principles. Deep venous thrombosis (DVT) and pulmonary embolism (PE), considered together as venous thromboembolism (VTE), remain common problems. The incidence of PE is in excess of 600,000 cases per year in the United States, and despite this frequency it remains a commonly missed diagnosis. Mortality of untreated PE is approximately 30%, whereas its diagnosis and proper treatment lower this rate more than 10-fold, to 2.5%. Up to 90% of PEs arise from the deep venous system of the legs, although they can form in the proximal thigh and iliac veins or inferior vena cava (IVC). Thrombosis and subsequent embolism can occur in the veins of the upper extremity, particularly in patients with central venous catheters and a history of congestive heart failure. The development of VTE is primarily related to stasis of blood flow, vascular wall damage, activation of the clotting system, and a hypercoagulable state.

II. Risk factors

A. Acquired risk factors. The most common are immobilization, surgery within the last 3 months (especially pelvis and hip), and malignancy. Other risks include a history of VTE, trauma to the lower extremity, congestive heart failure, therapeutic estrogen use, postpartum state, and obesity.

B. Inherited risk factors. The most common is activated protein C resistance resulting from a specific point mutation in the gene coding for coagulation factor V Leiden. More than 11 million persons in the United States and approximately 20% to 60% of patients with VTE have activated protein C resistance. Hyperhomocysteinemia, caused by a heterozygous cystathiene beta-synthase deficiency, the prothrombin variant 20210, and patients with the antiphospholipid antibody syndrome all are at increased risk. Less common inherited risk factors include deficiencies of antithrombin III, protein C, and protein S and abnormalities in plasminogen or tissue plasminogen activator.

III. Clinical presentation

A. Signs and symptoms. Leg swelling and tenderness are the most common signs and symptoms of DVT. However, 95% of patients with symptoms suggestive of DVT have another diagnosis, and 50% to 85% of patients with DVT present without symptoms. At least one of the following—dyspnea, tachypnea, pleuritic chest pain, or signs and symptoms of DVT—is seen in 97% of patients with PE. These findings are nonspecific, and almost all the presenting symptoms of PE are as likely to be present in those without PE. Syncope is an uncommon presenting symptom of PE. Only crackles on auscultation and tachypnea are present in more than half the patients with PE. An increased pulmonary second heart sound (P_2) and a fourth heart sound are more common in patients with PE but are found in fewer than 25% of these patients.

B. Radiographs, electrocardiograms, and arterial blood gases. The chest radiograph is abnormal in more than 80% of patients with PE. Consolidation, atelectasis, pleural effusions, and enlarged central pulmonary arteries with decreased pulmonary vasculature are common in patients with PE. The classic Hampton hump is uncommon.

The electrocardiogram is also commonly abnormal (70% or more) but the most common findings of sinus tachycardia and ST segment and T-wave changes are too nonspecific to be of value. The classic S_1-S_2-S_3 and S_1-Q_3-T_3 patterns are uncommon.

Arterial blood gases are commonly abnormal. In the Prospective Investigators of Pulmonary Embolism Diagnosis (PIOPED) trial, the mean partial pressure of arterial oxygen (P_aO_2) was 70 ± 16 mmHg in patients with PE, no different from those without PE, a finding reflecting the similarity in gas exchange abnormalities in conditions that commonly mimic PE. In fact, 15% of patients with proven PE had a P_aO_2 of 85 mm Hg or greater, and 10% to 15% of patients with PE had a normal alveolar-arterial gradient [(A-a) DO_2], a more sensitive test of gas exchange. An abnormal P_aO_2 or (A-a) DO_2 is compatible with PE, but when this value is normal, the diagnosis should not be excluded.

IV. Diagnosis of deep venous thrombosis

A. Venography. This is the reference standard for the diagnosis of DVT. It remains difficult to perform and requires expertise for interpretation. Complications include foot and calf pain, superficial phlebitis, DVT, and hypersensitivity reactions to radiocontrast media. Noninvasive tests have supplanted the venogram.

B. Impedance plethysmography. Impedance plethysmography (IPG) has an overall sensitivity and specificity of 83% and 92%, respectively. False-positive results may arise with tensing of the leg muscles, compression by an extravascular mass, elevated central pressure obstructing venous outflow, or reduced arterial flow. IPG is not sensitive to calf vein thrombosis. Studies demonstrate an initial negative test in 6% to 26% of symptomatic patients who develop an abnormal test result (DVT) with serial testing.

C. Real-time B-mode ultrasonography. Real-time imaging permits direct visualization of major vascular channels, and the Doppler signal provides an audible and graphic depiction of blood flow. Failure to collapse the vascular lumen completely with gentle probe pressure and the finding of intraluminal echogenic material resulting from clot are diagnostic of thrombosis. The sensitivity of duplex ultrasound for proximal DVT is 97%, and the specificity is 99%. False-positive tests may result from an inability to compress the femoral vein because of pregnancy or a pelvic tumor. False-negative tests may result from missing small clots or misinterpreting total occlusion of the femoral vein because of dilated collateral veins. Duplex ultrasound is less sensitive in identifying isolated calf vein thrombosis. The predictive value of duplex ultrasound is greater than that of IPG.

V. Diagnosis of pulmonary embolism

A. Ventilation-perfusion lung scans. The PIOPED trial was the first prospective trial to report on the value of the ventilation-perfusion (V/Q) scanning in acute PE. Criteria for interpretation of the scan were established by the PIOPED nuclear medicine investigators, and these have been used by many institutions to interpret the scans. Scans are categorized as normal, near-normal, intermediate, indeterminate, or high probability based on the number and size of the perfusion abnormalities present, and whether or not they are matched with abnormalities of ventilation. PIOPED investigators also assigned clinical probabilities of PE's presence before the scans' performance. The positive predictive value of a high-probability lung scan is approximately 88%. A prior history of PE decreased the positive predictive value to 74%. Conversely, a normal lung perfusion scan effectively rules out clinically important PE. Unfortunately, in PIOPED, a high-probability or normal/near-normal scan occurred in only 27%. Assigning prior probabilities was found to be helpful only in concordant situations, which was infrequent. A high clinical suspicion combined with a high-probability lung scan improved the diagnostic accuracy to 96%; a low clinical suspicion combined with a low-probability lung scan detected PE in only 4%.

In patients with underlying cardiopulmonary disease, in particular chronic obstructive pulmonary disease, the frequency of nondiagnostic scans is higher than in those without underlying disease. Similarly, in patients in an intensive care unit who are in respiratory failure, the clinical, radiographic, arterial blood gas and V/Q scan findings are unsatisfactory in making a diagnosis.

B. Pulmonary angiography. Angiography is the standard by which to diagnose PE. Intravascular filling defects and the trailing embolus sign are diagnostic. The procedure is safe, with a mortality risk of 0.1% to 0.5%. Cardiac perforation, hematoma, and contrast media reaction can all occur. A negative angiogram excludes the diagnosis of PE.

C. Investigational diagnostic studies. Magnetic resonance imaging has a high sensitivity and specificity for the diagnosis of pelvic and thigh venous thrombosis, but additional studies are required before this becomes a standard diagnostic technique. Magnetic resonance angiography also appears promising for the diagnosis of PE. A negative D-dimer agglutination test using a bispecific antibody (Simpli-Red) has a high negative predictive value of more than 95% for DVT and PE. A quantitative plasma D-dimer less than 300 to 500 ng/mL as assessed by an immunosorbent assay similarly has an excellent negative predictive value, particularly if noninvasive leg studies are negative or a lung perfusion scan is interpreted as low probability. Reliability of other D-dimer tests is not known. Contrast-enhanced helical computed tomography of the chest (spiral CT) appears to be promising in the diagnosis of PE. Its sensitivity for central emboli is approximately 95% (overall sensitivity 72%, specificity 95%). Emboli in segmental or small vessels occur with a frequency of 15% to 30% and may be missed by spiral CT. A negative study therefore may require additional investigation.

D. Algorithm for the diagnosis of pulmonary embolism. The limited utility of clinical findings and of the V/Q scan makes decision making difficult. Only a patient with a high-probability lung scan and a clinical impression that is suggestive of the diagnosis or is uncertain warrants treatment without additional investigation. The only situation that warrants a decision neither to treat nor to pursue further evaluation is a normal perfusion scan. In all other situations, PE is difficult to exclude, and additional diagnostic evaluation is required.

Diagnostic algorithms take advantage of the continuum of VTE; most PEs arise from DVT of the lower extremity. A noninvasive study (IPG, duplex) that finds evidence of DVT prompts anticoagulation. Noninvasive studies may be negative in up to 57% of patients with angiographically proven emboli. Therefore, a negative study does not exclude PE, and pulmonary angiography is warranted.

VI. Treatment

A. Heparin. Intravenous heparin is the therapy of choice for acute PE. Heparin interrupts the progression of the thrombotic process. An initial loading dose of 5,000 to 10,000 U is given on the basis of a strong clinical suspicion unless a high risk or contraindication to anticoagulation exists. Given the risk of heparin-induced thrombocytopenia, a platelet count should be obtained daily. After the loading dose, a continuous infusion of heparin is given at 1,300 U per hour. Adjustments are made using a nomogram, to achieve a thrombin clotting time (TCT) of 0.2 to 0.4 heparin U/mL, or an activated partial thromboplastin time (aPTT) 1.5 to 2.5 times mean normal range. The aPTT appears to be much less accurate than the TCT, and the latter should be used when the baseline aPTT is prolonged, such as seen with a lupus-type inhibitor. The risk of recurrent thromboembolism is increased if adequate anticoagulation is not achieved within 24 to 48 hours. The aPTT should be rechecked in 4 to 6 hours after bolus and then every 6 hours for the first 24 to 36 hours or until it is clear that the therapeutic range has been achieved. If, after the initial loading dose, there is little or no change in the TCT or aPTT, the patient should receive a second loading dose.

The most common complication of heparin therapy is bleeding, which occurs in 5% to 20%. A relationship between bleeding and higher levels of anticoagulation exists. Thrombocytopenia is relatively uncommon. In most patients, the platelet count falls only modestly. In a few patients, immunoglobulin G antibodies develop, and the platelet count can fall precipitously to less than 100,000 (often 40,000 to 60,000/mm^3). This condition must be recognized promptly and the heparin discontinued immediately because of the risk of venous and arterial thrombosis. Anticoagulation with warfarin is required, and if this cannot be achieved, nonheparin anticoagulants should be used, or consideration should be given to IVC interruption.

B. Low-molecular weight heparin. Prospective, randomized trials have found low-molecular-weight heparin to be as effective as unfractionated heparin in the treatment of acute DVT and PE. No difference was seen in recurrent VTE, bleeding, or mortality. Subcutaneous administration with a fixed dose, once or twice a day, and no need for laboratory monitoring make home therapy, after initial hospitalization, a viable option in certain patients.

C. Warfarin. Warfarin is initiated at the time of heparinization. Warfarin leads to the depletion of vitamin K–dependent coagulant proteins: factors II, VII, IX, and X. It also limits the carboxylation of anticoagulant proteins C and S. Because the biologic half-lives of the clotting factors are variable, the international normalized ratio (INR) may reach the therapeutic range quickly because of a decrease in factor VII, but other coagulant factors may be present in sufficient quantities to generate thrombin. Therefore, warfarin must be overlapped with heparin for 4 or 5 days. After this interval, heparin may be stopped once the INR is in the therapeutic range. Daily dosing is based on the INR, with the goal being 2 to 3. In patients with VTE who have the antiphospholipid antibody syndrome, a high recurrence of thromboembolism supports the need of an INR of 3.0 to 3.5.

The duration of warfarin therapy is 3 to 6 months, although data suggest that the course should be longer. If VTE recurs, the patient should receive anticoagulants for 1 year or longer. Hypercoagulable states, the presence of risk factors, and pulmonary hypertension dictate indefinite treatment. An alternative to warfarin is subcutaneous heparin given twice daily to achieve an aPTT of 1.5 times the mean control value midway between doses.

Bleeding, most commonly in the gastrointestinal and urinary tracts, complicates warfarin therapy in 4.3% to 6%. The risk is clearly influenced by the intensity of anticoagulant therapy (14% to 42% when the INR is ≥ 3) and with concomitant use of aspirin and with comorbid conditions (central nervous system, renal, hepatic and cardial disease).

D. Thrombolytic therapy. Thrombolysis is recommended for patients with acute, massive PE who are hemodynamically unstable despite fluid resuscitation and the use of vasopressors. No consensus exists on the use of thrombolytic therapy for acute DVT. When thrombolytic therapy is used, heparin is discontinued until the aPTT is ≤ 1.5 times control. Streptokinase is given, with a 250,000 IU loading dose and then 100,000 IU per hour for 24 hours; urokinase is given as a loading dose of 4400 IU/kg followed by 4,400 IU per hour; and tissue-type plasminogen activator, the easiest lytic to administer, is given as 100 mg over 2 hours. Heparin should be restarted when the aPTT has returned to 1.5 times control or less, followed by warfarin in usual fashion. Contraindications to therapy are identical to those for coronary thrombolysis.

E. Inferior vena cava interruption. Indications for IVC interruption are a contraindication to or complication of anticoagulation in a patient with or at high risk for VTE of the lower extremity, documented recurrent VTE despite adequate anticoagulation, chronic recurrent embolism with pulmonary hypertension, and pulmonary embolectomy. The most commonly used device, the Greenfield filter, is inserted through the femoral or internal jugular vein, and it has a 20-year efficacy rate of 95% and patency rate of 96%. If possible, anticoagulation should be resumed. IVC filters are effective in primary prophylaxis of thromboembolism in patients with a high risk of bleeding (extensive trauma, visceral cancer, and spinal cord injury). There is no benefit to insertion of a filter in patients with free-floating thrombi.

Thrombus at the site of insertion, migration of the filter, improper filter deployment, formation of clot proximal to the filter with proximal propagation and embolization, venous insufficiency, and IVC obstruction are all potential complications of an IVC filter. Rare complications include myocardial infarction, vessel perforation, pericardial tamponade, and cardiac arrhythmia.

F. Pulmonary embolectomy. The role of emergency embolectomy is unclear. Angiographically documented massive PE with hemodynamic instability and a contraindication to thrombolysis may be considered indications. Mortality rates range from 10% to 75%. Acute respiratory distress syndrome, acute renal failure, cardiac arrhythmias, mediastinitis, and severe neurologic sequelae are all complications of embolectomy.

G. Transvenous catheter extraction of emboli. A balloon-tipped catheter guided under fluoroscopy has been used for the suction extraction of proximal PE. Indications are similar to those for embolectomy. Success rates of up to 88% have been reported with a mortality rate of 27%. This procedure requires further evaluation.

Selected Readings

Aguilar D, Goldhaber SZ. Clinical uses of low-molecular weight heparins. *Chest* 1999; 115:1418.

Reviews the use of low-molecular-weight heparin for the prophylaxis and treatment of VTE in pregnancy and in selected cardiovascular conditions.

Goodman LR, Curtin JJ, Mewissen MW, et al. Detection of pulmonary embolism in patients with unresolved clinical and scintigraphic diagnosis: helical CT versus angiography. *AJR Am J Roentgenol* 1995;164:1369.

Despite its value in diagnosing proximal PE, the sensitivity of helical CT substantially declines in the diagnosis of PE in subsegmental vessels.

Greenfield LJ, Proctor MC. Current indications for caval interruption: should they be liberalized in view of improving technology? *Semin Vasc Surg* 1996;9:50.

The Greenfield filter is associated with a high degree of efficacy (95%) and caval patency (96%).

Hyers TM, Agnelli G, Hull RD, et al. Antithrombotic therapy for venous thromboembolic disease. *Chest* 1998;114:561S.

Recommendations from the fifth American College of Chest Physicians Consensus Conference on Antithrombotic Therapy.

Kearon C, Julian JA, Math M, et al. Noninvasive diagnosis of deep venous thrombosis. *Ann Intern Med* 1998;128:663.

An outstanding review. Provides evidence-based recommendations for the diagnosis of DVT in symptomatic, asymptomatic, and pregnant patients.

Khamashta MA, Cuadrado MJ, Mujic F, et al. The management of thrombosis in the antiphospholipid antibody syndrome. *N Engl J Med* 1995;332:993.

The risk of recurrent thrombosis in this syndrome is high. Long-term anticoagulation with a target INR greater than or equal to 3 is recommended.

PIOPED Investigators. Value of the ventilation/perfusion scan in acute pulmonary embolism: result of the prospective investigators of pulmonary embolism diagnosis (PIOPED). *JAMA* 1990;263:2753.

A landmark study, the first to evaluate prospectively the testing characteristics of the V/Q lung scan.

Prandoni P, Polistena P, Bernardi E, et al. Upper extremity deep venous thrombosis: risk factors, diagnosis, and complications. *Arch Intern Med* 1997;157:57.

Upper extremity DVT is associated with central venous catheters, thrombophilia, and a previous leg DVT. The diagnostic accuracy of the duplex scan is confirmed. PE is common (36%).

Rashke RA, Reilly BM, Guidry JR, et al. The weight based heparin dosing nomogram compared with a "standard care" nomogram: a randomized controlled trial. *Ann Intern Med* 1993;119:874.

A weight-based nomogram proved superior. More patients reached a therapeutic range sooner, and the risk of recurrent VTE was lower.

Schulman S, Rhedin AS, Lindmarker P, et al. The duration of oral anticoagulant therapy after a 2nd episode of venous thromboembolism. *N Engl J Med* 1997;336:393.

The risk of recurrent thrombosis with indefinite (versus 6-month) anticoagulation was lower, but the trend was toward an increased risk of major hemorrhage.

Stein PD, Coleman RE, Gottschalk A, et al. Diagnostic utility of ventilation/perfusion lung scans in acute pulmonary embolism is not diminished by pre-existing cardiac or pulmonary disease. *Chest* 1991;100:604.

The V/Q scan is more often nondiagnostic, but the testing characteristics of the scan are unchanged in patients with preexisting cardiac or pulmonary disease.

Stein PD, Hull RD, Salzman HA, et al. Strategy for diagnosis of patients with suspected pulmonary embolism. *Chest* 1993;103:1553.

Diagnostic strategies are presented using clinical evaluation, the V/Q scan, and evaluation for DVT. They may be able to decrease the need for angiography from 72% to 33%.

47. MANAGING HEMOPTYSIS

Oren P. Schaefer and Richard S. Irwin

I. **Overview.** Hemoptysis is the expectoration of blood derived from the lungs or bronchial tubes. It may be scant, with blood streaking of the sputum, or profuse. Massive hemoptysis is the expectoration of 600 mL of blood within 24 to 48 hours and occurs in 3% to 10% of patients with hemoptysis. Pseudohemoptysis is the expectoration of blood from a source other than the lower respiratory tract; from the oral cavity, nares, pharynx, or tongue; from the gastrointestinal tract; and from colonization of the oropharynx with the red pigment–producing *Serratia marcescens.*

II. **Etiology.** Hemoptysis is generally considered in two categories: nonmassive and massive (more than 600 mL in 24 hours). Patients in the intensive care unit (ICU) frequently have massive hemoptysis, and the spectrum of the causes of hemoptysis in these patients probably differs little from that reported in major series.

A. **Nonmassive hemoptysis.** Although bronchitis, bronchiectasis, lung carcinoma, and tuberculosis have always been among the most common causes of hemoptysis, their incidence varies depending on the study population. Table 47-1 lists some of the more common causes of hemoptysis.

B. **Massive hemoptysis.** Virtually all causes of hemoptysis may result in massive hemoptysis, but this condition is most frequently caused by infection, in particular, tuberculosis, mycetoma, bronchiectasis, lung abscess, and cancer. Diffuse intrapulmonary hemorrhage, usually from an immunologically mediated disease, is also considered in the differential diagnosis of massive hemoptysis in the ICU. Catastrophic, albeit rare causes of massive hemoptysis include rupture of a pulmonary artery from a balloon flotation catheter and tracheoarterial fistula.

C. **Idiopathic hemoptysis.** By using a systematic diagnostic approach, the cause of hemoptysis can be found in most instances. In 2% to 32% of patients, the cause may be idiopathic. Idiopathic or essential hemoptysis is seen most commonly in men between the ages of 30 and 50 years. Although it usually presents as nonmassive hemoptysis, it can be massive. Follow-up study almost always fails to reveal the source of bleeding, even though 10% of these patients have recurrent hemoptysis.

III. **Pathogenesis.** The bronchial arteries are the primary source of blood to the airways from the main stem bronchi to the terminal bronchioles, the supporting framework of the lung that includes the pleura, intrapulmonary lymphoid tissue, and large branches of the pulmonary vessels and nerves in the hilar regions. The pulmonary arteries supply the pulmonary parenchymal tissue, including the respiratory bronchioles. The systemic circulation is responsible for the bleeding in about 92% of cases. The pathogenesis of hemoptysis depends on the type and location of the disease. In general, if the lesion is endobronchial, the bleeding is from the bronchial circulation, and if the lesion is parenchymal, the bleeding is from the pulmonary circulation.

IV. **Diagnosis**

A. **Routine evaluation.** A detailed history and physical examination must be performed. Any history of anticoagulant use is important to elicit. The frequency, timing, and duration of hemoptysis may be helpful. For example, bleeding caused by bronchogenic carcinoma, generally a late finding, usually is of short duration. A specific travel history may suggest certain endemic fungal or parasitic diseases. Chronic sputum production before hemoptysis suggests a diagnosis of chronic bronchitis, bronchiectasis, or cystic fibrosis. With the presence of orthopnea and paroxysmal nocturnal dyspnea, one should consider the diagnosis of mitral stenosis or left ventricular failure. Pulmonary embolism, a commonly missed diagnosis, should always be considered. Trauma from suctioning through an endotracheal or tracheostomy tube, especially when coagulation is abnormal,

TABLE 47-1. Common causes of hemoptysis[a]

Tracheobronchial disorders
Acute tracheobronchitis
Bronchiectasis
Bronchogenic carcinoma
Chronic bronchitis
Cystic fibrosis
Gastric acid aspiration
Tracheobronchial trauma
Tracheoarterial fistula
Cardiovascular disorders
Congestive heart failure
Mitral stenosis
Pulmonary arteriovenous fistula
Pulmonary embolism
Hematologic disorders
Anticoagulant therapy
Thrombocytopenia
Disseminated intravascular coagulation
Localized parenchymal disease
Acute and chronic pneumonia
Aspergilloma
Lung abscess
Pulmonary tuberculosis
Diffuse alveolar hemorrhage
Goodpasture syndrome
Systemic lupus erythematosus
Trimellitic anhydride toxicity
Cocaine inhalation
Viral pneumonitis
Wegener granulomatosis
Bone marrow transplantation
Pulmonary capillaritis
Other
Idiopathic
Iatrogenic (e.g., bronchoscopy, cardiac catheterization)

[a] This list is not meant to be all inclusive. See Hemoptysis chapter in *Intensive Care Medicine,* 4th edition for an expanded list with references.

is a common cause of hemoptysis in the ICU. Tracheoarterial fistula fortunately is infrequent. The onset is usually 48 hours or more after tracheostomy. Sentinel bleeding occurs in up to 50%. Traumatic rupture of a pulmonary artery by a Swan-Ganz catheter is considered in the appropriate setting. Although patients with diffuse intrapulmonary hemorrhage typically have hemoptysis, its absence does not rule out substantial intrapulmonary bleeding. One should suspect this diagnosis in patients who have undergone recent bone marrow transplantation when they present with cough, dyspnea, hypoxemia, and diffuse pulmonary infiltrates.

B. Physical examination. Inspection of the skin and mucous membranes may show telangiectasias, suggesting hereditary hemorrhagic telangiectasia, or ecchymoses and petechiae, suggesting a hematologic abnormality. Pulsations transmitted to a tracheostomy cannula should heighten suspicion of a tracheoarterial fistula or the risk of one. Inspection of the thorax may show evidence of recent or old chest trauma, and unilateral wheeze or rales may herald localized disease such as bronchial adenoma or carcinoma. Crackles are heard diffusely on auscultation in congestive heart failure as well as diffuse intrapulmonary hemorrhage. Careful cardiovascular examination may rule in mitral stenosis, pulmonary artery stenosis, or pulmonary hypertension.

C. Laboratory studies. A *chest radiograph* must be obtained in every patient. It may suggest a diagnosis (e.g., tumor, congestive heart failure) and may help to localize the likely bleeding site. Up to 30% of patients with hemoptysis have normal chest radiographs. A *complete blood count* may suggest an infection, hematologic disorder, or chronic blood loss. *Urinalysis* may reveal hematuria and may suggest a systemic disease associated with diffuse parenchymal disease. *Coagulation studies* may uncover a primary or contributing hematologic disorder. The *electrocardiogram* may help suggest the presence of a cardiovascular disorder. A high-resolution chest *computed tomography* scan may enhance the yield of bronchoscopy in localizing a bleeding source and point to a diagnosis.

Bronchoscopy is invaluable for diagnosis and localization of the pulmonary hemorrhage. The best results are obtained when flexible bronchoscopy is performed during or within 24 hours of active bleeding, when the bleeding site can be localized in up to 91%. When the procedure is done within 48 hours, localization drops to 51%. After bleeding stops, this is reduced further. The flexible bronchoscope is usually the instrument of choice in diagnosing lower respiratory tract problems. Rigid bronchoscopy is preferred in cases of massive hemorrhage because patency of the airway is maintained more effectively during the procedure. Angiography has determined the site of bleeding in up to 90% of cases. When performed routinely, diagnostic angiography establishes a diagnosis not identified by bronchoscopy in only 4% of patients. A more specialized, disease-focused diagnostic evaluation may need to be systematically performed.

V. Treatment. Treatment of hemoptysis involves both supportive and definitive care. One should consider the cause, amount of bleeding, and patient's underlying lung function. The amount of hemoptysis should be quantitated; massive hemoptysis is associated with significant mortality and requires urgent evaluation and treatment.

A. Supportive care. Supportive care includes bed rest and mild sedation. Cough suppressants should not be used. An effective cough is necessary to clear blood from the airways and to avoid asphyxiation. Supplemental oxygen may be required. If bleeding continues and hypoxemia ensues, endotracheal intubation and mechanical ventilation may be necessary. To facilitate flexible bronchoscopy, an endotracheal tube with an internal diameter of 8.5 mm or greater should be used if possible. Fluid and blood resuscitation is administered as indicated. Chest physical therapy and postural drainage should be avoided.

B. Definitive care

1. **Nonmassive hemoptysis.** In patients with scant or submassive hemoptysis, treatment is directed at the specific cause.
2. **Massive hemoptysis.** Treatment is aimed not only at the specific cause but also toward stopping the bleeding. Death from massive hemoptysis is predominantly due to asphyxiation, and the likelihood of death is directly related to the rate of bleeding. Initial management requires protection of the uninvolved lung from aspiration of blood. The bleeding lung should therefore be kept dependent. Placement of a double-lumen endotracheal (Carlen) tube can effect bronchial isolation, but the tubes can be difficult to place, they are easily dislodged, and once in position their small diameter may prevent subsequent bronchoscopy. Rigid bronchoscopy performed with the patient under general anesthesia may be required to clear the airway of aspirated blood and for therapeutic maneuvers.

   A bronchoscopically positioned Fogarty balloon catheter can provide effective tamponade when the bleeding bronchial segment is located. Bronchoscopically directed iced saline lavage of the bronchi leading to the site of hemorrhage has been successful in stopping hemorrhage as well. Lasers have been used to control hemoptysis in patients with cancer, but recurrence of bleeding within a few weeks is typical, and no large studies of patients with massive hemoptysis have been reported.

   Angiography can identify the bleeding site and, when combined with embolization, has been successful in stopping bleeding in massive hemoptysis in more than 90% of cases. Rebleeding within 1 to 4 days can occur, and multiple procedures may be necessary. Twenty percent of patients bleed again within 6 months. Complications, including embolization of spinal arteries, or myelitis, are rare when the procedure is performed by experienced angiographers.

Rupture of the pulmonary artery after vessel catheterization is treated initially by balloon tamponade of the ruptured vessel. With the balloon deflated, the catheter is withdrawn 5 cm, the balloon is inflated with 2 mL of air, and the balloon is allowed to float back into the hemorrhaging vessel to occlude it. Because the catheter usually floats to the right pulmonary artery, when it is not known which pulmonary artery has been ruptured, one should place the patient in the right lateral decubitus position. Similarly, when tracheoarterial fistula is suspected, overinflation of the tracheostomy tube cuff may stop the hemorrhage and may prove lifesaving.

The role of emergency surgery remains controversial. The trials of therapy span different decades of practice, have widely differing causes of hemoptysis in their populations, and employ several different definitions of massive hemoptysis. Studies that advocate emergency surgery for all patients with massive hemoptysis when feasible cite statistics that suggest a significant survival benefit. More recent studies challenge this approach; mortality varies more with whether the patient is an operable candidate than with whether the patient undergoes surgery. Mortality also appears to be affected by diagnosis; it is negligible when hemoptysis is due to bronchitis, tuberculosis, bronchiectasis, or anticoagulation, whereas it is marked in patients with cancer and hemoptysis of more than 1 L per day.

Conservative, nonsurgical treatment has been advocated when hemoptysis has an infectious cause. In patients with cystic fibrosis, even with normal lung function, resection should be avoided because repeated episodes in other areas are likely to occur. A patient with a forced expiratory volume in 1 second (FEV_1) of less than 2 L or a maximum voluntary ventilation of less than 50% of predicted should not undergo surgery unless split lung function studies reveal that he or she is not likely to be left with a severe respiratory impairment ($FEV_1 \leq 800$ mL).

No one treatment can be recommended for all patients on the basis of reported studies. Therapy in a given patient depends on the cause of the bleeding, lung function, availability of resources, and local expertise. The following strategy is suggested. Patients who are not candidates for surgery because of poor pulmonary function, significant comorbid illness, or diffuse lesions should be treated with selective angiography and embolization. Resectional surgery should be performed in operable patients when surgery is the definitive treatment for the underlying disease. All potentially operable patients who continue to bleed at rates of more than 1 L per day despite supportive, conservative care should undergo either surgical resection or embolization. In patients with diffuse intrapulmonary hemorrhage, selective arterial embolization and surgery are not options. For immunologically mediated diseases such as Goodpasture syndrome or systemic lupus erythematosus, high-dose corticosteroids and cytotoxic agents are recommended to control progressive pulmonary hemorrhage and hypoxemia. High-dose steroids are recommended for the alveolar hemorrhage seen after bone marrow transplantation.

Selected Readings

Bobrowitz ID, Ramakrishna S, Shim Y-S. Comparison of medical vs. surgical treatment of major hemoptysis. *Arch Intern Med* 1983;143:1343.

Conservative, medical therapy appears effective in most patients. One should consider surgery if hemoptysis is uncontrolled after medical therapy or when aspiration is severe or progressive.

Conlan AA, Hurwitz SS, Krige L, et al. Massive hemoptysis: review of 123 cases. *J Thorac Cardiovasc Surg* 1983;85:120.

Iced saline lavage was effective in all 23 patients in whom it was used. Active tuberculosis and bronchiectasis made up the majority of the patients' illnesses.

Dweik RA, Stoller JK. Role of bronchoscopy in massive hemoptysis. *Clin Chest Med* 1999;20:89.

Bronchoscopy plays a central role in the diagnosis and treatment of massive hemoptysis. Bronchoscopy allows for lateralization and more specific localization of bleeding. Acute control of bleeding can be achieved through the bronchoscope by various techniques.

Garzon AA, Cerruti M, Golding ME. Exsanguinating hemoptysis. *J Thorac Cardiovasc Surg* 1982;84:829.

Twenty-four patients are described with bleeding of more than 1,000 mL (rate of more than 155 mL per hour). Surgical experience in these patients is reviewed; survival was 75%.

Green RJ, Ruoss SJ, Kraft SA, et al. Pulmonary capillaritis and alveolar hemorrhage: update on diagnosis and management. *Chest* 1996;110:1305.

A description of five cases and a comprehensive review of the subject.

Johnston H, Reiza G. Changing spectrum of hemoptysis: underlying causes in 148 patients undergoing diagnostic flexible fiberoptic bronchoscopy. *Arch Intern Med* 1989;149:1666.

Bronchitis and bronchogenic cancer were found to be more common than bronchiectasis and tuberculosis, a reversal from prior surveys.

McGuinness G, Beacher JR, Harkin TJ, et al. Hemoptysis: prospective high-resolution CT/bronchoscopic correlation. *Chest* 1994;105:1155.

Computed tomography was better for the diagnosis of bronchiectasis and aspergilloma, and bronchoscopy was better for bronchitis and mucosal lesions. The two studies are likely complementary.

Mullerworth MH, Angelopoulos P, Couyant MA, et al. Recognition and management of catheter-induced pulmonary artery rupture. *Ann Thorac Surg* 1998;66:1242.

Catheter-induced pulmonary artery rupture is uncommonly seen in the ICU; constant awareness is therefore essential. A plan of management is presented. Early pulmonary angiography is advocated for accurate diagnosis and to enable treatment by embolization.

Rabkin JE, Astafjev VI, Gothman LN, et al. Transcatheter embolization in the management of pulmonary hemorrhage. *Radiology* 1987;163:361.

Three hundred six patients underwent bronchial arterial embolization. The short-term success rate was over 90%, although hemoptysis recurred in 14%.

Saumench J, Escarrabill J, Padró L, et al. Value of fiberoptic bronchoscopy and angiography for diagnosis of the bleeding site in hemoptysis. *Ann Thorac Surg* 1989;48:272.

Bronchoscopy had an overall yield of 68% in localizing the site of bleeding. When it was done early, the yield was 91% (vs. 50%). Angiography added little to this.

Saw EC, Gottlieb LS, Yokoyama T, et al. Flexible fiberoptic bronchoscopy and endobronchial tamponade in the management of massive hemoptysis. *Chest* 1976;589.

Discussion of use of a Fogarty balloon catheter for endobronchial tamponade.

Schaefer OP, Irwin RS. Tracheo-arterial fistula: an unusual complication of tracheostomy. *J Intensive Care Med* 1995;10:14.

A complete review of this catastrophic complication of tracheostomy.

Stoll JF, Bettmann MA. Bronchial artery embolization to control hemoptysis: a review. *Cardiovasc Intervent Radiol* 1988;11:263.

A comprehensive review with emphasis on bronchial anatomy and technique.

Stoller JK. Diagnosis and management of massive hemoptysis: a review. *Respir Care* 1992;37:564.

A complete review of all aspects of massive hemoptysis.

48. ASPIRATION AND NEAR-DROWNING

Nicholas A. Smyrnios and Richard S. Irwin

I. Definitions. *Aspiration* is defined in *Webster's New Collegiate Dictionary* as "taking a foreign material into the lungs with the respiratory current." The foreign material can be particulate matter such as food particles, irritating fluids (e.g., hydrogen chloride, mineral oil), or oropharyngeal secretions containing infectious agents. Although infectious pneumonia may be caused by inhaling organisms in the airstream, aspiration of oropharyngeal contents is the primary means for bacterial pathogens to enter the lower respiratory tract.

In 1981, Modell proposed the following definitions for *drowning* and *near-drowning: drowning* means "to die from suffocation by submersion in water"; *near-drowning* means "to survive, at least temporarily, after suffocation by submersion in water." In practice, most authors require that the victim survive for at least 24 hours to be called a case of near-drowning. The term *immersion injury* is used to imply either entity.

II. Aspiration

A. Pathogenesis

1. **Normal upper gastrointestinal defenses against aspiration.** The following upper gastrointestinal structures normally work in a coordinated, synchronized fashion: teeth, tongue, hypopharyngeal muscles, epiglottis, vocal cords, upper esophageal sphincter, esophagus, and lower esophageal sphincter. The risk of aspiration is increased when the normal mechanisms fail to work in a coordinated manner. Some of the foregoing defenses may become impaired with increased age or during sleep.
2. **Normal respiratory defenses against aspiration.** Particles that are larger than 10 μm in diameter rarely reach the lower respiratory tract because they are removed from the airstream by aerodynamic filtration in the nose, mouth, and larynx. Particles between 2 and 10 μm in diameter can reach the airways, and those between 0.5 and 1.5 μm in diameter can reach the alveoli. Normally, mucociliary clearance removes large particles, and the alveolar macrophage and neutrophil clear the smallest ones. Cough provides a clearance function only when mucociliary clearance is inefficient or overwhelmed. As clearance is taking place, the infectious particles are detoxified by lysozyme and other proteases. Immunologic mechanisms augment the nonimmunologic mechanisms. Aspirated material will cause pulmonary disease if it cannot be effectively cleared and detoxified or if it is irritating (e.g., hydrogen chloride). Conditions that bypass aerodynamic filtration (e.g., intubation), overwhelm mucociliary clearance (large-volume aspiration), or impair alveolar phagocytes (e.g., alveolar hypoxia) may lead to the syndromes described in Table 48-1.

B. Diagnosis

1. **General considerations.** The possibility that an aspiration syndrome is causing any pulmonary problem should be considered in every patient, but especially in the elderly, debilitated, or sedated patient with unexplained deterioration in pulmonary status.
2. **Diagnostic protocol.** The diagnostic tests available are shown in Table 48-2. In addition to taking a history and performing a physical examination, the physician should watch the patient swallow from a glass of water. An obvious pharyngeal problem may be uncovered by watching the patient cough and sputter and tilt his or her neck and head in an unnatural posture. This test may not be sensitive in the critically ill patient, even when the evaluation is performed by speech and swallowing experts. The gag reflex has not been shown to predict the risk of aspiration.

TABLE 48-1. Aspiration syndromes

Mendelson syndrome
Foreign body aspiration
Bacterial pneumonia and lung abscess
Exogenous lipoid pneumonia
Recurrent pneumonias
Chronic interstitial fibrosis
Bronchiectasis
Mycobacterium fortuitum or *M. chelonei* pneumonia
Diffuse aspiration bronchiolitis
Tracheobronchitis
  Chronic persistent cough
  Bronchorrhea
  "Asthma"
Near-drowning

Expectorated sputum smears and cultures may be inadequate to assist with diagnosis. Quantitative cultures obtained with either protected brushing catheters or bronchoalveolar lavage by bronchoscopy may be more helpful. Lung biopsy may be necessary to confirm a diagnosis of exogenous lipoid pneumonia. Videofluoroscopic modified barium swallow examination seems to be the best study available to detect aspiration resulting from pharyngeal dysfunction. No available test has adequate sensitivity and specificity when one is attempting to diagnose aspiration in tube-fed patients.

C. Treatment

1. Mendelson syndrome. This syndrome is due to the parenchymal inflammatory reaction caused by a aspiration of liquid gastric contents. After aspiration, patients may develop the acute respiratory distress syndrome (ARDS). This should be anticipated in patients with a marked disturbance of consciousness, especially if a nasogastric tube has been placed. Consequently, most of these patients should be intubated for airway protection until they are awake. Elevation of the head of the bed also decreases gastroesophageal

TABLE 48-2. Diagnostic protocol for aspiration syndromes

History
Physical examination
  Baseline examination
  Observation of patient drinking water
Chest radiographs
Lower respiratory studies
  Expectorated samples
  Transtracheal aspiration
  Protected specimen brush with quantitative cultures
  Bronchoalveolar lavage
  Lung biopsy
Upper gastrointestinal studies
  Contrast films
  Endoscopy
  Motility
  Scintiscan
  24-hour esophageal pH monitoring
Bedside methods for detecting aspiration in tube-fed patients

reflux and aspiration. The management of ARDS is described in Chapter 41. Antibiotics are indicated only when the chemical pneumonitis is complicated by infection.

2. **Foreign body aspiration.** Aspiration of solid particles causes varying degrees of respiratory obstruction. Particles that reach the lower respiratory tract and do not totally obstruct the trachea can be removed by bronchoscopy. Those that totally obstruct the trachea must be removed immediately by subdiaphragmatic abdominal thrusts and finger sweeps in the unconscious patient or by chest thrusts in the markedly obese person and women in advanced states of pregnancy.
3. **Bacterial pneumonia and lung abscess.** Although aspiration bacterial pneumonias that are community acquired are most commonly due to *Streptococcus pneumoniae* and anaerobes, nosocomial aspiration bacterial pneumonias are most commonly (50% to 74% of cases) due to facultative, enteric gram-negative bacilli. This epidemiologic knowledge is helpful in selecting the appropriate antibiotic.
4. **Exogenous lipoid pneumonia.** This condition can be caused by aspiration of animal, vegetable, or mineral oil or of formula feedings. Its clinical presentation often cannot be distinguished from that of acute bacterial pneumonia. Although corticosteroids may be helpful in cases of acute lipid aspiration, exogenous lipoid pneumonias usually resolve on their own. The key is to prevent recurrences. Cricopharyngeus and esophageal achalasia and Zenker's diverticulum should be surgically repaired. Gastroesophageal reflux disease with aspiration can be treated with the following: 8-inch head-of-the-bed elevation; acid suppression; a high-protein, low-fat antireflux diet; nothing to eat or drink for 2 hours before bedtime and no snacking between meals; and prokinetic drugs. If these measures fail, surgery may be considered. Patients receiving nasogastric tube feedings should be positioned at a 45-degree angle. Patients with swallowing problems resulting from neuromuscular disease may require stoppage of oral feedings and can receive nutrition through a gastrostomy or jejunostomy. There is little agreement about what level of gastric residual volumes places a patient at increased risk of aspiration, although some authors limit infusions when residuals approach 200 mL in patients with nasogastric tubes and 100 mL in patients with gastrostomy tubes. No studies have proven that postpyloric tubes decrease the risk of aspiration when compared with prepyloric tubes.
5. **Tracheobronchitis.** Aspiration of small amounts of liquid gastric contents, oral feedings, or formula feeding solutions may cause airway consequences. Tracheobronchitis caused by aspiration should be suspected in hospitalized patients who have cough and wheeze or large amounts of sputum production. In general, postoperative, debilitated, and recently extubated patients stop aspirating and their bronchorrhea disappears when oral feeding and drinking are stopped. Oral intake should not resume until a modified barium swallow demonstrates the patient's ability to swallow without aspirating.

III. Near-drowning

A. Pathogenesis. Table 48-3 lists the common causes of near-drowning.

B. Pathophysiology. Most of the pathologic consequences of near-drowning are due to hypoxemia and hypothermia. Mechanisms that protect against hypothermia on land are ineffective in cold water. Freshwater and saltwater events produce nearly identical sequelae.

1. **Cardiac effects.** Near-drowning may cause heart rate and blood pressure increases, atrial and ventricular arrhythmias, and transient increases in central venous and pulmonary capillary wedge pressures and decreases in cardiac output.
2. **Pulmonary effects.** Both freshwater and saltwater events may lead to noncardiogenic pulmonary edema and ARDS. Bacterial pneumonia, barotrauma, trauma from cardiopulmonary resuscitation, chemical pneumonitis, centrally mediated apnea, and oxygen toxicity can contribute to respiratory deterioration.

TABLE 48-3. Causes of near-drowning

Alcohol
Inadequate adult supervision
Child abuse
Seizures
Boating accidents
Aquatic sports
Drugs
Voluntary hyperventilation

3. **Neurologic effects.** Severe anoxic encephalopathy with persistent coma, seizures, delayed language development, spastic quadriplegia, aphasia, cortical blindness, and death have been reported.
4. **Other organ systems.** The effect of near-drowning on the musculoskeletal, hematopoietic, and renal systems can be found in the chapter on near-drowning in the fourth edition of *Intensive Care Medicine.*

C. Diagnosis

1. **History and physical examination.** The patient's age, underlying cardiac, respiratory, or neurologic diseases, and medications used must be determined. One should also determine the activities precipitating the immersion, the duration of submersion, and the temperature and type of water in which it occurred.

   Tachypnea, tachycardia, signs of cerebral anoxia, and injuries that may have caused or resulted from the immersion are common physical findings. The classification system described in Table 48-4 is used to guide the initial neurologic assessment.
2. **Laboratory studies.** Hemoglobin, hematocrit, and serum electrolytes are usually normal. Arterial blood gas analysis commonly shows metabolic acidosis and hypoxemia. The blood alcohol level, prothrombin time, partial thromboplastin time, serum creatinine, urinalysis, and drug screen are obtained to help determine the cause of the accident and to assess for complications. Cervical spine radiography should be performed whenever a patient has evidence of trauma. An electrocardiogram should be obtained and continuous monitoring performed whenever a significant chance of dysrhythmia exists. Chest roentgenograms are abnormal in up to 80% of victims.

D. Treatment

1. **Initial resuscitation.** The initial resuscitation of victims is described in detail in the fourth edition of *Intensive Care Medicine.* Resuscitation must be continued at least until the patient has been rewarmed. In the field, passive external rewarming or inhalation of heated oxygen is used. In the hospital,

TABLE 48-4. Classification of neurologic status

Neurologic Category	Outcomes
A: awake and alert within 1 hour of arrival	100% intact neurologic survival
B: obtunded and stuporous but arousable	89–100% survival, rare neurologic deficit
C: comatose	Mortality high Neurologic dysfunction: common
C1: decorticate	
C2: decerebrate	
C3: flaccid	

cardiopulmonary bypass should be used in patients with severe hypothermia, especially those with circulatory collapse. When this is not possible, rewarming with warmed peritoneal lavage, hemodialysis, or heated oxygen can be attempted (see Chapter 55).

2. **Therapy of the underlying cause.** Ethanol or other drug intoxications, seizures, hypoglycemia, and severe electrolyte abnormalities are treated as described elsewhere in this manual. If any question of possible head or neck trauma exists, the patient's neck should be immobilized in a brace until cervical spine radiographs are available.
3. **Treatment of respiratory and other organ failure.** Initial management involves monitoring partial pressure of arterial oxygen (P_aO_2) and providing supplemental oxygen. The treatment of ARDS is described in Chapter 41. Nasal continuous positive airway pressure may be useful for patients with pulmonary edema. Serum electrolytes rarely require therapy. The treatment of renal failure in near-drowning may require the placement of a pulmonary artery catheter, and patients with extreme cases may require dialysis. The cardiac dysrhythmogenic effects of hypothermia are corrected by rewarming. Musculoskeletal contractures are treated with casts or splints; subluxed or dislocated hips can be approached with various operative procedures; and scoliosis is treated with bracing or spinal instrumentation.
4. **Neurologic resuscitation.** Maintaining adequate oxygenation and cerebral blood flow with mechanical ventilation and careful fluid management are the central foci of therapy for comatose victims. Hypothermic patients must be warmed to near-normal core temperature. Patients with seizures should be treated with phenytoin or phenobarbital.

Selected Readings

Donner MW, Silbiger ML. Cinefluorographic analysis of pharyngeal swallowing in neuromuscular disorders. *Am J Med Sci* 1966;251:600.

Role of barium swallow in the diagnosis of aspiration.

Fandel I, Bancalari E. Near-drowning in children: clinical aspects. *Pediatrics* 1976; 58:573.

Review of clinical findings in pediatric victims.

Green GM. Pulmonary clearance of infectious agents. *Annu Rev Med* 1968;19:315.

Classic article describes pulmonary defense mechanisms against infection.

Huxley EJ, Viroslav J, Gray WR, et al. Pharyngeal aspiration in normal adults and patients with depressed consciousness. *Am J Med* 1978;64:564.

Seventy percent of patients with depressed consciousness aspirate. Aspiration occurs frequently in patients with depressed sensorium and in healthy adults during deep sleep.

Logemann JA. Swallowing physiology and pathophysiology. *Otolaryngol Clin North Am* 1988;21:613.

A comprehensive review of the swallowing mechanisms.

Lorber B, Swenson RM. Bacteriology of aspiration pneumonia: a prospective study of community and hospital acquired cases. *Ann Intern Med* 1974;81:329.

Epidemiologic findings useful in making treatment decisions.

Modell JH, Conn AW. Current neurological considerations in near-drowning. *Can Anaesth Soc J* 1980;3:197.

Provides commonly used classification system.

Schwindt WD, Barbee RA, Jones RJ. Lipoid pneumonia. *Arch Surg* 1967;95:652.

Description of the clinical findings of a common syndrome.

Torres A, Serra-Batlles J, Ros E, et al. Pulmonary aspiration of gastric contents in patients receiving mechanical ventilation: the effect of body position. *Ann Intern Med* 1992;116:540.

Elevating the head of the bed is a simple, effective, no-cost measure to prevent aspiration of gastric contents.

49. PULMONARY HYPERTENSION

Oren P. Schaefer and Lewis J. Rubin

I. Etiology. The cause of pulmonary artery hypertension (PAH) is grouped into one of three major pathophysiologic categories: (a) *passive,* resulting from elevated post-capillary pressure; (b) *active,* resulting from the constriction or obstruction of capillary or precapillary vessels that increases resistance to flow; and (c) *reactive,* in which PAH is initially passive, but the upstream pulmonary vasculature responds to chronic passive congestion by developing an active component superimposed on a passive component (Table 49-1). One can review the pathogenesis of PAH in *Intensive Care Medicine,* Fourth Edition. PAH is said to be present when mean pressure > 25 mmHg at rest or 30 mmHg during exercise.

A. Passive pulmonary hypertension. PAH results from the elevation of the pulmonary capillary wedge (PCW) pressure, which reflects postpulmonary capillary pressure. The pulmonary artery end-diastolic pressure (P_aED) rises passively because of the increased blood volume that can occur in left ventricular failure, mitral stenosis, or obstruction of the major pulmonary veins. As the P_aED and PCW pressures are both elevated, the (P_aED-PCW) pressure gradient remains normal (up to 5 cm H_20).

B. Active pulmonary hypertension. PAH results from vasoconstriction or anatomic restriction in the total cross-sectional area of the pulmonary vascular bed. Restriction can be at the precapillary or capillary level. In active PAH, the (P_aED-PCW) pressure gradient is elevated (greater than 5 mm Hg); the PCW pressure is normal. Diseases commonly causing active PAH are listed in Table 49-1. Causes of PAH from disorders of ventilation can be found in Table 49-2. The most important vasoconstrictive stimulus in the setting of chronic respiratory disease is alveolar hypoxemia, with resulting hypoxic vasoconstriction. Alveolar hypoxemia occurs in a number of different pulmonary diseases as a consequence of high altitude, alveolar hypoventilation, or ventilation-perfusion inequalities. Acidemia and hypercarbia cause pulmonary vasoconstriction directly, and both augment the effect of hypoxemia. Mechanical obstruction of precapillary vessels from thromboemboli, with associated hypoxemia and release of vasoactive substances, is responsible for PAH seen with pulmonary thromboembolism.

C. Reactive pulmonary hypertension. PAH results from a combination of passive and active mechanisms. Although the condition is initially due to passive congestion, pulmonary artery pressures subsequently rise out of proportion to post-capillary pressures as passive congestion becomes chronic. In reactive PAH, the (P_aED-PCW) pressure gradient is elevated, as is the PCW pressure. This situation most likely occurs in patients with mitral valvular disease, particularly mitral stenosis. It may also be present in pulmonary venoocclusive disease.

II. Diagnosis

A. Signs and symptoms. Exertional dyspnea is the most common symptom. In cases of nonprimary PAH, symptoms related to the underlying disease may predominate (e.g., productive cough in chronic obstructive pulmonary disease [COPD], orthopnea or paroxysmal nocturnal dyspnea in congestive heart failure, pleuritic chest pain in pulmonary thromboembolism). In patients with primary PAH, other complaints include fatigue, substernal chest pain, and exertional or postexertional syncope. The physical findings related solely to PAH are usually indicative of right ventricular (RV) pressure overload and include a large jugular venous A wave, left parasternal (RV) heave, pulmonic ejection click and murmur, enhanced pulmonic component of the second heart sound (P_2), RV fourth heart sound, and signs of RV failure (hepatomegaly, peripheral edema). These findings are usually not appreciable until the pulmonary artery systolic pressure is more than 55 mm Hg. With severe hypertension, one may also find prominent jugular venous V waves, an RV third heart sound, and murmurs

TABLE 49-1. Causes of pulmonary artery hypertension

Passive pulmonary hypertension
Left ventricular failure
Mitral valve disease
Congenital pulmonary vein stenosis
Acquired obstruction of major pulmonary veins
Left atrial myxoma or thrombus
Active pulmonary hypertension
Pulmonary embolism
Schistosomiasis
Primary pulmonary hypertension
Human immunodeficiency viral infection
Congenital heart disease (Eisenmenger reaction)
Disorders of ventilation
Collagen vascular disease
Sickle cell hemoglobinopathies
Portal hypertension
Ingestion of drugs and herbal remedies
Appetite-suppressant drugs (e.g., fenfluramine)
Pulmonary vasculitis
Reactive pulmonary hypertension
Mitral valve disease
Pulmonary venoocclusive disease
Toxic oil syndrome (rapeseed oil ingestion)
Eosinophila-myalgia syndrome (contaminated L-tryptophan ingestion)

TABLE 49-2. Pulmonary hypertension from disorders of ventilation

Vasoconstriction of precapillary and capillary vascular bed
Structurally normal pulmonary parenchyma and vascular bed
High-altitude pulmonary hypertension (residence at > 3,000 m)
Primary central hypoventilation
Obstructive sleep apnea
Obesity-hypoventilation syndrome
Paralytic poliomyelitis
Myasthenia gravis
Pulmonary parenchymal disease
Chronic obstructive pulmonary disease
Cystic fibrosis
Anatomic restriction of the pulmonary capillary bed
Diffuse parenchymal lung disease
Sarcoidosis
Progressive systemic sclerosis
Idiopathic interstitial pulmonary fibrosis
Acute respiratory distress syndrome
Extensive lung resection
Extensive fibrothorax
Vasoconstriction plus anatomic restriction of the vascular bed
Kyphoscoliosis
Chronic fibrotic tuberculosis

of tricuspid or pulmonic regurgitation. When PAH is not primary, signs of the underlying disease are likely prominent.

B. Chest roentgenogram. The routine chest radiograph is a useful test to screen for abnormalities of the pulmonary circulation. Certain roentgenographic findings are characteristic of PAH and are qualitatively similar in all forms of the disease, although they are most marked in patients with left-to-right shunts caused by congenital defects. These findings include marked enlargement of the main pulmonary artery segment, dilatation of the central hilar pulmonary artery branches to the origin of the segmental vessels, and constriction of the segmental arteries. These changes correlate with the decreased cross-sectional area of the vascular bed. The classic signs of passive PAH are the signs of pulmonary venous hypertension—prominence of the upper lobe vessels over the lower lobe vessels resulting from redistribution of pulmonary blood flow. The presence of interstitial edema and of alveolar edema is suggestive but not specific for pulmonary venous hypertension.

C. Electrocardiography. The electrocardiogram is reliable in predicting the presence of severe PAH with right axis deviation and RV hypertrophy. However, it is less predictive in the setting of COPD. With the downward displacement of the heart in the thorax from hyperinflation and with the degree of PAH often less severe, electrocardiographic evidence of RV hypertrophy is uncommon.

D. Echocardiography. A valuable, noninvasive modality to evaluate PAH, echocardiography can assess both RV and left ventricular function, exclude congenital heart disease, and assess for the presence of mitral valve disease and left atrial myxoma. Doppler examination of the regurgitant tricuspid jet can allow for estimation of the pulmonary artery systolic pressure. The values correlate well with those found by cardiac catheterization. The echocardiogram is also valuable for following changes after introduction of therapy. Transesophageal echocardiography can provide a better evaluation of the right heart, although is an invasive procedure. It may be useful in patients with COPD in whom hyperinflation makes transthoracic echocardiography technically difficult.

E. Pulmonary function tests. Spirometry, lung volumes, and diffusion capacity for carbon monoxide provide valuable information regarding underlying parenchymal or airway disease. In diffuse interstitial fibrosis, a vital capacity of up to 50% of predicted may suggest PAH at rest; when vital capacity is between 50% and 80% of predicted, PAH with exertion is suggested. In systemic sclerosis, a severely reduced diffusion capacity is a better predictor than vital capacity. In obstructive airway disease such as COPD, PAH is seen when the forced expiratory volume in 1 second (FEV_1) is less than 1 L, the partial pressure of arterial oxygen (P_aO_2) is less than 50 mm Hg, or the partial pressure of arterial carbon dioxide (P_aCO_2) is more than 45 mm Hg.

F. Cardiac catheterization. This is perhaps the single most important study in the evaluation of PAH. Right heart catheterization with a Swan-Ganz catheter not only documents elevated PA pressure, but also allows one to categorize it as active, passive, or reactive based on the (P_aED-PCW) gradient, or by the calculation of pulmonary vascular resistance. PCW pressure with a balloon flotation catheter may not be possible in these patients, however, and in the critically ill patient, the PCW may not accurately reflect left ventricular end-diastolic volume.

G. Other studies. Left heart catheterization can be valuable when the origin of PAH is not clear after the above testing. It is of particular value in the patient with congenital heart disease or when acquired obstruction of the main pulmonary veins is considered. Ventilation-perfusion lung scanning is valuable when considering a diagnosis of chronic thromboembolic PAH; perfusion scans are most often interpreted as high probability, whereas in primary PAH they are normal or low probability. Pulmonary angiography sometimes may be required to make the diagnosis.

III. Treatment. Treatment rests on proper identification of the underlying condition.

A. Passive pulmonary hypertension. This is clearly reversible if the underlying cause of pulmonary venous hypertension is corrected. Lowering pulmonary venous pressure, for example, by surgical correction of aortic or mitral valvular disease or removal of a left atrial myxoma, can reverse passive PAH. Passive PAH may be controlled in other patients with combination medical therapy such as preload- or afterload-reducing agents.

B. Active pulmonary hypertension. The most common cause of acute active PAH is pulmonary embolism, and it is reversible with anticoagulation (and time) or thrombolytic therapy; as the degree of vascular embolic obstruction and hypoxemia improves, pulmonary artery pressures decline. Patients with unresolved proximal vessel obstruction should be referred to a center experienced in performing pulmonary endarterectomy.

Primary PAH may in rare cases spontaneously regress. Oral warfarin anticoagulation appears to improve survival and should be used in all patients who do not have a contraindication. Some patients respond to vasoactive agents. Oxygen, intravenous prostacyclin, inhaled nitric oxide, and the oral calcium channel blocking agents nifedipine and diltiazem have been shown to improve pulmonary hemodynamics in certain patients, albeit inconsistently. Given that drug therapy is not a benign intervention, all patients considered for such should be carefully monitored with a Swan-Ganz catheter and a formal drug trial to ensure efficacy and to minimize complications. When one assesses the response to vasodilators, the overall effects on pulmonary and systemic hemodynamics, gas exchange, and oxygen transport must be considered. A favorable response is defined as a 20% decline in pulmonary vascular resistance, with an increase in cardiac output, but without any effect on gas exchange or systemic pressure. This response occurs only in 25% to 30% of patients. Use of the rapidly acting intravenous agents prostacyclin or adenosine, both powerful vasodilators with short half-lives, can have predictive value for the use of subsequent oral therapy. Continuous intravenous infusion of prostacyclin and the use of calcium channel antagonists in patients with primary PAH for periods ranging from months to years has been shown to improve symptoms, hemodynamics, and survival. Calcium antagonists should only be used in those patients demonstrating acute reactivity. For those patients who do not respond to a vasodilator drug trial, salt restriction, oxygen, digitalis, and diuretics are usually prescribed; there may be a role for prostacyclin in these nonresponders as well. Similar interventions can be considered for patients with PAH associated with human immunodeficiency virus, although the prognosis is poor. Lung or combined heart-lung transplantation should be considered in patients unresponsive to medical therapy and who have low cardiac output.

In patients with ventricular septal defect, patent ductus, and secundum atrial defects, treatment is surgical correction. This is best accomplished before severe (systemic level) PAH occurs. Once Eisenmenger syndrome has developed, patients should be evaluated for transplantation because surgical correction of the congenital defect is contraindicated.

Patients with ventilatory disorders are treated with specific intervention. Alveolar hypoxemia of any source must be aggressively sought and treated with supplemental oxygen. Flow rates that achieve arterial oxygen saturation of more than 90% are used. Respiratory center stimulants such as progesterone may be effective in primary central hypoventilation, although tolerance and side effects to the drug often develop. Nasal continuous positive pressure is effective for obstructive sleep apnea, and weight loss must be prescribed in morbidly obese patients. Supplemental oxygen has multiple benefits, including prolonged survival, for the hypoxemic patient with COPD. Interstitial fibrosis may be treated with oral corticosteroids or other immunosuppressive drugs, although response rates are variable and depend on the underlying disease.

C. Reactive pulmonary hypertension. Surgery for mitral valve disease is not contraindicated because the patient may have reactive PAH. Both components of PAH, reactive and passive, should resolve after mitral valve surgery. Treatment of pulmonary venoocclusive disease with various measures has been poorly responsive.

Selected Readings

Barst AJ, Rubin LJ, Long WA, et al. A comparison of continuous intravenous epoprostenol (prostacyclin) with conventional therapy for primary pulmonary hypertension. *N Engl J Med* 1996;334:296.

A randomized trial found therapy with prostacyclin to confer improvements in symptoms, hemodynamics, and survival.

D'Alonzo GE, Bower JS, Dantzker DR. Differentiation in patients with primary and thromboembolic pulmonary hypertension. *Chest* 1984;85:457.

One cannot distinguish the two entities by clinical characteristics (symptoms, examination, chest radiography, electrocardiography, and pulmonary function tests). Lung scans in patients with thromboembolic PAH were found to be high probability, whereas those with primary PAH were normal to low probability.

Fuster V, Steele PM, Edwards WD, et al. Primary pulmonary hypertension: natural history and the importance of thrombosis. *Circulation* 1984;70:580.

One hundred twenty patients with primary PAH were evaluated. In autopsy studies of more than half the deceased patients, the major histologic feature was thrombus. Anticoagulant therapy is recommended for patients with primary PAH.

Gaine SP, Rubin LJ. Primary pulmonary hypertension. *Lancet* 1998;352:719.

A timely review with a nice discussion on etiology and pathogenesis.

Galie N, Ussia G, Passarelli P, et al. Role of pharmacologic tests in the treatment of primary pulmonary hypertension. *Am J Cardiol* 1995;75:55A.

An excellent article outlining pharmacologic vasodilator testing in the evaluation of patients with primary PAH.

Kanemoto N, Furya H, Etoh T, et al. Chest roentgenograms in primary pulmonary artery hypertension. *Chest* 1979;76:45.

Description of roentgenographic findings seen in primary PAH.

Masuyama T, Kodama K, Kitabatake A, et al. Continuous-wave Doppler echocardiographic detection of pulmonary regurgitation and its application to noninvasive estimation of pulmonary artery pressure. *Circulation* 1986;74:484.

Estimates of pulmonary artery pressure by measuring regurgitant flow velocity in patients with PAH. Results correlate with those from right heart catheterization.

McLaughlin VV, Genthner DE, Panella MM, et al. Reduction in pulmonary vascular resistance with long-term epoprostenol (prostacyclin) therapy in primary pulmonary hypertension. *N Engl J Med* 1998;338:273.

Long-term therapy with epoprostenol was found to lower pulmonary vascular resistance beyond the level achieved in the short term with intravenous adenosine and had sustained efficacy in the 27 patients who were followed.

Moser KM, Daily PO, Peterson K, et al. Thromboendarterectomy for chronic, major-vessel thromboembolic pulmonary hypertension: immediate and long-term results in 42 patients. *Ann Intern Med* 1987;107:560.

From one of the world's leading centers performing thromboendarterectomy for chronic unresolved PAH. Surgery is feasible even in patients with severe disease and protracted hemodynamic impairment.

Rich S, McLaughlin VV. Lung transplantation for pulmonary hypertension: patient selection and maintenance therapy while awaiting transplantation. *Semin Thorac Cardiovasc Surg* 1998;10:135.

Lung transplantation is considered a definitive treatment of patients with advanced pulmonary vascular disease and PAH. With advances in medical management, the guidelines for patient selection for lung transplantation are constantly evolving and are reviewed here.

Rich S, Kaufman E, Levy PS. The effect of high dose calcium channel blockers on survival in primary pulmonary hypertension. *N Engl J Med* 1992;327:76.

High-dose therapy with diltiazem or nifedipine was found to prolong survival in a group of patients with primary PAH with demonstrated vasoresponsiveness, compared with those without primary PAH or patients in a primary PAH registry.

Shapiro SM, Oudiz RJ, Cao T, et al. Primary pulmonary hypertension: improved long-term effects and survival with continuous intravenous epoprostenol infusion. *J Am Coll Cardiol* 1997;30:343.

Patients receiving continuous infusion epoprostenol for treatment of primary PAH experience a decrease in pulmonary artery pressure and improved long-term survival compared with historical control subjects.

Whyte RI, Robbins RC, Altinger J, et al. Heart-lung transplantation for primary pulmonary hypertension. *Ann Thorac Surg* 1999;67:937.

Heart-lung transplantation results in survival comparable to that reported for single-lung or double-lung transplantation. Obliterative bronchiolitis is a significant cause of late death but seems to occur less frequently with heart-lung transplantation than with lung transplantation alone.

50. PLEURAL DISEASE IN THE CRITICALLY ILL PATIENT

Mark M. Wilson and Steven A. Sahn

I. General principles. Pleural disease itself is an unusual cause for admission to the intensive care unit (ICU). Exceptions are a large hemothorax for monitoring the rate of bleeding and hemodynamic status, a secondary spontaneous pneumothorax (PTX), and a large unilateral or bilateral pleural effusion causing acute respiratory failure. Pleural disease may be overlooked in the critically ill patient because it is usually overshadowed by the major reason for admission to the ICU. It is also often a subtle finding on clinical examination and chest radiography (i.e., the supine or semierect position of these patients changes the usual appearance of free pleural fluid and air).

II. Pleural effusions. Pleural effusions should be suspected if one sees increased homogeneous density over the lower lung fields compared with the upper lung fields. As the effusion increases in size, the increased radiodensity involves the upper hemithorax as well. Approximately 175 to 525 mL of pleural fluid results in blunting of the costophrenic angle on an erect chest radiograph (CXR). In most instances, this quantity of pleural fluid can be detected on a supine CXR as an increased homogeneous density over the lower lung field that does not obliterate normal bronchovascular markings, does not show air bronchograms, and does not show hilar or mediastinal displacement until the effusion is massive. Underlying diffuse parenchymal lung disease is common in patients in the ICU and makes the CXR diagnosis of pleural effusion problematic; ultrasonography or computed tomography scanning may be required.

Pleural effusions are most commonly caused by primary lung disease, but they may also result from systemic illnesses (Table 50-1). When a pleural effusion is suspected on examination and is confirmed by CXR, a diagnostic thoracentesis should be performed to establish the cause. Exceptions may be patients with a secure clinical diagnosis (e.g., atelectasis, uncomplicated congestive heart failure) or only a small amount of pleural fluid (less than 1 cm from the pleural line to the inside of the chest wall on the lateral decubitus CXR). When sampling of fluid is indicated clinically and the effusion is small, thoracentesis should be performed under ultrasound guidance. No absolute contraindications exist to thoracentesis; the major relative contraindications are an uncorrectable bleeding diathesis and an uncooperative patient. PTX, the most clinically important complication of thoracentesis, is no more likely to occur in the patient receiving mechanical ventilation than in the patient who is not (4% to 30% incidence, depending on experience of operator); however, if a PTX does develop, the patient receiving mechanical ventilation will likely develop a tension PTX (see later). Therapeutic thoracenteses are primarily indicated for the relief of dyspnea. Contraindications to therapeutic thoracentesis are similar to those for diagnostic thoracentesis. Complications of therapeutic thoracentesis are also similar to those for diagnostic thoracentesis, except there appears to be an increased risk of PTX, and three complications unique to therapeutic thoracentesis may be seen—hypoxemia, unilateral pulmonary edema, and hypovolemia. The relief of dyspnea cannot be adequately explained by changes either in lung volume or in the mechanics of breathing, but it may be the result of decreased stimulation of lung or chest wall receptors or both.

A. Atelectasis. Atelectasis is a common cause of small pleural effusions in the ICU in patients who are comatose or otherwise immobile, who have major bronchial obstruction (cancer, mucus plugging, foreign body), or who have had upper abdominal surgery. Atelectasis causes pleural fluid by decreasing local pleural pressure, thus favoring movement of fluid from the parietal pleural surface into the pleural space. Analysis of the pleural fluid reveals a serous transudate that dissipates over several days once atelectasis resolves.

TABLE 50-1. Causes of pleural effusions in the intensive care unit

Atelectasis
Congestive heart failure
Pneumonia
Hypoalbuminemia
Pancreatitis
Hepatic hydrothorax
Esophageal sclerotherapy
Postmyocardial infarction
Coronary artery bypass surgery
Esophageal rupture
Hemothorax
Chylothorax
Abdominal surgery
Acute respiratory distress syndrome
Pulmonary embolism
Iatrogenic

B. Congestive heart failure. Congestive heart failure is the most common cause of all transudative pleural effusions and is seen commonly in the ICU. Most patients have the classic signs and symptoms of congestive heart failure and have cardiomegaly and bilateral small to moderate effusions of similar size on CXR. They usually also have evidence of pulmonary congestion, with the severity of pulmonary edema correlating with the presence of pleural effusions. These effusions are classic transudates. Thoracentesis should only be performed if the diagnosis is in question or if the patient's course is other than expected (i.e., patient is febrile or has pleuritic pain, unilateral or disparate sized effusions, absence of cardiomegaly, or a partial pressure of arterial oxygen [P_aO_2] inappropriate for the degree of pulmonary edema). Therapy involves decreasing venous hypertension and improving cardiac output with preload and afterload reduction.

C. Hepatic hydrothorax. Pleural effusions occur in approximately 6% of patients with cirrhosis of the liver and clinical ascites as a result of movement of ascitic fluid through congenital or acquired diaphragmatic defects. Usually, the CXR reveals a normal cardiac silhouette and a right-sided pleural effusion in 70% of patients (left-sided in 15%, bilateral in 15%). The diagnosis is substantiated by demonstrating that pleural and ascitic fluids have similar protein and lactate dehydrogenase concentrations. Treatment is directed at resolution of the ascites with sodium restriction and diuresis. Care should be exercised with large-volume paracentesis or thoracentesis, because hypovolemia may occur with rapid evacuation of the fluid. Chemical pleurodesis is uniformly unsuccessful. Transjugular intrahepatic portosystemic shunt (to decrease formation of ascites by decompression of portal hypertension) and video-assisted thoracoscopy (to patch the diaphragmatic defect followed by talc poudrage) have been effective.

D. Parapneumonic effusions. Community-acquired and nosocomial pneumonia are common in critically ill patients. The CXR commonly shows a small to large pleural effusion ipsilateral to a new alveolar infiltrate. When the effusion is free-flowing on lateral decubitus CXR and thoracentesis shows a nonpurulent, polymorphonuclear neutrophil–predominant exudate (uncomplicated effusion), the patient has a high likelihood of resolution without sequelae over 7 to 14 days using antibiotics alone. If the CXR demonstrates loculation of fluid, and pus is aspirated at thoracentesis, then the diagnosis of empyema is established, and immediate drainage is needed. Draining the pleural space should also be considered in the case of free-flowing nonpurulent fluid, with a positive Gram stain or culture, or when the fluid pH is less than 7.20 (complicated effusion), given the associated increase in morbidity and mortality.

E. Pancreatitis. Pleural effusions are seen in 3% to 17% of patients with pancreatitis as a result of direct contact of the diaphragm with pancreatic enzymes (so-called sympathetic effusion), transfer of ascitic fluid through diaphragmatic defects, a fistulous tract between a pseudocyst and the pleural space, or retroperitoneal movement of fluid into the mediastinum with mediastinitis or rupture into the pleural space. The effusion is usually small and left-sided (60%), but it may be isolated to the right (30%) or bilateral (10%). The patient usually presents with abdominal symptoms of acute pancreatitis. The fluid is a polymorphonuclear neutrophil–predominant exudate with glucose values approaching those of the serum and amylase values greater than those of serum. No specific therapy is usually necessary; the effusion resolves as the pancreatic inflammation subsides.

F. Pulmonary embolism. Pleural effusions occur in 41% to 50% of patients with pulmonary embolism and are the result of increased capillary permeability, imbalance in microvascular and pleural space hydrostatic pressures, and pleuropulmonary hemorrhage. The usual finding is an exudative effusion; however, approximately 20% of patients with pulmonary embolism have transudates as a result of associated atelectasis. The CXR virtually always shows a small (less than one-third of the hemithorax), unilateral pleural effusion, and pleural fluid analysis is highly variable and nondiagnostic. The pleural fluid is hemorrhagic in two-thirds of patients and may occur in the absence of radiographic infarction. Effusions that progress with therapy should be evaluated for recurrent embolism, hemothorax from anticoagulation therapy, an infected infarction, or an alternate diagnosis. When consolidation is absent on CXR, resolution is usual in less than 1 week; with consolidation, resolution of effusions typically takes 2 to 3 weeks. Although the association of pleural effusion with pulmonary embolism does not alter therapy and the presence of a bloody effusion is not a contraindication to full-dose anticoagulation, evidence of active pleural space hemorrhage during therapy necessitates discontinuation of anticoagulation, tube thoracostomy, and placement of a vena caval filter.

G. Esophageal rupture. A potential life-threatening event, esophageal rupture requires immediate diagnosis and therapy. The history is usually of severe retching or vomiting or a conscious effort to resist vomiting. In some patients, the perforation may be silent or associated with instrumentation of the esophagus. PTX, present in 75% of patients with spontaneous rupture, indicates violation of the mediastinal pleura; 70% of PTXs are on the left, 20% are on the right, and 10% are bilateral. Mediastinal air (seen in less than half of patients) is seen early if pleural integrity is maintained, whereas pleural effusion (occurs in 75%) secondary to mediastinitis tends to occur later. A presumptive diagnosis should be confirmed immediately with lateral decubitus esophagrams. Early thoracentesis shows a sterile, serous exudate in patients without mediastinal perforation. Once the mediastinal pleura tears, amylase of salivary origin appears in the fluid in high concentration. As the pleural space is seeded with anaerobic organisms from the mouth, the pH falls rapidly and progressively to approach 6.00. The diagnosis of spontaneous esophageal rupture dictates immediate operative intervention; survival is greater than 90% if primary closure is achieved within the first 24 hours.

H. Hemothorax. An arbitrary, but practical, definition of hemothorax with regard to therapy is a pleural fluid-to-blood hematocrit ratio greater than 50%. Most hemothoraces result from penetrating or blunt chest trauma, but they can also be seen complicating invasive procedures (e.g., thoracentesis, closed pleural biopsy, central venous catheters), with pulmonary infarction, malignancy, or ruptured aortic aneurysm, or as a complication (rarely) of anticoagulation. In trauma patients, concomitant PTX has a high incidence (approximately 60%). Traumatic hemothorax should be treated with immediate, large-diameter tube thoracostomy. If bleeding continues, and depending on the individual circumstances, thoracotomy may be required.

I. Coronary artery bypass surgery. Small left pleural effusions are virtually always present after coronary artery bypass surgery. Associated left lower lobe atelectasis and elevation of the left hemidiaphragm are generally present on CXR as well. Left diaphragm dysfunction results from intraoperative phrenic nerve injury secondary to cold cardioplegia, stretch injury, or surgical trauma. Larger and grossly bloody effusions are associated with internal mammary artery grafting, which causes marked exudation of fluid from the arterial harvest site. Concomitant pleurotomy may increase pleural fluid accumulation by increasing fluid production and by decreasing lymphatic drainage from the pleural space. Large effusions that qualify as a hemothorax are best treated with tube thoracostomy. It is likely prudent to drain moderately large, bloody effusions, to avoiding the need for decortication later.

J. Abdominal surgery. Approximately half the patients undergoing abdominal surgery develop small unilateral or bilateral pleural effusions within 48 to 72 hours of surgery, especially after upper abdominal surgery, in patients with postoperative atelectasis, and in those with free ascitic fluid at the time of surgery. These effusions are usually exudative and are related to diaphragmatic irritation or atelectasis. Small effusions generally do not require diagnostic thoracentesis, are of no clinical significance, and resolve spontaneously.

III. Pneumothorax. PTX refers to the presence of free air in the confines of the chest cavity (i.e., pleural space).

A. Causes and pathogenesis. Spontaneous PTX occurs without an obvious cause as a consequence of the natural course of a disease process, either without clinical findings of lung disease (primary spontaneous PTX) or with clinically manifest lung disease (secondary spontaneous PTX) such as chronic obstructive pulmonary disease, status asthmaticus, interstitial lung disease, *Pneumocystis carinii* or necrotizing pneumonias, or cystic fibrosis. Traumatic PTX may result from penetrating or blunt chest trauma. Iatrogenic PTX, the most common cause of PTX in patients in the ICU, occurs as a consequence of barotrauma or invasive procedures (e.g., thoracentesis, central venous catheters). Cannulation of the subclavian vein is associated with a higher risk of PTX (less than 5%) than cannulation of the internal jugular vein (less than 0.2%). PTX is the most clinically important form of barotrauma and occurs in 1% to 15% of all patients receiving mechanical ventilation. The number of ventilation days, presence of underlying disease, and use of positive end-expiratory pressure (PEEP) affect the incidence of PTX.

The alveolar walls and visceral pleura normally maintain a fairly constant pressure gradient between the airways and the pleural space. When the transpulmonary pressure gradient is transiently increased, alveolar rupture may occur; air enters the interstitial tissues of the lung (i.e., interstitial emphysema) and may enter the pleural space or decompress to the mediastinum (i.e., pneumomediastinum). When PTX occurs, the elasticity of the lung causes it to collapse until the pleural defect seals or the pleural and alveolar pressures equalize. Should a ball-valve effect occur, permitting only egress of air from the lung into the pleural space, the progressive accumulation of air (and positive pressure) within the pleural space produces a tension PTX. Tension PTX compresses mediastinal structures, resulting in impaired venous return to the heart, decrease in cardiac output, and, at times, fatal cardiovascular collapse. When a PTX develops in the setting of mechanical ventilation, 30% to 97% of patients develop tension.

B. Diagnosis. Most iatrogenic PTXs occur at the time of the procedure from direct lung puncture, but delayed (up to 12 to 24 hours later) PTXs have been noted. In the supine patient, PTX gas migrates along the anterior surface of the lung, making detection on the anteroposterior CXR problematic. The base, lateral chest wall, and juxtacardiac areas should be carefully visualized for evidence of PTX. Accumulation of air along the mediastinal parietal pleura may simulate pneumomediastinum. An erect or decubitus (with the suspected hemithorax upward) CXR should be obtained to assess for the presence of a PTX.

PTX in the mechanically ventilated patient usually presents as an acute cardiopulmonary emergency with a mortality rate of 7% if it is rapidly diagnosed clinically, versus a mortality rate of 31% to 77% for delayed diagnoses. The diagnosis of tension PTX should be considered in any mechanically ventilated patient who develops a sudden deterioration characterized by apprehension, tachypnea, cyanosis, decreased ipsilateral breath sounds, subcutaneous emphysema, tachycardia, and hypotension. Hypoxemia, increasing peak and plateau airway pressures, decreasing compliance, and auto-PEEP may be some of the earlier signs of tension PTX. The most common CXR signs of a PTX under tension are contralateral mediastinal shift, ipsilateral diaphragmatic depression, and ipsilateral chest wall expansion. In patients receiving mechanical ventilation, little or no midline mediastinal shift may result from a tension PTX, and a depressed ipsilateral diaphragm is a more reliable sign of tension. A high index of suspicion for tension PTX in patients receiving mechanical ventilation is necessary to avoid potentially catastrophic situations because up to 30% of PTXs may not be detected initially, and many may then progress to tension PTX.

C. Treatment. Up to half of spontaneously breathing patients with needle-puncture (iatrogenic) PTX may be managed expectantly without the need for tube drainage. If the patient is receiving mechanical ventilation or if the PTX is large or has caused significant symptoms or gas exchange abnormalities, then tube thoracostomy should be performed as soon as possible. In fact, when the appropriate clinical signs and symptoms of tension PTX are noted in mechanically ventilated patients, treatment should not be delayed to obtain CXR confirmation. If a chest tube is not immediately available, placement of a large-bore needle into the anterior second intercostal space on the suspected side will be lifesaving and confirms the diagnosis; a rush of air is noted when the needle enters the pleural space.

Selected Readings

Bartter T, Mayo PD, Pratter MR, et al. Lower risk and higher yield for thoracentesis when performed by experienced operators. *Chest* 1993;103:1873.

A prospective study of 50 thoracenteses showing the dramatic effect of the level of training in reducing the risk of complications from this procedure.

Collins JD, Burwell D, Furmanski S, et al. Minimum detectable pleural effusions: a roentgen pathology model. *Radiology* 1975;105:51.

A small autopsy study that associated chest radiographic findings with specific quantities of pleural fluid.

Collins TR, Sahn SA. Thoracentesis: clinical value, complications, technical problems, and patient experience. *Chest* 1987;91:817.

A prospective study of 129 thoracenteses that highlights the clinical value and limitations of diagnostic thoracentesis.

Rohlfing BM, Webb WR, Schlobohm RM. Ventilator-related extraalveolar air in adults. *Radiology* 1976;121:25.

A descriptive study of the manifestations of extraalveolar air resulting from mechanical ventilation in 38 patients.

Sahn SA. Management of complicated parapneumonic effusions. *Am Rev Respir Dis* 1993;148:813.

A review of the management of complicated parapneumonic effusions that stresses the importance of early diagnosis and treatment to prevent development of this complication.

51. MECHANICAL VENTILATION: INITIATION

Ann E. Connolly and Richard S. Irwin

I. General principles. Negative-pressure ventilators such as the iron lung or tank ventilator were used until the mid-1950s, but because they were bulky and poorly tolerated, they have been almost entirely replaced by positive-pressure ventilators in both the home and acute settings. Positive-pressure ventilation creates a cyclic, superatmospheric pressure in the upper airway, resulting in a pressure gradient between the upper airway and the lungs that pushes gases through the airways. Positive-pressure ventilation is delivered through an endotracheal tube or tracheostomy tube or in a noninvasive manner through a face or nasal mask. Conventional positive-pressure ventilation is identified with respiratory rates up to 60 breaths per minute. High-frequency positive-pressure ventilation (HFPPV) is any mode of ventilation delivered at higher respiratory rates.

II. Types of positive-pressure ventilation. Conventional positive-pressure ventilation is commonly applied by means of volume-cycled or pressure-preset ventilation.

A. Volume-cycled ventilation. Volume-cycled ventilation delivers a set volume, regardless of the pressure generated (within limits) within the system. Volume-cycled ventilation has been the mode of choice for many years in the treatment of adults with acute respiratory failure. A predefined minute volume delivery is, with few exceptions, guaranteed. The limitations to this mode include the following: (a) changes in the mechanical properties of the lungs from atelectasis, edema, or bronchoconstriction may create high inflation pressures (perhaps increasing the risk of barotrauma); and (b) the patient cannot adjust the breathing pattern according to changes in ventilatory demand.

B. Pressure-preset ventilation. Pressure-preset ventilation delivers a predefined target pressure to the airway during inspiration, so the resulting tidal volume (V_T) and inspiratory flow profile vary with the impedance of the respiratory system and the strength of the patient's inspiratory efforts. Therefore, V_T decreases when lungs or chest wall become stiff, when the airway resistance increases, or when the patient's inspiratory efforts decline. The limitation to pressure ventilation is that an increase in respiratory system impedance can lead to a fall in minute ventilation ($\dot{V}_E$), hypoxemia, and carbon dioxide retention.

III. Means to activate a machine breath

A. Controlled mechanical ventilation. Controlled mechanical ventilation is a mode with rate, inspiratory-to-expiratory timing (I:E), and inspiratory flow (or pressure) determined entirely by machine settings. Because the settings cannot be altered by patient effort, the only indication for this mode is when the patient is apneic from sedation, neuromuscular blockade, or disease.

B. Assist/control ventilation. Assist/control ventilation mode is sensitized to respond to the patient's inspiratory effort. If the patient has no inspiratory effort, the machine cycles automatically and delivers a controlled breath. There are two mechanisms by which ventilators recognize patient effort and switch from expiration to inspiration. During pressure triggering, phase switching occurs whenever the airway pressure falls below a predetermined level. The flow-by mode, which is available on new-generation ventilators, is an alternative to conventional pressure-based machine triggering and allows a base flow of gas to be programmed through the circuitry, so change in flow is sensed by the machine. Differences between inspiratory and expiratory flows result in a machine breath. Compared with pressure triggering, flow-by reduces patient work necessary to initiate a breath.

Because although only a modest inspiratory effort is required to trigger the ventilator, many patients perform muscular work throughout the entire assisted breath. If it is determined that work of breathing is excessive or potentially fatiguing, the following measures should be attempted (before considering neuromuscular blockade): (a) lower the trigger sensitivity setting; (b) raise the inspiratory flow ($\dot{V}_I$); (c) evaluate oxygenation and alveolar ventilation; (d) assess the adequacy of machine backup rate and positive end-expiratory pressure (PEEP) settings; and (e) address sedation and pain control.

C. Intermittent mandatory ventilation. Intermittent mandatory ventilation is a combination of spontaneous ventilation and volume-cycled assisted ventilation. Between mechanically controlled breaths, the patient breathes spontaneously, and the ventilator serves as a source of warmed, humidified, and potentially oxygen-enriched gas. Virtually all modern ventilators use a synchronized intermittent mandatory ventilation mode that is sensitized to the patient inspiratory effort and eliminates the possibility of the patient's receiving a double breath. At intervals determined by the intermittent mandatory ventilation frequency setting, the machine becomes sensitized to the patient's inspiratory efforts and delivers a mechanically assisted breath. Between the assisted cycles, the patient breathes spontaneously (rate and depth determined by patient).

D. Pressure-support ventilation. Pressure-support ventilation, a form of pressure-preset ventilation, is intermittent positive-pressure breathing with a sensing device that only delivers the breath at the time the patient makes an inspiratory effort. It is an alternative to volume-cycled ventilation for alert patients with increased rate and respiratory drive.

E. Pressure-control ventilation. Pressure-control ventilation, a form of pressure-preset ventilation, differs from pressure-support ventilation in that the operator sets a machine backup rate and determines inspiratory time (T_I). If the patient has periods of apnea, the assist/control feature ensures ventilation. Because the patient does not have the same control over V_T and breathing patterns as with pressure-support ventilation, this mode is usually reserved for patients who are hypoxic and heavily sedated or paralyzed, when the need to match ventilator rate and timing with intrinsic respiratory rhythms is not an issue.

F. Noninvasive mechanical ventilation. Noninvasive mechanical ventilation encompasses all modes of ventilatory assistance that can be applied without an endotracheal or tracheostomy tube. Noninvasive mechanical ventilation has been shown to be effective initial therapy for patients with chronic obstructive pulmonary disease and overt hypercapnic respiratory failure. Other conditions for which noninvasive mechanical ventilation appears to be effective include (a) exacerbations of airways obstruction (early application in the emergency room may avert intubation) and (b) ventilatory insufficiency from chest wall disease, neuromuscular disease, and sleep-related disorders (initial rescue treatment). Noninvasive mechanical ventilation is relatively contraindicated in patients who cannot protect their airway or clear their secretions.

IV. Ventilator settings

A. Fraction of inspired oxygen. Fraction of inspired oxygen (F_iO_2) should initially be 100% for most adults started on mechanical ventilation. Subsequent adjustments in F_iO_2 are usually guided by pulse oximetry and arterial blood gas analyses. It is currently believed that an F_iO_2 lower than 0.6 is not injurious to the lungs even when it is used for days or weeks.

B. Tidal volume. V_T in a volume-cycled preset mode is set directly or follows from the minute volume and rate setting. When a pressure-preset mode is used, V_T is the consequence of the patient's respiratory system impedance, the pressure amplitude setting, and the duration over which the inflation pressure is applied. In the past, the recommendation was for a V_T of 10 to 12 mL/kg ideal body weight (appropriate for persons with normal or minimally impaired lung function). Because there is overwhelming evidence that inflation above total lung capacity can damage normal lung units, the current trend is to ventilate the lungs of patients with acute lung injury with a V_T of 6 mL/kg ideal body weight. Patients with chronic obstructive pulmonary disease and asthma should initially be started with a V_T of 8 mL/kg.

C. "Sighing." "Sighing" is a programmable setting in some ventilators. It is unknown whether sighs are needed to prevent atelectasis during mechanical ventilation with conventional VT and PEEP settings; therefore, most practitioners do not program sighs.

D. Inflation pressure setting. Inflation pressure setting is a dependent variable in volume-cycled ventilation, but it generally should not be allowed to increase without limit. A pressure limit or pop-off pressure (set on the control panel) should be imposed to avoid overinflation and possible lung rupture. Random pop-off cycles can be due to coughing or splinting; frequent popping off can be an indication of acute respiratory distress. In a pressure-preset mode, ventilators require an inflation pressure amplitude setting. This setting (often referred to as a pressure-control or pressure-support setting) determines the relative pressure increase during assisted ventilation and is an important determinant of peak lung volume and V_T. Peak pressures should generally be kept to less than 50 cm H_2O.

E. Respiratory rate. Respiratory rate in volume-cycled ventilation should be determined by considering the patient's actual rate demand in conjunction with the T_I or inspiratory-expiratory setting. The machine backup rate should always be set close to the patient's actual rate. If the actual rate is so high that effective ventilation cannot be achieved, the need for sedation and then paralysis should be considered.

F. Inspiratory flow. Inspiratory flow is generally adjusted by the respiratory therapist while observing patient-ventilator interactions. In pressure-preset mode, inspiratory flow is not a set variable, but is determined by patient mechanics and inspiratory effort as well as PEEP, pressure, amplitude, and T_I settings.

G. Minute ventilation. Minute ventilation ($\dot{V}_E$) is the consequence of the V_T and rate settings. Persons with normal pulmonary function maintain normocapnea with a resting ventilation of approximately 5 L per minute. (As a general rule, set $\dot{V}_E$ for patients with acute respiratory distress syndrome at approximately 15 to 20 L per minute until arterial blood gas analyses, airway pressure responses, and cardiovascular status guide further ventilator adjustments; patients with chronic obstructive pulmonary disease average 8 to 12 L per minute unless the disease is exacerbated by left heart failure, sepsis, or pneumonia).

H. Positive end-expiratory pressure. PEEP is the artificial maintenance of positive pressure after passive exhalation is complete and is compatible with positive-pressure mechanical ventilation in any mode. PEEP is usually titrated to the least amount necessary to achieve adequate blood gas tensions (e.g., arterial oxygen saturation 90% or greater or PO_2 greater than or equal to 60 mm Hg with F_IO_2 values less than 0.6). The major cardiovascular complication associated with PEEP is reduction in cardiac output.

For patients with hypoxemic respiratory failure, PEEP is used to raise lung volume to recruit collapsed and flooded alveoli and to improve oxygenation. It is useful in the treatment of pulmonary edema (noncardiogenic and cardiogenic); it increases P_aO_2 by decreasing pulmonary shunting and improving ventilation and perfusion matching.

For patients with obstruction, PEEP is used to minimize inspiratory work of breathing in dynamically hyperinflated patients. It is now appreciated that end-expiratory alveolar pressure can remain positive even when PEEP is not intentionally applied. This is auto-PEEP or intrinsic PEEP ($PEEP_i$) and is not readily apparent on the ventilator manometer. When disregarded, $PEEP_i$ can lead to serious errors in management. By adding extrinsic PEEP in ventilator-dependent patients with $PEEP_i$, the adverse effects of $PEEP_i$ (e.g., hypotension, fatigue of respiratory muscles, failure of machine to trigger) can be mitigated. Decreasing respiratory rate and VT in sedated or paralyzed patients may also help.

V. Mechanical Ventilation Strategies in the Management of Disease. See Table 51-1.

VI. Complications associated with positive-pressure ventilation. An improved understanding of patient-ventilator interactions and lung biology has led to a greater appreciation for the risk of barotrauma associated with positive-pressure ventilation. The classic manifestations of barotrauma include pulmonary interstitial emphysema with pneumomediastinum, subcutaneous emphysema, pneu-

TABLE 51-1. Mechanical ventilation strategies in the management of disease

Pathophysiology	Goal of Therapy	Suggested Initial Ventilator Strategies
Respiratory failure, (with near normal mechanics and gas exchange)	Maintain or restore adequate alveolar ventilation and oxygenation	Rate: 10–12 breaths/min Volume-cycled mode: V_T 10 mL/kg Pressure preset mode: pressure amplitude 10–15 cm H_2O applied for 0.75 to 1 sec
Status asthmaticus	Minimize dynamic hyperinflation and ensure adequate oxygenation Hypercapnia permissible Sedation and perhaps paralysis needed	V_T: ≤ 8 mL/kg Initial peak flow rate ≈ 60 L/min Rates: 12–16 breaths/min Keep V_{EI} < 20 mL/kg
Chronic obstructive pulmonary disease	Minimize hyperinflation and inspiratory work despite limited control over respiratory rate	V_T: 8 mL/kg Initial peak flow: 40–60 L/min Rate: below spontaneous rate PEEP: 5 cm H_2O
Acute respiratory distress syndrome	Minimize overdistention and sheer force injury Ensure adequate oxygenation Hypercapnia permissible.	Volume-cycled mode: V_T: 6 mL/kg Keep P_{plat} < 35 cm H_2O Pressure preset mode: P_{peak} setting: ≤ 40 cm H_2O Rate: 20–30 breaths/min unless patient paralyzed to tolerate hypercapnea or IRV PEEP: no upper limit, but rarely possible to ventilate sufficiently at cycling pressures between 20 cm H_2O PEEP and 35 cm H_2O P_{plat}; then consider sedation and paralysis and prone positioning
Head trauma	Avoid excessive intrathoracic pressures Provide sufficient ventilation to lower $PaCO_2$	V_T: 10 ml/kg Rate: 20–30 breaths/min Use oxygen supplementation to correct hypoxemia rather than PEEP
Myocardial ischemia, and congestive heart failure	Use PEEP to recruit flooded lung units and redistribute edema fluid from the alveolar to interstitial spaces	V_T: 8 mL/kg Rate: below spontaneous rate PEEP Avoid premature weaning trials that increase work of breathing and associated myocardial oxygen demand

IRV, inverse ratio ventilation; PEEP, positive end-expiratory pressure; P_{peak}, peak airway pressure; P_{plat}, plateau airway pressure; V_{EL}, volume at end inspiration, the volume of air above functional residual capacity that is in the patient's lungs after delivery of V_T. See the chapter on Mechanical Ventilation in *Intensive Care Medicine,* 4th edition for details.

moretroperitoneum, pneumoperitoneum, and pneumothorax with or without tension. In addition, investigators recognize many more subtle manifestations of ventilator-induced lung injury that were originally attributed to intrinsic disease. These range from capillary leak and noncardiogenic edema to alveolar hemorrhage and subpleural cyst formations and are thought to be causally related to overdistention and surfactant depletion from excessive tidal excursions. Large V_T can be injurious even when lung inflation beyond total lung capacity is avoided.

Strategies to minimize barotrauma and to optimize PEEP are important and require monitoring of a variety of physiologic parameters. See *Intensive Care Medicine,* 4th edition for details.

Selected Readings

Brochard L. Inspiratory pressure support. *Eur J Anaesth* 1994;11:29.
Good overview of pressure-support ventilation.

Brochard L, Mancebo J, Wysocki M, et al. Noninvasive ventilation for acute exacerbations of chronic obstructive pulmonary disease. *N Engl J Med* 1995;333:817.
In-depth discussion of the role of noninvasive mechanical ventilation.

Froese AB, Bryan AC. High frequency ventilation. *Am Rev Respir Dis* 1987;135:1363.
Concise overview of high-frequency ventilation.

Haake R, Schlichtig R, Ulstad DR. Barotrauma pathophysiology, risk factors, and prevention. *Chest* 1987;91:608.
A review of the pathophysiology, risk factors, clinical presentation, and strategies to manage barotrauma.

Marcy TW. Barotrauma: detection, recognition, and management. *Chest* 1993;104:578.
A concise discussion of barotrauma—clinical manifestations, pathogenesis, and ventilatory strategies.

Marini JJ. Evolving concepts in the ventilatory management of acute respiratory distress syndrome. *Clin Chest Med* 1996;17:555.
Offers an update on approaches to management of acute respiratory distress syndrome.

Marini JJ, Rodriguez RM, Lamb V. The inspiratory work-load of patient-initiated mechanical ventilation. *Am Rev Respir Dis* 1986; 134:902.
A look at the patient's component of mechanical workload during MV.

Pepe PE, Marini JJ. Occult positive end-expiratory pressure in mechanically ventilated patients with airflow obstruction. *Am Rev Respir Dis* 1982;126:166.
A discussion of the hemodynamic consequences of $PEEP_i$.

Ranieri VM, Eissa NT, Corbeil C, et al. Effects of positive end-expiratory pressure on alveolar recruitment and gas exchange in patients with the adult respiratory distress syndrome. *Am Rev Respir Dis* 1991;144:544.
Explanation of the application of PEEP.

Slutsky AS. Mechanical ventilation. *Chest* 1993;104:1833.
American College of Chest Physicians' Consensus Conference that covers the entire topic.

52. MECHANICAL VENTILATION: WEANING

Ann E. Connolly and Richard S. Irwin

I. General principles. For most patients (80% to 90%), weaning from mechanical ventilation (MV) is accomplished rapidly and without difficulty when the precipitating reason for respiratory failure is corrected or resolves. For others, however, a more gradual and systematic approach is required, and the process may be difficult and prolonged.

The most common methods of weaning are (a) trials of spontaneous breathing alternating with periods of full ventilatory support, (b) synchronous intermittent mandatory ventilation (SIMV), and (c) pressure-support ventilation (PSV). Extensive research has been conducted to determine the best method for weaning, but to date none has been shown to be superior. However, two randomized, controlled clinical trials have shown that SIMV is inferior to spontaneous breathing and PSV weaning modes. Consequently, SIMV is not discussed here. Evidence indicates that use of a systematic, team approach focused on addressing and correcting medical causes of weaning failure plays an important role in achieving success.

Numerous studies have evaluated a wide variety of physiologic indices to predict the patient's ability to sustain spontaneous ventilation without MV. These studies have yielded conflicting data and all have limitations, but some are useful as a means of assisting the clinician in determining the likelihood of success or failure in weaning patients from MV.

II. Pathogenesis of respiratory failure. The spectrum of respiratory failure ranges from lung (gas exchange) failure manifested by hypoxemia with normocapnea or hypocapnea to pump (ventilatory) failure manifested by hypoxemia and hypercapnea. Lung failure is commonly due to pulmonary edema (noncardiogenic or cardiogenic). Pump failure may be due to central nervous system depression (e.g., drug overdose, anesthesia) or respiratory muscle fatigue or both. Factors that may contribute to respiratory muscle fatigue are (a) central nervous system depression, (b) mechanical defects, (c) lung disease that increases the work of breathing, and (d) mediators of ongoing active diseases, such as sepsis, that adversely affect the respiratory muscles. There are potentially four reversible reasons for prolonged MV:

1. Inspiratory muscle fatigue (likely multifactorial) (Table 52-1).
2. Inadequate respiratory drive (may be due to nutritional deficiencies, sedatives, central nervous system abnormality, or sleep deprivation).
3. Inability of the lungs to carry out gas exchange (may occur if the underlying cause of respiratory failure has not sufficiently improved).
4. Psychologic dependency.

Although no studies have determined the relative importance of these factors, and combinations of these factors may be present, the literature suggests that pump failure resulting from inspiratory respiratory muscle fatigue is primarily responsible for failure to wean these patients from MV (Table 52-1).

III. Patient assessment. Weaning trials should be attempted when the patient is hemodynamically stable and improving (Table 52-2). Although physiologic indices have not been studied to determine when to initiate weaning trials, the index of rapid shallow breathing (f/V_T) and maximum inspiratory pressure (MIP), measured under the conditions described by Yang and Tobin, can be recommended as relatively accurate, although imperfect, predictors of weaning success or failure. Threshold values of f/V_T less than or equal to 105 (positive predictive value = 0.78 and negative predictive value = 0.95) and MIP less than or equal to –15 cm H_2O (positive predictive value 0.59 and negative predictive value 1.00) were those that discriminated best between patients who were successfully weaned and those in whom a weaning trial failed. Once weaning starts, if the patient deteriorates either

TABLE 52-1. Possible causes of inspiratory respiratory muscle fatigue

Nutritional and metabolic deficiencies (may be from hypokalemia, hypomagnesemia, hypocalcemia, hypophosphatemia, hypothyroidism)
Systemic diseases (decreased protein synthesis and increased degradation, decreased glycogen stores)
Persistently increased work of breathing (e.g., disease, ventilator)
Failure of the cardiovascular system (e.g., disease, ventilator)
Neuromuscular dysfunction/disease (drugs, critical illness polyneuropathy)
Combinations of the above[a]

[a]Also consider corticosteroids, chronic renal failure, hypoxemia and hypercapnea.

clinically or physiologically, the weaning trial should be terminated, and the MV should be resumed. Screening patients daily to identify those who can breathe spontaneously will reduce the duration of MV and the cost of intensive care. We attempt to avoid certain pitfalls by preparing patients psychologically to understand that a failed weaning trial has no bearing on their ultimate prognosis and by avoiding placing a weaning stress on patients with active ischemic heart disease. In general, we initiate only one weaning trial in a 24-hour period.

IV. Weaning process. Before initiating weaning trials, one should do the following:

1. When the patient is stable and improving, communicate that weaning trials will begin.
2. Obtain baseline values and monitor clinical parameters: heart rate, respiratory rate, subjective distress, pulse oximetry (S_aO_2), and cardiac rhythm.
3. Continue to monitor and record these values during the weaning trial.
4. Attempt to provide a calm atmosphere; offer the patient encouragement and support.
5. Avoid sedation to ensure maximal patient cooperation and effort.
6. Whenever possible, sit the patient upright in bed or in a chair.
7. Provide a fraction of inspired oxygen (F_iO_2) concentration 10% greater than when on the ventilator.

Because there are no consistently reliable predictors, the practitioner must rely on clinical judgment and signs of clinical deterioration. Evidence of clinical deterioration includes heart rate 30 beats per minute above baseline, development of ventricular ectopy or supraventricular tachyarrythmia, mean arterial blood pressure more than 15 mm Hg or less than 30 mm Hg of baseline, respiratory rate higher than 35 breaths per minute for at least 5 minutes, S_aO_2 less than 90%; and dyspnea rated by the patient as 5/10 or more. On the other hand, it is important not to terminate weaning trials prematurely because this can markedly prolong MV. The duration of the weaning trials depends on the patient population, the weaning mode, and local practice. Various approaches have been proposed (e.g., extubation after 2 hours of successful spontaneous breathing, extubation of stable patients on a pressure-support ventilation setting of 5 cm H_2O for 2 hours). To avoid the need for reintubation and its associated risks such as increased mortality, increased

TABLE 52-2. Criteria for initiating a weaning trial

Patient must be clinically stable and improving
Fraction of inspired oxygen requirement ≤ 0.50
Positive end-expiratory pressure (PEEP) requirement ≤ 5 cm H_2O
Minute ventilation <20 L/min
Maximum inspiratory pressure < -10 cm H_2O
$f/V_T < 100$

intensive care or hospital length of stay, or the need for transfer to long-term care or rehabilitation facilities, we do not place rigid limits on weaning trials and may continue weaning in weak patients for up to 24 hours before extubation.

V. Modes of weaning. General guidelines for weaning trials are presented in Table 52-3.

A. Spontaneous breathing trials. Machine support is withdrawn, and patients are closely observed as they breathe spontaneously. This can be accomplished by disconnecting the patient from the ventilator and connecting a T-piece adapter to the endotracheal tube. An alternative method is to use low levels of continuous positive airway pressure (CPAP). CPAP may reduce the work of breathing for patients with airflow obstruction, and it allows the clinician to take advantage of the ventilator alarm systems. Newer ventilators are equipped with flow-by systems, which can be used in conjunction with the CPAP mode. This option involves setting an adjustable base flow through the ventilator circuit, thus reducing the work associated with breathing through a demand flow system. In contrast to methods that involve gradual withdrawal of machine support, a spontaneous breathing trial permits the patient's cardiorespiratory response patterns to be assessed without the influence of machine settings. Rather than arbitrary termination of a weaning trial, it should be continued until the patient has clinical signs consistent with fatigue.

B. Pressure-support ventilation weaning. This method involves gradually decreasing the level of pressure support, thus making the patient responsible for a gradually increasing amount of ventilation. In this mode, a target pressure is applied to the endotracheal tube, which augments the inflation pressure exerted by the inspiratory muscles (P_{mus}) on the respiratory system. As the lungs inflate, inspiratory flow begins to decline, and as it reaches a threshold value (differs among machines), the ventilator switches to expiration. Enthusiasm for this method should be tempered by knowledge of potential adverse

TABLE 52-3. Guidelines for weaning

Spontaneous Breathing

Use one of following methods: (a) if the ventilator is equipped with flow-by, switch to CPAP 5 cm H_2O with flow-by or (b) fit the patient's endotracheal tube with a T-piece circuit and supply humidified oxygen-enriched gas. Continue the trial unless clinical findings, oxygenation, or cardiac monitoring suggest respiratory muscle fatigue or clinical deterioration. If the trial is terminated, place the patient on the preweaning MV settings. In general, we do not subject patients to more than one failed trial in a 24-hour period. If no history of lung disease and on ventilator less than 1 week, and the patient appears to be tolerating spontaneous breathing without dyspnea for 2 hours and maintains adequate oxygenation, extubate. For patients on prolonged MV or with COPD, we usually observe for up to 24 hours before extubating.

PSV Weaning

Switch to PSV mode or if already on PSV, decrease amount of pressure support. If on prolonged MV, or with COPD: begin at setting of 25 cm H_2O if switching from another mode. If on PSV, decrease the amount of support. Decrease airway inflation pressure by 2 to 4 cm every hour unless clinical findings, oxygenation, or cardiac monitoring suggest respiratory muscle fatigue or clinical deterioration. If the patient does not tolerate increased work of breathing, return to the previously tolerated level or higher until stable again. When the patient has been stable for 1 hour on PSV of 0 to 5 cm H_2O, fit with a T-tube or switch to CPAP with flow-by and observe for extended period before extubation. If no underlying lung disease, and on ventilator less than 1 week, decrease pressure at 30-minute intervals. If pressure of 0 to 5 cm H_2O is well tolerated for 2 hours, extubate.

COPD, chronic obstructive pulmonary disease; CPAP, continuous positive airway pressure; MV, mechanical ventilation; PSV, pressure-support ventilation.

TABLE 52-4. Ways to increase respiratory muscle strength and decrease muscle demand.

Increase Strength	Decrease Demand
Improve cardiovascular function (poor cardiac performance may contribute to decreased supply of oxygen to respiratory muscles)	Maximize treatment of systemic disease (e.g., infection) to decrease metabolic requirements
Discontinue sedative drugs whenever possible (may be responsible for central fatigue)	Use diuretics to keep patients with lung edema on the dry side to make lungs less stiff
Reverse malnutrition	Diagnose and treat underlying cardiac disorders
	If patient fails to wean and endotracheal tube size is small (< 7 mm), consider changing to a larger tube to avoid increased work of breathing

patient-ventilator interactions that include (a) pressure-support setting–induced central apneas and (b) dyssynchrony between patient and machine for patients with high intrinsic respiratory rates and reduced inspiratory pressure output and when ventilator support results in greater than normal tidal volumes. The diagnostic and prognostic significance of this dyssynchrony is uncertain.

VI. Management of weaning failure. The respiratory muscles play a significant role in the onset and perpetuation of respiratory failure. When patients have met the traditional indications for weaning but fail, this failure is predominately due to inspiratory respiratory muscle fatigue. In general, muscle fatigue occurs because of a decrease in the maximum force the muscles are capable of generating or an increase in the force required of the muscles to sustain ventilatory demand (supply vs. demand). Ways to increase respiratory muscle strength and to decrease muscle demand should be systematically instituted (Table 52-4).

VII. Conclusion. Advances have been made in our understanding of why patients fail to wean, and strategies have been developed to achieve successful weaning. When one is managing patients who fail to wean from MV, this failure is not likely due to the technology or mode, but rather results from their diseases and how well their diseases are managed. A number of studies support the use of protocol-directed, team approaches to achieve successful outcomes. Programs designed to incorporate methods to identify and correct factors that allow for the persistence of inspiratory respiratory muscle fatigue or weakness have been shown to improve the quality of care for patients receiving MV and to decrease intensive care unit length of stay and hospital costs.

Selected Readings

Brouchard L, Rauss A, Benito S, et al. Comparison of three methods of gradual withdrawal from ventilatory support during weaning from mechanical ventilation. *Am J Respir Crit Care Med* 1994;150:896.

This article is a well-known study comparing methods of weaning.

Cohen IL, Bari N, Strosberg MA, et al. Reduction of duration and cost of mechanical ventilation in an intensive care unit by use of a ventilatory management team. *Crit Care Med* 1991;19:1278.

This article provides more evidence that a team approach to weaning from MV leads to favorable outcomes.

Ely EW, Baker AM, Dunagan DP, et al. Effect of the duration of mechanical ventilation of identifying patients capable of breathing spontaneously. *N Engl J Med* 1996; 335:1864.

Randomized, controlled trial suggesting an organized team approach used for weaning can influence the duration of MV.

Epstein A, Frutos F, Tobin MJ, et al. Effect of failed extubation on the outcome of mechanical ventilation. Chest 1997;112:186.

A look at risks associated with reintubation.

Esteban A, Frutos F, Tobin MJ, et al. A comparison of four methods of weaning patients from mechanical ventilation. *N Engl J Med* 1995;332:345.

This article is a well-known study comparing methods of weaning.

Macklem PT. Respiratory muscles: the vital pump. *Chest* 1980;78:753.

This article provides insight into respiratory muscle fatigue.

Smyrnios N, Irwin RS, Connolly A, et al. A multidisciplinary ventilator management program: improvement in quality of care, ICU utilization, and economics at one year. *Am J Respir Crit Care Med* 1997;155:A19.

This article provides more evidence that a team approach to weaning from MV leads to favorable outcomes.

Yang KL, Tobin MJ. A prospective study of indexes predicting the outcome of trials of weaning from mechanical ventilation. *N Engl J Med* 1991;324:1445.

An evaluation of several indices proposed to predict weaning success or failure.

53. RESPIRATORY ADJUNCT THERAPY

Cynthia T. French and Richard S. Irwin

I. **General principles.** Aerosolized drugs are most commonly delivered by hand-held metered-dose inhalers (MDIs), updraft aerosol units (nebulizer devices that produce aerosol by constant gas flow without pressure regulation), or inhalation of fine powder. When used by properly trained spontaneously breathing patients and taken in equivalent doses, bronchodilator aerosols administered by MDIs are as effective as those delivered by nebulizer devices. For those patients who are unable to use their MDI properly because of poor hand-breath coordination or handicaps, reliable aerosol delivery can usually be achieved with the use of an aerosol holding chamber that attaches to the MDI. In intubated and mechanically ventilated patients, aerosols can also be delivered by small-volume sidestream nebulizers and MDIs with an aerosol holding chamber made for this purpose. Various therapeutic aerosols are described in this chapter.

A. **Bland aerosol.** The bland aerosol of sterile water is effective in humidifying inspired gas. In contradistinction to nonintubated patients in whom humidification is largely superfluous because gas is largely humidified and warmed by the upper respiratory tract, humidification and warming of inspired gases are imperative for intubated patients. Two devices that provide warming and humidification during mechanical ventilation are a heated waterbath humidifier and a heat and moisture exchange filter. A potential disadvantage of the heat and moisture exchange filter is that resistance of airflow through the device may progressively rise, thus increasing the work of breathing and conceivably impeding weaning from the ventilator.

B. **Mucolytic agents.** Theoretically, mucolytic agents facilitate expectoration of excessive lower airway secretions and improve lung function. Although *N*-acetylcysteine (Mucomyst) liquefies inspissated mucus plugs when it is administered by direct airway instillation, it is of questionable use when administered as an aerosol to nonintubated patients. Because mucolytic instillations of aerosols can induce bronchospasm in patients with airway disease, these agents should be administered to these patients in combination with a bronchodilator. Recombinant human DNase given as an aerosol once or twice a day to patients with cystic fibrosis has been described as helpful in some cases.

C. **Antimicrobial agents.** Although endotracheal instillation and aerosolization of antimicrobial solutions have been successful in tracheotomized patients and in patients with cystic fibrosis with tracheobronchial infections and colonization, little evidence supports the use of aerosolized antibiotics for acute bacterial pneumonia. Ribavirin (Virazole) aerosol is recommended for patients with severe lower respiratory tract disease or infants with chronic underlying conditions who have respiratory syncytial virus infection. Because the long-term effect of this drug to exposed health care workers is unknown, conservative safety practices must be followed.

D. **Racemic epinephrine.** Racemic epinephrine (Racepinephrine or Vaponefrin) is effective in decreasing laryngeal edema by causing vasoconstriction. The usual adult dose is 0.5 mL of a 2.25% solution diluted in 3 mL of normal saline every 4 to 6 hours. Because rebound edema frequently occurs, patients must be observed closely; because tachycardia is common during treatment, it may precipitate angina. The role of racemic epinephrine aerosol in epiglottitis is not known. Because racemic epinephrine is associated with potentially serious side effects, administration by inhalation of mixtures of helium and oxygen (see later) should be considered first to decrease airway resistance and therefore the work of breathing associated with laryngeal edema or other upper airway diseases.

E. Selective beta$_2$-sympathomimetic agents. Beta$_2$-sympathomimetics such as albuterol are the agents of choice for bronchodilation and mucociliary stimulation. The dose and frequency vary depending on the disease and the situation. The dose can vary from two puffs of albuterol by MDI every 4 to 6 hours in patients with chronic obstructive pulmonary disease (COPD) and stable asthma to four to eight puffs every 20 minutes up to 4 hours, then every 1 to 4 hours as needed or 2.5 to 5 mg of a solution by updraft nebulizer every 20 minutes for three doses, then 2.5 to 10 mg every 1 to 4 hours as needed, or 10 to 15 mg per hour continuously for severe asthma exacerbations. Some physicians have treated acute episodes of asthma in the emergency department in a dose-to-result fashion as follows: initially four puffs of MDI of a short-acting bronchodilator such as albuterol is followed by one additional puff every minute until the patient subjectively or objectively improves or side effects occur (e.g., tremor, tachycardia, arrhythmia). In mechanically ventilated patients with COPD, four puffs of albuterol by MDI with an appropriate holding chamber have to date provided the best combination of bronchodilator effect and safety. If large and frequent doses of beta$_2$-agonists are given, electrocardiogram and serum potassium monitoring are indicated. Nebulized albuterol can cause a prompt and significant decrease in plasma potassium concentration that is evident at 30 minutes and is sustained for at least 2 hours.

F. Anticholinergic agents. These agents appear to have a role in acute asthma when they are combined with sympathomimetic drugs, in exacerbations of COPD when given alone or with albuterol, in intubated patients to prevent or ameliorate bradycardia induced by suctioning, and in selected patients to decrease severe bronchorrhea. The usual adult dose of ipratropium bromide (Atrovent) is 0.5 mg of a nebulizer solution every 6 hours as needed or four puffs by MDI every 6 hours as needed. Ipraotropium and albuterol may be combined in the same nebulizer, and ipratropium and albuterol are also available as a combined MDI product (Combivent).

II. Lung expansion techniques. These include any technique that increases lung volume or assists the patient in increasing lung volume to greater levels than reached at his or her usual unassisted or uncoached inspiration, and these methods are meant to duplicate a normal sigh maneuver. Lung expansion techniques are indicated to prevent atelectasis and pneumonia in patients who cannot or will not take periodic hyperinflations, such as postoperative upper abdominal and thoracic surgical patients and patients with respiratory disorders resulting from neuromuscular and chest wall diseases. Techniques include coached sustained maximal inspiration with cough, incentive spirometry, volume-oriented intermittent positive-pressure breathing, intermittent continuous positive airway pressure (CPAP), or positive expiratory pressure mask therapy.

III. Augmentation of mucociliary clearance. Causes of ineffective mucociliary clearance and subsequent retention of tracheobronchial secretions include depression of the clearance mechanisms and oversecretion in the face of normal mucus transport. The most important consideration in improving mucociliary clearance is to remove the inciting cause (e.g., remove endotracheal tube, stop smoking, treat asthma, stop or reduce suctioning). Mucociliary clearance can be enhanced pharmacologically. Beta$_2$-agonists and aminophylline in the same dose as given for bronchodilation speed up mucus transport in patients with various chronic obstructive lung diseases.

IV. Augmentation of cough effectiveness. Cough assumes a major airway clearance role when mucociliary transport is ineffective. Pharmaceutical or mechanical protussive therapy may be indicated. Although hypertonic saline, amiloride, and terbutaline by aerosol after chest physical therapy have been shown to increase cough clearance, their clinical utility remains to be determined (e.g., reduce morbidity or mortality). Various mechanical measures improve cough effectiveness, including positive mechanical insufflation followed by manual compression of the lower thorax and abdomen in quadriparetic patients, an abdominal push maneuver that assists expiratory efforts in patients with spinal cord injuries, abdominal binding and muscle training of the clavicular portion of the pectoralis major in tetraplegic patients, and chest physical therapy or alternatives.

Chest physical therapy usually includes a combination of the following: therapeutic positioning, percussion to the chest wall over the affected area, vibration of the chest wall during expiration, and coughing. It is indicated in patients with cystic fibrosis and bronchiectasis, in the unusual patient with COPD who expectorates more than 30 mL of sputum each day, and in patients with lobar atelectasis. It is not effective in patients with a weak cough. Complications of chest physical therapy are infrequent but potentially severe and include problems such as massive pulmonary hemorrhage and decreased partial pressure of arterial oxygen (P_aO_2) from positioning the diseased lung downward in spontaneously breathing patients, rib fractures, increased intracranial pressure, decreased cardiac output and decreased forced expiratory volume in 1 second (FEV_1). Chest physical therapy does not work unless patients have an effective cough.

Use of a flutter mucus clearance device, positive expiratory pressure mask therapy, and autogenic drainage are all alternatives that have shown promise in augmenting secretion removal in patients with cystic fibrosis, chronic bronchitis, and bronchiectasis, as has the cough mechanical assist (insufflator/exsufflator) device in neuromuscular diseases.

Mechanical aspiration or suctioning, although routine in most hospitals, is the source of numerous potential complications such as tissue trauma, laryngospasm, bronchospasm, hypoxemia, cardiac arrhythmias, respiratory arrest, cardiac arrest, atelectasis, pneumonia, misdirection of catheter, and death. Complications are generally avoidable if proper technique and indications are adhered to strictly. *Intensive Care Medicine,* fourth edition should be consulted for further information regarding all types of suctioning.

V. Oxygen therapy. Administration of supplemental oxygen is indicated for acute myocardial infarction, bronchial asthma, sickle cell crisis, carbon monoxide poisoning, gas gangrene, cluster headaches, and respiratory failure. In the setting of hypercapnic respiratory failure (P_aO_2 less than 55 mm Hg; P_aCO_2 greater than 46 mm Hg), the goal of oxygen therapy is to increase the P_aO_2 to 55 to 60 mm Hg. The presence of hypercapnia should alert one to the possibility that too much oxygen may lead to carbon dioxide narcosis even though it uncommonly occurs. Therefore, one should avoid excessively rich oxygen mixtures. Barring abrupt decompensation for which intubation and mechanical ventilatory support must be used, controlled low-flow oxygen must be used. This consists of the provision of gas with a relatively low concentration of oxygen. To minimize the risk of inducing carbon dioxide narcosis, oxygen must be administered incrementally beginning with low concentrations. Two commonly used devices include the air entrainment mask (Venturi-type mask) and the nasal cannula. The Venturi-type mask is driven by pure oxygen and entrains varying amounts of room air. It consequently floods the patient's face with gas of a precisely calibrated concentration of 24%, 28%, 31%, 35%, 40%, or 50% oxygen. In the hypercapnic, hypoxemic patient, therapy can begin with the 24% or 28% Venturi masks. If the P_aO_2 remains less than 55 mm Hg 30 minutes later, administration of progressive increments of inspired gas is undertaken. Arterial blood gases are measured at frequent intervals, usually every 30 minutes for the first 1 to 2 hours or until it is certain the P_aO_2 is 55 mm Hg or greater and carbon dioxide narcosis is not developing. Carbon dioxide narcosis is present only when hypercapnia and acidemia progress and are associated with confusion, stupor, and coma. If progressive hypercapnia and mental status changes occur, endotracheal intubation should be considered, or supplemental oxygen should be decreased (not discontinued) in a stepwise fashion.

The second type of low-flow delivery system is the nasal cannula (nasal prongs). Although the Venturi-type masks deliver the most precise doses of oxygen, they may be uncomfortable. Major advantages of nasal prongs include the ability of patients to eat, drink, cough, and talk without removing the device. Even though it is not possible to predict precisely the delivered concentration of oxygen for a given oxygen flow rate by nasal cannula (the delivered concentration depends on multiple factors, such as minute ventilation, tidal volume, respiratory rate, and peak inspiratory flow demand), oxygen must still be administered by progressive increments starting from a low flow rate. Flow rates of 0.5 to 1 L per minute by nasal prongs approximate an F_iO_2 of 0.24, and a rate of 2 L per minute approximates 0.28.

In nonhypercapnic respiratory failure (P_aO_2 less than 55 mm Hg), the goal of oxygen therapy is to increase P_aO_2 to 60 mm Hg or greater. This criterion is greater than the minimum acceptable P_aO_2 of 55 mm Hg cited for hypercapnic patients because acute hypoxemia is less well tolerated than chronic hypoxemia, and carbon dioxide narcosis is not a concern. To achieve the desired P_aO_2, therapy can be delivered initially by nasal prongs or a Venturi-type mask. The appropriate flow rate or F_iO_2 is adjusted based on serial pulse oximetry or arterial blood gas results. When hypoxemia is caused by a lung disease other than COPD, pulse oximetry or arterial blood gases can be monitored every 7 minutes, rather than every 30 minutes. When oxygen is delivered by nasal prongs at flow rates up to 4 to 5 L per minute, the gas must be routed through a humidifier to prevent drying. If higher flow rates are necessary, higher concentration Venturi-type masks (up to 50%) should be given. If a well-fitted 50% Venturi-type mask fails to achieve an oxygen saturation of at least 90% or a P_aO_2 of 60 mm Hg or greater, the patient usually has severe cardiogenic pulmonary edema, acute respiratory distress syndrome, overwhelming pneumonia, or a cardiac or pulmonary vascular shunt. In these settings, a 100% nonrebreathing mask is recommended. When properly worn, it has the potential to deliver the most predictable oxygen concentration (approximately 90%) of all the high-concentration delivery mask devices (e.g., aerosol masks, partial rebreathing masks, or face tents), and it can reveal the presence of a right-to-left shunt. If the P_aO_2 is 60 mm Hg or less in the face of an F_iO_2 of approximately 0.90, a right-to-left shunt of approximately 40% of the cardiac output is present. If the chest radiograph in this setting demonstrates diffuse pulmonary infiltrates and the patient does not improve rapidly with diuretics, adequate oxygenation is not possible without intubation and mechanical ventilation with positive end-expiratory pressure.

In adults, the major potential complications of oxygen therapy include decreased mucociliary clearance, tracheobronchitis, and pulmonary oxygen toxicity. Mucociliary clearance is decreased by 40% when 75% oxygen is breathed for 9 hours and by 50% when 50% oxygen is breathed for 30 hours. Symptomatic tracheobronchitis is caused consistently by the inhalation of high concentrations of oxygen (90% or greater) for 12 hours or more; it is manifested by substernal pain, cough, and dyspnea. To avoid clinically significant pulmonary oxygen toxicity, prolonged administration of concentrations greater than 50% should be restricted, whenever possible, to 48 hours. It is best avoided by restricting delivery of oxygen to the lowest concentration and shortest duration absolutely necessary to achieve a satisfactory P_aO_2. Even if prebronchodilator arterial blood gases fail to reveal hypoxemic respiratory failure (P_aO_2 less than 55 mm Hg), all patients with acute asthma treated in the emergency department or hospital should receive supplemental oxygen by nasal prongs or Venturi-type mask in an effort to minimize the paradoxic postbronchodilator hypoxemia that may occur because of worsening ventilation-perfusion ratios.

On occasion, a patient may be encountered who receives oxygen on a long-term basis by transtracheal catheter. Respiratory failure can be caused by the catheter if it is obstructed by a mucus ball. See *Intensive Care Medicine,* fourth edition, for further reading about this possibility.

VI. Administration of helium-oxygen (heliox). Because helium is less dense than nitrogen, it has the potential to improve airflow when airflow is likely to be turbulent. This is the case in large airways, especially when an upper airway obstructing lesion is present. Heliox has successfully decreased airway resistance in patients with postextubation upper airway obstruction, in children with severe croup who were refractory to inhaled racemic epinephrine, and in upper airway obstruction from tracheal tumors or extrinsic compression. The effect of increasing concentrations of helium in decreasing airway resistance is linear, but most reduction takes place when the concentration of helium reaches 40%. Therefore, heliox mixtures should contain a minimum of 40%, helium with the balance of the mixture being oxygen. For instance, for patients in respiratory distress with little hypoxemia because of laryngeal edema, a heliox mixture of 79% helium and 21% oxygen suffices. For patients in respiratory distress with profound hypoxemia resulting from pulmonary edema associated with laryngeal edema, a heliox mixture of 40% helium and 60% oxygen is most advantageous. Heliox may also improve gas exchange and decrease the work of breathing in some patients with status asthmaticus and acute bronchiolitis when conventional therapies have failed.

VII. Nasal continuous positive airway pressure. Nasal CPAP has been shown to be effective in the treatment of obstructive sleep apnea-hypopnea syndrome and left ventricular failure. Patients usually respond to 3 to 15 cm of H_2O. Prior uvulopalatopharyngoplasty may compromise nasal CPAP therapy by increasing the mouth air leak and reducing the maximal level of pressure that can be tolerated. Multiple nasal delivery devices are available that may improve patient comfort and compliance. Uncommon serious complications include bilateral conjunctivitis, massive epistaxis, and worsening obstruction in a patient with a large, lax epiglottis. For patients with sleep apnea syndrome who cannot tolerate nasal CPAP because of the sensation of excessive pressure, a nasal ventilator that provides bilevel positive pressure during inspiration and expiration may be tolerable.

Selected Readings

Bach JR. Update and perspective on noninvasive respiratory muscle aids. Part 2. The expiratory aids. *Chest* 1994;105:1538.

An excellent overview by a leading specialist in the use of noninvasive respiratory muscle aids. Includes information regarding the cough in-exsufflator device.

Coates AL, MacNeish CF, Meisner D, et al. The choice of jet nebulizer, nebulizer flow, and addition of albuterol affects the output of tobramycin aerosols. *Chest* 1997; 111:1206.

Demonstrates important issues related to delivery.

Dhand R, Tobin, MJ. Inhaled bronchodilator therapy in mechanically ventilated patients. *Am J Respir Crit Care Med* 1997;156:3.

Excellent overview of issues affecting this mode of drug delivery.

Hillberg RE, Johnson DC. Noninvasive ventilation. *N Engl J Med* 1997:337;1746.

Review article.

Hollman G, Shen G, Zeng L, et al. Helium-oxygen improves clinical asthma scores in children with acute bronchiolitis. *Crit Care Med* 1998;26:1731.

The efficacy of heliox was shown in this randomized, double-blind, placebo-controlled trial.

Hudgel DW. Treatment of obstructive sleep apnea. *Chest* 1996;109:1346.

Detailed review of current treatment options.

Irwin RS, French CT, Mike RW. Respiratory adjunct therapy. In: Irwin RS, Cerra FB, Rippe JM, eds. *Intensive care medicine,* 4th ed. Philadelphia: Lippincott–Raven, 1999:763.

Origin of this text.

Irwin RS, Boulet LB, Cloutier MM, et al. Managing cough as a defense mechanism and as a symptom: a consensus panel report of the American College of Chest Physicians. *Chest* 1998;114[Suppl];133S.

Consensus panel report.

Konstan MW, Stern RC, Doershuk CF. Efficacy of the flutter device for airway mucous clearance in patients with cystic fibrosis. *J Pediatr* 1994;124;689.

Good description of and explanation of use of the flutter device.

Kudukis TM, Manthous CA, Schmidt GA, et al. Inhaled helium-oxygen revisited: effect of inhaled helium-oxygen during the treatment of status asthmaticus in children. *J Pediatrics* 1997;130:217.

The efficacy of heliox was shown in this randomized, double-blind, placebo-controlled trial.

Newhouse M, Dolovich M. Aerosol therapy: nebulizer vs metered dose inhaler. *Chest* 1987;91:799.

Supporting editorial by experts.

Salathe M, O'Riordan TG, Wanner A. Treatment of mucociliary dysfunction. *Chest* 1996;110:1048.
Excellent review of treatment of mucociliary dysfunction.

Scanlan CL, Thalken R. Medical gas therapy. In:Scanlan CL, Spearman C, Sheldon RL, et al, eds. *Fundamentals of respiratory care,* 6th ed. St. Louis: CV Mosby, 1995:702.
A classic respiratory care text with an excellent description of oxygen masks and other delivery devices.

Shults RA, Baron S, Decker J, et al. Health care worker exposure to aerosolized ribavirin: biological and air monitoring. *J Occup Environ Med* 1996, 38:257.
Source: National Institute of Occupational Safety and Health.

Turner MO, Patel A, Ginsburg S, et al. Bronchodilator delivery in acute airflow obstruction. *Arch Intern Med* 1997;157:1736.
Metaanalysis, conclusions supporting the use of MDI with spacer.

US Department of Health and Human Services. *Guidelines for the diagnosis and management of asthma.* NIH publication no. 97-4051. Bethesda, MD: National Heart, Lung, and Blood Institute: National Asthma Education and Prevention Program, 1997.
Expert panel advice.

Vater M, Hurt PG, Aitkenhead AR. Quantitative effects of respired helium and oxygen mixtures on gas flow using conventional oxygen masks. *Anaesthesia* 1983:38:879.
Solid article.

54. ACUTE INHALATIONAL INJURY

Mark M. Wilson and Peter J. Jederlinic

I. **Overview.** Inhalational injury can result in a variety of acute respiratory syndromes with widely differing pathogenic mechanisms. For example, acute lung injury after inhalation of respiratory irritants results from a direct toxic effect of rapid onset, whereas hypersensitivity-induced lung injury is immunologically mediated and may require days or months to develop. A single agent may cause several different syndromes, depending on the intensity and duration of exposure. The patient's occupation may offer important clues to the diagnosis of acute inhalational injury. Although many environmental respiratory problems are the result of workplace exposure, natural disasters may have similar results.

Agents that cause inhalational injury may be inhaled as gases, vapors, solid particles, or liquid aerosols. Large particles and droplets (more than 5μ in diameter) deposit in the nose and air passages, whereas smaller particles reach and affect the terminal bronchioles and alveoli. The smallest particles may not deposit at all, but they can still exert their toxic effect. Disease is caused by asphyxia, direct toxicity, or systemic reactions (immunologic or nonimmunologically mediated).

II. **Asphyxiants.** Simple asphyxiants include carbon dioxide (CO_2), nitrogen (N_2), and methane (CH_4), which are normally present in the atmosphere and can be fatal in increased concentrations. Toxic asphyxiants are present in the atmosphere in minute amounts or are released by manufacturing processes or combustion; they asphyxiate at low concentration and include carbon monoxide (CO), hydrogen cyanide (HCN), acrylonitrile (vinyl cyanide), hydrogen sulfide (H_2S), and carbon disulfide (CS_2).

Approximately 5,600 deaths are attributed to CO poisoning in the United States each year. Of these, fewer than half these deaths are suicides, and the rest are accidental. This colorless, odorless, tasteless, nonirritating gas is the most common cause of poisoning and is responsible for 80% of smoke inhalation–related fatalities.

A. **Etiology.** CO_2 accumulates in sealed or poorly ventilated areas. N_2 is found in increased amounts in mines; if present with increased amounts of CO_2, it causes significant reductions in ambient partial pressure of oxygen (PO_2). CH_4 is a highly explosive gas released during the breakdown of organic matter. It occurs naturally in the crust of the earth and is also present in mines. Cyanide is encountered as inorganic salts in metallurgy, electroplating, and photoprocessing; in the combustion of natural (wood, silk) and synthetic polymers (nylon, polyurethane). Morbidity related to H_2S (as found in sewage processing, petrochemical plants, and leather and rubber processing) inhalation is minimal because of the characteristic forewarning "rotten egg" odor that is appreciated at low concentrations. CO is generated during the combustion of any carbon-containing fuel. Cigarette smoke contains about 4% CO, and active smoking has a significant impact on the interpretation of CO levels.

B. **Pathophysiology.** Simple asphyxiants displace oxygen (O_2) from inspired air. Cyanide blocks the final step of oxidative phosphorylation and mitochondrial O_2 utilization. H_2S alters the O_2-carrying capacity of the blood by binding to hemoglobin and also poisons the respiratory enzymes of the cell, similar to the action of cyanide.

The affinity of CO for hemoglobin is 250 times that of O_2. CO readily and reversibly binds to hemoglobin; its high affinity for hemoglobin makes even low concentrations of CO toxic. The formation of carboxyhemoglobin (COHb) causes a reduction in the total O_2-carrying capacity of the blood, a left shift of the oxyhemoglobin dissociation curve, and an increased affinity for O_2 at the remaining binding sites. The net effect on O_2 delivery, therefore, is greater than that expected from the decreased O_2-carrying capacity alone. Because of the increased affinity of CO for fetal hemoglobin, infants and fetuses are at greater risk for poisoning.

C. Diagnosis. Symptoms of hypoxia (breathlessness, tachycardia, headache and diaphoresis, bounding pulse, syncope, and cardiac arrest) characterize exposure to the simple asphyxiants; they vary in severity depending on exposure intensity. Victims of cyanide exposure give off a distinctive "bitter almond" odor, but its detection is unreliable, and the correct diagnosis is better reached by careful history of the circumstances involved.

A careful history is also important in CO intoxication because the clinical features are protean and depend on the duration of exposure, the concentration involved, and the underlying health of the victim. Increasing severity of symptoms correlates with COHb level. Subacute intoxication frequently results in flulike symptoms. Acute CO intoxication causes rapid loss of consciousness without warning. Neurologic and cardiovascular impairments predominate, reflecting the high O_2 requirement of these organ systems. Breathlessness is uncommon initially, and cyanosis, previously thought to be uncommon, is actually seen more frequently than the "cherry-red" skin color. Signs and prognosis of acute poisoning correlate poorly with COHb levels obtained on arrival at the hospital.

Toxicology screens help to rule out other causes of these presenting symptoms. Arterial blood gas analysis helps alert the clinician to the possibility of CO or HCN exposure. In both, metabolic acidosis is present, and arterial O_2 (P_aO_2) tension is normal or near normal. In HCN poisoning, arterial and venous O_2 pressures (PO_2) are nearly the same. In CO poisoning, although P_aO_2 is normal or near normal, measured O_2 saturation and content are reduced. COHb levels are readily available and are essential to the diagnosis of CO intoxication; interpretation must take into account baseline COHb levels and time elapsed since exposure. COHb levels of less than 10% are not usually associated with symptoms; levels of 10% to 20% (mild exposure) are associated with headaches, tinnitus, dizziness, nausea, and slight behavioral abnormalities; levels of 20% to 40% (moderate exposure) can present with coma and seizures; levels higher than 40% suggest severe exposure and increased risk of cardiac arrest.

D. Treatment. The principles of basic management for any asphyxiation include 100% O_2, support of respiratory and circulatory systems (cardiopulmonary resuscitation as needed), and treating complicating conditions such as burns and alcohol or drug intoxication.

Therapy for cyanide poisoning was based in the past on the use of agents that compete with cytochrome oxidase for cyanide, such as intravenous or inhaled nitrites (amyl nitrite). These agents form complexes with hemoglobin and result in the formation of methemoglobin, which is subsequently converted to thiosulfate. Sodium thiosulfate can also be administered directly intravenously. Dicobalt edentate, a chelated cobalt, is the newest, most effective, and least toxic competitive agent available. It is given intravenously as a 600-mg, slowly pushed dose with a repeat dose of 300 mg if there is no improvement.

O_2 is the major therapy for CO poisoning, because it can be rapidly instituted and because it decreases the half-life of COHb to 40 to 60 minutes or less (vs. 240 minutes breathing room air) by competing with CO for hemoglobin binding sites. Hyperbaric O_2 (HBO) therapy reduces general morbidity of CO poisoning and the development of neurologic sequelae in particular. O_2 at 2.5 atmospheres reduces the half-life of COHb to 22 minutes and, furthermore, increases the dissolved O_2 concentration in the blood to a level that will supply the body's needs without hemoglobin. The limited availability of HBO therapy often prevents its applicability, and many patients are treated adequately using 100% O_2 alone. Patients with severe poisoning (COHb greater than 40%) or with cardiac or neurologic symptoms should undergo HBO therapy if available; otherwise, 100% O_2 should be used, and if improvement is not noted within 4 hours, patients should be transferred to an HBO facility. Admission is required for those with a COHb greater than 25% and those with lower levels with signs of cardiac ischemia or neurologic impairment.

III. Toxic gases. Various agents (possibly accounting for 10% of all occupational lung disease) act as toxic irritants to the upper and lower respiratory tract and cause mucosal edema, impaired mucociliary function, and diffuse alveolar damage with pulmonary edema with high concentration exposures. Agents in this class include ammonia (NH_3, and ammonium hydroxide in solution), chlorine (Cl_2), phosgene ($COCl_2$, which hydrolyzes to form hydrochloric acid [HCl]), nitrogen dioxide (NO_2), sulfur dioxide (SO_2), formaldehyde, cadmium, mercury, the salts of vanadium and osmium, paraquat, and the metal hydrides (arsine, phosphine, silane, diborane).

A. Etiology. Major uses of NH_3 include fertilizer production, chemicals, plastics, dye manufacture, and refrigeration. The industrial uses of Cl_2 are in the production of alkali bleaches and disinfectants and in paper and textile processing. Most exposures result from industrial spills. Uses of $COCl_2$ include the production of isocyanate, pesticides, dyes, and pharmaceuticals. Firefighters, welders, and paintstrippers are exposed to heated chlorinated hydrocarbons, and $COCl_2$ is released in these settings. Because $COCl_2$ is less irritating to the eyes and mucous membranes than Cl_2 or HCl and may be inhaled for prolonged periods without discomfort, the risk of serious injury to the lower respiratory tract is greatly increased. Oxides of N_2 are used in dye and fertilizer manufacture and are generated during nitric acid use, arc welding and braziering, engraving, metal work, and combustion of nitrogenous compounds, as well as in fresh silage.

B. Pathophysiology. Many of the irritant gases discussed cause similar pathologic changes. NH_3, SO_2, and HCl have high water solubility and tend to be highly irritating to conjunctivae, mucous membranes, and upper air passages. Laryngospasm, bronchospasm, and mucous membrane necrosis ensue. Less water-soluble agents (oxides of N_2, $COCl_2$) can penetrate more deeply into the respiratory tree and can cause damage at the alveolar and lower airway levels, resulting in pulmonary edema and bronchospasm. The absence of immediate symptoms with these less water-soluble agents can prolong exposure. In addition to concentration and solubility, extremes of pH and chemical reactivity influence the amount of damage inflicted. HCl, SO_2, and $COCl_2$ are acidic, whereas Cl_2 and oxides of N_2 are highly alkaline. Toxicity is enhanced if particulates (soot) are present, to help carry irritants further down the airways.

C. Diagnosis. A careful situational history cannot be overemphasized because these disorders usually occur in the setting of an industrial or transport-related accident. This helps to establish which agents are involved, relative concentrations, the site of exposure (closed space or outdoors), and duration. Patients present in acute respiratory distress with the following: evidence of burn injury; skin lesions; intense edema, erythema, and ulceration of the conjunctival and mucous membranes; and possible laryngeal obstruction. Auscultation of the chest may reveal stridor, crackles, and expiratory wheezing, depending on the time elapsed since exposure. The typical bat-wing distribution of cardiogenic pulmonary edema is less likely on chest radiograph (CXR) than the diffuse or patchy infiltrates of noncardiogenic pulmonary edema. Anaphylaxis and angioneurotic edema with bronchospasm can have similar presentations, but severe mucous membrane inflammation and ulceration are not prominent features of those disorders.

D. Treatment. The mainstay of management for any gas exposure is removal of the victim from the site of exposure and immediate administration of O_2. Airway patency should be ensured because of the risk of progressive laryngeal edema over several hours. Bronchospasm is treated with bronchodilators. Intravenous fluids are necessary because of fluid losses secondary to mucosal edema and sloughing and associated burn injury. Empiric antibiotics are not indicated, and the early use of corticosteroids remains controversial.

IV. Hypersensitivity pneumonitis. Hypersensitivity pneumonitis (HP) results from an immunologic reaction to inhaled antigens that affects the alveoli and interstitium of the lung but not the airways.

A. Etiology. Exposure to antigens (especially thermophilic actinomycetes) dispersed by contaminated humidification and by climate control systems is the common causative agents encountered. Fungal antigens, animal antigens (excrement and extracts), amebas, insects, and chemicals may also cause HP.

B. Pathophysiology. The unifying features of agents causing HP are their ability, based on particle size, to penetrate to the distal airways and alveoli, leading to the development of alveolitis.

C. Diagnosis. The clinical presentation of HP varies depending on intensity, duration, and recurrence of exposure. Brief, intermittent exposures result in fever (up to 40°C), chills, malaise, cough, and dyspnea within 4 to 10 hours of exposure, with the severity of these symptoms dependent on the intensity of exposure. On examination, patients appear acutely ill, and chest auscultation usually reveals end-inspiratory crackles. A neutrophilic leukocytosis of up to 25,000/mm^3 with left shift is common; however, eosinophilia is rare. The erythrocyte sedimentation rate is elevated. Arterial blood gas analysis demonstrates mild to moderate hypoxemia and hypocapnia. Serum immunoglobulins (IgG, but not IgE) are elevated. The CXR in acute or subacute forms of HP can be normal, show a diffuse nodular or reticulonodular pattern sparing the costophrenic angles and apices, or reveal diffuse patchy infiltrates without any associated adenopathy. When the patient is severely affected, the CXR may suggest noncardiogenic pulmonary edema. The lack of response to antibiotics and the recurrent nature of acute HP are helpful in distinguishing this disorder from infectious pneumonia. In chronic HP, CXR findings are pulmonary fibrosis with reduced lung volumes, coarse linear or reticular interstitial infiltrates, and honeycombing.

D. Treatment. Acute management of HP includes supplemental O_2 when hypoxemia is evident. Limited courses of corticosteroids may speed resolution in acute and subacute forms, but is of limited effect in established fibrosis in the chronic stage. Only leaving the exposure permanently will help prevent disabling pulmonary fibrosis.

V. Smoke inhalation. The victim of smoke inhalation presents a unique challenge to the physician because of the complex nature of the fire environment and the frequent association with significant surface burns, trauma, and the delayed sequelae of infection and multiorgan system failure. Approximately 80% of fire-associated deaths (with or without surface burns) are attributed to smoke inhalational injury. Inhalational injury exerts a synergistic lethal effect when surface burns are present, with a mortality exceeding 50% (vs. a 4% mortality for surface burns only).

A. Etiology. Cigarettes remain the major cause of house fire deaths, but carelessness with matches, wood stoves, heaters, and appliances and heating system malfunctions also contribute significantly.

B. Pathophysiology. Respiratory injuries in fire victims with smoke inhalation can be the result of asphyxia, heat, and exposure to toxic products of incomplete combustion (TPCs). Most deaths are the result of asphyxia. CO and HCN are the two major asphyxiants and frequently occur together. The TPCs liberated in a given setting are determined by the type of fuel, the temperature, the rate of heating, the presence or absence of O_2, and the distance from the source. With an ever-increasing list of new synthetic materials in use, a wide variety of TPCs may be encountered, and synergistic toxicity from combinations of TPCs is a definite problem. Many of the considerations discussed earlier with regard to toxic gases apply here.

Although hot particulates, hot gases, and steam can result in injury to the lower respiratory tract, direct heat injury is usually limited to the upper respiratory tract, as a result of reflex apnea from intense heat exposure. Edema formation is related to release of O_2-free radicals and thromboxanes and causes upper airway obstruction in up to 30% of burn patients. Frank pulmonary edema is a rare sequela of smoke inhalation (up to 8.8%), but it has an associated high mortality (83%).

Pulmonary complications of inhalation injury can be subdivided based on time of occurrence as early (CO poisoning, upper airway obstruction, tracheobronchial obstruction), delayed for 2 to 5 days (upper airway obstruction, pulmonary edema, pneumonia), and late (pulmonary edema, pneumonia, pulmonary embolism).

C. Diagnosis. Whether or not surface burns are present, it is essential to consider smoke inhalation in any victim retrieved from an accident scene. Classic predictors of smoke inhalation injury include the following: a consistent exposure history; respiratory signs and symptoms (dyspnea, hoarseness, wheezing, stridor); cervical, facial, and oropharyngeal burns, especially between the nose and mouth; and expectoration of carbonaceous sputum. Initial evaluation should focus on recognition and treatment of CO poisoning and airway obstruction, the major early problems. A delay in symptom onset (hours to days) is not uncommon. Lung examination is inconsistent and may not be abnormal until 24 hours later.

Arterial blood gas analysis and cooximetry for COHb level are essential in the management of victims of smoke inhalation. High COHb levels are markers of the potential for inhalation of other toxins and suggest the need for immediate measurement and institution of empiric therapy for cyanide poisoning. Unexplained metabolic acidosis or a lactate concentration greater than 10 mM/L in the presence of normal or mildly elevated COHb levels and normal P_aO_2 also suggests cyanide exposure. A CXR should be obtained routinely, but a normal radiograph has little predictive value for subsequent inhalation injury.

D. Treatment. Control of the airway is the initial priority. Endotracheal intubation is indicated for stridor, for facial burns and smoke inhalation with central nervous system depression, for mucous membrane burns, for full-thickness burns of the nose and lips, for full-thickness burns of the neck, and when signs and symptoms suggest impending obstruction (e.g., drooling, hoarseness). Nasotracheal intubation may be preferred over orotracheal intubation in the presence of mouth burns, because the latter may predispose to contractures of the mouth. An endotracheal tube 8 mm or greater in internal diameter is preferable, because frequent therapeutic bronchoscopies may be necessary in the presence of inspissated secretions, plugs, and casts that obstruct the airway repetitively. Bronchodilators may be useful for the management of bronchospasm after smoke inhalation. Corticosteroids have been associated with increased mortality resulting from infection, and their routine use has not been recommended.

Selected Readings

Dolan MC. Carbon monoxide poisoning. *Can Med Assoc J* 1985;133:392.

This article provides an excellent overview of CO poisoning and its management.

Fink J. Hypersensitivity pneumonitis. In: Marchant JA, ed. *Occupational respiratory disease.* Washington, DC: US Department of Health and Human Services, 1986:481.

Frank R. Acute and chronic respiratory effects of exposure to inhaled toxic agents. In: Marchant JA, ed. *Occupational respiratory disease.* Washington, DC: US Department of Health and Human Services, 1986:571.

Goldfrank LR, Bresnitz EA. Toxic inhalants including cyanide. In: Goldfrank LR, Flomenbaum NE, Lewin NA, et al, eds. *Toxicologic emergencies.* Norwalk, CT: Appleton & Lange, 1990:737.

The foregoing three book chapters provide detailed information on asphyxiants, toxic gases, and hypersensitivity pneumonitis–related acute inhalational injuries.

Haponik EF. Smoke inhalation. *Am Rev Respir Dis* 1988;138:1060.

A summary of an American Thoracic Society symposium on the presentation, diagnosis, pathophysiology, and treatment of this complex syndrome.

Olson KR. Carbon monoxide poisoning: mechanisms, presentation, and controversies in management. *J Emerg Med* 1984;1:233.

This article provides an excellent overview of CO poisoning and its management.

55. DISORDERS OF TEMPERATURE CONTROL: HYPOTHERMIA

Mark M. Wilson and Frederick J. Curley

I. General principles. In healthy, resting persons, the equilibrium between heat production and heat loss is tightly regulated, producing an average oral temperature of 36.6±0.38°C. Hypothermia, in which core temperature is less than 35°C (95°F), may occur in patients of all ages. The overall mortality from hypothermia in the United States has been conservatively estimated at 17 deaths per 1 million population per year. The mortality rate for treated hypothermia ranges from 12% to 73%.

Humans generate body heat from the energy released in the dissociation of high-energy bonds during the metabolism of dietary fats, proteins, and carbohydrates. Shivering or an increase in muscle tone produces a fourfold rise in net heat production, whereas vigorous exercise may cause a sixfold increase. Heat may be exchanged with the environment by radiation, conduction, convection, or evaporation. *Radiation*—the transfer of thermal energy between objects with no direct contact—accounts for 50% to 70% of heat lost by humans at rest in a neutral environment (i.e., 28°C). *Conduction* involves the direct exchange of heat with objects in direct contact with the body. When the body is submerged in water, large quantities of heat may be lost rapidly. *Convection*—the exchange of heat with the warmer or cooler molecules of air that pass by the skin—may produce rapid heat exchange in the setting of greater temperature differences between the skin and the air and with rapid air flow (i.e., the wind chill factor). *Evaporation* of sweat from the skin results in net heat loss from the body. Unlike the other methods of heat exchange, evaporative heat loss occurs even when the skin is surrounded by a warmer environment.

The anatomy and regulation of the system that controls body temperature are reviewed in depth elsewhere and are only briefly described here. The hypothalamus directly senses local temperature and integrates this information with afferent data to make appropriate adjustments in autonomic tone, and perhaps endocrine function, to maintain body temperature homeostasis. When the hypothalamus perceives a temperature decrease it modulates autonomic tone to cause the following changes: (a) sweat production decreases or ceases entirely; (b) the cutaneous vasculature constricts; and (c) muscle tone increases involuntarily, and shivering begins.

Voluntary responses also play an important role in thermoregulation. Impairment of the ability to alter our environment in response to thermal stress (e.g., adding or removing clothes, changing posture or level of activity, moving to a different climate) predisposes to an imbalance in heat exchange. The ability to regulate temperature effectively declines with age, probably as a result of deterioration in sensory afferents.

II. Causes and pathogenesis. The most frequent causes of hypothermia appear to be exposure to cold, use of depressant drugs, and hypoglycemia. A more detailed list of the causes of hypothermia is presented in Table 55-1.

The incidence of hypothermia doubles with every 5°C drop in ambient temperature. Wet clothing effectively loses up to 90% of its insulating value. Convective heat loss because of the wind may increase to more than five times baseline values. Victims of hypothermia resulting from exposure frequently display inappropriate behavior that compounds the hypothermia.

Depending on the patient population studied, alcohol contributes to hypothermia in 14% to 91% of cases. Because alcohol has been shown to impair the perception of cold, to cloud the sensorium, and to act as a direct vasodilator, persons under the influence of alcohol are less likely to perceive danger or to respond appropriately to cold; moreover, they are unable to conserve heat properly by vasoconstriction. Most sedative-hypnotic drugs cause hypothermia by inhibiting shivering and impairing capability for voluntary control of temperature.

TABLE 55-1. Causes of hypothermia

Unintentional
- Normal aging
- Exposure to cold
- Drugs (alcohol, phenothiazines, barbiturates, paralytic agents, antibiotics, bromocriptine, neuroleptics)
- Endocrine dysfunction (hypoglycemia, diabetic ketoacidosis, hyperosmolar coma, hypothyroidism, panhypopituitarism, adrenal insufficiency)
- Central nervous system disorders (stroke, primary/metastatic neoplasm, luetic gliosis, sarcoidosis, carbon monoxide poisoning, thiamine deficiency, Wernicke-Korsakoff syndrome, anorexia nervosa, multiple sclerosis)
- Spinal cord transection
- Skin disorders (psoriasis, ichthyosis, erythroderma, extensive third-degree burns)
- Debility (lymphoma, lupus, sepsis, severe cardiac or renal or hepatic failure)
- Trauma

Intentional/Iatrogenic
- Exposure to cold (operating and recovery rooms)
- Infusion of cool/cold blood products or fluids
- Continous ultrafiltration at high flow rates
- Central cooling techniques to assist cardiothoracic surgery

Table 55-2 outlines some of the profound metabolic alterations that occur in response to hypothermia. The shivering phase of hypothermia generally occurs in the range of 35°C to 30°C and is characterized by intense energy production resulting from increased muscle tone and the powerful rhythmic contractions of small and large muscle groups. In the nonshivering phase (less than 30°C), metabolism slows dramatically, at times causing multiple organ failure.

Increasing degrees of hypothermia produce a tendency for malignant dysrhythmias, depressed cardiac function, and hypotension. The electrocardiogram (ECG) in mild hypothermia may show bradycardia with prolongation of the PR interval, QRS complex, and QT interval. At temperatures lower than 30°C, first-degree block is not unusual, and at 20°C, third-degree block may be seen. At temperatures

TABLE 55-2. Effects of hypothermia

- Metabolic depletion (catabolism in shivering phase, followed by hypometabolism)
- Cardiac dysrhythmias (bradycardia, heart-blocks, atrial or ventricular fibrillation, asystole)
- Hypotension
- Decreased minute ventilation/apnea
- Dehydration
- Hyperosmolarity
- Stupor/coma
- Granulocytopenia
- Hemoconcentration/hyperviscosity
- Anemia
- Thrombocytopenia
- Ileus
- Pancreatitis
- Hepatic dysfunction
- Hyperglycemia
- Increased susceptibility to infection (pneumonia, sepsis)
- Altered drug clearance

lower than 33°C, the ECG commonly shows a characteristic J point elevation. As temperature drops, the J wave increases in prominence and is almost always present at core temperatures lower than 25°C. Atrial fibrillation is extremely common at temperatures of 34°C to 25°C, and ventricular fibrillation (VF) frequently occurs at temperatures lower than 28 °C. Asystole is common when core temperatures drop to less than 20°C. Although blood pressure is initially maintained by an increase in vascular resistance, systemic resistance falls, and hypotension is common at temperatures lower than 25°C.

Pulmonary mechanics and gas exchange appear to change little with hypothermia. Although the ventilatory response to an elevation in carbon dioxide tension (PCO_2) may be blunted, no clear decrease in hypoxic drive occurs. Both tidal volume and respiratory rate decline as core temperature lowers. At 25°C, respirations may be only three or four per minute; at temperatures less than 24°C, respiration may cease.

As blood pressure decreases during the nonshivering phase, glomerular filtration rate and renal blood flow may decrease by 75% to 85%, without a significant change in urine production. This process is termed *cold diuresis* and is due to a defect in tubular reabsorption. The net result is dehydration and a relatively hyperosmolar serum.

The brain tolerates hypothermia extremely well; complete neurologic recovery has been described in hypothermic adults after 20 minutes of complete cardiac arrest and after up to 3.5 hours of cardiopulmonary resuscitation. The mechanism by which hypothermia has a seemingly protective effect is far from understood.

Hypothermia affects white blood cells, red blood cells, platelets, and perhaps coagulation mechanisms. Although the white blood cell count in mild hypothermia remains normal to slightly elevated, it may drop severely at temperatures lower than 28°C. The hematocrit usually rises in hypothermic patients at a temperature of 30°C, a reflection of hemoconcentration from dehydration and from splenic contraction. Platelet counts drop as temperature decreases (hepatic sequestration), and prolongation of the bleeding time has been noted at 20°C. Platelet levels and function return to normal on rewarming. Although deep venous thrombosis and disseminated intravascular coagulation have been reported in hypothermia, there is no clear evidence of a coagulopathy associated with hypothermia.

Ileus is frequently present at temperatures higher than 30°C and is almost always present at lower temperatures. Subclinical, asymptomatic pancreatitis also appears to be common. Hepatic dysfunction occurs commonly and involves both synthetic and detoxification abnormalities.

Although it is generally assumed that acute hypothermia blunts endocrine function, only the effect on insulin metabolism has been clearly described. Hypothermia directly suppresses the release of insulin from the pancreas and increases resistance to insulin's action in the periphery. Elevations in blood glucose, however, are usually mild. Changes in thyroid and adrenal function also occur, but they are less well defined.

III. Diagnosis. The diagnosis of hypothermia may be suggested by a history of exposure or immersion, a high-risk patient profile (e.g., elderly, alcoholic, diabetic, quadriplegic, or severely debilitated), clinical examination, and laboratory abnormalities. Cool skin, muscle rigidity, some degree of shivering or muscle tremor, and acrocyanosis are present in most noncomatose patients. Although mental status changes vary widely among patients, they follow a typical pattern: between 35°C and 32°C, the patient may be stuporous or confused; between 32°C and 27°C, the patient may be verbally responsive but incoherent; and at temperatures less than 27°C, most patients are comatose but able to respond purposefully to noxious stimuli. Deep coma is an uncommon complication of hypothermia, but when present it may be difficult to distinguish from death. Reflexes remain normal until body temperature is lower than 27°C, when they become depressed or absent. Pupillary reflex may be difficult to detect at temperatures less than 30°C and may become fixed at temperatures lower than 27°C. The criteria for death cannot be applied to patients with the foregoing findings until their core temperature is back near 37°C.

Because the symptoms of hypothermia frequently mimic those of other disorders, the diagnosis may be missed unless the patient has a clear history of exposure or an accurate temperature reading is taken. Thermometers calibrated to record temperatures lower than 35°C are necessary, and sites that reflect core temperature must be used (e.g., bladder, rectal, tympanic, esophageal, or great vessel sites are preferable).

ECG changes are almost always present. Because of an increased solubility of carbon dioxide and oxygen, blood gases reported at 37°C may show a value of PO_2 + PCO_2 greater than 150 mm Hg on room air, a biochemical impossibility at euthermia. An elevated hematocrit, a good output of dilute urine with hypotension, ileus, and an elevated amylase are helpful but nonspecific indicators of hypothermia.

IV. Treatment. Treatment of hypothermia should be aggressive. The field management of hypothermia from exposure or immersion is clearly limited but nonetheless important. Wet clothes should be removed and replaced with dry ones if available. The victim should be insulated from cold and wind as much as possible. Sharing the body heat of another person and the consumption of hot drinks offer no advantages and are no longer encouraged. Patients should not be transported upright because seizures may result from orthostatic hypotension. Rough handling must be avoided; even minor manipulations can induce VF.

Early death from hypothermia is generally due to hypotension and dysrhythmias. Fluid resuscitation, preferably through a central vein, should be attempted in all patients in hypothermic shock. Slightly hypotonic crystalloid fluids should be given after warming to at least room temperature. Pressor agents and procedures (e.g., intubation or catheter placement) have been safe in these patients and should not be withheld because of a fear of dysrhythmia.

The management of dysrhythmias must be approached in a nontraditional manner because many pharmacologic agents, pacing efforts, and defibrillation attempts do not work in the hypothermic patient. Because atrial dysrhythmias and heart block generally resolve spontaneously on rewarming, therapy is usually unnecessary. For supraventricular tachyarrhythmias, digitalis should be avoided (efficacy is unclear and toxicity increases with rewarming), and calcium channel blockers have not been shown to be efficacious. In hypothermic patients experiencing VF, both procainamide and lidocaine have been of little benefit. Bretylium appears to be the drug of choice and has been shown to both decrease the incidence of VF and increase the likelihood of successful cardioversion. Electrical defibrillation should probably be attempted at least once, but it is unlikely to succeed until the patient's core temperature surpasses 30°C. Prophylactic insertion of pacemaker wires should be avoided in otherwise stable patients because of the risk of inducing VF. The role of pacing in established fibrillation is unclear.

Despite complex changes in acid-base status with hypothermia, PCO_2 and pH values uncorrected for temperature may be used accurately to assess these patients. However, because of a decrease in oxygen solubility on warming the arterial blood sample to 37°C, measured PO_2 values may be substantially higher that their actual value in colder patients. Therefore, PO_2 values must be corrected for temperature, or the presence of hypoxemia may be overlooked. The following formula may be used: decrease the PO_2 measured at 37°C by 7.2% for each degree that the patient's temperature is lower than 37°C.

Diseases known to predispose to hypothermia should be diagnosed and treated early. If hypoglycemia is documented, the patient should be given 25 to 50 mg of glucose as a 50% dextrose solution. Because of the ineffective action of insulin and the relatively high serum osmolarity from cold diuresis in hypothermia, treatment with highly concentrated glucose solutions should be delayed until the blood glucose level is measured. The possibility of alcohol or sedative-drug overdose is usually indicated by the patient's history and is confirmed by toxicology. No reports indicate adverse effects of naloxone or thiamin in hypothermia; these agents should routinely be given if coma is present.

Rewarming methods may be divided into three categories: passive external rewarming, active external rewarming, and active central rewarming. Passive external rewarming is the least invasive and slowest rewarming technique. It requires only that the patient be dry, sheltered from wind, and covered with blankets to decrease heat loss, thereby allowing thermogenesis to restore normal temperature. Temperature increase varies inversely with the patient's age; the average rate of temperature increase with this method is only 0.38°C per hour.

Active external rewarming is by far the most controversial method. It involves raising the core temperature by heating the skin with hot blankets, electric heating pads, and hot water bottles (thereby circulating warmed air immediately adjacent to the skin) or immersion in a tub of warm water. These methods do work; however, mortality appears to be higher than with the other two methods. In contrast, use of warmed air circulated through a plastic blanket surrounding the patient (i.e., Bair Hugger) has proven safe and effective in rewarming postoperative patients and appears to work well with other types of hypothermia. Although further study is needed, this may prove an excellent primary therapy or a useful temporary therapy while interventions for active central rewarming are prepared.

Active central rewarming is the fastest and most invasive warming technique available. Safe and effective methods include the following: oxygen that has been humidified and heated to 40°C to 46°C delivered by face mask or endotracheal tube (raises temperature slightly less than 1°C per hour); peritoneal lavage with saline or dialysate fluid heated to 38°C to 43°C and exchanged every 15 to 20 minutes (raises temperature by 2°C to 4°C per hour); and hemodialysis or cardiopulmonary bypass (raises temperature by 1°C to 2°C per hour). Gastric lavage is also an effective method; however, this method involves the risk of aspiration and VF during tube insertion. The desired rate of rewarming varies according to the patient's cardiopulmonary status and underlying disease. The rewarming methods selected must be appropriate for the individual patient.

Selected Readings

Buckley JJ, Bosch OK, Bacaner MB. Prevention of ventricular fibrillation during hypothermia with bretylium tosylate. *Anesth Analg* 1971;50:587.

A small animal study (31 dogs) that served as the basis for the current choice of bretylium as the first-line antidysrhythmic agent in hypothermia.

Cabanac M. Temperature regulation. *Annu Rev Physiol* 1975;37:415.

This article lays the basic groundwork for discussions of hypothermia.

Herity B, Daly L, Bourke GJ, et al. Hypothermia and mortality and morbidity: an epidemiologic analysis. *J Epidemiol Community Health* 1991;45:19.

The results of a 7-year survey of hospital admissions and deaths in Ireland.

Kurtz KJ. Hypothermia in the elderly: the cold facts. *Geriatrics* 1982;37:85.

This article lays the basic groundwork for discussions of hypothermia.

Raheja R, Puri BK, Schaeffer RC. Shock due to profound hypothermia and alcohol ingestion. *Crit Care Med* 1984;9:644.

A case report highlighting the effects of alcohol-associated hypothermia.

Thompson R, Rich J, Chmelik F, et al. Evolutionary changes in the electrocardiogram of severe progressive hypothermia. *J Electrocardiol* 1977;10:67.

Another case report focused on the characteristic ECG changes seen in hypothermia.

Wagner JA, Robinson S, Marino RP. Age and temperature regulation of humans in neutral and cold environments. *J Appl Physiol* 1974;37:562.

This article lays the basic groundwork for discussions of hypothermia.

56. DISORDERS OF TEMPERATURE CONTROL: HYPERTHERMIA

Mark M. Wilson and Frederick J. Curley

I. **Overview.** This chapter reviews three of the major hyperthermic syndromes: heat stroke, malignant hyperthermia, and neuroleptic malignant syndrome (NMS). A fourth syndrome, drug-induced hyperthermia, is less well described and is only briefly discussed. Our knowledge of these conditions arose from the more common and better understood syndrome of heat stroke in which most deaths from hyperthermic syndromes result.

II. **Heat stroke.** Heat stroke is a syndrome of acute thermoregulatory failure in warm environments characterized by central nervous system depression, core temperatures usually higher than 40°C, and typical biochemical and physiologic abnormalities. Mortality in some series has reached 70%. During a warm summer in the United States, approximately 4,000 deaths may occur as a direct result of heat stroke.

A. **Etiology.** Exertional heat stroke is typically seen in younger persons who exercise at higher than normal ambient temperatures. Although thermoregulatory mechanisms are typically intact, they are overwhelmed by the thermal challenge of the environment and the great increase in endogenous heat production. Nonexertional ("classic") heat stroke affects predominantly elderly or sick persons and occurs almost exclusively during a heat wave. These patients frequently have some impairment of thermoregulatory control, and temperatures rise easily with thermal challenge. Causes of heat stroke fall into two categories: increased heat production and impaired heat loss.

Endogenous heat production during exertion ranges from 300 to 900 kcal per hour. Even in conditions favoring the maximal evaporation of sweat, only 500 to 600 kcal may be lost per hour. In these conditions, even a healthy person with intact regulatory mechanisms may be overwhelmed. Fever, thyrotoxicosis, and the hyperreactivity associated with amphetamine or hallucinogen use are other causes of an increased endogenous heat production.

Impaired voluntary control (as seen in schizophrenic, comatose, senile, or mentally deficient patients) increases the risk of heat stroke when ambient temperatures are high. These patients may fail to perceive a temperature rise, to move to a cooler location, or to change to lighter clothes.

Dehydration and impaired cardiovascular performance also predispose to heat stroke because they may decrease skin or muscle blood flow and may jeopardize any movement of heat from the core to the environment. On the other hand, acclimatization to higher ambient temperatures can greatly increase heat tolerance by increasing cardiac output, decreasing peak heart rate, and lowering the threshold necessary to induce sweating, to increase the volume of sweating, to expand extracellular volume, and to minimize sweat sodium loss.

Skin disorders that impair sweat gland function (e.g., cystic fibrosis, chronic idiopathic anhidrosis) and central nervous system lesions (e.g., hypothalamic lesions) that impair thermoregulation may predispose to heat stroke. Anhidrosis has been reported in some series in up to 100% of classic heat stroke victims. However, some persons do perspire profusely, a finding indicating that sweat gland malfunction is not inherent to the pathogenesis of this syndrome.

The increased risk of heat stroke in the elderly is primarily the result of their inability to sweat effectively. These patients are also more likely to have a compromised cardiovascular response to heat exposure, to have deficient voluntary control and poor acclimatization, and to take drugs that may adversely affect thermoregulation.

B. **Pathophysiology.** The primary injury in heat stroke is direct cellular toxicity of temperatures higher than 42°C. Above this temperature (called the critical thermal maximum), mitochondrial activity ceases, enzymatic reactions are dysfunctional, and cell membrane integrity becomes unstable. Factors such as dehydration, metabolic acidosis, and local hypoxia potentiate the damage. Muscle degeneration and necrosis result directly from the extremely high temperatures. Significant muscle enzyme elevation and severe rhabdomyolysis occur commonly in exertional heat stroke but rarely in classic heat stroke. Direct thermal toxicity to the brain and spinal cord rapidly produces cell death, cerebral edema, and local hemorrhage. These changes may lead to profound stupor or coma, almost universal features of all the hyperthermic syndromes. Seizures secondary to edema and hemorrhage are not uncommon. Moreover, ataxia, dysmetria, and dysarthria may be seen acutely and in survivors of hyperthermia.

Cardiac output is usually high in response to increased demands, low peripheral vascular resistance secondary to vasodilation, and dehydration. Hypotension occurs commonly as a result of either high output failure or temperature-induced myocardial hemorrhage and necrosis with subsequent cardiac depression and failure.

Some renal damage occurs in nearly all hyperthermic patients; it is potentiated by dehydration, cardiovascular collapse, and rhabdomyolysis. Acute renal failure occurs in 5% of patients with classic heat stroke, but it is seen in up to 35% of cases of exertional heat stroke. Urine findings include a characteristic "machine oil" appearance.

The combination of direct thermotoxicity and relative hypoperfusion of the intestines frequently leads to ischemic intestinal ulcerations and possibly frank bleeding. The liver appears to be particularly sensitive to temperature damage; hepatic necrosis and cholestasis occur in nearly every case and cause death in 5% to 10% of cases.

White blood cell counts are typically elevated from release of catecholamines and hemoconcentration. Anemia and a bleeding diathesis are frequently present. Disseminated intravascular coagulation is present in most cases of fatal hyperthermia and usually appears on the second or third day after the insult.

In heat stroke, sweating involves the active excretion of potassium from the body and produces normal to low serum potassium levels. With severe cell injury in exertional heat stroke, potassium levels may be extremely elevated from cell lysis. Hypophosphatemia and hypocalcemia also occur commonly.

Direct thermal injury to the pulmonary vascular endothelium may lead to cor pulmonale or acute respiratory distress syndrome. This and the tendency for myocardial dysfunction make pulmonary edema common.

C. Diagnosis. Heat stroke should be expected in any patient exercising in hot weather (ambient temperatures generally greater than 25°C) or in susceptible persons during heat waves (ambient peak temperatures exceed 32°C and minimum temperatures do not fall below 27°C). Coma or profound stupor is nearly always present, but the other traditional criteria of anhidrosis and core temperature higher than 41°C may be absent (profuse sweating is typical in exertional heat stroke). Diagnostic criteria for heat stroke includes a core temperature higher than 40°C, severely depressed mental status or coma, elevated serum creatine kinase levels, and a compatible history.

D. Treatment. Primary therapy includes cooling and decreasing thermogenesis. Cooling by either evaporative (placing a nude patient in a cool room, wetting the skin with water, and encouraging evaporation with fans) or direct external methods (immersing the patient in ice water or packing the patient in ice) has proved effective.

External methods suffer from inconvenience and the possibility that cold skin may vasoconstrict, thus limiting heat exchange from the core. Rarely, peritoneal lavage with iced saline, gastric lavage, hemodialysis or cardiopulmonary bypass with external cooling of the blood may be necessary to reduce the temperature. Temperature should be continuously monitored and cooling efforts stopped as it approaches 39°C.

Dysrhythmias, metabolic acidosis, and cardiogenic failure complicate the early management of hyperthermic crises. Hypotension should be treated initially with normal saline and, if necessary, isoproterenol. Dopamine and alpha-adrenergic agonists should be avoided because of their tendency for peripheral vasoconstriction. Digitalis should be avoided because of the likelihood of hyperkalemia.

Arterial blood gas analysis should be done early in treatment, and when blood is drawn in patients with core temperatures higher than 39°C, values should be corrected for temperature resulting from altered solubilities of oxygen and carbon dioxide. The net effect is that the patient is more acidotic and less hypoxemic than the uncorrected values imply. For clinical purposes, the following formulas may be used to correct arterial blood gas values measured at 37°C: for each 1°C the patient's temperature exceeds 37°C, one should increase the oxygen tension 7.2%, increase the carbon dioxide tension 4.4%, and lower the pH 0.015 units.

Morbidity and mortality are directly related to the peak temperature reached and the time spent at an elevated temperature. Delays in treatment of as little as 2 hours may increase the risk of death up to 70%. When heat stroke is swiftly recognized and aggressively treated, mortality should be minimal.

III. Malignant hyperthermia. Malignant hyperthermia is a drug- or stress-induced hypermetabolic syndrome characterized by vigorous muscle contractions, an abrupt increase in temperature, and cardiovascular collapse. It occurs, on average, in 1 of every 15,000 patients receiving anesthesia and has a mortality between 10% and 30%.

A. Etiology. Similar to exertional heat stroke, increased thermogenesis is responsible for overwhelming the patient's ability to dissipate heat. Here, however, a defect of calcium metabolism in skeletal muscles causes development of repeated or sustained contractions after specific exposures.

Although halothane and succinylcholine are involved in more than 80% of cases, many other agents have been implicated as well (e.g., enflurane, decamethonium, gallamine, diethyl ether, ketamine, phencyclidine, cyclopropane). Stress, anoxia, viral infections, and lymphoma have also been reported to trigger malignant hyperthermia.

B. Pathophysiology. Direct thermal injury is the predominant cause of toxicity resulting from sudden increases in temperature, frequently exceeding 42°C. Pathophysiologic changes parallel those of exertional heat stroke.

Vigorous muscle contractions almost immediately precipitate severe metabolic acidosis and increased carbon dioxide production. High elevations of creatine kinase, aldolase, and lactate dehydrogenase are virtually universal in full-blown episodes, a reflection of ongoing rhabdomyolysis. Hyperkalemia occurs in minutes to hours and, in combination with tissue hypoxia and acidosis, makes ventricular dysrhythmias more common.

Cerebral edema and hemorrhage from direct thermal injury produce coma. Seizures occur in most patients with uncontrolled cases. Renal failure from pigment load frequently occurs in malignant hyperthermia. Dehydration and low cardiac output contribute to this later as the syndrome progresses. Because higher maximal temperatures are usually seen in malignant hyperthermia, hepatic failure and gastrointestinal tract bleeding are more prominent than in heat stroke.

C. Diagnosis. The metabolic predisposition to malignant hyperthermia appears in general to be inherited in an autosomal dominant fashion with variable penetrance and expressivity. Because there is no one suitable noninvasive screening test, screening of family members (i.e., muscle biopsy for drug challenge) of proven cases remains the best method of identifying susceptible persons before hyperthermic crisis.

Early signs of hyperthermic crisis vary with the agent administered, but they include muscle rigidity (masseter contractures after succinylcholine), sinus tachycardia, supraventricular tachydysrhythmias, mottling or cyanosis of the skin, increased carbon dioxide production, and hypertension. Hyperthermia is typically a late sign in an acute crisis and is rapidly followed by hypotension, acidosis, peaked T waves on the electrocardiogram from hyperkalemia, and malignant ventricular dysrhythmias. Although malignant hyperthermia is not difficult to diagnose late in a full-blown crisis, early recognition may be difficult. Increased end-tidal carbon dioxide (from increased muscle metabolism) and masseter spasm are two signs that may be diagnostically helpful preceding hyperthermia.

Because malignant hyperthermia occurs almost exclusively in the perioperative setting, the differential diagnosis is generally limited. Thyroid storm (now infrequent) and pheochromocytoma may be difficult to distinguish from malignant hyperthermia in the anesthetized patient. The temperature rise in pheochromocytoma is typically much slower than in malignant hyperthermia. Hyperthermia from narcotic administration in patients taking monoamine oxidase inhibitors should also be considered in the differential diagnosis.

D. Treatment. Direct pharmacologic intervention to decrease thermogenesis is mandatory. Dantrolene acts by uncoupling the excitation-contraction mechanism in skeletal muscle and by lowering myoplasmic calcium. In an acute crisis, 1 to 2.5 mg/kg of fresh dantrolene should be given intravenously every 5 to 10 minutes; most authorities advise not to exceed 10 mg/kg. Oral or intravenous dosages of 1 to 2 mg/kg every 6 hours should continue for 24 to 48 hours.

Evaporative cooling, iced saline lavage (gastric, peritoneal), and infusion of chilled solutions may be helpful. Direct external cooling methods are helpful, but management of associated problems becomes almost impossible. Aggressive external cooling may be necessary if dantrolene fails to slow thermogenesis promptly.

Ventricular fibrillation with cardiovascular collapse is the most common cause of death in the early stages of the syndrome. Procainamide increases the uptake of myoplasmic calcium and should be given prophylactically as soon as malignant hyperthermia is diagnosed.

Because seizures occur nearly universally, prophylactic treatment with phenobarbitol is strongly recommended.

IV. Neuroleptic malignant syndrome. NMS results primarily from an imbalance of central neurotransmitters, and may be diagnosed in any patient with (a) an unexplained temperature elevation, (b) muscular rigidity and characteristic extrapyramidal signs, and (c) a history of recent neuroleptic drug use. Mental status changes, coma, and catatonia are common. Most current knowledge is derived from case reports rather than from systematic study. Incidence rates for NMS from long-term prospective studies in inpatient psychiatric hospitals range from 0.07% to 2.2% and appear to be declining.

A. Etiology. In all reports of NMS, patients either were receiving agents that decrease dopaminergic hypothalamic tone or the syndrome appeared after withdrawal of dopaminergic agents. Butyrophenones (haloperidol), phenothiazines, thioxanthenes, and dibenzoxazepines are believed to act as dopamine receptor blocking agents. Atypical antipsychotic drugs (risperidone, molindone, clozapine, fluoxetine) and dopamine blockers used to treat gastrointestinal tract disease (metoclopramide, domperidone) have also caused NMS. Drugs acting at the D_2 dopamine binding sites appear to have the greatest potential for causing the syndrome.

B. Pathophysiology. The increase in muscular rigidity, akinesia, mutism, and tremor are thought to be due to hypothalamic dopaminergic imbalance. Motor abnormalities vary, but in general they are typical of the parkinsonian type of extrapyramidal reactions. The central origin of the muscle spasm is further suggested by its resolution with the use of centrally acting dopaminergic agents (bromocriptine, amantadine, L-DOPA).

The hyperthermia of NMS results from an increase in endogenous heat production, impaired heat dissipation, loss of voluntary temperature regulation, and possibly an elevation of the hypothalamic setpoint. The finding that the degree of temperature increase varies directly with the severity of muscular rigidity strongly suggests that muscle contracture is responsible for increased thermogenesis; in this sense, NMS is similar to malignant hyperthermia. The syndromes are, however, clearly different in the following ways: (a) the causative agents are dissimilar; (b) in NMS the driving force to increased temperature is a change in hypothalamic tone, whereas in malignant hyperthermia it is a calcium transport defect in skeletal muscle metabolism; (c) malignant hyperthermia does not have prominent extrapyramidal symptoms; and (d) NMS lacks a hereditary predisposition.

Because of the relatively low maximal temperatures (39.9°C on average; only 40% are higher than 40°C) in NMS compared with the other hyperthermic syndromes, direct thermal injury occurs less often. Rhabdomyolysis is usually mild and may occur in up to one-third of patients. Renal failure, from myoglobin-induced acute tubular necrosis and dehydration from diaphoresis, occurs in 9% to 30% of patients and is usually transient and mild, but it is associated with substantially increased mortality. Any hematologic or hepatic alterations are also mild. Seizures occur only rarely.

Pulmonary complications, from extrapyramidal actions, are probably the most serious frequent sequelae of NMS. These include copious sialorrhea leading to aspiration pneumonia and the need for mechanical ventilation.

C. Diagnosis. Onset of symptoms occurs within hours of the initial dose up to 4 weeks later, but primarily within the first 2 weeks. Early symptoms usually include dysphagia or dysarthria, pseudoparkinsonism, dystonia, and catatonic behavior. Muscle rigidity generally precedes (59%) or is concurrent (23%) with hyperthermia. Autonomic signs of hypermetabolism (diaphoresis, tachycardia, tachypnea, changes in blood pressure) suggest the onset of hyperthermia, and peak temperatures are usually reached within 48 hours of onset of symptoms.

A thorough examination and diagnostic evaluation for other causes of hyperthermia should be conducted. Patients without classic symptoms of NMS are more likely to have another cause of hyperthermia. Heat stroke must be considered in patients who take neuroleptic agents during periods of high ambient temperature or after vigorous exercise. Unlike NMS, however, heat stroke is usually accompanied by flaccid obtundation, and muscular rigidity is rare. Malignant hyperthermia more closely resembles NMS in that both conditions have increased thermogenesis from muscular rigidity and similar laboratory findings, and both respond to dantrolene. In most cases, an adequate history should clearly separate the two syndromes. Additionally, the symptoms of malignant hyperthermia are much more rapid in onset and more severe.

D. Treatment. The goal of treatment of NMS is to reduce the temperature, to reverse extrapyramidal side effects, and to prevent sequelae such as renal failure and pneumonia. Specific agents used to decrease thermogenesis (by reducing muscle contracture) include dantrolene, curare, pancuronium, amantadine, bromocriptine, and L-DOPA. Paralysis should produce a prompt decrease in temperature, but this requires mechanical ventilation and extensive support. Bromocriptine (2.5 mg three times daily), amantadine (100 to 200 mg twice daily), and carbidopa/L-DOPA (10 to 100 mg three times daily) increase central dopaminergic tone, decreasing the central drive for muscular rigidity and thermogenesis. These agents also act directly to reduce extrapyramidal side effects.

By minimizing rhabdomyolysis and by aggressive hydration and diuresis, acute tubular necrosis and renal failure may be avoided. Prophylactic intubation should be strongly considered for patients with excessive sialorrhea, swallowing dysfunction, or coma.

The best treatment regimen for NMS remains to be determined. The duration of treatment must be adjusted according to the metabolism of the inciting agent, but in most cases it can be tapered over 1 to 2 weeks. Although mortality rates as high as 20% to 30% are reported, this can probably be reduced to less than 10% with appropriate support.

V. Drug-induced hyperthermia. Numerous drugs (e.g., cocaine, phencyclidine, amphetamine, lysergic acid diethylamide) may cause hyperthermia through excessive muscular contracture or hypermetabolism. The so-called serotonin syndrome (SS) is the result of drugs that directly or indirectly elevate central nervous system serotonin neurotransmission (e.g., tricyclic antidepressants, amphetamines, meperidine, dextromethorphan, monoamine oxidase inhibitors, and the serotonin reuptake inhibitors). SS is primarily (greater than 85% of cases) due to combination drug therapy and most commonly presents with muscle rigidity, autonomic nervous system dysfunction, and hyperthermia. These reactions appear to be idiosyncratic; they are infrequent in comparison to the total number of persons using the drug and may occur after low-dose use or massive overdose. Treatment in general parallels that for exertional heat stroke and is usually associated with a favorable prognosis. In all cases, treatment should be directed at minimizing the toxicity of the causative drug, aggressive supportive care, and consideration for use of a specific serotonin receptor antagonist such as cyproheptadine.

Selected Readings

Caroff SN, Mann SC. Neuroleptic malignant syndrome. *Med Clin North Am* 1993; 77:185.

A well-written general overview of NMS.

Gillman PK. The serotonin syndrome and its treatment. *J Psychopharmacol* 1999; 13:100.

A recent, thorough review of what is known of the serotonin syndrome.

Gronert GA. Malignant hyperthermia. *Anesthesiology* 1980;53:395.

A detailed and readable early review of malignant hyperthermia.

Kilbourne EM, Choi K, Jones S, et al. Risk factors for heat stroke: a case-control study. *JAMA* 1982;247:3332.

A case-control study of 156 subjects and 462 matched controls that helped identify important factors associated with heat stroke.

Knochel JP. Environmental heat illness: an eclectic review. *Arch Intern Med* 1974; 133:841.

Knochel JP. Heat stroke and related heat disorders. *Dis Mon* 1989;35:306.

Two classic reviews of environmental heat stress illnesses by one of the world's foremost authorities.

Strazis KP, Fox AW. Malignant hyperthermia: a review of published cases. *Anesth Analg* 1993;77:297.

A compilation and review of the epidemiology, associated various drugs, and mortality rates for the 503 reported cases of malignant hyperthermia reported in the literature to that date.

57. SEVERE UPPER AIRWAY INFECTIONS

Oren P. Schaefer, Richard S. Irwin, and Teresa E. Jacobs

I. General principles. The upper airway consists of the nose, mouth, nasopharynx, oropharynx, and hypopharynx; it communicates with the paranasal sinuses. Although minor infections in these areas are common, deep neck infections can be fatal.

II. Supraglottitis (epiglottitis). Supraglottitis is an acute, usually bacterial inflammation of the supraglottic structures—the epiglottis, aryepiglottic folds, and arytenoids—that can progress to abrupt and fatal airway obstruction. The condition is well recognized in children, in whom the presentation and course are usually fulminant. In adults, the course is often more indolent, and the mortality is higher, largely because of misdiagnosis and unexpected airway obstruction.

Haemophilus influenzae type B has been identified most often in both pediatric and adult cases. In the past, about 60% of children had documented bacteremia, nearly always from *H. influenzae.* Blood cultures in adults are positive in only 15%. With the introduction of the *H. influenzae* B vaccine, this infection in children has become uncommon. Various other bacteria, viruses, and *Candida* species have also been described.

A. Diagnosis

1. History and physical examination. In the young child, sore throat, then dysphagia, is followed within hours by stridor. The child leans forward and is usually pale and frightened. Breathing is slow, and drooling is characteristic. The progression to respiratory depression and arrest may be sudden. In adults, the frequency of misdiagnosis is as high as 75%. Adults present with a sore throat, with or without dysphagia, and less commonly with respiratory difficulty, muffled voice, drooling, fever, and stridor. Most patients have a preceding upper respiratory tract infection. The duration of symptoms is variable, ranging from hours to almost a week. In older children and in adults, one should consider supraglottitis when sore throat and dysphagia are out of proportion to visible signs of pharyngitis.

Evaluation depends in part on age and severity of symptoms. In young children when the presentation is classic, pharyngeal examination should not be attempted. The patient may need an artificial airway established in the controlled setting of an operating room; the examination can be done at that time. In older patients without respiratory distress, examination of the larynx and supralaryngeal structures is recommended initially.

2. Diagnostic tests. A lateral soft tissue radiograph of the neck may be helpful to rule in acute supraglottitis. Epiglottic thickening (thumb sign), swelling of the aryepiglottic folds, ballooning of the hypopharynx, and narrowing of the vallecula are important radiologic findings. When the suspicion of supraglottitis is high, a normal radiograph is inadequate to exclude the diagnosis, and direct visualization of the structures should be pursued. Only in the stable child should a lateral neck radiograph be performed. Few laboratory tests are helpful at the time of initial evaluation. Blood cultures are essential. Throat cultures are of no value at presentation and correlate poorly with blood culture results and clinical outcome.

B. Treatment. Maintaining airway patency is paramount. In children, early placement of an artificial airway significantly reduces mortality. Intubation for adults is reserved for early signs of airway obstruction. All patients must be observed in an intensive care unit with immediate availability of equipment and personnel for emergency intubation. Humidification and mild sedation can be valuable. Antibiotic regimens must cover *H. influenzae* and also, in adults, *Staphylococcus aureus, Streptococcus pneumoniae,* and other streptococcal species and are initially given intravenously and continued by mouth for a

10- or 14-day course. Use of corticosteroids in patients with infectious supraglottitis is controversial.

III. Infections of the deep spaces of the neck. Knowledge of the anatomy is a prerequisite to understanding the etiology, manifestations, complications, and treatment of deep neck infections. The fascial planes both separate and connect distant areas, thereby limiting and directing the spread of infection. Suppurative processes in three cervical spaces—submandibular, lateral pharyngeal, and retropharyngeal—are considered life-threatening. The pertinent anatomy can be reviewed in the chapter on severe upper respiratory airway infections in the fourth edition of *Intensive Care Medicine.*

A. Etiology. Bacteria of the oral flora can become pathogenic when mucosal barriers are interrupted. Infections are often due to a mixture of anaerobic and aerobic organisms; the former predominate, with *Peptostreptococcus, Fusobacterium,* and *Bacteroides* most frequently isolated. Facultative gram-negative bacilli are less common causes of deep neck infections.

B. Submandibular space infection. Infection in the submandibular space is exemplified by Ludwig's angina. Most patients are young, otherwise healthy adults and present with neck pain and swelling, tooth pain, and dysphagia. Odontogenic infections are implicated in up to 90% of cases. Dyspnea, tachypnea, stridor, a muffled voice, drooling, and tongue swelling all can occur. Examination reveals bilateral, woody submandibular swelling, mouth distortion secondary to enlargement of the tongue, and fever. Trismus is not uncommon and indicates spread to the lateral pharyngeal space. Airway obstruction can result from obstruction by the swollen, displaced tongue, edema of the neck and glottis, extension to involve the epiglottis, and poor control of pharyngeal secretions.

C. Lateral pharyngeal space infections. Signs of anterior compartment involvement include unilateral trismus resulting from irritation of the internal pterygoid muscle, induration and swelling along the angle of the jaw, high fever, and medial bulging of the lateral pharyngeal wall. A history of recent upper respiratory infection, pharyngitis, or tonsillitis is often present. In posterior compartment infections, signs of sepsis are the cardinal features. Trismus and tonsillar prolapse are notably absent. Dyspnea may occur as edema involves the larynx and epiglottis. External swelling may be visible when it spreads to the parotid space, but most patients have no localizing signs.

Suppurative jugular venous thrombosis is the most common complication and is associated with bacteremia and septic emboli. Involvement of the carotid artery has a mortality of up to 40%. Because the carotid sheath is dense and not easily invaded, 1 or 2 weeks of illness usually precede arterial erosion. Signs suggestive of carotid sheath involvement include persistent tonsillar swelling, ipsilateral Horner syndrome, and cranial nerve palsies. Impending rupture of a carotid aneurysm may be signaled by "herald bleeds" from the nose, mouth, or ears.

D. Retropharyngeal space infections. Retropharyngeal space abscesses are uncommon and most often are seen in children less than 6 years of age. The lymph node chains in this space are the source of most retropharyngeal space abscesses; they regress by about the age of 4 years, a finding that explains the higher frequency in young children. Symptoms include fever, irritability, and refusal to eat. The neck is often held stiffly, sometimes tilted away from the involved side. Dyspnea and dysphagia may occur. Respiratory compromise can occur as the abscess protrudes anteriorly or ruptures into the airway, with aspiration and possible asphyxiation.

In adults, fever, sore throat, dysphagia, nasal obstruction, noisy breathing, stiff neck, and dyspnea are most common. Pain originating in or radiating to the posterior neck that increases with swallowing suggests the diagnosis. Severe respiratory distress, particularly if accompanied by chest pain or pleurisy, suggests mediastinal extension.

E. Descending infections. Any deep neck infection has access to the posterior mediastinum. Descending, necrotizing mediastinitis carries a mortality of more than 40%. It develops as soon as 12 hours or as late as 2 weeks from the onset of the primary infection and is manifested by widespread necrosis that extends to the diaphragm and occasionally into the retroperitoneal space. A ruptured mediastinal abscess may result in purulent pleural and pericardial effusions. Severe dyspnea and pleuritic or retrosternal chest pain occurring with or subsequent to the onset of an oropharyngeal infection are suggestive.

Cervical necrotizing fasciitis progresses superficially along the fascial planes of the neck and chest wall, and in its early course, the physical appearance may be deceptively benign. Skin erythema occurs initially and progresses to dusky skin discoloration, blisters or bullae, and, eventually, skin necrosis. Gas in the tissues can be readily seen by computed tomography (CT). Surgical exploration and wide excision are essential to determine the full extent of necrosis and to improve prognosis.

F. Diagnosis. It is important to distinguish the space or spaces involved in deep neck infections, to prevent potentially devastating complications and to perform early surgical therapy if necessary. Involvement of multiple spaces and interference with the examination by trismus can make evaluation difficult. Initial assessment should always include a lateral neck radiograph. This study is particularly valuable in evaluating retropharyngeal space infections; prevertebral soft tissue swelling and the loss or reversal of the normal cervical lordosis suggest infection. CT can define neck masses with excellent results and is indicated in all cases. Ultrasonography of the neck may be valuable to identify fluid-filled masses and to guide needle aspiration for culture and surgical drainage. Its specificity may not be high, and CT is preferable when it is available. Magnetic resonance imaging offers little advantage over CT. If carotid arterial involvement is suspected, carotid artery angiography is recommended.

G. Treatment. All deep neck infections require hospitalization for proper treatment. Therapy includes airway management, antibiotics, and timely surgical exploration.

1. **Airway management.** Upper airway obstruction most often complicates infections of the submandibular space. Endotracheal intubation can be difficult to perform because of trismus and intraoral swelling. Blind intubation is unsafe because of the risk of trauma to the posterior pharyngeal wall or rupture of an abscess in the lateral pharyngeal or retropharyngeal space. Intubation over a fiberoptic laryngoscope is recommended.
2. **Antimicrobial therapy.** Intravenous antibiotic therapy is required for all neck infections. Given the rising frequency of penicillin resistance among oral anaerobes, the combination of high-dose penicillin G and metronidazole is recommended. Agents active against gram-negative bacilli are used in patients at risk for prior colonization or if these pathogens are identified in culture. In patients with a history of penetrating trauma, vertebral disc disease, and intravenous drug use, coverage for *S. aureus* is necessary.
3. **Surgery.** Despite conservative therapy with antibiotics and selective needle aspiration, surgical intervention may be necessary. This is most important when infection involves the retropharyngeal space and the lateral pharyngeal space. The surgical approach to drainage is intraoral or extraoral, depending on the space involved, and is guided by imaging studies.

IV. Sinusitis. Sinusitis in the intensive care unit usually presents in two situations: (a) an uncommon, potentially fatal complication of a community-acquired sinus infection such as meningitis, osteomyelitis, orbital infection, or brain abscess; or (b) a hospital-acquired sinus infection.

A. Etiology. In community-acquired acute sinusitis, the most common causes are *H. influenzae, S. pneumoniae,* viruses, and in children, *Moraxella catarrhalis.* More than half the cases of hospital-acquired sinusitis are of polymicrobial origin, although anaerobes are relatively uncommon. Invasive rhinocerebral mucormycosis is seen most often in association with patients with diabetes mellitus and acidosis, burns, chronic renal disease, cirrhosis, and immunosuppression. *Aspergillus* species can be invasive in immunocompromised patients. Intracranial complications can occur as a result of expansile disease or pressure necrosis.

B. Diagnosis

1. **History and physical examination.** Failure of nasal symptoms to resolve after a typical cold, facial pain, and a change in nasal discharge from clear to purulent are the most common complaints in adults. Other complaints include postnasal drip, nasal obstruction, cough, and decreased smell. Maxillary toothache, poor response to decongestants, abnormal transillumination, and purulent nasal discharge are independent predictors of sinusitis. Sphenoid sinusitis is uncommon, but delay in diagnosis has been associated with increased morbidity and mortality. The presentation is one of a severe headache, often accompanied by fever and nasal discharge. Trigeminal hyperesthesia or hypesthesia occurs in 30%.

   Nosocomial sinusitis occurs in 5% to 8% of admissions to intensive care units. Orotracheal as well as nasotracheal airways, nasogastric tubes, and nasal packing are all risks for its development. Other contributing factors are a history of corticosteroid therapy, obtundation, immobility, supine positioning, and blood in the sinuses on admission.

2. **Radiology.** Sinus radiographs predict culture-positive antral aspirates in 70% to 80% of acute and more than 90% of chronic cases. Findings include an air-fluid level, opacification, and mucosal thickening of more than 5 mm in adults. CT scans of the sinuses are particularly useful for evaluating possible bony or soft tissue complications and when considering a diagnosis of sinusitis in the critically ill. This is particularly true for sphenoid sinusitis in which it is essential to exclude extension to nearby structures. Air-fluid levels are not always caused by infection.

3. **Antral aspirate.** Aspiration of the maxillary antrum is considered the standard technique by which to diagnose infectious maxillary sinusitis. Antral aspiration in critically ill patients can help to distinguish between infectious and noninfectious sinus involvement as well as to direct the most appropriate antibiotic therapy for nosocomial infections.

C. Treatment. Therapy of uncomplicated sinusitis includes antibiotics and decongestants. In acute sinusitis, coverage against *H. influenzae* and *Streptococcus* species and *M. catarrhalis* in children is required. Empiric treatment is appropriate, and sinus aspiration is reserved for complicated or refractory cases. Effective bacterial eradication can be achieved with 10 to 14 days of antibiotics. In chronic sinusitis, treatment reflects the preponderance of anaerobes and increased numbers of beta-lactamase–producing organisms. The duration of therapy is unclear, but a course of at least 3 weeks is preferred. Concomitant use of topical vasoconstrictors and oral decongestants is important to facilitate sinus drainage. Because reduction of mucosal swelling is important, antihistamines and often topical steroids are suggested, particularly in patients with an allergic component. With nosocomial sinusitis, removal of nasopharyngeal tubes should be attempted. Antibiotics must be effective against facultative gram-negative rods and *S. aureus* and are given intravenously for 2 weeks. Response should be rapid, within 48 to 96 hours. Surgical drainage is reserved for patients who do not respond to medical therapy or, in the case of sphenoid sinusitis, who develop neurologic signs while receiving appropriate antibiotic therapy.

D. Complications. Complications of acute sinusitis are rare but can be fatal. Orbital complications include cellulitis and abscess, subperiosteal abscess, and cavernous sinus thrombosis. The last complication has a mortality of more than 20%. Intracranial complications include osteomyelitis, meningitis and epidural abscess, subdural empyema, and brain abscess, and they have an overall mortality of 40%.

Selected Readings

Balcerak RJ, Sisto JM, Bosack RC. Cervicofacial necrotizing fasciitis: report of three cases and literature review. *J Oral Maxillofac Surg* 1988;46:450.

The key to successful management of such infections is early diagnosis of the disease process with prompt surgical and medical intervention.

Barratt GE, Koopman CF, Coulthard SW. Retropharyngeal abscess: a ten-year experience. *Laryngoscope* 1984;94:455.

Eight cases are described with a discussion of anatomy, bacteriology, radiology, treatment, and complications.

Bert F, Lambert-Zechovsky N. Microbiology of nosocomial sinusitis in intensive care unit patients. *J Infect* 1995;31:5.

Infections were often polymicrobial and the common pathogens, S. aureus, Pseudomonas aeruginosa, Acinetobacter baumannii, *and* Enterobacteriaceae, *often drug resistant.*

Blomquist IK, Bayer AS. Life-threatening deep fascial space infections of the head and neck. *Infect Dis Clin North Am* 1988;2:237.

A concise review of the three major deep space neck infections.

Clayman GL, Adams GL, Paugh DR, et al. Intracranial complications of paranasal sinusitis: a combined institutional review. *Laryngoscope* 1991;101:234.

Subdural empyema, brain abscess, venous sinus thrombosis, and osteomyelitis are all potential complications of paranasal sinusitis. A discussion of these true medical and surgical emergencies is presented.

Dzyak WR, Zide MF. Diagnosis and treatment of lateral pharyngeal space infections. *J Oral Maxillofac Surg* 1984;42:243.

Four cases are reviewed with an excellent discussion of anatomy, pathophysiology, therapy, and complications of lateral pharyngeal space infection.

Estrera AS, Landay MJ, Grisham JM, et al. Descending necrotizing mediastinitis. *Surg Gynecol Obstet* 1983;157:545.

Ten patients with mediastinitis complicating oropharyngeal infection are described in detail.

Gidley PW, Ghorayeb BY, Stiernberg CM. Contemporary management of deep neck space infections. *Otolaryngol Head Neck Surg* 1997;116:16.

The operative techniques and antibiotics used are discussed. The main complications of jugular vein thrombosis, carotid artery rupture, and mediastinitis are described.

Mayo-Smith MF, Spinale JW, Donskey CJ, et al. Acute epiglottitis: an 18-year experience in Rhode Island. *Chest* 1995;108:1640.

Four hundred seven cases were identified in children and adults. Epiglottitis now occurs almost exclusively in adults, often with less severe symptoms and a lower incidence of H. influenzae *infection.*

Rothrock SG, Pignatiello GA, Howard RM. Radiologic diagnosis of epiglottitis: objective criteria for all ages. *Ann Emerg Med* 1990;19:978.

Various measurements on the soft tissue lateral neck radiograph are described in adults and children and are found to have excellent sensitivity for the radiologic diagnosis of epiglottitis.

Solomon P, Weisbrod M, Irish JC, et al. Adult epiglottitis: the Toronto Hospital experience. *J Otolaryngol* 1998;27:332.

Soft tissue lateral neck radiographs were abnormal in 88%, but they had a 12% false-negative rate. A rapid clinical course (less than 12 hours), evidence of tachycardia, and positive pharyngeal or blood cultures were factors that selected for a group of patients requiring formal airway intervention.

Talmor M, Li P, Barie PS. Acute paranasal sinusitis in critically ill patients: guidelines for prevention, diagnosis, and treatment. *Clin Infect Dis* 1997;25:1441.

Nosocomial sinusitis is common, is usually caused by gram-negative bacilli or is polymicrobial, and is best evaluated by CT scanning of all paranasal sinuses.

Thadepall H, Mandall AK. Anatomic basis of head and neck infections. *Infect Dis Clin North Am* 1988;2:21.

An excellent review of pertinent anatomy.

58. ACUTE INFECTIOUS PNEUMONIA

Oren P. Schaefer and Michael S. Niederman

I. General principles. With more than 4 million cases in the United States annually and ranking as the sixth leading cause of death, pneumonia remains a significant health problem. Up to 20% of patients with community-acquired pneumonia (CAP) require hospitalization. Of patients hospitalized for other reasons, 10% to 20% develop nosocomial pneumonia, and the percentage is higher in patients with the acute respiratory distress syndrome. Underlying comorbidity and certain medical interventions not only increase the risk for pneumonia, but also increase the morbidity and mortality from it (Table 58-1).

II. Pneumonia in the intensive care unit

A. Severe community-acquired pneumonia. A few patients present from the community with severe pneumonia. Mortality rates for patients admitted to the intensive care unit (ICU) with CAP range from 21% to 54%. Although there is no uniform definition, the American Thoracic Society (ATS) guideline on CAP, as well as other guidelines, have suggested criteria for severe CAP. Such criteria may be overly sensitive, but their presence suggests the likelihood of more significant disease with an associated increased mortality risk, and the clinician should consider admitting the patient to an ICU. (See Selected Readings.) The use of early and effective empiric therapy and ICU admission can improve survival in severe CAP.

B. Nosocomial pneumonia. Pneumonia is the infection most likely to contribute to death of hospitalized patients. Risk factors for nosocomial pneumonia are grouped into 4 categories: underlying acute illness that predisposes to secondary pneumonia; coexisting medical illness; factors associated with therapies frequently used in the ICU; and malnutrition. The most important risk factor for nosocomial pneumonia is intubation with mechanical ventilation, which increases the risk 7- to 21-fold. Antibiotic use adds to the risk, as does colonization with bacteriologically virulent pathogens such as *Pseudomonas aeruginosa* and *Acinetobacter* sp. Other conditions associated with an increased risk include general surgery, acute respiratory distress syndrome, head injury, advanced age, obesity, cardiac or pulmonary disease, renal failure, malignancy, diabetes mellitus, tracheostomy, nasogastric tubes use, and use of corticosteroids, antibiotics and H_2 antagonists.

III. Pathogenesis. An understanding of normal host defense mechanisms and impairments and the pathogenesis of pneumonia are important in evaluating and managing the patient. Many diseases increase the risk of pneumonia as a result of disease-associated dysfunction of respiratory host defenses. A full discussion is beyond the scope of this manual, but one is referred to the chapter on acute infectious pneumonia in the fourth edition of *Intensive Care Medicine.*

IV. Etiology

A. Community-acquired pneumonia. Despite an extensive and costly diagnostic evaluation, the agent causing pneumonia can be identified in only approximately 50% of cases. Organisms identified as causing severe CAP include those that also cause less severe disease. The most common organism is *Streptococcus pneumoniae,* followed by *Legionella pneumophila, Haemophilus influenzae, Mycoplasma pneumoniae, Chlamydia pneumoniae,* and, less commonly, *Staphylococcus aureus,* anaerobes, and enteric gram-negative bacilli. The frequency of viral infection causing CAP is not known, but it likely is as high as one-third of all cases. The incidence of each pathogen depends on many factors including the age and comorbidities of the patient as well as the severity of the acute illness. In specific clinical settings, certain pathogens may be more common.

TABLE 58-1. Conditions and interventions that increase risk, morbidity, and mortality of pneumonia[a]

Condition	Intervention
Age >65 yr	Antibiotic therapy
Cardiac disease	Gastric acid suppression
Chronic obstructive pulmonary disease	Endotracheal intubation
Diabetes mellitus	Medications
Renal disease	Corticosteroids
Hepatic disease	Immunosuppressants
Malnutrition	Central nervous system depressants
Bronchiectasis	
Malignancy	
Splenic dysfunction	
Immunosuppressive illness	

[a] Underlying comorbidities and certain medical interventions noted in the table not only increase the risk for pneumonia but also increase the morbidity and mortality from it.

B. Nosocomial pneumonia. When pneumonia develops in hospital patients, the predominant pathogens are enteric gram-negative bacilli, particularly when pneumonia is of late onset (on or after day 5 of admission). These organisms are more likely to be drug resistant; similarly, *S. aureus* is more likely to be methicillin resistant. The latter is particularly common in patients with underlying chronic obstructive pulmonary disease or prior antibiotic use or in patients receiving mechanical ventilation. These situations, as well as chronic corticosteroid use, are risk factors for *P. aeruginosa.* In intubated, mechanically ventilated patients, polymicrobial infections are not unusual. Methicillin-sensitive *S. aureus, Streptococcus pneumoniae,* and *H. influenzae* are more common in early-onset (before day 5) nosocomial pneumonia.

V. Clinical presentation

A. Community-acquired pneumonia. The signs and symptoms of pneumonia depend on both host and bacterial factors. Acute onset of fever and chills, pleuritic chest pain, and productive cough are classic symptoms of pneumonia. Some patients, especially the elderly, may have a more indolent presentation with preceding upper respiratory tract symptoms, fever without chills, nonproductive cough, headache, and myalgias. The presentation depends on the host's inflammatory response, and patients with altered immune function have a more subtle clinical presentation. Elderly patients may present with only mental status changes.

B. Nosocomial pneumonia. In the ICU, it is difficult to determine when hospital-acquired pneumonia is present. Clinical diagnosis has been notoriously poor. A weighted scoring system using six clinical variables—fever, white blood cell count and differential, the presence of pathogens in the sputum, purulence of sputum, radiographic changes, and changes in oxygenation—may be helpful. Elderly and immunosuppressed patients may have few clinical findings when pneumonia develops in the hospital. Conversely, patients receiving mechanical ventilation who have infectious tracheobronchitis may have purulent secretions, fever, and pathogens colonizing the sputum, but not pneumonia.

VI. Approach to the patient with overwhelming pneumonia. Three groups of patients are seen by the critical care physician: the community patient with life-threatening pneumonia; the compromised host either in the hospital already or coming from the community or a nursing home; and the patient already in the ICU, often receiving mechanical ventilation, who deteriorates with a nosocomial lower respiratory tract infection.

A. Historical information. Comorbid illness, medication use, history of immunosuppression, geographic and travel history, and exposure to animals are most pertinent.

B. Physical examination. The examination may not itself be specific for a diagnosis of pneumonia, but it is valuable in conjunction with other data. Findings may help to predict the severity of disease. One should look for evidence of pleural effusion or metastatic infection. Dermatologic findings such as erythema nodosum or ecthyma gangrenosum may suggest a specific pathogen or group of organisms.

C. Diagnostic testing

1. **Routine laboratory tests.** A relatively streamlined evaluation is recommended. Chest radiograph, complete blood count, routine chemistry studies, blood cultures, and an assessment of oxygenation should be performed on all patients considered for hospitalization. Most laboratory results are best used to predict disease severity.
2. **Serology.** Routine serologic testing is not recommended. Acute antibody titers are rarely elevated, and the rise in convalescent titers can take weeks. Serologic evaluation is reserved for retrospective epidemiologic purposes to document viral and atypical pathogen infection. Urinary *Legionella* antigen may be valuable in those with severe CAP, with a yield of approximately 50%; it is only positive in serogroup I infection.
3. **Chest radiography.** Although radiographic patterns may suggest a specific pathogen, they are not diagnostic. Multilobar involvement carries a worse prognosis. One should examine the radiograph for pleural effusions and evidence of cavitation. In the ICU, the limitations of chest radiography must be recognized. Coexisting and preexisting lung disease may obscure the findings of pneumonia, and many noninfectious processes can mimic pneumonia.
4. **Sputum examination.** Routine sputum Gram stain and culture remain controversial; results often do not affect empiric therapy. Up to 30% of patients admitted with pneumonia do not produce sputum, and when it is obtained, its interpretation depends on the quality of the sample and the expertise of the reader. Sputum evaluation may be valuable in the patient at risk for infection with an atypical or opportunistic or resistant organisms or tuberculosis.
5. **Culture.** A definitive diagnosis of a specific pathogen is certain only if cultures of blood, pleural fluid, or spinal fluid are positive. Bacteremia is uncommon, occurring in only 15% of patients with CAP and in only 8% to 15% of patients with nosocomial pneumonia. Expectorated or suctioned sputum can be cultured, but the results are difficult to interpret because of the problem in separating infection from colonization in the critically ill.

D. Invasive diagnostic culture techniques. Techniques that avoid the overgrowth by colonizing rather than pathogenic organisms have been devised. *Transtracheal aspiration* by puncture of the cricothyroid membrane has limited value and is no longer practiced. *Transthoracic needle aspiration* of the lung is limited by a high false-negative rate and a risk of pneumothorax and hemoptysis of 30% and 10%, respectively. The role of *flexible bronchoscopy* in evaluating patients with severe CAP has expanded. Bronchoscopically directed *protected specimen brush* (PSB) catheters and *bronchoalveolar lavage* (BAL) are of value in both patients with CAP and those with nosocomial pneumonia. Quantitative cultures of PSB can give accurate estimates of the numbers and types of bacteria present in lung tissue when more than 10^3 organisms/mL are isolated. BAL remains most valuable in establishing nonbacterial causes of infection, especially in the immunocompromised host or the patient with acquired immunodeficiency syndrome. The use of bronchoscopy in the diagnosis of ventilator-associated pneumonia (VAP) remains controversial. The visualization of purulent secretions seen surging from distal bronchi during exhalation may be predictive of VAP. *Open lung biopsy* is the unequivocal standard for the diagnosis of infection and is most often used in the immunocompromised host with rapidly progressing lung infection, particularly when invasive fungal or viral species are considered.

VII. Differential diagnosis. A differential diagnosis for pneumonia exists. In the patient who is critically ill, diseases that mimic pneumonia may be more common, as discussed in the article by Lynch and Sitrin.

VIII. Treatment

A. Supportive therapy. The role of supportive therapy is critical because the use of antibiotics may not alter outcome during the first 24 hours of treatment.

1. **Nutritional therapy.** Nutritional evaluation and support early in the course of pneumonia are recommended. Enteral nutrition is the preferred route because data suggest better preservation of immune function. Although small-bore tubes placed in the jejunum may theoretically minimize aspiration risk, no data prove this hypothesis.
2. **Chest physical therapy.** There is little to support its routine use in patients with an effective cough and minimal secretions. This technique is best reserved for patients with pneumonia along with bronchiectasis, cystic fibrosis, and diseases associated with bronchorrhea.
3. **Aerosols and humidity.** Humidification to reduce mucus viscosity has little if any impact and may provoke cough. Mucolytics such as *N*-acetylcysteine can precipitate bronchospasm and therefore must be used selectively. Beta$_2$-adrenergic bronchodilators can enhance mucociliary clearance and ciliary beat frequency, although they are best reserved for treatment of patients with chronic obstructive pulmonary disease or asthma and pneumonia.

B. Antibiotic therapy. Effective antibiotic therapy has been shown to improve survival in patients with severe CAP. Empiric antibiotic therapy is indicated but can be modified as dictated by the results of the diagnostic investigation. Both the ATS and the Infectious Disease Society of America have published guidelines for management and treatment of severe CAP. (See Selected Readings.)

1. **Severe community-acquired pneumonia.** Initial therapy should consist of a third-generation cephalosporin, ceftriaxone or ceftizoxime, plus a macrolide, such as erythromycin or azithromycin, given intravenously. In a clinical setting in which *P. aeruginosa* may be more common, an antipseudomonal penicillin or ceftazidime and an aminoglycoside should be used. If *L. pneumophila* is identified, rifampin, 600 mg per day, should be added.

   The frequency of penicillin resistance among *S. pneumoniae* in the United States has increased nearly fourfold since the early 1990s. Pneumococcal isolates with minimal inhibitory concentrations of up to 0.06, 0.1 to 1.0, and ≥ 2 μg/mL represent strains that are susceptible, intermediate (partially resistant), and highly resistant, respectively. These isolates often have diminished susceptibility to other antibiotics. The newer-generation quinolones (e.g., levofloxacin) appear to retain good activity against *S. pneumoniae* regardless of penicillin resistance. Ampicillin-resistant *H. influenzae*, 15% to 20% overall, and *Moraxella catarrhalis*, (80+% resistance) are also problematic. Although resistance levels are rising, they have not been clearly associated with increased mortality in those patients with CAP.
2. **Nosocomial pneumonia.** In addition to treating the commonly recognized pathogens, consideration must also be given to the patterns of bacterial infection found in the hospital, to resistance patterns, and to the patient's recent history of antibiotic use. Patients with hospital-acquired pneumonia are categorized on the basis of disease severity, risk factors for specific pathogens, and time of onset (early or late). Treatment can be based on this information (Table 58-2). Although combination therapy is considered standard, data support the safe and effective use of monotherapy with a broad-spectrum antibiotic for infections by organisms without significant resistance. Patients at risk for pseudomonal infection or infection with a highly resistant gram-negative pathogen should be treated with combination therapy until culture data demonstrate the absence of such organisms.

TABLE 58-2. Antibiotic therapy in nosocomial pneumonia

Severity of Illness	Likely Organisms	Therapy[c]
Mild to moderate, no risk factors[a] or severe, early onset, no risk factors	Core organisms[b]	Second- or-third-generation cephalosporin, beta-lactam/beta-lactamase inhibitor
Mild to moderate, specific risk factors[a]	Core + specific pathogens	Above antibiotics modified for consideration of specific pathogen
Severe, early onset specific risk factors	Core + *Pseudomonas aeruginosa,* MRSA, resistant gram-negative bacilli, *Acinetobacter* sp.	Combination antipseudomonal therapy[d] Consider vancomycin
Severe, late onset ± risk factors	Same	Same

MRSA, methicillin-resistant *Staphylococcus aureus.*

[a] Risk factors for specific pathogens (e.g., anaerobes after recent abdominal surgery).

[b] Core pathogens: *Streptococcus pneumoniae,* methicillin-sensitive *S. aureus,* nonresistant gram-negative bacilli.

[c] Suggested therapy for hospital acquired pneumonia based on severity, timing, and risk factors for specific pathogens.

[d] Aminoglycoside or ciprofloxacin with an antipseudomonal beta-lactam.

Selected Readings

Allen RM, Dunn WF, Limper AH. Diagnosing ventilator-associated pneumonia: the role of bronchoscopy. *Mayo Clin Proc* 1994;69:962.

A discussion of the two diagnostic procedures used most frequently to obtain uncontaminated lower airway secretions during bronchoscopy—PSB and BAL.

Bartlett JG, Breiman RF, Mandell LA, et al. Community acquired pneumonia in adults: guidelines for management. *Clin Infect Dis* 1998;26:811.

Consensus guidelines from the Infectious Disease Society of America. Complements nicely the ATS statement on CAP.

Campbell GD, Neiderman MS, Broughton WA, et al. Hospital-acquired pneumonia in adults: diagnosis, assessment of severity, initial antimicrobial therapy, and preventative strategies. *Am J Respir Crit Care Med* 1996;153:1711.

The ATS consensus statement on hospital-acquired pneumonia, including microbiology, diagnostic studies, and therapy, with an excellent discussion on response to therapy and prevention.

Fagon JY, Chastre Y, Hance AJ, et al. Detection of nosocomial lung infection in ventilated patients: use of a protected specimen brush and quantitative culture technique in 147 patients. *Am Rev Respir Dis* 1988;138:110.

Pulmonary infiltrates and purulent tracheal secretions do not always predict VAP. Bronchoscopic techniques with quantitative culture can be valuable and can allow one to avoid unnecessary antibiotics.

Heyland DK, Cook DJ, Marshall J, et al. The clinical utility of invasive diagnostic techniques in the setting of ventilator-associated pneumonia: Canadian Critical Care Trials Group. *Chest* 1999;115:1076.

The use of bronchoscopy with PSB and BAL cultures in the mechanically ventilated patient with suspected VAP may increase physician confidence in the diagnosis and may allow for greater ability to limit or discontinue antibiotic treatment.

Lynch JP, Sitrin RG. Noninfectious mimics of community-acquired pneumonia. *Semin Respir Infect* 1993;8:14.

A comprehensive review of the mimics of CAP, perhaps a more common problem in patients in the ICU.

Neiderman MS, Bass JB, Campbell GD, et al. Guidelines for the initial management of adults with community acquired pneumonia: diagnosis, assessment of severity, and initial antimicrobial therapy. *Am Rev Respir Dis* 1993;148:1418.
The ATS consensus statement on CAP.

Niederman MS, Craven DE, Fein AM, et al. Pneumonia in the critically ill hospitalized patient. *Chest* 1990;97:170.
A excellent discussion by experts in the field on topics concerning severe nosocomial pneumonia.

Neill AM, Martin IR, Weir R, et al. Community acquired pneumonia: aetiology and usefulness of severity criteria on admission. *Thorax* 1996;51:1010.
The criteria of the British Thoracic Society for severe CAP performed well as a severity indicator at admission (sensitivity 95%, sensitivity 71%). A 36-fold risk of death was found when 2 of the following were present: respiratory rate greater than 30 per minute, diastolic blood pressure less than 60 mm Hg, blood urea nitrogen greater than 7 mmol/L, and confusion.

Pallares R, Linares J, Vadillo M, et al. Resistance to penicillin and cephalosporin and mortality from severe pneumococcal pneumonia in Barcelona, Spain. *N Engl J Med* 1995;333:474.
Despite an overall frequency of resistance to penicillin and cephalosporins by S. pneumoniae *of 29% and 6%, respectively, there was no associated increased mortality in patients with a resistant strain of severe pneumococcal pneumonia.*

Pugin J, Aukenthaler R, Mili N, et al. Diagnosis of ventilator-associated pneumonia by bacteriology analysis of bronchoscopic and nonbronchoscopic "blind" bronchoalveolar lavage fluid. *Am Rev Respir Dis* 1991;143:1121.
"Blind" BAL can be of value in clinical practice; its sensitivity is slightly lower than for bronchoscopic BAL. Clinical scoring criteria for predicting VAP are described.

Torres A, González J, Ferrer M. Evaluation of the available invasive and non-invasive techniques for diagnosing nosocomial pneumonia in mechanically ventilated patients. *Intensive Care Med* 1991;17:439.
A complete review of the invasive and noninvasive techniques to diagnose VAP, including bronchoscopic PSB and BAL, as well as percutaneous lung needle aspiration.

V. RENAL PROBLEMS IN THE INTENSIVE CARE UNIT

59. METABOLIC ACIDOSIS AND METABOLIC ALKALOSIS

David M. Clive

I. Normal acid-base physiology. The pH of extracellular fluid is tightly regulated and normally runs between 7.36 and 7.44. This regulation is made possible largely by the bicarbonate buffer system. Preservation of this buffer reserve depends, in turn, on two renal physiologic processes: (a) reclamation of filtered bicarbonate, most of which occurs in the proximal tubule; and (b) the disposal of 50 to 100 mEq of metabolically produced hydrogen ion each day. These hydrogen ions are actively secreted by pumps throughout the nephron. They are buffered either by filtered buffers such as phosphate anion, or by ammonia, produced by the deamination of glutamine in the proximal tubule.

II. Metabolic acidosis. Metabolic acidosis is defined as an abnormally low plasma pH (also called acidemia) accompanied by a fall in the serum bicarbonate concentration. Metabolic acidoses are broadly classified by the presence or absence of an expanded anion gap. The anion gap (AG in the following equation) is the difference between the plasma concentrations of the predominant cation (sodium) and anions (chloride and bicarbonate):

$$AG = Na^+ - [Cl^- + HCO_3^-]$$

A. Acidosis with an expanded anion gap. Lactic acidosis is a paradigm example of acidosis with an expanded anion gap. Lactic acid is composed of a hydrogen ion and an anion, lactate. As lactic acid accumulates in the plasma, each hydrogen ion titrates a bicarbonate anion. Therefore, for each one milliequivalent fall in the bicarbonate level, a lactate anion is added to the plasma. Lactate is normally present in minuscule amounts in the plasma (up to 1.0 mmol/L). Because lactate is an *unmeasured anion,* that is, not appearing in the anion gap calculation, its retention causes an apparent increase in the anion gap. Lactate levels higher than 4.0 mmol/L are considered diagnostic of lactic acidosis.

The high anion gap acidosis of renal failure is caused by retention of metabolic waste acids that would be filtered and excreted under normal circumstances. Of these, sulfuric acid is the most prevalent. Tubular abnormalities of ammonia production, hydrogen ion secretion, and bicarbonate reabsorption may contribute a normal-gap component to the acidosis of renal failure (see later).

Diabetic ketoacidosis (DKA), as the name implies, is characterized by an overabundance of ketoacids such as acetoacetic acid and beta-hydroxbutyric acid in the blood. In the recovery phase of DKA, these ketoacids provide substrate for the regeneration of lost bicarbonate. Because ketoacids are excreted in the urine during the evolution of DKA, their loss may be viewed as loss of potential bicarbonate. Thus, even when ketoacids vanish from the plasma during the recovery phase, the acidosis may convert to normal-gap acidosis because of persistent bicarbonate deficiency.

Certain toxic ingestions may be associated with the development of a high-gap metabolic acidosis. Most notoriously, these include ethylene glycol and methanol. In both cases, the expansion of the anion gap is related to accumulation of acid metabolites of each toxic alcohol, oxalic acid in the case of ethylene glycol and formic acid in the case of methanol.

B. Acidosis with a normal anion gap. In normal-gap acidosis, the decrement in plasma bicarbonate concentration is matched by an increase in chloride. For this reason, normal-gap acidoses are often referred to as *hyperchloremic acidosis.* This substitution of chloride for bicarbonate can come about as follows: (a) addition of exogenous HCl, or its equivalent, to the body; (b) bicarbonate loss, which may occur either from the gastrointestinal tract or kidney; and (c) retention of hydrogen ions. Diarrhea and the renal tubular acidoses are the most common causes of hyperchloremic acidosis. Table 59-1 shows the major causes of hyperchloremic acidosis and their mechanisms.

C. Clinical presentation. On physical examination, patients may demonstrate Kussmaul respirations, which are not so much rapid as deep and represent the response of the respiratory center to acidosis. Hypotension is often present in severe acidosis. It is often argued that acidosis reduces vascular tone and myocardial contractility, but these effects are debated. Acidotic states often occur in association with other factors, such as hypovolemia, which may also contribute to a lower blood pressure. Hyperkalemia, when present, probably reflects egress of potassium from cells as hydrogen ions enter.

D. Diagnosis. This is a simple laboratory diagnosis made on the basis of a low blood pH in association with a reduced plasma bicarbonate concentration.

1. **Respiratory compensation.** Respiratory compensation for metabolic acidosis is caused by chemical stimulation of the brainstem respiratory centers. To determine whether compensation meets the expected degree, the following formula may be used:

$$\text{Expected } P_{CO_2} \text{ (mm Hg)} = [(1.5 \times HCO_3^-) + 8] \pm 2$$

A quicker estimate may be made by comparing the last two digits of the pH (i.e., those to the right of the decimal point) with the carbon dioxide pressure (P_{CO_2}); by mathematical coincidence, these numbers should be approximately equal.

2. **Multiple acid-base disturbances.** Multiple acid-base disturbances are not uncommon. Metabolic alkalosis and metabolic acidosis can occur simultaneously. For example, a patient who has been vomiting copiously may then develop ketoacidosis. Because these two acid-base imbalances tend to offset each other, such a patient may have near-normal blood pH and bicarbonate concentration. The presence of the acidosis is disclosed by the expanded anion gap. The alkalosis, suggested by the history of vomiting, manifests itself as a serum bicarbonate level higher than that expected for the degree of expansion of the anion gap. In other words, the magnitude of the drop in serum bicarbonate (ΔHCO_3) resulting from the acidosis is much less than the magnitude of the expansion of the anion gap (ΔA.G.) Note that the so-called "Δ/Δ" ratio (the ratio of anion gap increase to bicarbonate decrease) is usually greater than 1.0, even in simple metabolic acidosis. Only when the ratio is greater than 1.6 does a mixed disturbance need be invoked. When respiratory alkalosis is superimposed on metabolic acidosis, the P_{CO_2} is lower

TABLE 59-1. Causes of metabolic acidosis with a normal anion gap

Cause of Hyperchloremic Acidosis	Cause	Mechanism
Hydrogen chloride overload	Cholestyramine	Intraintestinal exchange of chloride for bicarbonate
	Parenteral alimentation	Exogenous hydrogen chloride loading
Bicarbonate loss	Type 2 renal tubular acidosis	Inadequate proximal tubular bicarbonate reabsorption
	Diarrhea	Bicarbonate loss from gut
H^+ retention	Type 1 renal tubular acidosis	Failure of distal nephronal proton pumps
	Type 4 renal tubular acidosis (hypoaldosteronism)	Impaired ammonia production

than would be expected based on simple respiratory compensation alone; the pH is much closer to normal than in compensated metabolic acidosis.

3. **Multiple superimposed metabolic acidoses.** If, for example, a patient with diarrhea develops DKA, the simultaneous presence of hyperchloremic normal-gap acidosis (resulting from the diarrhea) and high-gap acidosis (from the ketoacidosis) is revealed by a drop in bicarbonate far exceeding the extent to which the anion gap has widened. In summary, the recognition of complex acid-base disturbances necessitates attention to anion gap, pH, bicarbonate level, and P_{CO_2} (Table 59-2).

   An interesting characteristic of ketoacidosis is that, in this particular form of acidosis, the Δ/Δ ratio is usually no greater than 1.0, reflecting the loss of ketoacids, which otherwise could expand the anion gap, in the urine.

4. **Urinary anion gap.** The urinary anion gap (UAG in the following equation) is calculated as follows:

$$UAG = (Na^+ + K^+) - Cl^-$$

   The urinary anion gap is expected to be negative in patients with metabolic acidosis, because large amounts of ammonium are excreted as a urinary buffer and act as unmeasured cations. A neutral or positive urinary anion gap in an acidotic patient therefore bespeaks a problem in urinary acidification or ammoniagenesis.

E. Treatment. Invariably, the best approach to therapy of metabolic acidosis is to treat its underlying cause. Supplementation of bicarbonate should not be considered unless blood pH is less than 7.20 or serum bicarbonate levels are less than 12 mEq/L. Even in these settings, alkali administration is unlikely to help unless the predisposing circumstances are addressed. Bicarbonate deficit may be calculated as follows:

$$HCO_3^- \text{ deficit} = LBM\ (0.5)\ (24 - HCO^-_{3\,obs})$$

where LBM is the lean body mass in kilograms, 0.5 is the "bicarbonate space" in liters per kilogram, and $HCO^-_{3\,obs}$ is the observed serum bicarbonate. In severe acidosis, or when ongoing bicarbonate losses are severe, the bicarbonate space may increase to more than 0.7.

Specific approaches to the therapy of DKA, lactic acidosis, the acidoses associated with toxic ingestions, and the acidosis of renal failure are found elsewhere in this text (Chapters 61, 62, 86, and 106).

III. Metabolic alkalosis. The findings of an elevated plasma pH and bicarbonate concentration establish the diagnosis of metabolic alkalosis. The pathogenesis of metabolic

TABLE 59-2. Recognition of some common complex acid-base disturbances

Disturbance	P_{CO_2}	HCO_3	pH	ΔHCO_3 vs. Δ Anion Gap
Metabolic acidosis with metabolic alkalosis	Normal or near normal	Normal or near normal	Normal or near normal	$\Delta HCO_3 <$ Δ anion gap
Compound metabolic acidosis	↓↓	↓↓↓	↓↓↓	$\Delta HCO_3 >$ Δ anion gap
Mixed respiratory alkalosis with metabolic acidosis	↓↓↓	↓↓	Normal or near normal	—

alkalosis has two phases, a *generative phase* and a *maintenance phase.* Metabolic alkalosis can be generated in three ways:

1. Loss of hydrogen ion in gastric juice or urine.
2. Exogenous bicarbonate loading.
3. Loss of fluid with a higher chloride-to-bicarbonate ratio than that of normal extracellular fluid. This phenomenon, widely referred to as *contraction alkalosis,* usually only results in modest hyperbicarbonatemia.

Normally, excess bicarbonate is disposed of rapidly. Sustained hyperbicarbonatemia therefore means that a pathophysiologic process is allowing the retention of accumulated bicarbonate, that is, permitting the maintenance of alkalosis. The most common causes of failure to correct a bicarbonate surplus are *hypokalemia* and *hypovolemia.* Because of the powerful capacity of the kidneys to excrete bicarbonate, metabolic alkalosis from exogenous alkali loading is uncommon and usually occurs only if renal insufficiency is present.

A. Classification. Metabolic alkaloses are usually defined as being *chloride resistant* or *chloride responsive.*

1. Chloride-responsive alkalosis. Chloride-responsive alkalosis, as the name implies, results from chloride loss. Most commonly, this occurs with diuretic use or vomiting. Loop and thiazide diuretics enhance delivery of sodium to the distalmost segments of the nephron, where sodium–hydrogen ion exchange occurs. Under the presence of aldosterone, stimulated by the diuretic, this exchange is potentiated. The lost hydrogen ion is likely to be excreted with chloride anion. Vomiting and nasogastric suction cause loss of fluid rich in hydrogen and chloride ions, and this loss leads directly to bicarbonate excess. Less directly, bicarbonate retention in this setting is favored by the paucity of hydrogen ion reaching the duodenum, a situation that lessens the stimulus for pancreatic secretion of bicarbonate into the intestinal lumen.

A transient form of alkalosis known as *posthypercapnic alkalosis* occurs after the resolution of compensated respiratory acidosis. Bicarbonate levels rise in a state of sustained hypercapnia; once the hypercapnia resolves, the accumulated bicarbonate is excreted in the urine. Until this bicarbonate "dumping" process is complete, a state of metabolic alkalosis obtains.

With the cessation of vomiting, nasogastric suctioning, or diuretic therapy and the replacement of lost chloride, alkalosis of this type is permanently correctable with chloride repletion. Because potassium deficits are usually present, potassium chloride is the preferred supplement.

2. Chloride-resistant alkalosis. Chloride-resistant alkalosis is seen in association with obligate losses of hydrogen ion or chloride in the urine. Ongoing diuretic therapy falls into this category, and the mechanism is as described earlier. Mineralocorticoid excess states, such as hyperaldosteronism and Bartter syndrome, are characterized by enhanced distal tubular sodium–hydrogen ion exchange. Patients with Bartter syndrome may also have intrinsic impairment of tubular chloride reabsorption.

B. Clinical presentation. Alkalemia itself is relatively free of adverse clinical effects. Most of the symptoms, such as muscle spasm, paresthesias, and weakness, are more directly attributable to the commonly associated electrolyte imbalances such as hypokalemia, reduced ionized calcium level, and sodium depletion (hypovolemia).

C. Diagnosis. History is key in uncovering the cause of metabolic acidosis. Patients should be questioned for vomiting and diuretic use. Bulimic patients and persons who abuse diuretics may not yield this information willingly. The presence of hypertension in a patient with hypokalemic alkalosis should raise suspicion of a mineralocorticoid excess state such as primary hyperaldosteronism. A lifelong history of muscle weakness and of polyuria in a normotensive patient with hypokalemic alkalosis suggests Bartter syndrome. The urine chloride concentration may be useful in differentiating among the causes of alkalosis (Table 59-3). Finding < 15 mEq/L is typical of chloride-responsive alkalosis, > 20 mEq/L of chloride-resistant.

TABLE 59-3. Chloride concentration in metabolic alkalosis

Urine chloride concentration	
< 15 mEq/L	> 20 mEq/L
Vomiting	Mineralocorticoid excess states
Nasogastric suction	Exogenous alkali loading[a]
Recent diuretic use	Ongoing diuretic use
Posthypercapnia	Severe hypokalemia
Exogenous alkali loading[a]	Bartter syndrome and related disorders

[a] The level of chloride excretion in these states depends on whether bicarbonate retention is associated with intrinsic renal tubular damage is present (high urine chloride) or simply hypovolemia (low urine chloride).

D. Treatment. Emergency treatment of metabolic alkalosis is rarely necessary because of the relative paucity of adverse effects associated with this disorder. Only when blood pH is extremely high, such as higher than 7.55, need urgent therapy be contemplated. For chloride-responsive metabolic alkalosis, chloride replacement is the cornerstone of treatment. This may be accomplished in several ways.

1. **Chloride-responsive alkalosis.** *Chloride-containing solutions* may be administered, the specific nature of the fluid dictated by the clinical situation. Because hypovolemia and metabolic alkalosis frequently coexist, it may be necessary to replace much of the chloride deficit as sodium chloride. Most patients with metabolic alkalosis also have a potassium deficit and at are risk for ongoing potassium wasting, particularly if they are receiving sodium chloride. Potassium chloride may be administered at rates of up to 20 mEq per hour with proper monitoring.

   For patients with persistent vomiting or those receiving continuous nasogastric suctioning, loss of hydrogen chloride may be attenuated by medications such as H_2 blockers that reduce gastric acid output.

   For patients in whom it would be undesirable to administer a large sodium or potassium load, there are other means for achieving a more favorable chloride-bicarbonate balance. *Acetazolamide* (250 mg intravenously or orally one to four times daily) may be given. Another option, particularly useful in severe degrees of alkalemia, is to give isotonic hydrochloric acid. This solution should only be administered through a large vein, and at a rate of up to 100 mEq per 6 hours. Ammonium and arginine hydrochloride are alternatives to hydrochloric acid, but they should be avoided in patients with liver or kidney disease, who are at risk of encephalopathy. The dose of hydrogen ion may be calculated using the following equation (which is the mirror image of the "base deficit" equation introduced earlier in the discussion of metabolic acidosis):

   $$HCO_3^- \text{ excess} = 0.5 \text{ (body weight) } (HCO^-_{3\text{ obs}} - HCO^-_{3\text{ desired}})$$

   Severe alkalosis in patients with renal failure may be treated by dialysis with *chloride-rich dialysis solutions.*

2. **Chloride-resistant alkalosis.** Therapy of chloride-resistant metabolic alkaloses has two components. *Potassium chloride* administration is generally necessary. Definitive therapy, however, should be aimed at the cause of the problem. Hypertensive patients should be investigated for primary aldosteronism. If the diagnosis is secured, treatment with *spironolactone,* or, in the case of aldosterone-producing adenoma, *surgery,* may be undertaken. Bartter syndrome is usually approached with nonsteroidal antiinflammatory drugs, amiloride, triamterene, and angiotensin-converting enzyme inhibitors in various combinations.

Selected Readings

Adrogue HJ, Madias NE. Management of life-threatening acid-base disorders (two parts). *N Engl J Med* 1998; 338:26 and 107.

Practical guide for approaching acid-base emergencies.

Battle DC, Hizon M, Cohen E, et al. The use of the urinary anion gap in the diagnosis of hyperchloremic metabolic acidosis. *N Engl J Med* 1988;318:594.

Shows how to use urinary anion gap in differentiating among forms of renal tubular acidosis as well as nonrenal acidosis.

Black RM. Metabolic acidosis and metabolic alkalosis. In: Irwin RS, Cerra FB, Rippe JM, eds. *Intensive care medicine,* 4th ed. Philadelphia: Lippincott–Raven, 1999:926.

Source material for this chapter.

Emmett M, Narins RG. Clinical use of the anion gap. *Medicine* 1977;56:38.

Another classic, which provides conceptual framework for understanding the use of the anion gap, as well as brief descriptions of major clinical anion-gap acidoses.

Friedman BS, Lumb PD. Prevention and management of metabolic alkalosis. *J Intensive Care Med* 1990;5[Suppl]:S22.

A practically oriented review.

Garella S, Dana CL, Chazan JA. Severity of metabolic acidosis as a determinant of bicarbonate requirements. *N Engl J Med* 1973;289:121.

This article introduced the concept of expansion of the bicarbonate space in profound metabolic acidosis.

Madias NE. Lactic acidosis. *Kidney Int* 1986;29:752.

A thorough exploration of the pathophysiology of lactic acidosis and the complex issues surrounding its proper therapy.

Seldin DW, Rector FC. The generation and maintenance of metabolic alkalosis. *Kidney Int* 1972;1:306.

The classic treatise on the pathophysiology of metabolic alkalosis.

Smulders YM, Frissen J, Slaats EH, et al. Renal tubular acidosis: pathophysiology and diagnosis. *Arch Intern Med* 1996;156:1629.

Concise, lucid review of a challenging subject.

60. DISORDERS OF PLASMA SODIUM AND PLASMA POTASSIUM

Eric S. Iida and David M. Clive

I. Disorders of plasma sodium. Managing disorders of plasma sodium requires an appreciation of the relationship between plasma sodium and osmolality. Maintenance of normal plasma osmolality depends on (a) the ability of the kidneys to eliminate excess water and (b) intact thirst sensation with access to water. Osmolality is estimated as follows:

$$\text{Posm} = 2 \times \text{plasma Na}^{+} \text{ concentration} + \text{glucose} / 18 + \text{BUN} / 2.8$$

where BUN is blood urea nitrogen. Therefore, plasma sodium concentration is the major determinant of plasma osmolality. Solutes that can raise the measured osmolality but do not result in fluid movements across semipermeable membranes (termed "ineffective" osmoles) include ethanol, ethylene glycol, and methanol. A plasma osmolality increase of 1% to 2% or, more important, a blood pressure or volume decrease of 7% to 10%, stimulates antidiuretic hormone (ADH). A decline in plasma osmolality of 1% to 2% suppresses ADH and results in dilute urine.

A. Hyponatremia

1. **Causes.** Causes of hyponatremia are outlined in Table 60-1. The syndrome of inappropriate ADH (SIADH) is characterized by the following: euvolemia; plasma hypoosmolality; urine osmolality greater than 100 to 150 mOsmol/kg; urinary sodium concentration greater than 20 mEq/L; normal adrenal, renal, and thyroid function; and normal potassium and acid-base balance. Table 60-2 lists major causes of SIADH.
2. **Clinical presentation.** Symptoms of hyponatremia include lethargy, confusion, nausea, vomiting, and, in severe cases, seizures and coma. The likelihood of symptoms relates to the level of hyponatremia and the rapidity with which it develops.
3. **Assessment of volume status.** Assessment of volume status is essential. The plasma osmolality, if elevated relative to the calculated value, indicates pseudohyponatremia. A urine osmolality greater than 100 mOsmol/kg demonstrates defective urinary dilution; lower values suggest primary polydipsia. Typically, the urine sodium is less than 20 mEq/L with effective volume depletion and more than 40 mEq/L with SIADH. The findings of metabolic alkalosis and hypokalemia in cases of hyponatremia suggest diuretic use; metabolic acidosis and hypokalemia suggest diarrhea or laxative abuse; and metabolic acidosis and hyperkalemia suggest adrenal insufficiency. Hypouricemia (less than 4 mg/dL) and a low BUN-to-creatinine ratio can be seen in SIADH or cerebral salt wasting; in volume depletion, these values are typically normal or elevated.

   To estimate the amount of sodium needed to raise the plasma concentration, multiply total body water times the difference between the desired sodium level (a target of about 120 mEq/L is usually adequate) and the current level. Lean body weight times 0.6 for men or 0.5 for women approximates total body water. Actual serum sodium concentration should be monitored during the correction phase. Take into account any potassium repletion when calculating the amount of sodium to be given because it, too, is osmotically active.
4. **Treatment.** Salt therapy, usually as isotonic saline, is appropriate in patients with true volume depletion or adrenal insufficiency (along with cortisol replacement). Patients with sodium levels less than 115 mEq/L or symptoms may need hypertonic saline given through central access. In asymptomatic patients, one should aim for a rate of rise of plasma sodium not faster than 12 mEq per day (0.5 mEq per hour). With symptomatic patients,

TABLE 60-1. Causes of hyponatremia

- Impaired water excretion (Uosm >100 mosm/kg and usually >300 mosm/kg)
  - Hypovolemic states
    - True volume depletion (by gastrointestinal, skin, or renal losses)
    - Edematous states with reduced effective circulating blood volume (advanced liver and heart disease)
  - Diuretics
  - Advanced renal failure
  - Endocrine deficiencies (hypothyroidism and hypoadrenalism)
  - SIADH
  - Cerebral salt wasting
  - Reduced solute intake (Uosm <100 mosm/kg)
- Normal water excretion (Uosm <100 mosm/kg)
  - Primary polydipsia
    - Psychiatric disorders (particularly with phenothiazines)
    - Hypothalamic disorders
- Hyponatremia without hypoosmolality
  - Normal Posm
    - Pseudohyponatremia (hypertriglyceridemia, hyperproteinemia, genitourinary tract irrigation)
  - Increased Posm
    - Hyperosmolar hyponatremia (hyperglycemia, mannitol infusion in renal failure)
    - Azotemia (effective osmolality is reduced)

Posm, plasma osmolality; SIADH, syndrome of inappropriate antidiuretic hormone.

one can use an initial rate of correction of 1.5 to 2.0 mEq per hour for the first 3 to 4 hours or longer if the patient remains symptomatic. After initial treatment, one should slow the rate of correction to achieve 12 mEq net over the initial 24 hours.

Edematous hyponatremic patients should be treated by water restriction, as should those with SIADH, primary polydipsia, and advanced renal failure. Other modalities include loop diuretics and demeclocycline (although azotemia may develop), angiotensin-converting enzyme inhibition in congestive heart failure, and salt tablets or hypertonic saline for patients with symptomatic hyponatremia in liver disease. In primary polydipsia, water restriction may result in a dramatic rise in plasma sodium levels.

TABLE 60-2. Major causes of the syndrome of inappropriate antidiuretic hormone secretion

- Pulmonary diseases of any cause
- Neurologic diseases affecting the central nervous system
- Ectopic production (carcinoma, especially small cell lung)
- Drugs (intravenous cyclophosphamide, carbamezapine, chlorpropamide, NSAIDs, cisplatin)
- Following major surgery (pain-induced, after mitral commissurotomy for mitral stenosis)
- Exogenous antidiuretic hormone or oxytocin
- HIV infection (from central nervous system, pulmonary, and malignant causes)
- Idiopathic (monitor periodically for underlying disorders)
- Cerebral salt wasting

HIV, human immunodeficiency virus; NSAIDs, nonsteroidal antiinflammatory drugs.

Osmotic demyelination ("central pontine myelinolysis") can occur when chronic hyponatremia is corrected too rapidly. Imaging studies may not be positive for up to 4 weeks. Symptoms develop from 1 day to several days after correction and include mental status changes, dysarthria, dysphagia, paraparesis or quadriparesis, coma, and, uncommonly, seizures. Raising the plasma sodium more than 20 mEq/L in the first 24 hours or to more than 140 mEq/L incurs the greatest risk. Treatment is supportive.

Severe, symptomatic, or resistant SIADH often requires salt administration. To elevate the plasma sodium, the osmolality of the fluid given must exceed that of the urine. A loop diuretic may help to lower the urine osmolality. Demeclocycline (300 to 600 mg twice a day), an increase in dietary solute intake, or, all else failing, 30 g urea per day comprise alternative strategies.

In 25% to 30% of cases of SIADH, and in certain other conditions, the hypothalamic osmostat is reset downward and is manifested by asymptomatic, stable, chronic mild hyponatremia. A reset osmostat does not require treatment and is unlikely to respond to intervention.

B. Hypernatremia. Table 60-3 lists major causes of hypernatremia.

1. **Clinical presentation.** Symptoms of hypernatremia include lethargy, weakness, irritability, and, with acute elevations in the plasma sodium to more than 158 mEq/L, potentially irreversible twitching, seizures, and coma. Chronic hypernatremia rarely induces symptoms; however, if the condition is corrected too aggressively, significant neurologic complications caused by cerebral edema may ensue.
2. **Diagnosis.** Diagnosis relies on the history and measurement of urine osmolality. In patients with intact hypothalamic and renal function, the urine osmolality will be greater than 700 to 800 mOsmol/kg, a finding implicating unreplaced free water losses, sodium overload or, rarely, a primary defect in thirst. The urine sodium is low (less than 20 mEq/L) with water loss and volume depletion and high (more than 100 mEq/L) after hypertonic salt ingestion. A urine osmolality less than that of the plasma suggests either central (ADH-deficient) or nephrogenic (ADH-resistant) diabetes insipidus. Nephrogenic diabetes insipidus with polyuria can occur with long-term lithium use, hypercalcemia, and severe hypokalemia. A historical clue to central diabetes insipidus is that the associated polyuria is often abrupt in onset. The water-restriction test can confirm the diagnosis. In this test, the patient discontinues water intake for several hours to stimulate ADH release and to cause the kidney to retain free water, thus leading to a rise in urine osmolality. If no response occurs, one should administer 1-deamino-8-D-arginine vasopressin (DDAVP, a synthetic ADH substitute); if the urine osmolality rises, the patient has central diabetes insipidus. In practice, results may be obscured by incomplete defects, whether central or nephrogenic; direct measurement of the ADH level may be helpful in this situation.

TABLE 60-3. Major causes of hypernatremia

- Unreplaced water loss
  - Insensible and sweat losses
  - Gastrointestinal losses
  - Central or nephrogenic diabetes insipidus
  - Hypothalamic lesions affecting thirst or osmoreceptor function:
    - Primary hypodipsia
    - Essential hypernatremia
    - Reset osmostat in mineralocorticoid excess
- Water loss into cells: severe exercise or seizures
- Sodium overload: intake of hypertonic sodium solution

3. Treatment. To treat hypernatremia caused by water loss, estimate the water deficit as:

CBW[plasma Na / 140 – 1]

where CBW = current (observed) body water = 60% lean body mass.

The formula only applies to the current free water deficit and not to any simultaneous volume deficit. The water should be given intravenously in a 5% dextrose solution or orally at a rate of correction not exceeding 0.5 mEq per hour.

In patients with diabetes insipidus, the goal is to decrease urine output. For central diabetes insipidus, prescribe DDAVP by nasal spray (5 to 20 mg once or twice a day). Potential risks of treatment are water retention and hyponatremia. Other treatment options include chlorpropamide, carbamazepine, and clofibrate. Treatment of nephrogenic diabetes insipidus aims to correct the underlying disorder or to remove the offending drug, although lithium-induced nephrogenic diabetes insipidus may be irreversible. Thiazide diuretics and amiloride diminish polyuria in nephrogenic diabetes insipidus; however, thiazides may lead to increased tubular lithium absorption and toxic levels. Nonsteroidal antiinflammatory drugs may be helpful by promoting the effect of ADH. A low-sodium, low-protein diet limits solute excretion and thus urine output at any given urine osmolality. Finally, because some patients have incomplete nephrogenic diabetes insipidus, supraphysiologic levels of ADH may ameliorate symptoms.

II. Disorders of plasma potassium. Plasma potassium levels depend on the net balance of intake, shifts between plasma and intracellular compartments, and excretion. Intake of potassium includes dietary and intravenous sources. Movement of potassium into cells is primarily mediated through insulin and beta-adrenergic stimulation. Conversely, a relative absence of insulin or beta-adrenergic stimulation prevents potassium movement into cells. Urinary excretion occurs almost exclusively through secretion in the distal tubule and is stimulated by high potassium levels, aldosterone, and a high rate of distal urine flow. Alternate routes of excretion, such as through insensible losses or the gastrointestinal tract, can be significant at times.

A. Hypokalemia. Table 60-4 list major causes of hypokalemia.

1. Clinical presentation. Manifestations include electrocardiogram (ECG) changes such as T-wave depression, prominent U waves, and eventually frank arrhythmias. Muscle weakness, cramps, and paresthesias occur usually with plasma levels below 2.5 mEq/L. Rhabdomyolysis and impaired respiratory muscle function can also complicate severe hypokalemia. Renal manifestations include polyuria.

2. Diagnosis. Diagnostic maneuvers include measurement of urinary potassium losses; otherwise healthy persons lower potassium excretion to less than 25 to 30 mEq per day during hypokalemia. Low urinary excretion rates suggest gastrointestinal loss or prior diuretic use. If metabolic acidosis is present, look for lower gastrointestinal losses; if metabolic acidosis accompanies potassium wasting, the diagnoses most often responsible include diabetic ketoacidosis, renal tubular acidosis, and a salt-wasting nephropathy. Metabolic alkalosis with a low urinary excretion rate suggests surreptitious vomiting or diuretic use. In alkalotic patients, urinary electrolyte (sodium, potassium, and especially chloride) measurement may distinguish the effects of vomiting from those of diuretic use or Bartter syndrome. Finally, in alkalotic patients with hypertension and potassium wasting, one should consider renovascular disease, surreptitious diuretic therapy with underlying hypertension, or primary mineralocorticoid excess.

3. Treatment. Therapy of loss is replacement. In diabetic ketoacidosis, potassium therapy is usually begun once the plasma potassium is 4.5 mEq/L or less (if the patient is making urine) because treatment with fluids and insulin shifts potassium back into cells. Otherwise, plasma levels between 3 and 3.5 mEq/L generally produce no symptoms, except in patients with

TABLE 60-4. Major causes of hypokalemia

Decreased intake
Increased entry into cells
- An elevation in extracellular pH
- Increased availability of insulin
- Elevated beta-adrenergic activity (e.g., high catecholamine states)
- Hypokalemic periodic paralysis
- Marked increase in blood cell production
- Hypothermia

Increased gastrointestinal losses
Increased urinary losses
- Diuretics
- Primary mineralocorticoid excess
- Loss of gastric secretions
- Nonreabsorbable anions (e.g., HCO_3^- in renal tubular acidosis, beta-hydroxybutyrate in diabetic ketoacidosis, hippurate [glue sniffing], penicillin derivatives from high-dose therapy)
- Metabolic acidosis
- Hypomagnesemia
- Amphotericin B
- Salt wasting nephropathies (e.g., Bartter syndrome, tubulointerstitial disease, hypercalcemia)
- Polyuria

Increased sweat losses
Dialysis

heart disease (especially if taking digitalis) or advanced liver disease, and they can be treated initially with 60 to 80 mEq per day. One should also treat any underlying disorder and hypomagnesemia. With ongoing diuretic therapy, one can alternately use relatively high doses of a potassium-sparing diuretic; concurrent potassium supplementation requires careful monitoring and should be avoided if renal insufficiency is present.

Generally, chloride-based preparations correct potassium deficits fastest. One should use bicarbonate or citrate-based supplements when acidosis is present, such as in chronic diarrheal states or renal tubular acidosis. Potassium-rich foods are generally less effective. Intravenous therapy with a saline solution is preferable to a dextrose-based solution because the latter can stimulate insulin release. Concentrations of potassium greater than 60 mEq/L can cause pain and sclerosis of peripheral veins.

In patients with severe or symptomatic hypokalemia, oral replacement can transiently raise plasma levels as much as 1 to 1.5 mEq/L after 40 to 60 mEq and by 2.5 to 3.5 mEq/L after 135 to 160 mEq. Careful monitoring is required, and more potassium should be given as necessary. A patient with a plasma concentration of 2 mEq/L, for example, may have a potassium deficit of 400 to 800 mEq. Generally, the maximum rate of intravenous administration is 10 to 20 mEq per hour. Higher rates require central access, can disturb cardiac conduction and should be considered only in extreme circumstances.

B. Hyperkalemia Table 60-5 lists major causes of hyperkalemia. To develop persistent hyperkalemia, a defect must develop in urinary excretion from a reduction either in aldosterone effect or in the delivery of sodium and water to the distal secretory site. Table 60-6 lists major causes of hypoaldosteronism.

1. **Clinical presentation.** Manifestations include cardiac conduction disturbances, paresthesias, muscle weakness, and paralysis. Severe symptoms occur when plasma concentrations are greater than 7.5 mEq/L, but sub-

TABLE 60-5. Major causes of hyperkalemia

Increased potassium release from cells
- Pseudohyperkalemia
- Metabolic acidosis
- Insulin deficiency, hyperglycemia, and hyperosmolality
- Increased tissue catabolism
- Beta-adrenergic blockade
- Exercise
- Other
  - Digitalis overdose
  - Hyperkalemic periodic paralysis
  - Succinylcholine
  - Arginine hydrochloride

Reduced urinary potassium excretion
- Hypoaldosteronism
- Renal failure
- Effective circulating volume depletion
- Selective impairment of potassium excretion

Drugs
- Dapsone
- Sulfa/trimethoprim
- Nonsteroidal antiinflammatory drugs
- Angiotensin-converting enzyme inhibitors
- Spironolactone and other potassium sparing diuretics

stantial interpatient variability exists. ECG abnormalities follow a characteristic progression in patients with plasma levels greater than 6.5 mEq/L: symmetric peaking of T waves, reduced P-wave voltage and widening of the QRS complexes, and ultimately a sinusoidal pattern. However, the ECG may not show changes despite higher levels, especially if the rate of rise of potassium has been slow.

2. **Treatment.** One can treat an asymptomatic patient without ECG changes and with a plasma potassium level of 6.5 mEq/L with a cation exchange resin such as sodium polystyrene sulfonate (Kayexalate). With a level of less than 6.0 mEq/L, diuretics alone may suffice. General measures to implement include a low-potassium diet and the discontinuation of offending drugs. Specific treatments of severe or symptomatic hyperkalemia vary in their

TABLE 60-6. Major causes of hypoaldosteronism

Hyporeninemic hypoaldosteronism
- Renal disease, most often diabetic nephropathy
- Nonsteroidal antiinflammatory drugs
- Angiotensin-converting enzyme inhibitors
- Cyclosporine
- HIV infection, including trimethoprim administration

Primary adrenal insufficiency

Potassium-sparing diuretics (trimethoprim may act similarly)

Heparin

Congenital adrenal hyperplasia (21-hydroxylase deficiency is most common)

Isolated impairment in aldosterone synthesis

Pseudohypoaldosteronism (end-organ resistance)

Severe illness

HIV, human immunodeficiency virus.

onset of action and mechanism. *Calcium* (1 ampule of 10% calcium gluconate) stabilizes cell membranes. It acts within minutes but is short-lived in effect. Calcium should not be given in bicarbonate-containing solutions, or precipitates may form. It should be prescribed only when absolutely necessary in patients taking digoxin, because hypercalcemia can induce digitalis toxicity. *Insulin* (10 U of regular) and glucose (50 mL of 50% solution) can decrease potassium levels by 0.5 to 1.5 mEq/L. The effect begins in 15 minutes and lasts for several hours. In a hyperglycemic diabetic patient, one should use insulin alone. *Sodium bicarbonate* (1 ampule of a 7.5% sodium bicarbonate solution) works best in patients with metabolic acidosis but is less effective in renal failure. It starts acting within 30 to 60 minutes, and the effect lasts for several hours. *Albuterol* (20 mg in 4 mL of saline by nasal inhalation or 0.5 mg by intravenous infusion) can lower the plasma potassium concentration by 0.5 to 1.5 mEq/L within 30 to 60 minutes. Tachycardia or angina can occur; beta-adrenergic agonists should probably be avoided in susceptible patients. Loop or thiazide *diuretics* remove potassium from the body. Cation exchange *resins* such as Kayaxelate remove potassium in exchange for sodium and can be given orally or by retention enema. Intestinal necrosis and volume overload can potentially complicate treatment. One should consider *dialysis* if the foregoing measures fail, the hyperkalemia is severe, or the patient has marked tissue breakdown with release of large amounts of potassium. Hemodialysis removes potassium many times faster than peritoneal dialysis.

Selected Readings

Black RM. Disorders of plasma sodium and plasma potassium. In: Irwin RS, Cerra FB, Rippe JM, eds. *Intensive care medicine,* 4th ed. Philadelphia: Lippincott–Raven, 1999:941.

Source material for this chapter.

Gennari FJ. Hypokalemia. *N Engl J Med* 1998;339:451.

A good review.

Lauriat SM, Berl T. The hyponatremic patient: practical focus on therapy. *J Am Soc Nephrol* 1997;8:1599.

Good discussion of risks and issues surrounding treatment, although the approach is more aggressive than presented here.

Miller M, Kalkos T, Moses A, et al. Recognition of partial defects in antidiuretic hormone secretion. *Ann Intern Med* 1970;73:721.

Description of the water-deprivation test and its interpretation.

Scheinman SJ, Guay-Woodford LM, Thakker RV, et al. Genetic disorders of renal electrolyte transport. *N Engl J Med* 1999:340:1177.

Summarizes advances in defining mechanisms of some less common but important disorders that alter potassium and sodium balance such as Bartter syndrome.

Weiner ID, Wingo CS. Hyperkalemia: a potential silent killer. *J Am Soc Nephrol* 1997; 9:1535.

A good review of the subject.

61. ACUTE RENAL FAILURE IN THE INTENSIVE CARE UNIT

Claire A. Scanlon and David M. Clive

I. Overview. A sudden decline in kidney function is termed *acute renal failure* (ARF). It is often diagnosed when azotemia and oliguria are noted. ARF may stem from any of three types of insults: impaired renal perfusion, injury to the renal parenchyma, or obstruction of the urinary tract. Thus, renal failure is often classified as *prerenal, renal (also intrinsic or parenchymal),* or *postrenal* (Table 61-1).

A. Prerenal azotemia and autoregulatory failure. Prerenal azotemia is the result of decreased renal perfusion caused by extrarenal factors such as hypovolemia, reduced effective circulating volume, selective renal hypoperfusion, and autoregulatory failure (Table 61-2). Correction of these factors usually restores renal function. The hallmark of prerenal conditions is intense renal conservation of salt and water, typically reflected in the urine composition with urine sodium concentration (U_{Na}) less than 10 mEq/L, fractional excretion of sodium (FE_{Na}) less than 1%, and urine osmolality (U_{osm}) greater than 500 mOsmol/kg; FE_{Na} is the fractional excretion of Na = 100 × (urine sodium / plasma sodium) / (urine creatinine / plasma creatinine). The BUN-to-creatinine ratio may rise from the normal 10:1 to greater than 20:1; however, this finding is not pathognomonic of prerenal states (Table 61-3).

B. Intrinsic renal disease. Injury to any component of the renal parenchyma may cause ARF.

1. Glomerular and vascular disease. Causes of ARF include the following: vasculitis; acute glomerulonephritis; diseases of either the main renal vessels or their branches, such as renal artery or renal vein thrombosis; and microscopic occlusion of smaller vessels, as occurs in a variety of disorders such as atheroembolic renal disease, thrombotic thrombocytopenia purpura/hemolytic-uremic syndrome, scleroderma, and malignant hypertension. Diseases of the main renal vessels are discussed in further detail later.

2. Tubulointerstitial diseases

a. Acute tubular necrosis. Acute tubular necrosis (ATN) may result from renal ischemia or exposure to nephrotoxins (aminoglycoside antibiotics, radiocontrast agents, heavy metals, myoglobin). A suggestive history is elicited in 80% of patients with ATN. Classic urinary findings consist of sloughed renal tubular epithelial cells, epithelial cell casts, and muddy brown granular casts. In contrast to prerenal azotemia, the FE_{Na} is generally high (more than 1%), a finding suggesting tubular damage with impaired sodium reabsorption. Urinary concentration is also impaired, generally resulting in U_{osm} of approximately 300 mOsmol/kg.

b. Acute interstitial nephritis. Acute interstitial nephritis is characterized by inflammation of the renal interstitium and tubules. It is often drug induced, with features of allergy: fever, rash, and eosinophilia.

C. Postrenal azotemia. This term refers to azotemia caused by obstruction of urine flow from the kidneys. The most common causes of outflow obstruction are prostatic enlargement, stones, urinary infections, and tumors. For obstruction to cause azotemia, both kidneys must be involved, or unilateral obstruction in a patient with only one functioning kidney must occur. A precipitous decline in urine output or complete cessation of urine flow (anuria) is highly suggestive of complete obstruction of the urinary tract. However, partial obstructions, even high-grade ones, may not be associated with low urine output. Obstruction is usually easily detected by sonography, with hydronephrosis evident. Depending on the site of obstruction, immediate treatment may involve the placement of an indwelling urinary catheter, ureteral stents, or nephrostomy drainage until the underlying cause can be treated.

TABLE 61-1. Causes of acute renal failure

Prerenal azotemia
- Hypovolemia
- Reduced effective circulating volume
- Autoregulatory failure

Intrinsic renal disease
- Glomerular diseases
- Vascular diseases (main renal artery and microcirculation)
- Tubulointerstitial disease
- Acute tubular necrosis
- Acute cortical necrosis

Postrenal failure
- Ureteric obstruction (bilateral or solitary kidney)
- Lower tract obstruction (bladder neck or urethra)

TABLE 61-2. Causes of prerenal azotemia

Hypovolemia
- Gastrointestinal losses
  - Vomiting
  - Diarrhea
  - Surgical drainage
- Renal losses
  - Osmotic agents
  - Diuretics
  - Renal salt wasting disease
  - Adrenal insufficiency
- Skin losses
  - Burns
  - Excessive diaphoresis
- Hemorrhage
- Translocation of fluid ("third-spacing")
  - Postoperative
  - Pancreatitis

Reduced effective circulating volume
- Hypoalbuminemia
- Hepatic cirrhosis
- Left ventricular cardiac failure
- Peripheral blood pooling (vasodilator therapy, anesthetics, anaphylaxis, sepsis, toxic shock syndrome)
- Renal artery occlusion
- Small vessel disease (malignant hypertension, toxemia, scleroderma)
- Renal vasoconstriction (hypercalcemia, hepatorenal syndrome, cyclosporine, pressor agents)

Autoregulatory failure
- NSAIDs (preglomerular vasoconstriction)
- CEIs (postglomerular vasodilation)

CEIs, converting enzyme inhibitors; NSAIDs, nonsteroidal antiinflammatory drugs.

TABLE 61-3. Causes of blood urea nitrogen or serum creatinine elevation without reduction of glomerular filtration rate

Increased biosynthesis of urea
Gastrointestinal bleeding
Drug administration
Corticosteroids
Tetracycline
Increased protein intake
Amino acid administration
Hypercatabolism and febrile illness
Increased biosynthesis of creatinine
Increased release of creatinine from muscle (rhabdomyolysis)
Drug-interference with tubular creatinine secretion
Cimetidine
Trimethoprim
Spuriously elevated creatinine colorimetric assay
Ketoacids (diabetic ketoacidosis)
Cephalosporins

II. Clinical syndromes. Two-thirds of inpatients with ARF are likely to have either ATN or prerenal azotemia. ATN usually requires a more profound ischemic insult than does prerenal azotemia.

A. Ischemic acute renal failure. The most common cause of ARF in the intensive care unit is renal hypoperfusion. Frequently, more than one causal factor is required to induce ARF. Treatment is aimed at correcting the underlying cause.

B. Nephrotoxicity and drug-induced acute renal failure. Endogenous and exogenous agents can cause renal toxicity in a large proportion of patients in the intensive care unit.

1. **Myoglobinuria and hemoglobinuria.** Myoglobinuric ARF occurs as a result of the nephrotoxic effects of the intracellular protein, myoglobin, which is released into plasma during skeletal muscle injury (rhabdomyolysis). The diagnosis is suggested by serum creatine kinase levels greater than 5,000 μ/L. Specific therapy is aimed at reducing tubular toxicity by increasing nephronal flow rates and optimizing urinary dilution and alkalinization. Administration of isotonic bicarbonate-rich fluids (e.g., 3 ampules of bicarbonate in 1 L of 5% dextrose in water) and diuretics (e.g., mannitol or loop diuretics) is recommended. Mannitol, however, may cause volume overload if the kidneys are unable to effect diuresis. Hemoglobin is also capable of inducing ARF. Renal failure, however, is relatively rare, occurring with massive intravascular hemolysis (e.g., fulminant transfusion reactions, hemolytic crises).
2. **Tumor lysis syndrome.** The sudden release of tumor cell contents, including phosphates, uric acid, and purine metabolites, in response to induction chemotherapy is termed tumor lysis syndrome. ARF is caused by diffuse nephronal microobstruction by these products. This syndrome occurs in patients with hematologic and lymphoproliferative malignancies, especially of large tumor burden. Patients at risk should routinely receive prophylaxis before chemotherapy, including volume expansion, maintenance of diuresis, alkalinization of the urine, and pretreatment with allopurinol. Once established, the syndrome is difficult to treat, and interim dialytic therapy is often required in oliguric patients.
3. **Radiocontrast-induced nephropathy.** The administration of intravenous radiocontrast is associated with rapidly developing, and typically oliguric, ARF. Serum creatinine generally peaks around 4 days after the procedure, and renal function returns to baseline within 7 to 14 days. Because no specific therapy exists, preventive measures are emphasized, especially for

patients at increased risk. Risk factors include preexisting renal insufficiency, diabetic nephropathy with renal insufficiency, volume depletion, large contrast dose (more than 2 mL/kg), age greater than 60 years, hyperuricemia, hepatic failure, and multiple myeloma. Modest hydration before the procedure (0.45% saline, 0.5 to 2.0 mL/kg per hour to start 2–6 hours before contrast administration) and to continue 6 hours afterward is advocated. Diuretics are to be avoided during this period. There may be a benefit to the use of nonionic, low-osmolality radiocontrast media in at risk patients.

4. **Drug-induced syndrome.** There are four major syndromes of drug-induced ARF.
   a. **Acute tubular injury.** Drugs exerting direct toxic effects, typically to the proximal tubular epithelium, cause this syndrome. Agents include aminoglycoside antibiotics, certain cephalosporins, cisplatin, amphotericin B, and foscarnet. Predisposing risk factors for tubular injury include volume contraction, preexisting renal insufficiency, and liver disease. ARF is usually reversible with drug discontinuation.
   b. **Intratubular microobstruction.** Selected drugs, such as acyclovir, methotrexate, sulfamethoxazole, and low-molecular-weight dextran may precipitate in and obstruct the nephrons. Prevention of tubular obstruction necessitates optimal hydration of the patient and maintenance of high urine flow rate. The syndrome is usually reversible and short-lived.
   c. **Acute interstitial nephritis.** An ever-enlarging list of drugs can cause acute interstitial nephritis (Table 61-4). Among the most common culprits are penicillins, sulfa drugs, thiazide diuretics, and allopurinol. Cases vary widely in the time of onset after exposure to the agent (days to years), the dose-risk relationship, the severity of the renal failure, and the time to reversal after drug discontinuation. The urine sediment typi-

TABLE 61-4. Drugs most often implicated in acute interstitial nephritis

Antibiotics
Penicillinase-resistant penicillins
Cephalosporins
Ampicillin
Amoxicillin
Penicillin G
Sulfonamides and sulfa-trimethoprim
Rifampin
Ethambutol
Tetracycline
Diuretics
Furosemide
Thiazides and related compounds
Nonsteroidal antiinflammatory drugs
Ibuprofen
Indomethacin
Fenoprofen
Naproxen
Phenylbutazone
Mefenamic acid
Tolmetin
Miscellaneous drugs
Diphenylhydantoin
Cimetidine
Alpha-methyldopa
Allopurinol
Captopril

cally shows red and white cells, often including eosinophils. Renal recovery should occur on discontinuation of the drug. Protracted cases may benefit from a short course of steroids.

d. **Autoregulatory failure.** Two patterns of hemodynamically mediated, drug-induced renal failure may occur. When the main action of the drug is to permit afferent arteriolar vasoconstriction, such as with nonsteroidal antiinflammatory drugs or vasopressors, failure to autoregulate renal blood flow ensues, and prerenal azotemia develops. If a drug causing efferent arteriolar vasodilatation, such as a converting enzyme inhibitor, is given to a patient with a fixed impediment to blood flow (e. g., bilateral renal artery stenosis), a sharp reduction in glomerular filtration rate (GFR) may occur. Unless severe renal ischemia has occurred, renal failure is reversible after withdrawal of the drug.

C. **Renal vascular disease**

1. **Renal artery occlusion.** Generally, ARF is seen only if a thromboembolic event involves both kidneys or a solitary functioning kidney. Renal artery emboli typically occur in the setting of cardiac disease, such as arrhythmia, myocardial infarction, or valvular disease. Clinical hallmarks include acute flank pain, oliguria, and hematuria. Radiologic techniques, including nuclear imaging, computed tomography, and arteriography can confirm the diagnosis. Arteriography is the most invasive study and associated with the greatest risks, but it yields the most anatomic information. Therapy is most effective if performed within 24 hours. Options include surgical thrombectomy, supportive care with anticoagulation, and possibly use of fibrinolytic agents.
2. **Renal vein thrombosis.** Situations in which renal vein thrombosis may occur include the nephrotic syndrome, renal cell carcinoma, hematologic disorders characterized by hypercoagulability, sickle cell disease, pregnancy, use of oral contraceptives, and trauma. As in renal artery occlusion, ARF seldom occurs unless both kidneys are simultaneously involved; clinical features are similar as well. Duplex venography and computed tomography can confirm the diagnosis. Treatment involves anticoagulation and possibly fibrinolytic therapy.
3. **Atheroembolic renal disease (cholesterol emboli).** Showers of cholesterol emboli occur in patients with severe aortic atherosclerosis, typically after a precipitating event such as aortography, major vascular surgery, or blunt trauma to the abdomen; they may also develop spontaneously or in association with anticoagulant therapy. In addition to the kidney, the spleen, pancreas, bowel, retina, brain, and extremities may also be affected. Often, the diagnosis is overlooked unless peripheral signs of involvement, such as blue distal digits, a mottled appearance of the lower extremities (livedo reticularis), and Hollenhorst plaque in the retinal vessels, are evident. Laboratory testing may reveal eosinophilia, hypocomplementemia, and a nondiagnostic urine sediment. There is no specific management for cholesterol emboli; anticoagulant use may worsen the course of the disease. Patients may suffer minor degrees of azotemia or may progress to irreversible renal failure requiring dialysis.

D. **Renal dysfunction in patients with liver disease.** Although prerenal azotemia is the most common renal syndrome in patients with advanced liver disease, hepatorenal syndrome is the most feared. Hepatorenal syndrome refers to the development of progressive oliguria and azotemia in patients with advanced hepatic dysfunction. It is characterized by severe sodium retention unresponsive to volume loading or diuretics. Although hepatorenal syndrome is generally irreversible barring a recovery of liver function, reports exist of reversal of renal dysfunction with infusions of salt-poor albumin or fresh frozen plasma and peritovenous or portosystemic shunting procedures.

The management of patients with cirrhosis and sodium retention is challenging. A tenuous balance must be maintained between control of ascites or edema and the avoidance of hypovolemia or severe prerenal azotemia. Standard treatment involves dietary sodium restriction, diuretic regimens including spironolactone, and paracentesis. Colloid infusion should be performed simultaneously with large-volume paracentesis to minimize the risk of hypovolemia and its consequences.

Electrolyte and acid-base disturbances are common. Primary respiratory alkalosis is frequently observed. A mixed acid-base disturbance of respiratory alkalosis and metabolic acidosis often develops in patients who suffer an additional insult such as sepsis or renal failure. Both potassium depletion and metabolic alkalosis should be avoided because they enhance ammonia synthesis and aggravate hepatic encephalopathy.

III. Diagnosis

A. History and physical examination. The history can be helpful because it may establish the chronicity of the problem, reveal underlying previous renal or urinary abnormalities, or identify exposure to nephrotoxic agents or ischemic events. The physical examination may provide diagnostic information. For example, orthostatic hypotension, diminished skin turgor, and dry mucous membranes suggest a diagnosis of prerenal azotemia; bladder distention and prostatic enlargement point to obstructive uropathy.

B. Urine tests. The laboratory workup should commence with urinalysis. The urine dipstick test provides information regarding the presence of heme pigments and protein. When the test is positive, it should raise the suspicion of intrinsic renal pathology. Microscopic analysis of the urine should also be done because formed elements in the urine can yield information about the nature of the renal failure.

C. Blood tests. Serum chemistry studies should be monitored closely to aid in the management of critical acid-base and electrolyte abnormalities. Complete blood count may identify anemia or eosinophilia, pointing to the chronicity of renal failure or the diagnosis of acute interstitial nephritis, respectively. Serologic tests should be ordered only if there is appropriate suspicion of the underlying disorder.

D. Radiography. Various radiographic techniques may assist in the evaluation of ARF. In general, renal ultrasound should be the first radiologic test ordered, because it is a safe, quick, and high-yield procedure. It permits the identification and measurement of the kidneys as well as characterization of the parenchyma and collecting systems. Computed tomography offers similar benefits, but it should be performed without contrast in the patient with ARF to avoid the added nephrotoxicity of intravenous radiocontrast. Likewise, intravenous pyelography has little role in the evaluation of ARF, because of concerns about radiocontrast-induced nephrotoxicity. Retrograde pyelography is reserved for patients in whom there is strong concern for urinary tract obstruction. Isotopic renal scanning is a safe and effective method to assess renal perfusion as well as function.

E. Renal biopsy. Renal biopsy is reserved for patients who are thought to have parenchymal renal disease. The procedure should be considered when azotemia is of recent onset and unknown cause, when the possibility exists that the patient has a renal disease that may require specialized drug treatment such as steroids or immunosuppressive medication, or when the biopsy may be of prognostic importance.

IV. Consequences.

Regardless of the cause, the consequences of ARF are similar. The physician should carefully assess and monitor the patient for acute complications.

A. Hyperkalemia. This is the most immediately life-threatening electrolyte imbalance encountered in patients with ARF. Sources of potassium, endogenous or exogenous, need to be identified and regulated if possible. Endogenous sources include tissue breakdown, cell lysis, and hematoma reabsorption. Exogenous sources include diet, intravenous fluids, and medications. Medications that interfere with potassium regulation, such as nonsteroidal antiinflammatory drugs, heparin, and angiotensin-converting enzyme inhibitors, should be discontinued. Specific medical interventions besides dietary restriction include diuretics to increase urine flow rate, potassium binding resins, and dialysis if hyperkalemia is severe or refractory to the foregoing interventions (see Chapter 62).

B. Metabolic acidosis. Metabolic acidosis that results from reduced tubular hydrogen excretion normally produces hyperchloremic or low anion gap acidosis. When the GFR is severely impaired, retention of acidic wastes in the extracellular fluid may produce high anion gap acidosis. Mild metabolic acidosis (serum bicarbonate level no less than 16 mEq/L) does not require therapy. More marked acidosis requires correction with bicarbonate therapy. Severe acidosis (serum pH less than 7.20) requires therapy with parenteral sodium bicarbonate; however, the patient's volume status must be monitored carefully because the sodium salt may lead to volume overload, particularly if the patient is oliguric. Acidosis that cannot be treated medically is an indication for dialysis.

C. Abnormal salt and water metabolism. Patients with ARF can neither conserve nor excrete sodium or water maximally; hence they are at risk for derangements of water and sodium balance. Hyponatremia and volume overload are common.

D. Abnormal calcium and phosphorus metabolism. When the GFR falls below one-third of normal, the kidneys' ability to excrete phosphorus is impaired, resulting in phosphorus retention. High serum phosphorus levels lead to the formation of insoluble calcium phosphorus salts that may precipitate in soft tissue; if the product of the serum calcium and phosphorus concentrations exceeds 70, this is likely. Phosphate binders, such as calcium carbonate, should be used to decrease intestinal absorption of phosphate in patients with elevated phosphorus levels. If the calcium × phosphorus product exceeds 70, aluminum hydroxide gels should be used preferentially until the product is decreased.

E. Uremia. Accumulation of endogenous toxins in the body results in uremia. In general, the syndrome manifests itself when the GFR is less than 10 mL per minute. Uremia may present as vague symptoms such as lethargy, malaise, anorexia, and nausea. Other less subjective manifestations constitute stronger indications for prompt initiation of dialysis, including bleeding diathesis, seizures, coma, and the appearance of a pericardial rub.

TABLE 61-5. Predialysis management of acute renal failure

Fluid balance
- Weigh patient daily
- Monitor input and output
- In volume-depleted patients replace extra cellular fluid with isotonic saline (or bicarbonate)
- In normovolemic or edematous patients, restrict fluid intake (~1,500 mL/d) and sodium intake (<2 g/d)
- Only use diuretics in oliguric patients who are either normovolemic or hypervolemic

Acid/base and electrolyte balance
- Avoid water overload and hyponatremia (restrict free water intake, particularly in oliguric patients)
- Restrict potassium intake (<2 g/d) and treat hyperkalemia
- Supplemental bicarbonate for serum level <15mM
- Use phosphate binders to maintain serum phosphorus <5.0 mg/dL

Drugs
- Avoid nephrotoxins when possible
- Adjust doses of all drugs excreted by the kidneys
- Withhold NSAIDs and CEIs in patients with prerenal azotemia
- Avoid magnesium-containing drugs (antacids, milk of magnesia)

Nutrition
- Restrict protein intake to <0.5 g/kg/d to prevent increased urea synthesis
- Ensure calorie intake to >400 kcal/d to reduce tissue catabolism

Reduction of infectious risks
- Remove indwelling urinary catheter in oliguric, nonobstructed patients
- Strict aseptic technique and rapid removal, when feasible, of vascular catheters

CEIs, converting enzyme inhibitors; NSAIDs, nonsteroidal antiinflammatory drugs.

F. Abnormal drug metabolism. A careful review of all medications is imperative in the care of the patient with ARF. Drugs that are excreted almost entirely by the kidneys will need adjustment in drug dose or dosing intervals. If dialysis is initiated, adjustments may need to be made to account for clearance with dialysis.

V. Treatment. The predialysis management of ARF is outlined in Table 61-5. These simple procedures are applicable for any patient with ARF and may be critical for the patient's survival. In general, dialysis therapy should be reserved for patients in whom fluid and biochemical parameters cannot be controlled through medical means alone or in patients who develop uremic symptoms. The use of dialysis is discussed in depth in Chapter 62.

VI. Prognosis and outcome. Overall, the mortality rate from ARF ranges from 25% to 64%. In general, nonoliguria is associated with the best odds of recovery of renal function and approximately half the mortality of oliguric ARF. Recovery of renal function, however, can be expected in most patients who survive ARF, except those who have acute bilateral cortical necrosis or other irreversible forms of parenchymal renal disease.

Selected Readings

Battaller R, Sort P, Gines P, et al. Hepatorenal syndrome: definition, pathophysiology, clinical features and management. *Kidney Int* 1998;53[Suppl 66]:S47.

A current review of this challenging disease.

Berns AS. Nephrotoxicity of contrast media. *Kidney Int* 1989;36:730.

An excellent discussion on the epidemiology, pathophysiology, and prevention of contrast-induced nephrotoxicity.

Clive DM, Cohen AJ. Acute renal failure in the intensive care unit. In: Rippe JM, Irwin RS, Fink MP, et al, eds. *Intensive care medicine,* 4th ed. Boston: Little, Brown, 1998:969.

An extensive review of this subject.

Dubrow A, Flamenbaum W. Acute renal failure associated with myoglobinuria and hemoglobinuria. In: Brenner BM, Lazarus JM, eds. *Acute renal failure,* 2nd ed. New York: Churchill Livingstone, 1988:279.

A good review of pigment-induced ARF.

Eknoyan G. Acute tubulointerstitial nephritis. In: Schrier RW, Gottschalk CW, eds. *Diseases of the kidney,* 6th ed. Boston: Little, Brown, 1997:1249.

A thorough and well-written review of the topic.

Hou S, Bushinsky DA, Wish JB. Hospital-acquired renal insufficiency: a prospective study. *Am J Med* 1983;74:243.

A prospective study concluding that there is a substantial risk of developing renal failure in hospitalized patients and an associated high mortality rate.

Hricik DE, Dunn MJ. Angiotensin-converting enzyme inhibitor–induced renal failure. *J Am Soc Nephrol* 1990;1:845.

A review of the speculated mechanisms and consequences of converting enzyme inhibitor–induced renal failure in patients with renovascular disease.

Rose BD. Acute renal failure. In: Rose BD, ed. *Pathophysiology of renal disease.* New York: McGraw-Hill, 1981:55.

A basic review of the causes of ARF, with emphasis on prerenal azotemia and ATN.

Smith MC, Ghose MK, Henry AR. The clinical spectrum of renal cholesterol embolization. *Am J Med* 1981;71:174.

A good review of the topic.

Solomon R, Werner C, Mann D, et al. Effects of saline, mannitol, and furosemide on acute decreases in renal function induced by radiocontrast agents. *N Engl J Med* 1994;331:1416.

An important study, the basis for the current recommendations for prevention of contrast-induced nephrotoxicity.

Swan SK, Bennett WM. Nephrotoxic acute renal failure. In: Brenner BM, Lazarus JM, eds. *Acute renal failure,* 3rd ed. New York: Churchill Livingstone, 1993:357.

An in-depth review of various nephrotoxic drugs and the general mechanisms by which they induce ARF.

62. DIALYSIS THERAPY IN THE INTENSIVE CARE SETTING

David M. Clive

I. **Background.** The technical foundations for both major forms of renal replacement therapy, hemodialysis and peritoneal dialysis, were in place in the first half of the twentieth century. Nonetheless, the ability to use these treatments in a practical and repeatable fashion is a more recent development. Dialysis is used in the treatment of chronic, or end-stage, renal failure, as well as in acute renal failure (ARF). Most patients with renal failure who are in intensive care units are in the latter category, and they are receiving dialysis on an interim basis.

Most cases of ARF resolve without requiring dialysis. However, intensively ill patients with ARF have a high mortality. Dialysis in this context is fraught with technical considerations and challenges.

A. **Hemodialysis.** Hemodialysis uses an artificial kidney or dialyzer and a dialysis machine, comprising mechanical pumps pushing blood and dialysate through their respective channels in the dialyzer. Typically, the blood flow rate is 300 mL/min, and that of dialysate is 500 mL/min. Dialysate passes through the system once and is discarded. The high flow rate and single-pass method enhance the gradient favoring transfer of permeant molecules from blood to dialysis. Membrane composition and surface area also influence clearances, with the newer, higher-porosity membranes achieving high clearances even of solutes with molecular weights exceeding 300 daltons. Two parameters for determining the "dose" of dialysis given to a patient are as follows:

1. $Kt / V =$ the volume adjusted fractional clearance of urea

   where K is the dialyzer urea clearance, t is time of the dialysis treatment, and V is the volume of distribution of urea.
2. URR or urea reduction ratio, defined mathematically as

   $[1 \times (\text{post-} \div \text{pre-blood urea nitrogen concentration})] \times 100$

These parameters were developed to optimize dialysis prescriptions in patients receiving long-term hemodialysis; their use in ARF is still being defined.

B. **Hemofiltration and hemodiafiltration.** Hemofiltration and hemodiafiltration employ extremely high-porosity dialyzers that permit transmembrane filtration of large volumes of plasma ultrafiltrate. They are generally run as continuous procedures and thus collectively are classified as *continuous renal replacement therapy (CRRT).* Solute movement occurs by convection. In continuous arteriovenous hemofiltration (CAVH), an arteriovenous circuit is used. Blood flow in CAVH is driven entirely by the patient's own hemodynamics, the filtrate being wholly or partially replaced with a physiologic replacement solution. Continuous venovenous hemofiltration is similar to CAVH, but it uses a venovenous circuit in conjunction with a blood pump. Several modifications of hemofiltration are used including slow continuous ultrafiltration, in which ultrafiltrate is removed relatively slowly and is not replaced, and high-volume hemofiltration, in which a certain portion of the ultrafiltrate is replaced with physiologic crystalloid. High-volume hemofiltration permits substantial convective solute clearance. In addition, dialysis solution may be infused slowly into the membrane cartridge in CRRT to allow *hemodiafiltration,* an extremely effective form of renal replacement therapy in ARF.

C. **Peritoneal dialysis.** Peritoneal dialysis, like hemodialysis, affords gradient-driven solute clearance. The gradient may be optimized by using maximal dialysis dwell volumes; 2 to 3 L is typical in an adult patient. Ultrafilitration in peritoneal dialysis is engendered by the osmolality of the dialysate, generally a dextrose-containing solution.

II. Indications for and timing of dialysis

A. Absolute indications. Absolute indications include severe fluid and electrolyte imbalances, such as hyperkalemia, hypervolemia, and metabolic acidosis, unmanageable through more conservative medical means. Uremic symptoms are usually relative indications (see later), with the exception of uremic pericarditis and severe uremic encephalopathy. These uremic manifestations are life-threatening and militate in favor of urgent dialysis.

B. Relative indications. Relative indications include more minor uremic symptoms, such as nausea and lethargy, bleeding believed to be exacerbated by uremic platelet dysfunction, and non–life-threatening chemical imbalances such as moderate hypercalcemia and hypermagnesemia.

C. Timing. Timing of dialysis has traditionally been a subject of considerable controversy. Some experts believe that early, even preemptive dialysis improves survival in ARF. Others challenge this and express concern that dialysis itself may lengthen the course of ARF. This area is still under investigation, and until firm recommendations are available, clinicians are advised to individualize their approach to each case.

III. Hemodialysis and hemofiltration

A. Dialyzers. Dialyzers for hemodialysis and hemofiltration are plastic cylinders encasing a bundle of parallel, hollow-fiber capillary tubes through which the blood flows. The dialysate runs countercurrent through the encasing jacket. The two major characteristics to be considered in choosing a dialyzer are, first, the ultrafiltration coefficient (K_{uf}), a function of its aggregate membrane surface area, and permeability. CRRT techniques demand extremely high K_{uf} membranes. Also important is the membrane type. Conventional dialyzers employ cellulose acetate or related cellophane-like membranes. The newer polymers, polyacrylonitrile, polymethylmethacrylate, and polysulfone, offer the potential advantage of "biocompatibility," that is, they do not lead to complement activation and cytokine production. This feature is important from several standpoints. Biocompatible membranes engender fewer host side effects such as pyrogenic reactions. Second, they have the propensity to adsorb proinflammatory substances such as bradykinin, interleukin-1, and tumor necrosis factor, still only a theoretic advantage. Third, patients with ARF receiving dialysis with biocompatible membranes may have better outcomes than those dialyzed with conventional dialyzers.

B. Dialysates. Dialysates for hemodialysis are physiologic fluids. Although there is some variation among solutions, glucose concentrations in dialysates are in the normoglycemic range. Sodium concentration ranges between 135 and 140 mEq/L. In some dialytic protocols, the sodium concentration may be varied as the treatment progresses (sodium "modeling" or "profiling"). This modification helps to control osmolar shift symptoms such as leg cramps, headaches, and dysequilibrium. Potassium content of dialysate solutions is usually prescribed at the time of treatment, particularly in patients receiving short-term dialysis. Potassium removal is an objective of most dialysis treatments. The kinetics of intradialytic potassium transfer is such that transient hypokalemia is to be expected within the first 5 hours after a dialysis session and should not be supplemented. Patients at risk for arrhythmias from hypokalemia, such as those receiving digitalis glycosides, should be dialyzed against a potassium concentration of 3 to 4 mEq/L, unless these patients are floridly hyperkalemic at the outset. Bicarbonate has supplanted acetate as the buffer base in virtually all hemodialysis solutions. The typical concentration of bicarbonate is 30 to 35 mEq/L. The treatment objectives regarding divalent cations in most patients undergoing dialysis are to engender positive calcium balance and modestly negative magnesium balance. Thus, dialysis concentrations of 3.5 and 1.0 mEq/L, respectively, are employed.

When dialysis is to be performed in conjunction with CRRT, peritoneal dialysis fluid is generally used. Custom modifications of these fluids, with varied the calcium content, are available for patients for patients with calcium imbalances. The standard buffer base in peritoneal dialysis stock solutions is lactate; in patients with impaired ability to metabolize lactate, this may pose a problem.

C. Replacement solutions. Replacement solutions for CRRT are isotonic solutions. Ringer's lactate is popular for this purpose because it contains the full range of physiologic solutes. Its use is limited in patients with specialized problems such as severe metabolic alkalosis or lactate intolerance. In such cases, custom-made solutions should be obtained from the hospital pharmacy.

D. Anticoagulation. Anticoagulation for hemodialysis and CRRT is made necessary by the thrombogenic potential of most dialyzer membranes. Patients who are anticoagulated at baseline or patients with severe bleeding problems may need little or no anticoagulation. Anticoagulation for the typical hemodialysis treatment involves systemic heparinization with a 2,000- to 5,000-U bolus of heparin, followed by an infusion of 1,000 U per hour for the duration of the treatment. The goal is to keep the activated clotting time approximately 50% over baseline. "Tight" and "fractional" heparinization protocols target an activated clotting time of 15% and 25% over baseline, respectively. Controlled heparinization protocols must be employed in patients at enhanced risk of bleeding. The safest form of anticoagulation, yet a challenging one to perform, is regional heparinization, in which sodium citrate is infused at low rates into the arterial line of the dialyzer circuit. By chelating calcium, the citrate achieves anticoagulation in the dialyzer; its effect is reversed at the venous end by the infusion of calcium chloride. This technique is used only in the most extreme cases of bleeding risk including:

1. Patients with active bleeding or within 14 days of major operative procedure or intracranial surgery.
2. Patients within 72 hours of a needle or forceps biopsy of a visceral organ.
3. Patents with pericarditis.
4. Patients within 72 hours of a minor surgical procedure.
5. Patients anticipated to receive a major surgical procedure within 8 hours of hemodialysis.

Anticoagulation in CRRT poses the same basic issues as for hemodialysis, except the anticoagulation, like CRRT, is continuous. The partial thromboplastin time in the arterial line is kept at 50% higher than control. Hemofilters are notoriously prone to thrombosis, probably because of the high protein concentrations they achieve during the ultrafiltrative process. CRRT therefore may not be feasible for patients at heightened risk for bleeding.

E. Angioaccess. Angioaccess for dialytic procedures in the intensive care unit usually involves the placement of a large-bore, dual-lumen catheter. In long-term maintenance hemodialysis, fistulas or arteriovenous grafts are the accesses of choice. They cannot be accessed as soon as they are implanted, obviating their use in patients with ARF. Furthermore, the easy removability of access catheters makes sense in patients with potentially reversible renal dysfunction. Catheters may be placed in the femoral, internal jugular, or subclavian location. Femoral venous catheters limit the patient to the supine position and are associated with a high risk of venous thrombosis and infection, and they are not recommended for use for more than a few days at a time. Subclavian catheters do not pose the same positional problems as femoral catheters, but they may induce the development of venous stenoses and thromboses. The internal jugular location is gaining in popularity for this reason. The basic technique for placing a catheter in any location is to employ sterile technique and local anesthesia. The vessel is cannulated with an introducer needle, and a guidewire is inserted through the needle. The catheter is ultimately passed over the wire (Seldinger technique). Care must be taken to avoid hitting arterial structures. In upper extremity locations, the risk of pneumothorax must be considered. Double-lumen catheters draw from and return into the same vein through different lumina.

Vascular access for CRRT is achieved in a similar fashion to that described in the previous paragraph. In CAVH, however, separate arterial and venous catheters are used.

IV. Peritoneal dialysis

A. Peritoneal dialysates. Peritoneal dialysates are less diversified than hemodialysis solutions. The major therapeutic consideration is choosing the dextrose concentration of the dialysate, because this is the method for controlling ultrafiltration. Three strengths are in common use: 1.5%, 2.5%, and 4.25% dextrose. The choice depends on the particular patient's ability to "clear fluid" during peritoneal dialysis; 4.25% dialysate is appropriate for clinically fluid overloaded patients with ARF. Diabetic patients undergoing peritoneal dialysis must have serum glucose concentrations followed closely.

B. Peritoneal access. Peritoneal access can be established on an emergency basis using a rigid catheter passed over a stylet. The patient's urinary bladder must be emptied to avoid perforation, because the access site is in the midline between the umbilicus and the symphysis pubis. More electively, soft, Dacron cuffed catheters (e.g., Tenckhoff catheter) are placed surgically.

V. Dose of dialysis. Adequacy of dialysis appears to affect outcomes in ARF, just as it does in chronic renal failure. Although the specific needs of patients with ARF have not yet been elucidated, it should be assumed they are at least equal to those of patients with chronic renal failure. This means a Kt/V greater than or equal to 1.2 or a URR greater than or equal to 70%.

VI. Continuous versus intermittent dialysis therapy. Nephrologists generally believe that CRRT offers advantages over intermittent hemodialysis in the treatment of ARF. CRRT is better tolerated hemodynamically, may be modified easily from minute to minute, and can be tailored to match a patient's changing daily fluid input. CRRT is fairly labor intensive. As already mentioned, it necessitates higher anticoagulation exposure. Further, outcome studies have yet to prove any benefit of CRRT over intermittent treatment. The choice should be made by the physician.

VII. Discontinuation of dialysis. Most patients with ARF become dialysis independent within several weeks. There are several indicators that this time may be at hand. Although the correlation between urine output and glomerular filtration rate is poor, an increase in the urine output in a previously oliguric patient is a favorable sign. In patients undergoing intermittent dialysis, a spontaneously falling serum creatinine level or one that fails to rise between treatments betokens a return of renal function. Discontinuation of dialysis may also be contemplated under less fortunate circumstances, that is, in patients with persistent renal failure who languish or fail despite intensive medical care. Such decisions should reflect close communication between patients (or their representatives) and physicians.

VIII. Choosing the optimum dialysis modality for a patient. The major considerations inherent in choosing one dialytic modality over another have already been discussed. Table 62-1 summarizes the relative advantages of each method.

IX. Complications of hemodialysis. Cardiovascular complications occur more frequently with hemodialysis than with the other blood purification techniques. Hypotension is the most common complication. Its pathophysiology is multifactorial, relating to the following:

1. Osmotic shifts.
2. Immunologic and vasomotor responses to dialysis membranes.
3. Alteration of autonomic function in the uremic state.
4. Myocardial ischemia, which may be "silent," that is, not accompanied by angina pectoris.
5. Dialysis-induced hypoxemia.

Hypotension of hemodialysis can be controlled or prevented by cooling of dialysate, which promotes vasoconstriction and improved myocardial contractility, and careful volumetric control of ultrafiltration.

Dysequilibrium syndrome refers to the series of neurologic symptoms, most commonly dizziness and headache, which result from a disparity in solute concentration between the cerebrospinal fluid and the vascular space. Osmolar clear-

TABLE 62-1. Choice of dialytic modality

Therapeutic Objective	IH	PD	CRRT
Large ultrafiltrate removal (target volume of removal ≥10% body weight)	√		√
Solute clearance	√		√
Rapid correction of solute or fluid overload	√		
Avoidance of anticoagulation	√		
Least hemodynamic instability		√	√
Avoidance of need for vascular access		√	
Allowance for mobility of patient	√	√	
Avoidance of cerebral edema and osmotic dysequilibrium (e.g., neurosurgery patient)		√	√
Allowance for large-volume alimentation fluid			√
Minimized need for nursing support		√	
Rapid removal of drugs or toxins	√		
Allowance for abdominal lavage (e.g., in fulminant pancreatitis)		√	

CRRT, continuous renal replacement therapy, IH, intermittent hemodialysis; PD, peritoneal dialysis. (From Lau TW, Chertow GM, Owen WF. Dialysis therapy in the intensive care setting. In: Irwin RS, Cerra FB, Rippe JM, eds. *Intensive Care Medicine*, 4th ed. Philadelphia: Lippincott–Raven, 1999.)

ance occurs rapidly from the vascular space and renders it hypoosmolal with respect to the brain. Water enters brain parenchyma in these circumstances, leading to cerebral edema. Paradoxic cerebrospinal fluid acidosis may also occur. These problems can be attenuated by mitigating the rate of solute clearance during dialyses, especially during the first few treatments.

Hypoxemia occurs commonly. It is attributed to alveolar hypoventilation and intrapulmonary leukostasis triggered by dialysis membranes. This is rarely a problem, except for patients with significant cardiopulmonary disease.

Technical errors such as air embolism and contamination of blood or dialysate lines are unusual given a rigorous quality control program in the dialysis unit.

Bleeding is the most greatest problem with CRRT and mandates a cautious approach to anticoagulation, as already noted.

Among patients on peritoneal dialysis, peritonitis is the predominant complication of therapy. These infections arise from introduction of pathogens into the dialysis system during dialysate exchanges. Tunnel infections arise at the catheter exit site and may track subcutaneously into the peritoneum. The most commonly isolated pathogens are *Staphylococcus aureus* and *S. epidermidis*. Gram-negative bacteria and fungi are occasionally culpable. When a patient is suspected of having peritonitis associated with peritoneal dialysis, it is recommended to begin therapy with broad-spectrum antimicrobial coverage, to be narrowed once culture reports are received.

Selected Readings

Daugirdas JT. Dialysis hypotension: a hemodynamic analysis. *Kidney Int* 1991;39:233.
An analysis of the pathophysiology of hemodynamic instability during hemodialysis.

Himmelfarb J, Hakim RM. The use of biocompatible dialysis membranes in acute renal failure. *Adv Ren Replace Ther* 1997;4:72.
Explores the concept of biocompatibility of dialysis membranes and their impact on outcomes in cases of dialysis-dependent ARF.

Kaplan AA, Longnecker RE, Folkert VW. Continuous arteriovenous hemofiltration: a report of six months' experience. *Ann Intern Med* 1984;100:358.
The report that publicized CAVH in the United States and ultimately led to widespread use of CRRT in ARF.

Lau TW, Chertow GM, Owen WF. Dialysis therapy in the intensive care setting. In: Irwin RS, Cerra FB, Rippe JM, eds. *Intensive care medicine,* 4th ed. Philadelphia: Lippincott–Raven, 1999:1024.

Source material for this chapter.

Lohr JW, Schwab SJ. Minimizing hemorrhagic complications in dialysis patients. *J Am Soc Nephrol* 1991;2:961.

A thorough discussion of principles of safe anticoagulation in renal replacement therapy.

Lowrie E, Lew N. The urea reduction ratio (URR):a simple method in evaluating hemodialysis treatment. *Contemp Dial Nephrol* 1991;12:11.

Introduces the concept of adequacy of dialysis therapy as determined by objective parameters.

Pastan S, Bailey J. Dialysis therapy. *N Engl J Med* 1998;338:1428.

A good review of the fundamentals of hemodialysis and peritoneal dialysis.

Tenckhoff H, Schechter H. A bacteriologically safe peritoneal access device. *Trans Am Soc Artif Intern Organs* 1968;14:181.

The soft, tunneled, cuffed peritoneal dialysis catheter was a historic development that made both ambulatory and long-term peritoneal dialysis possible.

VI. INFECTIOUS DISEASE PROBLEMS IN THE INTENSIVE CARE UNIT

63. APPROACH TO FEVER IN THE INTENSIVE CARE PATIENT

Marie J. George, Jennifer S. Daly, and Richard H. Glew

I. General principles. Fever is a common problem in the intensive care unit. This chapter discusses both noninfectious and infectious causes of fever and provides a diagnostic framework for evaluation.

II. Pathophysiology. Fever has been recognized as a sign of disease for centuries. The principal mediator of fever is the cytokine interleukin-1 (IL-1), although others, including tumor necrosis factor (TNF) and interleukin-6 (IL-6) have been shown to be similar effectors of fever. Cytokines interact with receptors in the preoptic anterior hypothalamic thermoregulatory area, causing synthesis and release of prostaglandins, which reset the thermoregulatory set point of the hypothalamus. Prostaglandins coordinate other adaptive responses such as shivering and peripheral vasoconstriction.

III. Measurement and fever patterns. No single normal body temperature exists, and temperatures measured at different body sites may vary. A person's body temperature varies physiologically; it is lowest in the morning and elevates with marked activity such as exercise or seizures. The febrile response to pyrogenic stimuli may be blunted or even absent in the elderly, in patients with azotemia or congestive heart failure, and in those receiving therapy with antipyretics or corticosteroids. Debilitated patients may exhibit a flattened, but minimally elevated temperature plot without the normal diurnal variation.

Despite medical folklore, fever patterns generally are not helpful in suggesting or establishing specific diagnoses. First, in many hospitalized patients, insufficient data exist to establish a pattern of fever, often because of the brevity of illness or the administration of confounding medications. Moreover, there is no relation between specific diagnoses and the occurrence of so-called intermittent, remittent, or hectic fevers. Similarly, although rigors are considered to suggest the presence of severe bacterial infection, shaking chills may also be seen in various nonbacterial disease states, including viral infections, drug reactions, other inflammatory conditions, and lymphoma.

IV. Noninfectious causes of fever. Although acute bacterial infections are among the most common and serious causes of fever in patients in the intensive care unit (ICU), fever may be a prominent manifestation of noninfectious illness. Fever can be a major symptom in patients critically ill with an acute vasculitis, subarachnoid hemorrhage, dissection of an aortic aneurysm, mesenteric ischemia, heat stroke, or hyperthyroidism. Fever may appear in the patient in whom the stress of surgery unmasks adrenal insufficiency or in the patient in whom malignant hyperpyrexia develops during surgery or after administration of nonanaesthetic agents such as phenothiazines. Bilateral adrenal hemorrhage, noted to occur in patients with a history of thromboembolic disease, recent surgery, or anticoagulant therapy, can present with fever and abdominal pain. Fever can be associated with acute alcohol withdrawal, although it is necessary to exclude infection. Likewise, fever after seizures must be differentiated from possible underlying causes of seizure, such as meningitis, encephalitis, or brain abscess. Fever occurring several days after hospital admission and restriction to bed can signal the development of deep venous thrombosis or pulmonary embolism. A common cause of nosocomial fever is adverse reaction to medications and blood products. Fever occurs with certain malignant diseases, such as lymphoma, hypernephroma, and liver neoplasia.

V. Infectious causes of fever. Nosocomial infections are an endemic problem in the ICU. The most common sources of bacterial infection in the ICU include the urinary tract, respiratory tract, and wounds. Secondary bacteremia can complicate infection in these sites but can also develop as a consequence of vascular invasion through intravenous lines, intraarterial monitors, temporary transvenous pacemakers, and intraaortic assist devices. The gastrointestinal tract can serve as the source for severe nosocomial infections as well. Acute acalculous cholecystitis may occur after surgery and severe trauma. Another cause of fever and abdominal pain in the ICU patient is antibiotic-associated pseudomembranous colitis, caused by *Clostridium difficile,* mesenteric ischemia, or intraabdominal abscess.

VI. Diagnosis. Fever in patients in the ICU or coronary care unit warrants immediate assessment because of the following: (a) patients requiring ICU support are severely ill, with complex underlying illnesses, and thereby are less likely than other hospitalized patients to survive serious nosocomial infections; and (b) the organisms common in nosocomial infections, *Staphylococcus aureus,* gram-negative bacilli, and fungi, may cause necrotizing destruction of tissue and blood infections, and they are relatively resistant to antibiotics. If the patient can communicate, he or she should be interviewed concerning localizing complaints. The patient, hospital chart, and caregivers should be reexamined for a history of relevant antecedent problems and information such as duration of vascular cannulation, quantity and purulence of sputum or wound drainage, changes in skin condition, apparent abdominal or musculoskeletal pain or tenderness, difficulty in handling respiratory secretions and food, and changes in ventilator support requirements. Family members may be helpful in recalling preexisting exposures or illnesses when fever occurs within the first 24–48 hours after admission.

Physical examination of the febrile patient in the ICU should be thorough. Skin examination may demonstrate findings suggestive of drug reaction, vasculitis, or endocarditis. All intravenous and intraarterial line sites should be inspected. Spreading erythema, warmth, and tenderness that appear to indicate cellulitis of an extremity can also be the hallmarks of deep venous phlebitis, pyarthrosis, or gout. After the first 24 hours postoperatively, wound dressings should be removed and examined. Fundoscopic lesions of disseminated candidiasis may be the first identifiable sign of this elusive pathogen. Purulent sinusitis can occur in the nasally or orally intubated patient and may have a paucity of associated symptoms. Oral lesions of recrudescent herpetic stomatitis are common in the ICU setting and may be ulcerated and necrotic.

Examination of the lungs can be difficult in the ICU patient. More sensitive (though nonspecific) indicators of pneumonia include the chest roentgenogram and the finding of unexplained deterioration in arterial oxygenation. Unfortunately, pulmonary infiltrates and arterial hypoxemia also can be seen with congestive heart failure, acute respiratory distress syndrome, reactions to medications, and pulmonary hemorrhage. Cardiac examination may demonstrate a pericardial friction rub resulting from Dressler syndrome or a new or changing murmur possibly caused by endocarditis.

Abdominal findings can be misleadingly unremarkable in the elderly, in the patient with diminished sensorium, and in the patient receiving potent analgesics. They may be confoundingly positive in the patient with recent abdominal or thoracic surgery. Examination of the genitals and rectum may demonstrate unsuspected epididymitis, prostatitis, prostatic abscess, or perirectal abscess.

VII. Laboratory studies. Initial laboratory evaluation of fever in the ICU patient should include urinalysis and culture, two blood cultures (each obtained from a separate venipuncture or intravascular catheter), and chest roentgenogram. While we believe that efforts should be made to routinely obtain sputum for Gram stain and culture, not all agree (see Chapter 58). Culture of sputum without concomitant Gram stain examination is virtually worthless, because most ICU patients exhibit pharyngeal colonization with gram-negative bacilli within a few days of hospitalization, and culture alone cannot distinguish colonization from infection. The growth from sputum of even formidable pathogens such as *Pseudomonas aeruginosa* is not an indication for antibiotic therapy unless parenchymal pulmonary infection is evidenced by the presence of fever, unexplained hypoxemia, grossly or microscopically purulent sputum, or pulmonary infiltrates. See Chapter 58 on pneumonia for a more in-depth discussion of diagnosing pneumonia.

In general, all abnormal fluid collections (pleural effusion, joint effusion, ascites) should be sampled for microscopic and chemical analysis and culture. Microbiologic yield from ascites culture has been shown to be greater when ascitic fluid is placed into blood culture or fungal isolator media. Except in cases of head trauma, neurosurgery, or high-grade bacteremia with invasive pathogens such as *S. aureus* or gram-negative bacilli, meningitis is an uncommon nosocomial infection. Sampling of cerebrospinal fluid usually need not be considered in the initial workup of nosocomial fever. However, lumbar puncture should be considered in the febrile ICU patient with sudden, unexplained change in mental status or in the febrile patient who has undergone recent neurosurgery or head trauma and whose mental status is difficult to evaluate. Symptomatic complaints or physical findings referable to the abdomen dictate the need for determination of liver chemistry studies and serum amylase, as well as abdominal diagnostic imaging.

VIII. Approach to initial presumptive antibiotic therapy. In the acutely ill, unstable patient in the ICU, it may be necessary to begin empiric broad-spectrum antibiotic therapy before an infectious cause is established. Subsequently, positive cultures may permit narrowing of the spectrum of antibiotic coverage or may dictate that additional organisms need to be covered by added antimicrobial therapy. Negative cultures in a patient who is unimproved yet stable on broad-spectrum therapy indicate that antibiotics should be discontinued and the patient reevaluated. Negative cultures, laboratory findings, and radiologic exams in a febrile patient who is unimproved or worsened may be a clue to disseminated fungal infection, and empiric antifungal therapy should be considered.

Once efforts have been made to determine the most likely site or sites of infection, one can make a reasonable estimate of infecting pathogens. In an ICU patient, one should assume that in addition to the usual expected pathogens, infection is likely to involve more opportunistic, hospital-associated pathogens such as *S. aureus,* coagulase-negative staphylococci (usually *S. epidermidis*), gram-negative enteric bacilli, and lactose nonfermenting gram-negative bacilli (e.g., *P. aeruginosa, Acinetobacter* species). Patients with intravascular lines and suspected bacteremia should have blood cultures obtained and their lines removed if possible (see Chapter 67).

Empiric antibiotic therapy for the febrile ICU patient should be initiated according to generally accepted principles based on likely pathogens followed by culture-directed therapy. (See Chapters 65–74 for specific diagnosis and sites of infections.) However, such guidelines must be interpreted in light of the types of organisms and patterns of drug resistance prevalent in the specific institution and intensive care unit. Ultimately, definitive antibiotic therapy is determined by review of the final microbiologic data with identification of the infecting microorganism and its antibiotic susceptibilities. Chapter 64 has a discussion of antimicrobial agents for specific infections and dosing of antimicrobials in ICU patients.

Selected Readings

Arbo MJ, Fine MJ, Hanusa BH, et al. Fever of nosocomial origin: etiology, risk factors, and outcomes. *Am J Med* 1993;95:505.

This study looked at 100 patients and found that many had causes of fever other than infection.

Clarke DE, Kimelman J, Raffin TA. The evaluation of fever in the intensive care unit. *Chest* 1991;100:213.

Review of the fever workup.

Mackowiak PA, LeMaistre CF. Drug fever a critical appraisal of conventional concepts. *Ann Intern Med* 1987;106:728.

Drug fever is common in hospitalized patients, and the diagnosis may be elusive.

Mackowiak PA, Bartlett JG, Bordon EC, et al. Concepts of fever: recent advances and lingering dogma. *Clin Infect Dis* 1997;25:119.

Transcript of a symposium that gives details regarding pathophysiology as well as reviewing causes of fever in selected groups of patients.

Musher DM, Faintein V, Young EJ, et al. Fever patterns: their lack of clinical significance. *Arch Intern Med* 1979;139:1225.

Fever patterns may not be useful in narrowing the differential diagnosis.

Sayer CB, Breder CD. The neurologic basis of fever. *N Engl J Med* 1994;330:1880.

Review of the pathophysiology of fever.

64. USE OF ANTIMICROBIALS IN THE TREATMENT OF INFECTION IN THE CRITICALLY ILL PATIENT

Jennifer S. Daly and Richard H. Glew

I. **General principles.** This chapter reviews antimicrobial agents used in the treatment of bacterial, viral, fungal, and protozoan infections. A summary of important considerations in using each of the agents is given.

II. **Penicillin G.** Penicillin G continues to be highly active against streptococci, meningococci, and most mouth anaerobes. Resistance of *Streptococcus pneumoniae* to penicillin is increasingly prevalent and limits the usefulness of this agent as empirical therapy. Treatment of severe enterococcal endocarditis (other than cases due to penicillin-resistant isolates of *Enterococcus faecium*) mandates the addition of an aminoglycoside, preferably gentamicin, to achieve synergistic bactericidal effect. Dosage adjustments should be made in patients with severe renal insufficiency (Table 64-1).

III. **Penicillinase-resistant semisynthetic penicillins.** Nafcillin and oxacillin are interchangeable: both exhibit excellent *in vitro* activity against most isolates of *Staphylococcus aureus,* except methicillin-resistant strains. Because of hepatic clearance, no adjustment in dose is necessary in patients with renal insufficiency (Table 64-1).

IV. **Anti–gram-negative penicillins.** Ampicillin and the antipseudomonal penicillins have been developed for use against gram-negative organisms. In light of its restricted spectrum, ampicillin has limited usefulness in the intensive care unit (ICU) and should not be relied on for gram-negative coverage, but it may be used as an alternative to penicillin in the treatment of enterococcal infections. Because of their broader spectrum, piperacillin and mezlocillin, usually in combination with an aminoglycoside, generally are used to treat suspected or documented infection resulting from gram-negative bacteria including *Pseudomonas aeruginosa* (Table 64-1)

V. **First-generation cephalosporins.** Cefazolin is active against staphylococci *(S. aureus)* but not against enterococci, *Listeria monocytogenes,* methicillin-resistant *S. aureus,* and many coagulase-negative staphylococci. Community-acquired strains of *Escherichia coli, Proteus mirabilis,* and *Klebsiella pneumoniae* often are susceptible, but nosocomial isolates of Enterobacteriaceae frequently are resistant. Cefazolin is the drug of choice for prevention of postsurgical wound infection in cardiac surgery.

VI. **Second-generation cephalosporins.** Cefoxitin and cefotetan exhibit moderately good activity *in vitro* against anaerobes, including a majority of *Bacteroides fragilis* isolates. Cefuroxime exhibits good activity against gram-positive cocci and *Haemophilus influenzae.*

VII. **Third-generation cephalosporins.** The third-generation cephalosporins exhibit an expanded spectrum and increased potency against gram-negative organisms compared with older cephalosporins. The activity of most third-generation cephalosporins against *P. aeruginosa* is variable and unpredictable; ceftazidime and cefepime are more potent against this organism than other cephalosporins, but resistance is increasing, and these agents generally should be used in combination with an aminoglycoside to treat *P. aeruginosa.* In ICU patients, the cephalosporins should be employed, at least initially, at maximal doses and frequencies (Table 64-1). In patients with severe impairment of renal function, dosages of cephalosporins, except ceftriaxone, must be adjusted to avoid accumulation.

VIII. **Penems.** The two penem antibiotics, imipenem and meropenem, have the broadest antibacterial spectrum among available beta-lactams. Dosage adjust-

TABLE 64-1. Examples of parenteral beta lactams

Antibiotic	Dose Based on Creatinine Clearance			
	>80 mL/min (normal)	50–80 mL/min	10–50 mL/min	<10 mL/min
Penicillins				
Penicillin G	3–4 million U q4h	3–4 million U q4h	3 million U q4h	2 million U q6h
Nafcillin or oxacillin	2 g q4h	2 g q4h	2 g q4h	2 g q4h
Piperacillin	3 g q4h or 4 g q6h	3 g q4h or 4 g q6h	3–4 g q8h	3–4 g q12h
Cephalosporins				
Cefazolin	1–2 g q8h	1–2 g q8h	1 g q8–12h	1–2 g q24h
Cefoxitin	1–2 g q6h	1–2 g q6h	1–2 g q6h	1 g q24–48h
Cefotetan	1–2 g q12h	1–2 g q12h	1–2 g q24h	1 g q48h
Cefotaxime	1–2 g q6–8h	1–2 g q6–8h	1 g q8–12h	1–2 g q24h
Ceftriaxone	1–2 g q12–24h	1–2 g q24h	1–2 g q24h	1–2 g q24h
Ceftazidime	1–2 g q8h	1–2 g q8h	1–2 g q12–24h	1 g q48h
Cefepime	1–2 g q8–12h	1–2 g q8–12h	1 g q12–24h	0.5 mg–1 g q24h
Monobactams and Penems				
Aztreonam	1–2 g q6–8h	1–2 g q6–8h	1 g q8–12h	1–2 g q24h
Imipenem/cilastatin	0.5–1 g q6h	0.5–1 g q6–8h	0.5–1 g q12h	0.25–0.5 g q12h
Meropenem	1 g q8h	1 g q8–12h	1 g q12h	1 g q24h

ment (Table 64-1) is necessary in patients with renal dysfunction because serum level–related myoclonus and seizures can occur, particularly when these drugs are used at higher doses, in elderly patients with impaired renal function, or in patients with a history of seizures. Treatment of highly resistant gram-negative bacilli with imipenem or meropenem generally should involve coadministration of an aminoglycoside.

IX. Monobactam. Aztreonam, a monobactam, has little cross-allergenicity with the beta-lactams leading to its role in the treatment of gram-negative infections in patients allergic to penicillins or cephalosporins. It exhibits a spectrum and potency against gram-negative bacteria much like that of the third-generation cephalosporins, but aztreonam has no antibacterial activity against gram-positive or anaerobic bacteria.

X. Beta-lactamase inhibitor combinations. Clavulanic acid, sulbactam, and tazobactam are beta-lactamase inhibitors, and the combination of one of these compounds with ampicillin, ticarcillin, or piperacillin results in a drug combination that is active against beta-lactamase–producing strains of *S. aureus, Bacteroides* species, *H. influenzae,* and enteric gram-negative bacilli. These combinations are ineffective against many isolates of *P. aeruginosa, Enterobacter cloacae, Citrobacter freundii,* and *Serratia marcescens.* Three beta-lactamase combination formulations are available parenterally: ampicillin-sulbactam (Unasyn), ticarcillin-clavulanate (Timentin), and piperacillin-tazobactam (Zosyn).

XI. Aminoglycosides. Although more toxic than penicillins and cephalosporins, the aminoglycosides provide the broadest range of potent, bactericidal antibiotic activity against gram-negative bacilli, particularly when multiply resistant enteric gram-negative bacilli species are considered possible pathogens, as in severely ill, hospitalized patients. These agents commonly are employed in the ICU as part of combination therapy together with an extended spectrum beta-lactam antibiotic. In addition, gentamicin in combination with ampicillin, penicillin, or vancomycin is indicated for treatment of endocarditis caused by enterococci or viridans group streptococci, and it may be used with vancomycin and rifampin for treatment of prosthetic valve endocarditis caused by coagulase-negative staphylococci. Recommended dosage schedules and serum concentrations for the aminoglycosides appear in Table 64-2.

XII. Fluoroquinolones. Fluoroquinolones are broad-spectrum agents highly active against enteric gram-negative bacilli (including enteric pathogens such as *Campylobacter, Salmonella,* and *Shigella* species) and *H. influenzae.* They are also active against other gram-negative bacteria such as *P. aeruginosa* and *Acinetobacter* species, but therapy of these organisms is problematic because resistance may develop during treatment even when quinolones are used as part of a multidrug regimen. In general, streptococci exhibit poor susceptibility to quinolones, although levofloxacin and newer compounds have good potency *in vitro* and may prove to be effective clinically. Against anaerobes, only trovafloxacin has activity, but this compound has been found to cause severe liver toxicity that limits its use. The fluoroquinolones are indicated in the treatment of complicated urinary tract infections, prostatitis, bacterial diarrhea of diverse causes, invasive (malignant) external otitis, gram-negative bacterial pneumonia, and intraabdominal and intrapelvic infections (in combination with anaerobic coverage). Resistance to fluoroquinolones is becoming increasingly common among *S. aureus* isolates and among gram-negative bacilli, especially *P. aeruginosa.*

XIII. Vancomycin. Vancomycin is used in the therapy of infections due to *S. aureus* resistant to semisynthetic penicillins and infections due to coagulase-negative staphylococci, especially infection of prosthetic heart valves and endovascular infections in patients undergoing long-term hemodialysis. Although most enterococci are inhibited by low concentrations of vancomycin, bactericidal killing of these organisms requires the addition of an aminoglycoside such as gentamicin. Resistance to vancomycin is an emerging problem, particularly in strains of *E. faecium.* The first *S. aureus* with reduced susceptibility to vancomycin was first reported in 1997 from Japan; it has now emerged in the United States. Oral

TABLE 64-2. Recommended dosage regimens and serum concentrations of gentamicin and tobramycin in patients in the intensive care unit based on calculated creatinine clearance[a]

Drug/Renal Function	Route	Loading Dose (mg/kg)	Regimen (mg/kg)	Serum Concentration (μg/mL)		
				Peak[c]	Trough[c]	8 h after Dose
Traditional regimen: Gentamicin, tobramycin						
> 80 mL/min	i.v.	2–2.5	1.3–1.7 q8h	4–8	1–1.5	
60–79 mL/min		2–2.5	1.3–1.7 q12h	4–8	1–1.5	
40–59 mL/min		2–2.5	3 q24h	4–8	1–1.5	
30–39 mL/min		2–2.5	2 q24h	4–8	1–1.5	
10–29 mL/min	i.v.	2–2.5	2–3 q48h[d]	4–8	1–1.5	
< 10 mL/min		2–2.5	1–2 q48h[d]	4–8	1–1.5	
Once-daily dosing[b]: Gentamicin, tobramycin						
> 80 mL/min	i.v.	Not needed	5–7 q24h	> 20	undetectable (<0.3)	2–6
60–79 mL/min	i.v.	Not needed	5–7 q36–48h (based on serum concentration at 6–14 h after dose)	> 20	undetectable (<0.3)	6–11

[a] Creatinine clearance = $\frac{(140 - \text{age})\,(\text{weight in kg})}{72\,(\text{serum creatinine level})}$ (for women, multiply the result by 0.85)

[b] Patient exclusions: age <12 yr, pregnancy, burns > 20% body surface area, ascities, dialysis, endocarditis, creatinine clearance < 60 mL/min.

[c] Serum for peak levels should be drawn 30 min after a 30-min infusion, and trough levels should be obtained within the 30 min before the next dose.

[d] Serum levels must be followed every 48h if renal function is decreasing.

vancomycin is employed only in patients with antibiotic-associated colitis caused by *Clostridium difficile.* Oral metronidazole is preferred for this infection to reduce the selective pressure toward vancomycin-resistant organisms.

XIV. Metronidazole. Metronidazole is highly active against obligate anaerobes. Although orally administered metronidazole is absorbed nearly completely, critically ill patients with the possibility of erratic gastrointestinal absorption should receive therapy by the intravenous route. Metronidazole is metabolized by the liver; no dose adjustment is required in patients with renal insufficiency, but dosages must be reduced in patients with severe hepatic insufficiency.

XV. Clindamycin. Clindamycin is active *in vitro* against a wide variety of anaerobic bacteria. It has been used with great success in the treatment of anaerobic infections of the head, neck, and lungs and pleural space, as well as in intraperitoneal infections. Some authorities suggest the use of clindamycin in addition to penicillin in the treatment of necrotizing fasciitis caused by beta-hemolytic streptococci because of its apparent activity against organisms present in extremely high inoculum.

XVI. Macrolides. The most common use of erythromycin or azithromycin is to treat community-acquired, non–life-threatening infections in normal hosts: primary atypical pneumonia, pharyngitis due to *Streptococcus pyogenes, Bordetella pertussis* infections, and enteritis due to *Campylobacter* species. In addition, azithromycin or erythromycin is the drug of choice for legionellosis. Erythromycin is excreted primarily in the bile, so dosage adjustment is not necessary in patients with renal impairment.

XVII. Amphotericin B. Amphotericin B is effective against most species of fungi that are pathogenic in humans and is the initial drug of choice for life-threatening, invasive, or systemic infections. Whereas *Candida albicans* generally is susceptible to amphotericin B and to imidazoles, non-*albicans* species of *Candida* often are less susceptible, and variable activity is evident against species of *Aspergillus* and Zygomycetes species, *Pseudallescheria boydii,* and *Fusarium* species. The combination of amphotericin B plus flucytosine is synergistic against *Candida* species and *Cryptococcus neoformans.*

Amphotericin B usually is given intravenously by infusion once daily over 2 to 6 hours, at a concentration of 0.1 mg/mL. Daily and total dosage are adjusted according to the fungal species, sites and extent of infection, and the individual tolerance of the patient. A test dose of 1 mg (in 25 to 100 mL 5% dextrose) is infused over 30 minutes. For patients who are critically ill with apparently rapidly progressive fungal disease, the full daily dose of 0.5 to 1 mg/kg can be given immediately after the test dose. For patients exhibiting intolerance with the test dose or subsequent increased doses, amphotericin B doses can be increased in a gradual fashion, with increase in the dose by 5 to 10 mg daily, until the final daily dose (0.4 to 0.6 mg/kg for candidiasis) is reached. The usual duration of amphotericin B therapy for systemic mycoses is 4 to 12 weeks, to a total of 1 to 2 g. For infections caused by less susceptible fungi (e.g., *Aspergillus,* Zygomycetes species *[Mucor],* and *Coccidioides immitis*), treatment warrants daily doses of up to 1 to 1.5 mg/kg and a total dose of 2 g or sometimes more. Preparations of amphotericin B complexed with cholesteryl sulfate (Amphotec), liposomal vesicles containing phosphatidylcholine, distearoylphosphatidylglycerol and cholesterol (AmBisome), a bilayered lipid membrane (Abelcet), and a colloidal dispersion (Amphocil) are available. The newer formulations are more expensive than amphotericin B deoxycholate but may be advantageous in patients with renal insufficiency that worsens during treatment with amphotericin B.

XVIII. Fluconazole. Fluconazole is available for intravenous and oral use and exhibits good activity *in vitro* against *Candida* species and *C. neoformans.* Oral absorption is excellent, resulting in serum levels nearly as high as with intravenous administration, and is independent of gastric acidity. Fluconazole penetrates well into bodily fluids, including cerebrospinal fluid, and has a long (30-hour) half-life; because of its renal clearance, adjustments must be made in dosing in patients with renal impairment. Fluconazole (usual dosage 100 to 400 mg per day) has a role in the treatment of systemic or invasive candidiasis due to *C. albicans*. For severe systemic mycoses (i.e., coccidioidomycosis, cryptococcosis) the usual daily dosage is 200 to 800 mg per day. Side effects of fluconazole are relatively minor and uncommon. Mild, transient elevation of serum transaminase levels occurs occasionally. Unlike ketoconazole, fluconazole does not affect adrenal function or androgen synthesis, but it does inhibit the metabolism and potentiate the effects of warfarin, phenytoin, cyclosporine, tacrolimus, and oral hypoglycemic agents.

XIX. Itraconazole. Itraconazole is a broad-spectrum antifungal with notable activity against *Aspergillus* species, *Histoplasma capsulatum, C. immitis, Sporothrix schenckii,* and the agents of chromomycosis. It is available for oral or IV use. Itraconazole is widely distributed in most tissues, but with poor levels in cerebrospinal fluid. Daily dosage is 200 to 400 mg orally, but higher doses are indicated in patients with central nervous system infection. Clearance is by hepatic metabolism, and no adjustment of dosage is required in patients with renal failure.

XX. Acylovir and related compounds. Acyclovir is used to treat infections due to herpes simplex virus (HSV) and varicella-zoster virus and is available for oral administration and as an intravenous preparation. Dosage varies according to the condition under treatment. Because 85% of clearance is renal, dosage must be reduced in patients with impaired renal function. Intravenous acyclovir at 10 to 12 mg/kg every 8 hours is the drug of choice for HSV encephalitis (for a course of 10 to 14 days), for congenital HSV infection (10 to 14 days), and for varicella-zoster infections (chickenpox or shingles) (7 to 10 days). Acyclovir at 5 mg/kg intravenously every 8 hours is effective against mucocutaneous HSV. Acyclovir or valacyclovir is used prophylactically in patients undergoing bone marrow or organ transplantation. Valacyclovir, a prodrug for acyclovir, is more completely absorbed than acyclovir and is rapidly hydrolyzed to acyclovir in the intestinal wall and the liver. Concomitant use of cimetidine decreases renal clearance and increases plasma concentrations of valacyclovir.

XXI. Ganciclovir. Ganciclovir is effective in the treatment of cytomegalovirus (CMV) retinitis, gastrointestinal infection, and pneumonitis in patients with acquired immunodeficiency syndrome (AIDS) and patients who have undergone solid organ or bone marrow transplantation. However, in patients undergoing bone marrow transplantation, the drug often is used in combination with intravenous CMV hyperimmune globulin for the treatment of CMV pneumonitis. It is used prophylactically in high-risk transplant patients. Treatment with ganciclovir usually involves induction therapy with 5 mg/kg intravenously twice daily for 14 to 21 days, followed by maintenance therapy (5 to 6 mg/kg once daily 5 days per week) in patients with AIDS. Dosage adjustments must be made in patients with renal impairment, especially in light of the relationship between drug serum levels and myelosuppression.

XXII. Foscarnet. Foscarnet has been demonstrated to be effective in the therapy of CMV retinitis in patients with AIDS. However, foscarnet is more expensive than ganciclovir and is associated with a significant (25%) incidence of nephrotoxicity. Dosage adjustment is required in patients with renal impairment. Nonrenal adverse effects include nausea, vomiting, anemia, seizures, and metabolic abnormalities.

XXIII. Trimethoprim-sulfamethoxazole. Trimethoprim-sulfamethoxazole (cotrimoxazole) can be used in the therapy of gram-negative infections in the patient in the ICU. Sometimes this agent is effective against beta-lactam–resistant nosocomial bacteria. The dose for serious gram-negative infections is 8 to 10 mg/kg per day, divided every 6 to 12 hours. Cotrimoxazole is the agent of choice in the treatment of *Pneumocystis carinii* pneumonia (see Chapter 71).

XXIV. Quinupristin/dalfopristin (Synercid). Quinupristin/dalfopristin is a new streptogramin antibiotic approved for treatment of infections due to *E. faecium* (including vancomycin-resistant strains) and complicated skin and soft tissue infections due to *S. aureus*. Use of this drug should be guided by results of laboratory susceptibility testing. Synercid is available as an IV preparation and may cause local reactions at the infusion site.

Selected Readings

Anonymous. Antimicrobial prophylaxis in surgery. *Med Lett* 1997;39:97.
Standard recommendations classified by surgical procedure.

Balfour HH. Antiviral drugs. *N Engl J Med* 1999;340:1255.
Good review of current antivirals.

Bisno AL, Steven DL. Streptococcal infections of skin and soft tissues. *N Engl J Med* 1996;334:240.
This review includes information about controversies regarding treatment of streptococcal disease.

Campbell GDJ, Silberman R. Drug resistant *Streptococcus pneumoniae. Clin Infect Dis* 1998;26:1188.
Review of epidemiology and treatment of patients with this pathogen, which is difficult to treat.

Hellinger WC, Brewer NS. Carbapenems and monobactams: imipenem, meropenem, and aztreonam. *Mayo Clin Proc* 1999;74:420.

Marshall FW, Blair JE. The cephalosporins. *Mayo Clin Proc* 1999;74:187.
Compares and contrasts available agents.

Patel R. Antifungal agents. Part I. Amphotericin B preparations and flucytosine. *Mayo Clin Proc* 1998;73:1205.
Review of the various preparations of amphotericin B.

Smith TL, et al. Emergence of vancomyin resistance in *Staphylococcus aureus. N Engl J Med* 1999;340:493.
A review of the newest, "most feared" pathogen.

65. BACTERIAL MENINGITIS

Alan L. Rothman

I. General principles. Despite advances in our knowledge of bacterial meningitis, morbidity and mortality from this disease remain substantial. Admission to the intensive care unit is therefore appropriate for any patient with bacterial meningitis.

A. Pathogenesis. Bacteria usually reach the cerebrospinal fluid (CSF) from the blood, except in meningitis after head trauma or neurosurgery. The bacteria that most commonly cause meningitis have developed strategies to escape host defenses at mucosal surfaces and in the blood. In the central nervous system, interactions between bacterial components and cells in the brain and meninges cause infiltration of leukocytes, altered cerebral blood flow, and disruption of cerebral function.

B. Etiology. *Streptococcus pneumoniae* is the most common cause of community-acquired bacterial meningitis in developed countries. *Neisseria meningitidis* is next most common, particularly in older children and young adults, and it can cause outbreaks of disease. *Haemophilus influenzae* was the most common cause in young children, but it has become much less common in countries where infants are routinely immunized against this pathogen. *Listeria monocytogenes* is most often a cause of infection in compromised hosts, including infants (less than 3 months of age), older adults (more than 50 years of age), and patients with alcoholism, immunosuppression, or general debility. Nosocomial bacterial meningitis is most often caused by those bacteria that colonize the skin or are common in the hospital environment, such as staphylococci and aerobic gram-negative bacilli.

C. Prognosis. The case-fatality rate and frequency of neurologic complications vary according to the pathogen, ranging from 10% to 50% or higher. The prognosis can be predicted on the basis of three clinical variables: hypotension, alteration in consciousness, and seizures. The outcome was favorable in 91% of patients who had none of these factors but in only 43% of patients who had two or more factors.

II. Diagnosis. The need to begin treatment rapidly in patients with bacterial meningitis requires that the clinical evaluation be compressed. The major objectives are to recognize the diagnosis and to define the likely pathogens.

A clinical history of the acute onset of fever with headache, photophobia, or stiff neck suggests bacterial meningitis. The diagnosis should also be considered in any patient with altered consciousness, even if another cause has been identified. Patients should also be asked about alcohol use, previous head trauma, recent use of antibacterial drugs, illnesses in contacts, and immunosuppressive disorders.

On physical examination, nuchal rigidity and altered consciousness suggest meningitis when these signs are present, but their absence does not exclude the diagnosis. Papilledema or focal neurologic deficits indicate that lumbar puncture should be delayed until a mass lesion can be excluded. Petechiae suggest infection with *N. meningitidis,* but they can be seen in other infections; Gram stain of material from skin lesions can help to identify the pathogen.

Most blood tests are of limited value for the diagnosis of bacterial meningitis, but they may help to identify complications. Blood cultures yield the infecting organism in 30% to 80% of patients with community-acquired infection and should be collected before initiation of antibacterial therapy.

Examination of CSF is invaluable for the diagnosis and management of bacterial meningitis, and it should be performed promptly. The CSF white blood cell count is typically greater than 1,000 cells/mm^3. Neutrophils predominate in most cases, and often constitute more than 85% of the white blood cells present. CSF glucose levels lower than 20 mg/dL are strong evidence of bacterial meningitis; however, up to 40% of patients have normal values (greater than or equal to 40%

to 50% of serum glucose). The CSF protein is usually greater than 100 mg/dL; markedly elevated levels help to distinguish bacterial from viral meningitis.

Gram stain of CSF is positive in at least 75% of community-acquired infections in the absence of prior antibacterial therapy. Gram stain should be performed even if there is minimal CSF pleocytosis. Bacteria are isolated from the CSF on routine culture in more than 90% of patients with community-acquired infection, except when antibacterial drugs were given before lumbar puncture. Susceptibility testing should be performed on all isolates from CSF. Bacterial antigen detection tests rarely add to the information obtained from Gram stain, but they may be useful when the patient has taken antibacterial drugs prior to presentation. Stains and cultures for fungi or mycobacteria are of low yield and can be reserved for patients with immunosuppression, those with a history suggesting chronic meningitis, or when the clinical situation raises the suspicion for these diseases (e.g., lymphocytic CSF pleocytosis with negative routine culture).

Cranial computed tomography or magnetic resonance imaging before lumbar puncture is rarely of value. These studies should be reserved for patients with focal neurologic deficits or another reason to suspect intracranial mass lesion.

III. Treatment

A. Antibacterial therapy. Empiric therapy should be started as early as possible after the diagnosis of bacterial meningitis is suspected. However, the short amount of time required for obtaining blood cultures and lumbar puncture is acceptable and important for patient management. If lumbar puncture cannot be performed immediately, therapy should be started as soon as blood cultures are obtained.

Ceftriaxone (usual adult dose, 2 g intravenously every 12 hours) is the mainstay of initial empiric therapy of community-acquired bacterial meningitis. Cefotaxime (usual adult dose, 2 g intravenously every 6 hours) may be used interchangeably. Both agents penetrate well into CSF and have excellent activity against *S. pneumoniae, N. meningitidis,* and *H. influenzae.* Vancomycin (usual adult dose, 2 g intravenously every 12 hours) should be added to ceftriaxone if the Gram stain of CSF shows gram-positive cocci or is negative, to provide improved coverage for penicillin-resistant *S. pneumoniae.* Ampicillin (usual adult dose, 2 g intravenously every 4 hours) should be given in addition to the foregoing to provide coverage for *L. monocytogenes* to patients less than 3 months or more than 50 years of age, those with immunosuppression, alcoholism, or debilitation, or if the CSF Gram stain shows gram-positive bacilli.

The preferred empiric therapy for patients with bacterial meningitis after neurosurgery is vancomycin (dose listed earlier) plus ceftazidime (usual adult dose, 2 g intravenously every 8 hours), to provide coverage for methicillin-resistant staphylococci and gram-negative bacilli including *Pseudomonas aeruginosa.* This recommendation may require modification based on local patterns of antimicrobial resistance.

There are few good alternatives for treatment of bacterial meningitis in patients with allergies to the foregoing agents. Therefore, a trial of ceftriaxone is warranted unless there is documented serious cephalosporin intolerance. Vancomycin is the preferred alternative for treatment of *S. pneumoniae.* Trimethoprim-sulfamethoxazole is the preferred alternative for treatment of *L. monocytogenes* and is also effective against *N. meningitidis.*

Once the results of CSF culture are known, therapy can be targeted based on the identity and tested susceptibility of the organism. For treatment of *S. pneumoniae* infection, the following guidelines have been suggested. Penicillin G may be used if the penicillin minimum inhibitory concentration (MIC) is less than or equal to 0.1 mg/L. Ceftriaxone as a single agent is appropriate if the ceftriaxone MIC is less than or equal to 0.5 mg/L (fully susceptible). If the ceftriaxone MIC is greater than 0.5 mg/L but less than or equal to 2.0 mg/L (intermediately resistant), ceftriaxone plus either vancomycin or rifampin should be used. If the ceftriaxone MIC is greater than 2.0 mg/L (fully resistant), combination therapy involving vancomycin, rifampin, and ceftriaxone has been recommended. However, optimal therapy is not well defined. Repeat lumbar puncture is warranted in patients infected with intermediately or fully resistant strains. If the CSF culture remains positive, consideration should be given to intrathecal administration of vancomycin (with continued intravenous therapy) or use of meropenem or alatrofloxacin as alternatives.

High-dose antibacterial therapy must be continued for the full course of therapy. Seven days' therapy is sufficient for infections caused by *N. meningitidis* or *H. influenzae*. For *S. pneumoniae* infection, a longer duration (10 to 14 days) is probably warranted, especially for strains not fully susceptible to ceftriaxone. Longer durations of therapy are also recommended for meningitis caused by *L. monocytogenes* (14 to 21 days) and gram-negative bacilli other than *H. influenzae* (21 days).

B. Corticosteroids. Dexamethasone (0.15 mg/kg intravenously every 6 hours for 2 to 4 days) hastened normalization of CSF glucose and reduced the frequency of neurologic complications of meningitis in several studies of children. Opinions vary on whether this agent should be given to all patients with community-acquired bacterial meningitis or reserved for more severe cases (e.g., patients with markedly increased intracranial pressure). Therapy with dexamethasone should be begun as early as possible; some experts recommend administering dexamethasone immediately before initiation of antibacterial therapy.

C. Supportive care. Careful fluid management and early recognition and treatment of complications are essential. The potential neurologic complications include seizures and increased intracranial pressure. Possible systemic complications include hypotension, disseminated intravascular coagulation, hypoxemia, and metastatic infection.

D. Infection control. Patients infected with *N. meningitidis* or *H. influenzae* should be placed in respiratory isolation for 24 hours after initiation of therapy. Household and day care contacts of patients with *N. meningitidis* infection, as well as intimately exposed hospital personnel (e.g., those who performed unprotected intubation), should receive chemoprophylaxis with rifampin, ciprofloxacin, or ceftriaxone. Chemoprophylaxis with rifampin is recommended for contacts of patients infected with *H. influenzae* if the household includes an unvaccinated child less than 4 years old or an immunocompromised child of any age.

Selected Readings

Aronin SI, Peduzzi P, Quagliarello VJ. Community-acquired bacterial meningitis: risk stratification for adverse clinical outcome and effect of antibiotic timing. *Ann Intern Med* 1998;129:862.

A retrospective study of 269 cases of bacterial meningitis that provides a model for the prediction of clinical outcome.

Coant PN, Kornberg AE, Duffy LC, et al. Blood culture results as determinants in the organism identification of bacterial meningitis. *Pediatr Emerg Care* 1992;8:200.

A study of the yield of blood cultures in 169 cases of bacterial meningitis in children.

Doern GV, Pfaller MA, Kugler K, et al. Prevalence of antimicrobial resistance among respiratory tract isolates of *Streptococcus pneumoniae* in North America: 1997 results from the SENTRY antimicrobial surveillance program. *Clin Infect Dis* 1998; 27:764.

Susceptibility data on 1,047 pneumococcal isolates from the United States and Canada. Overall, reduced susceptibility to penicillin and cefotaxime was detected in 28% and 4% of isolates from the United States, respectively.

Durand ML, Calderwood SB, Weber DJ, et al. Acute bacterial meningitis in adults: a review of 493 episodes. *N Engl J Med* 1993;328:21.

The largest review of clinical features and outcome in meningitis in adults, extending over a 27-year period.

Harvey DR, Stevens JP. What is the role of corticosteroids in meningitis? *Drugs* 1995;50:945.

Odio CM, Faingezicht I, Paris M, et al. The beneficial effects of early dexamethasone administration in infants and children with bacterial meningitis. *N Engl J Med* 1991;324:1525.

Dexamethasone, begun before the first dose of cefotaxime, reduced the frequency of neurologic sequelae in this clinical trial involving children with predominantly H. influenzae meningitis.

Paris MM, Ramilo O, McCracken GH Jr. Management of meningitis caused by penicillin-resistant *Streptococcus pneumoniae. Antimicrob Agents Chemother* 1995;39:2171.

A review of clinical and experimental data on the management of this important problem.

Quagliarello V, Scheld WM. Bacterial meningitis: pathogenesis, pathophysiology, and progress. *N Engl J Med* 1992;327:864.

An excellent review of the current understanding of the pathogenesis of bacterial meningitis.

Quagliarello VJ, Scheld WM. Treatment of bacterial meningitis. *N Engl J Med* 1997; 336:708.

An excellent review of all aspects of the treatment of bacterial meningitis, with detailed recommendations.

Rockowitz J, Tunkel AR. Bacterial meningitis: practical guidelines for management. *Drugs* 1995;50:838.

An excellent review of all aspects of the treatment of bacterial meningitis, with detailed recommendations.

Schuchat A, Robinson K, Wenger JD, et al. Bacterial meningitis in the United States in 1995. *N Engl J Med* 1997;337:970.

A picture of the epidemiology of bacterial meningitis in the United States after introduction of the H. influenzae conjugate vaccines.

Spanos A, Harrell FE Jr, Durack DT. Differential diagnosis of acute meningitis: an analysis of the predictive value of initial observations. *JAMA* 1989;262:2700.

This analysis of 422 cases derives a model to differentiate bacterial and viral meningitis.

Tauber MG, Moser B. Cytokines and chemokines in meningeal inflammation: biology and clinical implications. *Clin Infect Dis* 1999;28:1.

A detailed review of this important class of mediators of inflammation and their role in the pathogenesis of meningitis.

Townsend GC, Scheld WM. The use of corticosteroids in the management of bacterial meningitis in adults. *J Antimicrob Chemother* 1996;37:1051.

A nice review of clinical and experimental studies of adjunctive corticosteroid therapy for meningitis.

Tunkel AR, Scheld WM. Acute bacterial meningitis. *Lancet* 1995;346:1675.

A nice review of clinical and experimental studies of adjunctive corticosteroid therapy for meningitis.

66. INFECTIVE ENDOCARDITIS

Sarah H. Cheeseman and Karen C. Carroll

I. Definition. Infective endocarditis is infection of the endothelial lining of the heart, characterized on pathologic study by vegetations. Subacute bacterial endocarditis (SBE), most often caused by alpha-hemolytic (viridans) streptococci, has an insidious onset and smoldering course and usually affects valves with preexisting abnormalities, whether congenital, rheumatic, or degenerative (myxomatous) in origin. Acute bacterial endocarditis presents as fulminant infection, with abrupt onset and high fever, and it may have a rapid downhill course with respect to both valve destruction and systemic toxicity. Acute bacterial endocarditis is most frequently secondary to *Staphylococcus aureus* and may occur on previously normal valves.

II. Pathogenesis. The central pathophysiologic lesion is a vegetation, which develops when a fibrin-platelet thrombus formed at a site of turbulent flow becomes a trap for bacteria, which enter the blood from normal, everyday events such as brushing teeth, defecation, and manipulation of furuncles or other breaks in the skin. The clinical features of endocarditis derive from the erosion of normal tissue by this infected mass, with perforation of valve cusps and burrowing myocardial abscesses, and by embolization of the material in the vegetation to distant sites, such as the brain, viscera, and extremities. Immune-complex phenomena, as well as frank emboli, account for some of the skin lesions and renal disease. Patients with subacute bacterial endocarditis develop the anorexia and anemia characteristic of any chronic inflammatory process. In prosthetic valve endocarditis, the valve sewing ring is the nidus of infection, leading to valve dehiscence and myocardial abscess.

III. Diagnosis. The keys to diagnosis of endocarditis are suspecting the infection and obtaining adequate culture of blood. The working diagnosis for fever in an injection drug user or a patient with a prosthetic valve is endocarditis until proven otherwise. The clinician should suspect endocarditis in patients with fever with severe musculoskeletal pain, stroke, acute unexplained renal failure, persistent bacteremia, and bacteremia with organisms that commonly cause endocarditis in the absence of an obvious primary focus. These organisms are alpha-hemolytic (viridans) streptococci and the members of the HACEK group (normal oral flora), *Streptococcus bovis, Enterococcus,* and *S. aureus.*

Two or three separate blood cultures (drawn at different sites and times) with 20 mL of blood per culture should be obtained before any antibiotic is started. No amount of subsequent testing can compensate for omission of proper blood cultures.

Echocardiography plays an important role in providing anatomic definition of the lesion of endocarditis and following its progress, but the absence of a demonstrable vegetation does not disprove the diagnosis. Transesophageal studies are more sensitive than transthoracic studies and are particularly helpful in the management of prosthetic valve endocarditis. The Duke Criteria for the diagnosis of endocarditis accept the following echocardiographic findings as evidence of endocardial involvement and as major criteria for the diagnosis: an oscillating intracardiac mass on a valve or supporting structures or in the path of regurgitant jets or on implanted material, in the absence of an alternative anatomic explanation, *or* an abscess, *or* new partial dehiscence of a prosthetic valve.

The physical finding of greatest importance is new valvular regurgitation. A new regurgitant murmur (but not a change or an increase in one previously present) satisfies the Duke criterion for endocardial involvement and places the patient at risk of acute congestive failure. Characteristic physical findings include retinal hemorrhages, conjunctival and buccal mucosa petechiae, splinter hemorrhages, cutaneous petechiae, Osler nodes and Janeway lesions, and splenomegaly, but these may be absent. Fever is almost always present. In following the patient clinically, the clinician should seek signs of congestive heart failure, major vessel embolization, and new valvular regurgitation. In cases involving the aortic valve, serial electrocardiograms should be obtained to look for heart block.

IV. Treatment. The American Heart Association Committee on Rheumatic Fever, Endocarditis, and Kawasaki Disease recommendations for antimicrobial therapy are summarized here and should be consulted. Endocarditis caused by streptococci with a penicillin minimum inhibitory concentration (MIC) less than or equal to 0.1 μg/mL may be treated with 4 weeks of intravenous penicillin (12 to 18 mU per day, either continuously or in six equally divided doses) or ceftriaxone (2 g per day as a single dose); addition of gentamicin (1 mg/kg every 8 hours) to either of these regimens permits shortening the course to 2 weeks. If the MIC to penicillin exceeds 0.1 μg/mL, 4 weeks of penicillin (18 mU per day) or cefazolin (2 g every 8 hours), combined with 2 weeks of gentamicin, is recommended. Vancomycin (15 mg/kg every 12 hours) is the alternative for patients allergic to both penicillins and cephalosporins; concomitant gentamicin is not required. Therapy of enterococcal endocarditis requires synergistic combinations of penicillin (18–30 mU per day), ampicillin (12 g per day), or vancomycin plus gentamicin (1 mg/kg every 8 hours) for the entire 4- to 6-week course. For methicillin-susceptible staphylococci, nafcillin or oxacillin (2 g every 4 hours) or cefazolin (2 g every 8 hours) are given for 4 to 6 weeks. Addition of gentamicin does not alter the overall outcome but speeds defervescence and clearance of bacteremia; when not contraindicated, gentamicin is given for the first 5 days of therapy. Vancomycin is the only drug with proven efficacy in methicillin-resistant staphylococcal endocarditis and may also be used in cases of beta-lactam allergy. For staphylococcal prosthetic valve endocarditis, gentamicin is added to the foregoing regimens for the first 2 weeks, and concomitant rifampin (300 mg orally every 8 hours) is given for the entire course, a minimum of 6 weeks and often longer. Ceftriaxone is the drug of first choice for endocarditis caused by organisms of the HACEK group.

Endocarditis was uniformly fatal in the preantibiotic era and still carries an appreciable mortality rate. Infectious disease consultation is suggested for all cases and mandatory in those involving unusual or resistant organisms and prosthetic valve endocarditis.

Surgery plays an important role in the modern treatment of endocarditis and is recommended for virtually all cases of prosthetic valve infection due to *S. aureus*. Clear-cut indications for valve replacement in native valve endocarditis are microbiologic failure (inability to clear blood cultures) and the development of congestive heart failure requiring more than simple therapy. Once indications have been met, there is no advantage to delay, because it may be impossible to stabilize these patients by medical means, and the operative risk increases in the face of progressive heart failure. Multiple emboli, certain echocardiographic features, and conduction defects (in aortic valve disease) may also warrant early surgery, but in making this decision, one should note that the risk of emboli decreases markedly after the first 5 days of antibiotic therapy. It is wise to obtain a cardiac surgery consultation early for any patient with endocarditis caused by *S. aureus* or fungi or any patient with prosthetic valve endocarditis. Right-sided *S. aureus* endocarditis in injection drug users usually responds well to medical therapy alone.

Selected Readings

Abrams B, Sklaver A, Hoffman T, et al. Single or combination therapy of staphylococcal endocarditis in intravenous drug abusers. *Ann Intern Med* 1979;90:789.
The original clinical trial of combination therapy for staphylococcal endocarditis demonstrating that synergistic killing in the laboratory did not result in improved outcome in patients.

Birmingham GD, Rahko PS, Ballantyne F. Improved detection of infective endocarditis with transesophageal echocardiography. *Am Heart J* 1992;123:774.
A careful study of the incremental value of transesophageal over transthoracic echocardiography.

Chambers HF, Korzeniowski OM, Sande MA, et al. *Staphylococcus aureus* endocarditis: clinical manifestations in addicts and nonaddicts. *Medicine* 1983;62:170.
Classic study defining the differences in staphylococcal endocarditis between injection drug users and all others.

DiNubile MJ: Surgery in active endocarditis. *Ann Intern Med* 1982;96:650.
Superb and not-yet-outdated review of indications for cardiac surgery in active endocarditis.

Durack DT, Lukes AS, Bright DK, et al. New criteria for the diagnosis of infective endocarditis: utilization of specific echocardiographic findings. *Am J Med* 1994;96:200.
The latest set of diagnostic criteria for endocarditis and the first to incorporate echocardiographic findings. These may be more appropriate for retrospective classification than for prospective decision making.

John MDV, Hibberd PL, Karchmer AW, et al. *Staphylococcus aureus* prosthetic valve endocarditis: optimal management and risk factors for death. *Clin Infect Dis* 1998; 26:1302.
Single-center review documenting mortality of 42% with multivariate analysis showing that cardiac but not central nervous system complications increase the risk of death and valve replacement surgery decreases it.

Korzeniowski O, Sande MA, National Collaborative Study Group. Combination antimicrobial therapy for *Staphylococcus aureus* endocarditis in patients addicted to parenteral drugs and in nonaddicts. *Ann Intern Med* 1982;97:496.
Carefully done study as valuable for its documentation of the pace of response to treatment as for demonstrating that combined therapy produces nephrotoxicity as well as confirming lack of benefit.

Larbalestier RI, Kinchla NM, Aranki SF, et al. Acute bacterial endocarditis: optimizing surgical results. *Circulation* 1992;86 [Suppl II]:68.
Large series arguing for valve replacement before the occurrence of severe heart failure.

Middlemost S, Wisenbaugh T, Meyerowitz C, et al. A case for early surgery in native left-sided endocarditis complicated by heart failure: results in 203 patients. *J Am Coll Cardiol* 1991;18:663.
Series of 203 cases with early valve replacement.

Sexton DJ, Tenenbaum MJ, Wilson WR, et al. Ceftriaxone once daily for four weeks compared with ceftriaxone plus gentamicin once daily for two weeks for treatment of endocarditis due to penicillin-susceptible streptococci. *Clin Infect Dis* 1998;27:1470.
Data on once-daily therapy (using gentamicin at 3 mg/kg once daily).

Stinson EB. Surgical treatment of active endocarditis. *Prog Cardiovasc Dis* 1979;22:145.
Series of patients with infective endocarditis operated on for the indication of critically severe progressive heart failure with unexpectedly good outcome.

Stinson EB, Griepp RB, Vosti K, et al. Operative treatment of active endocarditis. *J Thorac Cardiovasc Surg* 1976;71:659.
An early report of valve replacement during active endocarditis stressing lack of correlation between duration of antibiotic treatment before operation and either operative outcome or bacteriologic findings.

Wilson WR, Karchmer AW, Dajani AS, et al. Antibiotic treatment of adults with infective endocarditis due to streptococci, enterococci, staphylococci and HACEK microorganisms. *JAMA* 1995;274:1706.
An authoritative statement on treatment regimens, with full explanation of the rationale and references.

67. INFECTIONS ASSOCIATED WITH VASCULAR CATHETERS

Suzanne F. Bradley and Carol A. Kauffman

I. General principles and definitions. Most of the approximately 200,000 nosocomial bacteremias that occur each year are catheter related. *Catheter-related infection* is defined as symptoms or signs of local or systemic infection without another obvious source and microbiologic evidence implicating the catheter. Approaches to catheter-related infection vary widely, and many accepted practices have little scientific basis.

II. Pathogenesis. Fibrin-platelet aggregates that accumulate on all intravascular catheters increase with prolonged catheterization and allow adherence of microorganisms. Microorganisms gain entry primarily along the insertion site; however, contamination of the hub and subsequently the internal catheter lumen may also occur. Catheter-related infections occur least often as a result of hematogenous seeding from a distant focus. To limit the tracking of bacteria from the skin insertion site along the catheter, subcutaneous tunneling and Dacron cuffs have been used for semipermanent central venous indwelling catheters.

The site of catheter insertion has an influence on the risk of infection. Catheters inserted into the internal jugular vein become infected more often than those in the subclavian vein as a result of difficulties in dressing the area and contamination with respiratory secretions. Catheter insertion in the groin should be avoided unless no other site exists because of difficulties in keeping the site clean. Catheter insertion in the lower extremities should also be avoided, except in children, because of poor blood flow with increased risk of infection.

Arterial catheters have rates of complications similar to those for venous catheters: thrombosis in 19% to 38% and infection in 4% to 9% of patients. Multilumen central venous catheters, particularly with prolonged insertion, have been associated with a higher rate of colonization and infection than single-lumen catheters. Major complications of catheter-related infection include septic shock, suppurative thrombophlebitis, metastatic infection, endocarditis, and arteritis.

III. Diagnosis. Cultures of the insertion site that yield 15 colonies or more may predict catheter-related infection; a negative surface culture greatly reduces the likelihood of catheter-related infection. Positive blood cultures, in the absence of another source of infection, strongly suggest catheter-related infection. Culture of the catheter itself provides further evidence that it is the source of infection. The optimum segment of catheter to culture is controversial. Most laboratories request that the catheter tip be sent in a sterile container, and this catheter segment is then rolled on an agar plate to determine the number of microbes. Growth of 15 colonies or more significantly correlates with the presence of local inflammation and signs and symptoms of septicemia.

IV. Microbiology and treatment. Coagulase-negative staphylococci are most commonly implicated in catheter-related infections, followed by *Staphylococcus aureus,* gram-negative bacilli, and *Candida* species. *Candida* species are found most often in infections of central venous catheters; *S. aureus* and coagulase-negative staphylococci cause infection of both peripheral and central catheters.

When infection occurs, the catheter should be removed because it serves as a persistent nidus of infection. For patients who have limited vascular access and semipermanent catheters, treatment of catheter-associated infection with antibiotics can be attempted. Successful treatment has been noted with coagulase-negative staphylococcal infections; however, infections due to *S. aureus, Candida,* and gram-negative bacilli almost always require catheter removal. Tenderness, swelling, and redness along the insertion site of a semipermanent catheter may portend tunnel infection, which is often impossible to treat medically.

In a patient with suspected catheter-related sepsis, initial treatment should consist of antimicrobial agents that cover both gram-positive cocci and gram-negative bacilli. Empiric therapy should consist of vancomycin, because it is consistently active against methicillin-resistant strains of *S. aureus* and coagulase-negative staphylococci, and an aminoglycoside or broad-spectrum penicillin or cephalosporin for treatment of gram-negative bacilli. When the organism is identified, the most appropriate agent based on susceptibility testing results should be used.

For catheter-associated coagulase-negative staphylococcal bacteremia, 7 to 10 days of nafcillin or cefazolin for a methicillin-susceptible organism and vancomycin for a methicillin-resistant organism are appropriate. *S. aureus* infection should be treated with a penicillinase-resistant penicillin or a first-generation cephalosporin for methicillin-susceptible organisms, and vancomycin is the best choice if the patient is allergic to beta-lactam antibiotics or the organism is methicillin-resistant. There is considerable debate concerning the appropriate length of therapy for catheter-associated *S. aureus* bacteremia. Patients with bacteremia or fever persisting more than 3 days after catheter removal and initiation

TABLE 67-1. Prevention of catheter-related infection

Intervention	Comments
Central catheter insertion	Sterile technique required: use masks, caps, sterile drapes, gowns, gloves
Cutaneous antisepsis Chlorhexidine Povidine-iodine Isopropyl alcohol	Routine use recommended during insertion; allow to dry; chlorhexidine may be most effective
Antimicrobial ointments Polymyxin B/neomycin Bacitracin Povidine-iodine Mupirocin Chlorhexidine-impregnated patch	Often used to decrease colonization at insertion site, but not proven effective in decreasing infection
Insertion site dressing	Sterile transparent vs. gauze dressing, no differences in infection rates shown: transparent: easier monitoring; gauze: less moisture buildup
Hub care/lumen disinfection	Not recommended at this time; not proven effective for prevention of infection
Systemic antibiotics	Not recommended; not proven effective for prevention of infection
Duration of catheter use[a]	
Peripheral venous catheters	Replace every 72 h
Pulmonary artery catheters	Replace every 5 d
Central venous catheters	Use for weeks to months; routine change by guidewire or new site not recommended
Arterial catheters	> 4 d higher risk of infection
Midline catheter (3–8″)	Use for several weeks
Percutaneous inserted central venous catheters (PICCs)[b]	Use for weeks to months
Semipermanent catheters[b]	Use for months
Antimicrobial-impregnated catheters	Consider for patients at high risk and for short-term use; expensive

[a] The optimal duration of insertion for each catheter type is listed above. Any catheter should be removed if erythema, pain, or purulent discharge develops at the insertion site. Distal emboli or hemorrhage may suggest arterial catheter infection.
[b] Requires insertion by specially trained personnel.

of antibiotics are at high risk for complications, including endocarditis, and they require 4 to 6 weeks of therapy. Short-course (2-week) intravenous therapy is appropriate only if the catheter is removed immediately, the patient's fever resolves promptly, resolution of bacteremia is documented by repeatedly negative blood cultures, and no metastatic foci are found. In the patient with preexisting cardiac valvular disease and increased risk of endocarditis, short-course therapy should probably not be used, and transesophageal echocardiography is strongly recommended. Patients should be followed closely for relapse or symptoms, such as back pain, suggesting metastatic infection.

Catheter-related sepsis from gram-negative bacilli requires treatment with antibiotics to which the microorganisms have been shown to be susceptible. Organisms such as *Pseudomonas* species and *Stenotrophomonas* species may be especially difficult to treat, particularly in the immunocompromised host. In general, an aminoglycoside, third-generation cephalosporin, or extended-spectrum penicillin is required, and for many patients, combination therapy is appropriate.

C. albicans often seeds distant sites, especially the retina and bones. All patients with catheter-associated candidemia should receive an antifungal agent. Outcome is improved if the catheter is removed promptly. Although both amphotericin B and fluconazole are effective, fluconazole has fewer side effects. The daily dosages are 400 mg of fluconazole and 0.5 to 0.7 mg/kg of amphotericin B. Patients with *C. glabrata* or *C. krusei* infection should be treated with amphotericin B. Treatment should continue for 2 weeks after blood cultures become negative. Metastatic complications of catheter-related candidemia require prolonged therapy with 1 to 2 g of amphotericin B or 3 to 6 months of fluconazole.

For guidelines to prevent catheter-related infection, see Table 67-1.

Selected Readings

Arnow PM, Quimosing EM, Beach M. Consequences of intravascular catheter sepsis. *Clin Infect Dis* 1993;16:778.

Large, retrospective analysis of complications of catheter-related bacteremia or fungemia.

Cobb DK, High KP, Sawyer RG, et al. A controlled trial of scheduled replacement of central venous and pulmonary-artery catheters. *N Engl J Med* 1992;327:1062.

Controlled trial addressing routine replacement of central venous catheters and the use of guidewires.

Darouiche RO, Raad II, Heard SO, et al. A comparison of two antimicrobial-impregnated central venous catheters. *N Engl J Med* 1999;340:1.

Controlled comparative trial of two antimicrobial-impregnated catheters demonstrating efficacy in preventing infection.

Goetz AM, Wagener MM, Miller JM, et al. Risk of infection due to central venous catheters: effect of site of placement and catheter type. *Infect Control Hosp Epidemiol* 1998;19:842.

Addresses the risks of catheter insertion sites and catheter types.

Hasaniya NWMA, Angelis M, Brown MR, et al. Efficacy of subcutaneous silver-impregnated cuffs in prevention of central-venous catheter infections. *Chest* 1996; 109:1030.

Large, randomized controlled trial assessing the protective benefit of attachable cuffs in preventing catheter infections in patients in the intensive care unit.

Lecciones JA, Lee JW, Navarro EE, et al. Vascular catheter-associated fungemia in patients with cancer: analysis of 155 episodes. *Clin Infect Dis* 1992;14:875.

A 10-year analysis of episodes of fungemia and their outcomes at the National Cancer Institute.

Maki DG, Ringer M, Alvarado CJ. Prospective randomised trial of povidine-iodine, alcohol, and chlorhexidine for prevention of infection associated with central venous and arterial catheters. *Lancet* 1991;338:339.

Controlled trial addressing the optimum method of cutaneous antisepsis before catheter insertion.

Pearson ML, Abrutyn E. Reducing the risk for catheter-related infections: a new strategy. *Ann Intern Med* 1997;127:304.

Editorial comment on the use of antimicrobial-impregnated catheters.

Pearson ML, Hospital Infection Control Practices Advisory Committee. Guideline for prevention of intravascular-device–related infections. *Infect Control Hosp Epidemiol* 1996;17:438.

Centers for Disease Control and Prevention guidelines for care of intravascular devices.

Raad II. Vascular catheters impregnated with antimicrobial agents: present knowledge and future direction. *Infect Control Hosp Epidemiol* 1997;18:227.

Overview of antimicrobial-impregnated catheters and their use.

Raad II. Intravascular-catheter-related infections. *Lancet* 1998;351:893.

Reviews pathogenesis and prevention of catheter-related infection.

Raad II, Sabbagh MF. Optimal duration of therapy for catheter-related *Staphylococcus aureus* bacteremia: a study of 55 cases and review. *Clin Infect Dis* 1992;14:75.

Retrospective analysis of managment and outcome of S. aureus bacteremia.

Raad II, Davis S, Khan A, et al. Impact of central venous catheter removal on the recurrence of catheter-related coagulase negative staphylococcal bacteremia. *Infect Control Hosp Epidemiol* 1992;13:215.

Assessment of the impact of catheter-removal on outcome from coagulase-negative staphylococcal bacteremia.

Raad II, Hohn DC, Gilbreath J, et al. Prevention of central venous catheter-related infections by using maximal sterile barrier precautions during insertion. *Infect Control Hosp Epidemiol* 1994;15:231.

Demonstrates the importance of sterile technique during central catheter insertion.

68. URINARY TRACT INFECTIONS IN THE INTENSIVE CARE UNIT

Jennifer S. Daly and Steven M. Opal

I. General principles. Urinary tract infection (UTI) remains the most common nosocomially acquired infectious disease in the United States. UTI is the most frequently recognized source of gram-negative bacteremia, which constitutes a major cause of mortality in the critically ill patient. The progressive development of resistance to antimicrobial agents by urinary pathogens and the difficulties attendant to the management of patients with indwelling urinary catheters remain major challenges in current critical care practices. Those UTIs of sufficient severity to require intensive care management and the problems associated with urinary catheters are the focus of this chapter.

II. Pathophysiology and microbiology. Most UTIs arise from ascending infection by enteric organisms that colonize the perineum and distal urethra. Because *Escherichia coli* is the most common enteric gram-negative aerobic bacterium in the human colon, it most frequently contaminates the lower urinary tract and results in ascending infection. Virulence properties in *E. coli* that are thought to contribute to UTI include specialized clones that colonize the uroepithelium such as those with specific uropathogenic O antigen, those with an iron assimilation system and hemolysin production, and those that possess adhesions. Adhesions allow the organism to attach and persist within the urinary tract and thereby avoid elimination during micturition.

Although UTIs are primarily caused by *E. coli,* other genera of the Enterobacteriaceae, including *Klebsiella, Enterobacter, Serratia, Proteus,* and *Providencia* species, are encountered in patients in the intensive care unit (ICU) who receive antibiotics or who have anatomic or functional abnormalities in urine flow. Gram-positive bacterial species occasionally cause UTIs. Coagulase-negative staphylococci such as *Staphylococcus saprophyticus* cause UTIs in sexually active women. Enterococci and hospital-acquired coagulase-negative staphylococci such as *S. epidermidis* cause UTIs in patients with long-term urinary catheters or those with structural abnormalities of the urinary tract including delayed emptying often found in elderly patients. *S. aureus,* on the other hand, when found in the urine should prompt a search for extrarenal sources of staphylococcal infection and is frequently seen in patients who have staphylococcal bacteremia. *Candida* species and other fungal organisms often complicate urinary catheterization. *Candida* in the urine may be associated with hematogenous dissemination (the urinary tract seeded from the blood) or UTI acquired by ascending infection from perineal surfaces.

Acute pyleonephritis or infection of the kidney may warrant ICU admission when this disorder is complicated by bacteremia and septic shock, urinary obstruction, papillary necrosis, or other local suppurative complications. Most patients respond within 72 hours to appropriate antimicrobial therapy and supportive measures. Functional or mechanical obstruction to urine flow is the principal underlying cause of treatment failure. Alleviation of obstruction is often essential to eradicate infection and to effect a cure. If patients do not respond promptly to conventional therapy, a search should be undertaken for suppurative complications. These complications include papillary necrosis, pyonephrosis, focal bacterial nephritis, and abscess.

III. Diagnosis. The clinical diagnosis of acute upper tract urinary infection is usually straightforward. Patients have a history of urinary frequency, dysuria, and sometimes costovertebral tenderness and signs of systemic toxicity. Urinalysis is dipstick positive for leukocyte esterase and nitrate, and the urinary sediment has large numbers of leukocytes or bacteria. Cultures should be performed before the initiation of antimicrobial therapy, which confirms the diagnostic impression and helps to direct appropriate antimicrobial therapy. Blood cultures also should be obtained to document whether the patient is bacteremic. Although the finding of more than 10^5 colony-forming units/mL is diagnostic of UTI, symptomatic women may have acute UTI with as few as 10^2 pathogenic organisms per milliliter. The absence of pyuria and bacteriuria does not exclude the possibility of UTI. Patients with neutropenia may not have white blood cells, and urine cultures may be negative in acute obstruction when the urine does not reach the bladder. Radiologic methods such as renal ultrasound, computed tomogroaphy, magnetic resonance imaging, intravenous pyelography, or cystoscopy and retrograde studies may be necessary to make the diagnosis.

IV. Treatment. Medical management of a patient with a UTI severe enough to require ICU admission consists of stabilization of the patient's hemodynamic parameters, supportive measures for septic shock, and empiric antimicrobial therapy directed toward the most likely urinary pathogens. The use of an extended-spectrum beta-lactam antibiotic (a third-generation cephalosporin or an extended-spectrum penicillin) in combination with aminoglycoside has become the standard therapeutic regimen in UTIs associated with septic shock caused by gram-negative bacilli. If the patient is not immunocompromised, has arrived to the ICU from the community, or has not received prior antimicrobial agents, then therapy with a third-generation cephalosporin, extended-spectrum penicillin, or quinolone alone is acceptable while awaiting culture results. Parenteral therapy is usually administered until the patient has been afebrile for 24 to 48 hours, clinical and laboratory parameters are improving, and the patient is taking oral food and medications. Therapy may then be administered orally and should be given for a total of about 2 weeks. If enterococcal UTI is suspected or documented, traditional therapy has included ampicillin with or without an aminoglycoside. If the organism is resistant to ampicillin, then vancomycin is needed. If the patient is infected with an enterococcus resistant to ampicillin and vancomycin, then the organism will need to be tested against a variety of available and investigational antimicrobial agents to find effective therapy.

V. Catheter-related urinary tract infections. Urinary catheters interfere with physiologic host defense mechanisms against UTI. Bacteria may gain access to the urinary tract during the insertion of the catheter, along the external surface after insertion, or through the lumen of the catheter. Most microbial pathogens enter from along the external surface of the catheter and have previously colonized the perineum or vagina. The presence of the foreign body interferes with antimicrobial agents, which may fail to kill microorganisms adherent to catheter materials. Infections are diagnosed by the presence of high-grade pyuria (more than 50 white blood cells per high-power field), fever, and urine culture. It is sometimes difficult to differentiate infection from colonization by symptoms and culture alone. The best treatment is removal of the urinary catheter. If bacteriuria persists after catheter removal, the patient should be treated with a short course of an appropriate antimicrobial agent. If the patient is systemically ill, treatment is warranted even if the catheter must remain in place and should be directed at the infecting organism. Long-term catheterization in men may lead to prostatitis, prostatic abscess, epididymitis, and other urethral complications.

VI. Candiduria. Isolation of *Candida* from the urine is problematic in that this may occur as contamination or as infection. The spectrum of infection ranges from cystitis alone to life-threatening systemic candidiasis or locally invasive *Candida* infection with the possibility that fungus balls will obstruct urinary flow. Unfortunately, quantitative cultures yielding *Candida* species do not have the same diagnostic and prognostic implications as quantitative cultures yielding a pathogenic bacterium. Recurrent isolation of *Candida* species in patients with unexplained fever and pyuria suggest *Candida* UTI. The infection may be treated with bladder instillation of amphotericin B, oral antifungal agents such as triazoles, or systemic amphotericin B. Fluconazole is a water-soluble antifungal agent that is excreted in the urine in high concentrations and is available in intravenous and oral preparations. A short course starting with 200 mg of fluconazole, followed by 100 mg a day orally for 4 days, is often effective. Resistance in *Candida* species other than *C. albicans* is a concern, and agents such as amphotericin B may be needed to treat serious infections caused by species such as *C. krusei* and *C. glabrata.*

Selected Readings

Abrutyn E, Mossey J, Berlin JA, et al. Does asymptomatic bacteriuria predict mortality and does antimicrobial treatment reduce mortality in elderly ambulatory women? *Ann Intern Med* 1994;120:827.

Even though ICU patients may have previous positive culture at a nursing home, treatment of asymptomatic patients in long-term care facilities is not useful.

Fisher JF, Newman CL, Sobel JD. Yeast in the urine: solutions for a budding problem. *Clin Infect Dis* 1995;20:183.

This article gives a practical approach to Candida UTI with an algorithm for management.

Harding GKM, Nicolle LE, Ronald AR, et al. How long should catheter-acquired urinary tract infection in women be treated? A randomized controlled study. *Ann Intern Med* 1991;114:713.

This article suggests short course therapy for catheter-acquired UTI, a protocol that is useful at discharge from the ICU.

Jacobs LG, Skidmore EA, Freeman K, et al. Oral fluconazole compared with bladder irrigation with amphotericin B for treatment of fungal urinary tract infections in the elderly. *Clin Infect Dis* 1996;22:30.

Comparison of two treatment approaches.

Kunin CM, White LV, Hua TH. A reassessment of the importance of "low-count" bacteriuria in young women with acute urinary symptoms. *Ann Intern Med* 1993;119:454.

This article reviews the culture "colony count" as an indication of infection.

Lipsky BA. Urinary tract infection in men: epidemiology, pathophysiology, diagnosis and treatment. *Ann Intern Med* 1989;110:138.

This article has information on treatment of recurrent bacteremia, prestatitis, and diagnostic evaluation needed in men with UTI.

Stamm WE, Hooton TM. Management of urinary tract infections in adults. *N Engl J Med* 1993;329:1328.

Overview that includes patients with complicated UTI.

Stapleton A, Moseley S, Stamm WE. Urovirulence determinants in *Escherichia coli* isolates causing first-episode and recurrent cystitis in women. *J Infect Dis* 1991;163:773.

This study looks at E. coli from outpatients with UTI for adhesions, hemolysin, and fimbriae.

69. TOXIC SHOCK SYNDROME, TICK-BORNE ILLNESSES, AND POSTSPLENECTOMY INFECTION

Debra D. Poutsiaka

I. General principles. Several bacterial infections exist that arise in the community, are rapid in onset, are fulminant in course, and possess a relatively high rate of mortality. Their presentation, typically in an emergency room and often nonspecific, should prompt suspicion and frequently admission to an intensive care unit. Several entities are presented here.

II. Toxic shock syndrome

A. General principles. Toxic shock syndrome (TSS) is a toxin-mediated multisystem disease characterized by the rapid onset of high fever, hypotension, diffuse macular erythroderma, mucous membrane inflammation, severe myalgia, vomiting, diarrhea, headache, and nonfocal neurologic abnormalities. Complications include prolonged hypovolemic shock, acute respiratory distress syndrome, acute renal failure, electrolyte and acid-base disturbances, cardiac dysrhythmia, and diffuse intravascular coagulation. TSS occurs in the setting of infection or colonization with toxin-producing strains of *Staphylococcus aureus* or group A streptococci.

Staphylococcal TSS occurs most commonly in menstruating women using tampons, but it also occurs with *S. aureus* infections in a variety of settings, such as surgical wound infections, postpartum infection, focal cutaneous lesions, and abscesses. Streptococcal TSS also occurs in patients with varied underlying infections.

B. Diagnosis. Five categories of clinical features are needed for diagnosis of staphylococcal TSS: (a) fever, (b) skin manifestations, (c) desquamation 1 to 2 weeks after the onset of illness, (d) hypotension, and (e) evidence of multisystem organ involvement in three or more areas (gastrointestinal, muscular, mucous membranes, renal, hepatic, hematologic, central nervous system). Laboratory features are nonspecific.

S. aureus and streptococci can be visualized by Gram stain and cultured from bodily fluids. Blood cultures are usually negative in *S. aureus* TSS but are positive in streptococcal TSS.

C. Treatment. It is essential to correct hypovolemic shock rapidly. Large doses of both a beta-lactamase–resistant antistaphylococcal antimicrobial agent, such as oxacillin, and penicillin should be instituted for coverage of staphylococci and streptococci until the bacteriologic diagnosis is confirmed. Alternatives include a first-generation cephalosporin, such as cefazolin, or vancomycin. Any infected areas should be surgically drained, and foreign bodies should be removed. The administration of intravenous immunoglobulin has been useful for the amelioration of the toxicity observed in TSS. In streptococcal TSS, the addition of clindamycin is sometimes recommended as a strategy to halt the production of streptococcal toxins.

III. Tick-borne illnesses

A. Rocky Mountain spotted fever

1. **General principles.** Rocky Mountain spotted fever (RMSF) is a potentially severe multisystem illness characterized by fever, rash, and tick bite. It is a tick-borne infection caused by *Rickettsia rickettsii.* Most cases occur during the late spring, summer, and early fall. Areas of recent high endemicity are the southeastern United States, primarily North Carolina, and mountainous regions of Oklahoma and Arkansas.
2. **Diagnosis.** Diagnosis is frequently made on historical and clinical grounds. A history of a tick bite is not always present, but the occurrence of other risk factors (exposure to dogs, time spent in wooded areas) may aid in diagnosis. Clinical findings include fever, rash, finding of tick infestation, neurologic

involvement, pneumonitis, lymphadenopathy, hepatomegaly, and splenomegaly. Multisystem organ failure can occur.

Laboratory features are nonspecific. Two-thirds of patients have an abnormal cerebrospinal fluid profile. The only rapid laboratory approach to specific diagnosis is the demonstration via immunofluorescence of *R. rickettsii* in skin biopsy specimens. A fourfold rise in specific antibody titers is also considered diagnostic.

3. **Treatment.** Treatment is with tetracycline or doxycycline. Pregnant women, children less than 8 years of age, and persons with hypersensitivity to tetracycline should receive chloramphenicol.

B. Babesiosis. Babesiosis in the United States, endemic in the Northeast, is caused by the protozoan, *Babesia microti,* transmitted by the tick vector, *Ixodes dammini.* In high-risk groups, such as the elderly and asplenic persons, the disease can pursue a fulminant and frequently fatal course characterized by multisystem organ failure. Diagnosis is made by thick and thin smears of the peripheral blood. Treatment is with quinine and clindamycin or azithromycin and atovaquone. Exchange transfusion may also be effective.

C. Ehrlichiosis. Ehrlichiosis is caused by the intracellular pathogens, *Ehrlichia chaffeensis* and *E. equi,* transmitted by tick vectors. In severe presentations, ehrlichiosis can be mistaken for septic shock, TSS, acute viral infection, or thrombotic thrombocytopenic purpura. Diagnosis is serologic or by the identification of morulae in peripheral blood leukocytes. Treatment is with tetracycline.

IV. Postsplenectomy infection

A. General principles. In its most fulminant form, known as *overwhelming postsplenectomy infection,* postsplenectomy infection is rapidly progressive, initially manifested by nonspecific symptoms, and frequently accompanied by disseminated intravascular coagulation, multiple organ failure, and death. Serious postsplenectomy infections are generally bacterial and are caused by organisms such as *Streptococcus pneumoniae, Haemophilus influenzae, Neisseria meningitidis, Escherichia coli, Pseudomonas aeruginosa, Staphylococcus aureus,* and others.

B. Diagnosis. Postsplenectomy infections should be considered in any person presenting with signs of sepsis with a history or surgical scar suggestive of splenectomy or in patients with conditions associated with functional asplenia.

Classically, overwhelming postsplenectomy infection is heralded by a prodrome consisting of fever, chills with rigors, pharyngitis, myalgias, nausea, and vomiting. It rapidly progresses to hypotension, disseminated intravascular coagulation, purpura, and respiratory distress with additional complications such as adrenal hemorrhage, gangrene, and coma. Death can ensue in less than 24 hours. Other common presentations include meningitis and pneumonia.

Laboratory features are nonspecific. Evidence of bacterial meningitis may be present. The appearance of bacteria, particularly pneumococci, on peripheral blood smears in patients with overwhelming postsplenectomy infection has been noted. Cultures of blood and other sterile sites are frequently positive for the offending bacteria.

C. Treatment. Initiation of broad-spectrum antibiotics, such as a third-generation cephalosporin, is essential.

Selected Readings

Dummler JS, Bakken JS. Ehrlichial diseases of humans. *Clin Infect Dis* 1995;20:1102.

This detailed review should be required reading for those who want to learn about ehrlichiosis or who may find themselves considering the diagnosis of ehrlichiosis in their patients.

Gelfand JA, Poutsiaka DD. Babesia. In: Mandell GL, Bennet JE, Dolan R, eds. *Principles and practice of infectious diseases,* 5th ed. New York: Churchill Livingstone, 2000:2899–2902.

This chapter provides a detailed description of the clinical aspects of babesiosis and includes the latest in treatment options.

Lynch AM, Kapila R. Overwhelming postsplenectomy infection. *Infect Dis Clin North Am* 1996;10:693.

This informative review is complete in its description of overwhelming postsplenectomy infection and includes discussions of the immunology of the spleen, and the epidemiology, bacteriology, and clinical aspects of overwhelming postsplenectomy infection.

Stevens DL. The toxic shock syndromes. *Infect Dis Clin North Am* 1996;10:727.

This review is a complete discussion of streptococcal and staphylococcal TSS, including case definitions, pathogenesis, clinical presentation, and treatment.

Walker DH. Rocky mountain spotted fever. *Clin Infect Dis* 1995;20:1111.

This detailed review provides an overview of RMSF and includes discussions of the tick vector life cycles and the difficulties in the diagnosis of RMSF.

70. ACUTE INFECTIONS IN THE IMMUNOCOMPROMISED HOST

Richard H. Glew and Raul Davaro

I. **General principles.** Advances in the management of leukemia, lymphoma, and solid tumors have resulted in a growing population of persons with defects of natural and specific immunity who are at increased risk of infections caused by a wide variety of different organisms.

II. **Pathogenesis.** In an immunocompromised patient with a suspected infection, the diagnostic plan begins with consideration of the nature and severity of predisposing immune defects. The immune system may be altered by derangements arising from the primary disease, the medical and surgical treatment of the condition, or a combination of these factors. Understanding of the immunologic defect helps to narrow the differential diagnosis (Table 70-1). Microorganisms capable of producing infections in immunocompromised patients are common pathogens and organisms once considered nonpathogenic and include species of viruses, pyogenic bacteria, bacteria that produce granulomatous infections, fungi, protozoa, and helminths.

III. **Sites of infection and organisms**

A. **Sites.** The most common sites of infection in the immunocompromised host are the blood, lung, and mucosal surfaces. Bacteremia and fungemia typically occur without an obvious source, although the gastrointestinal tract is the most likely origin of occult infection as a result of disruption of mucosal integrity and gut defenses by chemotherapy and neutropenia. Lung infections are difficult diagnostic challenges because of the lack of specificity and sensitivity of symptoms and signs and imaging studies. Oral mucositis is a frequent complication of neutropenia, chemotherapy, and trauma, and it also may be caused by Herpes simplex virus or thrush caused by *Candida* species. Genitourinary tract infection should be suspected in patients with indwelling urinary catheters and in patients with ureteral obstruction resulting from tumor, postirradiation scarring, or stones. Except in patients with impaired cell-mediated immunity and after neurosurgery, central nervous system infections are infrequent in immunocompromised patients.

B. **Organisms.** In immunocompromised patients, the predominant bacterial pathogens are gram-negative bacilli such as *Pseudomonas aeruginosa, Escherichia coli,* and *Enterobacter* species, followed by gram-positive cocci such as *Staphylococcus aureus,* including methicillin-resistant *S. aureus,* coagulase-negative staphylococci, and streptococci. Fungal infections have become more common with prolonged neutropenia and therapy with broad-spectrum antibiotics. Infections due to *Candida* species are common in patients with acute leukemias, cytotoxic chemotherapy, corticosteroids, and broad-spectrum antibiotic use and can produce mucositis, urinary tract infections, and fungemia or disseminated candidiasis. In patients with defective T-cell immunity (e.g., lymphoma, acquired immunodeficiency syndrome, corticosteroid therapy, or transplantation), infections with *Pneumocystis carinii* (interstitial pneumonia; PCP), *Cryptococcus neoformans* (meningitis), and *Toxoplasma gondii* (encephalitis) occur.

IV. **Diagnosis.** Physical findings in patients with neutropenia and infection often are obscured by diminished inflammation. Thus, a thorough history and physical examination must be performed initially and repeated daily, with special attention to the oropharynx, anorectal region, lungs, skin, optic fundi, recent surgical wounds, and vascular catheter sites.

Initial laboratory studies include the following: (a) cultures of blood and urine; (b) culture of sputum in patients with evidence of pulmonary disease; (c) swab, aspiration, or biopsy of suspicious skin or mucous membrane lesions for smears (Gram stain, fungal preparation), cultures (routine, fungal, and viral), and pathologic examination; (d) semiquantitative culture of intravenous catheters in place when fever develops (subcutaneously tunneled device removal can be deferred if

TABLE 70-1. Relationship between primary immune defect and infectious agents

Underlying Disease	Host Defect	Infectious Agent
Acute nonlymphocytic leukemia	Neutropenia	Enterobacteriaciae *Staphylococcus aureus, Streptococcus* spp. Fungi such as *Aspergillus, Candida*
Chronic lymphocytic leukemia	Abnormal humoral and cell-mediated immunity	Encapsulated bacteria *Streptococcus pneumoniae, Haemophilus influenzae, Neisseria* spp.
Hodgkin lymphoma Acquired immuno-deficiency syndrome	Depressed cell-mediated immunity	Mycobacteria, *Pneumocystis, Cryptococcus, Toxoplasma,* Herpes simplex, Herpes zoster Cytomegalovirus
Myeloma	Abnormal humoral immunity	Encapsulated bacteria *S. pneumoniae, H. influenzae, Neisseria* spp.

no local signs of infection are present pending result of blood cultures); (e) chest roentgenography; and (f) serum chemistry studies to detect visceral involvement caused by disseminated infection and to serve as baselines for monitoring possible adverse reactions to antimicrobial therapy.

Patients with defects in cell-mediated immunity often develop infections best diagnosed by histologic examination or special culture techniques (e.g., for mycobacteria, herpes viruses) of tissue by biopsy, bronchoalveolar lavage or transbronchial biopsy, gastrointestinal endoscopy, or surgery. Localizing symptoms and signs may indicate the need for computed tomography, magnetic resonance imaging, or nuclear medicine scans.

V. Treatment

A. Fever and neutropenia without obvious source. Empiric broad-spectrum antibiotic therapy has been the mainstay in the initial management of fever in neutropenic patients. Because of the high risk of life-threatening infections, all febrile patients with neutrophil counts of less than 500/mm^3, and those with counts of 500 to 1,000/mm^3 and falling should be treated promptly with broad-spectrum bactericidal antibiotics by the intravenous route and at high dosages.

In choosing the initial antibiotic regimen, consideration should be given to the type, frequency, and antibiotic susceptibilities of the bacterial isolates found in similar patients in the hospital. In most hospitals, a two-drug regimen is employed in patients requiring intensive care (Table 70-2) before the cause of the infection is known. At institutions where fulminant gram-positive bacterial infections are common, vancomycin may be incorporated in the initial therapeutic regimens in selected patients and discontinued 3 to 4 days later if such infection is not identified. In patients with indwelling central venous catheters, indications for catheter removal are as follows: (a) bacteremia due to *Corynebacterium jeikeium, Bacillus* species, *Pseudomonas* species, *Candida* species, *Fusarium* species, and vancomycin-resistant enterococci; (b) evident exit site infection or tunnel infection; (c) blood cultures persistently positive after 72 hours of appropriate therapy; and (d) the presence of septic thrombophlebitis.

In the patient for whom an infection has been documented clinically or microbiologically and in whom fever has resolved, antibiotics should be continued until all the following conditions have been met: (a) 3 days or more without fever, (b) at least 7 days of total antibiotic therapy, (c) clearance of clinical and

TABLE 70-2. Empiric regimens for initial therapy of the febrile adult neutropenic patient with cancer

Piperacillin, 12–18 g/d i.v. (divided q4–6h), plus tobramycin or gentamicin, 5 mg/kg/d or amikacin 20–25 mg/kg/d (divided q8h) i.v.

Ceftazidime, 3–6 g/d i.v. (divided q8h) plus or minus tobramycin or gentamicin, 5 mg/kg/d or amikacin 20–25 mg/kg/d (divided q8h) i.v.

Imipenem/cilastatin, 2–4 g/d i.v. (divided q6h).

Aztreonam, 3–6 g/d i.v. (divided q8h), plus vancomycin, 2 g/d (divided q12h), plus tobramycin or gentamicin 5 mg/kg/d or amikacin 20–25 mg/kg/d (divided q8h) i.v. (for patients allergic to penicillin and cephalosporin)

laboratory signs of infection, and (d) a total neutrophil count of at least 500/mL. If infection is considered likely and no organism has been isolated, treatment with the initial antibiotic regimen should be continued until the neutrophil count is higher than 500/mL and for more than 7 days.

Fever that extends beyond 3 days in patients without clinical and microbiologic evidence of infection suggests (a) a nonbacterial infection, (b) a bacterial infection with organisms resistant to antibiotics in use, (c) the emergence of a new bacterial infection involving organisms resistant to antibiotics in use, or (d) drug fever. Reassessment includes physical examination, chest roentgenogram, inspection of catheter sites, reculture of blood, and imaging of any organ or system with signs or symptoms of inflammation. Should fever persist for 7 days during neutropenia and despite antibiotic therapy, it is customary to begin empiric antifungal therapy with amphotericin B, the mainstay of therapy for infections caused by *Aspergillus* species and other filamentous fungi. However, imidazoles can be administered in selected patients with infections caused by *Candida* species.

B. Fever and pulmonary infiltrates. The differential diagnosis of pulmonary disease in immunocompromised patients is broad: infections from bacteria, fungi, protozoa, viruses, and helminths; congestive heart failure; acute respiratory distress syndrome; pulmonary hemorrhage; bronchiolitis obliterans with organizing pneumonia; radiation injury; malignant disease; and hypersensitivity or toxicity reactions to medications (e.g., methotrexate, busulfan) and blood products).

Focal or multifocal infiltrates tend to indicate infections by bacteria and those caused by *Aspergillus* species or Zygomycetes. Diffuse disease is more characteristic of viruses (herpes simplex virus and cytomegalovirus), PCP, or noninfectious processes (drug toxicity, lymphangitic carcinomatosis, and radiation pneumonitis). Cavitary disease can be seen with gram-negative bacilli, such as *P. aeruginosa,* as well as *S. aureus,* anaerobes, *Nocardia* species, and fungi *(Aspergillus* and the Zygomocetes genus *Mucor).*

In patients with diffuse pulmonary infiltrates and unrevealing physical examination and sputum analysis, bronchoscopy is indicated. Patients with fever, neutropenia, and pulmonary infiltrates should be started promptly on antibiotics such as a combination of a quinolone or a newer macrolide (azithromycin) with a third-generation cephalosporin. In patients with T-cell deficiency or recent high-dose corticosteroid therapy, consideration should be given to starting trimethoprim-sulfamethoxazole to cover PCP, followed promptly by diagnostic bronchoscopy. In the absence of clinical improvement or a definite diagnosis, empiric antifungal therapy and bronchoscopy or open lung biopsy should be considered.

A new pulmonary infiltrate that appears during recovery from neutropenia heightens awareness for the possibility of pulmonary aspergillosis and less common filamentous fungi (e.g., Zygomocetes, such as *Rhizopus,* and *Fusarium* species). Isolation of *Aspergillus* from respiratory tract cultures in persistently febrile neutropenic patients receiving broad-spectrum antibiotic therapy suggests the need to consider empiric treatment with high-dose amphotericin B (1 to 1.5 mg/ kg per day), especially in the setting of persistent or progressive pulmonary infiltrates.

VI. Prophylaxis. Oral quinolone administration has been studied in patients with prolonged neutropenia. These agents reduce levels of aerobic gram-negative bacilli within the gut lumen, the major reservoir for dissemination of infection in the immunocompromised host. Potential disadvantages include the development of resistant bacterial strains and an increase in infections caused by gram-positive species and fungi. Antifungal prophylaxis with oral azoles has proven effective in reducing infections by *Candida* species in patients undergoing bone marrow transplantation; however, increasing evidence of azole-resistant *Candida* species is a problem in many institutions.

Antiviral prophylaxis with acyclovir has been shown to reduce mucocutaneous infections caused by herpes simplex both in transplant recipients and in patients with acute leukemia. Prophylaxis against PCP with trimethoprim-sulfamethoxazole is necessary in patients with cancer who are undergoing intensive chemotherapy with regimens that have been specifically associated with a high incidence of PCP.

There is increasing interest in the routine use of hematopoietic growth factors such as granulocyte colony-stimulating factor for patients with neutropenia. Although the use of this factor has reduced the length of neutropenia, the final impact on cost and survival is marginal.

Selected Readings

Hughes WT, Armstrong D, Bodey GP, et al. 1997 guidelines for the use of antimicrobial agents in neutropenic patients with unexplained fever. *Clin Infect Dis* 1997;25:551.

Issued by the Infectious Disease Society of America, this article offers guidelines for a vast array of clinical situations in patients with fever and neutropenia.

Pizzo PA. Management of fever in patients with cancer and treatment-induced neutropenia. *N Engl J Med* 1993;328:1323.

Thorough review of the approach to fever and neutropenia in patients with neoplasia.

Shelhamer JH, moderator. Respiratory disease in the immunosuppressed patient. *Ann Intern Med* 1992;117:415.

Thorough diagnostic approach to the patient with immune suppression and lung disease.

Shelhamer JH, moderator. The laboratory evaluation of opportunistic pulmonary infections. *Ann Intern Med* 1996;124:585.

Consensus guidelines on laboratory evaluation.

71. INTENSIVE CARE OF PATIENTS WITH HIV INFECTION

Sarah H. Cheeseman and Mark J. Rosen

I. General principles. Therapies for human immunodeficiency virus (HIV) infection introduced in the last few years have resulted in a substantial reduction in the number of cases of acquired immunodeficiency syndrome (AIDS) and in mortality from AIDS. Patients with HIV who require treatment in an intensive care unit (ICU) for opportunistic infections now and in the future are more likely to be those who have not been diagnosed or in whom antiretroviral therapy has failed. We can also anticipate more admissions for complications of therapy and for the same reasons that bring uninfected persons to the ICU. For instance, it now seems possible that the protease inhibitors used to treat HIV may increase the risk of coronary artery disease by causing hyperlipidemia. Patients with lactic acidosis with hepatic steatosis, a rare, life-threatening toxicity of the nucleoside analog reverse transcriptase inhibitors, present to the ICU as suspected sepsis (and this condition may reverse with riboflavin). This chapter focuses on managing patients on antiretroviral therapy in the ICU and the diseases that lead to respiratory failure in HIV-infected patients.

II. Pathogenesis and management of the underlying disease. HIV infection results in progressive loss of CD4 cells and consequent susceptibility to certain infectious agents, termed opportunistic because they generally do not cause disease, or at least not severe disease, in immunologically normal hosts. When current combination antiretroviral therapy suppresses viral replication, the loss of CD4 cells may be prevented, and there may be remarkable increases in absolute CD4 count. This effect has been accompanied by a notable drop in the frequency of such infections as cytomegalovirus retinitis and disseminated *Mycobacterium avium* complex. Even incomplete viral response to therapy may result in considerable improvement in CD4 counts and protection from opportunistic infection. Nonadherence to antiretroviral therapy, particularly in patients taking less than the optimal dose of any of the agents in a regimen, or continuing two drugs while stopping the third, leads to drug resistance and loss of response. Admission to an ICU provides numerous opportunities for disruption of these regimens: the drugs are administered orally, and, for many of these agents, absorption is highly dependent on their being taken when the patient is either fed or fasted. Current regimens contain a minimum of three agents, and most include either a protease inhibitor or a nonnucleoside reverse transcriptase inhibitor. Members of these classes are inducers or inhibitors of the P-450 cytochrome oxidase pathway and thus are extremely prone to drug-drug interactions with a variety of medications. Every effort should be made to continue a patient's established regimen in the ICU, with reference to the latest available information on administration, prevention of toxicity (e.g., provision of 1.5 L or more of fluid per day to prevent crystalluria in patients receiving indinavir), and drug-drug interactions. If the oral route cannot be used or if contraindicated concomitant medications are required, all the antiretroviral drugs should be stopped. Prophylaxis against opportunistic infection, such as trimethoprim-sulfamethoxazole to prevent *Pneumocystis carinii* pneumonia (PCP) and clarithromycin or azithromycin to prevent disseminated *Mycobacterium avium* complex, should be continued (or started) in those patients for whom they are indicated.

III. Respiratory disease. PCP is still probably the most common cause of admission to ICU for persons with HIV. Bacterial infections, including pneumonia, are also important causes of mortality even among HIV-infected patients who do not meet diagnostic criteria for AIDS, and these infections often lead to patients' admission to ICU for respiratory failure and sepsis syndrome. The risk of bacterial pneumonia increases as the CD4 lymphocyte count declines and is higher in injection drug users than in patients in other HIV transmission categories. *Streptococcus pneumoniae* is the most notable cause of bacterial pneumonia in HIV-infected persons, but *Pseudomonas aeruginosa* is a significant problem in patients with far-advanced disease, with a history of prior opportunistic infections or CD4 counts less than 50/µL. Coinfection with HIV and *Mycobacterium tuberculosis* has fueled the resurgence of tuberculosis and the outbreak of multidrug-resistant tuberculosis. Fungal pneumonia may result either from new acquisition or reactivation of latent disease. Cryptococcal disease occurs in any locale; almost all patients with AIDS and cryptococcal pneumonia have meningitis and disseminated disease, and CD4 counts are typically less than 100/µL. *Aspergillus* affects even more severely immunosuppressed persons, with CD4 counts lower than 30/µL. Histoplasmosis produces miliary disease and dissemination, with the appearance of sepsis, in patients from the Ohio and Mississippi River valleys, the Caribbean, and Latin America. Coccidioidomycosis must be considered in patients from Arizona and central California.

IV. Diagnosis. The initial differential diagnosis is usually between bacterial pneumonia and PCP, but the possibility of tuberculosis must always be considered. Cavitation, hilar and mediastinal adenopathy, and pleural effusions may be valuable clues to the diagnosis of tuberculosis, but in patients with severe immunosuppression, diffuse infiltrates, miliary patterns, or normal chest radiographs are seen commonly. Bacterial pneumonias usually present in a typical fashion, with high fever, shaking chills, cough productive of purulent sputum, and localized areas of consolidation on chest radiography. However, this constellation of findings may occur in infections with other pathogens, such as mycobacteria and fungi. PCP occasionally presents as an acute illness with rapid development of respiratory failure over a few days, but more often it progresses gradually, with increasing cough and dyspnea over weeks or even months. Radiographically, the diagnosis is suggested by perihilar or diffuse granular opacities, but this pattern is not specific for PCP, and other presentations include pneumatoceles, pneumothorax, nodules, lobar consolidation, and a normal radiograph.

Definitive diagnosis of PCP requires demonstrating the organism in respiratory specimens. Sputum induced with 3% saline delivered by ultrasonic nebulization has a diagnostic yield of 50% to 80%. When sputum is negative, fiberoptic bronchoscopy and bronchoalveolar lavage are warranted. Transbronchial biopsy is usually not performed in patients receiving mechanical ventilation or those with uncorrectable coagulopathy, but this biopsy may be diagnostic when lavage is negative in PCP, as well as providing rapid diagnosis of mycobacterial, fungal, and noninfectious pulmonary diseases. Respiratory specimens from HIV-infected patients should always be examined for acid-fast bacilli by smear and culture.

V. Treatment. Initial therapy for HIV-infected patients with respiratory failure should be appropriate for *Streptococcus pneumoniae, Haemophilus influenzae,* and PCP (e.g., ceftriaxone, trimethoprim-sulfamethoxazole, and prednisone; Table 71-1 gives doses and alternatives for PCP). Adjunctive corticosteroid therapy given at the start of anti-*Pneumocystis* treatment reduces the likelihood of respiratory failure, deterioration of oxygenation, and death in patients with moderate to severe pneumonia. In patients already in respiratory failure at the initiation of therapy, the goal is to prevent the worsening of gas exchange that typically occurs during the first few days of therapy, presumably as a result of the inflammatory reaction to killed organisms. Response to an empiric regimen does not diminish the importance of establishing a specific diagnosis whenever possible; otherwise, patients will be committed to a prolonged course of potentially toxic antimicrobials and corticosteroids for a disorder that they do not have.

TABLE 71-1. Treatment of moderate to severe[a] *Pneumocystis carinii* pneumonia

Drug	Dose	Comments
Trimethoprim-(TMP) sulfamethoxazole (SMX)	15–20 mg/kg TMP, 75–100 mg/kg IV SMX i.v. or p.o. in three or four divided doses	Drug of choice, but toxicity (rash, fever, nausea, leukopenia) is frequent
Pentamidine isoethionate	3–4 mg/kg i.v. daily	Toxicity: dysglycemia, renal failure, QT interval prolongation, arrhythmias, pancreatitis, hypotension; 50% dextrose must be available
Trimetrexate	45 mg/m^2 i.v. daily (plus folinic acid, 20 mg/m^2 i.v. or p.o. q6h)	Not as effective as trimethophrim-sulfamethoxazole, but better tolerated
Clindamycin plus primaquine	600 mg q.i.d. 30 mg q.d.	Screen for glucose-6-phosphate dehydrogenase deficiency in appropriate patients
Prednisone	40 mg p.o. b.i.d., days 1–5 20 mg p.o. b.i.d., or 40 mg p.o. q.d., days 6–10 20 mg p.o. daily, days 11–21	Recommended as adjunctive therapy along with an anti-*Pneumocystis* agent for all patients with *P. carinii* pneumonia who meet criteria for moderate to severe disease

[a] $P_aO_2 \leq 70$ mm Hg, or $P_{(A-a)}O_2 \geq 35$–45 mm Hg breathing room air.
Intensive Care Medicine, 4th ed. Philadelphia: Lippincott Williams & Wilkins, 1998, Table 91-2, p. 1152.

Selected Readings

Baron AD, Hollander H. *Pseudomonas aeruginosa* bronchopulmonary infection in late human immunodeficiency virus infection. *Am Rev Respir Dis* 1993;148:992.

Early report describing both the overwhelming sepsis presentation and an indolent pattern like that seen in patients with cystic fibrosis.

Chaisson RE, Schecter GF, Theuer CP, et al. Tuberculosis in patients with the acquired immunodeficiency syndrome: clinical features, response to therapy, and survival. *Am Rev Respir Dis* 1987;136:570.

Groundbreaking population-based study highlighting atypical chest radiographs and extrapulmonary disease in patients with AIDS and tuberculosis.

De Palo VA, Millstein BH, Mayo PH, et al. Outcome of intensive care in patients with HIV infection. *Chest* 1995;107:506.

Experience of one medical center with critically ill patients with HIV infection.

Dropulic LK, Leslie JM, Eldred LJ, et al. Clinical manifestations and risk factors of *Pseudomonas aeruginosa* infection in patients with AIDS. *J Infect Dis* 1995;171:930.

Case-control study identifying risk factors as central venous or urinary catheters and steroid therapy.

Fouty B, Frerman F, Reves R. Riboflavin to treat nucleoside analogue-induced lactic acidosis. *Lancet* 1998;352:291.

First report of reversal of this syndrome with riboflavin, but cases were mild.

Henry K, Melroe H, Huebsch J, et al. Severe premature coronary artery disease with protease inhibitors. *Lancet* 1998;351:1328.

Initial report of this potentially life-threatening complication of therapy.

Hirschtick RE, Glassroth J, Jordan MC, et al. Bacterial pneumonia in patients infected with human immunodeficiency virus. *N Engl J Med* 1995;333:845.

A multicenter prospective study of 1,353 subjects, controlled for transmission group and HIV infection.

Keiper MD, Beumont M, Elshami A, et al. CD4 lymphocyte count and the radiographic presentation of pulmonary tuberculosis. *Chest* 1995;107:74.

Series demonstrating occurrence of atypical chest radiographs in patients with tuberculosis and CD4 counts of less than 200/μL.

Kovacs JA, Ng V, Masur H, et al. Diagnosis of *Pneumocystis carinii* pneumonia: improved detection in sputum with use of monoclonal antibodies. *N Engl J Med* 1988;318:589.

Description of high yield with immunofluorescent staining.

Luzzati R, Del Bravo P, Di Perri G, et al. Riboflavine and severe lactic acidosis. *Lancet* 1999;353:901.

Another report of successful treatment, in a sicker patient.

National Institutes of Health-University of California Expert Panel for Corticosteroids as Adjunctive Therapy for Pneumocystis Pneumonia. Consensus statement on the use of corticosteroids as adjunctive therapy for *Pneumocystis* pneumonia in the acquired immunodeficiency syndrome. *N Engl J Med* 1990;323:1500.

The official recommendation for steroids in moderate to severe PCP.

Rosen MJ, De Palo VA. Outcome of intensive care for patients with AIDS. *Crit Care Clin* 1993;9:107.

A literature review on critical care in AIDS.

Shafer RW, Edlin BR. Tuberculosis in patients infected with human immunodeficiency virus: perspective on the past decade. *Clin Infect Dis* 1996;22:683.

Superb review of all aspects of this problem.

Sundar K, Suarez M, Banogon PE, et al. Zidovudine-induced fatal lactic acidosis and hepatic failure in patients with acquired immunodeficiency syndrome: report of two patients and review of the literature. *Crit Care Med* 1997;25:1425.

Excellent review of this entity.

Wachter RM, Luce JM, Hopewell PC. Critical care of patients with AIDS. *JAMA* 1992;267:541.

A pessimistic view from the dark days of the epidemic.

72. INFECTIOUS COMPLICATIONS OF SUBSTANCE ABUSE

Brian J. Mady and Neil M. Ampel

I. **General principles.** Drug abuse is a growing and pervasive problem in our society and is attended by an increased risk of infection. Some of the more common infections associated with parenteral drug use include bacteremia, skin and soft tissue infections, vascular infections, endocarditis, skeletal infections, pneumonia, nervous system infections, and infection with human immunodeficiency virus (HIV).

II. **Bacteremia.** Bacteremia is a frequent occurrence in the febrile parenteral drug user. Approximately 60% of these bacteremias are due to causes other than endocarditis. Most are caused by skin or soft tissue infections or vascular infections.

There is geographic variation in the types of organisms isolated in these patients. However, drug users have an increased incidence of staphylococcal carriage, and *Staphylococcus aureus* is the most common blood culture isolate. Methicillin-resistant *S. aureus* infections are encountered with increasing frequency in some geographic locations. Streptococci are the second most frequent isolates and are commonly associated with skin and soft tissue infections. Gram-negative aerobic bacilli are the third most commonly isolated organisms, with *Pseudomonas aeruginosa* frequently reported. Polymicrobial bacteremia occurs in about 10% of cases, and in these cases approximately two-thirds have *S. aureus* as one of the organisms. Bacteremia and other infections caused by facultative anaerobic organisms including *Eikenella corrodens* are associated with drug users who contaminate the needle or injection site with saliva.

Empiric antibiotic therapy should be based on local experience but should include agents against *S. aureus* and streptococci as well as aerobic gram-negative bacilli. If methicillin-resistant *S. aureus* is prevalent in the parenteral drug–using community, vancomycin should be considered.

III. **Skin and soft tissue infections.** Skin and soft tissue infections are frequent occurrences in the parenteral drug user. Such infections are often polymicrobial and appear to be derived from either the skin or the oral cavity. The most common skin infections are simple cellulitis and localized abscesses. Simple cellulitis usually requires only antibiotic therapy directed against *S. aureus* or streptococci. In addition, localized soft tissue abscesses should be incised and drained.

Soft tissue infections may be indistinguishable from simple cellulitis in their early stages. The presence of vesicles or bullae, an area of central necrosis within a larger area of erythema, and the presence of subcutaneous crepitation in a patient with systemic toxicity suggest necrotizing fasciitis. Gas seen in soft tissues on radiographs also indicates deep infection. Necrotizing fasciitis requires immediate, aggressive debridement in association with parenteral antibiotics. Gram stain and culture are imperative to guide antimicrobial therapy because the number of potential pathogens is large. Empiric therapy should be directed against *S. aureus,* streptococci, anaerobes, and aerobic gram-negative bacilli.

IV. **Peripheral vascular infections.** Many different vascular complications may result from parenteral drug use. Septic thrombophlebitis is common and typically presents with fever, bacteremia, and swelling over the involved vein. When the injection site is into the deep tissues of the groin or neck, it may be difficult to distinguish involvement of vascular structures from simple cellulitis, soft tissue abscesses, or fasciitis. If there is a diagnostic dilemma, angiography should be performed to determine whether the vasculature is involved. Septic thrombophlebitis can often be treated with antibiotics alone, although incision, drainage, and removal of the vein are sometimes necessary. Anticoagulation is generally not needed.

Mycotic aneurysm is another frequent vascular complication that results when the user injects a drug directly into the artery. Patients typically present with fever and a tender, pulsatile mass, usually in the groin or the neck. Vascular surgical consultation should be obtained before any exploration of the lesion is performed. Angiography confirms the site and extent of the aneurysm. The most common organisms include *S. aureus* and streptococci and occasional aerobic gram-negative bacilli. Ligation and excision of the involved arterial segment are usually successful.

V. Endocarditis. Endocarditis in the parenteral drug user differs in several respects from endocarditis in the nonaddict. It is more likely to occur in persons without underlying valvular heart disease, to involve the tricuspid valve, to be due to *S. aureus,* and to have a more benign outcome. However, endocarditis accounts for fewer than 15% of all cases of fever in parenteral drug users who present to the hospital.

Patients with tricuspid valve endocarditis typically present with fever and chills of less than 1 week's duration, pleuritic chest pain, and occasional hemoptysis. A systolic murmur may or may not be present on admission but often develops during therapy. Signs of peripheral embolization are uncommon. On chest radiograph, multiple patchy infiltrates indicative of pulmonary emboli strongly suggest the diagnosis. Blood cultures are almost invariably positive, and *S. aureus* is usually isolated. Negative blood cultures in a patient with the appropriate clinical syndrome should raise the possibility that the patient has recently taken antibiotics. Left-sided endocarditis may also occur in parenteral drug users. Streptococci and *S. aureus* are the most frequent isolates. In addition to staphylococci and streptococci, various other organisms have been associated with endocarditis in the parenteral drug user including aerobic gram-negative bacilli, particularly *P. aeruginosa,* and fungi, most notably *Candida* species; polymicrobial endocarditis also occurs.

Empiric therapy of endocarditis in parenteral drug users should be directed against staphylococci, streptococci, and aerobic gram-negative bacilli. Nafcillin, oxacillin, or cefazolin is a reasonable choice if methicillin resistance in *S. aureus* has not been encountered. Aminoglycosides such as gentamicin or tobramycin should also be added both for initial therapy of aerobic gram-negative bacilli and for synergism against the staphylococci.

The prognosis of tricuspid valve *S. aureus* endocarditis is good, with a mortality of less than 10%. Various therapies have been used to treat *S. aureus* tricuspid valve endocarditis in the parenteral drug user, in addition to the standard treatment for left-sided endocarditis. Limited data suggest that parenteral drug users with methicillin-susceptible *S. aureus* endocarditis limited to the right heart valves may be treated with a 2-week course of nafcillin or oxacillin plus an aminoglycoside. In a small study of right-sided *S. aureus* endocarditis, a course of 4 weeks of ciprofloxacin plus rifampin was found to be efficacious. For patients with isolated tricuspid valve involvement and intractable infection, valvulotomy is successful in most cases.

Left-sided endocarditis secondary to *P. aeruginosa* has a poor outcome, with a mortality rate of nearly 70%. A course of 6 weeks of an antipseudomonal beta-lactam antibiotic plus an aminoglycoside and early surgical removal of the involved valve is often required. *Candida* endocarditis also has an extremely high mortality rate even with prompt valve replacement and systemic antifungal therapy.

VI. Skeletal infections. Infections of the bone and joints represent a distinct clinical syndrome in the parenteral drug user. Vertebral osteomyelitis is the most frequent skeletal infection reported. The lumbar, cervical, and thoracic spine is involved, in that order. Patients generally present with weeks to months of pain, often without high fevers, and many are afebrile. Typically, tenderness is found over the involved vertebral body, and there is often radiographic evidence of osteomyelitis. Septic arthritis in this group of patients often involves the sacroiliac and sternoarticular joints and the symphysis pubis. Patients usually have had weeks to months of pain and tenderness to palpations. Radiographs are usually normal at presentation.

The bacteriology of skeletal infections among drug users is most commonly with aerobic gram-negative bacilli and gram-positive cocci such staphylococci and streptococci. In addition, skeletal infections due to *Candida* species may also occur alone or as part of a dissemination syndrome. Because of the varied microbiology, biopsy or needle aspiration of the involved bone or joint is imperative to direct therapy.

VII. Human immunodeficiency virus infection. Injection drug use represents the second most common risk behavior for infection with HIV in the United States. The spectrum of HIV-related complications among injection drug users differs from that in other HIV-infected populations. Bacterial infections, especially pneumonia, endocarditis, and sepsis, are frequent occurrences. The incidence of bacterial pneumonia in HIV-infected drug users is four times higher than in HIV-negative drug users. Other complications in this patient population include tuberculosis and various opportunistic infections.

VIII. Nervous system infections. Epidural abscess is one of the most frequent central nervous system infections in the parenteral drug user. Pain associated with radicular symptoms is the most common presentation, and symptoms are often indolent. These infections are usually secondary to underlying vertebral osteomyelitis. Computed tomography and magnetic resonance imaging are useful in defining the extent of the infectious process. Staphylococci are the most frequent cause, although other pathogens, including *P. aeruginosa* and *Mycobacterium tuberculosis,* have also been recognized. Surgical decompression is often required, and therefore, neurosurgical consultation should be obtained.

Brain abscesses may occur usually as a result of embolization from either endocarditis or mycotic aneurysm. They are typically multiple and generally are secondary to *S. aureus.* More unusual causes have been described, including mucormycosis, and therefore a microbiologic diagnosis is imperative.

IX. Pulmonary infections. Pneumonia in parenteral drug users may be from inhalation or hematogenous spread. Bacterial pneumonia may be due to typical community pathogens such as *Streptococcus pneumoniae, S. aureus, Haemophilus influenzae,* and *Klebsiella pneumoniae.* If there is a recent history of unconsciousness, suggesting aspiration, anaerobes should also be considered. Septic pulmonary embolism, from endocarditis or vascular infections, is described earlier. Clinicians must maintain a high index of suspicion for tuberculosis in drug users, particularly if they are infected with HIV. In addition, with HIV infection, bacterial pneumonia, *Pneumocystis carinii* pneumonia, and other opportunistic infections must also be considered, depending on the level of immunosuppression.

Selected Readings

Chambers HF, Miller RT, Newman MD. Right-sided *Staphylococcus aureus* endocarditis in intravenous drug abusers: two-week combination therapy. *Ann Intern Med* 1988;109:619.

A small study demonstrating 94% efficacy with 2 weeks of antibiotics.

Dworkin RJ, Lee BL, Sandy MA, et al. Ciprofloxacin with rifampin: a predominately oral regimen for right sided *S. aureus* endocarditis in intravenous drug abusers. *Lancet* 1989;2:1071.

A small study demonstrating efficacy with an oral regimen possibly helpful for those patients refusing intravenous treatment.

Levine DP, Cran LR, Zervos MJ. Bacteremia in narcotic addicts at the Detroit Medical Center. II. Infectious endocarditis: a prospective comparative study. *Rev Infect Dis* 1986;8:374.

A classic two-part series on bacteremia in narcotic addicts.

Marantz PR, Linzer M, Feiner CJ, et al. Inability to predict diagnosis in febrile intravenous drug abusers. *Ann Intern Med* 1987;106:823.

The frequently quoted article showing the need for hospitalization of intravenous drug abusers.

O'Connor PG, Selwyn PA, Schottenfeld RS. Medical care for injection drug users with human immunodeficiency virus infection. *N Engl J Med* 1994;331:450.

A well-written review touching on multiple aspects of caring for the injection drug user with HIV.

73. TUBERCULOSIS IN THE INTENSIVE CARE UNIT

Jennifer S. Daly and Randall R. Reves

I. General principles and overview. The changing epidemiologic features of tuberculosis in the United States have had important implications for all health care providers, including those in the intensive care unit (ICU). Prompt recognition of tuberculosis and early institution of effective therapy will achieve the goals of successful treatment of the patient and the prevention of tuberculosis transmission.

II. Pathogenesis. The pathogenesis of tuberculosis is a two-stage process. The first is the development of tuberculosis infection, and the second is the progression to tuberculosis disease. In the susceptible host, the tubercle bacilli multiply to produce a localized pneumonia and spread to involve hilar lymph nodes. Tubercle bacilli then enter the blood and disseminate. This initial period of primary infection is usually clinically inapparent but may be recognized as primary tuberculosis, especially in children. The development of cell-mediated immunity brings the infection under control in most persons over a period of weeks. The tuberculin skin test usually becomes positive 2 to 10 weeks after the onset of the infection. The second stage or the development of active tuberculosis occurs in about 10% of immunocompetent individuals over their lifetime. About half these cases develop within the first 1 to 2 years after the initial infection with *Mycobacterium tuberculosis.* The pathologic features in immunocompetent people are characterized by the development of a granulomatous inflammatory process. In patients with defects in cell-mediated immunity, the risk of progressive primary or disseminated disease is increased. For instance, the annual risk of developing tuberculosis is 5% to 7% among HIV-infected persons with *M. tuberculosis* infection. Paralleling the decline in cell-mediated immunity is a decrease in the extent of granulomatous inflammation and an increase in the number of acid-fast bacilli in the tissues.

III. Diagnosis. The key to the diagnosis of tuberculosis in the ICU is consideration of the diagnosis in appropriate patients. Table 73-1 shows factors that should prompt consideration of tuberculosis in the differential diagnosis of patients in the ICU. Patients may present to the ICU with life-threatening tuberculosis as the primary disease or as active tuberculosis presenting as a coincidental illness in patients treated for another condition. As the primary diagnosis, tuberculosis can present as respiratory failure from fulminant tuberculosis pneumonia, as disseminated tuberculosis, or as the adult respiratory distress syndrome. Alternatively, patients may present with pericardial tamponade from pericardial tuberculosis, tuberculous meningitis with neurologic deterioration, or complications of gastrointestinal tract involvement. Patients with untreated or treated tuberculosis may present with life-threatening hemoptysis. Tuberculosis may also present as a secondary diagnosis as reactivation tuberculosis in patients with defects in cell-mediated immunity.

A. Chest radiography. Routine chest radiography is an invaluable diagnostic and screening test for patients at risk for tuberculosis. Patients with intact immunity and pulmonary tuberculosis usually have an abnormal chest radiograph; however, patients with HIV infection may occasionally have culture-positive pulmonary tuberculosis despite normal pulmonary radiographs. The usual radiographic pattern of primary tuberculosis is a lower lobe infiltrate with ipsilateral hilar adenopathy in primary tuberculosis (especially in children) or, in reactivation disease, a classic pattern of fibrotic and cavitary infiltrates in the apical segment of the upper lobe and superior segment of the lower lobes. It is important for clinicians to recognize the radiographic patterns of upper lobe parenchymal scars or calcified granulomas representing fibrotic foci of healed inactive tuberculosis. In contrast, in patients with miliary tuberculosis, radiographs may initially be normal or may show miliary nodules 1 to 3 mm in diameter.

TABLE 73-1. Factors that should prompt consideration of tuberculosis in the differential diagnosis

History of tuberculosis infection (positive tuberculin test)
History of tuberculosis disease, particularly if never or inadequately treated
Contact with known or suspected tuberculosis case
Presence of fibrotic lung lesions or upper lobe scars compatible with inactive tuberculosis
Immigration from countries with high risk of tuberculosis
Advanced age
Medically underserved populations
Alcohol or other drug use
Institutional exposure (congregate living)
Known or suspected HIV infection
Other immunosuppressed states

HIV, human immunodeficiency virus.

B. Microbiology. To make a timely diagnosis of tuberculosis, one must first consider the diagnosis, and then one must use modern rapid diagnostic methods. A positive tuberculin skin test indicates the presence of tuberculous infection, but it cannot be used to confirm or to exclude the diagnosis of active tuberculosis. Sputum microscopy remains the most important diagnostic tool in providing a presumptive diagnosis of tuberculosis. Sputum samples positive by auramine-stained smear or Ziehl-Neelsen stain may be examined with direct nucleic acid amplification tests to distinguish *M. tuberculosis* from nontuberculous mycobacteria. Acid-fast bacilli stains and cultures of gastric aspirates, other body fluids, and blood may be diagnostic as well as cultures and histologic features of involved tissue biopsy specimens. Although the mycobacterial pathogens grow slowly, current techniques using liquid media often detect *M. tuberculosis* within 2 to 6 days radiometrically, and then identification may be done promptly with genetic probes, within 1 to 3 weeks, rather than the usual 4 to 8 weeks for growth on routine solid media. Obtaining rapid drug susceptibility testing (within 1 to 3 weeks for acid fact bacilli smear–positive sputum specimens) can be achieved by submitting specimens to a laboratory that performs direct susceptibility testing. Laboratories that only perform initial isolation and then send isolates to reference laboratories often generate additional weeks of delays in providing susceptibility data to clinicians.

IV. Treatment. To reduce infectivity rapidly and to effect a cure without the risk of acquired drug resistance, patients should be started (when possible) on a four-drug combination of isoniazid, rifampin, pyrazinamide, and either ethambutol or streptomycin as a standard initial 8 weeks of therapy. Equally important as the choice of antimicrobial regimens is the issue of adherence to therapy after hospital discharge. Referral to an outpatient program capable of providing directly administered therapy for tuberculosis should be considered in every patient with tuberculosis because this mode of therapy achieves higher cure rates and nearly eliminates the risk of acquired resistance. Patients in whom drug-resistant strains are suspected or documented require initial treatment with a minimum of three and preferably four drugs to which the organism is susceptible and that have not been previously used. Cure rates of more than 95% can be achieved with a 6-month regimen among patients with drug-susceptible organisms (isoniazid and rifampin for the last 4 months). Patients with tuberculosis with strains resistant to isoniazid and rifampin require therapy or 18 or 24 months. These patients should be referred to an expert in the treatment of tuberculosis. In patients with renal failure, isoniazid and rifampin may given in standard doses. Ethambutol, pyrazinamide, aminoglycosides, and fluoroquinolones require dose adjustments. Rifampin, aminoglycosides, and fluoroquinolones may given intravenously. Isoniazid may be given intramuscularly. Corticosteroids may play a useful role in the adjunctive therapy in tuberculosis by reducing the inflammatory response.

Corticosteroids have been shown to lower the mortality and morbidity of patients treated for tuberculous meningitis and have some benefit in patients with tuberculous pericarditis.

V. Infection control and respiratory isolation. One of the major concerns about tuberculosis in the ICU is that of preventing nosocomial transmission. Infection-control measures to prevent the transmission of tuberculosis in health care settings are published by the United States Centers for Disease Control and Prevention. The Occupational Health and Safety Administration has adopted these guidelines as regulations, and both agencies continue to review the documents. There are three levels of the hierarchy of controls. The first two levels are the administrative and engineering controls designed to minimize the areas within health care facilities where exposure to cases of tuberculosis occurs. Early recognition of tuberculosis is the most important step in preventing transmission because this allows the appropriate use of respiratory isolation and the prompt initiation of treatment. The infectiousness of tuberculosis begins to decrease within days of the initiation of effective therapy. The safest approach in a patient receiving treatment in the hospital is to isolate the patient until three sputum smears are negative for acid-fast bacilli. The second priority is use of negative-pressure isolation rooms with at least six air changes per hour. Additional measures that may be of benefit in the intubated patient with tuberculosis include the use of closed-suctioning systems to avoid generation of infectious aerosols and the use of submicron filters for air exhausted from ventilated patients. The third level of the hierarchy of controls is the use of personal protective devices for the health care workers who will be in contact with the patient. Periodic tuberculin testing of hospital personnel should be continued as a means of monitoring the effectiveness of these measures and should allow evaluation of the tuberculin skin test converter with the provision of preventive therapy when appropriate.

Selected Readings

American Thoracic Society, Centers for Disease Control and Prevention. Treatment of tuberculosis and tuberculosis infection in adults and children. *Am Rev Respir Dis* 1994;149:1359.

This is the reference on which current therapy is based. Revisions are under way (according to the American Thoracic Society) but will become available by May 2000.

Centers for Disease Control and Prevention. Prevention and treatment of tuberculosis among patients infected with human immunodeficiency virus: principles of therapy and revised recommendations. *MMWR Morb Mortal Wkly Rep* 1998;47:1.

National guidelines outlining therapy and prophylaxis in HIV-infected patients. The recommendations consider the use of antiretrovirals and drug interactions with medications used to treat tuberculosis and mycobacterial infection.

Christie JD, Calihan DR. The laboratory diagnosis of mycobacterial diseases. *Clin Lab Med* 1995;15:279.

Review of laboratory methods.

Comstock GW. Epidemiology of tuberculosis. Am Rev Respir Dis 1982;125:8.

Review of traditional studies of epidemiology.

Guidelines for preventing the transmission of *Mycobacterium tuberculosis* in health-care facilities, 1994. *MMWR Morb Mortal Wkly Rep* 1994;43:1.

This is the standard guideline on which institutional infection control policies are based.

Hill AR, Premkumar S, Brustein S, et al. Disseminated tuberculosis in the acquired immunodeficiency era. *Am Rev Respir Dis* 1991;144:1164.

Tuberculosis may be difficult to diagnose and may present in organs other than the lungs in patients with HIV infection.

Horsburgh CR, Feldman S, Ridzon R. Quality standards for the treatment of tuberculosis. *Clin Infect Dis* 2000, in press.

Ten essential practice guidelines for the treatment of active and latent tuberculosis infection.

Iseman MD. Treatment of multi-drug resistant tuberculosis. *N Engl J Med* 1993; 329:784.

Review of therapeutic strategies, medications, and rationale for the treatment of patients with multidrug-resistant tuberculosis.

Weis SE, Slocum PC, Blais FX, et al. The effect of directly observed therapy on the rates of drug resistance and relapse in tuberculosis. *N Engl J Med* 1994;330:1179.

Review of data supporting the current recommendation for directly observed therapy for patients with tuberculosis.

74. BOTULISM AND TETANUS

Nelson M. Gantz

I. Botulism

A. General principles. Botulism is a rare disease requiring prompt diagnosis and early treatment to decrease the case fatality rate. Disease results from the action of potent neurotoxin produced by *Clostridium botulinum* and is classified into four types: foodborne botulism, wound botulism, infant botulism, and adult infectious botulism as a result of intestinal colonization with the organism.

B. Etiology. The causative agent of botulism is *C. botulinum,* an anaerobic gram-positive bacillus that produces spores. The property that distinguishes *C. botulinum* from other clostridial species is its ability to produce a potent neurotoxin, which causes paralysis by acting on the peripheral nervous system. Disease in humans is caused by strains that produce toxin: types A, B, E, and, rarely, F and G. Both the vegetative form of the organism and the toxins are heat labile and are destroyed in 10 to 15 minutes at 80°C. The spores, in contrast, are highly heat resistant and can survive boiling for hours. However, spores do not germinate and grow unless conditions are favorable.

C. Epidemiology. The organism and its spores are ubiquitous in nature, so foods are often contaminated. Under suitable conditions, such as improperly preserved food, toxin production can occur. Most of the cases of botulism are foodborne and involve home-canned or home-processed foods. Many recent cases have been associated with restaurants. Food contaminated with toxin, especially type E, may appear and taste normal. Sometimes, disease associated with toxin types A or B spoils the food and results in gas production and swollen cans. Wound botulism should be considered in parenteral abusers of black tar heroin who present with neurologic symptoms such as dysphagia, dysphonia, and wound infection.

D. Pathogenesis. In foodborne botulism, the preformed toxin in the food is ingested and is absorbed from the small intestine. The toxin acts at the neuromuscular junctions, where it inhibits the release of acetylcholine at the cholinergic synapses. Wound botulism occurs when *C. botulinum* infects a wound and produces toxin. In adults, intestinal colonization with the organism may occur after intestinal surgery and antibiotic therapy. Death from botulism results from respiratory paralysis.

E. Clinical presentation. The onset of symptoms and signs after the ingestion of the contaminated food may be as soon as 6 hours or as long as 8 days, with a usual interval of 18 to 36 hours. Botulism should be suspected in a patient who develops bilateral cranial nerve impairment with descending paralysis or weakness. Gastrointestinal complaints, which include nausea, vomiting, and abdominal cramps, often precede the neurologic manifestations. Frequent neurologic symptoms include dysphagia, diplopia, dysarthria, upper and lower extremity weakness, and blurred vision. Dizziness, dyspnea, fatigue, and dry mouth also occur commonly. The physical findings typically show an alert, afebrile patient with ptosis, upper and lower extremity weakness, and a hypoactive gag reflex. Ocular findings are common, and, in addition to ptosis, they include extraocular palsies, nystagmus, and dilated, poorly reactive, or fixed pupils. The symptoms and signs in wound botulism are identical to those seen with foodborne botulism, except fever secondary to the wound infection may be present, and there is no epidemiologic evidence to implicate a food. Gastrointestinal complaints usually do not occur. The incubation period in wound botulism varies from 4 to 14 days.

F. Diagnosis. The diagnosis of botulism, suspected on the clinical presentation, can be confirmed by demonstrating the presence of the botulinal toxin in the patient's serum or feces or incriminating food. The diagnosis can also be established by isolating the organism, *C. botulinum,* from the stool, wound, or suspected food. Another test that can be used to establish the diagnosis of botulism is the performance of repetitive nerve stimulation. Routine laboratory findings, including complete blood count, electrolytes, serum enzymes, and cerebrospinal fluid, are normal unless there are secondary complications. Some of the disorders that are most often confused with botulism include Guillain-Barré syndrome, myasthenia gravis, cerebrovascular accidents, other cases of food poisoning, carbon monoxide poisoning, drug reactions, tick paralysis, poliomyelitis, diphtheria, and Eaton-Lambert syndrome.

G. Treatment. The diagnosis and institution of specific therapy for botulism must be based on the clinical evidence, because laboratory confirmation is often delayed. One goal of therapy is to remove unabsorbed toxin from the gastrointestinal tract using a nasogastric tube for lavage and a cathartic or a tap water enema. A second goal is to administer as soon as possible trivalent antitoxin (A, B, E) to neutralize any circulating antitoxin in the serum. The toxin is of equine origin, and the patient should be skin tested for hypersensitivity to the product. One vial containing type A, type B, and type E antitoxins is administered intravenously. The third goal is meticulous nursing and medical supportive care. Pulmonary complications are the principal cause of death. Elective intubation should be performed when the vital capacity approaches 30% of the predicted value. Wound botulism is treated with debridement and high-dose intravenous penicillin G (3 million U intravenously every 4 hours) as well as antitoxin. The case fatality rate of foodborne botulism is about 15%.

II. Tetanus

A. General principles. Tetanus is a preventable disease. In spite of the availability of tetanus vaccine, approximately 50 cases occur yearly in the United States. Once tetanus has occurred, meticulous medical and nursing care in an intensive care unit are critical for survival.

B. Etiology. Tetanus is caused by *C. tetani,* a large, spore-forming, anaerobic gram-positive bacillus. The vegetative forms of the organism are easily destroyed by heat and disinfectants, in contrast to the spores, which are extremely resistant to physical and chemical disinfection. The manifestations of the disease result from the action of tetanospasmin, a potent exotoxin produced by the vegetative forms of the organism.

C. Epidemiology. The spores of *C. tetani* are found worldwide in soil. The source for the organisms is the feces of most warm-blooded animals. The incidence of the disease depends on the tetanus immunization status of the population. In a susceptible person, almost any wound may serve as a portal of entry for the organism. Cases have also been reported after gastrointestinal surgery, obstetric delivery and abortions, and injections, particularly in drug addicts. Tetanus-prone wounds may be minor and may not appear infected. Excluding neonates, the median age of patients with tetanus is about 50 years. The disease is limited almost exclusively to inadequately immunized persons.

D. Pathogenesis. After a puncture wound or laceration, which may be minor, spores introduced at the injury site are converted to the vegetative form of the organism. The organism proliferates only under anaerobic conditions usually associated with local vascular damage or trauma with tissue necrosis. The organism does not produce tissue injury or evoke an inflammatory reaction; rather, it produces a toxin, tetanospasmin, which is responsible for the disease. The toxin acts at the motor end plates of the skeletal muscles, the spinal cord, the brain, and the sympathetic nervous system. The toxin acts on the spinal cord to block the inhibitory nerve fibers, with resulting muscle stiffness and spasms. The toxin also acts on the sympathetic nervous system and causes profuse sweating, blood pressure fluctuations, tachycardia, and cardiac arrhythmias.

The incubation period for tetanus is usually 7 days but ranges from 1 to 54 days. Ninety percent of cases begin within 2 weeks of the injury.

E. Clinical presentation. Three forms of the disease are described: local, cephalic, and generalized. Cephalic tetanus is a variant of the local form of the disease, with patients having paralysis of the cranial nerves; the incubation period for this type of disease is usually 1 to 2 days and follows an injury to the scalp, face, or neck. Local tetanus is present when the muscle spasms are limited to those at or near the site of injury. The generalized form of the disease is the most common presentation. Local tetanus results in muscle spasms and increased muscle tone confined to the muscles adjacent to the injury site. Patients with generalized tetanus usually complain of trismus or lockjaw and have diffuse muscle spasms. Spasms of the facial muscles result in a grinning expression called *risus sardonicus.* Spasms of the neck and back muscles may result in opisthotonos. Laryngeal spasms may result in cyanosis and respiratory arrest. Generalized seizures occur and are often triggered by a variety of mild external stimuli. The sympathetic nervous system stimulation results in profuse perspiration, tachycardia, labile hypertension, and cardiac arrhythmias. The patient's mental status is usually not impaired.

F. **Diagnosis.** The diagnosis of tetanus is based on the characteristic clinical picture of a patient with trismus or other signs or tonic muscle spasms. A preceding history of a traumatic wound may or may not be present. The patient's susceptibility to tetanus based on the tetanus immunization history is critical. Tetanus is extremely unlikely in a patient with a prior history of receiving a course of tetanus immunization. Sera can be assayed for tetanus antitoxin. It is important to draw the sera before the administration of tetanus immune globulin. Wounds should undergo Gram staining and should be cultured anaerobically for *C. tetani,* which can be identified in about one-third of cases. Table 74-1 lists certain other conditions that may be confused with tetanus, which are part of the differential diagnosis of trismus. Rabies and hypocalcemia tetany may also be confused with tetanus.

G. **Treatment.** As soon as the disease is recognized, the patient should be transferred to the intensive care unit, because respiratory problems are the principal causes of death. A quiet area should be selected. The patient should be given 500 U intramuscularly of human hyperimmune antitetanus globulin. The wound should be surgically debrided, and a 10-day course of penicillin (2 million U intravenously every 4 hours) should be administered to eradicate any organisms. Patients allergic to penicillin can be given metronidazole or a cephalosporin if they have no history of an immediate reaction to penicillin.

The mainstay of therapy is the provision of meticulous intensive care. An asotracheal tube or an oral endotracheal tube should be inserted promptly to manage the copious pharyngeal secretions and to prevent airway obstruction. Once the airway is secure, drugs are needed to control the spasms and the seizures. Muscle relaxation can usually be obtained using a benzodiazepine. Some patients require neuromuscular blockade with an agent such as vecuronium. A prolonged induced coma may be required. The discontinuation of the sedation is determined by trial

TABLE 74-1. Causes of trismus

Local
Abscesses (alveolar)
Parotitis
Fractures
Infected upper molar teeth
Cervical lymphadenopathy
Temporomandibular joint arthritis
Systemic
Phenothiazines
Strychnine poisoning
Trichinosis
Other
Cerebrovascular accidents
Acute hysteria

and error. Problems with cardiac arrhythmias are not uncommon and demand close attention. The hypertension caused by the increased catecholamines often requires treatment with labetalol. The outcome of a patient with tetanus depends on the quality of the supportive care. The overall case fatality rate is about 11%. Prevention is most important. Patients presenting with an injury with an inadequate tetanus immune status should receive tetanus immunoglobulin (250 U intramuscularly) as well as tetanus toxoid.

Selected Readings

Faust RA, Vicker OR, Cohn I Jr. Tetanus: 2,449 cases in 68 years at Charity Hospital. *J Trauma* 1976;16:704.
Clinical features include muscle spasms and no sensory deficits.

Hughes JM, Blumenthal JR, Merson MH, et al. Clinical features of type A and B food-borne botulism. *Ann Intern Med* 1981;95:442.
Clues to the diagnosis include symmetric neurologic findings, no sensory deficits, and the absence of fever.

Shapiro RL, Hatheway C, Swerdlow D. Botulism in the United States: a clinical and epidemiologic review. *Ann Intern Med* 1998;129:221.
This review notes that treatment consists of supportive care and trivalent equine antitoxin.

Weinstein L. Tetanus. *N Engl J Med* 1973: 289:1293.
This review describes diagnosis and management.

VII. GASTROINTESTINAL AND HEPATOBILIARY PROBLEMS IN THE INTENSIVE CARE UNIT

75. GASTROINTESTINAL BLEEDING: PRINCIPLES OF DIAGNOSIS AND MANAGEMENT

Chandra Prakash

I. **General principles.** Acute gastrointestinal (GI) bleeding is a common clinical emergency. Early recognition of clinical and endoscopic prognostic signs helps in the triage to the intensive care unit of patients at risk of rebleeding. The mortality rate from GI bleeding has remained steady at 6% to 12%. Newer nonsurgical therapies may improve survival.

II. **Initial approach**

A. **Rapid evaluation.** Mental confusion, agitation, diaphoresis, mottled skin (livedo reticularis), and cold extremities accompany hypotension with hemorrhagic shock. A quantitative estimate of the amount of bleeding is helpful, because the initial blood count may not reflect the degree of blood lost. Nevertheless, initial blood testing should be performed urgently, to obtain baseline values and to type and crossmatch blood for transfusion. Abdominal pain is not common with GI bleeding and may indicate the presence of hemobilia, intestinal infarction, or perforation. Chest pain may imply a superimposed myocardial infarction or dissecting aneurysm. Previous vascular surgery adds aortoenteric fistula to the differential diagnosis.

B. **Resuscitation.** Resuscitation of the unstable patient takes precedence over other treatments. Recognizing and aggressively treating intravascular volume depletion are of the highest priority and should proceed concurrently with the initial diagnostic evaluation. Intravenous access with large-bore peripheral catheters or a central venous catheter is needed for aggressive administration of fluids or blood products. Ongoing massive hematemesis may require endotracheal intubation for airway protection before endoscopy. Exsanguinating hemorrhage may require immediate surgical management, at times with assistance of limited endoscopy to help direct the surgical approach.

III. **Diagnosis**

A. **Clinical presentation.** Repeated passage of liquid bloody stool indicates ongoing or recurrent bleeding, because fresh blood has laxative properties. As bleeding stops, stool consistency normalizes, and its color darkens. Melena can persist for several days, and the stool may remain positive for occult blood for up to 2 weeks after GI bleeding has ceased.

B. **Nasogastric aspiration.** Passage of a nasogastric tube may help to detect upper GI bleeding in patients with an obscure bleeding site. Further use of the nasogastric tube for lavage to control bleeding is unsubstantiated, although lavage may help to remove clots from the stomach in preparation for endoscopy.

C. **Endoscopy.** When a bleeding site proximal to the jejunum is suspected, esophagogastroduodenoscopy is the diagnostic procedure of choice. Endoscopy is performed when the patient is hemodynamically stable, but resuscitation is usually ongoing at the time of the procedure. When a lower GI bleeding source is suspected, sigmoidoscopy or colonoscopy may be helpful after bowel preparation. These procedures may help to detect and treat colonoscopic bleeding sources or to localize fresh blood to a segment of colon and to direct other therapeutic measures. The tests typically are performed, however, after the bleeding has ceased or in patients with subacute bleeding. Common causes of upper and lower GI bleeding are listed in Table 75-1.

D. **Imaging studies.** A technetium-99m–labeled red blood cell scan can detect bleeding rates as low as 0.1 mL per minute and is a reasonable initial imaging test in the patient with signs of active bleeding distal to the upper GI tract. If active bleeding is found, angiography is often indicated for confirmation of the site and administration of intraarterial vasopressin for bleeding control. Patients who

TABLE 75-1. Causes of gastrointestinal (GI) bleeding

	Common causes	Uncommon causes
Upper GI Bleeding	Duodenal and gastric ulcers Esophageal and gastric varices Gastritis and erosions Mallory-Weiss tears Esophagitis	Cancer Angiodysplasia Dieulafoy lesions Hemobilia Portal gastropathy Cameron erosions
Lower GI Bleeding	Diverticulosis Angiodysplasia Cancer and polyps Ischemic colitis Inflammatory bowel disease Hemorrhoids	Stercoral ulcers Anal fissure Postpolypectomy bleeding Solitary rectal ulcer syndrome Infectious colitis Vasculitis Radiation proctitis/colitis Colonic varices Meckels diverticulum Marathon runner's bleeding Endometriosis Intussusception Aortoenteric fistula

continue to bleed in spite of intraarterial vasopressin may require surgical management. Barium studies are avoided in the setting of acute bleeding.

IV. Treatment

A. Acid suppression. Rationale for using acid suppression in acute upper GI bleeding is based on the coagulopathy resulting from an acid milieu. Intravenous histamine-2-receptor antagonists are prescribed frequently for patients with GI bleeding with limited proof of efficacy. A randomized trial showed that the proton-pump inhibitor omeprazole (40 mg orally every 12 hours for 5 days) significantly decreased the incidence of recurrent bleeding and surgery in hospitalized patients with peptic ulcers; the study was restricted to patients who had duodenal ulcers with high likelihood of recurrent bleeding, yet none underwent any commonly performed endoscopic therapies. Whether acid suppression has a routine role in acute upper GI hemorrhage managed conventionally remains conjectural.

B. Endoscopy. Endoscopic therapy, using thermal devices (heater probe, electrocoagulation, laser), injection therapy (sclerosing solutions, hypertonic saline, epinephrine), or banding devices, offers a convenient and expedient method of treating upper GI bleeding from many causes. These treatments can decrease further bleeding, shorten hospital stay, decrease transfusions, decrease emergency surgery, and lower costs in acute upper GI bleeding. Recurrent bleeding occurs in up to 30% of patients with bleeding ulcers despite successful endoscopic therapy, and continued observation for up to 72 hours is recommended. Endoscopic therapy is of use for some colonic bleeding sites, such as angiodysplasia.

C. Angiographic therapy. Intraarterial vasopressin has been used for angiographic management of bleeding from sites throughout the GI tract, but control of bleeding duodenal ulcers has been disappointing; bleeding stops in fewer than 50% of these patients. Vasopressin use is attended by risk of cardiovascular complications. Gelfoam or metal coil emboli cause localized thrombosis and vessel occlusion, an approach usually reserved for situations with limited alternatives. Tissue ischemia and perforation can result, especially in the colon. Although angiographic therapy may be first-line therapy in lower GI bleeding from diverticula or angiodysplasia, the approach is usually reserved for patients with bleeding peptic ulcer disease in whom endotherapy has failed or who are ineligible for this endotherapy and who have a prohibitive surgical risk.

D. Surgery. Surgical consultation should be obtained early in patients with clinical and endoscopic risk factors for high morbidity and mortality. Patients with massive ongoing hemorrhage that overwhelms the resuscitative effort need urgent surgical assessment. Patients failing to respond to endoscopic or angiographic management also need surgical assessment. Arterial embolization and percutaneous shunts for variceal bleeding are alternatives in high-risk surgical candidates.

Selected Readings

Branicki FJ, Boey J, Fok PJ, et al. Bleeding duodenal ulcer: a prospective evaluation of risk factors for rebleeding and death. *Ann Surg* 1989;211:411.

Recurrent bleeding and mortality were significantly higher with bleeding duodenal ulcers larger than 1 cm in diameter.

Cook DJ, Guyatt GH, Salena BJ, et al. Endoscopic therapy for acute non-variceal hemorrhage: a meta-analysis. *Gastroenterology* 1992;102:139.

A metaanalysis of acute nonvariceal upper GI bleeding showing significant reduction of recurrent bleeding, need for surgical intervention, and mortality after endoscopic hemostatic therapy.

Jensen DM, Machicado GA. Colonoscopy for diagnosis and treatment of severe lower gastrointestinal bleeding: routine outcomes and cost analysis. *Gastroenterol Endosc Clin North Am* 1997;7:477.

Indications, therapeutic potential, and outcomes of urgent colonoscopy in acute lower GI bleeding.

Khuroo MS, Yattoo GN, Javid G, et al. A comparison of omeprazole and placebo for bleeding peptic ulcer. *N Engl J Med* 1997; 336:1054.

A significant reduction in recurrent bleeding and need for surgery was noted in omeprazole-treated patients with bleeding peptic ulcers not managed with endoscopic hemostatic techniques.

Kollef MH, O'Brien JD, Zuckerman GR, et al. BLEED: a classification tool to predict outcomes in patients with acute upper and lower gastrointestinal hemorrhage. *Crit Care Med* 1997;25:1125.

An outcome measure based on clinical and laboratory evaluation that, when applied at emergency room presentation, predicts hospital outcomes and likelihood of recurrent bleeding in patients with acute upper and lower GI bleeding.

Longstreth GF. Epidemiology and outcome of patients hospitalized with acute lower gastrointestinal hemorrhage: a population-based study. *Am J Gastroenterol* 1997; 92:419.

Diverticulosis is identified as the leading cause of acute lower GI bleeding, and annual incidence rates, recurrence, and mortality are characterized.

MacLeod IA, Mills PR. Factors identifying the probability of further haemorrhage after acute upper gastrointestinal haemorrhage. *Br J Surg* 1982;69:256.

Risk of recurrent bleeding was higher from esophageal varices or peptic ulcers, in patients with shock, or anemia, or absence of alcohol consumption at presentation, and in patients who are more than 60 years of age.

Miller LS, Barbarevech C, Friedman LS. Less frequent causes of lower gastrointestinal bleeding. *Gastrointest Clin North Am* 1994;23:21.

Uncommon and rare causes of lower GI bleeding are reviewed.

Pennoyer WP, Vignati PV, Cohen JL. Management of angiogram positive lower gastrointestinal hemorrhage: long term follow-up of non-operative treatments. *Int J Colorectal Dis* 1996;11:279.

Angiotherapy with vasopressin infusion or embolization is highly effective in controlling massive lower GI bleeding and has a low recurrence rate.

Peura DA, Lanza FL, Gostout FL, et al. The American College of Gastroenterology bleeding registry: preliminary findings. *Am J Gastroenterol* 1997;92:924.

A wealth of demographic and etiologic information on both upper and lower GI bleeding, including current practice standards.

Reinus JF, Brandt LJ. Vascular ectasias and diverticulosis: common causes of lower intestinal bleeding. *Gastroenterol Clin North Am* 1994;23:1.

An excellent review of the common causes of lower GI bleeding.

Robinson P. The role of nuclear medicine in acute gastrointestinal bleeding. *Nucl Med Commun* 1993;14:849.

Appropriateness of patient selection and timeliness of the study are critical in the use of nuclear medicine studies in the investigation of acute GI bleeding.

Saeed ZA, Ramirez FC, Hepps KS, et al. Prospective validation of the Baylor bleeding score for predicting the likelihood of rebleeding after endoscopic hemostasis of peptic ulcers. *Gastrointest Endosc* 1995;41:561.

Validation of a three-component scoring system to identify patients at increased risk of bleeding from peptic ulcer disease.

Zuckerman GR, Prakash C. Acute lower intestinal bleeding. Part I. Clinical presentation and diagnosis. Part II. Etiology, therapy and outcomes. *Gastrointest Endosc* 1998;48:606–616;1999;49:228–238.

A comprehensive well-referenced two-part review on current concepts in acute lower GI bleeding.

Zuckerman GR, Trellis DR, Sherman TM, et al. An objective measure of stool color for differentiating upper from lower gastrointestinal bleeding. *Dig Dis Sci* 1995; 40:1614.

An objective pocket-sized color card with five stool colors helps to differentiate upper from lower GI bleeding.

76. STRESS ULCER SYNDROME

Chandra Prakash

I. Definition. The term *stress ulcer* is used to define erosive or ulcerative mucosal abnormalities of the upper gastrointestinal tract in the face of extreme physiologic stress. Endoscopy demonstrates that as many as 52% to 100% of patients admitted to intensive care units (ICUs) have evidence of gastric mucosal injury within the first 24 hours, but most are asymptomatic. *Stress ulcer syndrome* is the term used when the mucosal lesion is associated with clinical bleeding or perforation.

II. Pathogenesis

A. Mucosal damage. Gastric acid is essential for stress ulceration. The typical patient, however, has normal or even decreased gastric acid secretion, a finding suggesting that a breakdown of the mucosal defense mechanisms is also required. Defense mechanisms include (a) the mucus and mucus-bound bicarbonate that provide an anatomic barrier and buffer the intraluminal hydrogen ions, (b) intact intramucosal blood flow that brings systemic bicarbonate to prevent intramural pH shifts, and (c) mucosal cell restitution that allows for rapid restoration of the mucous-cell layer when the epithelium is damaged. Stress results in mucosal ischemia, leading to drops in intramucosal pH from back-diffused hydrogen ions that is compounded by a deficit of systemic bicarbonate buffer and oxygen. Subsequent reperfusion contributes to the formation of toxic oxygen-derived free radicals and superoxides while decreasing the synthesis of cytoprotective prostaglandins. These effects create a favorable situation for mucosal damage. The role of *Helicobacter pylori* in the pathogenesis remains unknown.

B. Risk factors. A statistically significant predisposition to stress ulceration has been demonstrated in patients in the ICU who have coagulopathy or who require prolonged mechanical ventilation. Other contributory risk factors include major surgery, hemorrhagic shock, hypotension, trauma, and sepsis. The incidence of gastrointestinal bleeding increases with each risk factor up to two; additional risk factors do not further increase the incidence (Table 76-1). Mortality rates can be as high as 50% to 80% in patients who bleed, although death is usually attributed to the underlying disease.

III. Diagnosis. Stress ulcers come to clinical attention when they bleed. Significant stress ulcer bleeding occurs in 2% to 6% of critically ill patients and presents within 14 days of the onset of physiologic stress or ICU admission as hematemesis, gross blood from the nasogastric tube, or melena. Patients with thermal injury from burns or with acute intracranial disease including head trauma and coma appear to be at increased risk (Curling ulcers and Cushing ulcers, respectively) (Table 76-1). On endoscopy, the earliest mucosal changes are found in the most proximal part of the stomach and include pallor, mottling, and submucosal petechiae. These lesions coalesce to form superficial linear erosions and ulcers, eventually involving the antrum and sometimes the duodenum. The result is a diffuse area of mucosal damage that can ooze blood and occasionally lead to massive hemorrhage or perforation.

IV. Treatment. The risk of bleeding from stress ulcers and the overall prognosis are related to the severity of underlying illness, aggressive management of which should always take precedence. When patients at risk for stress ulceration are identified early in the ICU stay, mucosal integrity can be pharmacologically enhanced using prophylactic agents (see the next section of this chapter). For clinically significant bleeding, upper GI endoscopy helps to establish the diagnosis and to determine the need for endoscopic thermal or injection therapy. If endoscopic measures fail, angiography can be attempted, using intraarterial vasopressin or embolization if the bleeding site can be demonstrated. If multiple bleeding lesions are present, continuous gastric lavage with 5 to 10 L of ice-cold lactated Ringer's solution over 1 to 2 hours has been advocated. Surgical therapy is reserved for severe, life-threatening hem-

TABLE 76-1. Risk factors for gastrointestinal bleeding and perforation in stress ulcer syndrome

Patient categories presumed at high risk
- Burns on more than 50% of body surface area
- Acute intracranial lesions, including tumor, trauma, infection, stroke
- Fulminant hepatic failure
- Sepsis, especially pulmonary and intraperitoneal sources
- Major trauma
- Postoperatively, especially following abdominal, cardiovascular, thoracic, or neurologic surgery
- Intensive care patients with superimposed complications: shock, prolonged mechanical ventilation (>3 d), acute renal failure, jaundice, coagulopathy
- Multiorgan system failure

Patient categories presumed not at high risk
- Burns on less than 35% of body surface area (unless shock or sepsis superimposed)
- Chronic brain disease
- Chronic obstructive pulmonary disease or transient respiratory illnesses
- Dialyzed chronic renal failure
- Cardiac disease, including myocardial infarction, arrhythmias, and congestive heart failure

orrhage unresponsive to all other measures. The mortality of total gastrectomy approaches 100% in these critically ill patients, whereas subtotal gastrectomy can be associated with rates of recurrent bleeding approaching 50% from the remnant gastric mucosa. Vagotomy and oversewing of any remaining ulcers during subtotal gastrectomy may decrease the high rate of recurrent bleeding.

V. Prophylaxis. The logic of prophylaxis lies in the assumptions that the formation of stress ulcers can be prevented or that, once these ulcers are formed, the progression from ulcer to bleeding or perforation can be halted.

A. Antacids. Antacids (10 to 80 mL) can be administered through a nasogastric tube every 1 to 2 hours and ideally titrated to keep the gastric pH greater than 4.0, measured 1 hour after administration. Some antacids may cause diarrhea, may be contraindicated in renal failure, and may affect the bioavailability of oral medications. Their use involves expensive and time-consuming processes of frequent administration and monitoring of gastric pH. Nevertheless, antacids have demonstrated efficacy in the prophylaxis of stress ulcer syndrome.

B. Antisecretory drugs. Histamine-2-receptor antagonists are administered intravenously, either as a standard intermittent bolus or by continuous infusion. Continuous infusion more effectively maintains the desired gastric intraluminal pH. Patients with a creatinine clearance of less than 30 mL per minute should receive half the recommended dose, and caution should be exercised in patients with thrombocytopenia. The optimal gastric pH level is unknown, and the need for 24-hour pH control is not essential for a prophylactic effect. Although controlled studies are lacking, proton pump inhibitors in usual doses can also be used.

C. Sucralfate. Sucralfate, the aluminum salt of sulfated sucrose, coats the early shallow mucosal lesions and protects them from further acid and pepsin damage without altering gastric pH. It is usually delivered in the form of a slurry through a nasogastric tube at a dose of 4 to 6 g per day. Although it is safe for long-term use in critically ill patients, sucralfate should be used with caution in patients with chronic renal insufficiency. Some clinicians prefer sucralfate because of its low side effect profile and cost and because of some evidence that sucralfate results in fewer cases of nosocomial pneumonia.

D. Other agents. Prostaglandins, free radical scavengers such as dimethylsulfoxide and allopurinol, and the bioflavin meciadanol have also been used for stress ulcer prophylaxis with varying results. Retrospective studies on burn patients and patients receiving assisted ventilation suggest that upper GI bleeding may be reduced by enteral feeding.

E. Complications of prophylaxis. Nosocomial pneumonia as a complication of stress ulcer prophylaxis is a growing concern. Gastric alkalinization and colonization with gram-negative bacilli are thought to play a causal role, and, consequently, some studies suggest a higher incidence of nosocomial pneumonia in patients who receive antisecretory drugs. Further studies are needed before one prophylactic agent can be confidently recommended over another.

Selected Readings

Cook D, Guyatt G, Marshall J, et al. A comparison of sucralfate and ranitidine for the prevention of upper gastrointestinal bleeding in patients requiring mechanical ventilation: Canadian Critical Care Trials Group. *N Engl J Med* 1998;338:791.
A multicenter randomized blinded placebo-controlled trial showing a significantly lower rate of gastrointestinal bleeding in mechanically ventilated critically ill patients treated with intravenous bolus ranitidine as compared with nasogastric sucralfate.

Cook DJ. Stress ulcer prophylaxis: gastrointestinal bleeding and nosocomial pneumonia. Best evidence synthesis. *Scand J Gastroenterol Suppl* 1995;210:48.
This metaanalysis concludes that all stress ulcer prophylactic agents are effective in decreasing the incidence of stress ulcer bleeding, but sucralfate may be associated with a lower risk of nosocomial pneumonia and mortality.

Cook DJ, Fuller HD, Guyatt GH, et al. Risk factors for gastrointestinal bleeding in critically ill patients. *N Engl J Med* 1994;330:377.
This prospective multicenter cohort study identified respiratory failure and coagulopathy as two strong independent risk factors for stress ulcer bleeding.

Cook DJ, Reeve BK, Scholes LC. Histamine-2-receptor antagonists and antacids in the critically ill population: stress ulceration versus nosocomial pneumonia. *Infect Control Hosp Epidemiol* 1994;15:437.
In critically ill patients, sucralfate results in a lower incidence of nosocomial pneumonia than either antacids or histamine-2-receptor antagonists.

Cook DJ, Reeve BK, Guyatt GH, et al. Stress ulcer prophylaxis in critically ill patients: resolving discordant meta-analysis. *JAMA* 1996;275:308.
Histamine-2-receptor antagonists reduce clinically significant stress ulcer bleeding, but data are insufficient to determine the advantage of one medical approach over another.

Driks MR, Craven DE, Celli BR, et al. Nosocomial pneumonia in intubated patients given sucralfate as compared with antacids or histamine type 2 blockers. *N Engl J Med* 1987;317:1376.
A randomized trial showing that sucralfate may be preferable to antacids and histamine-2-receptor blockers in mechanically ventilated patients.

Hubert JP, Kiernan PD, Welch JS, et al. The surgical management of bleeding stress ulcers. *Ann Surg* 1980;191:672.
Surgery carries a high mortality in bleeding stress ulcers; near-total gastrectomy and total gastrectomy are most effective in controlling bleeding.

Langtry HD, Wilde MI. Lansoprazole: an update of its pharmacological properties and clinical efficacy in the management of acid-related disorders. *Drugs* 1997;54:473.
Preliminary studies of lansoprazole show promise in patients at risk for stress ulcers.

Levy MJ, Seelig CB, Robinson NJ, et al. Comparison of omeprazole and ranitidine for stress ulcer prophylaxis. *Dig Dis Sci* 1997;42:1255–1259.
A prospective randomized trial concluding that oral omeprazole is safe, effective, and clinically feasible for stress ulcer prophylaxis.

Metz CA, Livingston DH, Smith S, et al. Impact of multiple risk factors and ranitidine prophylaxis on the development of stress related upper gastrointestinal bleeding: a prospective multicenter double-blind randomized trial. *Crit Care Med* 1993;21:1844.
Two concomitant risk factors increased risk for stress ulcer bleeding, but additional risk factors were not detrimental.

Ortiz JE, Sottile FD, Sigel P, et al. Gastric colonization as a consequence of stress ulcer prophylaxis: a prospective randomized trial. *Pharmacotherapy* 1998;18:486.

Bacterial colonization was increasingly likely in patients with a persistently alkaline gastric pH.

Raff T, Germann G, Hartmann B. The value of early enteral nutrition in the prophylaxis of stress ulceration in the severely burned patient. *Burns* 1997;23:313.
Early enteral nutrition prevented stress-related upper gastrointestinal bleeding in burn patients.

Tryba M, Cook DJ. Gastric alkalinization, pneumonia and systemic infections: the controversy. *Scand J Gastroenterol Suppl* 1995;210:53.
Gastric alkalinization significantly increases the risk of nosocomial pneumonia in patients receiving long-term mechanical ventilation, but only selected patients benefit from acid-independent stress ulcer prophylaxis relative to nosocomial pneumonia.

Tryba M, Cook D. Current guidelines on stress ulcer prophylaxis. *Drugs* 1997;54:581.
A review article emphasizing that improvement of oxygenation and microcirculation in the ICU play an important role in preventing stress ulcers.

Zuckerman GR, Shuman R. Therapeutic goals and treatment options for prevention of stress ulcer syndrome. *Am J Med* 1987;83 [Suppl 6A] :29.
The basis and goals of prophylactic therapy for stress ulcers are reviewed.

77. VARICEAL BLEEDING

Chandra Prakash

I. General principles. Acute variceal bleeding occurs in at least 20% of all patients with cirrhosis and varices. The mortality of an acute bleeding episode approaches 30% to 50%. When bleeding ceases spontaneously, it recurs in 60% of patients within 10 days. Decompensation from liver disease, aspiration, hepatic encephalopathy, hepatorenal syndrome, septicemia, alcohol withdrawal, and exsanguination all contribute to a poor outcome. Early accurate diagnosis, stabilization of hemodynamics, and immediate hemostasis are critical, as are prevention of recurrent bleeding and prevention and treatment of superimposed complications.

II. Pathophysiology. The cause of portal hypertension in nearly all cases is mechanical obstruction to portal venous flow. Although typically resulting from cirrhosis, reversible portal hypertension can also occur in the setting of acute hepatitis. Other causes include portal vein and hepatic vein thrombosis, as well as unusual disorders such as congenital hepatic fibrosis and schistosomiasis. Secondary hemodynamic changes associated with cirrhosis, including peripheral vasodilatation, decreased systemic vascular resistance, increased cardiac output, and splanchnic hyperemia, contribute to increased portal pressure. A collateral circulation develops to decompress the portal venous system, the most clinically significant locations being the junctions of squamous and columnar mucosae (gastroesophageal, anal, and peristomal). These collateral vessels progressively enlarge to form varices. Risk factors for variceal rupture include a portosystemic pressure gradient greater than 12 mm Hg, large variceal size, and progressive hepatic dysfunction.

III. Diagnosis. Variceal bleeding is typically brisk, presenting as hematemesis, melena, and varying degrees of hemodynamic instability. Acute bleeding is self-limited in 50% to 60% of cases. Approximately half the patients with stigmata of chronic liver disease who present with acute upper gastrointestinal bleeding have nonvariceal sources of hemorrhage, and endoscopic verification is required. On endoscopy, a fresh fibrin clot may be seen protruding from a varix. Detecting blood pouring from a variceal rent is unlikely; more often, nonbleeding varices are the only findings. In such cases, banding or sclerotherapy is warranted because of the high rate of early recurrent bleeding.

IV. Treatment

A. Initial resuscitation. Appropriate resuscitative efforts should be initiated without delay, even before endoscopic evaluation (see Chapters 75 and 146). Nasogastric aspiration may be necessary when the diagnosis of an upper gastrointestinal hemorrhage is in doubt; fears of trauma to a varix from the tube are largely unfounded, but good lubrication and careful technique should be exercised. Packed red blood cell transfusion, fresh frozen plasma, and platelet infusion may be necessary before endoscopy, depending on initial laboratory test results. Airway protection with endotracheal intubation is mandatory in the massively bleeding or obtunded patient. Patients with alcoholism should receive thiamin and should be monitored closely for alcohol withdrawal.

B. Endoscopic therapy. Sclerotherapy and band ligation are the two techniques used for endoscopic control of bleeding varices. Sclerotherapy confers a long-term survival advantage over medical management. A sclerosant solution is injected into the variceal lumen or into the adjacent submucosa of the distal esophagus. Band ligation involves placing small elastic "O" rings over the varices. Subsequent strangulation of the vessel with sloughing and fibrosis of the adjacent esophageal tissues results in the obliteration of the varix. Active bleeding is controlled with either technique in 80% to 90% of patients after one or two treatments; risks of recurrent bleeding, duration of hospitalization, blood transfusion requirements, and survival are similar. Band ligation has gained acceptance as the endoscopic treatment of choice because of a lower incidence of esophageal ulceration, stricture formation, perforation, bacteremia, and respiratory failure. Serial scheduled endoscopic treatment sessions at weekly to monthly intervals ensure obliteration of the varices. Endoscopic therapy is frequently ineffective in *gastric variceal bleeding,* wherein early consideration of nonendoscopic therapy is warranted.

C. Octreotide. Octreotide is the pharmacotherapeutic agent of choice in acute variceal bleeding. This synthetic octapeptide shares structural and functional properties with somatostatin in reducing splanchnic blood flow and portal pressure. Aside from transient nausea and abdominal pain from bolus doses, significant adverse effects are rare. A bolus of 25 to 100 μg is followed by a continuous infusion of 25 to 50 μg per hour for 48 to 72 hours. Octreotide is effective in stopping active bleeding from varices and has an important role in the prevention of early recurrent bleeding after initial hemostasis.

D. Vasopressin. Vasopressin, when infused intravenously, is a potent vasoconstrictor that reduces splanchnic blood flow and portal pressure. Adverse effects from systemic vasoconstriction include hypertension and myocardial ischemia; electrolyte abnormalities can result from the antidiuretic effect of this pituitary hormone. The starting dose is typically 0.4 U per minute, titrated to a maximum of 1 U per minute if required for bleeding control. Adverse cardiac effects interfere with treatment in nearly 30% of patients and contribute to the limited success rate of this approach. Concurrent intravenous nitroglycerin infusion, titrated to maintain a systolic blood pressure of 100 mm Hg, is recommended. Nitroglycerin may prevent side effects from systemic vasoconstriction and does not compromise the desired clinical effect of vasopressin. Treatment with vasoconstricting agents should not be considered definitive therapy. The drugs, particularly octreotide, are safe and useful adjuncts that may allow delaying endoscopic therapy to a safer, more elective setting.

E. Transjugular intrahepatic portosystemic stent shunt. The transjugular intrahepatic portosystemic stent shunt (TIPSS), an iatrogenic fistula between radicals of the hepatic and portal veins, is created by interventional radiologists using ultrasonographic and fluoroscopic guidance. An expandable metal stent is left in place, and the portosystemic pressure gradient is reduced to less than 12 mm Hg. A TIPSS is commonly recommended if bleeding recurs after two or more endoscopic attempts at prevention, on an emergency basis in active uncontrolled bleeding, or if bleeding has occurred from gastric varices or portal hypertensive gastropathy. The technical success rate in constructing a TIPSS is more than 90%, with near-universal success in bleeding control, but 15% to 60% of patients develop some degree of shunt insufficiency within 6 months. Doppler ultrasound examination for determining shunt patency is recommended for postprocedure bleeding recurrence. The shunt can usually be revised with little morbidity. Twenty to thirty percent of patients develop transient deterioration of liver function after elective shunt placement, and up to one-fourth of patients may experience new or worsened hepatic encephalopathy.

F. Surgical shunts. Surgical shunts are considered in patients with good long-term prognosis who need portal decompression, such as patients with Child A cirrhosis and patients with noncirrhotic portal hypertension. The utility of surgical shunting in the acutely bleeding patient with cirrhosis is limited by high operative mortality and postprocedure encephalopathy.

G. Balloon tamponade. Gastric and esophageal balloon devices for direct tamponade of the bleeding varices (Sengstaken-Blakemore, Minnesota, and Linton-Nachlas balloons) may be required for patients with severe or persistent bleeding. Initial success approaches 90%, but rates of recurrent bleeding are high, and definitive plans for portal decompression should be made before deflating the balloon. Complications occur in 15% to 30% of patients; balloon-related deaths occur in up to 6%. Endotracheal intubation should precede balloon placement for airway protection.

H. Other measures. Nonshunting operations, such as the Sugiura procedure (mucosal transection and devascularization of the esophagus) are infrequently used, because varices recur, and bleeding recurs in more than 20% of patients. Embolization of the short gastric veins in gastric variceal bleeding and splenectomy in splenic vein thrombosis are other potential management options.

Selected Readings

Binmoeller KF, Soehendra N. Nonsurgical treatment of variceal bleeding: new modalities. *Am J Gastroenterol* 1995;90:1923.

A clinical review of the nonsurgical modalities available for the therapy of variceal bleeding.

Bosch J. Medical treatment of portal hypertension. *Digestion* 1998;59:547.

Significant advances in the pharmacotherapy of portal hypertension in the 1990s are outlined.

Burroughs AK, Planas R, Svoboda P. Optimizing emergency care of upper gastrointestinal bleeding in cirrhotic patients. *Scand J Gastroenterol Suppl* 1998;226:14.

Of the vasoactive drugs available, somatostatin is the best treatment option, based on metaanalysis of clinical studies.

De Franchis R, Banares R, Silvain C. Emergency endoscopy strategies for improved outcomes. *Scand J Gastroenterol Suppl* 1998;226:25.

This review emphasizes that pharmacotherapy in combination with endoscopic intervention is more effective than endoscopic treatment alone in patients with variceal bleeding.

Haddock G, Garden OJ, McKee RF, et al. Esophageal tamponade in the management of acute variceal hemorrhage. *Dig Dis Sci* 1989;34:913.

Balloon tamponade controlled variceal bleeding in 94%, but 6.4% had fatal complications from the procedure.

Idezuki Y. Transection and devascularization procedures for bleeding from oesophageal varices. *Baillieres Clin Gastroenterol* 1992;6:549.

A review discussing surgery for bleeding esophageal varices and its indications.

Imperiale TF, Teran JC, McCullough AJ. A meta-analysis of somatostatin versus vasopressin in the management of acute esophageal variceal hemorrhage. *Gastroenterology* 1995;109:1289.

Somatostatin is more efficacious with a lower risk of adverse effects when compared with vasopressin.

Patch D, Nikolopoulou V, McCormick A, et al. Factors related to early mortality after transjugular intrahepatic portosystemic shunt for failed endoscopic therapy in acute variceal bleeding. *J Hepatol* 1998;28:454.

Patients with uncontrolled bleeding, advanced liver disease, sepsis, and multiorgan failure have a high mortality despite immediate bleeding control by TIPSS.

Rossle M, Deibert P, Haag K, et al. Randomized trial of transjugular-intrahepatic-portosystemic shunt versus endoscopy plus propranolol for prevention of variceal rebleeding. *Lancet* 1997;349:1043.

The transjugular shunt was more effective than endoscopic treatment in prevention of recurrent variceal bleeding but resulted in encephalopathy in 36%; there was no survival difference.

Rossle M, Siegerstetter V, Huber M, et al. The first decade of the transjugular intrahepatic portosystemic shunt (TIPS): state of the art. *Liver* 1998;18:73.

A review of the indications, technical aspects, complications, and outcome of the TIPSS procedure.

Sanyal AJ, Freedman AM, Lake JR, et al. Transjugular intrahepatic portosystemic shunts for patients with active variceal hemorrhage unresponsive to sclerotherapy. *Gastroenterology* 1996;111:138.

TIPSS was highly effective as salvage therapy in 30 patients with continued bleeding despite urgent sclerotherapy.

Schoenfeld PS, Butler JA. An evidence-based approach to the treatment of esophageal variceal bleeding. *Crit Care Clin* 1998;14:441.

Evidence from randomized controlled trials indicates that band ligation is more effective than sclerotherapy, that beta-blockers and nitrates may prevent the initial episode of bleeding, and that somatostatin may decrease rebleeding rates with or without endoscopic therapy.

Schuman BM, Beckman JW, Tedesco FJ, et al. Complications of endoscopic injection sclerotherapy: a review. *Am J Gastroenterol* 1987;82:823.

A review of complications after sclerotherapy, including their prevention and management.

Steigmann GV, Goff JS, Michaletz-Onody PA, et al. Endoscopic sclerotherapy as compared with endoscopic ligation for bleeding esophageal varices. *N Engl J Med* 1992;326:1527.

Esophageal band ligation is associated with fewer treatment-related complications and better survival rates when compared with esophageal sclerotherapy for bleeding esophageal varices.

78. INTESTINAL PSEUDOOBSTRUCTION (ILEUS)

Chandra Prakash and Ray E. Clouse

I. General principles. The term *acute intestinal pseudoobstruction,* or ileus, is used to describe a syndrome of intestinal dilatation and other clinical features of obstruction without a mechanical explanation. The process can involve the small or large intestines and can result secondarily from practically any medical insult (Table 78-1), particularly life-threatening systemic diseases, drugs, infection, vascular insufficiency, surgery, and electrolyte abnormalities. Colonic dilatation in the presence of a competent ileocecal valve (Ogilvie syndrome) is given particular attention because of the potential for cecal rupture.

Chronic intestinal pseudoobstruction results from myopathic disorders or disorders involving the enteric nervous system. Strategic areas of the central nervous system may be involved as well. A more extensive form of chronic pseudoobstruction also involves other hollow viscera such as the urinary tract, reproductive system, and biliary tract. The list of known causes of chronic intestinal pseudoobstruction is long and includes collagen vascular disorders, endocrine abnormalities (such as diabetes mellitus), neurologic disorders (including Parkinson disease), and a variety of drugs.

II. Pathogenesis. In the intensive care setting, the pathogenesis of acute intestinal pseudoobstruction usually remains undefined, and most patients are severely ill from multiple disease processes. Insult to the enteric nervous system is the final common pathway resulting from direct trauma during surgery or disruption of intracellular function from electrolyte abnormalities, infection, vascular insufficiency, and other causes. Catecholamines are released within the wall of the intestine in postoperative ileus and act on alpha$_1$-adrenergic receptors to interfere with motor function. Trauma to the sacral nerve roots or compression by the postpartum uterus has been suggested as the underlying cause of this disorder after pregnancy or cesarean section.

III. Diagnosis

A. History. Patients with acute pseudoobstruction often have no history of past episodes. Inquiry into dysfunction of other hollow viscera—urinary, biliary, and reproductive tracts—is important in the chronic variety, as is a careful search for other features of known causes or a family history. Eye problems such as ptosis or ophthalmoplegia can be associated with visceral myopathies.

B. Physical examination. The abdomen is markedly distended and tympanitic on percussion, with absent or diminished bowel sounds, and the patient has relatively little abdominal pain, features that can also be seen with mechanical obstruction. Palpation or percussion tenderness and other peritoneal signs should alert the physician to a primary intraabdominal inflammatory process that may need immediate surgical attention or to ischemic damage to the colonic wall in cases of marked colonic dilatation.

C. Laboratory studies. Conventional laboratory tests may detect electrolyte imbalances that are easily corrected. Elevated amylase and lipase values direct attention to the pancreas, whereas a high white blood cell count suggests an infectious or inflammatory process.

D. Imaging studies. An obstructive series (supine and upright abdominal radiographs with a chest radiograph) is an essential early step to determine the distribution of intestinal gas and to assess the presence of free intraabdominal air. Mechanical bowel obstruction must always be considered and often requires exclusion using additional imaging studies including computed tomography with contrast, thin-film barium enema, or small bowel series. In the acute setting, serial plain radiographs may be sufficient to exclude a mechanical process, especially if the clinical setting favors pseudoobstruction.

E. Colonoscopy. Colonoscopy is both diagnostic and therapeutic when the large bowel is solely or dominantly involved, and it allows detection of obstructing

TABLE 78-1. Common causes of acute intestinal pseudoobstruction

Electrolyte abnormalities
Hypocalcemia, hypokalemia, hyperkalemia, hypomagnesemia, hypomanganesemia
Infections
Sepsis; pneumonia; viral illnesses (including viral hepatitis and viral pancreatitis); gastroenteritis (viral or bacterial); pelvic inflammatory disease; peritonitis; pseudomembranous colitis; AIDS enteropathy
Inflammation
Pancreatitis; cholecystitis; Crohn ileitis or colitis; ulcerative colitis; appendicitis; diverticulitis
Metabolic disorders
Diabetes mellitus and its complications; sickle cell crises; acute intermittent porphyria; renal failure; hypothyroidism
Pregnancy
Premature labor; placenta previa; cesarean section; postdelivery ileus
Drugs
Opiates; phenothiazines; tricyclic antidepressants; antiparkinsonian medications; $alpha_1$-adrenergic agonists (e.g., ephedrine sulfate, phenylpropanolamine); $alpha_2$-adrenergic agonists (e.g., clonidine); calcium channel antagonists; anticholinergics; interleukin-2
Trauma
Abdominal insult; trauma to the head (cerebrovascular accident or subarachnoid hemorrhage); back injury (pelvic or spinal fractures)
Postoperative ileus
Abdominal; urologic; orthopedic; other operations
Toxicities
Organophosphate poisoning; mushroom poisoning (*Amanita*); radiation sickness; heavy metal poisoning (lead, arsenic, mercury)

lesions such as colon cancer and decompressing massively dilated bowel or volvulus. When the cecum approaches 9 to 10 cm in diameter, the possibility of perforation begins to increase rapidly, and colonoscopic decompression may be needed urgently. The decision to proceed with colonoscopic decompression in suspected cases of pseudoobstruction is also influenced by the abdominal examination. If a nonmechanical cause is evident, it may be prudent to observe the patient while correcting precipitating factors before further investigation is undertaken.

IV. Treatment

A. General measures. Basic supportive measures and watchful waiting are sufficient in most cases of acute intestinal pseudoobstruction. Fluid replacement and correction of electrolytes are essential. If infection is a factor, prompt and appropriate antibiotic therapy is crucial. Many drugs alter gastrointestinal motility, including adrenergic agonists (e.g., clonidine), tricyclic antidepressants, sedatives, and opiates; withdrawal or decreasing doses of potentially offending medications may assist the return of gut function. Total parenteral nutrition may be necessary as a temporary measure in protracted cases. The ambulatory patient is encouraged to undertake short walks and exercise, although supportive data for these and many other commonly practiced maneuvers are scant.

B. Decompression. Use of a nasogastric tube attached to intermittent suction prevents swallowed air from passing through the gastrointestinal tract and partially controls intestinal accumulation. In chronic cases, a percutaneous endoscopic gastrostomy tube can be considered for decompression, especially if vomiting or gastric distention occurs. Rectal tubes assist in decompression of the rectosigmoid colon but have little impact on decompressing the proximal colon; turning the patient from side to side at frequent intervals may improve the benefit from rectal decompression.

When the pattern of colonic obstruction is present, colonoscopy is often used because of its dual diagnostic and therapeutic capabilities. Colonoscopic decompression should be considered when the cecal diameter approaches 9 to 10 cm, and it can be performed in the presence of retained stool. Distention with air during colonoscopy is kept to a minimum, and the procedure should be terminated in favor of surgery if signs of ischemia are clearly evident. Successful decompression can be expected in approximately 80% of patients with one procedure, but if dilatation recurs, repeat colonoscopy is usually successful. Successful decompression may be accomplished when the colonoscope only reaches the hepatic flexure, but less comprehensive procedures are usually ineffective. A fenestrated tube placed in the cecum or transverse colon may help to prevent recurrence until full recovery, largely through stenting the colonic lumen.

C. Surgery. Surgical consultation may be required during the initial evaluation, both for weighing the evidence favoring mechanical obstruction and for managing severe colonic distention, when present. For colonic distention, a cecostomy is occasionally required when colonoscopic decompression fails, but it is successful primarily in the absence of perforation or ischemic bowel changes. Exploration is reserved in acute cases for a strong indication such as peritoneal signs. Exploration is also occasionally required to clarify a clinically obstructed picture and may on occasion be curative. If no lesion is found during exploratory surgery in chronic cases, full-thickness biopsies should be obtained from the small and large intestines for histologic evaluation of nerve and muscle.

D. Medications. Pharmacotherapy has a limited role in acute intestinal pseudoobstruction. Neostigmine (2 mg IV slowly over 3–5 minutes) can rapidly reestablish colonic tone with resolution of pseudoobstruction in selected patients; mechanical obstruction is an absolute contraindication. Side effects include symptomatic bradycardia, syncope, abdominal pain, and excessive salivation. The use of laxative agents or suppositories is discouraged. Intravenous erythromycin acts as a motilin agonist and has been reported to stimulate motor activity in the stomach and proximal small intestine. This drug has been used with some benefit in refractory cases of postoperative ileus. Guanethidine (an adrenergic neuronal blocker), bethanechol (a cholinergic agonist), and metoclopramide have also been used in acute intestinal pseudoobstruction, with mixed results. Extreme caution must be exercised when considering use of prokinetic agents because they stimulate the upper gastrointestinal tract, have less effect on the lower tract, and increase the risk of perforation. Case reports suggest good results with cisapride, and the drug is beneficial for some patients with chronic syndromes. Tachyphylaxis is common.

Selected Readings

Camilleri M, Phillips S. Acute and chronic intestinal pseudoobstruction. *Adv Intern Med* 1991;36:287.

An excellent review of the pathophysiology, diagnosis, and treatment of acute and chronic intestinal pseudoobstruction.

Colemont LJ, Camilleri M. Chronic intestinal pseudoobstruction: diagnosis and treatment. *Mayo Clin Proc* 1989;64:60.

A comprehensive review of chronic intestinal pseudoobstruction focusing on pathophysiology, diagnosis, and management.

Dorudi S, Berry AR, Kettlewell MGW. Acute colonic pseudoobstruction. *Br J Surg* 1992;79:99.

A review article addressing the pathogenesis and surgical management of colonic pseudoobstruction.

Hutchinson R, Griffiths C. Acute colonic pseudo-obstruction: a pharmacological approach. *Ann R Coll Surg Engl* 1992;74:364.

When conservative management has failed, pharmacologic manipulation of the autonomic innervation of the colon with guanethidine and neostigmine may be beneficial in some patients.

Livingston EH, Pasaro EP. Postoperative ileus. *Dig Dis Sci* 1990;35:121.

Pathogenesis, diagnosis, and management of postoperative ileus are reviewed.

Murr MM, Sarr MG, Camilleri M. The surgeon's role in the treatment of chronic intestinal pseudoobstruction. *Am J Gastroenterol* 1995;90:2147.
Surgery has a therapeutic or palliative role in selected patients with chronic intestinal pseudoobstruction.

Stroder WE, Nostrant TT, Eckhauser FE, et al. Therapeutic and diagnostic colonoscopy in nonobstructive colonic dilatation. *Ann Surg* 1983;197:416.
Colonoscopy is a safe diagnostic and therapeutic tool in massive cecal dilatation without pneumoperitoneum or peritoneal signs.

Vanek VW, Al-Salti M. Acute pseudo-obstruction of the colon (Ogilvie's syndrome): an analysis of 400 cases. *Dis Colon Rectum* 1986;29:203.
Colonoscopic or operative decompression is indicated if the cecal diameter is more than 12 cm on plain abdominal radiographs or if conservative management is unsuccessful.

Verne GN, Eaker EY, Hardy E, et al. Effect of octreotide and erythromycin on idiopathic and scleroderma-associated intestinal pseudoobstruction. *Dig Dis Sci* 1995;40:1892.
Erythromycin and octreotide can relieve abdominal pain and nausea in selected patients with pseudoobstruction.

79. FULMINANT COLITIS AND TOXIC MEGACOLON

Chandra Prakash

I. General principles. *Fulminant colitis* implies a serious progression of mucosal inflammation, usually to deeper layers of the colon, resulting in severe bloody diarrhea, abdominal tenderness, and systemic toxicity. Colonic circular muscle paralysis can precipitate colonic dilatation or *toxic megacolon,* the term used to describe this entire sequence of events. Toxic megacolon is most commonly seen as a complication of ulcerative colitis, but can occur with both idiopathic and infectious colitis, Crohn disease, amebic colitis, pseudomembranous colitis, and other infections. Factors associated with increased mortality include age greater than 40 years, the presence of colonic perforation, and delay of surgery. Early recognition and treatment of toxic megacolon can substantially lower mortality from as high as 50% (with colonic perforation) to less than 15%.

II. Clinical presentation

A. History. Toxic megacolon usually occurs on the background of chronic inflammatory bowel disease. Although segmental colitis can be associated with toxic megacolon, the latter is more commonly seen with extensive colitis. Toxic megacolon typically occurs early in the course of ulcerative colitis, and 25% to 40% of cases present with the initial attack. Progressive diarrhea, bloody stool, and crampy abdominal pain are typical symptoms. A paradoxic decrease in stool frequency with passage of bloody membranes is an ominous sign. Manipulation of the inflamed bowel with diagnostic examinations such as barium enema or colonoscopy, medications (including vigorous laxatives, antidiarrheals, anticholinergics), electrolyte imbalances, and pH disturbances can contribute to the development of the condition. Corticosteroids can suppress signs of perforation and peritonitis, but whether these drugs can precipitate toxic megacolon is controversial.

B. Physical examination and laboratory studies. Systemic toxicity is heralded by fever, tachycardia, and leucocytosis, and it can progress to confusion, agitation, or apathy. Abdominal pain and distention, with diminished bowel sounds on auscultation, are common. Peritoneal signs indicate transmural inflammation or perforation, but they may be minimal or absent in elderly patients or in patients receiving corticosteroids. Anemia, hypokalemia, and hypoalbuminemia also can occur.

III. Diagnosis

A. Laboratory studies. Initial clinical evaluation and laboratory tests should assess the degree of systemic toxicity, fluid and electrolyte deficits, pH disturbances, and the need for blood transfusion. Stool should be sent for *Clostridium difficile* toxin and other pathogens.

B. Radiologic studies. Plain radiographs of the abdomen reveal loss of haustration and segmental or total colonic dilatation (usually only mild), with mucosal thumbprinting or pneumatosis cystoides coli in severe transmural disease. Free peritoneal air is an immediate indication for surgery. Small bowel ileus may accompany toxic megacolon and is a poor prognostic sign for conservative management. Discrepancies may exist between physical and radiographic findings.

C. Endoscopy. A limited proctoscopic examination may show extensive ulceration with friable, bleeding mucosa, but rarely the examination is normal. An abdominal radiograph after cautious proctoscopic air insufflation can provide a partial contrast study to define the proximal extent of disease. More extensive endoscopic examination is contraindicated.

IV. Treatment

A. General measures. Vigorous fluid, electrolyte, and blood replacement must be instituted early in the resuscitative effort, because hemodynamic instability is typical. Total body potassium depletion is common and needs urgent repletion.

Phosphate, magnesium, and calcium deficiency also should be corrected parenterally. Oral intake is discontinued and nasogastric suction is employed for small bowel ileus. Anticholinergic and narcotic agents should be stopped immediately.

B. Treatment of inflammatory bowel disease. When inflammatory bowel disease is diagnosed or suspected, use of parenteral corticosteroids or adrenocorticotropic hormone is essential. Augmented doses (hydrocortisone, 100 mg every 6 hours, or methylprednisolone, 6 to 15 mg every 6 hours) should be administered. A continuous infusion may help to maintain steady plasma levels. Aminosalicylates (mesalamine, sulfasalazine) have no role in the treatment of fulminant colitis or toxic megacolon and should be withheld until the patient has recovered and has resumed eating. Intravenous cyclosporine (4 mg/kg per 24 hours in a continuous infusion) can be used when severe ulcerative colitis without toxic megacolon fails to improve after 7 to 10 days of intensive intravenous hydrocortisone therapy. The role of cyclosporine in toxic megacolon is controversial.

C. Antibiotics. Broad-spectrum antibiotics are administered intravenously once toxic megacolon or transmural inflammation is suspected and are continued until the patient stabilizes over several days to a week. Broad-spectrum antibiotics should be followed by pathogen-specific therapy in infectious colitis. Metronidazole or vancomycin should be used if *C. difficile* infection is considered likely from the clinical presentation or proctoscopic findings.

D. Surgical indications. Surgical exploration for toxic megacolon is indicated if no improvement occurs despite 12 to 24 hours of intensive medical management. Delay of operative therapy may promote higher mortality. Evidence of colonic perforation is an unequivocal indication for emergency surgery. Other indications for emergency surgery include signs of septic shock and imminent transverse colon rupture (the most dilated region in most cases of toxic megacolon), especially if the diameter is greater than 12 cm. Hypoalbuminemia, persistently elevated acute-phase reactants, small bowel ileus, and deep colonic ulcers are poor prognostic factors for successful medical therapy. The absence of acute colonic dilatation may permit delay of surgical intervention in fulminant colitis. The potential for prolonged intensive medical management and complications must be balanced against early surgical intervention to reduce mortality and morbidity. Generally, medical management may be continued for at least 5 to 7 days in the absence of colonic dilatation, as long as the patient is stable or improving.

E. Surgical options. The type of operation performed for the treatment of fulminant colitis or toxic megacolon depends on the clinical status of the patient and the experience of the surgeon. Most surgeons prefer a limited abdominal colectomy with ileostomy, leaving the rectosigmoid as a mucous fistula, or oversewing the rectum, using a Hartmann procedure. This allows less operating room time in acutely ill patients yet leaves the option for a subsequent sphincter-saving ileoanal anastomosis. In older patients, a one-stage resection with ileostomy may be appropriate.

Selected Readings

Actis GC, Ottobrelli A, Pera A, et al. Continuously infused cyclosporine at low dose is sufficient to avoid emergency colectomy in acute attacks of ulcerative colitis without the need for high-dose steroids. *J Clin Gastroenterol* 1993;17:10.

Seven of eight patients with acute steroid-resistant ulcerative colitis went into clinical remission with 2 weeks of intravenous cyclosporine infusion.

Caprilli R, Vernia P, Colaneir O, et al. Risk factors in toxic megacolon. *Dig Dis Sci* 1980;25:817.

The severity of electrolyte imbalance and of metabolic derangement appears to be important in the progression of severe colitis to toxic megacolon.

Caprilli R, Vernia P, Latella G, et al. Early recognition of toxic megacolon. *J Clin Gastroenterol* 1987;9:160.

Persistent small bowel gaseous distention and severe metabolic alkalosis may predict the development of toxic megacolon in severe ulcerative colitis.

Carbonnel F, Lavergne A, Lemann M, et al. Colonoscopy of acute colitis: a safe and reliable tool for assessment of severity. *Dig Dis Sci* 1994;39:1550.

Colonoscopy in acute ulcerative colitis is generally safe and can provide prognostic information in some cases.

Chew CN, Noland DJ, Jewell DP. Small bowel gas in severe ulcerative colitis. *Gut* 1991;32:1535.

Presence of small bowel distention in severe ulcerative colitis predicts poor response to medical therapy.

Gore RM, Ghahremani GG. Radiologic investigation of acute inflammatory and infectious bowel disease. *Gastroenterol Clin North Am* 1995;24:353.

Plain abdominal radiographs, barium studies, and cross-sectional imaging are complementary to endoscopic evaluation in acute enterocolitis.

Lichtiger S, Present DH, Kornbluth A, et al. Cyclosporine in severe ulcerative colitis refractory to steroid therapy. *N Engl J Med* 1994;330:1841.

Intravenous cyclosporine is rapidly effective in some patients with severe, corticosteroid-resistant ulcerative colitis.

Marion JF, Present DH. The modern medical management of acute, severe ulcerative colitis. *Eur J Gastroenterol Hepatol* 1997;9:831.

The current medical arsenal and surgical experience in severe ulcerative colitis are reviewed.

Meyers S, Janowitz HD. The place of steroids in the therapy of toxic megacolon. *Gastroenterology* 1978;75:729.

The benefit of initiating steroid therapy for toxic megacolon in unclear; when this therapy is initiated, the patient needs to be watched carefully for signs of deterioration.

Present DH. Toxic megacolon. *Med Clin North Am* 1993;77:1129.

A comprehensive review of the presentation, precipitating factors, diagnosis, and management of toxic megacolon.

Roy MA. Inflammatory bowel disease. *Surg Clin North Am* 1997;77:1419.

A review of advances in the evaluation and treatment of complicated inflammatory bowel disease.

80. FULMINANT HEPATIC FAILURE

Chandra Prakash and Reem Ghalib

I. General principles. *Fulminant hepatic failure* (FHF) is defined as severe hepatic synthetic disfunction and encephalopathy occurring within an 8-week period in a patient without prior evidence of liver disease. The appearance of encephalopathy within 2 weeks of the onset of jaundice in the setting of acute hepatic dysfunction is also consistent with FHF, as long as the prothrombin time is prolonged.

II. Etiology. Causes of FHF include viral hepatitis, drugs, and toxins (e.g., acetaminophen, alcohol, halothane, isoniazid, ketoconazole, mushrooms, sulfonamides, nonsteroidal antiinflammatory drugs, phenytoin, sulfonamides), as well as other diseases (e.g., portal vein thrombosis, hepatic vein thrombosis, venoocclusive disease, ischemic hepatitis, Wilson disease, Reye syndrome, acute fatty liver of pregnancy). Identification of the cause is important for several reasons: (a) specific treatments are available for drug and toxin overdose; (b) infectious causes such as viral hepatitis A have important public health implications, including contact tracing and postexposure prophylaxis; and (c) prognosis varies with the cause. Better survival rates occur with acetaminophen toxicity and viral hepatitis A and B, whereas poor outcome results from idiosyncratic drug reactions, acute Wilson disease, halothane hepatitis, and non-A, non-B hepatitis.

Acetaminophen overdose is a common cause of drug-induced FHF. Toxicity is mediated by a metabolite formed from the parent compound by the cytochrome P-450 mixed-function oxidase system in the liver cell. Glutathione binds to this metabolite, which, when glutathione levels are depleted, binds to other hepatocyte molecules and results in hepatocyte necrosis. Hepatic injury is potentiated by alcohol, other hepatotoxic medications, and starvation. The usual lethal dose of acetaminophen is 10 to 20 g, but much lower doses are lethal in patients with chronic alcoholism and in patients taking medications that stimulate the cytochrome P-450 system.

III. Complications

A. Encephalopathy and brain edema. By definition, all patients with FHF have encephalopathy, but not all have cerebral edema. *Cerebral edema* is an increase in brain tissue water content, thought to result from either a breakdown in the blood-brain barrier or impaired cellular osmoregulation, that increases intracranial pressure (ICP). Typical manifestations include vomiting, headache, bradycardia, and papilledema. These findings may be absent or minimal in FHF, and a high index of suspicion must be maintained.

B. Cardiorespiratory complications. Hemodynamic changes in FHF mimic septic shock, including high cardiac output and low systemic vascular resistance. Arrhythmias are often a result of metabolic (hypokalemia, acidosis, hypoxia) or mechanical (Swan-Ganz catheter) events. Approximately 40% of patients with FHF have cardiogenic or noncardiogenic pulmonary edema. Arterial hypoxemia can result from bacterial infection, intrapulmonary hemorrhage, atelectasis, intrapulmonary shunting from liver disease, and noncardiogenic pulmonary edema. Hypoxemia can exacerbate cerebral edema and can precipitate multiorgan failure.

C. Coagulopathy. Patients with FHF typically have reduced synthesis of coagulation factors. Overt disseminated intravascular coagulation is unusual, but qualitative and quantitative defects in platelet function and elevated fibrin degradation product levels are often seen. Gross hemorrhage is rare; when it occurs, the gastrointestinal tract is the most common site. Other bleeding sites include skin puncture wounds, kidneys, retroperitoneum, lungs, nasopharynx, and endometrium.

D. Metabolic disorders. The most common metabolic disorder seen in FHF is lactic acidosis. Excess lactate production from tissue hypoxia is coupled with impaired hepatic uptake and metabolism. Lactic acidosis is difficult to correct with bicarbonate infusions and may require dialysis. Renal failure is an ominous complication that results from intravascular volume depletion, acute tubular necrosis, or hepatorenal syndrome.

E. Infections. Impaired neutrophil function, altered Kupffer cell function, and deficiency of opsonins play roles in the increased incidence of infections in FHF. Bacteremia occurs in 20% to 25% of patients, commonly with *Staphylococcus* species, *Streptococcus* species, gram-negative organisms, and fungi, especially *Candida* species. The recognition of sepsis is challenging, because the hemodynamic picture resembles septic shock even without infection.

IV. Treatment

A. General measures. Blood products and colloids (albumin, plasma, dextran) are preferred for treatment of hypovolemia. Hypoxemia is treated with supplemental oxygen or by mechanical ventilation when appropriate. Endotracheal intubation is often required to prevent aspiration and to assist in the management of cerebral edema.

B. Hepatic encephalopathy and cerebral edema. Frequent neurologic examinations are important to assess signs and symptoms of ICP. Some patients benefit from standard therapy for chronic encephalopathy (low protein diet, lactulose, neomycin). Computed tomography of the brain is neither sensitive nor specific for diagnosing increased ICP in FHF, but it helps to exclude other structural lesions that would alter clinical management. The most sensitive method for detecting raised ICP is a surgically placed intracranial transducer. Risks, including epidural or intracranial bleeding and infection, are balanced against the risk of death from cerebral herniation, which occurs in 30% to 50% of patients with FHF who do not undergo liver transplantation. The ICP is maintained at less than 15 mm Hg while the cerebral perfusion pressure (difference between mean arterial pressure and ICP) is kept at more than 50 mm Hg. Hyperventilation to maintain an arterial carbon dioxide partial pressure (PCO_2) of 25 to 30 mm Hg may help acutely lower ICP. Mannitol (0.5 to 1 g/kg) or thiopental (30 to 40 mg/kg loading dose, followed by 5 mg/kg as needed) intravenously has been used with variable success. Steroids are not beneficial. Patients should be maintained in a quiet, nonstimulated environment, and a 30-degree elevation of the head is optimal. Refractory or sustained intracranial hypertension with cerebral perfusion pressure lower than 40 mm Hg is associated with a high incidence of posttransplant neurologic deaths.

C. Metabolic management. In the presence of a rising creatinine concentration, placement of a Swan-Ganz catheter is generally required for fluid management. Nephrotoxic agents are avoided, and low-dose dopamine infusions (2 to 4 μg/kg per hour) to increase renal blood flow can be tried. Hemodialysis may be ultimately necessary for the treatment of both acute tubular necrosis and hepatorenal syndrome. Careful attention is given to correction of electrolyte imbalance. Prevention of hypoglycemia is essential for preservation of neurologic function. Frequent glycemic monitoring coupled with infusions of 5% to 50% dextrose solutions may be necessary.

D. Infections. Surveillance cultures of blood, sputum, and urine should be completed with a low threshold for the institution of antibiotics to prevent sepsis. The use of prophylactic antibiotics remains controversial.

E. Coagulopathy. Morbidity and mortality of FHF are not affected by prophylactic correction of coagulopathy. Fresh frozen plasma or platelet transfusions (keeping platelet counts higher than 50,000/mm^3) may be necessary for overt bleeding or for elective invasive procedures. Parenteral vitamin K (10 mg for 3 days) should be administered to differentiate vitamin K deficiency from hepatic failure.

F. Acetaminophen toxicity. Early identification of acetaminophen as the cause of FHF can be lifesaving, because *N*-acetylcysteine can be administered to prevent hepatic glutathione depletion. The decision to administer *N*-acetylcysteine is based on a nomogram of serum levels and time after ingestion. This agent is highly effective in preventing massive hepatic necrosis when it is used within 10 hours of an overdose, but beneficial effects have been noted when treatment occurs as long as 36 hours after ingestion of acetaminophen. Signs of poor prognosis include prothrombin time longer than 100 seconds, serum creatinine higher than 3.4 mg/dL, and arterial pH less than 7.3.

G. Liver transplantation. Liver transplantation is an important therapeutic modality in patients with FHF, and survival rates exceed 50% in most series. Prognostic criteria help to select patients for liver transplantation. The single most important predictor of poor outcome in FHF is the degree of encephalopathy; other indicators of poor prognosis include non-A, non-B hepatitis, drug- or toxin-induced FHF (other than acetaminophen), age less than 10 or more than 40 years, duration of jaundice more than 1 week before the onset of encephalopathy, serum bilirubin greater than 18 mg/dL, and prothrombin time longer than 50 seconds. Patients with indicators of poor prognosis should be evaluated early and transferred to a facility capable of performing liver transplantation.

H. Experimental treatment. Hepatocyte transplantation and filtration devices are experimental modalities under investigation for supporting the liver while awaiting hepatocyte recovery or liver transplantation. Prostaglandin E_1 has been used with some success, but it has not been evaluated in controlled studies.

Selected Readings

Anand AC, Nightingale P, Neuberger JM. Early indicators of prognosis in fulminant hepatic failure: an assessment of the King's criteria. *J Hepatol* 1997;26:62.

Multivariate analysis showed prothrombin time, serum creatinine, white cell count, and abnormal potassium levels as independent predictors of mortality in acetaminophen-induced FHF.

Bernstein D, Tripodi J. Fulminant hepatic failure. *Crit Care Clin* 1998;14:181.

A review article outlining the causes, clinical features, and management of FHF.

Bernuau J, Rueff B, Benhamou J-P. Fulminant and subfulminant liver failure: definitions and causes. *Semin Liver Dis* 1986;6:97.

A discussion of the definitions and causes of subfulminant hepatic failure and FHF.

Bismuth H, Figueiro J, Samuel D. What should we expect from a bioartificial liver in fulminant hepatic failure? *Artif Organs* 1998;22:26.

A bioartificial liver could act as a bridge to liver transplantation in FHF, especially given donor organ shortage.

Dhiman RK, Seth AK, Jain S, et al. Prognostic evaluation of early indicators in fulminant hepatic failure by multivariate analysis. *Dig Dis Sci* 1998;43:1311.

Age greater than 50 years, prothrombin time longer than 100 seconds, and overt features of raised ICP at admission, as well as the onset of encephalopathy more than 7 days after the onset of jaundice, predict an adverse outcome in viral hepatitis–induced FHF.

Donovan JP, Schafer DF, Shaw BW Jr, et al. Cerebral oedema and increased intracranial pressure in chronic liver disease. *Lancet* 1998;351:719.

Cerebral edema contributes to poor outcome in chronic liver disease and may preclude liver transplantation.

Ede RJ, Gimson AES, Bihari D, et al. Controlled hyperventilation in the prevention of cerebral edema in fulminant hepatic failure. *J Hepatol* 1986;2:43.

Hyperventilation appears to delay the onset of cerebral herniation but cannot be recommended as a prophylactic measure.

Lidofsky SD. Liver transplantation for fulminant hepatic failure. *Gastroenterol Clin North Am* 1993;22:257.

This review discusses patient selection, outcomes, and management issues in liver transplantation for FHF.

Mendoza A, Fernandez F, Mutimer DJ. Liver transplantation for fulminant hepatic failure: importance of renal failure. *Transpl Int* 1997;10:55.

Pretransplant renal failure strongly predicts poor outcome from liver transplantation in FHF.

O'Grady JG, Alexander GJM, Hayallar KM, et al. Early indicators of prognosis in fulminant hepatic failure. *Gastroenterology* 1989;97:439.

Prognostic indicators are identified that best select candidates for liver transplantation in acetaminophen toxicity and other causes of FHF.

O'Grady JG, Langley PG, Isola LM, et al. Coagulopathy of fulminant hepatic failure. *Semin Liver Dis* 1986;6:159.
Specific coagulation abnormalities that have been identified in FHF are reviewed in detail.

Rolando N, Harvey F, Brahm J, et al. Prospective study of bacterial infection in acute liver failure: an analysis of fifty patients. *Hepatology* 1990;11:49.
This prospective study characterizes the high incidence and poor prognosis of bacterial infection in acute liver failure and emphasizes the need for a high index of suspicion and prompt therapy, perhaps even prophylactic therapy.

Williams R, Gimson AES. Intensive liver care and management of acute hepatic failure. *Dig Dis Sci* 1991;36:820.
A review of the principles of management and assessment of prognosis of FHF.

81. COMPLICATIONS OF CHRONIC LIVER DISEASE

Chandra Prakash

I. General principles. Chronic liver disease is associated with a variety of complications requiring admission to an intensive care unit. Patients with spontaneous bacterial peritonitis (SBP), intractable ascites, recurrent encephalopathy, or variceal bleeding may also need to be evaluated for liver transplantation. Identification and management of common complications are discussed in this chapter and in Chapters 61, 77, and 80.

II. Pathophysiology. Portal hypertension associated with chronic liver disease contributes to encephalopathy by diverting portal blood into the systemic circulation through the development of varices and spontaneous shunts. Patients with encephalopathy from chronic liver disease do not develop either the increased intracranial pressure or the cerebral edema encountered in fulminant hepatic failure. Ascites results from alterations in hepatic outflow and intrahepatic portal hypertension. Other events in its pathogenesis include primary renal sodium retention, diminished effective circulating volume with secondary renal sodium retention, and increased production of hepatic lymph. Bacteremia can seed ascitic fluid, causing SBP, a process exacerbated by abnormal immunologic defense mechanisms.

Hypersplenism from portal hypertension sequesters blood elements and results in pancytopenia. Platelets are usually functional unless uremia is present. When large portions of the hepatic parenchyma are replaced by fibrosis, synthesis of protein and of coagulation factors is compromised, manifesting as hypoalbuminemia and prothrombin-time prolongation (not corrected with vitamin K administration). Chronic liver disease also produces impaired renal water excretion, reduced concentrating ability, and renal acidification, in addition to altered sodium and potassium metabolism. These defects present as acute renal failure, hepatorenal syndrome, glomerulonephropathies, or chronic renal insufficiency.

III. Diagnosis

A. History. The medical history should focus on symptoms of liver disease, the presence of complications, and precipitants. Fatigue, poor concentration, daytime sleepiness with nighttime insomnia, jaundice, and increasing abdominal girth indicate hepatic dysfunction. Precipitants of encephalopathy include increased nitrogen load (gastrointestinal bleeding, excess dietary protein, azotemia, constipation), electrolyte imbalance, drugs (narcotics, tranquilizers, sedatives, diuretics), infection, surgery, superimposed acute liver disease, and progression of liver disease. One-third of patients with SBP have no specific abdominal symptoms, and a high index of suspicion must be maintained. Studies show that 10% to 27% of patients with ascites have SBP on presentation.

B. Physical examination. Mental status may wax and wane; accurate serial assessments are important. Asterixis and myoclonus, when elicited, are not specific for hepatic encephalopathy. Jaundice, easy bruising, spider nevi, ascites, fluid overload, and peripheral edema can be demonstrated on physical examination. Muscle wasting and apparent nutritional deficiencies despite adequate oral intake can result from poor synthetic function. Respiratory compromise occurs from tense ascites and sympathetic pleural effusions. Liver size is variable, but splenomegaly may be found in patients with portal hypertension. Clinical evidence of active or occult gastrointestinal bleeding should be sought. The abdominal examination is often deceptively benign in SBP.

C. Laboratory studies. Identifying metabolic abnormalities (hypoglycemia or hyperglycemia, electrolyte imbalance, hypophosphatemia, hypoxemia) and assessing volume status are of primary importance. Hepatorenal syndrome is diagnosed by measuring urine sodium concentration (less than 10 mEq/L) and urine osmolality (urine osmolality more than 100 mOsmol higher than plasma osmolality), calculating the ratio of urine creatinine to plasma creatinine (greater than 30:1), and evaluating urine sediment (usually normal). Liver function tests, including serum protein and albumin, transaminases, alkaline phosphatase, and prothrombin time are performed at the initial evaluation and serially, as indicated. Viral serologic tests help to exclude superimposed viral hepatitis; a normal alpha-fetoprotein level in conjunction with an unremarkable ultrasound examination will help to exclude hepatocellular cancer. A toxicology screen should be considered. Particular attention should be given to obtaining cultures of blood, urine, sputum, and ascites, especially in patients with suspected encephalopathy and SBP. The issue of pursuing a lumbar puncture in a patient with encephalopathy should be individualized; coagulopathy may increase the risk of this procedure.

D. Diagnostic paracentesis. When ascites is identified, a diagnostic paracentesis is essential for determining its nature and for excluding SBP. Paracentesis is relatively safe, even in the setting of severe coagulopathy. Ultrasonographic localization of ascites is occasionally required to direct paracentesis. The risk of complication is low, with infection estimated at 0.6% from entrance of the needle into bowel and bleeding from coagulopathy at 1%. Fluid should be sent for cell count and differential, culture, albumin, and cytologic examination. Bacterial culture is performed by inoculating two blood culture bottles at the patient's bedside; cultures for acid-fast organisms and fungi should also be obtained. Other tests occasionally used include triglycerides (for diagnosing chylous ascites), carcinoembryonic antigen (for malignant ascites), and amylase (for pancreatic ascites). SBP is diagnosed when more than 250 neutrophils/mm^3 are present.

IV. Treatment

A. Encephalopathy. Treatments include dietary adjustments, medications, and liver transplantation for intractable symptoms. Modest protein reductions (40 to 60 g per day) may suffice; commercial products rich in branched-chain amino acids are reserved for refractory situations. Lactulose, an artificial nonabsorbable disaccharide, is metabolized to small organic acids in the colon and creates an acidic environment, osmotic diarrhea, and decreased nitrogen delivery to the liver. Lactulose is administered orally (15 to 45 mL every 4 to 6 hours titrated to three to four soft bowel movements per day) or as an enema (300 mL lactulose plus 700 mL water every 4 to 6 hours). Neomycin (500 to 1,000 mg orally every 6 to 12 hours) and metronidazole (250 to 500 mg orally three times a day) are also effective. Nephrotoxicity and neurotoxicity may limit their use. Recurrent uncontrolled encephalopathy can warrant liver transplantation.

B. Ascites. Restriction of sodium is an essential step in the management of ascites. Administration of intravenous fluids and crystalloid solutions should be minimized. Spironolactone (50 to 400 mg daily in divided doses) inhibits sodium reabsorption in the distal tubules and collecting ducts by blocking the effects of aldosterone. Loop diuretics (furosemide, bumetanide) can complement the action of distal tubular diuretics. Large-volume paracentesis is well tolerated by patients with cirrhosis; concomitant albumin infusion may have a role in selected patients with extremely low serum albumin levels and intravascular volume depletion. Complications have dampened enthusiasm for use of peritoneovenous shunts. Transjugular intrahepatic portosystemic shunts manage refractory ascites with variable success, and refractory ascites remains an indication for liver transplantation.

C. Spontaneous bacterial peritonitis. The most common organisms implicated in SBP are gram-negative bacilli (*Escherichia coli* and *Klebsiella* account for about 50%); other pathogens include gram-positive cocci (*Streptococcus* and *Staphylococcus* species) and anaerobes. The drug of choice without bacteriologic identification is a third-generation cephalosporin (e.g., cefotaxime, 2 g intravenously every 8 hours; ceftriaxone, 1 g intravenously every 12 hours), dose-adjusted for renal dysfunction. Duration of therapy is not standardized, but a course of

5 days of intravenous antibiotic therapy typically is adequate. Repeat paracentesis 48 hours after initiation of therapy should demonstrate a 50% drop in neutrophil count and negative cultures. Trimethoprim-sulfamethoxazole (one double-strength tablet 5 days of each week) is effective prophylaxis for preventing recurrences.

D. Hepatorenal syndrome. Patients with hepatorenal syndrome may be managed temporarily with dialysis or hemofiltration, but they require liver transplantation for long-term survival. Renal function corrects after liver transplantation.

E. Other management aspects. The coagulopathy of chronic liver disease is usually refractory to vitamin K administration, but a 3-day trial of parenteral vitamin K (10 mg subcutaneously daily) is indicated at presentation. Platelet transfusion is reserved for patients with active bleeding or prophylaxis before invasive procedures. Hepatocellular carcinoma carries a poor prognosis, but small lesions may be amenable to surgical excision in patients with well-compensated cirrhosis. Abstinence from alcohol should be emphasized, to retard progression of chronic liver disease.

Selected Readings

Bataller R, Gines P, Guevara M, et al. Hepatorenal syndrome. *Semin Liver Dis* 1997; 17:233.

Diagnostic criteria and advances in therapy of hepatorenal syndrome are reviewed.

Boyer TD, Warnock DG. Use of diuretics in the treatment of cirrhotic ascites. *Gastroenterology* 1983;84:1051.

Guidelines for diuretic use in patients with ascites.

Hoefs JC. Diagnostic paracentesis: a potent clinical tool. *Gastroenterology* 1990;98: 230.

A discussion of laboratory tests performed on ascitic fluid and their clinical relevance.

Inadomi J, Sonnenberg A. Cost-analysis of prophylactic antibiotics in spontaneous bacterial peritonitis. *Gastroenterology* 1997;113:1289.

Patients with ascitic fluid protein less than 1 g/dL or a previous history of SBP benefit most from prophylaxis.

Mesquita MA, Balbino EP, Albuquerque RS, et al. Ceftriaxone in the treatment of spontaneous bacterial peritonitis: ascitic fluid polymorphonuclear count response and short-term prognosis. *Hepatogastroenterology* 1997;44:1276.

Ceftriaxone is safe and effective in SBP.

Rimola A, Soto R, Bory F, et al. Reticuloendothelial system phagocytic activity in cirrhosis and its relation to bacterial infections and cirrhosis. *Hepatology* 1984;4:53.

Depression of reticuloendothelial system phagocytic activity in patients with decompensated cirrhosis increases the risk of bacteremia.

Riordan SM, Williams R. Current concepts: treatment of hepatic encephalopathy. *N Engl J Med* 1997;337:473.

A review article outlining the grading system, differential diagnosis, precipitating events, and management of hepatic encephalopathy.

Runyon BA. Paracentesis of ascitic fluid: a safe procedure. *Arch Intern Med* 1986;146: 2259.

The likelihood of complications is minimal with carefully performed paracentesis.

Runyon BA. Management of adult patients with ascites caused by cirrhosis. *Hepatology* 1998;27:264.

The development of ascites represents a landmark in the natural history of cirrhosis, but treatment regimens are effective in 90% of patients.

Runyon BA, McHutchison JG, Antillon MR, et al. Short-course versus long-course antibiotic treatment of spontaneous bacterial peritonitis: a randomized controlled study of 100 patients. *Gastroenterology* 1991;100:1737.

A 5-day course of intravenous antibiotics is as effective as a 10-day course.

Singh N, Gayowski T, Yu VL, et al. Trimethoprim-sulfamethoxazole for the prevention of spontaneous bacterial peritonitis in cirrhosis: a randomized trial. *Ann Intern Med* 1995;122:595.

Use of trimethoprim-sulfamethoxazole is a cost-effective method of preventing SBP.

Strauss E, da Costa MF. The importance of bacterial infection as precipitating factors of chronic hepatic encephalopathy in cirrhosis. *Hepatogastroenterology* 1998;45:900.
Bacterial infection is the precipitant in one-third of cases of hepatic encephalopathy.
Tito L, Rimola A, Gines P, et al. Recurrence of spontaneous bacterial peritonitis in cirrhosis: frequency and predictive factors. *Hepatology* 1998;8:27.
The 1-year recurrence rate of SBP is nearly 70%, with a 38% 1-year survival
Wong F, Blendis L. Pathophysiology and treatment of hepatorenal syndrome. *Gastroenterologist* 1998;6:122.
This review discusses the hemodynamics in the pathogenesis of hepatorenal syndrome.

82. DIARRHEA

Chandra Prakash

I. General principles. Diarrhea frequently complicates the course of the critically ill patient. If untreated, it can produce serious fluid and electrolyte imbalance, skin breakdown and local infection, and difficulty with nutritional management. The differential diagnosis of diarrhea in patients in the intensive care unit (ICU) differs considerably from that in the general population; investigation is focused and limited to tests safely performed in the critically ill patient. Diarrhea is the most common nonhemorrhagic gastrointestinal complication in the ICU setting.

II. Etiology. Three principal categories should be considered when determining the cause of diarrhea: iatrogenic causes, diarrhea secondary to underlying diseases, and diarrhea as a primary manifestation of the disease (Table 82-1).

A. Medications. Medications, especially antibiotics, are perhaps the most common cause of iatrogenic diarrhea in the ICU. Alterations in intestinal flora, breakdown of dietary carbohydrate products, and prokinetic effects (e.g., from erythromycin) are all postulated mechanisms for antibiotic-related diarrhea. Additionally, *Clostridium difficile* toxin production can be implicated in 15% to 20% of cases. The toxin produces changes in brush border function, intestinal fluid transport, and gastrointestinal peristalsis. Several other medications that can cause diarrhea are listed in Table 82-1.

B. Enteral feeding. In most instances, diarrhea in enterally fed patients is also associated with concurrent antibiotic use. Osmolarity of the enteral solution can play a role in some instances, as can bolus feeding distal to the pylorus. Enteral formulas high in lactose or fat content may precipitate diarrhea in susceptible patients.

C. Other causes. Hypoalbuminemia can change Starling forces sufficiently to inhibit intestinal fluid absorption, but this is not a uniform occurrence, even in severe cases. Immunosuppression, gastrointestinal bleeding, intestinal ischemia and fecal impaction can also result in diarrhea in the ICU setting. Other common diseases seen in the ICU that are directly or indirectly associated with diarrhea are listed in Table 82-1.

III. Diagnosis

A. Clinical assessment. Attention to historical data (e.g., onset, relation to antibiotic usage or enteral feeding) may lead to prompt diagnosis and management. *C. difficile*—related diarrhea may occur up to 8 weeks after the offending antibiotic is discontinued. Abdominal pain suggests ischemia, infection, or inflammatory conditions such as vasculitis or graft-versus-host disease (GVHD), depending on the clinical setting. Bloody diarrhea may indicate overt gastrointestinal bleeding, ischemic colitis, or occasionally, pseudomembranous colitis. Passage of frequent small-volume stools with urgency or tenesmus suggests distal colonic involvement, whereas passage of less frequent, large-volume stools suggests a more proximal process. Physical examination is usually nonspecific but helpful in assessing severity of volume loss. Skin rashes or mucosal ulcerations can point toward GVHD, inflammatory bowel disease, or vasculitis; other extraintestinal manifestations of diseases associated with diarrhea should be noted. An abnormal rectal examination may be the only sign of a partially obstructing fecal impaction.

B. Laboratory studies. Left untreated, severe diarrhea causes hyperchloremic metabolic acidosis and prerenal azotemia, along with other serious electrolyte imbalances. Leukocytosis may suggest infection or ischemia, and gastrointestinal bleeding may be associated with a falling hematocrit.

C. Stool studies. Fresh stool specimens should be sent for *C. difficile* toxin assay and culture. Immunosuppressed patients may need more extensive stool tests, including ova and parasite evaluation and concentration for isolation of *Cryptosporidium, Microsporidium,* or *Isospora belli.* The stool osmolar gap, which is

TABLE 82-1. Differential diagnosis of diarrhea in the intensive care unit

Iatrogenic Causes
- Medications: antibiotics (especially erythromycin, ampicillin, clindamycin, cephalosporins), antacids (magnesium containing), magnesium and phosphorus supplements, lactulose, colchicine, digitalis, quinidine, theophylline, levothyroxine, aspirin, nonsteroidal antiinflammatory agents, cimetidine, misoprostol, diuretics, beta-blocking agents, chemotherapeutic agents
- Enteral feeding
- Pseudomembranous colitis

Diarrhea secondary to underlying diseases
- Infections and neoplastic disease in immunosuppressed patients
- Gastrointestinal bleeding
- Neutropenic enteropathy
- Ischemic bowel disease
- Postsurgical diarrhea (after cholecystectomy, gastric surgery, pancreatectomy, and in short bowel syndrome)
- Fecal impaction
- Opiate withdrawal

Diarrhea as a primary manifestation of disease
- Diabetic diarrhea
- Renal failure
- Sepsis
- Adrenal insufficiency
- Graft-versus-host disease
- Vasculitis
- Inflammatory bowel disease
- Infectious diarrhea
- Celiac sprue
- Cirrhosis with portal hypertension

the difference between expected stool osmolarity $\{[(\text{stool Na}^+) + (\text{stool K}^+)] \times 2\}$ and measured stool osmolarity, may help to distinguish between osmotic and secretory causes when diarrhea is severe or protracted and no diagnosis is apparent; an elevated stool osmolar gap (greater than 70 mOsmol) suggests osmotic causes. Additionally, high-volume stool output that persists with fasting supports a secretory origin. A Sudan stain for fecal fat or stool pH is occasionally helpful (pH is decreased in carbohydrate malabsorption).

D. Imaging studies. Plain abdominal radiographs can detect partial obstruction, perforation, or changes associated with enteritis or colitis and are recommended in the presence of pain or an abnormal abdominal examination. Contrast studies including computed tomography and intestinal radiographs may be required in difficult or protracted cases.

E. Endoscopy. Flexible sigmoidoscopy is useful in diagnosing pseudomembranous colitis, ischemic colitis, cytomegalovirus colitis, herpetic proctocolitis, or GVHD and is usually considered in the presence of bright red rectal bleeding or other indicators of distal colitis. Mucosal biopsies are helpful on occasion when endoscopic findings are nonspecific or absent.

IV. Treatment

A. General measures. Correction of fluid and electrolyte imbalance needs immediate attention. Central venous access and monitoring may be necessary in patients with severe fluid loss. Proper patient hygiene and skin care should be maintained, and patient isolation with enteric precautions should be instituted when indicated. Iatrogenic causes of diarrhea are corrected by withdrawal of the offending medications. Enteral feedings suspected of causing diarrhea should be reduced in volume, diluted, given by continuous infusion, or temporarily discontinued. A change in formula to an elemental diet may be indicated in patients with short bowel syndrome, pancreatic insufficiency, radiation enteritis, fistula, or inflammatory bowel disease. In severe cases, total parenteral nutrition may be necessary as a temporary measure.

B. Specific treatment. Specific or pathogen-related treatment should be administered whenever possible in both immunocompromised and immunocompetent hosts. If *C. difficile*—related diarrhea is suspected, the offending antibiotic should be discontinued when possible; spontaneous improvement often results from this measure alone. Oral metronidazole (250 to 500 mg three times daily) and oral bacitracin (25,000 units four times daily) are as effective as oral vancomycin (125 to 500 mg four times daily), yet they are less expensive. Vancomycin should typically be reserved for treatment failures and severe cases. Response is expected within 24 to 48 hours with improvement in diarrhea, pain, fever, and leukocytosis, but treatment should be continued for 7 to 14 days. As many as 24% patients have a relapse, and longer retreatment courses are required. Anion exchange resins such as cholestyramine or colestipol are reportedly useful as adjunctive measures in mild cases or in relapses, but they are rarely required. These agents can bind vancomycin. Antimotility agents should not be used, because they may lengthen the course of the illness.

C. Symptomatic measures. When a cause of diarrhea is not found, palliative treatment lessens fluid losses, patient discomfort, and morbidity. Antimotility agents may decrease the frequency and severity of diarrhea, but monitoring for complications is required (e.g., central nervous system side effects, gut hypomotility). These drugs include loperamide (4 mg initially, and up to 16 mg per day), diphenoxylate with atropine (20 mg of diphenoxylate four times daily initially, then decrease and titrate to symptoms) and deodorized tincture of opium (6 to 12 gtt two to four times daily). Octreotide can be used for palliation of diarrhea in patients with acquired immunodeficiency syndrome, GVHD, hormone-producing tumors, and other causes of secretory diarrhea.

Selected Readings

Bartlett JG. Management of *Clostridium difficile* infection and other antibiotic-associated diarrhoeas. *Eur J Gastroenterol Hepatol* 1996;8:1054.

Investigation and therapy of antibiotic-associated diarrhea are outlined in this review.

Brown E, Talbot GH, Axelrod P, et al. Risk factors for *Clostridium difficile* toxin-associated diarrhea. *Infect Control Hosp Epidemiol* 1990;11:283.

Age greater than 65 years, ICU admission, gastrointestinal procedures, and administration of antibiotics for more 10 days were associated with C. difficile–associated diarrhea.

Cataldi-Betcher EL, Seltzer MH, Slocum BA, et al. Complications occurring during enteral nutritional support: a prospective study. *JPEN J Parenter Enteral Nutr* 1983;7:546.

Tube feedings are safely tolerated in most patients, but complications must be recognized and treated promptly.

Dark DS, Pingleton SK. Nonhemorrhagic gastrointestinal complications in acute respiratory failure. *Crit Care Med* 1989;17:755.

Diarrhea is the most common nonhemorrhagic gastrointestinal complication in the ICU, occurring more frequently in critically ill patients who are administered antacids.

Fekety R. Guidelines for the diagnosis and management of *Clostridium difficile*–associated diarrhea in colitis. *Am J Gastroenterol* 1997;92:739.

Practical guidelines for the management of C. difficile diarrhea.

Guenter PA, Settle RG, Perlmutter S, et al. Tube feeding–related diarrhea in acutely ill patients. *JPEN J Parenter Enteral Nutr* 1991;15:277.

Antibiotic usage was the factor most strongly associated with diarrhea in acutely ill patients administered tube feedings.

Kelly TWJ, Patrick MR, Hillman KM, et al. Study of diarrhea in critically ill patients. *Crit Care Med* 1983;11:7.

Notes the significant incidence of diarrhea in critically ill patients, especially in association with nasogastric feeding.

Sakai L, Keltner R, Kaminski D. Spontaneous and shock-associated ischemic colitis. *Am J Surg* 1980;140:755.

Ischemic colitis carries a high mortality when it is associated with full-thickness necrosis; radiologic findings correlated well with clinical and pathologic evidence of full-thickness necrosis.

Teasley DG, Gerding DN, Olson M, et al. Prospective randomized trial of metronidazole versus vancomycin for *Clostridium difficile*–associated diarrhea and colitis. *Lancet* 1983;2:1043.

Metronidazole and vancomycin have equivalent efficacy and tolerance in treating C. difficile–associated diarrhea, but metronidazole is more economical.

83. SEVERE AND COMPLICATED BILIARY TRACT DISEASE

Chandra Prakash

I. **General principles.** A wide spectrum of biliary tract diseases can be seen in the intensive care unit (ICU), with presentations ranging from mildly abnormal blood chemistries to life-threatening septic shock. Access to the biliary tree for diagnosis and therapy of these diseases can be obtained endoscopically by cannulation of the ampulla in the duodenum by endoscopic retrograde cholangiopancreatography (ERCP); percutaneously through liver parenchyma by percutaneous transhepatic cholangiography (PTC); or operatively through the peritoneal cavity.

II. **Etiology**

A. **Biliary obstruction.** Common causes of biliary obstruction include gallstone disease, benign stricture, and malignancy; other causes are listed in Table 83-1. Biliary obstruction without cholangitis most commonly results from neoplasms.

B. **Bile leak.** Leakage of bile into the peritoneal cavity or pleural space can result from open or laparoscopic cholecystectomy, endoscopic or percutaneous biliary manipulations, and neoplastic disease. The resultant bile peritonitis produces dramatic pain, ascites, leukocytosis, and fever.

C. **Acalculous cholecystitis.** Acalculous cholecystitis, which is typically seen in critically ill patients, can result in significant morbidity and mortality. This entity warrants a high index of suspicion and aggressive management.

D. **Gallstone pancreatitis.** Acute pancreatitis often results from biliary stone disease as well as alcohol abuse and other known causes. Evidence suggests that stone passage or impaction at the ampulla is responsible for gallstone pancreatitis. This recurrent and treatable cause should be considered in all patients with acute pancreatitis.

III. **Diagnosis**

A. **Clinical assessment.** Physical examination may reveal icterus, hepatomegaly, ascites, or focal tenderness over the liver or gallbladder. Findings range from acute abdomen to nonspecific fever and ileus. Signs and symptoms of acute cholecystitis often are not readily apparent in the ICU patient.

B. **Laboratory tests.** In acutely ill patients, bilirubin elevation can result from sepsis, drug effects, hemolysis, or other nonbiliary causes. Alkaline phosphatase can be elevated from other tissues including bone and placenta; concomitant elevation of 5′nucleotidase or γ-glutamyl transferase helps confirm hepatobiliary origin of the enzyme. Although serum transaminase elevations are the hallmark of hepatocellular injury, elevated levels can also be seen with biliary disease, especially inflammatory and infectious conditions and acute biliary obstruction. It is important to remember that (*a*) significant biliary disease can present with *normal* laboratory values and (*b*) abnormal test results may be the first clue to biliary disease in the obtunded or otherwise compromised ICU patient.

C. **Plain radiographs.** Plain abdominal radiographs usually reveal nonspecific findings (e.g., ileus). Gallstones are radio opaque in 20% of cases. Air in the biliary tree can result from a prior sphincterotomy, spontaneous biliary–enteric fistula, biliary–enteric surgical anastomosis, and, rarely, infection with gas-producing organisms. Gas within the gallbladder wall is one sign of acute cholecystitis.

D. **Ultrasonography.** Ultrasonography is a sensitive test for detecting biliary ductal dilatation; it can detect cholelithiasis with an accuracy exceeding 95% and is easily performed in the ICU. Other diagnoses made readily by ultrasonography include acute cholecystitis, choledocholithiasis, liver lesions, pancreatic masses, abscesses, and ascites.

E. **Radionuclide scanning.** ^{99m}Tc hepatic iminodiacetic acid (HIDA) scans yield both physiologic and structural information regarding the biliary tract. Filling of the gallbladder confirms patency of the cystic duct and virtually excludes acute chole-

TABLE 83-1. Causes of Biliary Obstruction

Intrinsic lesions
Gallstones
Cholangiocarcinoma
Benign stricture
Sclerosing cholangitis
Periarteritis nodosa
Ampullary stenosis
Parasites
Extrinsic lesions
Pancreatic carcinoma
Metastatic carcinoma
Pancreatitis
Pancreatic pseudocyst
Visceral artery aneurysm
Lymphadenopathy
Choledochal cyst
Hepatic cyst or cysts
Duodenal diverticulum
Iatrogenic lesions
Postoperative stricture
Hepatic artery infusion chemotherapy

cystitis; delayed views and routine pretreatment with cholecystokinin increase the accuracy to more than 90%. False–positive results can be seen from chronic cholecystitis, prolonged fasting, and long-term parenteral hyperalimentation. Scanning has a limited role in patients with poor hepatocellular function, complete biliary obstruction, or cholangitis, each of which prevents adequate uptake and excretion of the radiopharmaceutical into the biliary tree. Significant bile leaks are also identified accurately with HIDA scanning.

F. Computed tomography (CT) and magnetic resonance imaging (MRI). CT is highly accurate for the detection of the level and cause of biliary obstruction, especially in the pancreatic head region. In patients with normal renal function, a spiral CT or a dual phase study (arterial and venous) with thin cuts through the pancreas is better for defining lesions in the pancreas. MRI techniques that incorporate cholangiopancreatography also provide highly useful images of the liver and entire biliary tree without requiring invasive procedures. These studies are impractical in many critically ill patients who are often too sick for transport to the scanners.

G. ERCP and PTC. ERCP and PTC can be performed emergently when necessary, both for diagnosis and therapy of biliary disorders (see below). Portable fluoroscopy equipment is required for bedside procedures in unstable or moribund patients.

IV. Management

A. Biliary obstruction. Biliary obstruction is an indication for decompression by either ERCP or PTC and broad-spectrum antibiotics if cholangitis is suspected. Definitive therapy for stone disease and palliative therapy for benign or malignant disease can be accomplished during either procedure. Surgical approaches are reserved for patients who are good operative candidates with resectable malignancy, have symptomatic cholelithiasis requiring cholecystectomy, or have duodenal or gastric outlet obstruction in the setting of unresectable malignancy.

B. Bile leaks. ERCP should be performed as soon as possible after a bile leak is identified. Small leaks can be managed definitively with biliary decompression and stent placement at ERCP. Larger leaks or those associated with ischemia, trauma, or surgical anastomosis may eventually require percutaneous drainage, surgical repair, or bypass. Broad-spectrum antibiotics protect against sepsis and abscess formation.

C. **Acute cholecystitis.** Percutaneous cholecystotomy under ultrasonographic guidance has become the therapy of choice in patients too unstable for operative cholecystectomy when acute cholecystitis does not respond to antibiotics. The cholecystotomy drainage catheter is left in place until acute symptoms resolve, at which time an elective surgical cholecystectomy can be scheduled. In patients with severe comorbid medical conditions, the tube may simply be removed with or without percutaneous stone extraction.

D. **Acute gallstone pancreatitis.** Although most patients with acute gallstone pancreatitis improve with conservative therapy for pancreatitis, early ERCP may be indicated for removal of impacted or retained common bile duct stones, limiting further pancreatic inflammation and preventing cholangitis. Definitive therapy with elective cholecystectomy (or percutaneous cholecystotomy or endoscopic sphincterotomy in nonoperative candidates) is indicated to prevent recurrences.

Selected Readings

Carpenter HA. Bacterial and parasitic cholangitis. *Mayo Clin Proc* 1998;73:473.

The epidemiology, pathogenesis, and clinical manifestations of bacterial and parasitic cholangitis are reviewed comprehensively.

Chang L, Lo SK, Stabile BE. Gallstone pancreatitis: a prospective study on the incidence of cholangitis and clinical predictors of retained common bile duct stones. *Am J Gastroenterol* 1998;93:527.

The best predictor of common bile duct stones in gallstone pancreatitis is serum total bilirubin on hospital day 2; cholangitis is uncommon in this setting.

Elsakr R, Johnson DA, Younes Z, et al. Antimicrobial treatment of intra-abdominal infections. *Dig Dis* 1998;16:47.

New concepts about the treatment of intraabdominal infections, the antibiotics recommended, and the role of invasive procedures are outlined in this well-referenced article.

Fulcher AS, Turner MA, Zfass AM. Magnetic resonance cholangiopancreatography: a new technique for evaluating the biliary tract and pancreatic duct. *Gastroenterologist* 1998;6:82.

Technical refinements allow rapid and comprehensive imaging of the entire biliary tree and pancreatic duct in fewer than 20 seconds using magnetic resonance cholangiopancreatography.

Hammarstrom LE, Stridbeck H, Ihse I. Effect of endoscopic sphincterotomy and interval cholecystectomy on late outcome after gallstone pancreatitis. *Br J Surg* 1998; 85:333.

Endoscopic sphincterotomy reduced the overall incidence of recurrent pancreatitis after an episode of gallstone pancreatitis.

Kalliafas S, Ziegler DW, Flancbaum L, et al. Acute acalculous cholecystitis: incidence, risk factors, diagnosis and outcome. *Ann Surg* 1998;64:471.

Acute acalculous cholecystitis is a potentially lethal condition in critically ill and postoperative patients that requires a high index of suspicion for accurate diagnosis.

Kavanagh PV, vanSonnenberg E, Wittich GR, et al. Interventional radiology of the biliary tract. *Endoscopy* 1997;29:570.

An excellent review of the techniques available to the interventional radiologist for management of patients with acute biliary tract disorders.

Leung JWL, Ling TKW, Chan RCY, et al. Antibiotics, biliary sepsis and bile duct stones. *Gastrointest Endosc* 1994;40:716.

Imipenem and ciprofloxacin have the highest antimicrobial activity; ciprofloxacin has the highest biliary concentration in patients with duct stones and infected bile.

Loperfido S, Angelini G, Benedetti G, et al. Major early complications from diagnostic and therapeutic ERCP: a prospective multicenter study. *Gastrointest Endosc* 1998;48:1.

Morbidity and mortality is higher with therapeutic ERCP, but results are better in referral centers. Potential risk factors for complications are identified.

Ramirez FC, McIntosh AS, Dennert B. Emergency endoscopic retrograde cholangiopancreatography in critically ill patients. *Gastrointest Endosc* 1998;47:368.
Of all ERCPs, 2% are performed on critically ill patients; mechanical ventilation does not compromise technical success.

Shepherd HA, Royle G, Ross APR, et al. Endoscopic biliary endoprosthesis in the palliation of malignant obstruction of the distal common bile duct: a randomized trial. *Br J Surg* 1988;75:1166.
Endoscopically placed biliary stents compare favorably with conventional surgical bypass in the palliation of extrahepatic biliary obstruction.

Soetikno RM, Carr-Locke DL. Endoscopic management of acute gallstone pancreatitis. *Gastrointest Endosc Clin N Am* 1998;8:1.
A summary of four randomized, controlled trials looking at early endoscopic intervention in acute gallstone pancreatitis.

Stage JG, Moesgaard F, Gronvall S, et al. Percutaneous transhepatic cholelithotripsy for difficult common bile duct stones. *Endoscopy* 1998;30:289.
Difficult bile duct and intrahepatic stones can be safely and successfully removed percutaneously under local anesthesia.

Sugiyama M, Atomi Y. Follow-up of more than 10 years after endoscopic sphincterotomy for choledocholithiasis in young patients. *Br J Surg* 1998;85:917.
Endoscopic treatment is safe and effective in choledocholithiasis and has a low incidence of complications.

Sugiyama M, Tokuhara M, Atomi Y. Is percutaneous cholecystotomy the optimal treatment for acute cholecystitis in the very elderly? *World J Surg* 1998;22:459.
Percutaneous cholecystotomy is a safe and effective treatment for acute cholecystitis in the elderly, either as interim treatment or definitive therapy.

84. THE BASIC PRINCIPLES OF NUTRITIONAL SUPPORT IN THE INTENSIVE CARE UNIT

Dominic J. Nompleggi

I. General principles. Severe protein-calorie malnutrition, unfortunately, is common in critically ill patients. In all patients with serious illness, appropriate measures to avoid substrate deficiency and to replete nutrient deficiency are best recognized promptly, and appropriate therapy instituted without delay.

II. Pathogenesis. Malnutrition, which is common in patients in the intensive care unit (ICU), can be present on admission or develop as a result of the metabolic response to injury. These changes in metabolic response are difficult to assess. Their assessment includes evaluation of clinical, anthropometric, chemical, and immunologic parameters reflecting altered body composition.

III. Diagnosis. The purpose of nutritional assessment is to identify the type and degree of malnutrition in order to devise a rational approach to treatment. Percentage weight loss in the last 6 months, serum albumin level, and total lymphocyte count, which are readily available, are commonly used measures to assess nutritional status. Weight loss of 20% to 30% suggests moderate caloric malnutrition; 30% or greater indicates severe protein-calorie malnutrition. Loss of 10% or more over a short period of time is considered clinically important as well. The general appearance of the patient, with emphasis on evidence of temporal, upper body, and upper extremity wasting of skeletal muscle mass, provides a quick, inexpensive, and clinically useful measure of nutritional status.

Serum albumin measures visceral protein stores; it is a useful and readily available indicator of kwashiorkor (protein malnutrition). However, it is not a sensitive indicator of malnutrition in ICU patients because its synthesis is influenced by numerous factors other than nutritional status (e.g., protein losing states, hepatic function, and acute infection or inflammation).

Malnutrition is closely correlated with alterations in immune response as measured by skin test reactivity and total lymphocyte count. A total lymphocyte count less than $1{,}000/mm^3$ is indicative of altered immune function and is associated with decreased skin test reactivity. Loss of skin test reactivity is a measure of impaired cellular immunity, which has consistently been found to be associated with malnutrition.

Subjective global assessment (SGA) is a method for evaluating nutritional status that uses clinical parameters such as history, physical findings, and symptoms. The SGA determines whether (*a*) nutritional assimilation has been restricted because of decreased food intake, maldigestion, or malabsorption; (*b*) any effects of malnutrition on organ function and body composition have occurred; and (*c*) the patient's disease process influences nutrient requirements. In hospitalized patients, SGA has been shown to provide reliable and reproducible results with more than 80% agreement when blinded observers assessed the same patient.

Critical depletion of lean tissue can occur after 14 days of starvation in severely catabolic patients. Nutrition support should be instituted in patients who are not expected to resume oral feeding for 7 to 10 days.

IV. Treatment

A. Enteral feeding Enteral feeding has been shown in clinical studies to reduce infection and to preserve gut integrity, barrier, and immune function. It is the preferred route of nutrient administration. Current recommendations support initiation of enteral nutrition as soon as possible after resuscitation. The only contraindication is a nonfunctioning gut.

Initiation of enteral feeding distal to the pylorus does not require active bowel sounds or the passage of flatus or stool. Small bowel feedings can be given in the presence of mild or resolving pancreatitis and low output enterocutaneous fistulas (< 500 ml/d). Worsening abdominal distention or diarrhea in excess of

1,000 ml/d, requires a medical evaluation. If distention is present, enteral feedings should be discontinued. If no infectious cause is found for the diarrhea, antidiarrheals can be administered and feedings continued. Standard isotonic polymeric formulations can meet most patients' nutritional needs. Elemental formulas should be reserved for patients with severe small bowel absorptive dysfunction. Specialty formulations have a limited clinical role.

B. **Parenteral feeding.** Parenteral nutrient administration is recommended when the gastrointestinal tract is nonfunctional or inaccessible or enteral feeding is insufficient. Although parenteral nutrient admixtures are not as nutritionally complete as enteral formulations, nutritional goals are achieved more often with the former than the latter.

C. **Macronutrients.** Energy adequate to promote anabolic functions is essential. Caloric requirements should be based on the usual body weight; a requirement of 25 kcal/kg is adequate for most patients.

In prescribing parenteral feeding, the protein requirement (1.2–1.5 g/kg/d) should be calculated first to assure protein sparing and maintain lean tissue mass. Next, approximately 15% to 30% of total calories should be given as fat. The remaining calories should be given as a carbohydrate.

The goal in prescribing enteral formulations is similar. Protein requirements should be provided first and should dictate the total daily volume needed. The remainder of macronutrients are in fixed proportions, depending on the formulation selected.

D. **Micronutrients: vitamins, trace minerals, and fluid.** Potassium, magnesium, phosphate, and zinc should be provided in amounts necessary to maintain normal serum levels. The absolute requirements for vitamins, mineral, and trace elements have not yet been determined. Normal serum and blood levels of vitamins have been established, but can vary with the laboratory in which the measurement is obtained. In general, patients should receive fluid at 25 ml/kg body weight to avoid dehydration.

V. **Summary.** The need for nutritional support is determined by the balance between endogenous energy reserves of the body and the severity of stress. The best clinical markers of stress are fever, leukocytosis, hypoalbuminemia, and a negative nitrogen balance. The enteral route should be used to provide nutrients if the gut is functioning. Provision of energy and protein should be tailored to the individual patient. During illness, hypoalbuminemia should be viewed as a marker of injury and not as an indicator of impaired nutrition. Normal concentrations are unattainable in many critically ill patients because of large fluid shifts and acute-phase protein synthesis. The goal of short-term nutritional support is to optimize the body's metabolic response to injury by improving immune function, reducing inflammation, maintaining gut barrier function, and minimizing nitrogen deficit.

Selected Readings

Baker JP, Detsky AS, Wesson DE, et al. Nutritional assessment: a comparison of clinical judgment and objective measures. *N Eng J Med* 1982;306:969.

This paper validated the accuracy of simple subjective assessment compared with complex objective measurements in nutritional assessment.

Cerra FB, Benitez MR, Blackburn GL, et al. Applied nutrition in ICU patients: a consensus statement of the American College of Chest Physicians. *Chest* 1997;111:769.

The single best reference on ICU nutrition.

Detsky AS, McLaughlin JR, Baker JP, et al. What is subjective global assessment of nutritional status? *JPEN* 1987;11:8.

This paper presents the concept of subjective global assessment as a valid method of nutritional assessment.

Grant JP, Custer PB, Thurlow J. Current techniques of nutritional assessment. *Surg Clin North Am* 1981;61:437.

Excellent review of the methods of nutritional assessment.

Kirby DF, Delegge MH, Fleming CR. American Gastroenterological Association medical position statement: guidelines for the use of enteral nutrition. *Gastroenterology* 1995;108:1282.

This paper gives guidelines for the use of enteral nutrition therapy, particularly with reference to the use of specialized formulas.

Klein S, Kinney J, Jeejeebhoy K, et al. Nutrition support in clinical practice: review of published data and recommendations for future research direction. *JPEN* 1997;21:133.

A state-of-the-art review of the clinical practice of nutrition support which outlines areas for further research.

Reilly JJ, Gerhardt AL. (Ravitch M, ser. ed.) Modern surgical nutrition. *Curr Probl Surg* 1985;22:1.

Nutrition assessment and therapy for surgical patients.

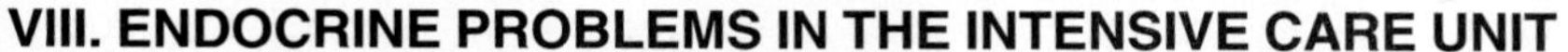

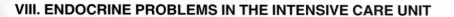

VIII. ENDOCRINE PROBLEMS IN THE INTENSIVE CARE UNIT

85. MANAGEMENT OF DIABETES IN THE CRITICALLY ILL PATIENT

Michael J. Thompson, Aldo A. Rossini, and John P. Mordes

I. **Diabetes in the critically ill patient.** Diabetes mellitus is a common problem in critically ill patients. It predisposes to cardiovascular, renal, and infectious complications that often require intensive surgical and medical care. Patients in the intensive care unit (ICU) with diabetes are particularly vulnerable to the adverse metabolic consequences of stress. Adequate control of diabetes minimizes the risk of iatrogenic metabolic complications, cardiovascular complications, poor wound healing, and infection.

II. **Pathogenesis**

A. **Glucose homeostasis.** Blood glucose concentration is tightly regulated, normally ranging only between 60 and 120 mg/dl. Regulation in large measure depends on the presence of appropriate quantities of circulating insulin. In the fed state, insulin secreted by pancreatic beta cells stimulates intracellular movement of glucose and inhibits gluconeogenesis and lipolysis. In the fasting state, insulin levels fall, enabling glycogenolysis, gluconeogenesis, lipolysis, and ketogenesis to occur. Even during prolonged fasting, however, a low concentration of circulating insulin continues to regulate the rates of each of these processes. The key to the ICU management of the patient with diabetes is achieving a consistent and appropriate degree of patient "insulinization" at all times.

B. **Types of diabetes mellitus.** Diabetes mellitus is not one disease, but a group of syndromes sharing the common feature of hyperglycemia. The most common diabetic syndromes are type 1 and type 2. Knowing the diagnosis can assist in ICU diabetes management.

1. **Type 1 diabetes** (formerly designated insulin-dependent, ketosis-prone, and juvenile diabetes) results from autoimmune destruction of pancreatic insulin-producing beta cells. These patients are totally deficient in insulin. They require exogenous insulin for survival. Discontinuation of insulin therapy, even for relatively brief intervals, can lead to serious metabolic complications.
2. **Type 2 diabetes** (formerly designated non–insulin-dependent or adult onset diabetes) is the result of relative, rather than absolute deficiency of insulin. It involves defects in both insulin action and insulin secretion. Some patients with type 2 diabetes can be treated with diet or oral agents, but others need insulin to control hyperglycemia. Infection, metabolic stress, and many medications commonly used in the ICU exacerbate type 2 diabetes and can lead to ketoacidosis, hyperosmolar coma, or lactic acidosis.
3. **Other types of diabetes** are less common. These can result from genetic defects of beta cell and insulin action and many other factors. Some conditions that can precipitate "secondary" diabetes are listed in Table 85-1.

III. **Diagnosis.** Appropriate treatment of the patient with diabetes in the ICU requires assessment of the type and duration of diabetes present, diabetes complications, and the degree of previous glycemic control. Patients with type 1 diabetes require exogenous insulin at all times, those with type 2 diabetes may not.

Long-standing diabetes is associated with complications that tend to be worse in patients whose condition is poorly controlled. Assessments of both cardiac function and peripheral circulation are necessary for all patients with diabetes. Diabetic neuropathy can affect the autonomic nervous system, with implications for management of blood pressure, heart rate, and voiding. Assessment of kidney function should include a urinalysis; proteinuria may precede abnormalities in blood urea nitrogen (BUN) and creatinine levels. Diabetic eye disease is not a contraindication to anticoagulation, but its severity should be assessed before instituting therapy.

A history of poor control of diabetes should alert the clinician to other potential problems. Poor control often implies poor nutrition. Infections to which individuals with diabetes are particularly susceptible include osteomyelitis, cellulitis, pyelone-

TABLE 85-1. Secondary forms of diabetes[a]

Etiology	Examples
Drug induced	Thiazide diuretics, loop diuretics (e.g. furosemide, ethacrynic acid, metolazone), antihypertensive agents (e.g. β-adrenergic blockers, calcium channel blockers, clonidine, diazoxide), hormones (e.g. glucocorticoids, oral contraceptives, α-adrenergic agents, glucagon, growth hormone), sympathomimetic drugs, antineoplastic agents (e.g. asparaginase, mithramycin, streptozocin), phenytoin, theophylline, niacin, cyclosporin, phenothiazines, lithium, isoniazid, pentamidine
Pancreatic diseases	Hemochromatosis, pancreatic cancer, pancreatitis, cystic fibrosis
Other endocrine disorders	Cushing's syndrome, pheochromocytoma, acromegaly, primary hyperaldosteronism, hyperthyroidism, polyendocrine autoimmune syndromes, POEMS syndrome (polyneuropathy, organomegaly, endocrinopathy, monoclonal gammopathy, skin changes)

[a] A partial listing of the causes of "secondary" diabetes. More exhaustive compilations and detailed descriptions are available in the references.

phritis tuberculosis, cholecystitis, cystitis, sinusitis, and gingivitis. Patients with type 2 diabetes are frequently hyperlipidemic and can develop pancreatitis when their diabetes is poorly controlled.

Abdominal pain accompanied by guarding and rebound tenderness is a common symptom of diabetic ketoacidosis. The diagnosis of diabetic ketoacidosis, on occasion, has been made at laparotomy, and this condition must be excluded in every patient being evaluated for an acute abdomen.

IV. Treatment methods

A. Goals of treatment. Blood glucose concentration in critically ill patients with diabetes is ideally maintained between 150 and 250 mg/dl. This degree of control provides a margin of safety to prevent hypoglycemia while precluding the metabolic, electrolyte, infectious, and cardiovascular consequences of persistent severe hyperglycemia. Treatment goals are summarized in Table 85-2.

B. Treatment of hyperglycemia in the critically ill

1. Insulin therapy. All patients in the ICU known to have type 1 diabetes and all other patients with blood glucose concentrations exceeding the critical care zone of 150 to 250 mg/dl should be treated with a **continuous intravenous** (IV) infusion of short-acting (regular) insulin.

Subcutaneous injections of intermediate-acting insulin should be avoided because absorption will vary with the adequacy of perfusion and because,

TABLE 85-2. Diabetes treatment goals in critically ill and surgical patients

Zone	Blood glucose concentration (mg/dl)
Hypoglycemia	<100
Safe but low margin for error	100–150
Critical care, surgical	150–250
Hyperglycemia	250–350
Severe hyperglycemia	>350

once given, dosage reduction is not possible. "Sliding scale" prescriptions for boluses of short-acting insulin should also be avoided because they amplify the risks of hypo- and hyperglycemia. Oral hypoglycemic agents should not be used in the ICU. Biguanide-class drugs such as metformin (Glucophage), in particular, should be discontinued in critically ill patients because of the risk of lactic acidosis.

Figure 85-1 indicates appropriate initial insulin infusion rates. Continuous insulin infusion requires frequent (every 1–2 hours) determinations of bedside blood glucose concentration.

2. **Adjusting insulin infusions.** Patients with diabetes in the ICU should receive continuous IV insulin until their clinical status is substantially improved and glycemic control is stable. Increasing insulin requirements can signal infection, myocardial infarction, tissue ischemia, hypoxemia, medications, or excessive carbohydrate feeding. Decreasing insulin requirements can signal hepatic failure, renal failure, or adrenal insufficiency.

   If blood glucose concentration falls below 200 mg/dl, a glucose infusion (D5W) should be started, and the insulin infusion rate adjusted to approximately 1.0 U/h to inhibit ketogenesis. Never stop insulin entirely during the

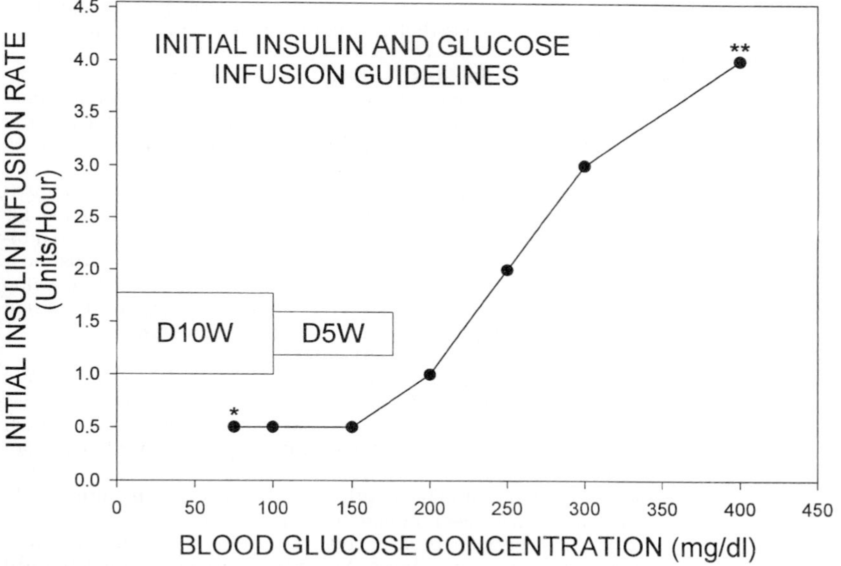

FIG. 85-1. Initial insulin and glucose infusion guidelines. **1.** Patients with type 1 diabetes should receive insulin at all times. **2.** Patients with blood glucose concentrations greater than 150 mg/dl in the ICU should be treated with a continuous insulin infusion. **3.** ICU patients with glucose concentrations less than 175 mg/dl should receive infusions of glucose as indicated.

*ICU patients who do not have type 1 diabetes generally require no insulin for glucose concentrations that are consistently less than 100 mg/dl. Patients with type 1 diabetes with values this low should be maintained on an insulin infusion of 0.5 U/h together with a glucose infusion at all times.

**The infusion rate needed to control extreme hyperglycemia cannot be predicted. We counsel starting with conservative infusion rates that can then be adjusted hourly as needed. If a blood glucose concentration greater than 400 mg/dl fails to respond to 4 U/h within 2 hours, the infusion rate should be doubled.

treatment of diabetes, even if the infusion rate is reduced to only 0.5 U/h or less. The half-life of IV infused insulin is only minutes. Hyperglycemia can recur rapidly in critically ill patients, as can ketoacidosis in the case of patients with type 1 diabetes.

3. **Transition to other forms of therapy.** When discharge from the ICU is contemplated, insulin therapy can be changed to twice daily injections of intermediate-acting insulin, with or without supplemental subcutaneous short-acting insulin. It is essential that the IV infusion of regular insulin be continued for 2 to 3 hours after the first subcutaneous injection of intermediate-acting insulin is given. Decisions regarding discontinuation of insulin or institution of oral hypoglycemia agents are often best left until the patient is no longer seriously ill.

C. **Surgery in the critically ill patient with diabetes.** Treatment of patients with hyperglycemia who are being prepared for urgent surgery in the emergency department can be initiated with either subcutaneous short-acting insulin or, preferably, a continuous insulin infusion, as described above. Critically ill patients with diabetes should be treated with an insulin infusion during surgery. The ICU patient with diabetes who requires surgery should be sent to the operating room or procedure suite with infusions of both insulin and 5% dextrose in half-normal saline. Frequent monitoring of blood glucose is essential. Intraoperative blood glucose concentrations should be maintained in the critical care surgical zone (Table 85-2). Anesthetic agents can exacerbate hyperglycemia. Regional and local anesthetics are preferable when appropriate.

D. **Special problems**

1. **Peritoneal dialysis and diabetes.** Critically ill patients with diabetes who are being treated with peritoneal dialysis, in general, should be maintained on a continuous, low-dose insulin infusion. Admixtures of glucose and insulin in the dialysate can lead to unpredictable alterations in glycemia in the presence of intercurrent severe stress.

2. **Hyperalimentation and diabetes.** Admixture of insulin with parenteral nutrition formulations, although a common practice, is not recommended for patients in the ICU. The ICU environment permits adjustment of insulin infusions to match both the nutritional load and overall metabolic status independently. If an obese patient receiving hyperalimentation should develop severe hyperglycemia and require large amounts of insulin, consideration should be given to reducing the amount of carbohydrate administered.

E. **Pearls: key points and pitfalls**

1. **Avoid sliding scales!** No role is seen for variable insulin boluses given only after hyperglycemia has occurred because the rapid changes in status that can occur in the critically ill can lead to fluctuating control. Patients with type 1 diabetes whose insulin is withheld until hyperglycemia occurs can quickly become ketoacidotic.

2. **Avoid sporadic insulin administration!** A patient begun on insulin should remain on a closely supervised infusion until the need for it has unequivocally disappeared. A previously normoglycemic patient who develops diabetes in the course of a severe illness should be treated continuously until the stress of the illness has been reduced enough to permit reassessment of the need for insulin. Very sporadic insulin administration can lead to high titers of antibodies and insulin resistance.

3. **Some patients are exquisitely sensitive to regular insulin!** Patients who have had type 1 diabetes for 15 years or more often develop extreme sensitivity to the effects of regular insulin. The reason is unclear, but such sensitivity frequently contributes to increased "brittleness" in these patients. Profound hypoglycemia can result from the use of as little as 5 to 10 U, given either subcutaneously or intravenously. When regular insulin is first given to patients who might be sensitive, the initial dose should be small (2–4 U). The response should be monitored by bedside blood glucose determinations.

4. **Be mindful of the diabetic kidney and radiographic contrast agents!** Nephropathy was commonly thought to render patients with long-standing

diabetes particularly susceptible to acute renal failure after angiographic procedures. With the advent of newer reagents and techniques, the risk of angiography may be no higher than in patients without diabetes. A prudent course of action, however, is to alert radiologists to the presence of diabetes, to hydrate diabetic patients before study, and to minimize dye loads.

Selected Readings

Alberti KG, Zimmet PZ. Definition, diagnosis and classification of diabetes mellitus and its complications. Part 1: diagnosis and classification of diabetes mellitus provisional report of a WHO consultation. *Diabet Med* 1998; 15:539.

General overview of diabetes by leading international authorities.

Choban PS, Burge JC, Scales D, et al. Hypoenergetic nutrition support in hospitalized obese patients: a simplified method for clinical application. *Am J Clin Nutr* 1997; 66:546.

Useful guidelines for nutritional management of the obese inpatient.

Ganda OP. Prevalence and incidence of secondary and other types of diabetes. In: Harris MI, Cowie CC, Stern MP, et al., eds. *Diabetes in America.* Bethesda: National Institutes of Health; 1995:69.

Comprehensive review of conditions that can lead to diabetes.

Hirsch IB, McGill JB, Cryer PE, et al. Perioperative management of surgical patients with diabetes mellitus. *Anesthesiology* 1991;74:346.

A detailed source of information on the management of diabetes in surgical patients.

Malmberg K. Prospective randomised study of intensive insulin treatment on long term survival after acute myocardial infarction in patients with diabetes mellitus. *BMJ* 1997;314:1512.

Evidence that glucose control can reduce cardiovascular mortality both short-and long-term.

Queale WS, Seidler AJ, Brancati FL. Glycemic control and sliding scale insulin use in medical inpatients with diabetes mellitus. *Arch Intern Med* 1997;157:545.

Evidence that the use of sliding scales leads to excessive hypo- and hyperglycemia in hospitalized patients.

Rossini AA, Thompson MJ, Gottlieb PA, et al. Management of diabetes in the critically ill patient. In: Irwin RS, Cerra FB, Rippe JM, eds. *Intensive care medicine,* 4th ed. Philadelphia: Lippincott–Raven; 1999:1258.

The full-length version of this chapter.

Zerr KJ, Furnary AP, Grunkemeier GL, et al. Glucose control lowers the risk of wound infection in diabetics after open heart operations. *Ann Thorac Surg* 1997;63:356.

Evidence that glucose control in the ICU after surgery is important.

86. THE DIABETIC COMAS

Michael J. Thompson, John P. Mordes, and Aldo A. Rossini

I. The four "diabetic comas." Four causes of stupor and coma are associated with disordered glucose metabolism.

- Diabetic ketoacidosis (DKA)
- Hyperosmolar hyperglycemic nonketotic coma (HHNKC)
- Alcoholic ketoacidosis
- Hypoglycemia

These four diagnoses should be considered during the evaluation of any patient with altered mental status.

II. Diabetic ketoacidosis

A. Pathophysiology. Diabetic ketoacidosis is caused by the total or near-total absence of circulating insulin. Without insulin, glucose no longer enters most types of cells and is neither stored nor metabolized. Glucagon secretion is increased and hepatic glucose production increases without restraint. Stress-responsive hormones accelerate catabolism. Lipolysis accelerates and large quantities of free fatty acids are metabolized to ketone bodies. Most threatening are the accumulation of hydrogen ions, loss of free water, and depletion of electrolytes.

B. Presentation and clinical findings. Any person with diabetes can develop ketoacidosis. It most often occurs in patients with type 1 diabetes who have either omitted their insulin or have an intercurrent infection. It occasionally occurs in patients with type 2 diabetes who have intercurrent severe infection, trauma, or myocardial infarction. Most patients in DKA are lethargic; approximately 10% are comatose. Postural hypotension is common, but shock is rare. Patients have rapid, deep (Kussmaul) respiration, and their breath has a sweet fruity odor. Patients in DKA are not febrile unless some other intercurrent disorder is present. The rare cases of hypothermia in DKA are associated with sepsis. Abdominal pain is common and can be accompanied by guarding with diminished bowel sounds. Patients in DKA may be nauseated and vomit guaiac-positive, coffee ground-like material. Pleuritic chest pain may be present. Hepatic enlargement with fatty infiltration can occur.

C. Laboratory

1. **Plasma glucose.** Plasma glucose concentration in the range of 400 to 800 mg/dl is typical in DKA. Occasionally, younger patients maintain blood glucose concentrations less than 300 mg/dl.
2. **Electrolytes**

   Sodium: Serum sodium concentration is variable; decreases occur due to osmotic diuresis and dilution by the osmotic effect of large amounts of extracellular glucose. The "corrected" serum sodium in a patient with a measured concentration of 135 mEq/L and a glucose concentration of 600 mg/dl is $1.6 \times (6 - 1) + 135$, or 143 mEq/L. Hypertriglyceridemia is a common cause of factitiously low sodium concentrations.

   Potassium: All patients in DKA are at risk for life-threatening hypokalemia during treatment, despite the fact that the serum potassium concentration is usually elevated at presentation. Total body potassium loss (in the range of 200–700 mEq) typically occurs. Normal or low concentrations of potassium early in ketoacidosis reflect a very severe potassium deficit.

   Phosphorous: Elevated serum phosphate concentrations are common in untreated DKA, After therapy, there is a precipitous decline to subnormal levels.
3. **Anion gap acidosis.** Arterial blood gas and pH measurements are essential in the management of severe DKA. Uncomplicated DKA presents as an

anion gap acidosis. More chronic ketoacidotic states can be associated with hyperchloremic acidosis, probably as a consequence of the loss of neutralized ketone body salts. Rare cases of DKA are complicated by intercurrent metabolic alkalosis, most often from severe vomiting.

4. **Plasma ketones.** Plasma ketone levels do not necessarily reflect the full extent of ketogenesis because the test measures only acetoacetate (AcAc) and acetone. β-Hydroxybutyrate (BOHB), a "ketone body" produced from AcAc, is actually an acid alcohol. It is not measured in assays for ketones. Normally, the BOHB:AcAc ratio is 3 : 1, but acidosis increases the ratio to 6 : 1 or even 12 : 1 as pH decreases. Ketone body measurements can rise initially because of conversion of BOHB back to AcAc. Clearance occurs slowly; measurement more often than every 12 hours is generally unnecessary.
5. **Mixed anion gap acidosis.** A mixed anion gap acidosis can occur in patients in DKA. It can be caused by, for example, intercurrent lactic acidosis or salicylate intoxication. To determine if a nonketone body anion is complicating DKA, multiply the highest positive ketone dilution by 0.1 mm/L to estimate AcAc concentration. Multiply the AcAc concentration by 3 to 6 (depending on the pH) to estimate the BOHB concentration. If the anion gap is greater than the estimated concentrations of AcAc plus BOHB, the presence of an additional unmeasured anion should be considered (e.g., lactate, salicylate, uremic compounds, methanol, or ethylene glycol).
6. **Other laboratory findings**

   Renal: The blood urea nitrogen (BUN) of patients in DKA is typically elevated because of prerenal azotemia and increased ureagenesis. AcAc interferes with some creatinine assays.

   Hematology: The hematocrit and hemoglobin are usually high. Low values suggest preexisting anemia or acute blood loss. A leukocytosis with a left shift often occurs in the absence of intercurrent illness.

   Lipids: A marked elevation is seen of serum triglyceride concentrations, which reverses with insulin therapy.

   Other: Serum amylase, lipase, and creatine kinase concentrations are sometimes elevated. Uric acid concentrations may be elevated. Ketone bodies interfere with certain transaminase assays.

D. Treatment. Treatment of DKA should be directed at four main problems: hypovolemia, electrolyte disturbances, insulin deficiency, and identification of the precipitating event.

1. **Correction of hypovolemia.** Patients in DKA are always hypovolemic. Fluid and electrolyte therapy always takes precedence over insulin therapy (which can worsen hypovolemia by shifting salt and water from the extracellular compartments to the intracellular space). The free water deficit generally ranges between 5 and 11 L. Initial fluid resuscitation should be with an infusion of 0.9% saline. Approximately 2 L should be given during the first hour to restore blood volume, stabilize blood pressure, and establish urine flow. Saline (1 L 0.9%) can typically be given again during the next 2 hours. During the first 24 hours, 75% of the estimated total water deficit should be replaced. Urine flow should be maintained at approximately 30 to 60 ml/h. A simple method for judging the efficacy of fluid therapy is frequent determination of body weight. After the first 2 L, consider changing to hypotonic 0.45% saline if hypernatremia is present.
2. **Electrolytes**

   Potassium: All patients in DKA are potassium depleted. Because serum potassium concentration does not accurately reflect total body potassium, replacement should be initiated early in treatment. The recommended initial repletion rate is 20 mEq/h as KCl or K_3PO4. If a patient in mild DKA is alert and able to tolerate liquids, potassium can be given orally. Potassium concentration often falls precipitously after starting therapy, shifting to the intracellular space in the presence of glucose and insulin, exchanging for buffered intracellular hydrogen as acidosis resolves, and excreted with ketones as potassium salts. Sudden reduction in serum potassium concentration can cause flaccid paralysis, respiratory failure, and life-threatening cardiac arrhythmias. An electrocardiogram should be obtained.

Phosphate: Initially, the concentration of phosphate is elevated, but levels can decrease to less than 1 mm/L with insulin treatment. Persistent severe hypophosphatemia can cause neurologic disturbances, arthralgias, muscle weakness, rhabdomyolysis, and liver dysfunction. Each vial of potassium phosphate contains 93 mg phosphorus and 4 mEq/ml potassium. It is rarely necessary to administer more than one 5-ml ampule of potassium phosphate to a patient in DKA. The hazards of parenteral phosphate administration include hypocalcemia and metastatic calcification. Unless hypophosphatemia is severe and persistent, generally no need is seen for treatment.

Bicarbonate: Most authorities suggest that bicarbonate replacement should be done only in patients with an arterial pH less than 7.1. Bicarbonate therapy can produce hypokalemia, paradoxical cerebrospinal fluid acidosis, and a shift of the oxygen dissociation curve to the left that results in tissue hypoxia and lactic acidosis. We recommend bicarbonate therapy (a) when the pH is persistently less than 7.1 after 2 to 3 hours of treatment; (b) when the initial pH is less than 7.0; (c) in cases complicated by depressed respiratory drive; and (d) when hypotensive shock is unresponsive to rapid fluid replacement. Administer sodium bicarbonate, 2 ampules totaling 88 mEq given over 1 hour. When the pH is greater than 7.2, treatment should be stopped.

Magnesium: Hypermagnesemia can occur early in the course of DKA. Mg^{2+} concentration generally returns to normal without treatment. In some patients, Mg^{2+} stores can be depleted and, in rare instances, lead to cardiac arrhythmia.

3. **Insulin.** Insulin therapy should be instituted only after fluid and electrolyte resuscitation is underway. We recommend an intravenous (IV) bolus of 10 U of regular insulin followed by a continuous IV infusion starting at 5 U/h. In children, the recommended initial bolus is 0.1 U/kg body weight and the infusion rate is 0.1 U/kg/h. Blood glucose concentration should be measured every 1 to 2 hours after starting the infusion. If the glucose concentration has not decreased by 100 mg/dl, the insulin infusion rate should be doubled. When glucose has fallen by more than 150 mg/dl, then the insulin infusion rate should be decreased by 50%, but it should never be stopped. If the blood glucose concentration falls below 200 mg/dl, a glucose infusion (D5W) should be started and the insulin infusion rate adjusted to 1.0 U/h to inhibit ketogenesis. Never stop insulin entirely during the treatment of DKA, even if the infusion rate is reduced to only 0.5 U/h or less.

   Identification of the precipitating event: Diabetic ketoacidosis may be the first sign of new-onset type 1 diabetes mellitus. Most cases, however, occur in patients known to have diabetes, and it is always necessary to ask why DKA has occurred in this setting. Common underlying causes of DKA include:

   Omission of insulin therapy
   Infection
   Major stressors (e.g., myocardial infarction, trauma)
   Medication (e.g., high-dose glucocorticoid therapy)

E. Pearls. Key points and pitfalls. Complications are not infrequent in cases of DKA; some are avoidable.

Never stop insulin completely! DKA can recur rapidly, especially in the presence of other intercurrent illnesses. Insulin infusions should always be continued, if only at 0.5 to 1 U/h, until the patient is well enough to be switched to subcutaneous injections of longer-acting insulin. The infusion can be stopped 2 to 3 hours after the first subcutaneous injection of intermediate-acting insulin is given.

Recurrent DKA: If ketoacidosis recurs in the intensive care unit (ICU) despite continued therapy with insulin, severe infection, a severe contra-insulin state (e.g., Cushing's syndrome), or medications (e.g., glucocorticoids) should be suspected.

Cerebral edema is a rare complication of DKA in adults, but it occurs occasionally in children. To avoid cerebral edema, the goal of DKA treatment during the first 24 hours is a blood glucose concentration not less than 200 mg/dl.

Persistent hypotension should prompt consideration of fluid shifts, bleeding, severe acidosis, arrhythmia, myocardial infarction, cardiac tamponade, sepsis, and adrenal insufficiency.

Renal complications include postrenal obstruction, atonic bladder, and acute tubular necrosis secondary to pyelonephritis.

Thrombosis of the cerebral vessels and stroke are recognized, but uncommon, complications of DKA.

III. Hyperosmolar hyperglycemic nonketotic coma

A. Pathophysiology. The pathophysiology of HHNKC involves three interrelated elements: (a) insulin deficiency, (b) renal impairment, and (c) cognitive impairment.

Relative lack of insulin is the fundamental defect. Patients have sufficient insulin to inhibit ketone body formation but not enough to prevent glycogenolysis and gluconeogenesis. The resulting hyperglycemia induces an osmotic diuresis, with resultant fluid and electrolyte losses.

Some degree of renal impairment accompanies all cases of HHNKC. Typical patients with the HHNKC syndrome are older and have reduced renal blood flow and glomular filtration rate. The underlying renal abnormalities in the HHNKC syndrome can be prerenal, renal, or postrenal. The common result is that affected patients are unable to compensate for the hyperglycemia with an osmotic diuresis.

Invariably, HHNKC involves acute or chronic impairment of cerebral function. Hyperglycemia leading to an osmotic diuresis and hyperosmolality normally activates a thirst response. A common history for HHNKC involves an elderly patient with impaired cognitive function from cerebrovascular disease, dementia, or central nervous system-depressant medications. Patients with trauma or burns are also susceptible to HHNKC.

B. Presentation and clinical findings. Patients who develop HHNKC are typically middle-aged or elderly. They often have a history of mild type II diabetes and a prodrome of progressive polyuria and polydipsia lasting days to several weeks. Most patients have underlying diseases; renal and cardiovascular disorders are common. Other intercurrent problems include infection, myocardial infarction, stroke, hemorrhage, and trauma. Additional factors include dialysis, hyperalimentation, and medications (e.g., thiazide diuretics, phenytoin, propranolol, immunosuppressive agents, and cimetidine).

Fever is a common finding in HHNKC even in the absence of infection, but infection must be rigorously excluded in all cases. Patients may have hypotension and tachycardia because of dehydration, and they frequently hyperventilate. Hyperventilation can reflect intercurrent lactic acidosis. Neurologic manifestations include tremors and fasciculations. Mental status abnormalities can range from mild disorientation to obtundation and coma. Up to a third of patients with HHNKC may seize.

C. Laboratory

1. **Plasma glucose** concentrations in HHNKC are generally higher than in DKA—usually greater than 600 mg/dl. Values as high as 2,000 mg/dl occur.
2. **Ketones.** Most patients in HHNKC are not ketonemic. Serum acetone levels are usually normal or only slightly elevated, seldom exceeding 1:2.
3. **Arterial pH.** Occasional patients in HHNKC will develop an intercurrent metabolic acidosis. Most patients in HHNKC are only mildly acidotic, the average pH being about 7.25 before treatment.

4. **Osmolality.** Serum osmolality in comatose patients usually exceeds 350 mOsm/kg. Dehydration induces prerenal azotemia.
5. **Sodium.** The serum sodium concentration in HHNKC at the time of presentation is variable, ranging between 100 and 180 mEq/L.
6. **Potassium.** Serum potassium concentration in HHNKC is also variable, ranging from 2.2 to 7.8 mEq/L.

D. Treatment. Treatment of HHNKC should be directed at four main problems: hypovolemia, electrolyte disturbances, insulin deficiency, and identification of the precipitating event.

1. **Correction of hypovolemia.** Patients with HHNKC, without exception, are profoundly dehydrated. Within the first 2 hours, 1 to 2 L of 0.9% saline should be given. Normal saline is recommended, even if hypernatremia is present, to expand the extracellular fluid compartment rapidly. After initial volume expansion and restoration of normotension, subsequent treatment for dehydration in this syndrome emphasizes free water replacement. The average patient requires 6 to 8 L of fluids during the first 12 hours of treatment.
2. **Electrolytes.** As soon as adequate urine flow has been established and the degree of hypokalemia estimated, potassium supplementation should be added to the IV fluids. A sudden fall in serum potassium concentration frequently accompanies the initial dose of insulin. Serum potassium concentration should be checked frequently and the electrocardiogram monitored for changes. Cardiac arrhythmias induced by hypokalemia may be irreversible, particularly in the elderly.
3. **Insulin.** Most patients with HHNKC are more sensitive to insulin than are patients with DKA. In addition, blood glucose concentration in HHNKC can fall precipitously when urine output is reestablished after volume expansion. Treatment with insulin is essential but should be instituted (a) with careful monitoring and (b) only *after* fluid and electrolyte resuscitation is underway. We do not recommend an initial IV insulin bolus. For the infusion, we recommend a starting dose of only 1 to 5 U/h, depending on individual circumstances. Attempt to maintain blood glucose concentration near 250 mg/dl for the first 24 hours. A rapid fall in blood glucose concentration can cause cerebral edema.
4. **Identification of the precipitating event.** HHNKC may be the first sign of newly recognized diabetes mellitus, but most cases occur in patients known to have glucose intolerance. Regardless of the previous glycemic history, it is always necessary to ask why HHNKC has occurred. Common and easily recognized underlying causes of DKA include infection and major stressors (e.g., myocardial infarction or trauma). Other precipitating events in the elderly can be more subtle. These can include drugs that depress the sensorium and inhibit the response to thirst (e.g., anxiolytics and sedatives), drugs that depress renal function (e.g., diuretics leading to prerenal azotemia), drugs that promote hyperglycemia (e.g., steroids) and other endocrine disturbances (e.g., hypothyroidism or apathetic thyrotoxicosis).

E. Pearls. Key points and pitfalls. Patients with HHNKC may be very sensitive to insulin! Do not be overly aggressive with insulin. Do not give insulin before volume restoration. When insulin is administered to patients with HHNKC syndrome, glucose shifts from the extracellular to the intracellular compartment. The rapid intracellular movement of free water can precipitate hypotension and shock. Rapid reduction in blood glucose is a major contributor to the development of cerebral edema and a fatal outcome in HHNKC.

IV. Alcoholic ketoacidosis

A. Pathophysiology. Ethanol metabolism consumes oxidized nicotinic acid dehydrogenase (NAD^+) and generates reduced nicotinic acid dehydrogenase (NADH). Sufficient ethanol ingestion can generate an unfavorable NADH/NAD^+ ratio, which in turn impairs gluconeogenesis. Hypoglycemia ensues when glycogen stores are exhausted, explaining the relationship of the disorder to nutritional state. Because of the hypoglycemia, insulin levels are low, which is permissive both to the release of free fatty acids from adipose tissue and to the formation of ketone bodies.

B. Presentation and clinical findings. Patients with this disorder may be stuporous or comatose. They are typically chronically alcoholic, but the disorder can occur after binge drinking in adults or accidental ingestion in children. Patients typically have not eaten for days and are susceptible to nausea, vomiting, and aspiration. Hypothermia and neurologic abnormalities, including trismus, seizures, hemiparesis, and abnormal tendon reflexes, may be observed. Evidence of inebriation is often absent.

The diagnosis depends on the demonstration of hypoglycemia in the setting of ketoacidosis. Definitive demonstration of hypoglycemia has three components:

1. Low plasma glucose concentration
2. Neuroglycopenic symptoms (e.g., hunger, headache, confusion, lethargy, slurred speech, seizures, coma) consistent with hypoglycemia
3. Resolution of those symptoms with administration of glucose

C. Laboratory

1. **Hypoglycemia.** Blood glucose concentrations can be as low as 20 mg/dl.
2. **Anion gap acidosis.** These patients are usually quite acidotic, with an arterial pH less than 7.2.
3. **Ketonemia and ketonuria.** Both ketoacids and lactate contribute to the unmeasured anion pool in this form of acidosis, but only the former is easily measured and detected.
4. **Other.** Liver function tests, amylase, and phosphate are typically normal.

D. Treatment

1. **Fluids and electrolytes.** Rehydration with IV fluids as appropriate.
2. **Glucose.** One ampule of D50W to correct hypoglycemia, being careful to avoid extravasation.
3. **Parenteral thiamine.** Give 100 mg to prevent Wernicke's encephalopathy.

E. Pearls. Key points and pitfalls.

1. By the time patients with this disorder are treated, the ethanol has often been metabolized and is no longer detectable.
2. Administration of sodium bicarbonate is generally not necessary. Treatment with glucose and fluids rapidly reverses the condition by raising the concentration of insulin, thereby inhibiting lipolysis and free fatty acid release.
3. Urinary ketones in a hypoglycemic patient generally excludes hyperinsulinemia as the cause of the low glucose concentration.
4. Persons with diabetes treated with insulin or sulfonylurea-class hypoglycemic agents who become intoxicated may develop life-threatening, profound hypoglycemia because of the metabolic synergy of ethanol and insulin.

V. Hypoglycemic coma. Hypoglycemia and hypoglycemic coma are discussed in Chapter 90.

Selected Readings

DeFronzo RA, Matsuda M, Barrett EJ. Diabetic ketoacidosis: a combined metabolic-nephrologic approach to therapy. *Diab Rev* 1994;2:209.
Comprehensive review that addresses common misconceptions about treatment.

Fulop M. Alcoholic ketoacidosis. *Endocrinol Metab Clin North Am* 1993;22:209.
Detailed review of the causes and treatment of alcoholic ketoacidosis.

Genuth SM. Diabetic ketoacidosis and hyperglycemic hyperosmolar coma. *Curr Ther Endocrinol Metab* 1997;6:438.
Extensive review of diabetic ketoacidosis and hyperglycemic hyperosmolar coma.

Ishihara K, Szerlip HM. Anion gap acidosis. *Semin Nephrol* 1998;18:83.
Detailed analysis of the diagnosis and analysis of anion gap acidoses.

Okuda Y, Adrogue HJ, Field JB, et al. Counterproductive effects of sodium bicarbonate in diabetic ketoacidosis. *J Clin Endocrinol Metab* 1996;81:314.
Concludes that bicarbonate therapy should be reserved for patients with severely depressed cardiovascular status.

Rossini AA, Mordes JP. The diabetic comas. In: Irwin RS, Cerra FB, Rippe JM, eds. *Intensive care medicine,* 4th ed. Philadelphia: Lippincott–Raven; 1998:1258.
The full-length version of this chapter.
Wilson HK, Keuer SP, Lea AS, et al. Phosphate therapy in diabetic ketoacidosis. *Arch Intern Med* 1982;142:517.
Concludes that phosphate therapy is usually not essential for diabetic ketoacidosis management.

87. THYROID EMERGENCIES

Alan P. Farwell and Charles H. Emerson

I. General principles. Thyroid storm and myxedema coma are life-threatening emergencies that represent the extreme ends of the spectrum of thyroid dysfunction in the decompensated patient. Their presentation is usually dramatic and is often precipitated by a non–thyroid-related illness or event. Both of these disorders are clinical diagnoses, as the thyroid hormone abnormalities do not differ significantly from uncomplicated thyrotoxicosis and hypothyroidism, respectively. As such, the recognition of these disorders requires a high degree of clinical suspicion and prompt institution of therapy.

II. Thyroid storm. Thyroid storm is an uncommon, but life-threatening complication of thyrotoxicosis in which a severe form of the disease is usually precipitated by an intercurrent medical problem. It occurs in untreated or partially treated thyrotoxic patients. Precipitating factors associated with thyroid storm include infections, stress, trauma, thyroidal or nonthyroidal surgery, diabetic ketoacidosis, labor, heart disease, iodinated contrast studies, thyroid hormone overdose, and radioiodine treatment (especially if not pretreated with antithyroid drugs). Although the cause of the rapid clinical decompensation is unknown, a sudden inhibition of thyroid hormone binding to plasma proteins by the precipitating factor, causing a rise in free hormone concentrations in the already elevated free hormone pool, may play a role in the pathogenesis of thyroid storm.

Thyroid storm is rare, accounting for less than 2% of all hospital admissions related to thyrotoxicosis. Historically, thyroid storm was frequently associated with surgery for hyperthyroidism. Because of better recognition of the disease and improved perioperative management with β-blockade, thyroid storm now is most often a result of untreated or poorly treated thyrotoxicosis, rather than a postoperative complication.

A. Clinical manifestations. Thyroid storm is primarily a clinical diagnosis. Clinical features are similar to those of thyrotoxicosis, but more exaggerated (Table 87-1). Cardinal features include fever (temperature usually > 38.5°C), tachycardia out of proportion to the fever, and mental status changes. Tachyarrhythmias, especially atrial fibrillation in the elderly, are common. Nausea, vomiting, diarrhea, agitation, and delirium are frequent presentations. Vascular collapse and shock, caused by dehydration and cardiac decompensation, are poor prognostic signs, as is the presence of jaundice. Coma and death may ensue in up to 20% of patients, frequently from cardiac arrhythmias, congestive heart failure, hyperthermia, or the precipitating illness.

Most patients display the classic signs of Graves' disease, the most common cause of thyrotoxicosis, including ophthalmopathy and a diffusely enlarged goiter. Thyroid storm also has been associated with toxic nodular goiters. However, in the elderly, severe myopathy, profound weight loss, apathy, and a minimally enlarged goiter may be observed. No distinct laboratory abnormalities are seen. Thyroid hormone levels are similar to those found in uncomplicated thyrotoxicosis; little correlation is seen between the degree of elevation of thyroid hormones and the presentation of thyroid storm. Abnormal liver function tests are common.

B. Diagnosis. The differential diagnosis of thyroid storm includes sepsis, neuroleptic malignant syndrome, malignant hyperthermia, and acute mania with lethal catatonia, all of which can precipitate thyroid storm in the appropriate setting. Clues to the diagnosis of thyroid storm are a history of thyroid disease, history of iodine ingestion, and the presence of a goiter or stigmata of Graves' disease. Clearly, the physician must have a high clinical index of suspicion for thyroid storm, as therapy must be instituted before the return of thyroid function tests in most cases.

TABLE 87-1. Clinical features of thyroid storm

Fever (usually greater than 41°C; 105.8°F)
Tachycardia/tachyarrhythmias
Delerium/agitation
Mental status changes
Congestive heart failure
Tremor
Nausea and vomiting
Diarrhea
Sweating
Vasodilatation
Dehydration
Hepatomegaly
Splenomegaly
Jaundice

C. Treatment. It should be emphasized that thyroid storm is a major medical emergency that must be treated in an intensive care unit (Table 87-2). Treatment includes supportive measures such as intravenous (IV) fluids, antipyretics, cooling blankets, and sedation. β-Adrenergic blockers (e.g., propranolol—oral or IV—and IV esmolol) are given for heart rate control. Calcium channel blockers can also be used to control tachyarrhythmias. Antithyroid drugs are given in large

TABLE 87-2. Treatment of thyroid storm

Supportive therapy
- Treatment of underlying illnesses
- Intravenous fluids
- Cooling blanket and/or antipyretics

β-adrenergic blocking drugs
- Propranolol—1 mg i.v./min to a total dose of 10 mg then 40–80 mg p.o. q6h, *or*
- Esmolol—500 mg/kg/min i.v. then 50–100 mg/kg/min, *or*
- Metoprolol—100–400 mg p.o. q12h, *or*
- Atenolol—50–100 mg p.o. daily

Antithyroid drugs
- Inhibition of thyroid hormone synthesis
  - Propylthiouracil (PTU)—800 mg p.o. first dose then 200–300 mg p.o. q8h, *or*
  - Methimazole—80 mg p.o. first dose then 40–80 mg p.o. q12h
- Block release of thyroid hormones from the gland
  - SSKI—5 drops p.o. q8h, *or*
  - Lugol's solution—10 drops p.o. q8h, *or*
  - Telepaque (Iopanoic acid)—1 g p.o. q.d., *or*
  - Lithium—800–1200 mg p.o. q.d.—achieve serum lithium levels 0.5–1.5 mEq/L
- Block T4 to T3 conversion
  - Corticosteroids—Dexamethasone 1–2 mg p.o. q6h
  - Most β-blockers—Propranolol 40–80 mg p.o. q6h
  - Propylthiouracil
  - Telapaque (iopanoic acid)
- Remove thyroid hormones from the circulation
  - Plasmapheresis, *or*
  - Peritoneal dialysis, *or*
  - Cholestyramine—4g p.o. q6h, *or*
  - Colestipol—20–30 mg p.o. q.d.

p.o., orally; q.d., every day; SSKI, saturated solution of potassium (K) iodide.

doses. PTU is preferred over methimazole because of its additional advantage of impairing peripheral conversion of T_4 to T_3. PTU and methimazole can be administered by nasogastric tube or rectally if necessary. Neither of these preparations is available for parenteral administration.

Iodides, orally or intravenously, can be used only after antithyroid drugs have been administered. The radiographic contrast dye iopanoic acid (Telepaque) is used to block thyroid hormone release and to inhibit T_4 to T_3 conversion. High-dose dexamethasone is recommended as supportive therapy, as an inhibitor of T_4 to T_3 conversion, and to manage possible intercurrent adrenal insufficiency. Orally administered ion-exchange resin (colestipol or cholestyramine) can trap hormone in the intestine and prevent recirculation. Plasmapheresis has also been used in severe cases. Finally, treatment of the underlying precipitating illness is essential to survival in thyroid storm.

Once stabilized, the antithyroid treatment should be continued until euthyroidism is achieved, at which point a final decision regarding antithyroid drugs, surgery, or ^{131}I therapy can be made.

III. Myxedema coma. Myxedema coma is a rare syndrome that represents the extreme expression of severe, long-standing hypothyroidism. It is a medical emergency; even with early diagnosis and treatment, the mortality rate can be as high as 60%. Myxedema coma occurs most often in the elderly and during the winter months; in a recent series, patients in 9 of 11 cases of myxedema coma were admitted in late fall or winter. In addition to cold stress, common precipitating factors include pulmonary infections, cerebrovascular accidents, trauma, surgery, and congestive heart failure. The clinical course of lethargy proceeding to stupor and then coma is often hastened by drugs, especially sedatives, narcotics, antidepressants, and tranquilizers. Indeed, many cases of myxedema coma have occurred in the undiagnosed hypothyroid patient who has been hospitalized for other medical problems.

A. Clinical manifestations. Cardinal features of myxedema coma are (a) hypothermia, which can be profound; (b) respiratory depression; (c) hypotension; and (d) unconsciousness (Table 87-3). Most patients have the physical features of severe hypothyroidism, including bradycardia; macroglossia; delayed reflexes; dry, rough skin; and myxedematous facies, which results from the periorbital edema, pallor, hypercarotinemia, periorbital edema, and patchy hair loss. Hypotonia of the gastrointestinal tract is common and often so severe as to suggest an obstructive lesion. Urinary retention caused by a hypotonic bladder is a related but less frequent finding. Pleural, pericardial, and peritoneal effusions may be present.

As with the diagnosis of thyroid storm, myxedema coma is a clinical diagnosis, as the thyroid hormone abnormalities are similar to those in uncomplicated hypothyroidism, with more than 95% of cases caused by primary hypothyroidism. Dilutional hyponatremia is common and may be severe. Elevated creatine kinase concentrations, sometimes markedly so, are encountered frequently and can misdirect the clinical picture toward cardiac ischemia. However, in most cases the MB fraction is normal and an electrocardiogram often shows the low

TABLE 87-3. Clinical features of myxedema coma

Mental obtundation
Hypothermia
Bradycardia
Hypotension
Coarse, dry skin
Myxedema facies
Hypoglycemia
Atonic gastrointestinal tract
Atonic bladder
Pleural, pericardial, and peritoneal effusions

voltage and loss of T waves that is characteristic of severe hypothyroidism. Elevated lactate dehydrogenase concentrations, acidosis, and anemia are common findings. Lumbar puncture reveals increased opening pressure and high protein content.

B. Diagnosis. The diagnosis of myxedema coma is based on the presence of the characteristic clinical syndrome in a patient with hypothyroidism. Because the patient is obtunded, a prior history of hypothyroidism must often be obtained from other sources. Friends, relatives, and acquaintances might have noted increasing lethargy, complaints of cold intolerance, and changes in the voice. Clues to the diagnosis include an outdated container of L-T_4 discovered with the patient's belongings, which suggests that he or she has been remiss in taking medication. The medical record may also indicate that the patient was to be taking thyroid hormone, or refer to previous treatment with radioactive iodine, or a thyroidectomy scar may be present.

Few of the signs and symptoms discussed above are unique to myxedema coma. Protein-calorie malnutrition, sepsis, hypoglycemia, and exposure to certain drugs and toxins, as well as cold exposure, can cause severe hypothermia. Hypotension and hypoventilation, other cardinal features of myxedema coma, occur in other disease states. Further, low thyroid hormone concentrations are commonly seen in the intensive care unit patient with the sick euthyroid syndrome (Chapter 91). Therefore, the diagnosis of hypothyroidism or myxedema coma cannot be made solely on the basis of a low free thyroxine index in an obtunded patient. What distinguishes myxedema coma from other disorders is the combination of laboratory evidence of hypothyroidism, the characteristic myxedema facies with periorbital puffiness, the skin changes, obtundation, and other physical signs characteristic of severe hypothyroidism. As with thyroid storm, the physician must have a high clinical index of suspicion for myxedema coma, because therapy must be instituted before the return of thyroid function tests in most cases.

C. Treatment. The mainstays of therapy are (a) supportive care, with ventilatory and hemodynamic support, rewarming, correction of hyponatremia and hypoglycemia, and treatment of the precipitating incident and (b) administration of thyroid hormone. All patients require continuous monitoring of the electrocardiogram and an IV access. Sedatives, hypnotics, narcotics, and anesthetics must be minimized or avoided altogether because of their extended duration of action and exacerbation of obtundation in the hypothyroid patient. Baseline thyroid function tests, serum cortisol, complete blood count, blood urea nitrogen, plasma glucose, and electrolytes are mandatory. Because of a 5% to 10% incidence of coexisting adrenal insufficiency in patients with myxedema coma, IV steroids (i.e., hydrocortisone 100 mg every 8 hours) are indicated before initiating T_4 therapy.

TABLE 87-4. Treatment of myxedema coma

Assisted ventilation for hypoventilation
Hemodynamic support for hypotension
Intravenous glucose for hypoglycemia
Water restriction or hypertonic saline for severe hyponatremia
Passive rewarming for hypothermia
Administer thyroid hormone intravenously
L-T4—200–300 μg loading dose, up to 500 μg in the first 24 h[a] and/or
L-T3—12.5 μg q6h[a]
Administer hydrocortisone i.v. (100 mg q8h)[a]
Treat underlying infection and other illnesses, if present
Avoid all sedatives, hypnotics, and narcotics

[a] Note that dosage must be individualized (see text).
i.v., intravenous.

Parenteral administration of thyroid hormone is necessary because of uncertain absorption through the gut. A reasonable approach is an initial IV loading dose of 200 to 300 μg L-T_4. If the state of consciousness, blood pressure, or core temperature inadequately improves during the first 6 to 12 hours after administration, another dose of L-T_4 should be given to bring the total dose during the first 24 hours to 0.5 mg. This should be followed by 50 to 100 μg IV every 24 hours until the patient is stabilized. Alternatively, in the most severe cases, some clinicians recommend using L-T_3 at a dosage of 12.5 to 25 μg IV every 6 hours until the patient is stable and conscious. Caution must be used to avoid overstimulation of the cardiovascular system. Once stable, the patient should be switched to L-T_4. The dose of thyroid hormone should be adjusted on the basis of hemodynamic stability, the presence of coexisting cardiac disease, and the degree of electrolyte imbalance.

Hypothermia is one of the hallmarks of myxedema coma and its severity can be underestimated if the thermometer is not shaken down or does not register below 30°C. At core temperatures below 28°C, ventricular fibrillation is a major threat to life. Despite its gravity, the management of the hypothermia of myxedema coma differs from the treatment of exposure-induced hypothermia in euthyroid subjects. In myxedema coma, the patient should be kept in a warm room and covered with blankets. Active heating should be avoided because it increases oxygen consumption and promotes peripheral vasodilation and circulatory collapse. Active heating is recommended only for situations of severe hypothermia where ventricular fibrillation is an immediate threat. In these cases, the rate of rewarming should not exceed 0.5°C/h, and the core temperature should be raised to approximately 31°C.

Although myxedema coma is associated with a high mortality rate, many patients can be saved by judicious therapy aimed at correcting the secondary metabolic disturbances and reversing the hypothyroid state. This must be done in a sustained but gradual fashion, however, because an effort to correct hypothyroidism too rapidly may completely negate the beneficial effects of the initial treatment.

Selected Readings

Arlot S, Debussche X, Lalau JD, et al. Myxoedema coma: response of thyroid hormones with oral and intravenous high-dose L-thyroxine treatment. *Intensive Care Med* 1991;17:16.

This study documents alternatives to oral administration of thyroid hormone.

Brooks MH, Waldstein SS. Free thyroxine concentrations in thyroid storm. *Ann Intern Med* 1980;93:694.

Burch HB, Wartofsky L. Life-threatening thyrotoxicosis. Thyroid storm. *Endocrinol Metabol Clin North Am* 1993;22:263.

Two in-depth reviews on the pathophysiology, presentation and management of myxedema coma and thyroid storm.

Candrina R, DiStefano O, Spandrio S, et al. Treatment of thyrotoxic storm by charcoal plasma perfusion. *J Endocrinol Invest.* 1989;12:133.

Hellman R, Kelly KL, Mason WD, et al. Propranolol for thyroid storm. *N Engl J Med* 1977;297:671.

Lazarus JH, Addison AJ, Richards AR, et al. Treatment of thyrotoxicosis with lithium carbonate. *Lancet* 1974;2:1160–1163.

Shakir KM, Michaels RD, Hays JH, Potter BB. The use of vile aced sequestrants to lower serum thyroid hormone concentrations in iatrogenic hyperthyroidism. *Ann Int Med* 1993;118:112–113.

Adjunctive therapies are important in the management thyroid storm. These four studies document several potentially useful therapeutic options.

Hickman PE, Sylvester W, Musk AA, McLellan GH, Harris A. Cardiac enzyme changes in myxedema coma. *Clin Chem* 1987;33:622.

Nee PA, Scane AC, Lavelle PH, et al. Hypothermic myxedema coma erroneously diagnosed as myocardial infarction because of increased creatinine kinase MB. *Clin Chem* 1987;33:1083.
These two studies show that creatine kinase elevations in myxedema coma are not due to myocardial ischemia.

Holvey DN, Goodner CJ, Nicoloff JT. Treatment of myxedema coma with intravenous thyroxine. *Arch Intern Med* 1964;113:89.
This study examines the use of intravenous administration of thyroid hormone.

Hylander B, Rosenquist U. Treatment of myxedema coma—factors associated with fatal outcome. *Acta Endocrinol* (Copenh) 1985;108:65.

Jordan RM. Myxedema coma. Pathophysiology, therapy, and factors affecting prognosis. *Med Clin North Am* 1995;79:185.
Two in-depth reviews on the pathophysiology, presentation and management of myxedema coma.

Pereira VG, Haron ES, Lima-Neto N, et al. Management of myxedema coma: report on three successfully treated cases with nasogastric or intravenous administration of triiodothyronine. *J Endocrinol Invest* 1982;5:331.
This study documents alternatives to oral administration of thyroid hormone.

Yeung SC, Go R, Balasubramanyam A. Rectal administration of iodide and propylthiouracil in the treatment of thyroid storm. Thyroid 1995;5:403.
This study documents alternatives to oral administration of antithyroid drugs.

88. HYPOADRENAL CRISIS AND THE STRESS MANAGEMENT OF THE PATIENT ON CHRONIC STEROID THERAPY

Christopher Longcope and Neil Aronin

I. Hypoadrenal crisis

A. General principles. The adrenal glands secrete five types of hormones, but only two of them are critical in the intensive care unit (ICU) setting. Mineralocorticoids (aldosterone being the principal hormone) have their major effects on electrolyte balance, and glucocorticoids (cortisol being the principle hormone) promote gluconeogenesis but have many other actions. Mineralocorticoids and glucocorticoids are life-maintaining and deficiency of either can result in a hypoadrenal crisis. By contrast, the other three types of adrenal hormones do not play a major role in this disorder.

Hypoadrenal crisis can occur as an acute event in individuals who give little background history of previous adrenal problems. A high index of suspicion is necessary because the diagnosis can be easily missed. To establish the diagnosis by biochemical testing requires time. It is wise to perform diagnostic testing procedures prior to initiating therapy but not to withhold therapy until the results are known.

1. Etiology. The most common cause of primary adrenal failure, Addison's disease, is autoimmune in nature. Other causes of adrenal failure include hemorrhage secondary to trauma, overwhelming sepsis, circulating anticoagulants, or anticoagulant therapy, tuberculosis, fungal disease, amyloidosis, the acquired immune deficiency syndrome (AIDS), antiphospholipid syndrome, infarction, irradiation, metastatic disease, and drugs.

The most common cause of secondary adrenal insufficiency is suppression of corticotropin (ACTH) release by prior glucocorticoid therapy. Pituitary tumors or hypothalamic disease can cause adrenal dysfunction.

2. Actions of mineralo- and glucocorticoids. The adrenal cortex secretes aldosterone from the zona glomerulosa and cortisol from the zona reticularis. Aldosterone, which promotes the reabsorption of sodium and the secretion of potassium and hydrogen in the renal tubule, is controlled mainly by the renin–angiotensin system.

Glucocorticoids promote gluconeogenesis and protein wasting, and increase the excretion of free water by the kidney. In large doses, glucocorticoids bind to mineralocorticoid receptors, thereby increasing sodium reabsorption and potassium and hydrogen ion excretion. Glucocorticoids act on numerous tissues, also affecting the sense of well-being, appetite, and mood. They directly inhibit the release of ACTH in the central nervous system. Glucocorticoids have a direct effect on the cardiovascular system and help maintain blood pressure, although the mechanisms are unknown.

The effects of excess glucocorticoids cause lymphopenia, leukocytosis, and eosinopenia. Excess glucocorticoids can lead to osteoporosis and reduction of hypercalcemia in certain diseases.

In primary adrenal failure, lack of aldosterone results in sodium wasting with concomitant loss of water and an increase in renal reabsorption of potassium. A decrease in plasma volume and dehydration occurs, with subsequent increases in blood urea nitrogen (BUN) and plasma renin activity.

The decrease in circulating levels of cortisol causes a marked increase in circulating levels of ACTH and a corresponding increase in β-lipotropin. Melanocyte-stimulating hormone activity increases and the skin, especially creases and scars, becomes pigmented. Hypotension develops, initially orthostatic, but can progress to frank shock in a crisis. Hypoglycemia and an increase in sensitivity to insulin are commonplace.

B. Diagnosis

1. Clinical. Clinical manifestations that suggest adrenal insufficiency can include a nonspecific history of increasing weakness, lassitude, fatigue, anorexia, vomiting, and constipation (with the hypoadrenal crisis, diarrhea can occur). Patients who present with adrenal hypofunction in crisis are hypotensive or in frank shock; they generally have a fever that can be high, show evidence of dehydration, and may be stuporous or comatose. In individuals whose loss of adrenal function occurs as a precipitous event (i.e.,:adrenal hemorrhage during the course of an infection, anticoagulant therapy, trauma, or after surgery), no hyperpigmentation is seen but flank pain is often present. Severely ill patients are often suspected of developing adrenal hypofunction, but the incidence and diagnosis of this entity are controversial.

In secondary adrenal failure caused by lack of ACTH, the signs and symptoms are primarily those of glucocorticoid deficiency, especially hypoglycemia. A deficit in overall pituitary secretion can lead to signs of other endocrine gland dysfunctions.

Although clinical signs of adrenal insufficiency can be important, the actual diagnosis of hypoadrenal function requires appropriate laboratory tests.

2. Adrenal function tests. In primary adrenal insufficiency, plasma levels of cortisol are usually low or in the low to normal range and do not rise after ACTH. This failure to respond to ACTH is the definitive test for primary adrenal hypofunction and should be carried out on anyone in whom the diagnosis is suspected. Severely ill patients with a serum cortisol less than 20 μg/dl should be suspected of having adrenal insufficiency and should be tested with intravenous (IV) ACTH. The ACTH stimulation is carried out by administering 250 μg of Cortrosyn (synthetic ACTH 1–24) IV, and plasma ACTH and cortisol levels are measured prior to and 30 to 60 minutes after the dose. A normal response is indicated by a stimulated cortisol level of more than 20 μg/dl. Although this is the standard test at present, an alternative test has been suggested in which only 1 μg synthetic ACTH is administered IV, with a normal response at 30 minutes of more than 18 μg/dl. With the low dose ACTH test, patients with secondary adrenal insufficiency show an increase in cortisol, although not to the same degree as those with normal hypothalamic-pituitary adrenal function. Because the analysis of plasma cortisol level cannot be done immediately, in critically ill patients dexamethasone (4 mg IV) can be given before the ACTH test.

In individuals who develop acute adrenal insufficiency as a result of adrenal hemorrhage, a computed tomography (CT) scan of the adrenal glands can be a very useful diagnostic tool. Individuals with adrenal hypofunction generally show varying degrees of hyponatremia and hyperkalemia and the sodium:potassium ratio is almost always less than 30.

C. Treatment. The management of suspected hypoadrenal crisis depends on the severity of the illness on presentation. The main objective of therapy is immediate administration of a glucocorticoid along with saline and glucose. Because large amounts of hydrocortisone are administered IV in salt-containing solutions, it is not necessary to administer a mineralocorticoid immediately. It is generally believed that individuals in the hypoadrenal state have an approximate 20% deficit of their extracellular fluid volume and should receive at least 3 L of glucose-containing saline in the first 24 hours.

In critically ill patients, the saline and glucose may have to be given in the first few hours. A bolus of 100 mg of hydrocortisone should be administered IV immediately and then 100 to 150 mg should be given IV over the next 24 hours. If the patient's condition is deemed sufficiently grave, 4 mg of dexamethasone sodium phosphate can be administered as initial therapy before carrying out the ACTH stimulation. However, because dexamethasone does not have potent salt-retaining activity, hydrocortisone should be used for continuing therapy.

After the initial 24 hours of therapy, the hydrocortisone can be decreased by 50%/d as the situation improves to reach a standard maintenance dose of

20 to 30 mg/d. As the maintenance dose is achieved, a mineralocorticoid (0.1 mg 9α-fluorohydrocortisone acetate) should be added.

In addition to therapy with glucocorticoids, saline, and glucose, any underlying infection should be treated vigorously.

II. Glucocorticoids and stress

A. General principles. In normal subjects, the secretion rate of cortisol increases from 10 mg/d to 50 to 150 mg/d during surgical procedures but rarely exceeds 200 mg/d. The degree of response depends, in part, on the extent and duration of surgery.

After the introduction of glucocorticoid therapy, several case reports linked withdrawal of steroids, adrenal suppression, and shock in patients on long-term steroid treatment.

The few studies available suggest that hypotension from inadequate adrenal function is uncommon. Thus, the development of shock in the acutely ill or surgical patient on steroid therapy (or after withdrawal within 1 year) should not be attributed solely to diminished adrenal responsiveness. Adrenal steroids can and should be administered, but other contributing causes of the hypotension should be sought. Suppression of the hypothalamic-anterior pituitary-adrenal axis can occur after only 5 days of glucocorticoid treatment. After long-term administration of corticosteroids, the adrenal axis may respond poorly to appropriate stimuli up to 1 year after steroid withdrawal. Adrenal suppression cannot be predicted based solely on glucocorticoid dosage and duration or a normal basal cortisol.

B. Diagnosis and treatment. Patients on glucocorticoid therapy for at least 4 weeks at either pharmacologic or replacement levels and those who have stopped glucocorticoids within the past year have the highest risk for adrenal suppression. Time permitting, a Cortrosyn test provides information on the adequacy of the adrenal response to stress. An adequate increase in plasma cortisol following corticotropin administration is interpreted to indicate the presence of an intact hypothalamic-anterior pituitary-adrenal axis, and patients who have a subnormal response to Cortrosyn also have a subnormal cortisol response to stress or surgery. For minor surgical procedures, the patient's usual dose of glucocorticoid is probably sufficient but a single dose of 25 mg hydrocortisone or its equivalent can be given instead. As the extent and duration of surgery increases, the glucocorticoid dose should be increased from 50 to 75 mg/d hydrocortisone or its equivalent for up to 2 days to 100 to 150 mg hydrocortisone or its equivalent for up to 3 days.

Hydrocortisone can be rapidly tapered and the patients returned to their usual dose of glucocorticoid if needed.

Selected Readings

Axelrod L. Glucocorticoid therapy. *Medicine* 1976;55:39.

A review of glucocorticoid action and effects on the hypothalamic-pituitary-adrenal axis; old but still useful.

Barquist E, Kirton O. Adrenal insufficiency in the surgical intensive care unit patient. *J Trauma* 1997;42:27.

Report on occurrence of acute adrenal insufficiency in ICU, including diagnostic steps, therapy, and prognosis.

Baxter JD, Tyrrell JB. Evaluation of the hypothalamic-pituitary adrenal axis: importance in steroid therapy, AIDS, and other stress syndromes. *Advances in Internal Medicine* 1994;39:667.

Review on evaluating patients for adrenal dysfunction, including tests that are being used and their interpretation.

Kehlet H, Binder C. Adrenocorticol function and clinical course during and after surgery in supplemented glucocorticoid-treated patients. *Br J Anaesth* 1973;45:1043.

Evaluation of adrenocorticol function and clinical course in glucocorticoid-treated patients during surgery.

Kehlet H, Binder C. Alteration in distribution volume and biological half-life of cortisol during major surgery. *J Clin Endocrinol Metabol* 1973;36:330.

Provides information on the changes in cortisol production and metabolism that occur during stress. One of the few reports giving secretion rates.

Kehlet H, Binder C. Value of an ACTH test in assessing hypothalamic-pituitary-adrenocortical function in glucocorticoid-treated patients. *BMJ* 1973;2:147.

Reports correlating results of prospective ACTH testing and later response to operative stress.

Lamberts SWJ, Bruining HA, de Jong FH. Corticosteroid therapy in severe illness. *N Engl J Med* 1997;337:1285.

Review of the normal adrenal response to stress and the treatment, during stress, of patients with adrenal dysfunction.

Magiakou MA, Chrousos GP. Corticosteroid therapy, nonendocrine disease, and corticosteroid withdrawal. In: Bardin CW, ed. *Current therapy in endocrinology*. St. Louis: CV Mosby, 1997:138.

Reviews adrenal suppression, stress, and therapy.

Masterson GR, Mostafa SM. Editorial II: Adrenocorticol function in critical illness. *Br J Anaesth* 1998;81:308.

Critical review of studies on adrenocorticol dysfunction and critical illness.

Oelkers W. Adrenal insufficiency. *N Engl J Med* 1996;335:1206.

Review of the general topic of adrenal insufficiency, both acute and chronic. Discusses the various tests to be used and treatment.

Salem M, Tainsh RE, Bromberg J, et al. Perioperative glucocorticoid coverage. *Ann Surg* 1994;219:416.

Excellent review of the physiology, diagnosis, and treatment of patients with absent or suppressed adrenocorticol function. Recommends lower doses of glucocorticoids than heretofore.

Streeten DHP. Shortcomings in the low-dose (1 μg) ACTH test for the diagnosis of ACTH deficiency states [Editorial]. *J Clin Endocrinol Metab* 1999;84:835.

Discusses the merits and demerits of low-dose ACTH testing. A thoughtful discussion of the article by Thaler and Blevins.

Szalados JE, Vukmir RB. Acute adrenal insufficiency resulting from adrenal hemorrhage as indicated by post-operative hypotension. *Intensive Care Med* 1994;20:216.

Reports on the incidence, diagnosis, and therapy of acute adrenal insufficiency caused by adrenal hemorrhage. This problem is being recognized more frequently than in the past.

Thaler LM, Blevins LS. The low dose (1-μg) adrenocorticotropin stimulation test in the evaluation of patients with suspected central adrenal insufficiency. *J Clin Endocrinol Metab* 1998;83:2726.

An endorsement for the low-dose ACTH test in the diagnosis of adrenocorticol dysfunction as proposed by Streeten.

Udelsman R, Ramp J, Gallucci WT, et al. Adaptation during surgical stress: a reevaluation of the role of glucocorticoids. *J Clin Invest* 1986;77:1377.

An argument against supraphysiologic glucocorticoid treatment during stress in adrenal insufficiency. The study was done using cynomolgus monkeys, but is applicable to humans.

89. DISORDERS OF MINERAL METABOLISM

Daniel T. Baran

I. General principles. Disorders of mineral metabolism occur frequently in patients admitted to intensive care units. These disorders are rarely the primary cause of admission, but they frequently exacerbate existing medical situations. Calcium, magnesium, and phosphate are instrumental for normal cellular function and neural signaling. Their metabolic balance is controlled by the interaction of parathyroid hormone (PTH), 1α, 25-dihydroxyvitamin D_3 (1,25 D), and calcitonin.

II. Pathogenesis of calcium disorders. Most total body calcium is located in bone. Less than 1% is found in extracellular fluids, where it is either free or bound to albumin or other anions. The free form of the calcium is biologically active. Changes in acid-base balance can affect the binding of calcium to albumin with alkalosis increasing binding and decreasing the free form. It is best to measure the free, ionized calcium directly when a question of altered calcium levels arises in the acutely ill patient.

Calcium balance depends on bone resorption and formation, intestinal absorption, and renal excretion. PTH increases bone resorption and renal calcium reabsorption directly, and indirectly enhances intestinal absorption by increasing 1,25 D levels. 1,25 D increases intestinal calcium absorption and bone resorption. Calcitonin inhibits bone resorption and increases renal calcium excretion.

III. Diagnosis of hypercalcemia. Hypercalcemia can result from increased bone resorption, decreased renal excretion, increased intestinal calcium absorption, or a combination of these mechanisms. The signs and symptoms of hypercalcemia can be divided into four groups: (a) mental, (b) neurologic, (c) intestinal and urologic, and (d) cardiovascular. The mental manifestations of hypercalcemia vary from stupor to coma. The neurologic effects include reduced muscle tone and reflexes. The intestinal and urologic signs include vomiting, polyuria, polydipsia, and constipation. The major cardiovascular effect of hypercalcemia is shortening of the QT interval on electrocardiogram (ECG). In the presence of ventricular ectopic beats, a shortened QT interval increases the potential for fatal arrhythmias.

The differential diagnosis of hypercalcemia includes malignancy and primary hyperparathyroidism. These two conditions account for 90% of all hypercalcemia cases. The malignancies most often associated with hypercalcemia include lung, breast, hematologic (myeloma and lymphoma), head and neck, and renal. Other causes of hypercalcemia include granulomatous disease, thyrotoxicosis, immobilization, vitamin D intoxication, Addison's disease, and familial hypocalciuric hypercalcemia.

An ionized calcium level is the most accurate marker of calcium levels. A total serum calcium level usually determines the diagnosis of hypercalcemia. Depending on the clinical situation, PTH and thyroid-stimulating hormone levels, along with urine protein electrophoresis and a bone scan, can help in establishing the cause of the hypercalcemia.

IV. Treatment of hypercalcemia. General measures in management involve attempts to (a) hydrate the patient and increase renal calcium clearance, (b) decrease bone resorption, and (c) decrease intestinal calcium absorption. Hydration plays a pivotal role in the management of the patient because response is rapid. Saline hydration creates a diuresis that increases renal calcium excretion. The aim of therapy is to achieve a urine output of 3 to 5 L/24 h. This usually requires 4 to 6 L/24 h of normal saline. Intravenous (IV) administration of furosemide (40–80 mg) prevents fluid overload and also inhibits renal distal tubular calcium reabsorption. Measurement of serum electrolytes is mandatory. Bone resorption can be decreased by administration of calcitonin (100 U subcutaneously every 6 hours) and pamidronate disodium (60 mg IV over 4 hours). Because of delay in the reduction of serum calcium with IV pamidronate, it has been used in conjunction with calcitonin to produce rapid and sustained decrements in serum calcium.

V. Diagnosis of hypocalcemia. The most frequent cause of hypocalcemia is low serum albumin concentrations in the critically ill patient. Ionized calcium is normal. True hypocalcemia (low ionized calcium) is usually caused by hypoparathyroidism, vitamin D deficiency, hyperphosphatemia, or magnesium deficiency. PTH, 25-hydroxyvitamin D_3, magnesium, and phosphate levels usually identify the cause. Abnormalities in liver function tests and impaired intestinal absorption can also be contributing factors.

VI. Treatment of hypocalcemia. Treatment of hypocalcemia depends on its severity and chronicity. Symptomatic patients should be treated with IV calcium. Either calcium gluconate (93 mg of elemental calcium in a 10-ml vial) or calcium chloride (272 mg of elemental calcium in a 10-ml vial) should be administered in 50 to 100 ml 5% dextrose in water over 10 to 15 minutes in the symptomatic patient. An infusion of 1 to 2 mg calcium/kg/h can be continued until the ionized calcium value is 4.5 mg/dl or the total calcium is 7 mg/dl. In the hypoparathyroid patient, calcium should be maintained between 8 and 8.5 mg/dl. In the absence of PTH, higher calcium levels are associated with hypercalciuria. Dietary supplements (1.5–2.5 g/d of elemental calcium) can be used for chronic therapy.

Vitamin D treatment is also usually required to maintain serum calcium levels in the hypoparathyroid patient. Ergocalciferol is usually given orally at a dose of 50,000 to 150,000 U/d. This preparation has a slow onset of action but has a wide safety margin. More rapid-acting preparations include 1α, 25-dihydroxyvitamin D_3 (0.25–1.0 μg/d). This active form of the vitamin is more potent but also more expensive for long-term management.

VII. Pathogenesis of magnesium disorders. Of extracellular magnesium, 30% circulates bound to albumin. Therefore, the albumin level should be known to interpret total magnesium levels. Levels are dependent on intestinal absorption and renal excretion. Hypomagnesemia usually results from decreased intestinal absorption (steatorrhea), increased renal excretion caused by an osmotic diuresis (hyperglycemia), or drugs (ethanol, aminoglycosides, cisplatin). Hypermagnesemia results in central nervous system depression, whereas hypomagnesemia is often attended by central nervous system hyperexcitability.

VIII. Diagnosis of hypermagnesemia. The most common cause of hypermagnesemia is renal failure, which can be aggravated by magnesium-containing antacids. Although serum magnesium may be elevated in diabetic ketoacidosis, this usually reflects dehydration and masks total body magnesium depletion.

IX. Treatment of hypermagnesemia. The neuromuscular depressant effects of elevated magnesium can be acutely antagonized by IV administration of 10 ml of 10% calcium gluconate (93 mg elemental calcium) diluted in 50 to 100 ml of 5% dextrose in water. Serum calcium must be monitored. In the presence of normal renal function, magnesium excretion can be increased by furosemide (40–80 mg IV) every 1 to 2 hours. Serum electrolytes need to be monitored. Dialysis is used to treat the symptomatic patient with hypermagnesemia when renal function is impaired.

X. Diagnosis of hypomagnesemia. Low serum magnesium levels are usually caused by a combination of decreased intake, decreased intestinal absorption, and increased renal excretion. Hypomagnesemia is frequently present in patients with malabsorption. Increased renal excretion is the most common cause of hypomagnesemia. Osmotic diuresis from hyperglycemia or hypercalcemia increases magnesium excretion. Hypomagnesemia is frequently encountered in the alcoholic patient. The central nervous system excitability seen in hypomagnesemic patients, in part, may be caused by hypocalcemia, which results from decreased PTH secretion and peripheral responsiveness to PTH.

XI. Treatment of hypomagnesemia. The patient with symptoms usually has a total body magnesium deficit of 1 to 3 mEq/kg body weight. Because of renal losses, replacement requires administration of 2 to 4 mEq/kg body weight. Magnesium (49 mEq; 6 ampules of 10% mg SO_4) can be given every 12 hours and administered IV over 3 to 6 hours. Serum magnesium and calcium levels need to be monitored. Oral therapy is adequate for mild magnesium deficiency.

XII. Pathogenesis of phosphorus disorders. Most of total body phosphate is found intracellularly. Because of shifts between compartments, serum phosphate does not reflect body stores. Acidosis causes a shift of phosphate from within cells to the extracellular compartment. Phosphate levels in the acidotic patient may be normal despite depletion of total body stores. Low serum phosphate directly stimulates renal production of 1α, 25-dihydroxyvitamin D_3. Phosphorus metabolism is closely linked to calcium and magnesium metabolism.

XIII. Diagnosis of hyperphosphatemia. Increased serum phosphate levels are most often encountered in the patient with renal failure or hypoparathyroidism. In both situations, hyperphosphatemia results from impaired renal excretion. Symptoms are usually caused by the accompanying hypocalcemia and not the hyperphosphatemia *per se*. Therapy should be directed at correction of the hypocalcemia.

XIV. Diagnosis of hypophosphatemia. Hypophosphatemia results from impaired intestinal phosphate absorption or increased renal excretion. Impaired absorption can result from phosphate-binding antacids or malnutrition, as seen in the alcoholic. Increased renal phosphate excretion is seen in hyperparathyroidism, vitamin D deficiency, and hyperglycemic states. The potential consequences of severe hypophosphatemia are impaired oxygen delivery to the tissues because of decreased 2,3-diphosphoglycerate levels, muscle weakness, and rhabdomyolysis.

XV. Treatment of hypophosphatemia. Severe hypophosphatemia (<1 mg/dl) requires parenteral therapy. Potassium phosphate for parenteral use contains 3 mmol/ml of phosphate. The phosphate (0.08–0.16 mmol/kg body weight) may be added to 5% dextrose in 50% normal saline and given over 6 hours. Doses should be 25% to 50% higher in the symptomatic patient and 25% to 50% lower if the patient is hypercalcemic. Parenteral therapy is contraindicated in the patient with renal failure or hypocalcemia. Intravenous phosphate in the patient with renal failure can cause hyperphosphatemia and worsen hypocalcemia. The usual oral dose of phosphate is 1 to 4 g/d in divided doses. Diarrhea is the most common side effect.

Selected Readings

Brody JJ, Bartl R, Burckhard T, et al. Current use of bisphosphonates in oncology. *J Clin Oncol* 1998;16:3890.

Discussion of the use of bisphosphonates in cancer patients and their indications for treatment of hypercalcemia of malignancy and metastatic bone pain, and for the prevention of the complications of multiple myeloma and metastatic bone disease, 68 references.

Bushinsky DA, Monk RD. Calcium. *Lancet* 1998;352:306.

A review of the mechanisms responsible for abnormalities in calcium homeostasis, the differential diagnosis of hypercalcemia and hypocalcemia, and appropriate therapy, 31 references.

Chan FK, Koberle LM, Thys-Jacobs S, et al. Differential diagnoses, causes, and management of hypercalcemia. *Curr Probl Surg* 1997;34:445.

Extensive discussion of recent advances in molecular biology and genetics that have facilitated the evaluation of patients presenting with hypercalcemia, 253 references.

Mundy GR, Guise TA. Hypercalcemia of malignancy. *Am J Med* 1997;103:134.

Clear description of the pathophysiology of hypercalcemia of malignancy, 81 references.

90. HYPOGLYCEMIA

Michael J. Thompson, John P. Mordes, and Aldo A. Rossini

I. Overview and definition. Hypoglycemia is frequently encountered in emergency departments and must be excluded in every patient with stupor or coma. Cases of refractory, prolonged hypoglycemia of unknown cause require admission to an intensive care unit (ICU). Severe hypoglycemia can lead to permanent neurologic damage.

No specific blood glucose concentration defines hypoglycemia. The physiologic definition of hypoglycemia is a blood glucose concentration sufficiently low as to cause the release of counterregulatory hormones (e.g., catecholamines) and impair the function of the central nervous system. Specifically, "Whipple's Triad" defines hypoglycemia as (a) documentation of a low blood glucose concentration; (b) concurrent symptoms of hypoglycemia; and (c) resolution of those symptoms after administration of glucose.

II. Pathophysiology. Hypoglycemia can be divided into fasting and nonfasting categories. "Nonfasting," "postprandial," "reactive" hypoglycemic states are not usually life-threatening and will not be discussed. "Fasting" hypoglycemia subsumes several subcategories: (a) states of overinsulinization, (b) states of impaired counterregulation, (c) states of inadequate endogenous glucose production, and (d) states in which gluconeogenic substrates are unavailable. Physiologically, most medication-induced hypoglycemia represents "fasting" hypoglycemia.

A. Hypoglycemia caused by excess insulin

1. **Insulin overdose.** Insulin overdose is the most common cause of hypoglycemia. In most cases, the overdose is inadvertent, the consequence of a missed meal or increased intensity of exercise. Patients with long-standing diabetes may be at increased risk of hypoglycemia because of increased sensitivity to regular insulin and defective counterregulatory responses. *Intentional overdoses* occur in both diabetic and nondiabetic individuals. Self-induced hypoglycemia should be suspected in anyone with access to insulin or oral hypoglycemic agents who experiences unexplained hypoglycemia.
2. **Sulfonylurea-class oral hypoglycemic agents.** This class of drugs enhances insulin secretion by pancreatic beta cells. Sulfonylurea overdose is the leading cause of hypoglycemia in diabetic persons aged more than 60 years. It typically occurs in the setting of acute or chronic starvation superimposed on mild to moderate liver or kidney failure. Accidental or intentional overdosage with sulfonylureas can also cause hypoglycemia in younger persons. Severe hypoglycemia has resulted from inadvertent substitution of an oral hypoglycemic agent for a different medication (e.g., chlorpropamide for chlorpromazine).
3. **Nonsulfonylurea-class oral hypoglycemic agents.** Oral hypoglycemic drugs of the biguanide class inhibit gluconeogenesis. Biguanide monotherapy is generally not a cause hypoglycemia. Drugs of the thiazolidinedione class and α-glucosidase inhibitors do *not* cause hypoglycemia when used as monotherapy, but these drugs can potentiate hypoglycemia caused by insulin or sulfonylureas.
4. **Drugs other than oral hypoglycemic agents.** In addition to sulfonylureas, a number of other medications can produce hypoglycemia by increasing circulating insulin concentration. Some of these are listed in Table 90-1.
5. **Insulinomas and other tumors.** Insulin-secreting pancreatic islet cell tumors are very rare. They classically cause fasting hypoglycemia. Paraneoplastic hypoglycemia can be caused by tumors that secrete insulinlike growth factors. Nesidioblastosis (nonmalignant islet cell adenomatosis) is another unusual cause of hypoglycemia from insulin use in children.
6. **"Autoimmune" or antibody-mediated hypoglycemia** is a rare condition in which endogenous autoantibodies bind to and activate the insulin receptor.

TABLE 90-1. Drugs and toxins associated with hypoglycemia[a]

Drugs that increase circulating insulin concentrations	Drugs that impair gluconeogenesis	Unknown mechanism of action
Direct stimulants of insulin secretion	Hepatotoxins (Amanitatoxin)	Acetazolamide (Diamox)
Acetohexamide (Dymelor)	Acetaminophen (Tylenol, Tempra)	Acetylsalicylic acid (Aspirin)
Chloroquine (Aralen)	Propoxyphene (Darvon)	Aluminum hydroxide (Dialume)
Disopyramide (Norpace)	Agents that decrease activity of gluconeogenic enzymes	Captopril (Capoten)
Glimepiride (Amaryl)	Metoprolol (Lopressor)	Chlorpromazine (Thorazine)
Glipizide (Glucotrol)	Nadolol (Corgard)	Cimetidine (Tagamet)
Glyburide (Micronase, Diabeta, Glynase)	Phenformin	Diphenhydramine (Benadryl)
Glibenclamide	Metformin (Glucophage)	Doxepin (Sinequan, Adapin)
Pentamidine (Pentam)	Pindolol (Visken)	Enalapril (Vasotec)
Quinidine	Propranolol (Inderal)	Ethylenediaminetetraacetic acid (EDTA, Versene)
Quinine	Hypoglycin	Haloperidol (Haldol)
Ritodrine (Yutopar)	Ethanol	Isoxsuprine
Terbutaline (Brethine, Bricanyl)		Lidocaine (Xylocaine)
Tolazamide (Tolinase)		Lithium (Eskalith)
Tolbutamide (Orinase)		Oxytetracycline (Terramycin)
Trimethoprim/sulfamethoxazole (Bactrim, Septra)		Paraaminobenzoic acid (PABA)
Agents that enhance the action of sulfonylureas		Paraaminosalicylic acid (PASA)
Bishydroxycoumarin (Dicoumarol)		Phenytoin (Dilantin)
Imipramine (Tofranil)		Ranitidine (Zantac)
Phenylbutazone (Butazolidin)		Sulfadiazine
		Sulfisoxazole (Gantrisin)
		Warfarin (Coumadin)

[a] Adapted from Seltzer HS: Drug-induced hypoglycemia: a review of 1418 Cases. *Endocrinol Metabol Clin of North Am,* 1989;18:163–183. A sampling of common trade names is shown in parenthesis; the enumeration of trade names is not exhaustive. Data for some listed agents may be very limited

B. Hypoglycemia associated with deficiencies in counterregulatory hormones

1. **Adrenal disease.** Glucocorticoid deficiency commonly causes hypoglycemia in children but not in adults.
2. **Pituitary disease.** Patients with hypopituitarism can develop hypoglycemia because of deficiencies of growth or thyroid hormone.
3. **Glucagon.** Glucagon deficiency is the rarest cause of hypoglycemia of endocrine origin.

C. Hypoglycemia from inadequate production of endogenous glucose

1. **Liver disease.** Hypoglycemia because of abnormal liver function generally does not occur until hepatic injury is severe. Hepatotoxins that can impair gluconeogenesis and cause hypoglycemia include carbon tetrachloride, the *Amanita phalloides* mushroom toxin, and urethane. Hepatic congestion because of severe congestive heart failure rarely causes hypoglycemia.
2. **Kidney disease.** Symptomatic hypoglycemia occurs in many diabetic patients undergoing dialysis. The cause may involve increased glucose-stimulated insulin release resulting from the high glucose concentration in the dialysate and impaired clearance of insulin because of the underlying renal disease. "Spontaneous" fasting hypoglycemia has been reported to occur in nondiabetic patients with end-stage renal disease.
3. **Ethanol-induced hypoglycemia (alcoholic Ketoacidosis).** Ethanol inhibits gluconeogenesis and the hepatic uptake of gluconeogenic precursors. Hypoglycemia can occur more than a day after the ingestion of a sufficient amount of ethanol. Ketonuria and ketonemia are usually present. Children and chronic alcohol abusers are most susceptible. The condition most commonly occurs in the setting of poor food intake and depleted glycogen stores. More information can be found in Chapter 86.
4. **Drugs.** Some of the many drugs and poisons that do not increase circulating insulin but nonetheless cause hypoglycemia are listed in Table 90-1. Beta blockers prevent the normal glycogenolytic and gluconeogenic response to hypoglycemia and can mask adrenergic symptoms. Salicylate intoxication causes hypoglycemia commonly in children but only rarely in adults. Hypoglycemia associated with angiotensin-converting enzyme inhibitors been reported in patients with diabetes.
5. **Sepsis** has occasionally been implicated as a cause of hypoglycemia. Septic hypoglycemic patients are often acidotic, and the fatality rate is high.
6. **Congenital enzymatic deficiencies** typically produce hypoglycemia in the context of glycogen storage disease or impaired hepatic gluconeogenesis. These uncommon conditions usually present in infancy.

D. Fasting hypoglycemia because of the unavailability of gluconeogenic substrate. The prototypic disease in which substrate deficiency leads to hypoglycemia is nonketotic hypoglycemia of childhood. The hallmark of the disease is a low basal blood concentration of the gluconeogenic precursor alanine.

III. Presentation and clinical findings

A. Adrenergic signs and symptoms are caused by counterregulatory hormones (catecholamines) released in response to hypoglycemia. The most prominent symptoms and signs are weakness, palpitations, anxiety, diaphoresis, tachycardia, peripheral vasoconstriction, and widening of the pulse pressure.

B. Neurologic signs and symptoms of neuroglycopenia include hunger, headache, confusion, slurred speech, and other nonspecific behavioral changes. These can progress to lethargy, obtundation, seizures, and coma.

IV. Laboratory. Obtain blood *and* urine samples from comatose hypoglycemic patients *when they are first seen.* This will allow appropriate assays for sulfonylureas or insulin to be performed later, if indicated.

A. Blood glucose concentration. The normal plasma glucose concentration is 60 to 120 mg/dl (3.3–6.7 mm). Whole blood glucose and capillary fingerstick glucose levels are 15% to 20% lower. Fingerstick blood glucose determinations can be less accurate at the lower end of their scale. Symptoms of hypoglycemia generally occur when the glucose concentration is less than 50 mg/dl (2.8 mm) in plasma or less than 40 mg/dl (2.2 mm) in whole blood. After approximately 48 hours of starvation, however, many individuals, particularly women, have a plasma glucose concentration of less than 50 mg/dl (2.8 mm). After 72 hours of fasting, the plasma glucose concentration can approach 40 mg/dl (2.2 mm) in asymptomatic individuals. Comparably "low" plasma glucose concentrations also occur in pregnancy during which the normal fasting plasma glucose concentration is 60 mg/dl or less (3.3 mm). "Factitious hypoglycemia" can occur as a result of storing blood samples at room temperature before testing. Glucose concentration in the test tube can decline at a rate of about 7%/h. The effect is enhanced if large numbers of white blood cells are present as the result of severe leukocytosis or leukemia.

B. Ketonuria. Low plasma glucose concentrations are associated with low circulating insulin levels that in turn promote lipolysis and ketogenesis. Hypoglycemia associated with ketonuria is unlikely to result from overinsulinization.

C. Detection of drugs and toxins. If oral agent abuse is suspected, *serum* and urine should be screened for sulfonylurea compounds. Not readily available as part of toxic screens, testing for sulfonylurea drugs must be requested specifically.

D. Detection of surreptitiously injected insulin. When abusive insulin self-administration is suspected, obtain simultaneous insulin and C-peptide blood concentrations during a hypoglycemic episode. Insulin and C-peptide are normally cosecreted by the pancreas in equimolar quantities, but the latter is not present in commercial insulin.

E. Insulinoma. Insulinomas are often small and difficult to visualize radiographically. In patients with suspected insulinoma, a fasting immunoreactive insulin (IRI, measured in μU/ml) and glucose (mg/dl) should be obtained. If the IRI-glucose ratio is greater than 0.3, the insulin concentration may be inappropriately high. Another useful test is the serum concentration of proinsulin, which is typically elevated to more than 30% of the insulin concentration in cases of insulinoma.

F. Other. Additional tests should be ordered as appropriate. In general, these should always include studies of hepatic and renal function. A cosyntropin test can be performed if adrenal insufficiency is suspected.

V. Treatment

A. Glucose. Treat presumed or documented hypoglycemia in the patient with stupor or coma with an intravenous (IV) injection of 50 ml of D50W over 3 to 5 minutes. The treatment is lifesaving in the presence of hypoglycemic coma and harmless when given to patients with coma from other causes. Avoid subcutaneous extravasation; the solution is hypertonic and can cause local tissue damage and pain. Treatment with D50W usually leads to improved mental status within minutes, but patients who are elderly or who have had very prolonged hypoglycemia may respond slowly.

If a patient is sufficiently alert and cooperative, oral carbohydrates (e.g., sucrose in orange juice or glucose tablets) can be given. Hypoglycemia in patients taking α-glucosidase inhibitors should be treated with *monomeric* glucose or fructose (e.g., fruit juice) because these drugs delay absorption of complex sugars, including sucrose.

The most common error in management is inadequate treatment leading to recurrence of symptoms. After the first bolus of D50W is given, an infusion of D5W or D10W glucose should be started in any patient whose hypoglycemic episode is not caused by exogenous short- or intermediate-acting insulin. Severe cases of unexplained hypoglycemia require intensive care monitoring. Blood glucose should be monitored every 1 to 3 hours and the serum glucose concentration maintained at a target level of at least 100 mg/dl.

To determine whether parenteral glucose is no longer needed, the infusion should be discontinued and blood glucose concentration measured every 15 minutes. If a patient is unable to maintain a blood glucose concentration more than 50 mg/dl or if the patient becomes symptomatic, reinstitution of glucose therapy is necessary.

When the cause of hypoglycemia is sulfonylurea ingestion, patients should usually be admitted to the hospital because continuous IV glucose is mandatory. The half-life of many drugs in this class is more than 24 hours. Meals should be provided if the patient can eat. It is particularly important that glucose infusions be continued while patients recovering from a sulfonylurea overdose are asleep. Patients with this condition may require 2 to 3 days of IV glucose therapy. The somatostatin analog, octreotide, which inhibits insulin secretion, can be used as an adjunct to the treatment of severe oral agent overdosage.

B. Glucagon. Glucagon is a useful drug, particularly in out-of-hospital treatment of hypoglycemia. It is useful in the emergency department or ICU if hypoglycemic coma occurs in a patient without IV access. It is most effective in patients with ample liver glycogen stores.

C. Agents that block insulin secretion. When refractory hypoglycemia is caused by an insulinoma or nesidioblastosis, it may be necessary on rare occasions to supplement glucose infusion therapy with drugs that inhibit insulin secretion. These include diazoxide and the somatostatin analog octreotide.

D. Steroids. When the cause of severe, refractory hypoglycemia is obscure, adrenocortical steroids can be given to increase gluconeogenic substrates and inhibit insulin action in the periphery.

E. Determine the precipitating factor. Glucose corrects hypoglycemia but not what causes it. The most common cause of hypoglycemia is inadvertent insulin overdosage because of changes in diet, increases in exercise, or injection of the wrong kind of insulin. Other causes of hypoglycemia include drugs and intercurrent illnesses, including renal or hepatic failure. A patient should not be discharged until one of these processes, outlined in the section on pathophysiology, is identified and an appropriate follow-up plan is formulated.

VI. Pearls. Key points and pitfalls.

A. Think about drugs! Many drugs cause hypoglycemia. In particular, persons with diabetes who become intoxicated can develop life-threatening, profound hypoglycemia from the metabolic synergy of ethanol and insulin.

B. Measure urinary ketones! Urinary ketones in a hypoglycemic patient generally excludes hyperinsulinemia as the cause of the low glucose concentration.

C. Beware of recurrent hypoglycemia! Many sulfonylurea-class oral hypoglycemic agents have a very long duration of action. Prolonged treatment is often required in cases of sulfonylurea overdose.

D. Be alert for "hypoglycemia unawareness!" Patients with diabetes may fail to perceive the symptoms of hypoglycemia, especially when it occurs precipitously. Hypoglycemia unawareness can result from frequent hypoglycemic episodes and medicines that interfere with recovery from hypoglycemia (e.g., beta blockers). Patients who have had diabetes for many years experience blunting of the normal counterregulatory response to hypoglycemia and may also become exquisitely sensitive to regular insulin (and therefore become hypoglycemic rapidly).

Selected Readings

Boyle PJ, Justice K, Krentz AJ, et al. Octreotide reverses hyperinsulinemia and prevents hypoglycemia induced by sulfonylurea overdoses. *J Clin Endocrinol Metab* 1993;76:752.

Useful information on this novel therapeutic agent.

Cryer PE. Hypoglycemia: the limiting factor in the management of IDDM. *Diabetes* 1994;43:1378.

Review of hypoglycemia by a leading international authority.

Klonoff DC, Barrett BJ, Nolte MS, et al. Hypoglycemia following inadvertent and factitious sulfonylurea overdosages. *Diabetes Care* 1995;18:563.

Excellent review of this common cause of hypoglycemia.

Mordes JP, Thompson MJ, Desemone J, et al. Hypoglycemia. In Irwin RS, Cerra FB, Rippe JM, eds. *Intensive care medicine,* 4th ed. Philadelphia: Lippincott–Raven; 1998:1297.

The full-length version of this chapter.

Seltzer HS. Drug-induced hypoglycemia. A review of 1418 cases. *Endocrinol Metab Clin North Am* 1989;18:163.

The most comprehensive reference on this subject.

Whipple AO. The surgical therapy of hyperinsulinism. *J Int Chirurgie* 1938;3:237.

The source article for the classic definition of hypoglycemia.

91. SICK EUTHYROID SYNDROME

Alan P. Farwell

I. General principles. Critical illness causes multiple alterations in thyroid hormone concentrations in patients who have no previously diagnosed intrinsic thyroid disease. These effects are nonspecific and relate to the severity of the illness. Despite abnormalities in serum thyroid hormone parameters, little evidence indicates that these patients have clinically significant thyroid dysfunction. Because a wide variety of illnesses tend to result in the same changes in serum thyroid hormones, such alterations in thyroid hormone indexes has been termed the "sick euthyroid syndrome." These changes are rarely isolated and often are associated with alterations in other endocrine systems, such as reductions in serum gonadotropin and sex hormone concentrations and increases in serum corticotropin (ACTH) and cortisol. Thus, the sick euthyroid syndrome should not be viewed as an isolated pathologic event but, instead, as part of a coordinated systemic reaction to illness that involves both the immune and endocrine systems.

II. Alterations in thyroid hormone economy with critical illness. The widespread changes in thyroid hormone economy in the critically ill patient occur as a result of (a) alterations in the peripheral metabolism of the thyroid hormones, (b) alterations in the regulation of the pituitary-thyroid axis, and (c) alterations in the binding of thyroid hormone to serum binding proteins.

A. Peripheral metabolic pathways. The major pathway of metabolism of T_4 is by sequential monodeiodination to generate 3,5,3′-triiodothyronine (T_3, activating pathway) or 3,3′, 5′-triiodothyronine (rT_3, inactivating pathway). One of the first alterations in thyroid hormone metabolism in acute illness is impairment in T_4 to T_3 conversion in peripheral tissues, which is affected by a wide variety of factors (Table 91-1). Because more than 80% of T_3 is derived from deiodination of T_4 in peripheral tissues, T_3 levels fall soon after the onset of acute illness. In contrast, inner ring deiodination of T_4 to produce rT_3 is unaffected by acute illness. However, degradation of rT_3 is impaired and levels of this inactive hormone rise in proportion to the fall in T_3 levels.

B. Pituitary-thyroid axis. Synthesis and secretion of thyroid hormone is under the control of the anterior pituitary hormone, thyrotropin (TSH), in a classic negative feedback system. Serum TSH levels are usually normal early in acute illness. However, TSH levels often fall as the illness progresses because of the effects of a variety of inhibitory factors that are common in the treatment of the critically ill patient (Table 91-2). Most common is the use of dopamine and the increased levels of glucocorticoids, either endogeneous or exogenous, both of which have a direct inhibitory effect on TSH secretion. Inhibitory signals from higher cortical centers can also play a role in decreasing TSH secretion and certain thyroid hormone metabolites that are increased in nonthyroidal illness.

C. Serum binding proteins. Both T_4 (99.97% bound) and T_3 (99.7% bound) circulate in the serum bound primarily to thyronine-binding protein (TBG), as well as several other proteins, all of which are synthesized in the liver. The binding of thyroid hormones to TBG is affected by a variety of factors in acute illness (Table 91-3). Essential to the understanding of the alterations of circulating thyroid hormones seen in critical illness is the "free hormone concept:" only the unbound hormone has any metabolic activity. Because of the high degree of binding of T_4 and T_3 to TBG, changes in either the concentrations of, or binding to, TBG would have major effects on the total serum hormone levels. However, because the pituitary responds to and regulates the circulating free hormone levels, minimal changes are actually seen in the free hormone concentrations and, thus, in overall thyroid function.

D. Pathogenesis. The cause of the alterations in thyroid hormone economy in critical illness is largely unknown. Cytokines have been shown to reproduce many

TABLE 91-1. Factors that inhibit T_4 to T_3 conversion in peripheral tissues

Acute and chronic illness
Caloric deprivation
Malnutrition
Glucocorticoids
β-adrenergic blocking drugs (e.g., propranalol)
Oral cholecytographic agents (e.g., iopanoic acid, sodium ipodate))
Propylthiouracil
Fatty acids
Fetal/neonatal period

of the features of the sick euthyroid syndrome in both animal and human studies, in particular, tumor necrosis factor α, IL-1, and IL-6, when administered in pharmacologic doses. Whether the sick euthyroid syndrome results from activation of the cytokine network or simply represents an endocrine response to systemic illness resulting from the same mediators that trigger the cytokine cascade remains to be determined.

III. Stages of the sick euthyroid syndrome. The changes in serum concentrations of thyroid hormone that are observed in critically ill patients represent a continuum of changes that depends on the severity of the illness (Fig. 91-1). Thus, the wide spectrum of changes observed often results from the differing points in the course of the illness that the thyroid function tests were obtained.

A. Low T_3 state. Common to all of the abnormalities in thyroid hormone concentrations seen in critically ill patients is a substantial depression of serum T_3 levels, which can occur as early as 24 hours after the onset of illness and can affect over half of the patients admitted to the medical service. The low T_3 state

TABLE 91-2. Factors that alter TSH secretion

Increase	Decrease
Chlorpromazine	Acute and chronic illness
Cimetidine	Adrenergic agonists
Domperidine	Caloric restriction
Dopamine antagonists	Carbamazapine
Haloperidol	Clofibrate
Iodide	Cyproheptadine
Lithium	Dopamine and dopamine agonists
Metoclopramide	Endogeneous depression
Sulphapyridine	Glucocorticoids
X-ray contrast agents	IGF-1
	Metergoline
	Methylsergide
	Opiates
	Phenytoin
	Phentolamine
	Pimozide
	Somatostatin
	Serotonin
	Surgical stress
	Thyroid hormone metabolites

TSH, thyroid-stimulating hormone.

TABLE 91-3. Factors that alter binding of T_4 to TBG

	Increase binding	Decrease binding
Drugs		
	Estrogens Methadone Clofibrate 5-Fluorouracil Heroin Tamoxifen	Glucocorticoids Androgens L-asparaginase Salicylates Furosemide Antiseizure medications (phenytoin, tegretol)
Systemic factors		
	Liver disease Porphyria HIV infection Inherited	Inherited Acute illness

TBG.

can be explained solely by the impairment of peripheral T_4 to T_3 conversion. Clinically, these patients appear euthyroid, although mild prolongation in Achilles tendon reflex time is found in some patients.

B. High T_4 state. Serum T_4 levels may be elevated early in acute illness because of either the acute inhibition of T_4 to T_3 conversion or increased TBG levels. This is seen most often in the elderly and in patients with psychiatric disorders. As the duration of illness increases, non-deiodinative pathways of T_4 degradation increase and return serum T_4 levels to the normal range.

C. Low T_4 state. As the severity and the duration of the illness increases, serum total T_4 levels may decrease into the subnormal range. Contributing to this decrease in serum T_4 levels are (a) a decrease in the binding of T_4 to TBG, (b) a decrease in serum TSH levels leading to decreased production of T_4, and (c) an increase in non-deiodinative pathways of T_4 metabolism. The decline in serum T_4 levels correlates with prognosis in the intensive care unit (ICU), with the

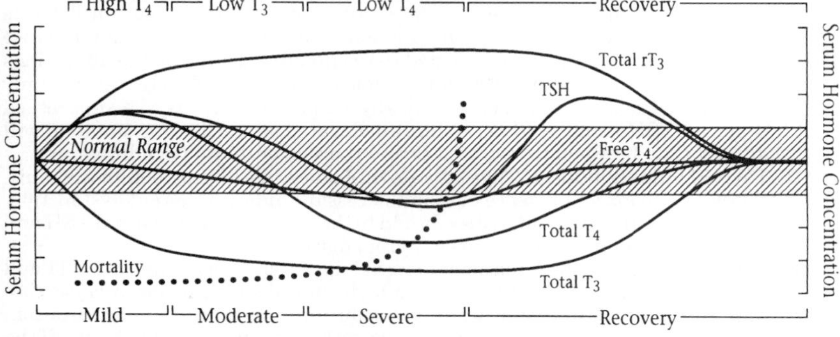

FIG. 91-1. Alterations in thyroid hormone concentrations with critical illness. Schematic representation of the continuum of changes in serum thyroid hormone levels in patients with nonthyroidal illness. These alterations become more pronounced with increasing severity of the illness and return to the normal range as the illness subsides and the patient recovers. A rapidly rising mortality rate accompanies the fall in total and free T_4 levels.

mortality rate increasing as serum T_4 levels drop below 4 μg/dl and approaching 80% in patients with serum T_4 levels less than 2 μg/dl. Despite marked decreases in serum total T_4 and T_3 levels to the hypothyroid range in the critically ill patient, the free hormone levels are often normal and most patients appear eumetabolic. Thus, the low T_4 state is more likely a marker of multisystem failure in these critically ill patients than a true hormone-deficient state.

D. Recovery state. As acute illness resolves, so do the alterations in thyroid hormone concentrations. This stage can be prolonged and is characterized by modest increases in serum TSH levels. Full recovery, with restoration of thyroid hormone levels to the normal range, can take up to several months after the patient is discharged from the hospital.

IV. Evaluation. The routine screening of an ICU population for thyroid dysfunction is not recommended because of the high prevalence of abnormal thyroid function tests and low prevalence of true thyroid dysfunction. Whenever possible, it is best to defer evaluation of the thyroid-pituitary axis until the patient has recovered from an acute illness. In principle, when thyroid function tests are ordered in a hospitalized patient, it should be with a high clinical index of suspicion for the presence of thyroid dysfunction. Because every test of thyroid hormone function can be altered in the critically ill patient, no single test can definitively rule in or rule out the presence of intrinsic thyroid dysfunction (Table 91-4).

A. TSH assays. The sensitive TSH assay is currently the best screening test for thyroid dysfunction in the healthy, ambulatory patient. The same does not hold true for the ill patient, as abnormal TSH values have been reported in up to 20% of hospitalized patients, more than 80% of which have no intrinsic thyroid dysfunction on followup testing when healthy. Thus, transient abnormalities in TSH secretion are commonplace in acute illness and abnormal TSH values require additional biochemical and clinical evaluation before a diagnosis of thyroid dysfunction can be made.

B. Free T_4 concentrations. Because abnormalities in binding to serum proteins are commonplace, total T_4 measurements alone are of little use in the acutely ill patient. Free T_4 concentrations are most frequently measured indirectly by the free T_4 index (FTI), which is determined by multiplying the total T_4 concentration by either the T_3- or T_4-resin uptake, which is an inverse estimate of serum TBG concentrations, or by the thyroid hormone binding ratio (THBR), which normalizes the resin uptake test. Methods to directly measure free thyroid hormone levels are also available; however, they may be no more accurate than the FTI and are often more expensive. The sensitivity of the FTI in hospitalized patients has been reported to be 92.3%, as compared with 90.7% for the sensitive TSH test.

C. Total T_3. No indication is seen for the routine measurement of serum T_3 levels in the initial evaluation of thyroid function in the critically ill patient, because serum T_3 concentrations are affected to the greatest degree by the alterations in thyroid hormone economy resulting from acute illness. This test should only be obtained if thyrotoxicosis is clinically suspected in cases of a suppressed sensitive TSH value. In this setting, an elevated serum T_3 concentration will differentiate between thyrotoxicosis and the sick euthyroid syndrome.

D. Thyroid autoantibodies. Thyroid autoantibodies (antithyroglobulin and antithyroid peroxidase) presence does not necessary indicate thyroid dysfunction. However, thyroid autoantibodies do add to the specificity of abnormal TSH and FTI values in diagnosing intrinsic thyroid disease.

E. Diagnostic approach. A reasonable initial approach is to obtain both FTI and TSH measurements in patients with a high clinical suspicion for intrinsic thyroid dysfunction. Assessment of these values in the context of the duration, severity, and stage of illness allows the correct diagnosis in most patients. If the diagnosis is still unclear, measurement of thyroid antibodies may be helpful as a marker of intrinsic thyroid disease. Only in the case of a suppressed TSH and a midnormal to high FTI is measurement of serum T_3 levels indicated.

V. Treatment for the sick euthyroid syndrome

A. General ICU patients. The question of whether the sick euthyroid syndrome in critically ill patients represents an adaptive or a pathologic response to illness

TABLE 91-4. Tests of thyroid function in the ICU

Tests	Typical normal range	Use	Limitation in acute illness
Thyroid-stimulating hormone (TSH)	0.4–5.0 mU/L	Best initial test to determine thyroid status in healthy patients	Loss of specificity, abnormal in up to 20% of hospitalized patients
Total T_4	4–12 μg/dl	Measures bound and free hormone in serum	Affected by alterations in serum-binding proteins
T_4- or T_3-resin uptake	25% to 35%	Estimate of the serum protein-binding sites	Affected by alterations in serum-binding proteins
Thyroid hormone binding ratio (THBR)	0.8–1.15	Estimate of the serum-protein binding sites	Affected by alterations in serum-binding proteins
Free T_4 index (FTI)	1–4 if use resin uptake 4–12 if use THBR	Estimate of free T_4 concentrations	Affected by alterations in serum-binding proteins
Free T_4, analog method	0.7–2.1 ng/dl	Direct measurement of free T_4 concentrations	May not be any more reliable than FTI
Free T_4, equilibrium dialysis method	0.7–2.1 ng/dl	Gold standard for measurement of free T_4 concentrations	Expensive, time consuming to perform, not readily available
Total T_3	75–180 ng/dl	Measures bound and free hormone in serum	Levels fall in all hospitalized patients, never a first line test
Free T_3	200–400 pg/dl	Direct measurement of free T_3 concentrations	No advantage to total T_3
Thyroid autoantibodies (anti-Tg, anti-TPO)	Negative	Determines presence of autoimmune thyroid disease	Second line test; may help predict presence of thyroid dysfunction

TPO, thyroid peroxidase; Tg, thyroglobulin.

remains unclear. What is clear is that supplemental thyroid hormone therapy, either in the form of L-T_4 or L-T_3, has no effect on morbidity or mortality. Thus, thyroid hormone replacement is not indicated in the routine ICU patient with the sick euthyroid syndrome.

B. Specialized patients. A theoretical basis exists for the use of T_3 to correct the acute drop in serum T_3 levels during cardiac bypass surgery. However, the clearly demonstrable benefit of T_3 repletion in animals has not been translated into similar benefit in humans undergoing coronary artery bypass in controlled clinical trials. Currently, no indication is seen for the routine use of T_3 in patients undergoing cardiac surgery. Similarly, the use of T_3 to "resuscitate" cardiac function in potential heart donors has been shown to have no effect if no antecedent cardiac dysfunction was present in the donor. A potential benefit has been shown with the use of T_3 in donors with preexisting cardiac dysfunction, suggesting that

T_3 may be beneficial to stabilize or improve cardiac function prior to cardiac transplantation. However, these studies have yet to be confirmed.

All premature infants have some degree of transient hypothyroxinemia because of the immaturity of thyroid function. Despite the potential theoretic benefit of normalizing T_4 in premature infants, studies have shown no beneficial effect on developmental outcome at 24 months. Thus, no indication is currently seen for the use of thyroid hormone treatment in premature infants.

Selected Readings

Braverman LE, Utiger RD, eds. *The thyroid,* 8th ed. Philadelphia: Lippincott Williams & Wilkins; 2000.

The most current and thorough text on clinical thyroidology.

Brent GA, Hershman JM. Thyroxine therapy in patients with severe nonthyroidal illnesses and low thyroxine concentration. J Clin *Endocrinol Metab* 1986;63:1.

Initial article demonstrating that L-T_4 replacement therapy in the sick euthyroid syndrome is of no benefit and may be harmful.

Farwell AP. Sick euthyroid syndrome. *J Intensive Care Med* 1997; 12:249.

Recent review with details of the points discussed in this chapter with extensive reference.

Hashimoto H, Igarashi N, Yachie A, et al. The relationship between serum levels of interleukin-6 and thyroid hormone in children with acute respiratory infection. *J Clin Endocrinol Metab* 1994;78:288.

Representative article on the attempts to link the development of the sick euthyroid syndrome to cytokine production during illness.

Kaptein EM, Weiner JM, Robinson WJ, et al. Relationship of altered thyroid hormone indices to survival in nonthyroidal illness. *Clin Endocrinol* (Oxf) 1982;16:565.

Classic article on the use of thyroid hormone indices as predictors of mortality in the critically ill patient.

Klemperer JD, Klein I, Gomez M, et al. Thyroid hormone treatment after coronary artery bypass surgery. *N Engl J Med* 1995;333:1522.

Examines the role of thyroid hormone replacement therapy in the sick euthyroid syndrome produced after coronary artery bypass surgery.

Novitzky D. Novel actions of thyroid hormone: the role of triiodothyronine in cardiac transplantation. *Thyroid* 1996;6:531.

Examines the role of T3 replacement therapy in the sick euthyroid syndrome following cardiac transplantation.

Slag MF, Morley JE, Elson MK, et al. Hypothyroxinemia in critically ill patients as a predictor of high mortality. *JAMA* 1981;245:43.

Classic article on the use of thyroid hormone indices as predictors of mortality in the critically ill patient.

Spencer CA. Clinical utility and cost-effectiveness of sensitive thyrotropin assays in ambulatory and hospitalized patients. *Mayo Clin Proc* 1988;63:1214.

This classic article documents the development and use of sensitive TSH assays by the investigators who developed them.

Spencer C, Elgen A, Shen D, et al. Specificity of sensitive assays of thyrotropin (TSH) used to screen for thyroid disease in hospitalized patients. *Clin Chem* 1987;33:1391.

This classic article documents the development and use of sensitive TSH assays by the investigators who developed them.

Surks MI, Chopra IJ, Mariash CN, et al. American Thyroid Association guidelines for the use of laboratory tests in thyroid disease. *JAMA* 1990;263:1529.

Guidelines published by the largest professional society of physicians and scientists dedicated to research and treatment of thyroid disease in the United States.

Van den Berghe G, de Zegher F, Lauwers P. Dopamine and the sick euthyroid syndrome in critical illness. *Clin Endocrinol* (Oxf) 1994;41:731.

Documents the effects of dopamine on TSH secretion, a major mediator of abnormal thyroid function tests in the ICU.

van Wassenaer AG, Kok JH, de Vijlder JJM, et al. Effects of thyroxine supplementation on neurologic development in infants born at less than 30 weeks gestation. *N Engl J Med* 1997;336:21.

Examines the role of thyroid hormone replacement therapy in the sick euthyroid syndrome produced by premature birth.

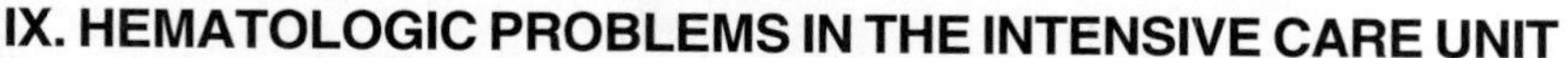

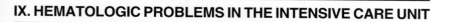

IX. HEMATOLOGIC PROBLEMS IN THE INTENSIVE CARE UNIT

92. ACQUIRED BLEEDING DISORDERS

Doreen B. Brettler and Robert V.B. Emmons

I. Platelet and coagulation physiology

A. Platelets. Platelet activation can be divided into three distinguishable events: adhesion, secretion, and aggregation. Adhesion is the property of stickiness whereby platelets interact with certain molecules (e.g., subendothelial collagen, and to a lesser extent, basement membrane and other subendothelial supporting elements). After adherence and cytoskeletal rearrangement, platelets are activated and secrete a number of substances including adenosine diphosphate (ADP), serotonin, coagulation factors, and platelet factor 4. Arachidonic acid is generated by activated platelets and channeled into thromboxane A_2 synthesis that mobilizes other platelets. Fibrinogen receptors are exposed, and platelets begin to aggregate in concert with the coagulation cascade and Von Willebrand factor to form a platelet thrombus.

B. Coagulation cascade. A sequential series of enzymatic reactions occurs at surfaces of activation between coagulation proteins that result in fibrin clot formation. Surfaces of physiologic importance in initiating clot formation appear to be collagen and subendothelial connective tissue that are exposed by injury, as well as platelet membrane phospholipids. All coagulation factor proteins are synthesized in the liver and factors II, VII, IX, and X require vitamin K for their normal synthesis. Vitamin K participates in a reaction that adds a carboxyl group to glutamic acid residues in the precursors of these factors responsible for calcium and phospholipid binding. Blockade of this reaction is the basis for the anticoagulation properties of warfarin. Von Willebrand factor, which is synthesized both by endothelial cells throughout the vascular system and by megakaryocytes, binds to platelets, the subendothelium, factor VIII, and fibrin.

C. Inhibition of clotting. A number of mechanisms limit the process of fibrin deposition, so that neither disseminated coagulation nor extensive local thrombosis occurs after injury. These mechanisms include self-inhibitors, specific inhibitors, and compartmentalization of reactions. Activated coagulation factors are rapidly cleared from the blood by cells of the reticuloendothelial system, primarily those in the liver. The major component of the fibrinolytic system is plasminogen, a serine protease that must be activated to plasmin by specific activators. Plasmin degrades fibrin clots as well as soluble fibrinogen to generate a number of fragments. These fibrin degradation products (FDPs) can inhibit additional fibrin monomer polymerization and thus predispose to poor clot formation and bleeding.

II. Laboratory evaluation of hemostasis

A. Platelets. Platelet number can be directly measured or estimated from the blood smear (one platelet per oil-immersion field is equivalent to ~ 10,000 platelets/µl). Platelet size on peripheral blood smear may also be helpful; large platelets suggest a shortened survival and rapid platelet turnover. Thrombocytopenia and platelet functional impairment can cause bleeding. The bleeding time measures various aspects of platelet function as well as vascular competency. The bleeding time is usually prolonged with any qualitative defect and thus has low specificity. Its value as a screening test to indicate the likelihood of bleeding as a result of a qualitative platelet disorder is low, and its use is not recommended for this purpose. However, it may be useful in specific disorders known to predispose to a long bleeding time (e.g., von Willebrand disease or uremia).

B. Coagulation cascade. The prothrombin time (PT) and partial thromboplastin time (PTT) are two general screening tests of the extrinsic and intrinsic coagulation systems, respectively. The PT and PTT are prolonged with one or more factor deficiencies or in the presence of acquired coagulation inhibitors. To determine whether a prolonged PT or PTT is attributable to a factor deficiency or an inhibitor, a mixing study is performed: the patient's plasma and pooled normal plasma are mixed in equal amounts and the appropriate test (PT or PTT) is performed on the mixture. Complete to nearly complete correction of the abnormality suggests a factor deficiency. Little or no correction immediately or a loss of correction after incubation favors the presence of an inhibitor. The finding of an abnormal PT or PTT is not uncommon in seriously ill, hospitalized patients. The thrombin time is a measure of the time required to convert fibrinogen to a fibrin clot after the addition of purified thrombin to plasma. It is often a helpful assay because it is prolonged in only three circumstances: deficient or functionally abnormal fibrinogen, heparin presence, or a high titer of FDP. FDP can also be measured using antibodies specific for cross-linked fibrin fragments (*d*-dimer). Traditional assays detect proteolytic fragments of fibrinogen or fibrin, whereas the *d*-dimer test specifically detects fibrin fragments. A positive *d*-dimer test indicates that thrombin was initially generated, that it converted fibrinogen to fibrin, and that plasmin acted on fibrin, meaning that intravascular coagulation with secondary fibrinolysis or disseminated intravascular coagulation (DIC) is present. A positive FDP finding does not discriminate between fibrinogen or fibrin proteolysis and, thus, between DIC and primary fibrinogenolysis.

III. Acquired qualitative platelet disorders

A. Drugs. The most common cause of qualitative platelet disorders is drugs. The main offenders are aspirin and other nonsteroidal antiinflammatory medications. Aspirin irreversibly acetylates and inactivates the enzyme cyclooxygenase, preventing the generation of prostaglandin intermediates and thromboxane A_2. These platelets no longer undergo release, bleeding time is prolonged, and secondary aggregation is poor or absent. One aspirin tablet (5 gr) is enough to prolong the bleeding time (1–2 times baseline) 2 hours later. In the patient who takes aspirin on a regular basis over several days, the bleeding time may take 7 to 10 days to normalize once aspirin is stopped. If bleeding is serious, platelet transfusions may be administered. A baseline and posttransfusion bleeding time should be obtained to assess the response. Other nonsteroidal antiinflammatory drugs cause a similar defect in cyclooxygenase activity, but the deficiency is reversible and lasts only as long as the drug is present in the circulation. Drugs specifically tailored to impair platelet function include the old drug, dipyridamole, and newer agents such as ticlopidine, clopidogrel, and specific platelet membrane IIb-IIIa inhibitors. A number of other drugs interfere with platelet function, many of which are commonly used in an intensive care setting. Table 92-1 lists the most likely offenders. None of these drugs is known for its tendency to induce spontaneous bleeding, use of any one can exacerbate or enhance underlying hemostatic defects or worsen traumatic bleeding. Correction of a drug-induced platelet defect requires cessation of the medication. The use of deamino-8-D-arginine vasopressin (DDAVP) has also been shown to improve the bleeding time in patients with some drug-induced qualitative platelet defects (see below). When drugs essential to the treatment of an individual cannot be easily discontinued, a risk-benefit assessment must be made carefully to determine whether to continue the drug in the face of bleeding.

B. Uremia. Uremia, a common cause of a functional platelet defect, is probably related to the accumulation of an uncleared metabolite. The bleeding time is often greater than 15 or 20 minutes. Peritoneal dialysis and, to a lesser extent, hemodialysis have been shown to improve the bleeding time. Infusions of cryoprecipitate or DDAVP in uremic patients have been successful in correcting the bleeding time, suggesting that von Willebrand factor (vWF) may be important in this defect, and DDAVP is known to increase the synthesis and plasma levels of factor vWF and VIII. Therapeutic improvement in the bleeding time has also been shown with the administration of estrogens, but the mechanism of this effect remains unknown. The infusion of donor platelets is not recommended in patients with uremia because the platelet defect results from the plasma environment and transfused platelets would be affected as much as endogenous platelets. If an invasive procedure is required in uremic patients whose bleeding time is prolonged, DDAVP at a dose of 0.3 μg/kg IV is indicated.

TABLE 92-1. Drugs that interfere with platelet functions

Classification	Examples
Antibiotics	Penicillin and derivatives Nitrofurantoin Hydroxychloroquine
Antihistamines and antitussives	Diphenhydramine and others Glycerol guaiacolate
Antiinflammatory agents	Aspirin and other nonsteroidal anti-inflammatory agents Corticosteroids
Antithrombotic agents	Heparin Dextran
Calcium channel blocking agents	Verapamil and others
Diuretics	Furosemide
Seritonin antagonists	Reserpine Cyproheptadine
Sympathetic blocking drugs	Alpha-blockers (phentolamine) Beta-blockers (propranolol)
Tranquilizers and antipsychotic agents	Phenothiazines and derivatives Tricyclic antidepressants
Vasodilators	Sodium nitroprusside Nitroglycerin
Xanthine derivatives	Theophylline, caffeine Dipyridamole
Miscellaneous	Clofibrate Ethanol

C. Myeloproliferative disorders. Myeloproliferative disorders are often associated with a qualitative platelet defect. The defect arises from a stem cell abnormality, resulting in the production of abnormal platelets. Most often, the release reaction is defective and results in an aspirinlike defect in platelet aggregation studies. Bleeding as well as thrombosis can be a problem. The former should be amenable to platelet transfusions, although the bleeding time does not always return to normal as expected.

D. Other disorders. Other conditions associated with functional platelet disorders include diseases associated with high plasma concentrations of FDP (e.g., DIC) and paraproteinemias (e.g., multiple myeloma). Both FDP and paraproteins interfere with reactions on the platelet surface, leading to poor platelet plug formation. Platelet transfusions are not indicated; correction of the defect depends on improvement of the underlying disease process and lowering the concentrations of FDP or paraproteins.

IV. Acquired coagulation disorders

A. Decreased production: vitamin K. It is rare to become vitamin K deficient on the basis of poor intake alone because the bacterial production of vitamin K is enough to maintain adequate factor production. Deficiency of the fat-soluble vitamin K occurs in patients with biliary disease and severely malnourished patients taking antibiotics that suppress the gut flora commonly seen in the intensive care unit. The characteristic laboratory findings in vitamin K deficiency include an initial prolongation of the PT caused by the short half-life and rapid decline of factor VII, and then a gradual prolongation of the PTT caused by depression of factor IX. A common clinical problem is the differentiation between liver impairment and vitamin K deficiency when both conditions may exist in a patient with a prolonged PT and PTT. Therapy depends on the severity of the coagulopathy. Parenteral vitamin K [10 mg intramuscular (IM), or 5 mg intravenous (IV)] corrects the PT in 12 to 24 hours. Fresh frozen plasma (initial dose 15–20 ml/kg followed by one third this dose every 8–12 hours) immediately replaces the vitamin K-dependent factors and corrects the PT. It should be used in a situation of abnormal coagulation studies with acute bleeding caused by vitamin K deficiency. When given IV, vitamin K must be administered slowly over several minutes watching for untoward effects. Vitamin K can be given subcutaneously with less side effects.

B. Decreased production: liver disease. Advanced liver disease is commonly associated with pathologic bleeding as a result of decreased factor synthesis, production of an abnormal factor, increased factor consumption, or, very rarely, primary fibrinolysis. The vitamin K-dependent factors are particularly sensitive to liver impairment, especially factor VII. The liver has great potential to produce fibrinogen, and its concentration is not depressed until late-stage liver failure occurs. Certain conditions (e.g., hepatomas, cirrhosis, chronic active liver disease, and acute hepatic failure) can produce dysfunctional fibrinogens. Many investigators have shown that the coagulation mechanism can be activated in liver disease. Activation is postulated to result from necrosis of hepatocytes and release of tissue thromboplastin, inadequate clearance of already activated factors by the liver's reticuloendothelial system, and depressed levels of naturally occurring inhibitors that are produced in the liver (e.g., antithrombin III). Coagulation results primarily in the consumption of factors II, V, VIII, XIII, and fibrinogen as well as the secondary activation of fibrinolysis and the generation of fibrin degradation products. Usually, multiple laboratory abnormalities occur, which may mimic DIC, including a prolonged PT, PTT, and TT and a mildly elevated FDP and even *d*-dimer. If portal hypertension exists, the spleen may be slightly enlarged and cause a mildly reduced platelet count because of hypersplenism. Treatment, which depends on the severity of the coagulopathy and the presence of bleeding, usually includes fresh frozen plasma. Treatment simply to correct an abnormal PT and PTT is not recommended because it takes a large volume of plasma to correct the abnormality, the correction is short-lived, and the protein load contained in the plasma may be enough to induce hepatic encephalopathy in a patient who is predisposed. Factor IX concentrates should be avoided because of the risk of thrombosis.

C. Accelerated destruction: DIC. Disseminated intravascular coagulation involves the pathologic activation of coagulation by an underlying disease process that leads to fibrin clot formation and secondary fibrinolysis, which then cause the consumption of coagulation factors, platelets, and red cells. It may not be apparent clinically, or it may be manifested by thrombosis, hemorrhage, or both, depending on the degree of activation and compensatory efforts of the body. The fulminant syndrome is most often a life-threatening bleeding disorder. Bleeding results from the developing factor deficiency (primarily I, II, V, VIII, and XIII), thrombocytopenia, excessive fibrinolysis, and high levels of FDP and *d*-dimer superimposed on a vascular system already damaged by diffuse microvascular thrombi. Bleeding is typically manifested by diffuse superficial hemorrhage in the form of ecchymoses and petechiae, as well as oozing from the gingiva, oral mucosa, gastrointestinal and urinary tracts, operative or IV line sites. The most common causes of DIC include gram-negative septicemia, certain malignancies, surgery, trauma, and obstetric complications. Acute promyelocytic leukemia is the neoplasm most commonly associated with DIC. The definitive diagnosis is established in the laboratory by a constellation of abnormalities. Factor consumption and high titers of FDP, which inhibit fibrin monomer polymerization, produce prolongations of the PT, PTT, and TT. The fibrinogen concentration is reduced and proteolytic fragments of fibrinogen and fibrin are elevated. The theoretic advantages of the *d*-dimer assay over the standard FDP assay may not add much to the clinical diagnosis of DIC. Thrombocytopenia and microangiopathic hemolytic anemia are usually evident. More sophisticated tests can be performed, looking specifically for fibrin monomer formation, fibrinopeptides, or activation of fibrinolysis, but they are seldom necessary to confirm the diagnosis in clinically significant cases of DIC. The most important factor in the treatment of DIC is correction of the underlying disease. Supportive measures include plasma and platelet transfusions to replace the deficient factors, antithrombin III and platelets. The often-cited danger of feeding the fire by replenishing these substances has never been clinically substantiated. Heparin use remains controversial. In certain specific conditions (e.g., purpura fulminans, where thrombosis is the main clinical manifestation, and acute promyelocytic leukemia) heparin may be helpful and should be considered. Otherwise, patients must be considered on an individual basis. If heparin is used, it should be started at low doses (5–10 U/kg/h) and given by constant infusion without a loading dose. Newer modes of therapy have been tested, but it is still too early to determine their efficacy or cost-effectiveness. These include concentrates of antithrombin III or protein C, low molecular weight heparin, specific thrombin inhibitors (e.g., hirudin), monoclonal antibodies to gram-negative endotoxin, or inhibitors of various modulators of coagulation. Efficacy of therapy can be monitored by looking for a decrease in FDP or *d*-dimer, an increase in fibrinogen concentration, or the normalization of the PT and PTT. No single laboratory parameter is definitive, however, and the overall clinical status of the patient must be continually assessed.

D. Accelerated destruction: fibrinolysis. Fibrinolysis occurs as a primary disorder when plasmin enzymatically attacks fibrinogen, producing high levels of FDP. Low levels of fibrinogen and high titers of FDP cause a prolongation of the TT, PT, and PTT. Plasmin also destroys factors V and VIII; however, other factors and the platelet count are normal and fibrin monomers and cross-linked fibrin fragments (*d*-dimer) are not detectable. Primary fibrinolysis occurs in tumors such as carcinoma of the prostate because of urokinase release and in extracorporeal open heart surgery. The therapeutic approach to fibrinolysis usually involves the use of a combination of heparin and epsilon-aminocaproic acid, as well as factor replacement with fresh frozen plasma. The combination is used because frequently a component of intravascular coagulation is present as well and epsilon-aminocaproic acid alone could provoke thromboses.

E. Cardiopulmonary bypass surgery. A complex hemorrhagic syndrome is seen in patients after cardiopulmonary bypass. The cause of bleeding is often multifactorial, including inadequate heparin neutralization, postneutralization rebound effect of heparin, thrombocytopenia, functional platelet defects, DIC, and excessive fibrinolysis. Much research has focused on functional platelet defects as the major cause of bleeding after bypass surgery, but extensive studies of DDAVP, a platelet function-enhancing agent, to reduce postoperative hemorrhage have shown it to be unsuccessful. In most cases of excessive bleeding after bypass surgery, it is often difficult to identify with certainty the abnormality that is predominantly responsible for the bleeding, so hemorrhage is usually attacked on multiple fronts. Of course, surgical bleeding is always a consideration; the identification of such bleeding is essential because it may require surgical reexploration.

F. Massive blood replacement. When the volume of blood transfused to a patient over a short interval approximates the patient's normal blood volume, dilutional deficiencies of platelets and labile coagulation factors (V and VIII) can cause bleeding. In these patients, 1 U of fresh frozen plasma should be given for every 5 U of blood transfused, although it is best to monitor hemostatic function and base replacement therapy on objective parameters. The platelet count should be monitored and platelet transfusions given only when serious thrombocytopenia attributable to dilution develops. A guideline to follow is to transfuse 1 to 2 U of platelets for every 5 U of blood transfused. Little firm evidence indicates that serious hypocalcemia develops with massive transfusion or that it plays a role in the coagulopathy. Therefore, routine infusions with calcium gluconate or calcium chloride are not recommended.

G. Inhibitors. Inhibitors of coagulation can be either antibodies or soluble fragments of fibrinogen or fibrin that interfere with coagulation and lead to bleeding. Antibodies directed toward factor VIII are the most common neutralizing factor-specific antibodies. They can be found in nonhemophilic individuals with autoimmune disorders, during the postpartum period, and in elderly individuals without demonstrable underlying disease. Factor VIII antibodies often have a strong affinity or neutralizing capacity that produces bleeding similar to severe hemophilia. Patients are notoriously difficult to treat when bleeding occurs because replacement therapy with factor VIII is ineffective. Immunosuppression with prednisone or other agents can be effective. The treatment of bleeding is problematic and a hematologist must be consulted. Much less frequently, acquired inhibitors have been described against fibrinogen and factors V, VII, XI, XII, and XIII as well as vWF. Streptomycin and isoniazid have been incriminated in the causes of inhibitors to factors V and XIII, respectively. Immunoglobulin usually of G (IgG) class that interacts with phospholipid is present in as many as 10% of patients with systemic lupus erythematosus (lupus inhibitor), as well as in a number of other disease states, including other autoimmune disorders, various malignancies, and human immunodeficiency virus (HIV-1 infection). It is also interacts with certain drugs, particularly those known to produce a lupuslike syndrome (e.g., procainamide, hydralazine, chlorpromazine). The in vivo significance of this inhibitor is minimal with regard to bleeding because patients generally do not manifest a bleeding tendency; however, they may exhibit a thrombotic tendency. This occurs more commonly in women, is associated with both venous and arterial thromboses, and is implicated as a cause of spontaneous abortions and intrauterine fetal death. Other manifestations include deep venous thromboses, pulmonary embolism, and strokes. Patients with a lupus inhibitor commonly have a prolonged PTT or a measurable antiphospholipid antibody, but neither test is 100% sensitive and both are much less specific for the clinical syndrome. A number of coagulation assays have been studied and recommended as screening and diagnostic tools for the identification of a lupus inhibitor. When detected, treatment is long-term oral anticoagulant therapy in most cases and aspirin therapy in others. However, the presence of a lupus inhibitor alone without clinical problems is not an indication for therapy.

Selected Readings

Ansell J, Klassen V, Lew R, et al. Does desmopressin acetate prophylaxis reduce blood loss after valvular heart operations? A randomized, double-blind study. *J Thorac Cardiovasc Surg* 1992;104(1):117.

Randomized trial showing that routine use of DDAVP during cardiopulmonary bypass does not alter blood loss or transfusion requirements.

Ansell JE, Kumar R, Deykin D. The spectrum of vitamin K deficiency. *JAMA* 1977; 238(1):40.

Review of 13 cases of vitamin K deficiency and clinical correlates.

Bick RL. Disseminated intravascular coagulation: objective clinical and laboratory diagnosis, treatment, and assessment of therapeutic response. *Semin Thromb Hemost* 1996;22(1):69.

Review of the pathophysiologic changes seen in DIC and criteria for defining severity and response to therapy.

Bick RL. Platelet function defects: a clinical review. *Semin Thromb Hemost* 1992; 18(2):167.

Clinical review of hereditary and acquired platelet dysfunction.

Harrington RA, Kleiman NS, Granger CB, et al. Relation between inhibition of platelet aggregation and clinical outcomes. *Am Heart J* 1998;136:S43.

The true relationship between the level of platelet inhibition and clinical outcome in a variety of circumstances is unknown. Work with certain platelet inhibitors suggests that inhibition greater than 80% is optimal but more data are needed. The current understanding is reviewed in this article.

Lind SE. The bleeding time does not predict surgical bleeding [see comments]. *Blood* 1991;77(12):2547.

Review of the poor predictive ability of surgical bleeding time.

Lucas RV, Miller ML. The fibrinolytic system. Recent advances. *Cleve Clin J Med* 1988; 55(6):531.

Review of the plasmin anticoagulation system and specific activators.

Mannucci PM. Desmopressin: a nontransfusional form of treatment for congenital and acquired bleeding disorders [see comments]. *Blood* 1988;72(5):1449.
Review of the utility of DDAVP in a variety of bleeding disorders.

Mannucci PM, Remuzzi G, Pusineri F, et al. Deamino-8-D-arginine vasopressin shortens the bleeding time in uremia. *N Engl J Med* 1983;308(1):8.
Randomized, double-blind trial of DDAVP versus placebo in uremic patients with bleeding tendencies.

Royston D. Coagulation in cardiac surgery. *Adv Card Surg* 1996;8:19.
Overview of the coagulation abnormalities during cardiac surgery and cardiac bypass.

93. THE CONGENITAL COAGULOPATHIES

Doreen B. Brettler and Robert V. B. Emmons

I. Hemophilia. Hemophilia A and B are clinically similar X-linked recessive bleeding disorders caused by decreased blood levels of properly functioning procoagulant factors VIII and IX, respectively. The incidence of the hemophilias is in the range of 10 cases per 100,000 live male births and 80% are hemophilia A. Men manifest the disease because the defective genes are located on the X chromosome. Female carriers of factor VIII or IX defects may exhibit mild hemophilia, especially after trauma or surgery, if their normal X chromosomes are randomly suppressed to a greater extent than normal (lyonization).

II. Clinical manifestations of hemophilia A and B

A. Severity. Severe hemophiliacs have factor VIII or IX levels no greater than 1% of normal (0.01 U/ml) and suffer severe bleeding. Factor levels greater than 5% of normal (>0.05 U/ml) usually cause hemorrhage only with trauma or surgery and are considered mild hemophilia. Patients with moderately severe disease fall somewhere between the two extremes. Within the kindred of a patient, clinical and laboratory severity of the disorder is constant.

B. Hemarthrosis. Joint hemorrhages, the most common manifestations of hemophilia, are seen in descending order of frequency in the knee, elbow, ankle, shoulder, hip, and wrist. Symptoms include pain, joint swelling, cutaneous warmth, and eventual severe limitation of motion, although the joint can return to normal over several weeks once the bleeding has stopped. Synovitis, which occurs after multiple bleeds into the joint, can predispose the joint to further bleeding and to the development of hemophilic arthropathy.

C. Hematoma. Large muscle hematomas, which can lead to severe sequelae through compression of vital structures, can produce fever, leukocytosis, severe pain, and low-grade hyperbilirubinemia caused by erythrocyte degradation. Hematoma mass effect can give rise to a variety of clinical presentations, depending on location. For instance, hematoma mass in the psoas can mimic appendicitis and cause femoral nerve palsy; in the muscles of the forearm or calf it can lead to nerve compression or ischemic contracture of the hand or ankle; and in the tongue or the muscles or soft tissues of the neck or throat it can rapidly obstruct the airway and require prompt aggressive therapy. Hemophilic cysts, or pseudotumors, begin as hematomas and may expand insidiously for several years, achieving huge dimensions, with a subsequent threat to life or limb.

D. Intracranial bleeding. Although relatively rare, intracranial bleeding accounts for 25% of hemorrhagic deaths in hemophilia. Sequelae such as mental retardation or seizures can also occur if such bleeds are not treated. A history of antecedent trauma is obtained from approximately 50% of the patients. Bleeding can be subdural, epidural, subarachnoid, intracerebral, or intraspinal.

E. Other sites of hemorrhage. Gastrointestinal bleeding is rare and should raise the suspicion of an organic gastrointestinal lesion. Prolonged gingival oozing is common, especially with dental changes or after instrumentation. If therapy is needed, several days of an antifibrinolytic agent (e.g., epsilon-aminocaproic acid or tranexamic acid) usually suffice. Urinary tract bleeding is usually painless unless a clot has formed in the ureter or the pelvis; it subsides after several days with conservative therapy such as increased intake of fluid. Inhibitors of fibrinolysis (e.g., epsilon-aminocaproic acid) should be *avoided* because they can increase clot formation in the collecting system and lead to renal colic. Epistaxis is not unusual in the hemophiliac.

F. Posttraumatic hemorrhage. Delayed bleeding that follows trauma is well documented in hemophilia and treatment with factor concentrate should be given after significant trauma regardless of whether evidence of hemorrhage is apparent.

III. General principles of replacement therapy

A. Factor VIII dose calculation. Each unit of factor VIII infused per kilogram body weight yields a 2% rise in plasma factor VIII level (i.e., 0.02 U/ml). The biologic half-life of factor VIII is between 8 and 12 hours. The minimal hemostatic level of factor VIII for most mild hemorrhages is thought to be 30% and 50% for advanced joint or muscle bleeding. Mild bleeding can be treated with one infusion but more severe bleeding may require repeating the infusion at 12-hour intervals at approximately 50% to 75% of the original dose infused to compensate for the residual in vivo level that remains from the initial dose. For the treatment of life-threatening bleeding in the intensive care unit or preoperatively, levels of 80% to 100% (40–50 U/kg) should be achieved, and the factor VIII level kept above the 40% to 50% range by appropriate doses of factor VIII infused at intervals of 8 to 12 hours. This more frequent infusion regimen decreases both the incidence of excessively low levels just before an infusion and the total amount of factor needed to maintain a given in vivo plasma level. Constant infusions of factor concentrate can also be given to keep a consistent level of greater than 30%, usually beginning with empiric dosing at 2 to 4 U/kg/h after a bolus of 50 U/kg intravenously (IV). Adequate supply for up to 4 weeks of replacement should be available prior to any elective surgery. For patients with major or life-threatening lesions, the measurement of in vivo factor VIII:C by standard laboratory assays is advisable because all of the above calculations are only approximations and PTT may be misleading.

B. Factor VIII source. In hemophiliacs who have not been exposed to any human blood-borne viruses, recombinant factor VIII should be considered as the therapy of first choice. All plasma-derived concentrates are virally inactivated by various methods. Because cryoprecipitate cannot be virally inactivated, a risk for viral transmission exists and, thus, it should not be used. The use of DDAVP (desmopressin) should be considered for the patient with mild hemophilia who needs treatment. The general rule is that 0.3 μg/kg IV over 30 minutes increases the factor VIII level threefold. Tachyphylaxis can occur after 3 to 4 days of use, and factor VIII levels should be checked periodically. Side effects include facial flushing, headache, and occasionally hyponatremia leading to seizures, especially in a patient not taking oral fluids who is receiving IV hydration, such as those in intensive care settings. Serum sodium levels should be checked intermittently in these patients. If tachyphylaxis develops or the patient does not have an adequate rise in factor VIII levels with DDAVP, recombinant factor concentrate should be used.

C. Factor IX dose calculation. Each unit of infused factor IX per kilogram of body weight yields a 1% rise in plasma IX level (i.e., 0.01 U/ml). The biologic half-life of factor IX is approximately 24 hours. A minimal level of 20% (20 U/kg) is usually targeted for most acute hemorrhages and 40% for more advanced bleeding. For major trauma or surgery, initial levels of 60% to 80% may be required, maintaining the level at above 40% through repeated infusions for several days, and then at levels above 20% for a total of 7 to 10 days. For major orthopedic surgery, considerably longer treatment periods may be needed. As with factor VIII concentrate, constant infusions can be used, which usually will decrease the total number of units consumed. It should be noted that with recombinant factor IX, 1.5 times the calculated dose must be given because of a reported decreased recovery.

D. Factor IX source. Recombinant factor IX is the treatment of choice for patients not previously transfused. For patients with severe or moderate factor IX deficiency, factor IX concentrates are the recommended treatment. As is true for factor VIII concentrates, the factor IX concentrates are accurate in their stated potency, virally inactivated, stable at 4°C for many months, and can be rapidly prepared for IV infusion. High-purity factor IX concentrates (AlphaNine, solvent detergent, Alpha Therapeutics, Los Angeles, CA; Mononine, Centeon, King of Prussia, PA) are available. They contain little, if any, factor II, VII, and X, and thus may have decreased thrombotic side effects in ill, bedridden patients. They are the concentrates of choice in a patient who is in the intensive care unit or undergoing surgery. Cryoprecipitate should *not* be used for factor IX-deficient patients because it does not contain any factor IX.

E. Side effects. Allergic reactions (e.g., urticaria or fever) to factor concentrates occur infrequently; they are very mild and anaphylaxis is rare. Changing to a different product lot number for subsequent infusions and antihistamine therapy is probably warranted. A major side effect of replacement therapy has been the human immunodeficiency virus (HIV) infection, and hepatitis, which may be of C, B, or A type. All newly diagnosed patients with hemophilia should be vaccinated for hepatitis B. Other new hepatitis viruses (e.g., hepatitis G) and transfusion-transmitted virus (TTV) have been found to be transmitted by plasma-derived concentrates and they are being investigated in the hemophilic population. Currently, approximately 20% of all hemophiliacs in the United States are HIV seropositive. Large doses of plasma-derived but not highly purified factor concentrate can cause hemolytic anemia in recipients with type A or B erythrocytes because of anti-A/B antibodies. Type O blood can be given if necessary. The administration of large doses of prothrombin complex concentrate (PCC) containing factors II, VII, IX, and X has been associated with clotting, including deep venous thrombosis, pulmonary embolism, disseminated intravascular coagulation (especially in patients with liver disease), and myocardial infarctions in young patients.

F. Inhibitors. An inhibitor antibody develops in 15% to 30% of patients with severe factor VIII deficiency and only in 10% of factor IX-deficient patients. Treatment of patients with inhibitors is problematic and they should avoid elective surgery. Low titer factor VIII inhibitor can sometimes be overcome with increased doses of the necessary concentrate. PCC is effective and it is usually given in large doses (70 U/kg body weight of factor IX activity. Activated PCC at doses of 70 U/kg have also been shown to be inconsistently effective. With both PCC and aPCC, no measurable factor VIII level is obtained, nor is shortening of the PTT seen. If the human inhibitor antibody titer is low (<20 U, Bethesda), empiric dosing of 100 to 300 U/kg of porcine factor VIII can result in measurable circulating factor VIII levels. Plasmapheresis, with columns that selectively remove IgG, while giving very high doses of human factor VIII concentrates can be tried. Recombinant factor VIIa is now also available (Novo-Seven, Novo, Denmark) and given at doses of 90 μg/kg every 2 hours. Eradication of the inhibitor using daily doses of factor VIII concentrate (immune tolerance) has been accomplished electively. Treatment of patients with factor IX inhibitor antibodies is problematic, with aPCC and recombinant factor VIIa being the only treatment modalities available. Plasmapheresis with replacement of high doses of factor IX as well as induction of immune tolerance may also be successful.

IV. Von Willebrand's disease

A. Overview. Von Willebrand's disease is the most common congenital coagulopathy, occurring in approximately 1 in 200 in the general population. Most patients have type 1 disease and are discovered on routine screening. Activated PTT is usually prolonged, as is the bleeding time, although the quantitative platelet count is normal. Factor VIII:C, von Willebrand factor (vWF) antigen, and ristocetin cofactor (RiCof) activity are all usually mildly reduced. Patients may have increased bruising, epistaxis, menorrhagia, or gingival bleeding. Patients with type 3 von Willebrand's disease are very rare and present with bleeding similar to that of a person with hemophilia. Patients with type 2 von Willebrand's disease have qualitative defects in their vWF structure and tend mostly to present with mild clinical symptoms.

B. Treatment. The patient with classic type 1 von Willebrand's disease responds very well to DDAVP at doses similar to those used in mild hemophilia (0.3 μg/kg IV over 30–40 minutes). DDAVP is also available as an intranasal preparation (Stimate) and minor surgery can be carried out 90 minutes after the adult patient takes two nasal puffs of the drug. Tachyphylaxis can occur after 3 to 4 days of use, and thus factor VIII levels should be checked periodically. DDAVP can be used also in type 2 Von Willebrand's disease, except in patients who have type 2B disease. Patients with type 3 von Willebrand's disease do not respond to DDAVP. For these patients and those with type 2B von Willebrand's disease, some hematologists use cryoprecipitate, which contains both factor VIII:C and vWF. However, cryoprecipitate is not yet virally inactivated and holds some risks for transmission of blood-borne viruses. Factor VIII concentrates have also been used. Some factor concentrates do contain vWF (Humate P, Centeon Lab, King of Prussia, PA; Alphaeight, Alpha Therapeutics, Los Angeles, CA), but the multimeric structure may be abnormal. These concentrates do not predictably shorten the bleeding time; thus, efficacy of treatment should not be judged on this parameter alone. For major bleeding resulting from surgery or severe trauma, correction of factor VIII:C levels is thought to be sufficient. If the patient has type 3 vWD, constant infusions of factor VIII:C concentrate may be necessary to maintain adequate levels. Dose calculations to maintain the factor VIII:C levels above 50% (calculated as in a patient with severe hemophilia A) should be done if surgery is to ensue or a significant injury has occurred. Factor VIII levels should checked repeatedly. If a patient with von Willebrand's disease, whether severe or mild, needs surgery or invasive intensive care unit monitoring, a hematologist skilled in coagulation problems must be consulted.

Selected Readings

Bona RD, Weinstein RA, Weisman SJ, et al. The use of continuous infusion of factor concentrates in the treatment of hemophilia. *Am J Hematol* 1989;32(1):8.

Reviews the methods used for continuous factor infusions to control bleeding in hemophilia.

Chavin SI, Siegel DM, Rocco Jr TA, et al. Acute myocardial infarction during treatment with an activated prothrombin complex concentrate in a patient with factor VIII deficiency and a factor VIII inhibitor. *Am J Med 1988;* 85(2):245.

Myocardial infarction is reported in a young patient receiving activated prothrombin complex.

Ghirardini A, Chistolini A, Tirindelli MC, et al. Clinical evaluation of subcutaneously administered DDAVP. *Thromb Res* 1988;49(3):363.

The dosing of DDAVP in mild hemophilia and von Willebrand disease is reviewed.

Hedner U, Glazer S, Pingel K, et al. Successful use of recombinant factor VIIa in a patient with severe haemophilia A during synovectomy [Letter]. *Lancet* 1988;2 (8621):1193.

Case report of the successful use of factor VIIa in a patient undergoing surgery.

Mannucci PM, Canciani MT, Rota L, et al. Response of factor VIII/von Willebrand factor to DDAVP in healthy subjects and patients with haemophilia A and von Willebrand's disease. *Br J Haematol* 1981;47(2):283.

The use of DDAVP is reviewed in a large population.

Mannucci PM, Gdovin S, Gringeri A, et al. Transmission of hepatitis A to patients with hemophilia by factor VIII concentrates treated with organic solvent and detergent to inactivate viruses. The Italian Collaborative Group [see comments]. *Ann Intern Med* 1994;120(1):1.

Case series of patients developing hepatitis A after factor concentrate infusion.

Mannucci PM, Tenconi PM, Castaman G, et al. Comparison of four virus-inactivated plasma concentrates for treatment of severe von Willebrand disease: a cross-over randomized trial. *Blood* 1992;79(12):3130.

The use of virally inactivated blood products to replace cryoprecipitate in the treatment of von Willebrand disease is reviewed.

Shopnick RI, Kazemi M, Brettler DB, et al. Anaphylaxis after treatment with recombinant factor VIII. *Transfusion* 1996;36(4)358.

Case report of a 5-week-old boy who developed anaphylaxis after treatment with recombinant factor VIII.

94. THROMBOCYTOPENIA

Janice Zaleskas and Ahmad-Samer Al-Homsi

I. General principles. Thrombocytopenia, or a platelet count of less than 100×10^9/L, is encountered in 25% to 60% of critically ill patients and is associated with a longer stay in the intensive care unit (ICU) and increased mortality. Thrombocytopenia among ICU patients may represent a manifestation of the presenting illness or, more commonly, be a complication of the hospital course. A schematic step-by-step approach to diagnosis and management of decreased platelet count in the ICU is recommended (Fig. 94-1).

II. Pseudothrombocytopenia is a laboratory artifact induced by EDTA-dependent platelet antibodies. Platelet aggregates are easily detectable on the peripheral blood smear. The true platelet count can be determined by using sodium-citrated blood. False thrombocytopenia can also result from rosette formation by platelets around white blood cells (satellitism) if samples are not readily processed.

III. A number of life-threatening diagnoses must immediately be considered in patients presenting with an acute fall in the platelet count. Correct diagnosis and appropriate management is lifesaving in these conditions. In addition, platelet transfusions, often intuitively ordered in the face of thrombocytopenia, are contraindicated in the first three of these four disorders.

A. Thrombotic microangiopathic syndromes. Thrombotic thrombocytopenic purpura (TTP) and its renal variant (hemolytic uremic syndrome or HUS), may be idiopathic or can be caused by (a) infection by verotoxin-producing *Escherichia coli* O157:H7 or *Shigella* species; (b) connective tissue disorders; (c) disseminated malignancy; (d) drugs, such as cyclosporin A, ticlopidine, mitomycin C, or pentostatin; or (e) human immunodeficiency virus (HIV) infection. Thrombotic microangiopathic syndromes can also complicate malignant arterial hypertension and pregnancy. Clinically, these disorders are defined by a pentad of manifestations including (a) fever; (b) direct antiglobulin test-negative hemolytic anemia characterized by presence of red blood cell fragments on the peripheral blood smear; (c) decreased platelet count; (d) renal failure; and (e) neurologic symptoms and signs. In addition, pregnancy-associated syndromes are often associated with abnormal liver function tests. However, most of patients have an incomplete clinical picture and a dyad of microangiopathic hemolytic anemia and fall in platelet count is sufficient for diagnosis. Coagulation profile is usually normal in thrombotic microangiopathic syndromes. Patients must be treated as soon as possible with plasma exchange. Treatment must be continued until clinical remission and normalization of platelet count is achieved. Cryopoor fresh frozen plasma can be used until plasma exchange is available. Aspirin and steroids are of no established value. Platelet transfusion may be harmful.

B. Heparin-induced thrombocytopenia (HIT). Type I HIT is a common nonimmunologic event in patients on heparin. It occurs during the first 3 days of therapy and is mild and self-limiting. Type II HIT is less common; it occurs in 1% to 3% of all patients treated with heparin. The incidence is even lower with low molecular weight heparins. Mediated primarily by antibodies to heparin/platelet factor 4 complex, type II HIT is characterized by a more than 25% drop in platelet count starting 5 to 15 days from initiation of treatment. Patients with *recent* (within 6–8 weeks) prior exposure to heparin, may develop HIT as early as hours after reexposure. Bleeding is uncommon in HIT. Indeed, HIT is a severe hypercoagulable state with up to 50% of patients developing venous or arterial thrombosis up to 30 days after diagnosis. Immunologic enzyme-linked immunosorbent assay (ELISA)-based and functional ^{14}C-serotonin release assays are available. However, false–negative and false–positive results are not uncommon. Thus, the diagnosis of HIT is

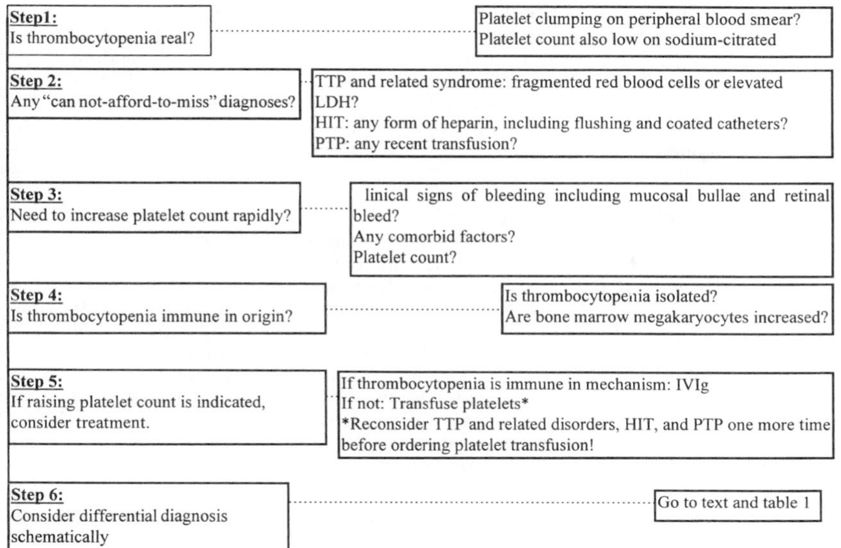

FIG. 94-1. Schematic approach to thrombocytopenia.

primarily *clinical* and must not be delayed by laboratory investigations. All forms of heparin must be stopped and anticoagulation with danaparoid or lepirudin should be instituted. Signs of recovery in platelet count within 48 hours support the diagnosis retrospectively. Warfarin use in HIT has been associated with limb gangrene and must be delayed until the platelet count recovers.

C. **Posttransfusion purpura (PTP)** is an unusual but devastating form of alloimmune thrombocytopenia. PTP is most often seen in older women who have had multiple pregnancies. Hemorrhagic manifestations and sudden severe drop in platelet count occur 7 to 10 days after receiving *any* form of blood products. Treatment is based on high doses of intravenous immunoglobulins (IVIg) and plasma exchange. Platelet transfusion is contraindicated.

D. **Disseminated intravascular coagulopathy (DIC)** is a hematologic complication of a wide variety of conditions including (a) tissue injury such as brain gunshot injury and extensive burns; (b) shock states and acute sepsis; (c) acute intravascular hemolysis; (d) obstetric complications, such as placental abruption, amniotic fluid embolism, and fetal retention; (e) acute leukemias and mucin-producing carcinomas; and (f) certain snake bites. In addition, chronic forms of DIC can be seen in patients with disseminated carcinomas. The clinical picture of DIC is a variable mixture of bleeding, often from preexisting punctures or wounds, and acral microvascualr thombosis. No *single* sensitive and specific laboratory test determines the diagnosis. Instead, it must rely on appropriate clinical setting and a variety of laboratory tests including low platelet count, prolonged prothrombin time (PT) and activated partial throbplastin time (aPTT), *decreasing* fibrinogen, elevated fibrinogen degradation products (FDP) and *D*-dimers, and depressed antithrombin III (ATIII). DIC is associated with a high mortality rate. Treatment must essentially focus on controlling the underlying condition. Platelets, fresh frozen plasma, and cryoprecipitates should be used meanwhile. AT III concentrates can be useful in selected cases. Heparin has no established role in the treatment of DIC.

IV. Assessment of risk of bleeding. Although thrombocytopenia is common in the ICU setting, it is rarely associated with life-threatening bleeding. Preexisting conditions (e.g., peptic ulcers, trauma, or surgery) increase the risk of bleeding. Physical examination provides additional indicators of risk of bleeding. Hemorrhagic bullae in the oral cavity and retinal bleeding are ominous signs. From a laboratory point of view, the risk of spontaneous bleeding does not increase until the platelet count falls below 15×10^9/L. Patients with autoimmune thrombocytopenia often tolerate well even lower numbers. Associated coagulation abnormalities must also be taken into account.

V. Mechanism of thrombocytopenia. Choosing a treatment aimed at raising platelet count must take into account the pathophysiology of thrombocytopenia. Therefore, before envisaging treatment, the mechanism of thrombocytopenia should be considered. In general, four general causes of decreased platelet count are seen: (a) lack of production; (b) immune-mediated destruction; (c) consumption and redistribution, such as in TTP and related disorders, DIC, and hypersplenism; (d) dilution after massive transfusions. Distinguishing between the different scenarios is usually possible on clinical grounds. Associated blood count abnormalities usually suggest central rather than peripheral mechanism. Bone marrow studies can further clarify the pathophysiology with megakaryocytes being decreased in central thrombocytopenia and normal or increased in peripheral thrombocytopenia.

VI. Emergency treatment of thrombocytopenia must be initiated if the risk of spontaneous bleeding is substantial or if the patient is already bleeding. Treatment of thrombocytopenia differs according to the causing illness. However, in general, patients with immune thrombocytopenia respond to high doses of IVIg. The most commonly used regimen is 0.4 g/kg/d for 5 consecutive days. Alternatively, 1 g/kg/d for a 2-day regimen may be used after IVIg platelet count recovers progressively within 24 or 48 hours. When an instant rise in platelet count is required, such as in patients with intracranial hemorrhage, platelet transfusions and emergency splenectomy must be considered. Patients with other types of thrombocytopenia (with the exceptions discussed above) are treated with platelet transfusions. Random pooled and single-donor pheresis platelet concentrates are available. Single-donor platelet concentrates carry a lower risk of transmission of infection and a lesser exposure to alloantigens. Platelet count must always be rechecked 1 hour after treatment.

VII. Differential diagnosis of thrombocytopenia

A. Acute sepsis is often associated with thrombocytopenia, even in the absence of DIC. Cytokine-induced platelet hemophagocytosis has been documented in approximately 60% of patients with sepsis syndrome. Monocytic and granulocytic ehrlichiosis are often associated with mild thrombocytopenia. In many patients, the buffy coat reveals the organism bundled in morula. Hantavirus pulmonary syndrome is characterized by rapidly developing noncardiac pulmonary edema. The hematologic picture includes increased white blood cells with more than 10% immunoblasts and thrombocytopenia. Finally, thrombocytopenia can result from direct bone marrow involvement by infections such as HIV, viral hepatitis C, or *Mycobacterium avium-intracellulare* (Table 94-1).

B. Drug-induced thrombocytopenia. The most commonly used drugs that have been associated with thrombocytopenia are listed in Table 94-2. In patients with unexplained thrombocytopenia, drugs that were introduced within 10 days from the appearance of thrombocytopenia must be substituted.

C. Massive transfusion and use of volume expanders are often associated by thrombocytopenia lasting 2 to 4 days and followed by rebound thrombocytosis.

D. Immune thrombocytopenic purpura (ITP) represents the most common cause of isolated thrombocytopenia in apparently healthy individuals. It is caused by platelet coating by antibodies and secondary clearance by tissue macrophages. ITP can be idiopathic or secondary to (a) connective tissue disorders; (b) lymphoproliferative disorders, including large granular lymphocytosis; (c) viral, including HIV, infections; and (d) drugs. Platelets are usually increased in size. However, giant platelets of the size of red blood cells are more suggestive of inherited platelet disorder. Megakaryocytes are typically normal or increased in the bone marrow. Nonetheless, the diagnosis can be established without

TABLE 94-1. Differential diagnosis of thrombocytopenia

Decreased platelet production	Primary bone marrow disorders Megaloblastic anemia Hemophagoytic syndrome Acute alcohol intoxication Drugs: Antineoplastic agents, cocaine, and the pill Radiation therapy
Increased platelet destruction	Acute sepsis Autoimmune thrombocytopenia Thrombotic microangiopathic syndromes Drugs: heparin, others PTP DIC
Platelet sequestration	Hypersplenism Extracorporal circulation Intravascular devices and catheters Hypothermic injury
Dilutional	Massive transfusion

PTP, posttransfusion purpura; DIC, disseminated intravascular coagulopathy.

bone marrow analysis, if physical examination, blood counts, and peripheral blood smear are all otherwise normal. Antinuclear antibody and HIV serology may be obtained. Patients with systemic lupus erythematosis may present with ITP long before any other evidence of disease. First-line treatment is based on steroids, although response can take up to 3 weeks. IVIg is an expensive form of therapy and should be viewed as temporary treatment in patients at high risk of bleeding. Intravenous anti-D antibodies can be used instead of IVIg in Rh (D)-positive unsplenectomized patients. The response, however, is slower and the increments are smaller. Splenectomy and immunosuppressive therapy are used as a second-line treatment.

TABLE 94-2. Commonly used drugs associated with thrombocytopenia

Heparins	
Nonsteroidial antiinflammatory drugs	
Antibiotics	Penicillins and cephalosporins Sulfonamides Rifampin Vancomycin
Hypoglycemics	Sulfonylureas
Cardiovascular drugs	Furosemide Thiazides Quinidine Procainamide Amrinone
Neuropsychiatric drugs	Phenytoin Carbamazepine Valproic acid
Miscellaneous	Glycoprotein IIb/IIIa inhibitors Gold Quinine H_2 blockers

Selected Readings

Baughman RP, Lower EE, Flessa HC, et al. Thrombocytopenia in the intensive care unit. *Chest* 1993:104:1243.
A study of the prevalence and risk factors associated with thrombocytopenia in ICU.

Boshkov LK, Warkentin TE, Hayward CPM, et al. Heparin-induced thrombocytopenia and thrombosis. Clinical and laboratory studies. *Br J Haematol* 1993;84:322.
A general discussion of clinical manifestations and diagnosis of heparin-induced thrombocytopenia.

Dabrow MB, Wilkins JC. Hematologic emergencies. *Postgrad Med* 1993;93:183.
A practical management review of disseminated intravascular coagulopathy and thrombotic thrombocytopenic purpura.

George NJ, Woolf SH, Raskob GE, et al. Idiopathic thrombocytopenic purpura. A practice guideline developed by explicit methods for the American Society of Hematology. *Blood* 1996;88:3.
Immune thrombocytopenic purpura diagnosis and management guidelines by a panel of experts.

Moake JL. Hemolytic uraemic syndrome. Basic science. *Lancet* 1994;343:393.
An easy-to-understand review of the pathophysiology of thrombotic microangiopathic syndrome.

Rutherford CJ, Frenckel EP. Thrombocytopenia. Issues in diagnosis and therapy. *Med Clin North Am* 1994;78:555.
A concise general review of thrombocytopenia.

95. ANTITHROMBOTIC THERAPY

Jean-François Lambert and Ahmad-Samer Al-Homsi

I. General principles. Antithrombotic agents such as platelet inhibitors, heparins, and warfarin are used to prevent *de novo* formation or progression of thrombi. Thrombolytic agents, on the other hand, are employed to hasten dissolution of *d* formed clots. These different classes of drugs are extremely useful in clinical practice, but if used carelessly, can also produce life-threatening complications.

II. Platelet inhibitors are mostly used in the prevention and acute treatment of arterial thrombosis such as in coronary artery disease and cerebral arteriosclerosis. The newer classes of medications are particularly helpful in acute coronary syndromes and in prevention of vascular lumen reocclusion after arterial angioplasty and stent introduction.

A. Aspirin irreversibly inhibits cyclooxygenase, thus blocking the prostaglandin synthesis necessary for platelet aggregation. Once discontinued, the effect of aspirin persists for the platelet life span (7–10 days). In contrast, nonsteroidal antiinflammatory agents show a reversible effect for a duration that is related to the drug half-life. Aspirin is used for primary and secondary prevention of myocardial infarction at a dose of 80 mg daily. Secondary (but not primary) prevention of cerebrovascular ischemic events has been proved with a similar dose.

B. Ticlopidin is a platelet aggregation inhibitor. Its effect is also irreversible. It is marginally superior to aspirin in prevention of ischemic strokes in patients with reversible ishemic attacks. Added to aspirin for 30 days, it reduces the incidence of reocclusion after coronary intraluminal stent placement. Ticlopidine is recommended at a dose of 250 mg twice daily. Blood counts must be monitored during therapy as absolute neutropenia occurs in 2% of patients. Furthermore, ticlopidin-induced thrombotic thrombocytopenic purpura has been described.

C. Glycoprotein IIb/IIIa inhibitors abciximab, eptifibatide, and tirofiban block the platelet glycoprotein IIb/IIIa and, therefore, impair fibrinogen binding and platelet aggregation. They are used in patients with refractory unstable angina and non–Q-wave myocardial infarction. When used within 2 to 4 days after a coronary event, these agents are associated with approximately 30% reduction in death. This effect seems to be sustained up to 6 months. In addition, abciximab has a somewhat drug-specific effect in the setting of percutaneous coronary revascularization with 58% reduction in 1-year mortality. Abciximab is administered as a bolus of 0.25 mg/kg followed by a continuous infusion at 10 μg/min for 12 hours. For acute coronary symptoms, eptifibatide is administered as a bolus of 180 mg followed by an infusion of 2 μg/kg/min. In the setting of percutaneous coronary revascularization, it is given as a 135-mg bolus followed by 0.5 μg/kg/min infusion. Tirofiban is given at dose of 0.4 μg/kg/min for 30 minutes followed by an infusion of 0.10 μg/kg/min for at least 48 hours. Bleeding is the major side effect of these drugs. A severe drop in platelet counts within hours or sometime days after infusion occurs in less than 0.1% of cases. This drop may be caused by the development of a new epitope on the platelet surface soliciting an immune response. The incidence appears higher on readministration of abciximab but without other sequelae.

III. Heparins

A. Unfractionated heparin is commercially extracted from bovine lung or porcine intestinal mucosa. Its anticoagulant effect is mediated through binding to antithrombin III, thus, enhancing binding and neutralization of serine protease coagulation factors, mainly IIa. Clinically, it is used in the prevention and treatment of venous and arterial thromboembolism. Heparin dosing must be weight-adjusted (Table 95-1) in order to attain prompt anticoagulation and reduce the frequency of recurrent thromboembolism. Warfarin can be started concurrently

TABLE 95-1. Weight-based heparin ordering

- Heparin bolus: 80 U/kg i.v.
- Heparin continuous IV: 18 U/kg/h
- Warfarin: 5 mg p.o. q.d. to start on first day of heparin
- Heparin dose adjustment (valid until heparin discontinued):

PTT (sec)	Additional bolus	Continuous infusion
<35	80 IU/kg i.v.	4 IU/kg/h increase
35″–45	40 IU/kg i.v.	2 IU/kg/h increase
46″–70	no	no change
71″–90	no	2 IU/kg/h decrease
>90	no	1 h stop and 3 IU/kg/h decrease

All dose adjustment should be made immediately with dose rounded to the nearest ml/h (40 U/h)
After any change: aPTT 6 hours later and further adjustment if needed.
If aPTT in therapeutic range (46 to 70): aPTT 6 hours later and every 24 hours.
i.v., intravenous; p.o., orally; q.d., every day; PTT, partial thromboplastin time; aPPT, activated partial thromboplastin time; sec, seconds.

with the initiation of heparin. Heparin must be continued for 5 days and until the target international normalized ratio (INR) has been achieved for 2 days. Despite close monitoring, heparin therapy increases the risk of bleeding. Approximately 5% to 10% of patients receiving heparin may have mild or moderate bleeding. The anticoagulant effect of a single bolus can be reversed by protamine sulfate, at a dose of 1 mg/100 U of heparin. If given after continuous heparin infusion, the protamine sulfate dose should be reduced by 50%, based on the hourly infusion dose. Heparin-induced thrombocytopenia is a common and serious complication of heparin treatment. Platelet counts must be followed twice a week during heparin therapy.

B. Low molecular weight heparins (LMWH) are fractionated derivatives of heparin with two- to fourfold enhanced anti-Xa to anti-IIa activity. LMWH have longer half-life and better bioavailability than heparin. For deep venous thrombosis (DVT) prophylaxis, LMWH are equal or superior to standard heparin or low-intensity warfarin regimens. In the surgical setting, the incidence of postoperative bleeding may be reduced by delaying treatment until 12 hours after surgery. In patients undergoing epidural or spinal anesthesia, LMWH must be held for 12 to 24 hours before needle placement or removal with subsequent doses delayed for 2 hours. In the treatment setting, meta-analyses of different clinical trials comparing LMWH with standard heparin suggest that LMWH are associated with lower rates of recurrence and possibly improved survival. Furthermore, LMWH are easier to use and require no monitoring of activity except perhaps in children and patients with renal failure where monitoring of anti-xa is suggested. Indeed, uncomplicated DVT can be treated in the outpatient setting with LMWH and warfarin at a substantial reduced cost. LMWH are also effective and safe in pulmonary embolism. Finally, LMWH compares favorably with unfractionated heparin and placebo in unstable angina and ischemic strokes (Table 95-2). Another advantage to LMWH over unfractionated heparin is the lower incidence of heparin-induced thrombocytopenia, perhaps because of lesser immmunogenicity and lack of platelet activation. However, LMWH use in patients with established heparin-induced thrombocytopenia is not advisable because of high cross-reactivity and currently available safe alternatives.

C. Danaparoid is a natural low molecular weight heparinoid with an anti-Xa to anti-IIa ratio of more than 20. Its half-life is approximately 24 hours. Danaparoid is approved for prevention of DVT after hip surgery. It has low cross-reactivity with unfractionated heparin and has been used successfully in patient with heparin-

TABLE 95-2. LMWH use

LMWH	DVT prophylaxis	Treatment of DVT or pulmonary embolism	Treatment of acute coronary ischemic syndromes
Enoxaparin	30 mg s.q. b.i.d. or 40 mg s.q. q24h	1.5 mg/kg s.q. q24h	1 mg/kg s.q. q12h
Dalteparin	Low risk: 2,500 IU s.q. q24h High risk: 5,000 IU s.q. q24h	100 IU/kg s.q. q12h	120 IU/kg q12h

LMWH, low molecular weight heparin; DVT, deep venous thrombosis; s.q., subcutaneously.

induced thrombocytopenia. For prophylaxis, danaparoid is given subcutaneously twice daily at a dose of 750 U for patients weighing less than 90 kg and 1,250 U subcutaneously twice daily for patients weighing more than 90 kg. For established thrombosis, treatment should be initiated with a bolus of 2,500 U, followed by continuous infusion at 400 U/h. The dose is reduced by 100 U/h every 4 hours until maintained at 150 to 200 U/h. Doses must be reduced in patients with impaired renal function. No need is seen to monitor therapy with anti-Xa activity, except perhaps in children and in patients with renal failure. Protamine sulfate is ineffective in reversing the danaparoid anticoagulant effect.

IV. Lepirudin and argatroban are direct thrombin inhibitors. Lepirudin is a recombinant protein similar to the natural hirudin. Argatroban is a synthetic molecule. They both have a short half-life. Lepirudin is approved for treatment in patients with heparin-induced thrombocytopenia. Argatroban has also been used in this setting. Lepirudin should be given as a bolus (0.4 mg/kg) followed by an infusion (0.15 mg/kg/h) targeting an activated partial thromboplastin time of 1.5 to 2.5. Although lepirudin doses need to be adjusted in renal failure, argatroban is metabolized by the liver and must be used cautiously in patients with impaired liver functions. Both agents affect prothrombin time (PT) and should be stopped several hours before measuring PT in patients being converted to warfarin.

V. Warfarin is an anti-vitamin K. Vitamin K is a necessary cofactor for posttranslational γ-carboxylation of glutamate, which allows coagulation factors to bind to Ca^{2+}, and thus, interact with phospholipid membranes. Vitamin K-dependent factors are II, VII, IX, X, and proteins C and S. Therapy with warfarin should be started only after therapeutic levels of anticoagulation with antithrombins have been achieved. A loading dose is unnecessary and not recommended. The starting dose must be reduced in poorly nourished patients and in those on wide-spectrum antibiotics. When starting therapy, the first factor to decrease is factor VII, so PT may increase early despite inadequate anticoagulation. After three consecutive doses, the anti-vitamin K dose can be adapted according to the INR (Table 95-3).

A. Prolonged PT and bleeding complications. Warfarin half-life ranges between 15 and 48 hours. It is affected by vitamin K intake, synthesis by intestinal flora and absorption, and by endless drug interactions. Drugs that bind to albumin can displace warfarin and increase its effects. The warfarin effect can be potentiated by reduced elimination by drugs metabolized by cytochrome P450. Therefore, close monitoring of PT (INR) is recommended when diet is modified or when introducing or discontinuing medications. For example, acetaminophen use is the most common cause of over anticoagulation with warfarin. The *Physicians Desk Reference* (PDR) contains a comprehensive list of drugs interacting with warfarin. In case of prolonged PT with an INR above the therapeutic range, small quantities of oral or subcutaneous vitamin K can be given without completely reverting the anticoagulation effect. Fresh frozen plasma and vitamin K (10 mg) sq are given for active bleeding. In case of limb- or life-threatening

TABLE 95-3. Guidelines for reversal of antivitamin K effect

INR	Treatment	Remarks
3.5–4.5—not bleeding	Hold treatment 24 h and reduce dose	Vit K if procedure planned may be considered
4.6–10—not bleeding	Vit K 1 mg p.o.	Recheck INR in 24 h
10.1–20—not bleeding	Vit K 5 mg p.o.	Recheck INR in 24 h
>20 or moderate bleeding	2–4 U FFP and Vit K 10 mg s.q.	The number of FFP units must be determined by repeated INR
Life-threatening bleeding	FFP or factor IX concentrates 25–50 U/kg[a] and vit K 10 mg s.q.	INR normalize; immediately recheck INR in 2 h

[a] More efficacious but may be thrombogenic.
INR, international normalized ratio; Vit K, Vitamin K; p.o., orally; FFP, fresh frozen plasma.

TABLE 95-4. Target therapeutic INR

Indications	Targeted INR
Prophylaxis and treatment of deep venous thrombosis and pulmonary embolism Tissue valves Atrial fibrillation	2.0–3.0
Mechanical heart valves Recurrent systemic embolism	2.5–3.5

INR, international normalized ratio.

TABLE 95-5. Thrombolysis checklist

Thrombolysis clinically indicated	❑ yes	❑ no
Age < 70 y[a]	❑ yes	❑ no
No active internal bleeding	❑ yes	❑ no
No recent cerebrovascular accident (2 mo.), head trauma (10 d), cerebral neoplasm or arteriovenous malformation	❑ yes	❑ no
No recent surgery (thoracic, abdominal 10 d), or central nervous system surgery (2 mo.)	❑ yes	❑ no
No recent spinal anesthesia or lumbar puncture (10 d)	❑ yes	❑ no
No gastrointestinal ulcerative lesions	❑ yes	❑ no
No severe uncontrolled hypertension (diastolic blood pressure > 125 mm Hg)	❑ yes	❑ no
No advanced retinopathy	❑ yes	❑ no
No known bleeding disorder	❑ yes	❑ no
Not pregnant or within 10 d postpartum	❑ yes	❑ no
No anticipated invasive procedure	❑ yes	❑ no

[a] Age is a relative contraindication with increased risk of bleeding. If all answers are yes, treatment may be given.

TABLE 95-6. Usage of thrombolytic agents

Thrombolytic agents	Deep venous thrombosis	Pulmonary embolism	Acute myocardial infarction	Acute ischemic stroke
Streptokinase	250,000 IU × 30′ then 100,000 IU/h × 24 h	250,000 IU × 30′ then 100,000 IU/h × 24 h	1.5×10^6 IU × 20′	—
Urokinase	4,400 IU/kg × 10′ then 4,400 IU/h × 24 h	4,400 IU/kg × 10′ then 4,400 IU/h × 24 h	2×10^6 IU bolus or 3×10^6 IU over 90′	—
Alteplase (rt-PA)	—	100 mg over 2 h	60 mg × 1 h (6–10 mg bolus) 20 mg over 2nd h and 20 mg over 3rd h	0.9 mg/kg (max 90 mg) 10% bolus followed by 90% over 1 h

bleeding, the use of concentrated factor IX and VII (20 to 50 U/kg) is the only treatment that provides immediate reversal of anticoagulation (Table 95-4). The use of high dose vitamin K results in a delay in reachieving anticoagulation.

VI. Thrombolytic therapy. In contrast to anticoagulants, thrombolytics are able to dissolve a clot after its formation. Streptokinase is purified from streptococci. It forms a 1:1 complex with plasminogen and efficiently activates plasminogen on the clot surface. Its use may be associated with allergic reactions. Urokinase is produced in renal epithelial cell cultures. It cleaves plasminogen into plasmin. It has no immunogenicity. Tissue plasminogen activator (t-PA) is the physiologic endothelial cell plasminogen activator. It specifically activates fibrin-bound plasminogen.

Thrombolytics are primarily used in myocardial infarction. They are also indicated in pulmonary embolism with hemodynamic changes and for patients with nonhemorrhagic strokes within 3 hours of onset of neurologic symptoms. In patients with DVT, thrombolytic therapy is associated with increased short-term clot dissolution without clear long-term benefit. If contraindications are complied with, the risk of bleeding with thrombolytics is not greater than with heparin anticoagulation (Table 95-5). Current recommended doses for thrombolytics in different indications are summarized in Table 95-6.

Selected Readings

Crowther MA, Donovan D, Harrison L, et al. Low dose oral vitamin K reliably reverses over-anticoagulation due to warfarin. *Thromb Haemost* 1998;79:1116.

A study providing a rationale for the use of low dose of vitamin K in patients with an excessive international normalized ratio.

Crowther MA, Ginsberg JB, Kearon C, et al. A randomized trial comparing 5-mg and 10-mg warfarin loading doses. *Arch Intern Med* 1999;159:46.

A well-designed, randomized trial discouraging the use of warfarin loading doses.

Makris M, Greaves M, Philips WS, et al. Emergency oral anticoagulant reversal: the relative efficacy of infusions of fresh frozen plasma and clotting factor concentrates on correction of the coagulopathy. *Thromb Haemost* 1998;77:477.

A paper favoring the use of factor concentrates over fresh frozen plasma when immediate reversal of warfarin is indicated.

Raschke RA, Reilly BM, Guidry JR, et al. The weight-based heparin dosing nomogram compared with a "standard care" nomogram in a randomized, controlled trial. *Ann Intern Med* 1993;119:874.

A randomized clinical trial favoring the weight-based dosing of heparin.

Topol EJ, Byzova TV, Plow EF. Platelet GPIIb-IIIa blockers. *Lancet* 1999;353:227.

An up-to-date review of mechanism of action and clinical use of GPIIb-IIIb blockers.

Weitz JI. Low molecular weight heparins. *N Engl J Med* 1997;337:688.

A comprehensive review of clinical trials supporting the use of low molecular weight heparins.

96. HYPERCOAGULABLE STATES

Gerald Alexander Colvin and Ahmad-Samer Al-Homsi

I. **General principles.** Hypercoagulable states are acquired or inherited conditions that alter blood coagulation, shifting the hemostatic balance toward inappropriate thrombosis. In most patients with inherited thrombophilic states, thrombosis is episodic with long asymptomatic periods. This pattern of occurrence indicates that some trigger exists for each event. Furthermore, the identification of an ever-increasing number of common and sometimes coexisting genetic risk factors, suggests that thrombotic disease is a polygenic condition with clinical syndromes brought out by different stress mechanisms.

II. **Acquired hypercoagulable states (Table 96-1).** Hypercoagulability in the intensive care unit (ICU) setting can be attributed to (a) decreased blood flow because of bedrest and depressed circulation; (b) increased procoagulant activity caused by tissue damage and release of tissue factor into the circulation; and (c) alterations in the homeostatic balance of coagulation with increased level of plasminogen activator inhibitor-1 (PAI-1), decreased antithrombin III (AT III) activity, and shutdown of the fibrinolytic system. Therefore, it is not surprising that markers of hypercoagulability are often found in critically ill patients (Table 96-2). Accordingly, in the absence of clear contraindication, patients in the intensive care unit must receive prophylactic treatment, such as subcutaneous heparin or a low molecular weight heparin (LMWH). Intermittent pneumatic compression devices can be used for added benefit.

A. **Sepsis, tissue damage, and inflammation** are common events that lead to a hypercoagulable state in critically ill patients. Cytokine-mediated activation of the coagulation system induces release of procoagulant substances and consumption of inhibitory factors such as AT III. Low levels of AT III, which can play an important role in promoting thrombosis in ICU patients, are associated with poor outcome. Indeed, Several randomized, placebo-controlled trials suggest that AT III replacement to a level above 70% results in accelerated recovery and a reduction in 30-day mortality in patients with acute sepsis and multiorgan failure.

B. **Antiphospholipid antibody syndrome (APLAS)** is mediated by antibodies to any of several negatively charged phospholipids. The syndrome can be idiopathic or secondary to an underlying connective tissue disorder. Antiphospholipid antibodies can also be detected in (a) acutely ill patients; (b) patients with the human immunodeficiency virus and other viral infections; (c) patients on certain medications, such as hydralazine, procainamide, quinine and phenytoin; and (d) substance abusers. However, the clinical relevance of antiphospholipid antibodies in these patients is questionable. The clinical manifestations of APLAS include (a) venous and *arterial* thrombosis; (b) cutaneous manifestations such as livedo reticularis and leg ulcers; (c) neurovascular manifestations and optic neuritis; (d) autoimmune thrombocytopenia; and (e) first trimester abortions or fetal loss syndrome. A combination of postpartum fever, pleuritic pain, and lung infiltrates has also been described. In addition, patients with APLAS may present with fulminant multisystem failure caused by widespread microvascular thrombi, with associated livedo reticularis and decreased platelet count. Many patients with this catastrophic presentation have preexisting connective tissue disorder and high titers of antiphospholipid antibodies. From a laboratory point of view, the diagnosis of APLAS is suggested by one or more of the following: (a) prolonged activated partial thromboplastin time (aPTT) not corrected by mixing studies; (b) lupus anticoagulant demonstrated by cephalin-kaolin or dilute Russell viper venom time (dRVVT); and (c) anticardiolipin antibodies. Lupus anticoagulant identified by dRVVT is more predictive of thromboembolic events. Furthermore, anti-β_2 glycoprotein I antibodies are more specific, in part because anticardiolipin

TABLE 96-1. Acquired hypercoagulable states

Stasis	Prolonged immobilization Varicose veins Congestive heart failure
Vessel injury	Trauma Hip and knee surgery Abdominal hysterectomy Previous thrombosis
Antiphospholipid antibody syndrome	
Metastatic adenocarcinomas	
Heparin-induced thrombocytopenia	
Acquired antithrombin III deficiency	Severe liver disease Nephrotic syndrome Disseminated intravascular coagulopathy (DIC) Pregnancy Treatment with heparin and L-asparaginase
Acquired protein C deficiency	Acute illness Severe liver disease DIC Treatment with warfarin and L-asparaginase
Acquired protein S deficiency	Severe liver disease Nephrotic syndrome Type I diabetes mellitus Pregnancy and birth control pill Treatment with warfarin
Hyperhomocysteinemia	
Hematologic disorders	Myeloproliferative disorders Paroxysmal nocturnal hemoglobinuria (PNH) Hyperviscosity states
Other drugs	Tamoxifen

antibodies associated with infectious diseases are not detected. However, the diagnosis of APLAS must never be solely based on abnormal laboratory tests.

C. Malignant tumors are associated with an increased incidence of thromboembolic events. Markers of hypercoagulability have been reported in half of all cancer patients and in up to 90% of patients with metastatic disease. In some patients, thrombotic manifestations precede any apparent malignant disease. The venous thrombosis associated with malignant tumors is often migratory, involving superficial as well as deep veins, frequently at unusual sites (e.g., arms and chest).

TABLE 96-2. Laboratory markers of hypercoagulable state in ICU patients

Increased levels	Thrombin-antithrombin III complex (TAT complex) Prothrombin fragments 1 and 2 Fibrinogen degradation products (FDP) PAI-1 *d*-Dimers
Decreased levels	T III

D. **Hyperhomocysteinemia,** which is common in the general population, is associated with an increased incidence of venous and *arterial* thrombosis. Hyperhomocysteinemia can be inherited as a result of an enzymatic defect (e.g., in thermolabile 5-methyltetrahydrofolate reductase) or associated with (a) certain medical conditions (e.g., systemic lupus erythematosus, chronic renal failure, psoriatic skin disease, and organ transplantation); (b) medications including thiazides, phenytoin, carbamazepine, nicotinic acid, and methotrexate; and (c) vitamin B_6, B_{12}, or folate deficiency. The diagnosis of hyperhomocysteinemia is based on determination of serum levels. The sensitivity of the test can be improved by ingestion of methionine (0.1 g/kg) 6 hours prior to level determination.

III. **Hereditary hypercoagulable states.** Well-established, inherited hypercoagulable states and their prevalence are summarized in Table 96-3. These disorders are transmitted in an autosomal dominant mode. Resistance to activated protein C (RAPC) results from a single point mutation in factor V coagulant. The original mutation was discovered in the city of Leiden. Other point mutations that also render factor V resistant to PC activity have since been described. Clinically, the severity of the different inherited thrombophilic conditions is disparate with AT III, protein C (PC), and protein S (PS) deficiency being more severe. In fact, whereas 80% of patients with AT III, PC, or PS deficiency are already symptomatic by the age of 45, only 25% of patients with RAPC experience symptoms by the age of 50. The hallmark of inherited thrombophilic conditions is *venous* thrombosis. This can be spontaneous or be provoked by added risk factors such as prolonged immobilization or surgery. Arterial thrombosis is very unusual in inherited thrombophilia, except in rare homozygous patients. Other clinical manifestations include warfarin-induced skin necrosis in patients with PC or PS deficiency treated without adequate coverage by an antithrombin and in purpura fulminans, which occurs at birth in homozygous patients with PC or PS deficiency. Finally, inherited thrombophilia recently has been linked to some of the pregnancy-related complications such as abruptio placentae, severe preeclampsia, fetal growth retardation, and stillbirth.

IV. **Diagnosis of hypercoagulable states.** Hypercoagulable states must be suspected in patients with thromboembolic events who (a) are aged less than 45 years; (b) have spontaneous and recurrent events; (c) present with events at unusual sites such as in upper extremities, chest wall, or mesenteric vasculature; or (d) have a suggestive family history. However, these criteria must not be considered exclusive. Indeed, patients with inherited disorders are commonly asymptomatic until late in life; they often present with provoked (rather than spontaneous) events and frequently have negative family history. The recommended initial workup for patients with suspected hypercoagulable states is summarized in Table 96-4. Pitfalls in interpretation of test results are also outlined.

V. **Management.** Patients with hypercoagulable states should receive optimal prophylactic treatment in the ICU setting. Indefinite anticoagulation is recommended

TABLE 96-3. Estimate of the frequency of inherited thrombophilia in the general population compared with individuals with spontaneous venous thrombosis

Defect	Frequency in the general population (%)	Frequency in patients with thrombosis (%)
Resistance to activated protein C	7 (White)[a]	20–60
Prothrombin G20210A allele	0.7–4	6
Antithrombin III deficiency	0.02–0.17	0.5–4.9
Protein C deficiency	0.2	4
Protein S deficiency	0.1	3
Hyperhomocysteinemia	10–40	15

[a] Less in other ethnic groups.

TABLE 96-4. Initial work-up in patients with suspected hypercoagulable states

Defect	Recommended screening test	Comments
General	Adroit H&P examination, CBC, PT, aPTT, and thrombin time	Prolonged thrombin time suggests dysfibrinogenemia
Malignant disease	Detailed H&P examination, CBC, blood chemistries, urinalysis, PSA (in men), and chest x-ray	Further workup as suggested by the initial studies
Antiphospholipid antibody syndrome	Lupus anticoagulant and anticardiolipin antibodies	Acutely ill persons often have slightly elevated titers of anticardiolipin antibodies. Testing must be repeated in 6 weeks
Hyperhomocysteinemia	Plasma homocystein level	Testing must not be done after acute thromboembolic events as levels may be falsely low
Resistance to activated protein C	Molecular PCR-based analysis or aPTT ratio with and without addition of PC	
Prothrombin G20210A allele	Molecular PCR-based analysis	
Antithrombin III deficiency	antithrombin III activity	AT III activity is depressed in DIC. Levels are also mildly decreased after acute thrombotic event and in patients on heparin. They return to normal 24–48 hours after therapy
Protein C deficiency	PC activity	PC activity is decreased in acute illness and in patients on warfarin. In patients on warfarin, testing must be delayed or levels must be compared with other vitamin K-dependent factors. Activity can be falsely low in patients with RAPC
Protein S deficiency	Total and free protein S antigen	PS antigen is depressed in patients on warfarin

H&P, history and physical; CBC, complete blood count; PT, prothrombin time; aPTT, actual partial thromboplastic time; PSA, prostate specific antigen; PCR, polymerase chain reaction; PC, protein C; DIC, disseminated intravascular coagulation; RAPC, resistance to activated PC.

in patients with APLAS after the first event, because recurrence within 5 years is seen in more than 50% of patients, if treatment has been discontinued. International normalized ratio (INR) must be maintained above 3 in these patients. However, it has recently been recognized that antiphospholipid antibodies can cause overestimation of INR. Therefore, treatment with LMWH may be a better choice, particularly during the first few weeks when the risk of recurrence appears particularly high. Immunosuppressive treatment is recommended in patients with catastrophic APLAS. Patients with underlying malignancy are often refractory to warfarin treatment and are best managed by LMWH. In patients with inherited hypercoagulability, life-long anticoagulation after a single thrombotic episode is not recommended, except perhaps after life-threatening events. This is particularly true if a transient precipitating factor is identifiable and can be removed. In case of AT III deficiency, higher than usual doses of heparin may be required to achieve therapeutic levels. Otherwise, AT III-independent antithrombins or AT III concentrates can be used. Warfarin must not be used in patients with PC or PS deficiency without therapeutic doses of antithrombins. Purpura fulminans must be treated during the acute phase with fresh frozen plasma or factor concentrates.

Selected Readings

Dahlbäck B. Resistance to activated protein C caused by the R506Q mutation ion the gene for factor V is a common risk factor for venous thrombosis. *J Intern Med* 1997; 242:1.

A thorough review of activated protein C resistance from factor V Leiden.

De Stefano V, Finazzi G, Mannucci PM. Inherited thrombophilia: pathogenesis, clinical syndromes, and management. *Blood* 1996;87:3531.

A thorough review of inherited thrombophilia, including management strategies.

Eby CS. A review of the hypercoagulable state. *Hematol Oncol Clin North Am* 1993; 7:1121.

An excellent basic review of acquired and inherited hypercoagulable states.

Eisele B, Lamy M, Thijs G, et al. Antithrombin III in patients with severe sepsis. *Intensive Care Med* 1998;24:388.

A randomized, placebo-controlled, multicenter trial, of AT III use in patients with severe sepsis.

Makris M, Rosendaal FR, Preston FE. Familial thrombophilia: genetic risk factors and management. *J Intern Med* 1997:242:9.

Basic review of inherited thrombophilia, including aood summary of incidence and occurrence data.

Rao AK, Kaplan R, Sheth S. Inherited thrombophilic states. *Semin Thromb Hemost* 1998;44:3.

Current and concise review of inherited thrombophilia.

Sähngen D, Whemeier A, Specker C, et al. Antiphospholipid antibodies in systemic lupus erythematosus and Sneddon's syndrome. *Semin Thromb Hemost* 1994;20:55.

A concise, clinical review of the antiphospholipid syndrome with emphasis on autoimmune-induced disease.

97. THE HEMOLYTIC ANEMIAS

Pamela S. Becker

I. General principles. Hemolytic anemias arise from destruction of red blood cells caused by intrinsic (largely inherited) or extrinsic defects. The breaking of the red blood cells can occur in the blood vessels, leading to intravascular hemolysis, or in the extravascular compartment, largely in the spleen and liver. Patients with chronic hemolytic anemia rely on increased erythroid production to compensate for the red blood cell destruction and, thus, are susceptible to three different types of "crises": aplastic, hemolytic, and megaloblastic. Parvovirus B19 is a classic cause of the aplastic crisis, and bacterial infections can cause hemolytic crises. Megaloblastoid crises arise because of relative folate deficiency, which can occur during adolescence (with growth spurts) or during pregnancy. Chronic hemolytic anemia is associated with pigment gallstones at an early age because of the chronic elevation of bilirubin in the bile and iron overload from chronic elevated absorption.

Hemolytic anemias can be of profound severity in the intensive care unit setting, because of severe autoimmune hemolytic anemia, overwhelming disseminated intravascular anticoagulation, or sepsis with an organism that carries a hemolytic toxin, among other causes. Hemolytic anemia should be suspected in the critically ill patient if the hematocrit fails to rise despite transfusion, an unexplained high lactate dehydrogenase (LDH) or bilirubin level is present, or hemoglobinuria without red cells is found on microscopic urinalysis. One confounding difficulty in the diagnosis is that the reticulocyte count may not be elevated in severely compromised patients because of bone marrow suppression.

II. Diagnosis. The signs and symptoms of hemolytic anemia as well as the laboratory features (Table 97-1) are a result of both the increased red cell destruction and compensatory red cell production. On physical examination, patients with hemolytic anemia may exhibit pallor and jaundice. Splenomegaly may be seen in patients with ongoing active hemolytic anemia. Individuals with chronic hemolytic conditions may have overexpanded marrow caused by erythroid hyperplasia, resulting in "chipmunk" facies (broad cheekbones, protruding maxillary bones), and extramedullary erythropoiesis, resulting in hepatosplenomegaly.

In cases of rapid intravascular hemolysis, there can be hemoglobinemia (pink colored plasma), hemoglobinuria (red colored urine), and hemosiderinuria. Haptoglobin binds free intravascular hemoglobin and is cleared through the liver, resulting in a low serum haptoglobin level. With both intravascular and extravascular hemolysis, serum bilirubin can be elevated, with most being indirect (unconjugated) bilirubin because the reticuloendothelial cells convert the hemoglobin released from destroyed red cells to bilirubin, and serum LDH is elevated because this enzyme is released from the destroyed red cells. The chronic elevation of serum bilirubin can result in pigment gallstones and cholecystitis.

An increased reticulocyte count reflects the compensatory overproduction of red cells. More specific tests can document or support the cause of the hemolytic anemia. For example, there is increased osmotic fragility in conditions leading to spherocytosis, such as hereditary spherocytosis or autoimmune hemolytic anemia. There is usually a positive Coombs test in autoimmune hemolytic anemia. The disseminated intravascular coagulation (DIC) screen (fibrin degradation products, *d*-dimer, and antithrombin III) is positive in DIC. The Ham's test and sucrose hemolysis tests are positive in paroxysmal nocturnal hemoglobinuria (PNH).

III. Treatment. One general supportive measure that should be instituted for all patients with hemolytic anemia is folic acid supplementation—1 mg daily for chronic hemolytic anemia; 5 mg daily during acute hemolytic crises. During times of exacerbations and hemodynamic compromise, patients may require transfusion support with red blood cells.

TABLE 97-1. Laboratory evaluation in hemolytic anemia

Test	Intravascular	Extravascular	Comment
Bilirubin, indirect	Yes	Yes	Elevated
Lactate dehydrogenase	Yes	Yes	Elevated
Reticulocyte count	Yes	Yes	Elevated
Plasma hemoglobin	Yes		Brisk intravascular
Osmotic fragility	Not prominent	Yes	Hereditary spherocytosis
Coomb's test	Yes, especially in cold autoimmune hemolytic anemia	Yes	Immune causes
Ham's test	Yes	—	PNH
Sucrose hemolysis	Yes	—	PNH
Urine hemosiderin	Yes	—	PNH, PCH
DIC screen	Yes	Yes	Positive in DIC
Blood smear			Abnormal forms
Hgb electrophoresis	Yes	Yes	S or C hemoglobin and others
Haptoglobin	Yes	Possibly	Low

DIC, disseminated intravascular coagulation; PNH, paroxysmal nocturnal hemoglobinuria; PCH, paroxysmal cold hemoglobinuria.

IV. Intrinsic disorders

A. Hemoglobinopathies

1. **Sickle cell disease.** Several complications of sickle cell syndromes can be life-threatening because of sickling and infarction in major organs. Approximately 10% of patients experience cerebrovascular accidents, usually in childhood. Initially, cerebral arterial thrombosis occurs, followed by aneurysm formation. Acute chest syndrome occurs in 40% of patients, a result of thrombosis in the pulmonary vessels leading to local hypoxia, then increased sickling, and eventually to hypoxemia in a progressive downward spiral. It can be difficult to distinguish pulmonary infarct from infection. Splenic sequestration crisis, also more common in children, can cause a profound drop in hematocrit and an exacerbation of hemolysis, as well as be associated with splenic infarct or rupture. Patients also are susceptible to sepsis from encapsulated organisms such as *Streptococcus pneumoniae* and *Escherichia coli,* because of an absent splenic function resulting from recurrent infarction by 1 to 2 years of age. Empiric antibiotic coverage should include medications that cover encapsulated organisms, such as cephalosporins. Patients with aplastic crisis related to parvovirus B19 infection will require red cell transfusion support until the reticulocyte count rises. Exchange transfusion should be considered for patients with acute central nervous system symptoms, cardiac symptoms, acute chest syndrome with hypoxia, or priapism; those undergoing eye surgery, surgery under general anesthesia, or angiography; or for those who have had a stroke, transfusion for a period of a few years after stroke. Exchange transfusion is performed by phlebotomy of 1 U at a time of whole blood, with replacement with packed red cell transfusions. The exchange should be down to the range of approximately 30% Hb S. Patients with extensive alloimmunization can have severe hemolytic transfusion reactions; red cell transfusion should be

used conservatively in these patients, and leukocyte depleted, phenotypically matched red cells should be administered.

Other complications of sickle cell disease include delayed growth and development; chronic hemolytic anemia with hematocrit in the range of 18 to 30; pain crises (especially abdomen, chest, joints) requiring narcotic administration with predisposing factors of dehydration, vasospasm, and infection; systolic ejection murmur due to hyperdynamic state; eventual right ventricle failure due to recurrent pulmonary infarction and pulmonary hypertension; inability to concentrate urine because of microinfarcts of the renal medulla; renal papillary infarcts resulting in hematuria, renal failure, recurrent joint effusions; osteomyelitis most likely caused by *Staphylococcus,* but can also be caused by *Salmonella* in these patients; recurrent bony infarcts leading to vertebral deformities, aseptic necrosis of femoral head, dactylitis (hand-foot syndrome); hepatic infarct; retinal infarcts and proliferative retinopathy; and chronic ankle ulcers. Compound sickle syndromes are seen (e.g., sickle-hemoglobin C and sickle β-thalassemia, both of which are associated with chronic sickling, but more mild anemia), and certain complications including splenomegaly, retinopathy, and avascular necrosis of the femoral head.

Treatments include penicillin prophylaxis in children; pneumococcal vaccine; folic acid supplementation (1 mg daily); hydration with hypotonic fluid, oxygen, analgesics; evaluation for infection and organ damage for sickle pain crisis; deferroxamine for iron overload; and hydroxyurea to increase hemoglobin F production and decrease crisis frequency.

2. **Thalassemia.** Thalassemia arises from insufficient synthesis of α or β globin. It can range in severity from the silent carrier state in α-thalassemia with deletion of a single α globin gene, to thalassemia major in patients who completely lack production of β globin. Patients with thalassemia major develop massive hepatosplenomegaly and chipmunk facies because of extramedullary erythropoiesis and complete transfusion dependence, with consequent development of transfusional iron overload, which leads to congestive heart failure and cirrhosis. The treatment is to transfuse to hemoglobin (10.5 g/dl) to prevent marrow expansion and splenomegaly, folate, splenectomy, deferroxamine, and bone marrow transplantation. Thalassemia minor is more mild and generally does not require transfusion support.
3. **Unstable hemoglobin disorders.** The unstable hemoglobin mutants have a chronic hemolytic anemia characterized by Heinz bodies composed of precipitated hemoglobin. They are treated with folate, red cell transfusions, avoidance of oxidants, and splenectomy.

B. Membrane defects. Several inherited defects of red cell membrane proteins lead to hereditary hemolytic anemia. The most frequent types are hereditary spherocytosis and hereditary elliptocytosis. Most cases are mild and splenectomy can ameliorate these conditions; however, severe forms can result in transfusion-dependent anemia despite splenectomy. Inherited defects of lipid synthesis (e.g., abetalipoproteinemia) can also lead to acanthocytosis (cells have irregular projections), and absent LDL can lead to vitamin E deficiency, oxidant sensitivity, and hemolysis.

C. Metabolic defects. These defects arise because of enzyme deficiencies critical to the Embden-Meyerhof or glycolytic pathway and the hexose monophosphate (HMP) shunt necessary for adenosine triphosphate (ATP) production or maintenance of the reduced state of the heme iron. Examples of these enzyme deficiencies include G6PD deficiency, which leads to hemolysis with infections or with use of certain oxidant drugs (e.g., primaquine, nitrofurantoin, sulfamethoxazole, chloramphenicol, phenacetin, dapsone, methylene blue, and vitamin K); glutathione synthetase deficiency; pyruvate kinase deficiency; glucose phosphate isomerase deficiency; triose phosphate isomerase deficiency; and phosphofructokinase deficiency. The G6PD deficiency can be managed by avoidance of oxidant drugs or ingestion of chemicals such as moth balls or foods such as fava beans; pyruvate kinase deficiency generally requires splenectomy.

D. Paroxysmal nocturnal hemoglobinuria (PNH). PNH is an acquired clonal stem cell disorder caused by a defect in synthesis of the phosphatidyl-inositol (PI) membrane anchor for a number of proteins, including decay accelerating factor (DAF—an inhibitor of C3 convertase). Because of the decreased binding of DAF, there is increased sensitivity to complement, which leads to intravascular hemolysis, resulting in variable hemoglobinuria, classically worse at night, and significant iron deficiency through urinary loss (a positive urine hemosiderin test). Patients also suffer from episodic abdominal pain attributed to venous thromboses (hepatic, portal, splenic, mesenteric v.) because of a defect in platelets. The disorder can evolve into aplastic anemia or acute leukemia and can be cured by allogeneic bone marrow transplantation. The diagnosis is by acid hemolysin (Ham test) or sucrose hemolysis (sugar water) test, which demonstrates the sensitivity to complement-mediated lysis, as well as flow cytometry that demonstrates a lack of proteins bound via the PI membrane anchor.

V. Extrinsic disorders

A. Autoimmune hemolytic anemia (AIHA). AIHA, which can be diagnosed by the direct Coombs' test, also known as the DAT (direct antiglobulin test), demonstrates immunoglobulin, complement, or both present on the red cell, or the indirect test that demonstrates antibody detected in the serum. About half of patients with warm AIHA exhibit both IgG and C′3 on the red blood cell count and a third only IgG; this type is often associated with other autoimmune disorders or malignancies and extravascular hemolysis. Cold agglutinin disease (cold AIHA) is characterized by antibodies that bind better at 4°C, usually because of an IgM antibody. Hemolysis is also primarily extravascular, but can be intravascular because of complement fixation. It is associated with infections such as *Mycoplasma pneumoniae* and infectious mononucleosis or malignancies. Drug-induced AIHA can arise by three mechanisms: (a) hapten (antibodies directed to the drug bound to the red blood cell membrane); for example, penicillin, with a positive DAT for IgG, indirect negative in the absence of drug; (b) immune complex–"innocent bystander" (circulating complexes of antibody-drug bound to serum protein); for example, quinidine, wherein an antibody is directed to the drug-protein complex which settles on red blood cells, fixing complement and leading to a positive DAT for C′3; and (c) drug-induced autoantibody (e.g., procainamide), usually with anti-Rh specificity, leading to a positive DAT for IgG and possibly, a positive indirect Coombs' test as well. The treatments for autoimmune hemolytic anemia include withdrawal of drug for the drug-induced variety, folate supplementation, and immunosuppression for the spontaneous warm and cold autoimmune hemolytic anemias or drug-induced autoantibody type. The immunosuppressives include steroids, cyclophosphamide, and azathioprine. In addition, danocrine and intravenous immune globulin can be effective. In cases of relapse after withdrawal of immunosuppressive medication or in severe hemolysis, splenectomy should be performed.

B. Microangiopathic hemolytic anemia

1. **DIC.** The blood vessels are partially occluded by fibrin deposition and the red cells become caught on fibrin strands, leading to fragmentation and hemolysis. Also occurring is consumption of platelets and coagulation factors, leading to thrombocytopenia and prolongation of the prothrombin time and partial thromboplastin time. The DIC screen demonstrates high fibrin degradation products, increased level of *d*-dimer, and low levels of antithrombin III. Management is largely supportive, with replenishment of red cells, platelets, fresh frozen plasma, and cryoprecipitate, and treatment of the underlying cause (sepsis, tissue necrosis, and so on) until resolution.
2. **Thrombotic thrombocytopenic purpura (TTP).** Five clinical features are seen in the presentation of TTP are fever, renal dysfunction, neurologic sequelae (including seizure), hemolytic anemia, and thrombocytopenia. The hemolytic anemia is manifested by an elevation in the reticulocyte count, LDH, and schistocytes present on the peripheral blood smear. The treatment is plasmapheresis.

3. **Hemolytic uremic syndrome (HUS).** Hemolysis and renal dysfunction are the most prominent features of HUS, although mild thrombocytopenia may also be present. Fragmented cells are also seen on the peripheral blood smear. HUS can be difficult to distinguish from TTP, but a recent study has found there to be a different pattern of von Willebrand factor multimers.
4. **Other vascular abnormalities.** Hemangiomas are focal proliferations of small blood vessels that can cause localized intravascular coagulation. Carcinomatosis occurs when metastatic deposits of cancer cells lodge in blood vessels. Renal vascular disorders (e.g., malignant hypertension) can lead to vessel narrowing or abnormal vessels in glomerulonephritis. Inflammation of small vessels can occur in polyarteritis nodosum or systemic lupus. All of these abnormalities of vessels can lead to shearing of red cells and hemolysis.

B. **Mechanical damage.** Red blood cells rupture under high shear stresses because of mechanical damage. This damage is reflected by abnormal shapes, including schistocytes, helmet cells, and fragments. The damaged cells are removed by the spleen.
   1. **"Waring blender" syndrome.** This syndrome occurs because of damage from prosthetic heart valves or stenotic, calcified heart valves, especially the aortic valve.
   2. **"March" hemoglobinuria.** The stomping of feet on hard surfaces over long distances causes red cell damage.

C. **Toxins.** Certain toxins and venoms result in profound hemolysis. Classic examples include *Clostridium welchii* sepsis, in which a phospholipase damages red blood cells phospholipid, leading to rapidly progressive and often fatal intravascular hemolysis, as well as snake or brown spider venoms.

D. **Chemical injury.** The red blood cell membrane can be injured by arsenic, copper, and high O_2 tension such as hyperbaric oxygen, presumed to be due to membrane oxidation.

E. **Burn injury.** Thermal burns cause direct damage to red blood cell membrane, resulting in spherocyte and schistocyte formation, especially when third-degree burns are sustained over greater than 20% of the body surface area.

F. **Malaria and babesiosis.** Malaria parasites directly invade red cells resulting in "knobs" formed on the membranes. These knobs lead to increased ion permeability, increased lipid fluidity, reduced deformability, increased oxidant production, and, ultimately, to hemolysis.

G. **Liver disease.** Severe liver disease results in spur cell anemia, characterized by acanthocytosis caused by the accumulation of unesterified cholesterol in the red blood cell membrane and hemolytic anemia with extravascular hemolysis. It is a late complication of liver dysfunction and augurs for a high mortality rate.

H. **Hypersplenism.** Splenomegaly from any cause can result in sequestration of blood cells and lead to a decline in any or all of the blood counts.

Selected Readings

Bunn HF, Forget BG. *Hemoglobin: molecular, genetic and clinical aspects.* Philadelphia: WB Saunders, 1986.
Provides a thorough discussion of all hemoglobin defects.

Engelfriet CP, Overbeeke MAM, von dem Borner AEG. Autoimmune hemolytic anemia. *Semin Hematol* 1992;29:3.
Reviews all of the different types of autoimmune hemolytic anemias with their occurrence in conjunction with systemic disease.

Gallagher PG, Forget BG. Spectrin genes in health disease. *Semin Hematol* 1993;30:4.
An overview of some inherited hemolytic anemias due to membrane defects.

Kazazian HH. The thalassemia syndromes: molecular basis and prenatal diagnosis in 1990. *Semin Hematol* 1990;27:209.
Reviews the details of the thalassemias.

Nathan DG, Orkin SH. *Hematology of infancy and childhood,* 5th ed., Philadelphia: WB Saunders, 1998.
Provides a thorough discussion of all aspects of inherited and childhood anemias.

Peters LL, Lux SE. Ankyrins: structure and function in normal cells and hereditary spherocytes. *Semin Hematol* 1993;30:85.
Reviews the molecular basis of hereditary spherocytosis.
Salama A, Mueller-Eckhardt C. Immune-mediated blood cell dyscrasias related to drugs. *Semin Hematol* 1992;29:54.
Reviews the mechanisms of drug-induced immune hemolytic anemias as well as other immune cytopenias.
Shinar E, Rachmilewitz EA. Oxidative denaturation of red cells in thalassemia. *Semin Hematol* 1990;27:70.
Covers all the oxidative hemolytic anemias.
Steinberg MH. Management of sickle cell disease. *N Engl J Med* 1999;340:1021.
Describes the detailed clinical features and treatment of sickle cell disease.

98. TRANSFUSION THERAPY: BLOOD COMPONENTS AND TRANSFUSION COMPLICATIONS

William V. Walsh

I. Blood component therapy

A. Red cell transfusions are generally provided as packed red blood cells (PRBC), rather than whole blood. The indication for PRBC transfusion is inadequate oxygen-carrying capacity in patients who are anemic or acutely bleeding. There is no generally accepted "transfusion trigger." A transfusion threshold of a hemoglobin concentration of 8 g/dl has been recommended by the Transfusion Practices Committee of the American Association of Blood Banks (AABB), and a threshold of 7 g/dl was recommended by both a 1988 NIH consensus conference and the Clinical Efficacy Assessment Project of the American College of Physicians. However, these guidelines referred to stable postoperative or medical patients, and may not be applicable to the critically ill.

Patients can compensate for severe anemia with fluid retention leading to intravascular volume expansion and increased cardiac output, lowered blood viscosity, and decreased hemoglobin affinity for oxygen, all resulting in increased oxygen delivery to tissues. A patient's ability to compensate is influenced by (1) how rapidly the anemia has evolved, (2) whether the patient has underlying atherosclerotic disease, and (3) whether acute bleeding has been stopped.

A rational approach to RBC transfusion therapy, therefore, focuses on signs and symptoms of inadequate tissue oxygenation (frequently myocardial or cerebral ischemia) or on physiologic data, such as decreased mixed venous oxygen saturation.

Anemia in the intensive care unit (ICU) patient is often partly caused by frequent diagnostic phlebotomies. Efforts are necessary to minimize these procedures or to limit the required volumes of blood.

B. Platelet transfusions are indicated for thrombocytopenic (platelet count < 50,000/mm^3) patients who are actively bleeding and, prophylactically, if invasive procedures are contemplated or if the risk of spontaneous hemorrhage is high (platelet count < 5,000/mm^3 or < 10,000/mm^3 with another risk factor for bleeding). Prophylactic platelet transfusions are most effective in patients with hypoproliferative thrombocytopenia (e.g., acute leukemia or after chemotherapy) and are seldom indicated in hyperproliferative conditions (e.g., idiopathic thrombocytopenic purpura). Frequently, in the ICU, both platelet consumption and bone marrow suppression contribute to thrombocytopenia. Platelet transfusions may be useful as a temporizing measure while specific therapies against the underlying cause of platelet consumption are instituted.

The dose of platelets is approximately 1 U/10 kg of body weight. Platelets are available as a pooled product from five to eight individual donors or, more commonly, as a pheresis pack harvested from an individual donor containing the equivalent of 7 to 10 U of pooled platelet concentrates. Pheresis packs convey less infectious risk and, potentially, less risk for alloimmunization. A single unit raises the platelet count of a healthy recipient by 5,000 to 10,000/mm^3. Fever, sepsis, disseminated intravascular coagulation (DIC), hypersplenism, and hemorrhage all shorten platelet survival and lessen the observed increment. Platelet counts are generally obtained 1 hour after transfusion and again 12 to 24 hours later, to measure efficacy.

C. Granulocyte transfusion is rarely performed because of both the difficulties in harvesting adequate amounts of functional granulocytes at pheresis and the high incidence of toxic reactions with their transfusion. Recent studies have shown that granulocyte colony-stimulating factor can be used to mobilize large numbers of functional granulocytes from donors. Granulocyte transfusions are generally reserved for profoundly neutropenic patients, without evidence of marrow recovery and with evidence of an advancing, usually fungal infection.

D. Fresh frozen plasma (FFP) is used to replete multiple clotting factor deficiencies that can occur with DIC, liver failure, vitamin K deficiency, or massive transfusion; more rarely, it is used to replace a single factor when no specific factor concentrate is available. Indications and usage are controversial, but an often quoted standard is a prothrombin time more than 1.5 times control in the presence of bleeding or in anticipation of an invasive procedure, when no specific therapy (e.g., vitamin K administration) is feasible. Another accepted indication is the use of FFP transfusion in conjunction with plasmapheresis to treat thrombotic thrombocytopenic purpura.

A solvent-detergent–treated FFP is now available, markedly reducing the risk of infectious complications.

E. Cryoprecipitate is generally used only to treat actively bleeding patients with hypofibrinogenemia associated with DIC. In emergencies, when specific factor concentrates are unavailable, it can also be used to treat patients with von Willebrand's disease. Generally, 8 to 10 bags of cryoprecipitate (each from an individual donor) are required, which represents an increased infectious risk.

F. Albumin has been used by some to increase both intravascular volume and oncotic pressure. However, many authorities feel that crystalloid is as effective in raising the intravascular volume and, because of rapid clearance, the effect of albumin on core pressure is often fleeting. Reactions to albumin and infectious complications are rare.

II. Complications

A. Immunologic complications

1. **Acute hemolytic transfusion reactions (HTR)** occur rarely (approximately 1 of every 20,000 U PRBC transfused) and are generally caused by a blood type A, B, or O (ABO) incompatibility. Clinical manifestations include gross hemoglobinuria, oliguric renal failure, hypotension, bronchospasm, and DIC. Initial symptoms and signs may include fever, backache, and flushing. Treatment involves immediate discontinuation of the transfusion and supportive measures such as crystalloid and diuretic use to maintain renal perfusion, vasopressors, bronchodilators, and steroids. Platelets and FFP may be necessary if the consumptive coagulopathy is severe. Mortality remains substantial.
2. **Delayed HTR** occur 1 to 3 weeks after transfusion. The incidence is once in several thousand transfusions. These reactions are caused by an anamnestic alloantibody to transfused RBC antigens. Anamnestic antibodies develop after previous remote sensitizations (e.g., pregnancy or prior blood transfusion), but are present in low titer and, therefore, are difficult to detect in screening. The antibody titers increase rapidly after reexposure to antigen and cause hemolysis. Clinical signs include fever and hemolytic anemia. Only 10% of these patients develop oliguria and renal failure. Most patients recover with supportive care.
3. **Febrile, nonhemolytic transfusion reactions** occur commonly and are generally innocuous. Patients present with fever and urticaria, which may necessitate interruption of the transfusion until more serious reactions are excluded. Their incidence can be reduced by premedication with acetaminophen, diphenhydramine, or both and by the use of leukocyte-depleted or plasma-depleted blood products. The pathophysiology is felt to involve either a recipient's reaction to contaminating leukocyte antigens in the product or an effect of leukocyte-derived cytokines which, during storage, accumulate in the plasma contaminating the product.
4. **Transfusion-related graft-versus-host disease (GVHD)** usually occurs in markedly immune compromised patients (e.g., patients with acute leukemia or premature infants) but has been occasionally reported in patients with normal immunity. Donor lymphocytes contaminating the blood product recognize recipient antigens as foreign and generate an immune reaction, leading to severe dermatitis, liver disease, gastroenteritis, and myelosuppression. Therapy involves immune suppressant drugs and supportive measures, but

GVHD is frequently fatal. GVHD usually can be prevented by irradiation of blood products, which abrogates the lymphocyte's ability to respond to mitogen without harming the other blood cells.

5. **Transfusion-related immunosuppression** is a controversial topic. Transfusions retrospectively have been associated with decreased rejection of renal allografts, possibly increased recurrence rates of colorectal cancer, and a modest increase in the rate of wound infections.
6. **Anaphylactic, nonhemolytic reactions** can develop in IgA-deficient patients with anamnestic class-specific antibodies to IgA in serum contaminating blood products. These patients should receive washed platelets or RBC, or FFP from IgA-deficient donors.
7. **Posttransfusion purpura,** which rarely has been induced by blood transfusion, generally occurs in women alloimmunized to platelet antigens during pregnancy. Although her platelets lack the offending antigen, the woman's antibody is apparently cross-reactive to her own platelets when produced in high titer. In severe cases, plasma exchange is necessary.

B. Infectious complications

1. **The risk of the human immunodeficiency virus (HIV) transmission** via blood transfusion is currently estimated at 1 of 800,000 U transfused. This remarkably low risk is because of self-exclusion or rejection of potential donors with risk factors for HIV infection, as well as to screening of donated units with the well-known enzyme-linked immunosorbent assay (ELISA) test (which detects HIV antibody) and the p24 antigen test (which markedly reduces the "window" after infection but prior to antibody production when units could test negative).

   An infected product will transmit virus to 79% of recipients. Untreated, 5% to 10% of recipients per year develop the acquired immune deficiency syndrome (AIDS).
2. **Human T lymphocyte virus (HTLV-1)** is a retrovirus that is transmitted with an efficiency of 20% to 40% by infected units. Of patients, 2% to 4% infected with HTLV-1 ultimately develop an acute T-cell leukemia; less than 1% develop a degenerative neurologic disease, tropical spastic paraparesis.
3. **The current risks** of transmission of hepatitis B and C are, respectively, 1 of 60,000 and 1 of 125,000. Acute posttransfusion hepatitis (PTH) develops 1 to 3 months after transfusion and is generally mild. However, almost half of patients with PTH develop chronic disease, and a significant proportion progress to cirrhosis, hepatoma, or both.
4. **Cytomegalovirus (CMV)** can be transmitted, although leukocyte depletion minimizes this risk. CMV can cause serious infections in immune compromised patients.
5. **Bacterial infections,** from contamination of the unit in processing, can be transmitted. These occur more commonly with platelet products, which are stored at room temperature, which facilitates bacterial growth.
6. **Malarial and protozoal infections** can occasionally be transmitted from asymptomatic donors recently arrived from regions where these agents are endemic.

C. Other complications

1. **Volume overload** occurs commonly. Each unit of PRBC or FFP may contribute 250 to 400 ml to intravascular volume. Multiple transfusions require careful attention to fluid management.
2. **Metabolic toxicity** is caused by the so-called "storage lesion" of blood products, in which the pH falls and the ammonia and potassium concentrations rise in stored products. With massive transfusion, patients can develop acidemia and clinically significant hyperkalemia or ammonia intoxication, as well as hypothermia if the products were refrigerated.
3. **Citrate** is used to anticoagulate blood products by chelating calcium. Massive transfusion can occasionally cause symptomatic hypocalcemia in neonates.
4. **Posttransfusion acute respiratory distress syndrome (ARDS)** can occur, especially in the setting of tissue trauma and hypotension. Whether blood products are causative is controversial. This syndrome is usually self-limited.

5. **Coagulopathy** can develop in heavily transfused patients. Once felt to be dilutional (because of transfusion of PRBC deficient in platelets and clotting factors), causation is now controversial. Clinical bleeding is rare. Policies mandating routine transfusion of FFP or platelets for every set number of PRBC transfusions are controversial.
6. **Iron deposition** leading to organ damage will occur in chronically transfused patients. This is a great concern in children with thalassemia and can be treated with chelation therapy.

II. Alternatives to random volunteer homologous blood product use

A. Preoperative autologous donation and perioperative blood salvage are the safest means of blood product support, but they may have limited relevance to the ICU setting.

B. Directed donations are discouraged by the American Red Cross and AABB, as theoretically they are slightly less safe than random volunteer-donated products, especially with regard to risk of GVHD.

C. Desmopressin (DDAVP), rather than cryoprecipitate or platelets, should be used for minor invasive procedures in patients with von Willebrand's disease or platelet dysfunction caused by uremia.

D. Recombinant erythropoietin will ameliorate anemia caused by renal insufficiency, AIDS, myeloma, and chemotherapy.

E. Care of patients who mandate "bloodless" approaches requires use of parenteral iron, vitamin B and folate supplements, and erythropoietin, as well as efforts to minimize blood loss.

Selected Readings

Autologous blood transfusions. *JAMA* 1986;256:2378.

American Medical Association position paper endorsing and describing autologous transfusions as well as cell-saver systems and hemodilution.

Consensus Conference. Perioperative red blood cell transfusion. *JAMA* 1988;260:2700.

Discuss indications for transfusion, morbidities of transfusion, and alternatives. Questions the then dogma that Hb concentrations less than 10 g/dl were associated with increased anesthesia risk and poor wound healing.

Gresens CJ, Holland PV. Current risks of viral hepatitis from blood transfusions. *J Gastroenterol Hepatol* 1998;13:443.

A comprehensive review of the topic.

Guidelines for counseling persons infected with human T-lymphotrophic virus type I (HTLV-I) and type II (HTLV-II). *Ann Intern Med* 1993;188:448.

Developed by the Centers for Disease Control, these guidelines discuss screening tests for HTLV-I and HTLV-II, associated diseases, and the transmission risk.

Heddle NM, Klama L, Meyer R, et al. A randomized, controlled trial comparing plasma removal with white cell reduction to prevent reactions to platelets. *Transfusion* 1999;39:231.

Plasma removal is more effective than poststorage white blood cell reduction in preventing reactions.

Mannucci PM. Desmopressin: a non-transfusional form of treatment for congenital and acquired bleeding disorders. *Blood* 1988;72:1449.

A comprehensive review of the use of DDAVP.

Petz LD, Swisher SN, Kleinman SK, et al, eds. *Clinical practice of transfusion medicine.* New York: Churchill Livingstone; 1995.

A comprehensive, yet quite readable textbook.

Savarese D, Waitkus H, Stewart FM, et al. Bloodless medicine and surgery. *Intensive Care Med* 1999;14:20.

The article considers various means of minimizing or eliminating the need for blood product support, prompted by the organized desires of Jehovah's Witness patients and others desiring a "bloodless" approach.

Thaler M, Shamiss A, Orgad S, et al. The role of blood from HLA-homozygous donors in fatal transfusion-associated graft-versus-host disease after open heart surgery. *N Engl J Med* 1989;321:25.

Describes the causative role played by transfusion of fresh blood from family members with a one-way HLA match in causing GVHD in immune competent patients.

Welch HG, Meehan KR, Goodnough LT. Prudent strategies for elective red blood cell transfusion. *Ann Intern Med* 1992;116:393.

Describes the research underlying the clinical guideline for RBC transfusion adopted by the American College of Physicians in 1992.

Wheatley T, Veitch PS. Effect of blood transfusion on postoperative immunocompetence. *Br J Anaesth* 1997;78:489.

An excellent, even-handed, brief review.

99. GRANULOCYTOPENIA

Diane M.F. Savarese and F. Marc Stewart

I. Definition. Granulocytopenia refers to an absolute decrease in granulocytes to less than 1,500 to 2,000 cells/mm^3. *Agranulocytosis* is a profound decrease in granulocytes, most often when the condition is drug-induced.

II. Differential diagnosis. The most common causes include drugs, sepsis, alcohol, nutritional deficiencies, and hemodialysis. The mechanism of granulocytopenia (Table 99-1) may be (a) decreased or ineffective marrow production, (b) increased destruction secondary to immune or nonimmune causes, or (c) redistribution from the circulating to the marginal pool.

With most chemotherapeutic agents, the granulocyte nadir occurs between 10 and 14 days after therapy. Other drugs such as melphalan, carmustine, and busulfan have a delayed nadir at 30 to 36 days; neutrophils may not recover for 6 weeks. Bone marrow transplantation patients can have a severe, prolonged period of neutropenia that can last from 12 days in an autologous stem cell transplant, to more than 25 days in a recipient of a matched, unrelated allogeneic transplant. Radiation of marrow proliferative areas such as pelvis, skull, ribs, spine, and sternum can also directly damage marrow stem cells. In large doses, alcohol can cause clinically significant neutropenia. In alcohol-related neutropenia, other factors such as folate deficiency and congestive splenomegaly from cirrhosis, can play a role. A variety of drugs can damage marrow stem cell production by an idiosyncratic reaction. A partial list is shown in Table 99-2.

Bacterial infections seldom cause neutropenia unless overwhelming septicemia is present. Viral infections can cause transient granulocytopenia. In patients with the acquired immune deficiency syndrome (AIDS), the frequency of leukopenia can be as high as 70%, and is commonly multifactorial. Cytomegalovirus (CMV)-associated neutropenia may be seen in organ and marrow transplant recipients. B19 parvovirus infections occasionally cause pure red cell aplasia and, in a few cases, neutropenia.

Transient granulocytopenia caused by peripheral consumption has been observed in patients with renal failure on hemodialysis. The granulocytopenia resolves within 1 to 2 hours after dialysis is stopped. Anaphylactic reactions to endotoxin or foreign proteins may stimulate complement activation, leading to transient neutropenia.

Acute leukemia can present as an isolated neutropenia; in most cases, however, patients are pancytopenic The diagnosis is easily confirmed by bone marrow aspirate or biopsy. Refractory anemia, preleukemia, paroxysmal nocturnal hemoglobinuria, and marrow infiltration by solid tumors can also cause neutropenia.

Increased destruction of neutrophils can occur on a nonimmune or an immune basis. Liver disease can produce splenomegaly and subsequent neutropenia. Collagen vascular diseases (e.g., systemic lupus erythematosus) can cause neutropenia on an immune basis, and Felty's syndrome may present with neutropenia.

III. Evaluation. A review of the history and the clinical setting should identify obvious precipitating factors; if not, the patient should be evaluated for occult infections or viral diseases. If neutropenia antedated admission to the intensive care unit, an attempt should be made to obtain previous blood counts to determine chronicity. Pulmonary infiltrates may prompt bronchoalveolar lavage (BAL) to assist in identifying pathogens such as *Pneumocystis carinii, Legionella sp, Mycobacteria sp,* and viral infections with CMV, herpes simplex, or zoster. Open lung biopsies occasionally give useful information to exclude invasive infection.

The peripheral blood smear and possibly the bone marrow must be examined to rule out a primary hematologic disorder. Chromosomal abnormalities may be diagnostic in patients with acute leukemia. Vacuolated bone marrow cells suggest a drug-induced idiosyncratic effect. Patients with a history of poor nutrition or those

TABLE 99-1. Mechanisms of neutropenia

Drug-induced
- *Decreased production*
  - Chemotherapy
  - Alcohol
  - Phenothiazines and other drugs (see Table 99-2)
  - Radiation
- *Increased destruction*
  - Penicillin
  - Quinidine
  - Procainamide

Not drug induced
- *Decreased production*
  - Viral infections (infectious mononucleosis, hepatitis, cytomegalovirus, measles, rubella, varicella)
  - Replacement of marrow by tumor or leukemia
  - Aplastic anemia
  - Leukemia
  - Human cyclic neutropenia
  - Chronic benign neutropenia
  - Congenital disease (Kostmann's syndrome)
  - B_{12} deficiency
  - Folate deficiency
- *Increased destruction*
  - *Nonimmune-mediated*
  - Hypersplenism
  - Renal dialysis
  - *Immune-mediated*
  - Autoimmune neutropenia
  - Felty's syndrome
  - Systemic lupus erythematosus
  - Paroxysmal nocturnal hemoglobinuria

who are maintained on mechanical ventilators for prolonged periods without folate supplementation should have serum and erythrocyte folate levels measured. Antinuclear antibodies or latex fixation studies may implicate collagen vascular diseases. Although assays for antineutrophil antibodies are relatively nonspecific, a positive test and characteristic bone marrow may suggest an autoimmune process.

IV. Management. Therapy depends on the cause and the degree of the neutropenia and whether fever is present. In patients with drug-induced neutropenia, any suspected drug should be withdrawn if possible. Most patients with drug-induced granulocytopenia recover spontaneously and uneventfully after 10 to 14 days.

In the absence of fever, prophylactic antibiotics need not be started. If an oral temperature of more than 38.2°C is present and the granulocyte count is less than 500 to 1,000/mm^3, blood and urine cultures should be obtained and broad-spectrum antibiotics initiated immediately. If CMV infection is suspected, "buffy coat" leukocyte cultures and urine cultures for CMV should be obtained.

The antibiotic regimen should include an antibiotic active against *Pseudomonas aeruginosa,* such as ceftazidime, often with an aminoglycoside. In patients allergic to penicillin or cephalosporins, a reasonable choice is ofloxacin with an aminoglycoside or aztreonam. Vancomycin can be added if there is a strong suggestion of a gram-positive infection, or if the patient has known colonization with methicillin-resistant staphylococci.

In an acute neutropenia secondary to chemotherapy or idiosyncratic drug reaction, antibiotic treatment should be continued until neutrophil recovery (> 500/mm^3). A

TABLE 99-2. Drugs that induce neutropenia by stem cell injury

Antiinfectives
Semisynthetic penicillins
Penicillin
Sulfonamides
Metronidazole
Vancomycin
Isoniazid
Ciprofloxacin
Beta-lactams
Nitrofurantoin
Zidovudine
Ganciclovir
Acyclovir
Antithyroid agents
Propylthiouracil
Methimazole
Anticonvulsants
Phenytoin
Carbamazepine
Cardiovascular agents
Captopril
Procainamide
Quinidine
Calcium channel blockers
Chlorothiazide
Hydrochlorothiazide
Antiinflammatory agents
Gold salts
Non-steroidal antiinflammatory agents
Penicillamine
Psychiatric agents
Phenothiazines
Meprobamate
Imipramine/desipramine
Selective serotonin reuptake inhibitors
Gastrointestinal drugs
Salicylazosulfapyridine (azulfidine)
Cimetidine/ranitidine
Metoclopramide

detailed algorithm for fever of unknown origin and granulocytopenia is shown in Figure 99-1. If an organism is isolated by culture and the patient remains neutropenic, broad-spectrum antibiotics should be continued, taking care that the isolated organism is adequately covered. If fever persists despite broad-spectrum antibiotics, especially if the patient is immunocompromised, fungal infection must be considered and empiric amphotericin-B added. Initial broad-spectrum antibiotic coverage should not be narrowed based on positive cultures until the neutropenia resolves.

In the setting of established febrile neutropenia, the reactive use of hematopoietic growth factors such as granulocyte colony-stimulating factor (G-CSF) and granulocyte-macrophage colony-stimulating factor (GM-CSF) is frequent but unsupported by the literature. No study has ever demonstrated improved survival despite a modest reduction in the number of days of neutropenia and the number of days of hospitalization when growth factors were added to antibiotic therapy in

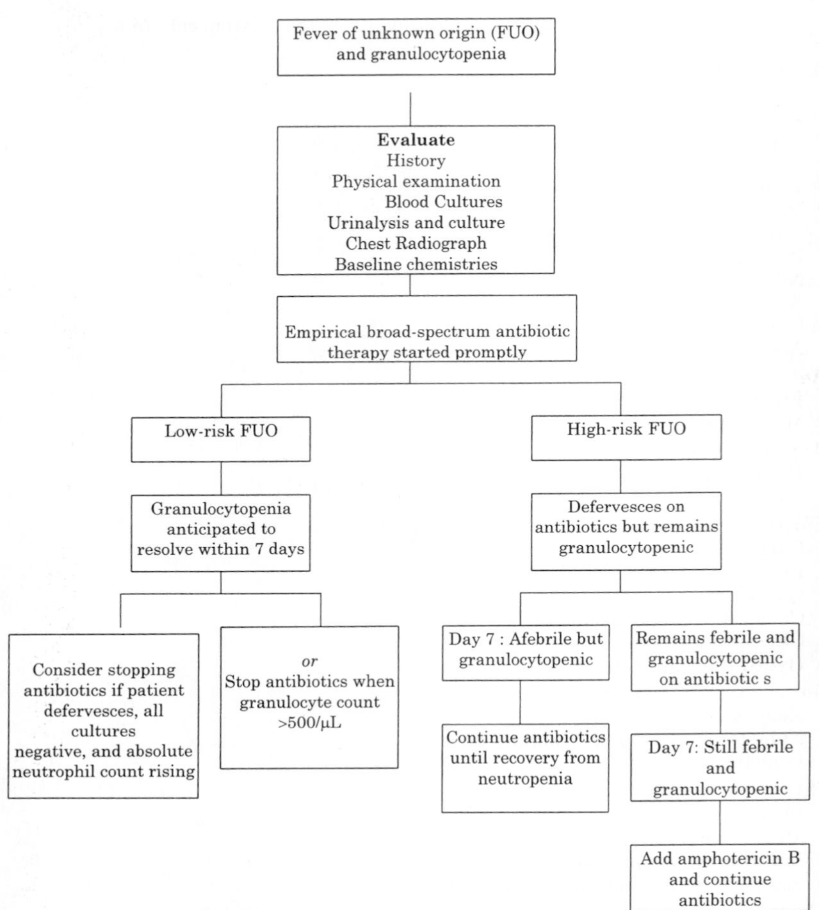

FIG. 99-1. Algorithm for managing fever of unknown etiology in the granulocytopenic patient. (Modified from Devita VT Jr., Hellman S, Rosenberg SA, eds. In: *Cancer, Principles & Practice of Oncology,* 5th ed. Philadelphia: Lippincott–Raven; 1997, with permission.)

patients with febrile neutropenia. Nevertheless, use of G-CSF or GM-CSF is a reasonable therapeutic maneuver in a patient who is profoundly and persistently neutropenic, and at high risk because of pneumonia, hypotension, multiorgan dysfunction, or fungal infection.

Anecdotal reports have suggested that drug-induced agranulocytosis responds to GM-CSF. In neutropenic human immunodeficiency virus (HIV)-positive patients, GM-CSF and G-CSF result in increases in neutrophil counts and augmentation of neutrophil function as well as increases in CD4+ lymphocytes; these are not sustained once growth factor is withdrawn.

Selected Readings

Coyle TE. Hematologic complications of human immunodeficiency virus infection and the acquired immunodeficiency syndrome. *Med Clin North Am* 1997:81:449.

Hematologic abnormalities are among the most common manifestations of advanced HIV infection. This excellent recent review is detailed and well written with an extensive background reference list.

Hathorn JW, Lyke K. Empirical treatment of febrile neutropenia: evolution of current therapeutic approaches. *Clin Infect Dis* 1997;24:S256.

This recent review of available therapeutic options for empiric antibiotic therapy presents a good historical perspective on the evolution of management approaches for febrile neutropenia.

Hughes WT, Armstrong D, Bodey GP, et al. 1997 guidelines for the use of antimicrobial agents in neutropenic patients with unexplained fever. *Clin Infect Dis* 1997;25:551.

This is the first in a series of practice guidelines commissioned by the Infectious Disease Society of America that provides evidence-based guidelines for diagnosis and management of neutropenic patients with unexplained fever.

Maher DW, Lieschke GJ, Green NM, et al. Filgrastim in patients with chemotherapy induced febrile neutropenia, a double-blind, placebo controlled trial. *Ann Intern Med* 1994;121:492.

This study randomized 218 patients with cancer and febrile neutropenia to receive granulocyte colony-stimulating factor (G-CSF) or placebo. Neutrophil recovery was accelerated with the granulocyte-macrophage colony-stimulating factor (GCSF) treatment and the duration of febrile neutropenia was shortened, resulting in a decreased risk for prolonged hospitalization.

Pizzo PA. Management of fever in patients with cancer and treatment-induced neutropenia. *N Engl J Med* 1993;328:1323.

This paper represents a seminal review of management of patients with cancer and treatment-induced neutropenia. It is well written, succinct, and presents excellent of guidelines for the management of patients—from initial presentation through resolution of neutropenia.

Rubin M, Hathorn JW, Marshall D, et al. Gram positive infections and the use of vancomycin in 350 episodes of fever and neutropenia. *Ann Intern Med* 1988;108:30.

The use of vancomycin for empiric coverage of febrile neutropenic patients is a controversial area. This paper provides support for withholding vancomycin in routine empiric therapy but adding it when clinical or microbiologic data suggest the need for it.

Vellenga E, Uyl-de Groot CA, de Wit R, et al. Randomized placebo-controlled trial of granulocyte-macrophage colony-stimulating factor in patients with chemotherapy-related febrile neutropenia. *J Clin Oncol* 1996;14:619.

This is a randomized, placebo-controlled trial of granulocyte-macrophage colony-stimulating factor (GMCSF) versus placebo in 134 patients with chemotherapy-related febrile neutropenia. This trial demonstrated that GMCSF shortens the period of neutrophil recovery but does not affect the number of days for resolution of fever or the duration of hospitalization.

100. THE LEUKEMIAS

Karen K. Ballen and F. Marc Stewart

I. General principles and definition. The use of chemotherapy has made many cancers, including acute myelogenous leukemia (AML) and acute lymphoblastic leukemia (ALL) potentially curable. Approximately 30% of adults with acute leukemia can be cured of their disease. High-dose chemotherapy followed by either autologous or allogeneic stem cell transplantation is now used as a curative therapy for patients with acute and chronic leukemia, lymphoma, myeloma, aplastic anemia, and it may be curative for more common diseases such as breast cancer and ovarian cancer.

II. Pathogenesis. Acute lymphoblastic leukemia occurs primarily in children, but it also occurs in adults. At presentation, patients will have leukemic involvement of the bone marrow, leading to pancytopenia. Patients may also have a mediastinal mass, leukemic meningitis, and testicular involvement. Acute myelogenous leukemia is more common in adults. The monocytic variants are associated with leukemic infiltration into the skin, gums, and meninges, and the promyelocytic variant can be associated with disseminated intravascular coagulation.

III. Diagnosis. Patients with acute leukemia often present with fatigue, shortness of breath, infection, and bleeding as a result of anemia, neutropenia, and thrombocytopenia. Diagnosis is made on bone marrow aspirate and biopsy. Acute leukemia is defined as greater than 30% blasts in the bone marrow. Lymphoblastic leukemia is distinguished from myelogenous leukemia on the morphology of the blast cells, histochemical stains, and flow cytometry.

IV. Treatment. Induction chemotherapy refers to chemotherapy used to achieve complete remission. For acute myelogenous leukemia, a common regimen is idarubicin and cytosine arabinoside (ARA-C). For acute lymphoblastic leukemia, a common regimen is asparaginase, prednisone, vincristine, and cyclophosphamide (Cytoxan). Consolidation chemotherapy refers to chemotherapy used to sustain complete remission. Allogeneic bone marrow transplantation is recommended for young patients with a matched donor who are at high risk of relapse with standard chemotherapy. This risk assessment is often based on cytogenetic abnormalities.

V. Medical complications of the acute leukemias

A. Leukostasis. Leukostasis can result when the white blood count, predominantly blasts, is greater than 100,000/mm^3. It is more common in acute myelogenous leukemia because the myeloblasts are larger than the lymphoblasts. Leukostasis can affect both the respiratory and central nervous system. The respiratory complications include pulmonary infiltrates and hypoxia. Central nervous system complications include visual and mental status changes. Central nervous system hemorrhage is more likely in patients with leukostasis. The treatment for leukostasis is prompt institution of chemotherapy to treat the leukemia, with the guidance of hematology and oncology consultation. Hydroxyurea, which is given orally, can lower the white count within 8 to 12 hours, while arrangements for definitive chemotherapy are underway. Leukopheresis can also be performed as a temporizing measure. Because elevation of the hematocrit increases viscosity and can worsen the manifestations of leukostasis, red blood cell transfusions should be used very cautiously.

B. Bleeding. Bleeding can occur as a result of either thrombocytopenia or disseminated intravascular coagulation. A platelet count below 10,000/mm^3 increases the risk of spontaneous bleeding and the patient should be treated with platelet transfusion. Patients who have received multiple transfusions can become alloimmunized and demonstrate poor response to platelet transfusion. Transfusion of HLA-matched platelets may be helpful. Family donors should not be used if the patient is a candidate for allogeneic bone marrow transplantation because of the risk of sensitization to donor antigens. All patients who are candidates for bone marrow transplantation should receive either cytomegalovirus (CMV)-negative blood products or filtered blood products (the filtration system also reduces the load of CMV) to reduce the risk of reactivation of CMV during the subsequent transplant. All patients with leukemia should receive irradiated blood products to reduce the risk of transfusion-associated graft-versus-host disease.

Disseminated intravascular coagulation is more common with the acute promyelocytic (M3) variant of AML. The granules in the promyeloblasts release procoagulants. Laboratory abnormalities include an elevated prothrombin time (PT) and partial thromboplastin time (PTT) and a decreased platelet count and fibrinogen level. Treatment is with fresh frozen plasma and platelet transfusion. Heparin use is controversial. The definitive treatment is chemotherapy to treat the leukemia.

C. Infection. Although the white blood count may be high, most patients with leukemia are functionally neutropenic—the white blood cells do not function normally. Chemotherapy suppresses normal hematopoiesis, further increasing the susceptibility to infection. Common infectious agents include staphylococcal and streptococcal organisms. The incidence of these gram-positive infections has increased with the widespread use of indwelling catheters. Gram-negative infections such as *Escherichia coli* and pseudomonas are more likely in cases of severe damage to the intestinal tract. Fungal infection is a serious infection in immunocompromised patients and may present with skin lesions (candida), sinus involvement (aspergillus), lung lesions (candida and aspergillus), or hepatitis (candida). Fungal infections are more common in patients who have had prolonged antibiotic therapy, have an indwelling catheter, and are receiving total parenteral nutrition. Patients with ALL who are on prolonged steroid therapy are also at risk for *Pneumocystis carinii* pneumonia.

Fever should always be treated immediately as a presumptive infection. The fever workup should consist of a careful history and physical examination, blood cultures for bacteria and fungus, urine culture, and a chest x-ray study. Antibiotics to treat gram-negative infection, including pseudomonas, should be

TABLE 100-1. Side effects from chemotherapy agents

Drug	Alopecia	Nausea/ Vomiting	Bone Marrow Suppression	Other
Cytosine arabinoside (ARA-C)	+	+	++	Fever, renal failure, cerebellar toxicity
Idarubicin Daunorubicin	++	++	++	Cardiac, mucositis, vesicant
Etoposide	+	+	+	Hypotension
All trans retinoic acid (ATRA)				Increased white blood cells Lung infiltrates
Cyclophosphamide (Cytoxan)	+	++	++	Hemorrhagic cystitis
Prednisone				Muscle weakness Edema, glucose intolerance
Vincristine		+		Neuropathy
Asparginase				Pancreatitis, coagulopathy

started promptly. A common regimen is ceftazidime with or without an aminoglycoside. If fever persists for 48 hours, additional coverage for gram-positive infections, such as vancomycin, should be added. If fever persists an additional 3 to 5 days, amphotericin should be added as antifungal coverage.

D. Metabolic disturbances. Patients with leukemia are susceptible to metabolic and electrolyte dysfunction, either from tumor lysis syndrome caused by the rapid destruction of tumor cells, from different medications (e.g., the potassium and magnesium wasting seen in patients on amphotericin), or from parenteral nutrition. The tumor lysis syndrome is characterized by a high uric acid level and a low calcium level. The hyperuricemia can progress to renal failure. To prevent this complication, patients should be treated with allopurinol, adequate hydration, and alkalinization of the urine, prior to the start of induction chemotherapy.

E. Side effects from chemotherapy agents are summarized in Table 100-1.

Selected Readings

Anttila V, Elonen E, Nordling S, et al. Hepatosplenic candidiasis in patients with acute leukemia: incidence and prognostic Implications. *Clin Infect Dis* 1997;24:375.
Review of 562 patients with acute leukemia, describing the incidence of serious candida infections.

Buchner T. Treatment of adult acute leukemia. *Curr Opin Oncol* 1997;9;18.
Overview of current chemotherapy treatment for acute myelogenous leukemia (AML) and acute lymphoblastic leukemia (ALL).

Chanock SJ, Pizzo PA. Infectious complications of patients undergoing therapy for acute leukemia: current status and future prospects. *Semin Oncol* 1997;24:132.
Comprehensive update of infectious complications in leukemic patients.

Cripe LD. Adult acute leukemia. *Curr Probl Cancer* 1997;21:1.
Excellent review of pathogenesis, diagnosis, and treatment strategies of acute leukemia.

Dutcher JP, Schiffer CA, Wiernik PH. Hyperleukocytosis in adult acute nonlymphocytic leukemia: impact on remission rate, duration, and survival. *J Clin Oncol* 1987;5:1364.
Description of the negative correlation between leukostasis and survival.

Forman SJ. Stem cell transplantation in acute leukemia. *Curr Opin Oncol* 1998;10:10.
Brief review of indications for transplantation in patients with acute leukemia.

Heckman KD, Weiner GJ, Davis CS, et al. Randomized study of prophylactic platelet transfusion threshold during induction therapy for adult acute leukemia: 10,000/μl versus 20,000/μl. *J Clin Oncol* 1997;15:1143.
No difference seen in bleeding episodes whether 10,000 or 20,000 platelets used as a threshold for transfusion.

Thomas ED, Clift RA, Feiffer F, et al. Marrow transplantation for the treatment of chronic myelogenous leukemia. *Ann Intern Med* 1986;104:155.
The classic reference describing one of the first diseases to be cured by bone marrow transplantation.

101. ONCOLOGIC EMERGENCIES

Diane M.F. Savarese

I. Superior vena cava (SVC) syndrome

A. Etiology. SVC syndrome may be caused by intrinsic obstruction by thrombosis or direct tumor invasion or by extrinsic SVC collapse from tumor compression. Cancer, especially lung and breast cancer and lymphoma, causes most cases of SVC; other causes are mediastinal or radiation fibrosis and thrombosis, especially in the setting of an indwelling central venous line.

B. Clinical manifestations. The common symptoms and signs of SVC syndrome (Table 101-1) are related to poor venous return, increased intravenous (IV) pressure, and collateral vessel engorgement.

C. Diagnosis. SVC syndrome is a clinical diagnosis. The chest radiograph is abnormal in more than 80% of patients (e.g., superior mediastinal mass, pleural effusion, hilar or right upper lobe mass). Contrast chest computed tomography (CT) scan may localize the mass and suggest other possible impending complications (e.g., vertebral spread). A superior vena cavagram is rarely necessary to confirm the diagnosis.

Most patients present without a known diagnosis of cancer. A specific tissue diagnosis should be made by the simplest, least invasive method, beginning with thoracentesis, bronchoscopy, mediastinoscopy, and proceeding to thoracoscopy and finally to limited thoracotomy if necessary. Routine diagnostic procedures carry little excess risk in patients with SVC syndrome and elevated venous pressures. However, patients with tracheal compression or stridor should be approached as a true medical emergency and treated immediately (see below).

D. Treatment. Nonspecific methods to decrease venous pressures include bedrest with reverse Trendelenburg position, diuretics (maintaining adequate intravascular volume), decreased salt intake, and oxygen. Steroids, although commonly prescribed, are of limited benefit. Although the role of anticoagulation and thrombolysis is unclear, they may be of benefit in patients with thrombosis, especially in those with an indwelling central venous catheter. Specific treatment of the malignancy may require radiation, chemotherapy, or both. Emergent radiation may be lifesaving in patients who present with tracheal compression or stridor.

II. Epidural spinal cord compression (ECC)

A. Etiology and pathophysiology. Although virtually any tumor can invade the spinal epidural space, the most common are lung, breast, prostate, kidney, lymphoma, and myeloma. ECC can result from increasing intradural pressure from enlarging vertebral body metastases, retroperitoneal lymphadenopathy extending through the paravertebral neural foramina, a pathologic vertebral collapse, or intradural metastases. Vascular compromise resulting in spinal cord infarction and rapid, irreversible loss of function follows.

B. Clinical presentation. Back pain is the initial symptom in more than 90% of patients. Motor weakness, varying from minimal to paralysis, often exists at presentation, progressing to paraplegia within hours occasionally. Sensory deficits are rarely the initial sign, but usually develop during the clinical course. Autonomic dysfunction, manifesting as loss of bowel and bladder control, is a late and poor prognostic sign. The degree of neural compromise has an enormous impact on prognosis. Patients who begin treatment paraplegic almost never regain ambulation. Thus, early diagnosis of ECC is essential to prevent paralysis.

C. Diagnosis. Initial evaluation should consist of a thorough neurologic examination and plain x-ray studies of the spine looking for pedicle loss, vertebral compression fractures, and osteoblastic or osteolytic bone lesions. In one study,

TABLE 101-1. Common symptoms and signs of superior vena cava syndrome

Symptom/sign	Incidence (%)
Facial swelling	43
Trunk and/or extremity swelling	40
Dyspnea	20
Chest pain	20
Cough	20
Dysphagia	20
Dizziness	10
Syncope	10
Visual disturbance	10
Thoracic vein distention	67
Neck vein distention	59
Facial edema	56
Tachypnea	40
Plethora of face	19
Cyanosis	15
Upper extremity edema	9
Paralyzed true vocal cord	3
Horner's syndrome	2

plain spine radiographs accurately predicted the presence or absence of spinal epidural metastases in 83% of cases with a sensitivity of 81% and a specificity of 86%. If either physical examination or x-ray study is abnormal, further spine imaging, such as with magnetic resonance imaging (MRI) or myelography is necessary to exclude ECC.

The procedure of choice for diagnosing the location and extent of ECC is MRI. Contrast-enhanced MRI is especially helpful in identifying leptomeningeal and intramedullary lesions. CT myelography may be necessary because of a lack of availability of timely MRI scanning in the emergency setting. Generally, contrast medium is introduced through the lumbar spine until an obstruction is encountered. The anatomy above an obstruction is then defined by a cisterna magna or cervical spinal tap. It is crucial to see the upper and lower extent of the lesion. Myelography carries a small risk of further neurologic deterioration in the presence of complete block.

D. Treatment. Radiation therapy is generally the treatment of choice. Laminectomy should be considered in the following settings: (a) recurrence after radiation therapy; (b) no prior diagnosis of malignancy and no more easily accessible site for biopsy; (c) symptoms progress during radiation therapy; (d) lesions rapidly progress over less than 24 hours; or (e) a need for spinal stabilization.

Corticosteroids are uniformly recommended and should be started as soon as ECC is suspected to diminish edema. Most physicians recommend dexamethasone (10 to 24 mg) IV bolus followed by 16 to 24 mg/d in divided doses every 6 hours. Higher dosages (100 mg/d for 3 days) with rapid tapering may enhance analgesia but no differences in neurologic outcome have been noted.

III. Hypercalcemia of malignancy

A. Etiology and pathophysiology. The solid tumors most often responsible for hypercalcemia caused by bone metastases are carcinoma of the breast, lung, and kidney. Hypercalcemia in the absence of bone metastases most frequently occurs with lung (squamous cell carcinoma), kidney, and pancreas cancer; it is caused by ectopic production of parathyroid hormone-related protein (PTHrP) by the tumor. Hypercalcemia in hematologic malignancies such as multiple myeloma can be produced by direct bone invasion or the local production of humoral factors such as osteoclast activating factor.

B. Clinical manifestations. The effects of hypercalcemia depend on the degree of elevation of ionized serum calcium and the rate of rise. Changes in mental status (e.g., lethargy or depression) can be subtle, but psychotic behavior, obtundation, and coma can develop. The spectrum of digitalis-toxic arrhythmias can develop more easily in a hypercalcemic patient. The most characteristic electrocardiographic changes of hypercalcemia are prolonged PR interval, occasionally producing high-grade atrioventricular block and shortened QT interval.

The earliest effect of hypercalcemia on the kidney is a decrease in concentrating ability with polyuria; dehydration and prerenal azotemia commonly follow. Tubular damage from nephrocalcinosis can produce acidosis, glycosuria, hypomagnesemia, and aminoaciduria. Gastrointestinal signs of hypercalcemia include anorexia, nausea, vomiting, constipation, and abdominal pain.

C. Diagnosis. Once the presence of hypercalcemia is established, many potential causes can be eliminated by the patient's history (Table 101-2).

Most laboratories report a total serum calcium level rather than the biologically active ionized calcium level. Approximately 40% of total serum calcium is bound to protein, primarily albumin. Because 1 g of albumin binds 0.8 mg of calcium, a decrease of each 1 g/dl in serum albumin concentration below the normal concentration of 4.0 g/dl can be corrected for by adding 0.8 mg/dl to the measured serum calcium to produce a corrected serum value. In multiple myeloma, hyperglobulinemia leads to increased binding of calcium so that total calcium levels are elevated, but ionized calcium may be normal.

D. Treatment. Because hypercalcemic patients are usually volume depleted, fluid replacement is necessary, usually with normal saline at 150 to 300 ml/h. Furosemide can be used in the euvolemic patient to maintain urine output, taking care to avoid further volume depletion. Total intake and output, weight, serum electrolytes, and urine electrolytes (at least within the first 12 hours) should be closely monitored.

Treatment options are summarized in Table 101-3. Intravenous phosphate therapy is effective in lowering markedly elevated calcium levels within several

TABLE 101-2. Differential diagnosis of hypercalcemia

Cancer
- With bone metastasis (solid tumor)
- Without bone metastasis (solid tumor)
- Hematologic (multiple myeloma, leukemia, lymphoma with bone involvement)

Primary hyperparathyroidism

Toxic
- Thiazides
- Milk-alkali syndrome
- Vitamin D or A toxicity

Endocrine
- Thyrotoxicosis
- Adrenal insufficiency
- Pheochromocytoma (usually in association with primary hyperparathyroidism)

Granulomatous disease
- Tuberculosis
- Sarcoidosis

Immobilization (especially with underlying bone disease)

Artifactual
- Hyperalbuminemia or hypergammaglobulinemia
- Venous stasis (prolonged tourniquet application)

TABLE 101-3. Management of hypercalcemia

Agent	Dose	Route	Onset of effect	Duration of effect	Adverse effects	Comments
Normal saline ± Furosemide		i.v.	<24 h			Must hydrate before giving Furosemide
Calcitonin	2–8 U/kg q 6–12 h 4 U/kg i.m. b.i.d. (common)	s.c. i.m.	4 h	–24 h	Nausea, hypersensitivity (give test dose)	Used for acute control Tachyphylaxis I.M. better absorbed
Mithramycin	25µg/kg over 4 h	i.v.	24–48 h	–5 days	Nausea, vomiting Renal toxicity Hepatoxicity Coagulopathy ↓ Platelets	*Vesicant*
Steroids	40–100 mg/d	p.o.	3–5 days	?	Many, both long- and short-term	Most effective for myeloma, breast cancer, lymphoma
Pamidronate	60–90 mg in 500 NS over 2–4 h	i.v.	24 h	Up to 14 days	Fever, ↓PO_4 ↑WBC, ↓Mg, ↓K	Maximal effect day 7
Gallium nitrate	200 mg/m^2 in 1 L NS over 24 h q.d. × 5	i.v.	24 h	2 weeks	Nephrotoxic Do not give unless creat ≤2.5	Maximal effect 4–5 days
Phosphate	1–3 g/d (Neutra-phos)	p.o.	24 h		*Diarrhea* Nausea	Useful for *mild* hypercalcemia
	50 mmol 6 h	i.v.	< 1 h		Hypotension, renal failure	*Toxic*
Dialysis						Last resort

i.m., intramuscularly; b.i.d., twice daily; q.d, every day; i.v., intravenously; s.c., subcutaneously; p.o., orally; NS, normal saline; WBC, white blood cell.

hours. Phosphates should not be given to patients who have elevated phosphate levels or significantly impaired renal function at the onset of therapy; concern over extraskeletal calcification has limited their usefulness. Although the frequency of complications can vary when an IV dose of phosphate is given slowly over 6 to 8 hours, rapid IV infusions have resulted in severe hypotension and hypocalcemia with extraskeletal calcifications. IV phosphates should be reserved for use in acute situations if other measures have not been successful or in the patient who is severely hypophosphatemic.

Bisphosphonates such as pamidronate have been shown to be effective in the acute treatment of the hypercalcemia of malignancy, with onset of action within 24 hours. Calcitonin causes rapid hypocalcemia by decreasing bone resorption and by increasing urinary calcium and phosphate excretion with onset of action of 4 hours. Concurrent use with steroids can delay development of tachyphylaxis. Mithramycin is best reserved for treatment of acute episodes because of toxicities and should be avoided in cytopenic patients. Steroids may be useful in the treatment of hypercalcemia associated with hematologic malignancies or breast cancer.

IV. Malignant pericardial disease

A. Etiology and pathogenesis. Primary pericardial tumors (sarcomas or mesotheliomas) occur rarely. Secondary pericardial involvement can occur as a result of direct invasion by adjacent tumors or by hematogenous or lymphatic metastatic spread, commonly from breast and lung cancer. Progressive disease can result in cardiac tamponade secondary to an enlarging effusion or restrictive or effusive disease from pericardial tumor growth or radiation fibrosis.

B. Clinical manifestations. Patients with cardiac tamponade present with pulsus paradoxus, venous hypotension, narrow pulse pressure, tachycardia, and, if cardiac tamponade is severe, with shock. Symptoms include facial swelling, dyspnea, and ill-defined chest discomfort.

Electrocardiographic abnormalities can include electrical alternans (rare in tamponade) or, more commonly, tachycardia, diffuse ST wave abnormalities, loss of voltage, T-wave inversions, or atrial arrhythmias. The chest x-ray film is nonspecific, although enlargement of the cardiac silhouette is commonly present.

C. Diagnosis. Echocardiography is the procedure of choice for the diagnosis of pericardial effusions. Chest CT may demonstrate pericardial thickening, and tumor extent and location. Cardiac catheterization is seldom needed to confirm the diagnosis.

D. Treatment. Cardiac tamponade requires prompt treatment. Supportive measures, such as IV volume expansion and supplemental oxygen, should be provided as needed while preparing for definitive therapy. Because of the decrease in diastolic filling attributable to the increased cardiac rate and chamber compression, medications that lower blood pressure, reduce preload, or decrease heart rate, (e.g. diuretics or beta-blockers) should be used with caution. Pericardiocentesis is the initial diagnostic procedure of choice in the workup of pericardial effusion of possible malignant origin and is therapeutic in patients with tamponade. The most common complications are right ventricular puncture, hemopericardium, and ventricular ectopy.

Prognosis of the patient with this condition is usually poor. Systemic tumor treatment can be considered for patients with chemotherapy-responsive cancers (breast, lymphoma). Radiation therapy can be useful in selected cases.

Mechanical interventions are usually recommended for definitive management. Indwelling intrapericardial catheters used in conjunction with systemic therapy or intrapericardial instillation of sclerosing agents such as doxycycline (0.5–1 g in 20 ml normal saline) or bleomycin (30–60 U) may prevent further symptomatic recurrence. Three available surgical approaches—subxiphoid pericardial window placement, limited thoracotomy with pleuropericardial window placement, and thoracotomy with pericardiectomy—provide alternative modes of treatment in a patient with an expected reasonable survival.

Selected Readings

Ahman FR. A reassessment of the clinical implications of the superior vena cava syndrome. *J Clin Oncol* 1984:2:961.

In a large series of 1,986 cases of superior vena cava syndrome are reviewed the safety of diagnostic procedures and the benefit of proceeding with a diagnostic study before embarking on treatment.

Bilezikian JP. Management of acute hypercalcemia. *N Engl J Medicine* 1992; 326: 1196.

This review article presents a succinct summary of modern management of hypercalcemia and a thorough discussion of available therapeutic options.

Byrne TN. Spinal cord compression from epidural metastasis. *N Engl J Med* 1992; 327:614.

This is an excellent recent summary of pathophysiology, presentation, diagnostic approaches, and state-of-the-art management of epidural spinal cord compression.

Liu G, Crump M, Goss PE, et al. Prospective comparison of the sclerosing agents doxycycline and bleomycin for the primary management of malignant pericardial effusion and cardiac tamponade. *J Clin Oncol* 1996;14:3141.

In this study, 27 patients were randomly assigned to intrapericardial instillation of bleomycin or doxycyline for the management of pericardial effusion after placement of a draining catheter. Although both were equally effective, bleomycin resulted in significantly less morbidity.

Rodichok LD, Harper GR, Ruckdeschel JC, et al. Early diagnosis of spinal epidural metastases. *Am J Med* 1981;70:1181.

This is a classic paper describing a study of 87 patients with back pain and a diagnosis of cancer. The use of the neurologic examination and plain radiographs of the spine to predict the risk for epidural cord compression is described.

Vaitkus PT, Herrmann HC, LeWinter MM. Treatment of malignant pericardial effusion. *JAMA* 1994;272:59.

This represents an excellent review of medical and surgical therapeutic modalities for the management of malignant pericardial effusion.

Wilkes JD, Fidias P, Baikus L, et al. Malignancy-related pericardial effusion. *Cancer* 1995:76:1377.

This paper reviews 127 cases of malignant pericardial effusion from the Roswell Park Cancer Institute, demonstrating that subxyphoid pericardiotomy is a safe intervention that effectively relieves pericardial effusion in 99% of cases with less than 10% recurrence and reoperation rates. An excellent review of surgical approaches to the management of pericardial effusion is provided.

X. PHARMACOLOGY, OVERDOSES, AND POISONINGS

102. APPLIED PHARMACOKINETICS

Erica L. Liebelt

I. **General principles.** Applied pharmacokinetics is the process of using measured drug concentrations, pharmacokinetic principles, and pharmacodynamic information to optimize drug therapy for individual patients. The change in drug concentration over time is related to the rate of drug absorption and administration, amount of drug administered, volume of distribution, rate of drug distribution from the central compartment to the tissue compartment, and rate of drug elimination.

II. **Drug administration and absorption.** The rate of drug absorption or administration influences or determines the time required to achieve therapeutic serum concentrations. Intravenous (IV) bolus, intermittent infusion, and continuous administration are three common methods of IV drug administration. Serum concentrations are assumed to have reached steady-state conditions after a drug has been administered for a period at least five times its half-life. Bioavailability is influenced by the fraction of active drug in its formulation, the rate of product dissolution, chemical properties of the dissolved drug, gastrointestinal (GI) motility, blood flow to the GI tract, blood pH, and surface area available for absorption, all of which can be altered by certain disease states, drugs, and surgery. For example, the absorption of acetaminophen can be enhanced with metoclopramide or delayed by the concomitant ingestion of an anticholinergic drug such as a phenothiazine.

First-pass effect or metabolism refers to the phenomenon whereby a proportion of an oral dose of a drug is metabolized by the liver or gut before it reaches the systemic circulation. In certain overdose situations, the first-pass metabolism can become saturated, with a resultant increase in the bioavailability of drugs. Examples include cyclic antidepressants, phenothiazines, opioids, and beta-blockers.

III. **Distribution.** The rate and extent of drug distribution depend on its chemical properties (protein and tissue binding, lipid solubility) and physiologic status of the patient. The volume of distribution (V_d) represents the theoretical volume into which a substance distributes in the body at equilibrium. It can be used to estimate the plasma drug concentration when a known amount of the drug has been ingested or given: V_d = dose/Cp where Cp is the plasma drug concentration. The larger the volume of distribution, the lower the serum drug's concentration relative to a dose and vice versa. Drugs with low V_d (< 1 L/kg) are distributed primarily in the extracellular fluid. Examples include aminoglycosides, phenobarbital, salicylates, and lithium. Drugs with large volumes of distribution (> 1 L/kg) have extensive tissue distribution and include digoxin, cyclic antidepressants, and phenytoin.

With first-order kinetics, the plasma or serum drug level declines at a rate equal to a constant fraction of the level per unit of time and can be characterized by a half-life, the time required for the drug level to decline by 50%. Most drugs have both a distribution (α) and elimination (β) phase half-life. The elimination half-life, $t_{1/2}$, equals $0.693/K_e$, where K_e is the elimination rate constant. Zero-order elimination occurs when a constant quantity of drug is eliminated per unit of time, of which ethanol, at intoxicating levels, is an example. Michaelis-Menten kinetics is a combination of first-order elimination kinetics at low drug concentrations and zero-order elimination at higher concentrations. It characterizes drugs that are eliminated by capacity-limited or saturable enzyme systems (e.g., aspirin and theophylline).

IV. **Protein binding.** The plasma proteins albumin and α-acid glycoprotein (AAG) are responsible for 95% of all drug binding. Only the unbound or free fraction of the drug is pharmacologically active. Decreased binding which occurs when protein levels are decreased or saturated (e.g., in overdoses) increases drug effects. Malnutrition, sepsis, burns, renal disease, and liver disease can all decrease albumin concentration and increase the percentage of free drug. Traumatic injuries, surgery, burns, psychiatric conditions, acute inflammation, and myocardial infarction are associated with large increases in AAG and, consequently, decrease circulating concentrations of free drug. Anionic drugs and weak acids (e.g., phenytoin, warfarin, and salicylates) tend to bind to albumin, whereas cationic drugs and weak bases (e.g., quinidine, propanolol, and lidocaine) usually bind to AAG.

V. Clearance. Clearance is a measurement of the body's ability to eliminate a substance from blood or plasma over time. Total body clearance is equal to the sum of all of the clearance processes—renal, hepatic, gastrointestinal, pulmonary, and artificial. It can be calculated by multiplying the rate constant of elimination by the volume of distribution ($Cl = K_e \times V_d$). If renal clearance accounts for 50% or more of total clearance, dosing regimens must be adjusted in patients with renal dysfunction to maintain appropriate serum drug concentrations. When a drug is freely filtered and neither secreted nor reabsorbed, renal clearance is equivalent to glomerular filtration rate (GFR). When renal function is stable, creatinine clearance (CrCl) and serum creatinine (SCr) are highly correlated and SCr can be used to estimate CrCl and, thus, GFR: CrCl (ml/min) = (140–age) × lean body weight/72 × SCr (multiply by 0.85 for women). Many disease states are associated with altered creatinine production, leading to poor correlation between SCr and GFR. In some instances, the actual CrCl should be measured using an 8-hour urine collection.

Hepatic clearance depends on blood flow to the liver, the intrinsic activity of hepatic enzymes, and the fraction of drug that is unbound and free to interact with these enzymes. Alterations in hepatic blood flow caused by drugs, surgical procedures, or disease states such as shock or heart failure cause significant changes in the rate of elimination of drugs such as aminoglycosides, lidocaine, meperidine, and ranitidine. The cytochrome mixed-function oxidase enzyme systems can be induced by specific drugs (phenobarbital, rifampin) and, thus, affect the metabolism of other drugs (acetaminophen, theophylline). Liver disease decreases the clearance of many drugs.

Selected Readings

Cockcroft DW, Gault MH. Prediction of creatinine clearance from serum creatinine. *Nephron* 1976;16:31.

Describes the formula used to predict creatinine clearance from serum creatinine, including its derivation and factors to correct for age and body weight.

Evans W, Schentag J, Jusko W, eds. *Applied pharmacokinetics: principles of therapeutic drug monitoring.* Vancouver, WA: Applied Therapeutics; 1990.

Extensive discussion on general aspects of pharmacokinetics and in-depth discussions on the pharacokinetics and dose—response data of various commonly monitored drugs.

Klotz U. Pathophysiological and disease-induced changes in drug distribution volume: pharmacokinetic implications. *Clin Pharmacokinet* 1976;1:204.

Reviews the effect of various disease states on a drug's volume of distribution and the clinical implications of these effects.

Pond SM, Tozer TN. First-pass elimination: basic concepts and clinical consequences. *Pharmacokinetics* 1984;9:1.

Detailed discussion of first-pass elimination, its effect on bioavailability of drugs, and implications on clinical and therapeutic effects.

Rosenberg J, Benowitz NL, Pond S. Pharmacokinetics of drug overdose. *Clin Pharmacokinet* 1981;6:161.

Detailed discussion of the pharmacokinetic differences that occur when drugs are taken in overdose. Several specific drugs are reviewed in this context.

Sue YJ, Shannon M. Pharmacokinetics of drugs in overdose. *Clin Pharmacokinet* 1992;23:93.

A review of the altered patterns of absorption, distribution, and metabolism or elimination that occur during drug overdose and a discussion of the clinical implications.

Tillement J, Lhoste F, Giudicelli JF. Diseases and drug protein binding. *Clin Pharmacokinet* 1978;3:144.

Discussion of diseases that decrease protein binding of drugs as a result of hypoalbuminemia and whether this reduction has clinically significant modifications on pharmacologic effects of drugs.

Winter ME, Koda-Kimble MA, Young LY, eds. *Basic clinical pharmacokinetics,* 2nd ed. Vancouver, Wa: Applied Therapeutics; 1988.

Simplified explanations of pharmacokinetic concepts and chapters on the calculation of doses for commonly monitored drugs, with multiple examples.

103. INDIVIDUALIZING AND MONITORING DRUG THERAPY

Jeffrey R. Tucker

I. General principles. Alteration in drug disposition can alter the response to pharmacotherapy. Drug disposition can be affected by many physiologic changes resulting from underlying disease, sepsis, or injury. Many pharmacokinetic and pharmacodynamic alterations can be anticipated by knowing the patient's physiologic status. Failing to appreciate the influence of dynamic changes results in greater variation in drug response and leads to a higher risk of treatment failure or serious drug-induced toxicity.

II. Dosage requirements. Variation in dosage requirements is not readily predictable by common organ function tests, such as serum creatinine or liver function tests. In contrast, estimates of cardiac output, oxygen delivery, and drug clearance can predict pharmacokinetic changes and allow for appropriate alterations in drug therapy. End-organ responses to illness or injury (e.g., oxygen clearance, cardiac output, serum proteins, vascular volume, extracellular fluid volume, metabolic rate, urinary urea nitrogen, urinary catecholamines, regional shunting in blood flow, amino acid utilization, and organ blood flow) can result in changes in drug disposition.

Three physiologic variables that the clinician can use to make qualitative assessments and inferences regarding a drug's disposition characteristics are the cardiac output, organ function, and serum protein concentration. The disposition of many drugs follows the changes in organ function, especially those agents that are dependent on organ blood flow for clearance. Drugs eliminated via the kidney by glomerular filtration generally appear to follow flow-limited characteristics. Dosage regimens of drugs primarily eliminated by the kidney must be adjusted accordingly. Quantitative approaches using serum drug measurements to calculate dosage regimens necessary to attain desired serum concentrations have been evaluated in clinical settings and have improved patient survival rates or significantly decreased intensive care unit (ICU) stay.

Drugs metabolized by various enzyme systems are generally more complex and less predictable than the flow-limited agents. Their clearance characteristics are categorized as capacity-limited, meaning clearance is not primarily dependent on blood flow to the organ, but rather on the intrinsic clearance capacity of the drug's enzyme system.

III. Pharmacokinetic changes. The qualitative pharmacokinetic changes for many of the pharmacologic agents used in the patient in the ICU can be anticipated knowing the patient's response to underlying diseases, fluid balance, injury, sepsis, and the drug's physiologic clearance properties. It is essential to identify the clinical parameters that describe the patient's hyperdynamic or hypodynamic state (including cardiac output and oxygen clearance) to assess the patient's physiologic or metabolic response. Classifying a patient as generally hypermetabolic or hypometabolic is useful to anticipate decreased or increased dosage requirements.

A patient with high cardiac output, oxygen clearance, or metabolic rate can be described as being hypermetabolic, a state that is secondary to injury-related changes and complications such as sepsis. Physiologic parameters (e.g., oxygen clearance, cardiac output, energy requirements, and blood flow to the kidney and liver) increase. As blood flow to the organ increases, drug clearance can also increase. In hypermetabolic states, blood flow increases secondary to the elevated cardiac output values and increased blood supply. The agents eliminated by the kidney via glomerular filtration or active secretion follow flow-limited characteristics. In hypermetabolic patients, drug deposition and dosage requirements can be affected and dosages may need adjustment to optimize therapy. Assessment of the patient's physiologic response can help determine whether a dosage adjustment is needed and what dosage adjustment is appropriate. In the hypermetabolic patient, drug clearance generally increases in parallel with the change in blood flow as long as the intrinsic function of the organ is not altered by medical complications, altered renal function, altered hepatic function, or drugs.

The patient with congestive heart failure or multiple system organ failure may have substantial decreases in organ function, such as cardiac output and organ blood flow. The functional capacity of the kidney or liver in removing drugs decreases markedly with the onset of changes in blood chemistry and clinical indicators of organ failure. The change in drug disposition can occur before the change in blood chemistry or other physiologic markers are evident.

The vascular and extracellular fluid volumes are known to be altered in postinjury patients and in those with underlying medical disease, such as congestive heart failure. Fluid shifts between physiologic spaces can occur and can affect the distribution of drugs to tissue compartments and the volume of distribution for many agents.

Serum proteins can demonstrate substantial changes secondary to underlying disease or after injury. The changes in serum protein concentrations affect the protein-binding characteristics of several drugs commonly used in the ICU and may be important factors determining patient response. Changes in protein concentration and total amount can alter the binding of drugs that are acids (e.g., phenytoin) or bases (e.g., lidocaine). Acidic drugs bind to albumin and basic agents to α_1-acid glycoprotein. The free fraction of acidic drugs such as phenytoin is higher for the same total serum concentration measured in these patients. The basic drugs have lower free fractions and, thus, less of the total drug available for the pharmacologic activity. The free fraction of the drug is both pharmacologically active and available for elimination. The patient's pharmacologic response and dosage requirements can also vary substantially during the hospital course.

Selected Readings

Abraham E. Host defense abnormalities after hemorrhage, trauma, and burns. *Crit Care Med* 1989;17:934.

Review article that provides an overview of the abnormalities of the immune system after significant stress (e.g., hemorrhage, trauma, or burns).

Bodenham A, Shelley MP, Park GR. The altered pharmacokinetics and pharmacodynamics of drugs commonly used in critically ill patients. *Clin Pharmacokinet* 1988;14:347.

A review article on the altered pharmacokinetics and pharmacodynamics of common drugs used in the ICU. Limited data show delayed drug clearance, altered volumes of distribution, and prolonged elimination half-lives, which may can affect the ICU course.

Boucher BA, Rodman JH, Jaresko GS, et al. Phenytoin pharmacokinetics in critically ill trauma patients. *Clin Pharmacol Ther* 1988;44:675.

This study of phenytoin pharmacokinetics of 12 patients to trauma intensive care showed a substantial clinically significant fall in serum concentrations. Possible mechanism may include changes in protein binding or induction of phenytoin metabolism.

Cloyd J. Pharmacokinetic pitfalls of present antiepileptic medications. *Epilepsia* 1991;32:S53.

A helpful review of the factors that cause fluctuations in antiepileptic drugs.

Durbin CG. Neuromuscular blocking agents and sedative drugs: clinical uses and toxic effects in the critical care unit. *Crit Care Clin* 1991;7:489.

A review article on the indications, contraindications, and toxicity of neuromuscular blocking agents, with a brief discussion of conditions that can affect dosing in the ICU.

Farina ML, Bonati M, Lapichino G, et al. Clinical pharmacological and therapeutic considerations in general intensive care: a review. *Drugs* 1987;34:662.

An extensive review of the clinical pharmacology in intensive care settings with a focus on a problem-oriented approach rather than a drug-focus review.

Griebel ML, Kearns GL, Fiser DH, et al. Phenytoin protein binding in pediatric patients with acute traumatic injury. *Crit Care Med* 1990;18:385.

A study of pediatric patients with acute head injury that demonstrated significant elevations in phenytoin-free fractions and recommended that monitoring both free and total serum phenytoin to prevent toxicity.

Hickling KG, Begg EJ, Perry RE, et al. Serum aminoglycoside clearance is predicted as poorly by renal aminoglycoside clearance as by creatinine clearance in critically ill patients. *Crit Care Med* 1991;19:1041.

A prospective study of 18 critically patient treated with gentamicin or tobramycin, which demonstrated individualized pharamcokinetic dosing is the only effective method of achieving target serum concentrations.

Mann HJ, Fuhs DW, Cerra FB. Pharmacokinetics and pharmacodynamics in critically ill patients. *World J Surg* 1987;11:210.

A review article on the pharmokinetic effects of cardiac, renal, and hepatic failure, with recommendations for the dosing of commonly used medications in the intensive care setting.

McLean AJ, Morgan DJ. Clinical pharmacokinetics in patients with liver disease. *Clin Pharmacokinet* 1991;21:42.

A review article on the pathology of liver disease and its effect on metabolism, with suggestions regarding modification of drug dosages.

Murray M. P450 enzymes: inhibition mechanisms, genetic regulation, and effects of liver disease. *Clin Pharmacokinet* 1992;23:132.

An overview of the importance of hepatic P450 enzymes and the effect of drug interaction and hepatic disease on their level of function.

Reed R, Wu A, Miller-Crotchett P, et al. Pharmacokinetic monitoring of nephrotoxic antibiotics in surgical intensive care patients. *J Trauma* 1989;29:1462.

A study demonstrating the importance of pharmacokinetic analysis of nephrotoxic antibiotics to maintain therapeutic levels in surgical intensive care patients.

Shelly MP, Mendel L, Park GR. Failure of critically ill patients to metabolize midazolam. *Anaesthesia* 1987;42:619.

Impaired ability of critically ill patients to metabolize midazolam was demonstrated in six patients with septic shock.

Shoemaker WC. Circulatory mechanisms of shock and their mediators. *Crit Care Med* 1987;15:787.

Discussion of the limitations of the traditional approach to circulatory physiology, and presents an approach founded on a model based on survival pattern.

Whipple J, Ausman R, Franson T, et al. Effect of individualized pharmacokinetic dosing on patient outcome. *Crit Care Med* 1991;19:1480.

Prospective, randomized clinical study showing that individualized pharmacokinetic and aminoglycoside dosing may improve the clinical outcome of ICU patients.

104. GENERAL CONSIDERATIONS IN THE EVALUATION AND TREATMENT OF POISONING

Richard Y. Wang

I. Evaluation. The diagnosis of poisoning is often made on the basis of a history of chemical exposure, a clinical course consistent with poisoning, and exclusion of other causes. Poisoning should always be considered in patients with metabolic abnormalities (especially, acid base disturbances), gastroenteritis, or changes in behavior or mental status of unclear cause. The "Poisindex" and "Material Data Safety" sheets can be used to identify drugs, chemicals, and pill forms. Plants, mushrooms, venomous insects, reptiles, and other animals can be identified by experts from local specialty societies, colleges, botanical gardens, and zoos.

II. Clinical manifestations Signs and symptoms of poisoning typically develop within minutes to an hour of an acute exposure, progress to a maximum within several hours, and gradually resolve over a period of hours to a few days.

The mental status and vital signs provide the most useful information for identifying the cause of poisoning. Using these parameters, the physiologic state can usually be characterized into one of four categories and a differential diagnosis can then be formulated (Table 104-1).

Chemicals with characteristic odors include arsenic (garlic), camphor, chloral hydrate (pears), cyanide (bitter almond), ethchlorvynol (plastic), hydrogen sulfide (rotten eggs), methyl salicylate (oil of wintergreen), naphthalene and paradichlorobenzene (mothballs), organophosphate insecticides (garlic), phosphine (fishy), and thallium (garlic).

Mydriasis can be caused by any agent or condition that results in physiologic excitation (Table 104-1). Miosis can be caused by opioids, cholinergic stimulants, and sympatholytic agents with α-adrenoreceptor blocking agents (e.g., phenothiazines). Visual disturbances suggest methanol, anticholinergic, cholinergic, digitalis, hallucinogens, and quinine poisoning. Vertical and rotary nystagmus are suggestive of phencyclidine intoxication. Lithium and phenytoin toxicity can cause nystagmus as well. Failure to respond to topical miotics is indicative of drug-induced pupillary dilatation by topical exposure.

Common causes of seizures are tricyclic antidepressants, cocaine, amphetamines, antihistamines, theophylline, and isoniazid. Poisoning by carbon monoxide, hypoglycemic agents, and theophylline can cause focal seizures. Central nervous system (CNS) hemorrhages are know complications of poisoning and should be investigated if focal signs and symptoms are present.

III. Laboratory findings. Serum chemistries, osmolality, and a urinalysis can provide important diagnostic clues and assist in the management of poisoned patients. Pregnancy testing is recommended in women of childbearing age. A low lactate, increased anion gap metabolic acidosis (AGMA) can be caused by ethylene glycol, methanol, or salicylate poisoning. Lactic acidemia is seen in biguanide (e.g., metformin) toxicity. An elevated serum osmolality (by freezing point depression) and crystalluria can be seen in ethylene glycol and methanol but not salicylate poisoning. Ketosis is commonly present in salicylate but not in ethylene glycol or methanol poisoning. Hypokalemia can be caused by barium salts, beta agonists, diuretics, methylxanthines, and toluene. Hyperkalemia can be caused by α-agonists, β-blockers, cardiac glycosides, and fluoride. Potential hepatotoxins include acetaminophen, ethanol, halogenated hydrocarbons (e.g., carbon tetrachloride), heavy metals, and mushrooms (e.g., *Amanita phalloides*). Renal dysfunction can be caused by ethylene glycol, agents causing rhabdomyolysis or hemolysis, nonsteroidal antiinflammatory drugs, and toluene.

IV. Electrocardiographic (ECG) clues. Ventricular tachydysrhythmias can result from myocardial irritation or reentry mechanisms. Myocardial irritants include sympathomimetics, cardiac glycosides, and halogenated hydrocarbons. Reentry

TABLE 104-1. Differential diagnosis of poisoning based on physiologic abnormalities and underlying mechanistic and specific causes

Excited[a]	Depressed[b]	Discordant[c]	Normal
Sympathomimetics	Sympatholytics	Asphyxiants	Agents with slow absorption
Amphetamines	α-Adrenergic antagonists	Cytochrome oxidase inhibitors	Agents that form concretions
Bronchodilators (β-agonists)	Angiotensin-converting enzyme inhibitors	Carbon monoxide	Anticholinergics
Catecholamine analogues	β-Adrenergic blockers	Cyanide	Carbamazepine
Cocaine	Calcuim channel blockers	Hydrogen sulfide	Digitalis preparations
Decongestants (α-adrenergic agonists)	Clonidine gestants	Inert (simple) gases	Dilantin Kapseals
Ergot alkaloids	Cyclic antidepressants (late, severe)	Irritant gases, fumes, vapors	Enteric-coated pills
Methylxanthines	Decongestants (imidazolone)	Methemoglobinemia	Lomotil (atropine and diphenoxylate)
Monoamine oxidase inhibitors	Digitalis	Oxidative phosphorylation inhibitors	Opioids
Thyroid hormones	Neuroleptics	Herbicides (nitrophenols)	Salicylates
			Sustained-release formulations
Anticholinergics	Cholinergics	Membrane active agents	Agents with slow distribution
Antihistamines	Bethanechol	Amantadine	Digitalis derivatives
Atropine (belladonna alkaloids)	Carbamate insecticides	Antiarrhythmics	Heavy metals
Cyclic antidepressants (early, mild)	Echothiophate	Beta-blockers	Lithium
Cyclobenzaprine	Myasthenia gravis therapeutics	Cyclic antidepressants (late, severe)	Salicylates
Muscle relaxants	Nicotine	Fluoride	Agents with active metabolites
Mydriatics (topical)	Organophosphate insecticides	Heavy metals	Acetaminophen
Nonprescription sleep aids	Physostigmine	Lithium	Chloramphenicol
Parkinson's disease therapeutics	Pilocarpine	Local anesthetics	Chlorinated hydrocarbons
Phenothiazines	Urecholine	Meperidine/propoxyphene metabolites	Ethylene glycol
Plants/mushrooms		Neuroleptics	Organophosphate insecticides (some)
		Quinine (antimalarials)	Methanol

- Hallucinogens
  - LSD/tryptamine derivatives
  - Marijuana
  - Mescaline/amphetamine derivatives
  - Psilocybin mushrooms
  - Phencyclidine
- Withdrawal syndromes
  - β-Adrenergic blockers
  - Clonidine
  - Cyclic antidepressants
  - Ethanol
  - Opioids
  - Sedative-hypnotics
- Opioids
  - Analgesics
  - Antidiarrheal drugs
  - Fentanyl and derivatives
  - Heroin
  - Opium
- Sedative-hypnotics
  - Alcohols
  - Anticonvulsants
  - Barbiturates
  - Benzodiazepines
  - Bromide
  - Ethchlorvynol
  - γ-hydroxybutyrate (GHB)
  - Glutethimide
  - Methyprylon
  - Muscle relaxants
- Low lactate increased anion gap metabolic acidosis
  - Alcoholic ketoacidosis
  - Ethylene glycol
  - Methanol (formaldehyde)
  - Paraldehyde
  - Metformin (biguanide hypoglycemics)
  - Salicylate
  - Sulfur/sulfate
  - Toluene
- CNS syndromes
  - Disulfiram
  - Extrapyramidal reactions
  - Isoniazid
  - Neuroleptic malignant syndrome
  - Serotonin syndrome
  - Strychnine
  - Volatile substances of abuse (hydrocarbons)
  - Methemoglobin inducers (some)
  - Paraquat
- Agents that inhibit metabolism
  - Disulfiram
  - Monoamine oxidase inhibitors
  - Salicylates
  - Thyroid hormone synthesis inhibitors
- Agents that inhibit nucleic acid synthesis
  - Amanita phalloides and related mushrooms
  - Cancer chemotherapeutic agents
  - Immunosuppressive agents
  - Podophylline
  - Viral antimicrobials
- Nontoxic exposure
- Psychogenic illness

[a]CNS simulation with increased vital signs.
[b]CNS depression with decreased vital signs.
[c]Mixed CNS and vital sign abnormalities.
CNS, central nervous system; GABA, γ-amino butyric acid.

dysrhythmias are caused by agents that trigger cardiac repolarization and depolarization abnormalities as manifest by an increased QRS duration and prolonged QTc interval, respectively. Toxins causing these effects include amantadine, types I and III antidysrhythmics, β-blockers, fluoride, heavy metals (e.g., arsenic, thallium), magnesium, normeperidine, organophosphate insecticides, potassium, cyclic antidepressants, antipsychotics, quinine, and related antimalarials.

Atrioventricular conduction abnormalities and bradydysrhythmias are commonly caused by β-blockers, calcium channel blockers, cardiac glycosides, organophosphate insecticides, and phenylpropanolamine.

V. Radiographic findings. Radiopaque agents are identified by the mnemonic CHIPE (chlorinated hydrocarbons, calcium salts, heavy metals, iron salts, iodinated compounds, phenothiazines, packets of drugs, and enteric coated tablets). The chest radiograph may demonstrate infiltrates following inhalation of irritant gases (e.g., chlorine, noncardiogenic pulmonary edema), fumes (e.g., metal oxides), vapors (e.g., isocyanates), and some ingestions (e.g., paraquat, salicylates).

VI. Toxicology testing. Comprehensive toxicology screens are often neither clinically useful nor cost-effective. They are not immediately available, can detect only a small fraction of all chemicals, and are not always reliable. A false–negative result can occur when the toxin is not included in the assay panel, or the concentration of the toxin is below the level of detection by the assay. The physician should speak directly with the laboratory technician to determine whether the assay is appropriate for the toxin being considered. Quantitative acetaminophen and salicylate levels, however, should be obtained in most patients suspected of overdose.

VII. Management. Supportive care remains the primary therapy for most poisoned patients; it includes monitoring (e.g., venous access, cardiac tracing, pulse oximetry, urine output, behavioral), respiratory care, cardiovascular therapy, and treatment of neuromuscular hyperactivity to limit rhabdomyolysis and thermogenesis. Prophylactic intubation may be required for patients with CNS depression to prevent aspiration of gastric contents. Antidotal therapy requires knowledge of the specific indications, contraindications, dosing, and potential complications (see subsequent chapters for details).

VIII. Cardiovascular therapy. Maintenance or restoration of a normal blood pressure, pulse, and sinus rhythm are the goals of therapy. Invasive hemodynamic (e.g., arterial, central venous, pulmonary artery pressure) monitoring may be necessary for optimal treatment. External or internal electrical cardiac pacing and intraaortic balloon pump counter pulsation or cardiopulmonary bypass should be used in patients unresponsive to routine therapy.

Hypotension (in the absence of an extremely fast or slow heart rate) should be treated with normal saline and then a direct-acting vasopressor with inotropic activity, (e.g., norepinephrine). Hypertension should be treated in the presence of chest pain, ECG evidence of ischemia, headache, papilledema, or encephalopathy. A nonselective sympatholytic (e.g., labetalol) or the combination of a α-blocker and a peripheral vasodilator (e.g., esmolol with nitroprusside) is preferred in patients with sympathomimetic poisoning. A vasodilator alone can be used if hypertension is associated with a normal heart rate or reflex bradycardia.

The treatment of ventricular tachydysrhythmias includes correction of electrolyte and metabolic abnormalities. Lidocaine is generally safe. Sodium bicarbonate, hypertonic saline, or hyperventilation may be effective for wide-complex tachycardias caused by antiarrhythmics, cyclic antidepressants, and possibly other membrane-active agents. Procainamide and other types IA and IC are contraindicated in patients with prolonged QRS and QT intervals.

Atropine and isoproterenol are the agents of choice in symptomatic bradycardia. Calcium and glucagon are effective for the treatment of calcium channel blocker and β-blocker poisonings.

IX. Neuromuscular therapy. Behavioral and muscular hyperactivity from sympathomimetic or hallucinogen poisoning and drug withdrawal should initially be treated with sedation. Benzodiazepines are preferred to neuroleptics (e. g., chlorpromazine, haloperidol) because the latter are more likely to cause hypotension.

Seizures are effectively managed with benzodiazepines and barbiturates. Administration of pyridoxine is necessary to stop seizures caused by isoniazid (INH).

X. Prevention of absorption. Decontamination is recommended in all patients, unless the exposure is clearly nontoxic. Body surfaces exposed to caustic agents should be immediately irrigated until the pH is between 5 and 8. For ingestions, gastrointestinal (GI) decontamination can be accomplished by activated charcoal administration, gastric lavage, emesis induction, whole bowel irrigation, and endoscopic removal of the ingested toxin. The treatment of choice is based on the actual and predicted severity of the poisoning and the relative efficacy, availability, risks, and contraindications of the different methods. The efficacy of all decontamination methods decreases with time. In most cases, such interventions are unlikely to be of benefit if more than 2 to 4 hours have elapsed since ingestions.

Activated charcoal is the recommended method of decontamination for most ingestions. It is easy to administer, relatively safe, and prevents absorption of ingested chemicals by binding them within the gut lumen. The recommended oral dose is at least 10 times the weight of the ingested toxin or a maximum of 1 to 2 g/kg of body weight. Activated charcoal is not recommended for ingestions of alkali, acids, and hydrocarbons with low systemic toxicity. It does not effectively bind inorganic salts (e.g., iron, lithium).

Gastric lavage prevents absorption by directly removing ingested toxins in the stomach. Gastric lavage may be of benefit for the removal of toxins that do not absorb well to charcoal and in patients with coma.

Syrup of ipecac, which removes ingested toxins from the stomach and proximal small intestine by inducing emesis, is reserved for home use.

Whole bowel irrigation (WBI), the oral administration of large volumes (0.5 L/h in children aged 6–12 years and 2 L/h for older patients) of a balanced electrolyte solution (e.g., Golytely), can prevent the absorption of ingested toxins by enhancing their GI elimination. WBI may be useful in patients with ingestions of enteric-coated or sustained release formulations, potentially toxic foreign bodies, and agents that are poorly adsorbed by activated charcoal. WBI is continued until the rectal effluent is clear, which takes approximately 2 to 4 hours.

Endoscopy can be used to remove foreign bodies or break up drug masses in the stomach. It should be reserved for patients with severe or potentially lethal poisoning, such as those with large amounts of heavy metal visible in the stomach on the radiograph and those who deteriorate or have rising drug levels despite attempts at gut decontamination by other methods.

Immediate surgery is indicated for patients who ingest packets of cocaine and develop signs of toxicity.

Cathartics have not been shown to prevent absorption and are recommended as an adjunct to charcoal to prevent constipation. Cathartics can cause water and electrolyte imbalance and are recommended only with the initial dose of charcoal. Cathartics are contraindicated in patients with caustic ingestions, not recommended in patients with renal insufficiency, and unnecessary in patients with diarrhea.

XI. Enhanced elimination. The elimination of some toxins by nonmetabolic routes can be enhanced by diuresis, alkalization of the urine, multiple-dose activated charcoal, WBI, and extracorporeal techniques. The choice of the technique is dependent on the actual or predicted severity of poisoning and its reversibility, the function of intrinsic detoxification mechanisms, and the potential risks of the intervention and its efficacy in removing the toxin.

Urinary alkalinization (urine pH above 7.5) can enhance the renal excretion of acidic chemicals (chlorphenoxyacetic acid herbicide 2,4-D, chlorpropamide, difluinisal, fluoride, phenobarbital, sulfonamides, and salicylates) by ion trapping. An alkalinizing solution for infusion can be created by adding 44 to 134 mEq of sodium bicarbonate to 1 L of D5W. It is administered at the same rate as the desired urine output. Acid-base, and electrolyte parameters and respiratory function must be carefully monitored during therapy.

Multiple-dose activated charcoal (MDAC) can enhance the elimination of previously absorbed chemicals by binding them within the GI tract as they are excreted in the bile, secreted by the stomach or intestine, or passively diffuse back into the gut lumen. Efficacy is likely to be greatest for toxins with high charcoal binding capacity, long intrinsic elimination half-life, and sustained-release formulations. MDAC can also enhance the elimination of agents administered parenterally. The recommended dose of activated charcoal is 0.5 to 1 g/kg every 2 to 4 hours.

Extracorporeal methods include hemodialysis, hemoperfusion, hemofiltration, plasmapheresis, peritoneal dialysis, and exchange transfusion. Hemodialysis can effectively remove barbiturates, bromide, chloral hydrate, ethanol, ethylene glycol, isopropyl alcohol, lithium, methanol, procainamide, theophylline, salicylates, and possibly, heavy metals. Patients should be monitored for a rebound (increase) in blood levels and clinical toxicity after the termination of extracorporeal therapies.

XII. Disposition. Patients with coma, hypotension, hypoventilation, seizures, or a nonsinus rhythm require further management in a critical care unit. Patients with severe agitation, extremes of temperature, hallucinations, hypertension, metabolic abnormalities, or enhanced elimination therapy may also require critical care. Those with intentional exposures require a psychiatric evaluation before discharge. Workplace exposures should be reported to the appropriate governmental agency (e.g., Occupational Safety and Health Administration, local health department), and workers should be warned to avoid reexposure.

Selected Readings

Berg M, Berlinger W, Goldberg M, et al. Acceleration of the body clearance of phenobarbital by oral activated charcoal. *N Engl J Med* 1982;307:642.

This human volunteer study demonstrated the ability of charcoal to inhibit enteroenteric circulation of phenobarbital to enhance drug elimination.

Frenia ML, Schauben JL, Wears RL, et al. Multiple-dose activated charcoal compared to urinary alkalinization for the enhancement of phenobarbital elimination. *J Toxicol Clin Toxicol* 1996;34:169.

This human volunteer study demonstrated increased phenobarbital elimination with urinary alkalinization and repeat dose activated charcoal therapy.

Goldfrank LR, Flomenbaum NE, Lewin NA, et al. Vital signs and toxic syndromes. In: Goldfrank KR, Flomenbaum NE, Lewin NA, et al, eds. *Toxicologic emergencies,* 6th ed. East Norwalk, CT: Appleton & Lange, 1988.

A discussion of the classic clinical manifestations of a variety toxicologic exposures.

Krenzelok E, Vale A. Position statements: gut decontamination. American Academy of Clinical Toxicology, European Association of Poisons Centres and Clinical Toxicologists. *J Toxicol Clin Toxicol* 1997;35:695.

This review discusses the role of various gut decontamination therapies in poisoned patients.

Kulig KW, Bar-Or D, Cantrill SV, et al. Management of acutely poisoned patients without gastric emptying. *Ann Emerg Med* 1985;14:562.

This study demonstrated the clinical benefit of gastric emptying in patients with serious overdoses when gastric lavage was accomplished within 1 hour of the ingestion.

Mofenson HC, Greensher J, Carraccio TR. Ingestions considered nontoxic. *Emerg Med Clin North Am* 1984;2:159.

A discussion of the nature of nontoxic exposures and their management.

Nice A, Leikin JB, Maturen A, et al. Toxidrome recognition to improve efficiency of emergency urine drug screens. *Ann Emerg Med* 1988;17:676.

The application of classic clinical manifestations correctly identified the drug or class causing intoxication in overdosed patients.

Olkkola K. Effect of charcoal-drug ratio on antidotal efficacy of oral activated charcoal in man. *Br J Clin Pharmacol* 1985;19:767.

This in vitro study demonstrated the effective drug:charcoal ratio to be 1:10 by weight.

Pond SM, Lewis-Driver DJ, Williams G, et al. Gastric emptying in acute overdose: a prospective randomized controlled trial. *Med J Aust* 1995;163:345.

This study failed to demonstrate clinical benefit from gastric emptying in all overdosed patients. However, when severity of illness was controlled for, patients with gastric emptying benefited.

Robertson WO. Syrup of ipecac: a slow or fast emetic? *Am J Dis Child* 1962;103:136.
This study demonstrated the effectiveness of ipecac as an emetic agent and its delayed onset.

Schwartz T. Toxicologic imaging. In: Goldfrank KR, Flomenbaum NE, Lewin NA, et al., eds. *Toxicologic emergencies,* 6th ed. East Norwalk, CT: Appleton & Lange, 1988.
A discussion of the role of radiologic imaging in the management of toxicologic exposures.

Smilkstein MJ, Steedle D, Kulig KW, et al. Magnesium levels after magnesium containing cathartics. *J Toxicol Clin Toxicol* 1988;26:51.
This study demonstrated increased serum magnesium concentrations in human volunteers with normal renal function who were administered magnesium cathartics in repeated fashion.

Tenenbein M, Cohen S, Sitar DS. Whole bowel irrigation as a decontamination procedure after acute drug overdose. *Arch Intern Med* 1987;147:905.
This human volunteer study demonstrated the effectiveness of whole bowel irrigation in decreasing drug absorption from the gut.

Winchester JF, Gelfand MC, Knepshield JH, et al. Dialysis and hemoperfusion of poisons and drugs—updates. *Transactions of the American Society of Artificial Internal Organs* 1977;23:762.
This review discussed the role of extracorporeal elimination in the poisoned patient.

105. ACETAMINOPHEN POISONING

Erica L. Liebelt

I. General principles. Acetaminophen (APAP) is the most common drug involved in intentional and unintentional overdoses in the United States. It is an active ingredient in hundreds of products, including combinations with opioid analgesics, antihistamines, and decongestants.

II. Toxicology. In therapeutic doses, approximately 90% of APAP is metabolized by hepatic conjugation with sulfate or glucuronide to form inactive metabolites. The remaining fraction undergoes oxidation by the cytochrome P-450 mixed function oxidases (CYPIIE1) to yield the toxic intermediate NAPQI (*N*-acetyl-para-benzoquinoneimine), which then reacts with reduced glutathione (GSH) to form inactive products that are excreted in the urine. NAPQI is a highly reactive electrophile that destroys both hepatocytes (centrilobular necrosis) and renal tubular cells. After overdose, the conjugation pathway becomes saturated, increasing the amount of APAP metabolized by the P-450 enzymes. GSH can then become depleted, allowing NAPQI to produce hepatotoxicity.

Single ingestions of more than 7.5 g in an adult and more than 150 mg/kg in children should be considered potentially toxic. Toxicity can also occur after repeated ingestions of therapeutic or slightly greater doses of APAP, especially in persons who have conditions associated with increased cytochrome P-450 activity (chronic alcoholics) or glutathione depletion (chronic malnutrition or recent ethanol use).

III. Clinical manifestations. Acute APAP toxicity can be divided into four phases based on the time after ingestion.

A. Stage 1 (0.5–24 hours). Patients may be asymptomatic, but may be experiencing nausea, vomiting, and malaise.

B. Stage 2 (24–48 hours). Patients have symptoms of hepatitis, including right upper quadrant abdominal pain, nausea, fatigue, and malaise. Elevation of aminotransferase levels usually occurs between 24 and 36 hours after ingestion, but in severe cases can occur by 16 hours. Complications during stage 2 are related to the degree of liver injury. Renal dysfunction may become evident by a rising creatinine level and active urinary sediment.

C. Stage 3 (72–96 hours). Liver injury becomes most pronounced, resulting in prolonged prothrombin time, elevated bilirubin, marked elevation of aminotransferases (> 1,000 IU/L), metabolic acidosis, and hypoglycemia. Clinical symptoms reflect the degree of liver injury and hepatic necrosis and can include jaundice and encephelopathy. Most patients go on to full recovery, even those with markedly elevated aminotransferase levels. Death can occur 3 to 7 days after ingestion as a result of intractable metabolic disturbances, cerebral edema, or exsanguination. Oliguric or anuric renal failure can result from renal tubular necrosis. Pancreatitis and myocardial necrosis have also been reported.

D. Stage 4 (4 days to 2 weeks). Patients who survive even with severe liver toxicity regain normal liver function. Recovery is often complete in 5 to 7 days in patients with minimal toxicity but can take 2 weeks or more in patients with more serious toxicity. No known cases have been seen of chronic or persistent liver abnormalities from APAP poisoning.

IV. Diagnostic evaluation. Obtain a serum APAP concentration between 4 and 24 hours after ingestion. If it falls on or above the treatment line on the Rumack–Matthew nomogram, the patient should be considered at risk for hepatotoxicity (Fig. 105-1). A single APAP concentration within the time period should be sufficient to plan appropriate therapy except in selected situations—to detect a rising level and define the peak value if the time of ingestion is unknown and if ingestion of the extended-release formulation is suspected. In the latter case, a second APAP level should be obtained 4 to 6 hours after the initial one.

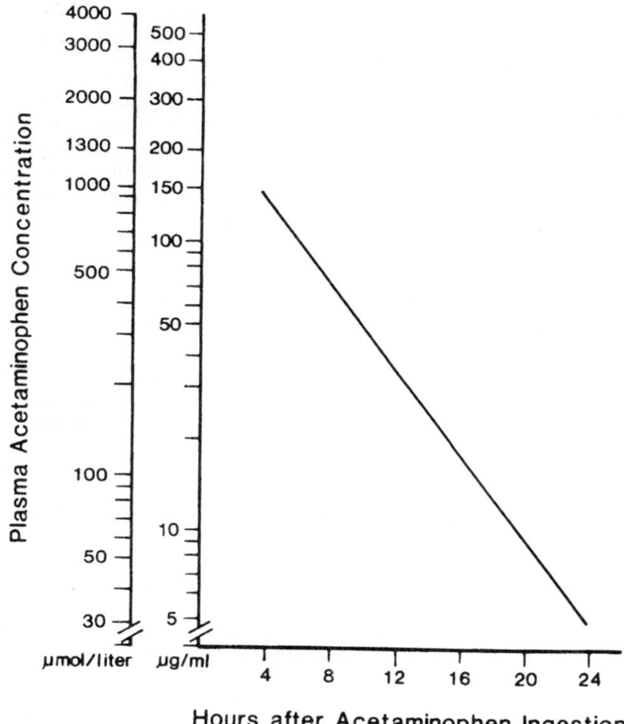

FIG. 105-1. Acetaminophen treatment nomogram. Patients with acetaminophen concentrations on or above the line require treatment with N-acetylcysteine.

If a patient is found to be at risk for toxicity, a complete blood count, electrolytes, blood urea nitrogen, creatinine, glucose, prothrombin and international normalized ratio (INR) time, aminotransferase levels, and bilirubin level should be obtained at admission and repeated every 24 hours until toxicity has resolved or been excluded.

V. Management

A. Gastrointestinal (GI) decontamination. Consider gastric lavage only if the patient ingested another highly toxic substance (cyclic antidepressant). Otherwise, activated charcoal alone should be administered if it can be given within 4 hours of the ingestion. Although the co-ingestion of charcoal and NAC (*N*-acetylcysteine) can decrease the amount of NAC absorbed in the GI tract, this decrease is clinically insignificant.

B. Antidotal therapy. The specific antidote for APAP toxicity is NAC. Although several mechanisms explain its benefit in preventing APAP-induced liver and renal injury, it primarily acts as a glutathione precursor and substitute. Begin NAC therapy after an acute overdose if the serum APAP concentration is in the toxic range on the nomogram, the ingested amount is potentially toxic and more than 8 hours have elapsed since ingestion, and if serum aminotransferases are elevated and the patient has a history of APAP ingestion. In the latter two instances, NAC can be continued or discontinued when the APAP level becomes available. The 72-hour treatment regimen uses oral NAC given as a

140 mg/kg loading dose followed by 17 doses of 70 mg/kg every 4 hours. The 20% NAC solution should be diluted at least 3 : 1 with a carbonated or fruit beverage.

C. Aggressive antiemetic therapy may be needed to treat APAP- or NAC-induced vomiting. Metoclopramide, droperidol, or ondansetron can be effective. NAC can also be given by a slow, continuous infusion through a gastric or duodenal tube. If vomiting occurs within 1 hour of any dose, that dose should be repeated. Intravenous (IV) NAC should be considered only in selected patients: those with refractory vomiting 12 to 16 hours after ingestion, GI bleeding, or fulminant hepatic failure. Although the oral preparation is not approved for IV administration, it has been reported to be safe and equally efficacious when given for 48 hours.

VI. Special considerations

A. Late treatment. Late NAC administration (> 24 hours) has shown clinical benefit in patients with APAP-induced fulminant liver failure.

B. Pregnancy. Pregnant women should be treated according to standard guidelines regardless of gestational age of the fetus.

C. Chronic overdose. The nomogram has no validity in chronic APAP overdose. Patients with elevated APAP levels and no hepatotoxicity can be treated with NAC until the APAP is negligible. Patients who develop hepatotoxicity should be given a full course of NAC.

Selected Readings

Cetaruk EW, Dart RC, Hurlbut KM, et al. Tylenol Extended Relief overdose. *Ann Emerg Med* 1997;30:104.

Case series of patients with overdoses of extended-release preparations of acetaminophen (APAP) that demonstrated peak levels after 4 hours, suggesting the need for another APAP level 4 to 6 hours after the first.

Harrison PM, Wendon JA, Gimson AE, et al. Improvement by acetylcysteine of hemodynamics and oxygen transport in fulminant hepatic failure. *N Eng J Med* 1991; 324:1852.

Study of patients with acetaminophen-induced fulminant hepatic failure that demonstrated increases in oxygen delivery and consumption in response to acetylcysteine, perhaps accounting for its beneficial effect on survival in these patients.

Keays R, Harrison PM, Wendon JA, et al. Intravenous acetylcysteine in paracetamol induced fulminant hepatic failure: a prospective controlled trial. *BMJ* 1991;303:1026.

A controlled trial of patients with paracetamol-induced fulminant hepatic failure demonstrating decreased cerebral edema and increased survival in those patients receiving intravenous N-acetylcysteine therapy compared to those who did not.

Mitchell JR, Thorgeirsson SS, Potter WZ, et al. Acetaminophen-induced hepatic injury: protective role of glutathione in man and rationale for therapy. *Clin Pharmacol Ther* 1974;16:676.

An animal study demonstrating that glutathionelike nucleophiles (e.g., cysteamine) protects hepatocytes from injury caused by the reactive acetaminophen metabolite.

Renzi FP, Donovan JW, Martin TG, et al. Concomitant use of activated charcoal and *N*-acetylcysteine. *Ann Emerg Med* 1985;14:568.

A human volunteer study showing no difference in N-acetylcysteine levels after oral consumption between those subjects who received charcoal and those who did not.

Rumack BH, Matthew H. Acetaminophen poisoning and toxicity. *Pediatrics* 1975; 55:871.

One of the first reviews to describe the toxicology of acetaminophen and proposals for treatment.

Rumack BH, Peterson RC, Koch GG, et al. Acetaminophen overdose: 662 cases with evaluation of oral acetylcysteine treatment. *Arch Intern Med* 1981;141:380.

One of the first and largest patient series to demonstrate the effectiveness of oral N-acetylcysteine treatment and the use of a nomogram to predict toxicity.

Smilkstein MJ, Bronstein AC, Linden C, et al. Acetaminophen overdose: a 48-hour intravenous *N*-acetylcysteine protocol. *Ann Emerg Med* 1991;20:1058.

A nonrandomized trial of acetaminophen-intoxicated patients who received 48 hours of intravenous N-acetylcysteine therapy, which was found to be both safe and effective and equal to the 72-hour oral regimen when started early.

Smilkstein MJ, Knapp GL, Kulig KW, et al. Efficacy of oral *N*-acetylcysteine in the treatment of acetaminophen overdose: analysis of the National Multicenter Sudy (1976–1985). *N Engl J Med* 1988;319:1557.

Outcome study of more than 2,000 patients with acetaminophen poisoning treated with oral N-acetylcysteine, demonstrating a time-dependent relationship for its maximal efficacy.

Whitcomb DC, Block GD. Association of acetaminophen hepatotoxicity with fasting and ethanol use. *JAMA* 1994;272:1845.

A retrospective case series of patients suggesting that acetaminophen hepatotoxicity appears to be enhanced by fasting and alcohol ingestion.

Yip L, Dart RC, Hurlbut KM. Intravenous administration of oral *N*-acetylcysteine. *Crit Care Med* 1998;26:40.

Recommended procedure and case series reporting the indications and adverse events associated with administration of the oral N-acetylcysteine preparation by the intravenous route.

106. ALCOHOLS AND GLYCOLS

Jeffrey R. Tucker

I. General principles. Ethanol (grain or beverage alcohol), methanol (wood alcohol), isopropanol (isopropyl or rubbing alcohol), and ethylene glycol are central nervous system (CNS) depressants. Isopropanol is more potent and methanol is less potent than ethanol in this regard. Ketoacidosis and hypoglycemia are caused by the hormonal, nutritional, metabolic, and intravascular volume changes caused by the consumption of ethanol. They can also be caused by the consumption of other alcohols. The formation of toxic metabolites by hepatic alcohol dehydrogenase is responsible for the renal toxicity of ethylene glycol, the ocular toxicity of methanol, and the increased anion gap metabolic acidosis (AGMA) caused by both. The most common sources of methanol and ethylene glycol are automotive windshield washer fluid, gasoline antifreeze, and radiator antifreeze, respectively. Because of their low molecular weight, high levels of an alcohol or ethylene glycol increase the serum osmolality. Hence, an elevated serum osmolality or osmolal gap is a clue to their presence.

II. Clinical presentation

A. Ethanol. Patients with acute ethanol intoxication can present with varying degrees of altered consciousness, including agitation, slurred speech, ataxia, stupor, and coma. Death from respiratory depression, aspiration, or cardiovascular collapse can occur in severe poisoning.

B. Isopropyl alcohol. Isopropanol produces an ethanol-like intoxication. Symptoms of gastritis (e.g., abdominal pain, nausea, vomiting, and possibly hematemesis) may also be present. Because its acetone metabolite causes a spurious increase in serum creatinine, an elevated creatinine level with normal blood urea nitrogen (BUN) can be a clue to the diagnosis.

C. Alcoholic ketoacidosis and hypoglycemia. Patients with alcoholic ketoacidosis usually present with a recent history of binge drinking, poor nutritional intake, vomiting, and little or no ethanol in their body. Laboratory findings include mild to moderate AGMA and mild ketonemia. Dehydration is invariably present. They may also exhibit signs and symptoms of withdrawal.

Hypoglycemia causes an altered mental status ranging from agitation to confusion and coma. Symptoms of increased sympathetic activity caused by catecholamine release (e.g., diaphoresis and tachycardia) can also be present.

D. Ethylene glycol and methanol. Ethylene glycol and methanol poisoning should be suspected in all patients with a history of ingesting alcohol substitutes or in those who have an unexplained AGMA. Initially, an ethanol-like intoxication along with nausea, vomiting, and occasionally seizures dominates the clinical picture. An increased serum osmolality and osmolal gap may also be present.

In ethylene glycol poisoning, cardiopulmonary effects (e.g, tachypnea, cyanosis, cardiogenic or noncardiogenic pulmonary edema) subsequently develop. Calcium oxalate crystalluria, proteinuria, and flank pain and tenderness may be present. Renal failure can ensue.

Neurologic, ophthalmologic, and gastrointestinal symptoms predominate in methanol toxicity. Patients are frequently alert on admission and complain of headache and dizziness. Visual symptoms are usually experienced acutely when the serum pH drops below 7.2. Blurred vision, photophobia, scotomata, eye pain, partial or complete loss of vision, and visual hallucinations (e.g., bright lights, "snowstorm,") have been reported. Methanol can produce hemorrhagic gastritis and pancreatitis, resulting in abdominal pain, nausea, vomiting, and diarrhea.

III. Evaluation. Patients with a history of ethanol ingestion and mild to moderate intoxication only need a serum ethanol level and a fingerstick blood sugar evaluation. Those with severe intoxication or an unreliable history should have electrolytes, BUN, creatinine, glucose, complete blood count, arterial blood gas, ethanol level, magnesium, calcium, phosphorus, liver function tests, prothrombin time, electrocardiogram, chest radiograph, and urinalysis.

Evaluation of known or suspected isopropanol poisoning should also include serum isopropanol and acetone serum levels. Evaluation of known suspected ethylene glycol and methanol poisoning should include quantitative serum levels of these compounds. Microscopic examination of the urine should also be performed.

IV. Management. Initial treatment includes supportive measures such as airway management, intravenous (IV) fluids, and cardiac monitoring. Gastric aspiration via a nasogastric tube should be done in patients with severe poisoning and within a few hours of isopropanol, ethylene glycol, or methanol ingestion. Activated charcoal should be considered when co-ingestants are suspected. Intravenous naloxone (2 mg) and thiamine hydrochloride (100 mg) should also be considered. If a bedside glucose test reveals hypoglycemia, IV dextrose (25–50 g) should be administered.

A. Alcoholic ketoacidosis and hypoglycemia. Intravenous fluids, glucose, and thiamine should be given for dehydration and to reverse the ketogenic process. Prolonged hospitalization and refeeding of malnourished patients may be required.

The IV bolus of dextrose should be followed by a high carbohydrate meal or an infusion of 10% dextrose in patients with hypoglycemia.

B. Ethylene glycol and methanol. Large doses of sodium bicarbonate may be required to treat metabolic acidosis. Antidotal therapy with ethanol (at a serum level of 100–150 mg/dl) or fomepizole can prevent the formation of toxic metabolites by alcohol dehydrogenase. Methanol and ethylene glycol are then eliminated slowly via pulmonary and renal excretion. Fomepizole offers numerous advantages over ethanol therapy: oral administration; twice daily dosing; lack of CNS depressant effects; no induction of hypoglycemia, hyperosmolality, or dilutional hyponatremia; and no need for frequent monitoring of drug levels.

Indications for antidotal therapy include an ethylene glycol or methanol level greater than 20 mg/dl; unexplained AGMA with an increased osmolar gap, low lactate level, visual disturbances or calcium oxalate crystalluria; and unexplained coma with a high osmolar gap and low ethanol levels.

Patients poisoned by ethylene glycol should receive pyridoxine (100 mg) and thiamine (100 mg) IV daily until ethylene glycol levels are unmeasurable and acidemia has cleared. Patients with methanol poisoning should be given intravenous IV leucovorin (1 mg/kg, maximal dose 50 mg) every 4 hours for a total of six doses.

Hemodialysis effectively removes ethanol, isopropanol, ethylene glycol, methanol, and their toxic metabolites and can correct metabolic abnormalities. It should be considered in severe poisoning unresponsive to other measures and should be used along with ethanol therapy in nearly all cases of ethylene glycol or methanol poisoning.

Selected Readings

Adams SL, Mathews JJ, Flatherty JJ. Alcoholic ketoacidosis. *Ann Emerg Med* 1987;16:90.

Case presentation and review of the clinical and laboratory features of alcoholic ketoacidosis.

Baud FJ, Galliot M, Astier A, et al. Treatment of ethylene glycol poisoning with intravenous 4-methylpyrazole. *N Engl J Med* 1988;319:97.

Case report of the clinical and kinetic data of ethylene glycol treated with intravenous 4-methylpyrazole.

Burns MJ, Graudins A, Aaron CK, et al. Treatment of methanol poisoning with intravenous 4-methylpyrazole *Ann Emerg Med* 1996;30:829.

First description of the effective treatment of methanol toxicity with the alcohol dehydrogenase inhibitor, 4-methylpyrazole with no generation of the toxic metabolite, formic acid.

Chamess ME, Simon RP, Greenberg DA. Ethanol and the nervous system. *N Engl J Med* 89;321:442.

An important review of the neurologic complications associated with ethanol abuse: intoxication, withdrawal, Wernicke's encephalopathy, dementia, cerebellar degeneration, and central pontine myelinolysis.

Dethlefs R, Naraqi S. Ocular manifestations and complications of acute methyl alcohol intoxication. *Med J Aust* 1978;2:483.

Clinical series of 24 men with methanol toxicity showing that the incidence of permanent ocular abnormalities correlated with metabolic acidosis.

Hoffman KS, Smilkstein MJ, Howland MA, et al. Osmol gaps revisited: normal values and limitations. *J Toxicol Clin Toxicol* 1993;31:81.

A study of 321 adults that evaluated the limitation of the osmol gaps in adults and concluded that small osmol gaps should not be used to eliminate an toxic alcohol ingestion.

Hoffman RS, Goldfrank LR. Ethanol-associated metabolic disorders. *Emerg Med Clin North Am* 1989;7:943.

An excellent review and discussion of the fluid, electrolytes, acid-base, glucose, and nutritional complications causes by elevated ethanol levels.

Jacobsen D, Hewlett TP, Webb K, et al. Ethylene glycol intoxication: evaluation of kinetics and crystalluria. *Am J Med* 1988;84:145.

A review of the two type of calcium oxalate crystals that are formed in the metabolism of ethylene glycol.

Jacobsen D, McMartin KE. Methanol and ethylene glycol poisonings: mechanism of toxicity, clinical course, diagnosis and treatment. *Med Toxicol* 1986;1:309.

A review article on methanol and ethylene glycol toxicity with excellent discussion of the similar clinically and biochemically characteristics that both compounds share.

Kruse JA, Cadnapaphorochni P. The serum osmole gap. *J Crit Care* 1994;9:185.

An in-depth review article on the different clinical indications for the use of osmole gap. Includes a helpful discussion regarding the limitations of its use.

LaCouture PG, Wason S, Abrams A, et al. Acute isopropyl alcohol intoxication: diagnosis and management. *Am J Med* 1983;75:680.

A review article focusing on the clinical presentation and management of isopropyl toxicity. Includes a helpful discussion of the differences between common toxic alcohols.

Martensson E, Olofsson U, Heath A. Clinical and metabolic features of ethanol-methanol poisoning in chronic alcoholics. *Lancet* 1998;1:327.

A study of 84 chronic alcoholic patients who ingested an ethanol-methanol suggesting that treatment should be based on the clinical presentation and acidosis and not solely on methanol blood concentrations.

Stokes JB, Aureon F. Prevention of organ damage in massive ethylene glycol ingestion. *JAMA* 1980;243:2065.

A case report that shows the importance of blocking the formation of the toxic metabolites in ethylene glycol toxicity.

107. ANTIARRHYTHMIC DRUG POISONING

Erica L. Liebelt

I. General principles. Antiarrhythmic drugs are classified into four categories based on their actions. A summary of the drugs' classification and their toxicity is shown in Table 107-1. The beta blockers (class II) and calcium channel blockers (class IV) are covered in other chapters.

II. Class IA agents. Quinidine, procainamide, disopyramide, and moricizine prolong the duration of the action potential by blocking rapid sodium channels, thereby slowing cardiac conduction and prolonging refractory periods. Cardiotoxic effects include QRS, JT, and QT interval prolongation, sinus bradycardia, sinus arrest, torsades de pointes, and depressed myocardial contractility resulting in hypotension. Conduction delays can occur at therapeutic doses.

Acute ingestions of quinidine can in result nausea, vomiting, and diarrhea. Quinidine can cause cinchonism (headache, tinnitus, deafness, diplopia, confusion), vertigo, visual disturbances (blurred vision, yellow vision), or delirium. Severe quinidine poisoning is manifest by lethargy, coma, seizures, and respiratory depression. Quinidine use can also cause potentially serious drug-to-drug interactions (e.g., increased digoxin concentrations).

Signs and symptoms of acute procainamide toxicity are similar to quinidine. Toxicity can result from prerenal azotemia induced by heart failure or overdiuresis causing toxic levels of its metabolite NAPA (*N*-acetylprocainamide). Drug levels should be monitored, especially when a change occurs in physiologic status. Therapeutic procainamide concentrations are between 4 and 8 μg/ml and those for NAPA 7 to 15 μg/ml. Long-term therapy can result in a lupuslike syndrome.

Anticholinergic side effects are common with disopyramide. In contrast to other class IA agents, it has a significantly more negative inotropic effect. Moricizine's side effects include dizziness, nausea, abdominal discomfort, and hypoesthesias. Experience with moricizine overdoses is limited.

III. Class IB drugs. Lidocaine, mexiletine and tocainide shorten action potential duration and reduce rate of depolarization selectively in ischemic cells. They have insignificant effects on conduction intervals at therapeutic doses. Most lidocaine toxicity is caused by errors in dosing and administration. Its metabolic clearance depends on liver blood flow; thus, some disease states such as congestive heart failure or shock are likely to cause drug accumulation. Neurologic toxicity, which usually precedes cardiotoxicity, includes lightheadedness, visual disturbances, paresthesias, tinnitus, drowsiness, confusion, and psychosis. Muscle twitching, tremor, ataxia, dysarthria, and seizures can occur. Massive overdose can result in seizures, coma, respiratory arrest, and cardiovascular collapse. QRS prolongation, atrioventricular (AV) block, bradycardia, and hypotension may also occur.

Massive tocainide overdose has caused toxicity similar to lidocaine with loss of consciousness, seizures, AV block, ventricular fibrillation, and asystole. Adverse effects are common; they include nausea, vomiting, diarrhea, paresthesias, confusion, ataxia, and tremor, the latter which may suggest the maximal tolerable dose has been achieved. Monitoring for agranulocytosis has been recommended.

Mexiletine's toxic profile is similar to lidocaine and tocainide. Hepatic impairment can significantly prolong the elimination half-life of this drug. Status epilepticus has been described, which may be caused by the drug's longer elimination half-life compared with lidocaine.

IV. Class IC drugs. Flecainide and propafenone cause marked slowing of cardiac conduction and small increases in refractory periods. The QRS and QT (but not the JT) intervals are typically prolonged. Flecainide toxicity is characterized by bradycardia, hypotension, coma, and, less commonly, tachycardia or seizures. Hypotension is less common than with class IA drugs. Propafenone overdose is similar to that of flecainide.

TABLE 107-1. Classes of antiarrhythmic drugs and adverse effects/toxicity[a]

Class	Effect on electrocardiogram	Adverse effects/toxicity
IA		
Quinidine	↑ QRS, ↑ QT, ±PR	Gastrointestinal upset Cinchonism Seizures, lethargy, coma Anticholinergic effects Hypotension, heart block Torsades de pointes Thrombocytopenia
Procainamide	↑ QRS, ↑ QT, ±PR	Fever Seizures, coma Lupuslike syndrome Hypotension Torsades de pointes
Disopyramide	↑ QRS, ↑ QT, ±PR	Seizures, coma Anticholinergic effects Hypotension, heart block Torsades de pointes
Moricizine	↑ QRS	Gastrointestinal upset Hypoesthesias, dizziness Hypotension
IB		
Lidocaine	None	Agitation, paresthesias, visual disturbances Seizures, coma Hypotension Cardiovascular collapse
Mexiletine	None	See lidocaine
Tocainide	None	Tremor, ataxia Seizures Agranulocytosis Hypotension
Phenytoin		See Chapter 109
IC		
Flecainide	↑PR, ↑ QRS	Hypotension AV Block, bradycardia Coma Neutropenia
Propafenone	↑PR, ↑ QRS	Seizures AV block, bradycardia Hypoglycemia
II. Beta-blockers	(See Chapter 112)	
III. Amiodarone	↑PR, ↑QRS, ↑ QT	Pulmonary fibrosis Hepatitis Photosensitive dermatitis Corneal microdeposits Hypo-/hyperthyroidism Peripheral neuropathy AV block, bradycardia
Sotalol	↑ QT	Hypotension Bradycardia
Bretylium	None	Hypotension Bradycardia
Ibutilide[b]		
IV. Calcium channel blockers	(See Chapter 113)	

[a] All agents are potentially proarrhythmic.
[b] Little reported toxicity.
AV, atrioventricular.

V. Class III drugs. Amiodarone and sotalol prolong the action potential and the refractory period by blocking potassium currents. Usually a JT (and hence QT) prolongation occurs without QRS changes. Sotalol is also a noncardioselective beta-blocker.

Serious acute toxicity with amiodarone has not been reported. Chronic toxicity from long-term therapy can result in pulmonary fibrosis, hyperthyroidism or hypothyroidism, peripheral neuropathy, tremor, corneal microdeposits, hepatitis, photosensitivity dermatitis, and blue-gray skin discoloration. In addition, it can cause ventricular arrhythmias or bradyarrhythmias.

Sotalol intoxication is characterized by bradycardia, hypotension, and torsades de pointes. The plasma half-life depends on glomerular filtration; thus, toxicity can occur in the presence of agents or medical conditions that alter kidney perfusion (e.g., nonsteroidal antiinflammatory agents).

VI. General management. Continuous electrocardiogram monitoring should be instituted as soon as possible. Advanced life support measures should be provided as necessary. Activated charcoal should be administered as soon as possible in acute ingestions.

Electrolytes, including calcium and magnesium, should be measured and any abnormalities corrected. Hypotension must be managed aggressively, initially with fluids and then with vasopressors. Invasive hemodynamic monitoring may be necessary to assess the cause of hypotension and to choose appropriate therapy. Excessive doses of inotropic agents should be avoided because they can precipitate ventricular tachyarrhythmias. Early consideration should be given to circulatory assist devices for patients with cardiogenic shock.

Specific treatment interventions for certain antiarrhythmic agents are summarized in Table 107-2. Boluses of hyptertonic sodium bicarbonate should be used to treat hypotension, QRS widening (> 100 msec), or ventricular tachyarrhythmias caused by class IA or IC drug toxicity. Type IA agents should not be used to treat cardiotoxicity caused by type IA, IC, and III drugs. Enhancement of drug elimination may be successful with either hemodialysis or hemoperfusion for selected drugs.

TABLE 107-2. Management of antiarrhythmic toxicity

- Enhance drug elimination
  - Hemodialysis—procainamide, NAPA (in presence of renal insufficiency), disopyramide, sotalol, tocainide
  - Hemoperfusion—disopyramide, NAPA, tocainide
- Hypotension
  - Isotonic fluid administration
  - Alkalinization and sodium loading (hypertonic $NaHCO_3$) for class I drugs
  - Inotropes, vasopressors
  - Circulatory assist devices (cardiopulmonary bypass, intraaortic balloon pump)
- Conduction abnormalities
  - Alkalinization and sodium loading (hypertonic $NaHCO_3$) for class I drugs
  - Pacing for atrioventricular block or bradycardia
- Ventricular arrhythmias
  - Torsades des pointes
    - Magnesium sulfate
    - Isoproterenol
    - Temporary pacing
  - Monomorphic ventricular tachycardia
    - Cardioversion if hemodynamically significant
    - Alkalinization and sodium loading (hypertonic $NaHCO_3$) for class I drugs
    - Lidocaine except for class IB drugs
    - Overdrive pacing

NAPA, *N* - acetylprocainamide.

Selected Readings

Atkinson Jr AJ, Krumlovsky FA, Huang CM, et al. Hemodialysis for severe procainamide toxicity: clinical and pharmacokinetic observations. *Clin Pharmacol Ther* 1976;20:585.

A case report showing the enhanced elimination of procainamide and N-acetylprocainamide with hemodialysis in addition to discussing the pharmacokinetics of this drug and its metabolite.

Hruby K, Missliwetz J. Poisoning with oral antiarrhythmic drugs. *Int J Clin Pharmacol Ther Toxicol* 1985;23:253.

Clinical and toxicologic data on several antiarrhythmic drugs, including quinidine and mexiletine.

Köppel C, Oberdisse U, Heinemeyer G. Clinical course and outcome in class IC antiarrhythmic overdose. *Clin Toxicol* 1990;28:433.

A case series of patients with class IC antiarrhythmic overdoses demonstrating that fatal outcome was caused by cardiac conduction disturbances progressing to electromechanical dissociation or asystole.

Kreeger RW, Hammill SC. New antiarrhythmic drugs: tocainide, mexiletine, flecainide, encainide, amiodarone. *Mayo Clin Proc* 1987;62:1033.

An excellent review of these drugs, including indications for use, pharmacology, and adverse effects.

Neuvonen P, Elonen E, Vuorenmaa T, et al. Prolonged QT interval and severe tachyarrhythmias: common features of sotalol intoxication. *Eur J Clin Pharmacol* 1981;20:85.

A case series that demonstrated prolonged QT interval, hypotension, bradycardia, and ventricular tachyarrhythmias in patients with sotalol overdoses.

Stratmann HG, Kennedy HL. Torsades de pointes associated with drugs and toxins: recognition and management. *Am Heart J* 1987;113:1470.

An excellent review of the pathophysiology of torsades de pointes and drugs or toxins that can precipitate this arrhythmia.

108. ANTICHOLINERGIC POISONING

Erica L. Liebelt

I. General principles. Anticholinergic poisoning can be precipitated by a variety of pharmaceutical agents including many over-the-counter preparations. In addition, several plants and mushrooms can also result in this toxicity as displayed in recent years by the widespread recreational use of jimson weed by adolescents (Table 108-1). This poisoning is manifested by a consistent and recognizable constellation of signs and symptoms—the anticholinergic toxidrome (Table 108-2). Although most cases result in only mild toxicity, the potential exists for serious and life-threatening toxicity.

II. Pharmacology. Anticholinergic compounds antagonize the effects of the endogenous neurotransmitter acetylcholine (ACh). Two types of ACh receptors—muscarinic and nicotinic—are distributed in the central nervous system (CNS), autonomic nervous system, and peripheral nervous system. Agents that block muscarinic cholinergic receptors, found predominantly in the parasympathetic terminals, lead to anticholinergic poisoning.

III. Clinical presentation. The anticholinergic toxidrome has been classically described by the mnemonic "Blind as a bat, Dry as a bone, Hot as Hades, Red as a beet, and Mad as a hatter." The most common clinical findings include sinus tachycardia, dry mucous membranes, dry and flushed skin, mydriasis, hypertension, urinary retention, and paralytic ileus. Other symptoms of CNS toxicity are confusion, disorientation, ataxia, and visual or auditory hallucinations. The most serious manifestations include agitation, delirium, hyperthermia, seizures, coma, and respiratory failure. The clinical presentation can be complicated by other pharmacologic actions of the ingested agent (tricyclic antidepressants) or the actions of co-ingestants (salicylates, sympathomimetics).

IV. Management. Initial management for the patient with anitcholinergic poisoning includes advanced life support measures. Monitoring for hyperthermia is important but often neglected in the agitated or uncooperative patient. An electrocardiogram should be obtained on all symptomatic patients to evaluate for conduction disturbances as well as arrhythymias. Routine laboratory tests should include electrolytes, blood urea nitrogen (BUN), creatinine, and creatine kinase (to evaluate for rhabdomyolysis). Toxicology testing can detect some but not all anticholinergic agents.

Gastrointestinal decontamination should be considered in all patients who present with anticholinergic poisoning following an acute ingestion. Because of delayed gastric emptying and impaired gut motility, administration of activated charcoal may prove beneficial even several hours after the ingestion. Repeated doses should not be given in the setting of an ileus or obstruction because of the risk of impaction or aspiration.

The decision to proceed with gastric emptying must take into consideration whether a potentially lethal substance exists that can be removed by gastric lavage. In addition, special attention must be given to protect the airway before lavage because of the CNS and respiratory depressive effects of the drug or co-ingestant.

Further interventions that may be indicated include placement of an indwelling catheter for bladder decompression, aggressive cooling for patients with hyperthermia, anticonvulsant therapy with benzodiazepines or phenobarbital, and correction of dehydration with intravenous (IV) fluids. Agitation and delirium should be controlled with benzodiazepines (phenothiazines, butyrophenones, and other agents with anticholinergic activity should be avoided).

Patients with minor toxicity (sinus tachycardia, dry mucous membranes) can be medically cleared if toxicity does not progress after 6 to 8 hours of observation. Patients presenting with progressive toxicity or moderate or severe toxicity should be admitted to a monitored setting.

A. Antidotal therapy. Physostigmine is an acetylcholinesterase inhibitor that can reverse the anticholinergic toxicity by increasing the amount of acetylcholine.

TABLE 108-1. Selected anticholinergic agents

Selected anticholinergic agents
Antihistamines (H_1-blockers)
Diphenhydramine
Hydroxyzine
Promethazine
Antiparkinsonian drugs
Benztropine
Trihexyphenidyl
Antipsychotics
Phenothiazines
Butyrophenones
Antispasmodics
Trihexyphenidyl
Belladonna alkaloids and related congeners
Atropine
Hyoscyamine
Ipatropium
Cyclic antidepressants
Muscle relaxants
Cyclobenzaprine
Mydriatics
Cyclopentolate
Tropicamide
Plants
Jimson weed
Bittersweet
Jerusalem cherry
Mushrooms
Amanita pantherina
Amanita muscaria

However, its use should be reserved for specific patients and clinical situations. The major indication for physostigmine use is CNS excitation (delirium, agitation, psychosis), which is often resistant to benzodiazepines and necessitates the use of physical restraint. It can also result in hyperthermia and its potential complications. Less common indications for physostigmine include seizures unresponsive to conventional treatment, severe hypertension resulting in acute symptoms, and hemodynamically significant supraventricular tachycardia.

Contraindications to the use of physostigmine include mechanical bowel or urogenital tract obstruction. It should be used cautiously in patients with asthma, diabetes, cardiovascular diseases, or any vagotonic state. Physostigmine should not be used in patients with suspected tricyclic antidepressant ingestions or any drug whose toxicity can result in cardiac conduction delays or arrhythmias. When administered to patients without anticholinergic toxicity, signs and symptoms of cholinergic excess (e.g., bronchospasm, bronchorrhea, seizures, and bradyarrhythmias) can occur.

Any patient receiving physostigmine must be placed on a cardiac monitor and continuously monitored. The dose for adults is 1 to 2 mg given as a slow IV infusion over 2 to 5 minutes. The dose for pediatric patients is 0.02 mg/kg, up to 0.5 mg. The dose can be repeated after 10 to 20 minutes if no reversal of anticholinergic effects has occurred. If excessive cholinergic effects occur with physostigmine's administration, they can be reversed with a titrating dose of atropine.

TABLE 108-2. Manifestations of the anticholinergic syndrome

Peripheral anticholinergic signs and symptoms
Tachycardia
Dry, flushed skin
Dry mucous membranes
Dilated pupils (variable)
Hyperpyrexia
Urinary retention
Decreased bowel sounds
Hypertension
Hypotension (may be late finding)
Central anticholinergic signs and symptoms
Confusion
Disorientation
Loss of short-term memory
Ataxia
Incoordination
Psychomotor agitation
Picking or grasping movements
Extrapyramidal reactions
Visual/auditory hallucinations
Frank psychosis
Coma
Seizures
Respiratory failure
Cardiovascular collapse

Modified from Kirk M, Kulig K, Rumack BH: Anticholinergics. In: Haddad LM, Winchester JE, eds: *Clinical management of poisoning and drug overdose,* 2nd ed. Philadelphia: WB Saunders, 1990;863; with permisssion.

Selected Readings

Blazer DG, Federspiel CF, Ray WA, et al. The risk of anticholinergic toxicity in the elderly: a study of prescribing practices in two populations. *J Gerontol* 1983;38:31.
This report describes the risk of anticholinergic poisoning in the elderly from the concomitant use of various medications with anticholinergic side effects prescribed by physicians to this cohort.

Brown JH. Atropine, scopolamine, and related antimuscarinic drugs. In: Gilman AG, Rall TW, Nies AS, et al, eds. *Goodman and Gilman's the pharmacological basis of therapeutics,* 8th ed. New York: Pergamon; 1990:150.
An overview of the pharmacology, adverse effects, and toxicity of antimuscarinic drugs.

Goldfrank L, Flomenbaum N, Lewin N, et al. Anticholinergic poisoning. *J Toxicol Clin Toxicol* 1982;19:17.
This article reports the clinical presentation of three patients poisoned with anticholinergic agents and discusses the diagnosis and treatment.

Hsu CK, Leo P, Shastry D, et al. Anticholinergic poisoning associated with herbal tea. *Arch Intern Med* 1995;155:2245.
This paper describes an outbreak of anticholinergic poisoning from herbal tea that contained belladonna alkaloids.

Shannon MW. Toxicology reviews: physostigmine. *Pediatr Emerg Care* 1998;14:224.
This review article presents two cases of anticholinergic toxicity in children and describes the clinical toxicity and indications for physostigmine.

109. ANTICONVULSANTS

Jeffrey R. Tucker

I. General principles

A. Phenytoin. Phenytoin is used in the treatment of generalized tonic-clonic, partial complex, and focal seizures. It blocks sodium channels in excitable cell membranes and prevents seizure foci from detonating adjacent areas. Phenytoin is a central nervous system (CNS) depressant with a propensity to cause cerebellar-vestibular dysfunction. It is a weak acid and is soluble only in alkaline media. The parenteral form has a pH of 10 to 12, and is dissolved in propylene glycol. Fosphenytoin, a prodrug of phenytoin, is soluble in water and can be administered intramuscularly. Therapeutic serum levels are 10 to 20 μg/ml. Phenytoin is metabolized by the liver. At low serum levels, metabolism is first-order kinetics. When plasma levels exceed 10 μg/ml metabolism follows zero-order elimination kinetics and the average half-life increases from 22 hours to more than 50 hours.

B. Valproic acid. Valproic acid is used to treat simple and complex absence seizures. It is thought to act by blocking the metabolism of the inhibitory neurotransmitter γ-aminobutyric acid (GABA), thereby increasing GABA levels in the CNS. Sprinkle and enteric-coated formations of divalproex (Depakote), the sodium valproate salt of valproic acid, are slowly absorbed and can cause delayed toxicity after overdose. Therapeutic serum levels are 50 to 100 μg/ml. Valproic acid is metabolized predominantly by the liver to several metabolites. It is a CNS depressant but lacks the cerebellar toxicity of other anticonvulsants. Valproic acid disrupts fatty acid and amino acid metabolism and can cause hepatoxicity with chronic use. Metabolic effects can contribute to CNS toxicity after acute overdose.

C. Carbamazepine. Carbamazepine is used in the treatment of generalized tonic-clonic, simple partial, and complex partial seizures. It is a CNS depressant with anticholinergic and cerebellar-vestibular activity. Tegretol, a trade brand, behaves like a sustained-release formulation. After overdose, absorption can be prolonged and erratic, resulting in delayed and cyclic coma. Therapeutic serum levels are 4 to 12 μg/ml. Carbamazepine is predominantly metabolized in the liver, with 40% converted to an active carbamazepine-10,11-epoxide metabolite. This pathway becomes saturated at toxic drug levels and the half-life increases from approximately 10 to 20 hours.

II. Clinical presentation

A. Phenytoin. Phenytoin initially depresses cerebellar and vestibular function. With increasing toxicity, cerebral function is affected. At blood levels of 20 and 40 μg/ml, dizziness, slurred speech, ataxia, tremor, vomiting, blurred vision, and nystagmus (in all directions) are noted. As levels increase, confusion, hallucinations, and sometimes psychosis can develop. At levels greater than 90 μg/ml, coma and respiratory depression occur. Patients who are chronically taking phenytoin are affected less than those who are not. Paradoxical intoxication with dystonia, choreoathetoid movements, decerebrate rigidity, and seizure activity has been reported in patients with underlying neurologic deficits. Hypotension and arrhythmias can occur during intravenous (IV) drug administration. These reactions are caused by propylene glycol toxicity and occur with rapid infusion rates. Cardiac toxicity from oral phenytoin is rare.

B. Valproic acid. Valproic acid causes CNS depression with or without metabolic abnormalities. Patients with an underlying seizure disorder may have breakthrough seizures. Serum levels of 180 μg/ml are usually associated with coma. Nausea, vomiting, and diarrhea are common but hypotension and cardiotoxicity are rare. Anion gap acidosis, hypocalcemia, hyperosmolality, hypernatremia, and thrombocytopenia may be present. Hyperammonemia associated with vomiting, lethargy, and encephalopathy can occur at therapeutic as well as toxic drug levels.

C. Carbamazepine. Signs and symptoms of poisoning include hypotension, hypothermia, CNS and respiratory depression, diminished or exaggerated deep tendon reflexes, and dysarthria. Cerebellar-vestibular dysfunction is manifest by nystagmus, ataxia, ophthalmoplegia, diplopia, absent doll's eye reflex, and absent caloric reflexes. Anticholinergic findings include hyperthermia, sinus tachycardia, hypertension, urinary retention, mydriasis, and ileus. Conduction abnormalities such as prolongation of the PR, QRS, and QT intervals and complete heart block can occur. Paradoxical agitation, combativeness, irritability, hallucinations, or seizures have also been reported.

III. Treatment

A. General. Patients should have a rapid evaluation of respiratory status followed by intubation if hypoxia or risk of aspiration is present. Intravenous access should be established and cardiac monitoring initiated. Gastrointestinal tract decontamination is performed by giving enteral activated charcoal. Multiple-dose activated charcoal can increase the rate of elimination of these agents. Seizures should be treated with benzodiazepines or barbiturates. Laboratory evaluation includes a complete blood count (CBC), electrolytes, blood urea nitrogen (BUN), creatinine, glucose, and liver function tests.

Drug levels should be followed every 4 hours until they peak and 12 to 24 hours thereafter. Because absorption can be delayed, a prolonged observation period is necessary. Patients with serious acute poisoning may require several days for recovery.

B. Phenytoin. Hypotension and arrhythmias that occur during phenytoin infusion should be treated by discontinuing the infusion. Crystalloids can also be given for hypotension; vasopressors are rarely necessary. Cardiac arrhythmias can be treated according to standard advanced cardiac life support protocols if necessary.

C. Valproic acid. Naloxone has increased the level of consciousness in some patients; the response is inconsistent. Severely poisoned patients can be treated with extracorporeal removal, such as hemodialysis or hemoperfusion. An ammonia level may be useful in assessing the CNS effects of metabolic derangements. A coagulation profile assists in evaluating hepatotoxicity. In addition, serum amylase and lipase levels should be obtained to rule out pancreatitis.

D. Carbamazepine. Hemoperfusion should be considered in patients who are unresponsive to supportive care.

Selected Readings

Alberto G, Erickson T, Popiel H, et al. Central nervous system manifestations of valproic acid overdose responsive to naloxone. *Ann Emerg Med* 1989;18:889.

A case report of valproic acid toxicity poisoning in which there was a clinical response to naloxone. The clinical presentation was similar to the opiod toxidrome of miosis, coma, and respiratory depression.

Apfelbaum JD, Caravati EM, Kems WP, et al. Cardiovascular effects of carbamazepine toxicity. *Ann Emerg Med* 1995;25:631.

A retrospective review of 72 patients with carbamazepine overdose showing a low incidence of significant cardiovascular toxicity.

Chadwick DW. Concentration-effect relationships of valproic acid. *Clin Pharmacol* 1985;10:155.

Excellent discussion of the limitations of monitoring of valproic acid because of its pharmacokinetic and pharmacodynamic effects.

Dezeeuw HA, Westenberg HGM, Van der Kleijn E, et al. An unusual case of carbamazepine poisoning with a near-fatal relapse after two days. *Clin Toxicol* 1979;14:263.

Case report of a relapse of neurologic symptoms which demonstrates the importance and toxicity of the active metabolite carbamazepine-epoxide.

Dupuis RE, Liditman SN, Pollack GM. Acute valproic acid overdose, clinical course and pharmacokinetic disposition of valproic acid and metabolites. *Drug Saf* 1990;5:65.

A case report of a toddler with significant cerebral edema, followed by a discussion of the metabolites of valproic acid and their toxicologic significance.

Durelli L, Mussazza U, Cavallo R. Carbamazepine toxicity and poisoning: incidence, clinical features, and management. *Med Toxicol Adv Drug Exp* 1989:4:95.
Discussion of carbamazepine poisoning with an emphasis on pharmacology, side effects, and toxicity.

Eamest MP, Marx JA, Drury LR. Complications of intravenous phenytoin for acute treatment of seizures: Recommendations for usage. *JAMA* 1983;249:762.
Discussion of the potential complications of parenteral phenytoin administration. Guidelines are based on a prospective study of 200 patients.

Farrar HC, Herald DA, Reed MD. Acute valproic acid intoxication: enhanced drug clearance with oral-activated charcoal. *Crit Care Med* 1993;21:299.
A case report showing increase elimination of valproic acid treated with a continuous infusion of activated charcoal.

Gill MA, Kem JW, Kaneko J, et al. Phenytoin overdose kinetics. *West J Med* 1978; 128:246.
A case report of phenytoin overdose followed by a review of the differences between pharmacokinetics and toxiokinetics of phenytoin.

Patel H, Crichton JU. The neurologic hazards of diphenylhydantoin in childhood. *J Pediatr* 1968;73:676.
An early review of 13 cases of phenytoin intoxication in children, with 70% caused by chronic toxicity. No sequelae reported in this series.

Stiliman N, Masden JC. Incidence of seizures with phenytoin toxicity. *Neurology* 1985;35:1769.
A retrospective study of phenytoin intoxicated patients with a 10% incidence of seizures.

Weaver DF, Camfield P, Fraser A. Massive carbamazepine overdose: clinical and pharmacologic observations in five episodes. *Neurology* 1988;38:755.
Clinical and pharmacologic observation demonstrating four distinct stages and the importance of the epoxide metabolite in causing toxicity.

Wyte CD, Berk WA. Severe oral phenytoin overdose does not cause cardiovascular morbidity. *Ann Emerg Med* 1991;20:508.
A retrospective review of severe phenytoin overdose showing no evidence of cardiovascular complications and no deaths.

110. ANTIHYPERTENSIVE AGENTS

Richard Y. Wang

I. **General principles.** β-adrenergic receptor antagonists and calcium channel blockers are discussed in Chapters 112 and 113.

II. **Loop diuretics (Table 110-1)** are used in the treatment of edema associated with congestive heart failure (CHF), cirrhosis, and renal disease. These agents decrease renal water reabsorption, increase renal blood flow, and enhance solute (e.g., sodium, chloride, potassium, hydrogen ion, calcium, magnesium, ammonium, bicarbonate, and phosphate) excretion. Acutely, they increase venous capacitance by dilating large veins.

Auditory toxicity is enhanced when these agents are used with aminoglycosides and cisplatin. Injectable formulations for parenteral use are available for furosemide and bumetanide.

III. **Thiazide and related diuretics (Table 110-2)** are used as monotherapy or with other agents. Thiazides enhance renal excretion of sodium, chloride, and water. Acutely, they lower the blood pressure by reducing plasma volume and cardiac output. They should be used with caution in patients with renal disease. Thiazide-induced hypokalemia and hypomagnesemia can predispose to cardiac glycoside toxicity.

IV. **Potassium-sparing diuretics (Table 110-3)** are used to enhance the effects of other diuretics and to counteract their kaliuretic action. They should not be used in patients with renal insufficiency because of potential hyperkalemia. Concurrent administration of angiotensin-converting enzyme (ACE) inhibitors or potassium can also result in hyperkalemia.

V. **Angiotensin-converting enzyme inhibitors (Table 110-4)** are used to treat congestive heart failure (CHF) as well as hypertension. These agents also inhibit bradykinin metabolism and enhance prostaglandin synthesis, effects thought to contribute to unwanted side effects such as cough, urticaria, and angioedema. Patients with sodium or volume depletion and those taking diuretics are at increased risk for hypotension and renal failure.

VI. **Antiotensin II receptor antagonists (Table 110-5)** can be useful for CHF as well as hypertension. Angiotensin II-type 1 receptor blockade results in vasodilation, decreased aldsoterone secretion, and enhanced sodium and water excretion. Volume or sodium depletion and concomitant diuretic use increase the risk of excessive blood pressure reduction.

VII. **Centrally active antiadrenergic agents (Table 110-6)** are generally used in conjunction with a diuretic. These agents stimulate postsynaptic α2-adrenergic receptors in the CNS, resulting in decreased sympathetic outflow and decreased peripheral and renal vascular resistance and heart rate. Increased norepinephrine release following abrupt discontinuation can result in rebound hypertension.

VIII. **Postganglionic sympathetic inhibitors (Table 110-7)** are generally reserved for hypertension refractory to other drugs because of their potential to cause orthostatic hypotension, syncope, impotence, and explosive diarrhea. These agents deplete norepinephrine from postganglionic sympathetic nerve terminals and inhibit the release of norepinephrine from sympathetic nerves.

IX. **Nitroglycerin** is used to treat hypertension associated with encephalopathy, aortic dissection, myocardial ischemia, and acute renal failure and to manage acute valvular insufficiency, low cardiac output states, and CHF. It relaxes vascular smooth muscle by increasing cyclic guanosine monophosphate. The venous circulation is affected most. A continuous infusion is initiated at a rate of 5 to 10 μg/min. The dosage is increased by 5 to 10 μg/min every 5 to 10 minutes until a response is noted.

X. **Nitroprusside** has the same indications and action as nitroglycerin. It is metabolized to cyanide, which combines with thiosulfate to form thiocyanate. Thiocyanate

TABLE 110-1. Dosing guidelines for the loop diuretics in the treatment of hypertension

	Furosemide[a–c]	Bumetanide[a–c]	Torsemide[a–c]	Ethacrynic acid[a–c]
Starting dose	10–20 mg p.o. b.i.d.	0.5 mg p.o. q.d.	5 mg p.o. q.d.	25–50 mg p.o. q.d.
Usual maintenance dose	20–40 mg p.o. b.i.d.	1–2 mg p.o. q.d.	5–10 mg p.o. q.d.	25–50 mg p.o. b.i.d.
Maximum dose	160–240 mg p.o. b.i.d.	5 mg p.o. b.i.d.	10 mg q.d.	100 mg p.o. b.i.d.
Relative potency	1	~40	~4	0.6–0.8

[a] The hypotensive effect of antihypertensive agents may be enhanced during concomitant loop diuretic administration. The dosage of the antihypertensive agent should be reduced when a loop diuretic is added to an existing antihypertensive regimen.
[b] The loop diuretics are contraindicated in patients with anuria.
[c] Patients with renal disease and liver disease may require higher doses of the loop diuretics.
p.o., by mouth; b.i.d., twice daily; q.d., every day.

TABLE 110-2. Available preparations and the oral dosing guidelines for the thiazide and related diuretics for the treatment of hypertension

Diuretic	Preparations	Starting dose	Maintenance dose	Maximal dose (mg/d)
Chlorothiazide	250, 500/mg tablets; 250 mg/5 ml oral suspension	250–500 mg/d	250–1000 mg/d	1000
Hydrochlorothiazide	25, 50, 100 mg tablets; 50 mg/5 ml, 100 mg/ml oral solution	50–100 mg/d	25–100 mg/d	200
Bendroflumethiazide	5, 10 mg tablets	5–20 mg/d	2.5–15 mg/d	20
Cyclothiazide	2 mg tablets	2 mg/d	2–4 mg/d	6
Methyclothiazide	2.5, 5 mg tablets	2.5–5 mg/d	2.5–5 mg/d	5
Benzthiazide	50 mg tablets	25–50 mg b.i.d.	25–50 mg b.i.d.	200
Hydroflumethiazide	50 mg tablets	50 mg b.i.d.	50–100 mg/d	200
Trichlormethiazide	2, 4 tablets	2 mg/d	2–4 mg/d	4
Polythiazide	1, 2, 4 mg tablets	2 mg/d	1–4 mg/d	4
Quinethazone	50 mg tablets	50–100 mg/d	50–100 mg/d	200
Metolazone	2.5, 5, 10 mg extended tablets	2.5–5 mg/d	2.5–5 mg/d	10
	0.5 mg prompt tablets	0.5 mg/d	0.5–1 mg/d	1
Chlorthalidone	25, 50, 100 mg tablets	25 mg/d	25–50 mg/d	100
Indapamide	2.5 mg tablets	2.5 mg/d	2.5–5 mg/d	5

TABLE 110-3. Dosing guidelines for the potassium sparing diuretics

	Spironolactone[a,b]	Triamterene[a,b]	Amiloride[a,b]
Starting dose	25–100 mg p.o. q.d.	50–100 mg p.o. b.i.d.	5 mg p.o. q.d.
Usual maintenance dose	50–100 mg p.o. q.d.	50–100 mg p.o. q.d.–b.i.d.	5–10 mg p.o. q.d.
Maximal dose	200 mg p.o. q.d.	150 mg p.o. b.i.d.	20 mg p.o. q.d.

[a] Take with food.
[b] When used in conjunction with other diuretics, reducing the doses of these agents may be required.
p.o., orally; q.d., every day; b.i.d., twice daily.

is eliminated by the kidneys. Cyanide toxicity can occur when thiosulfate body stores are depleted. It is most likely to occur early in treatment, at elevated doses, and in patients with poor nutrition, chronic disease, recent surgery, or chronic diuretic use. An elevated blood cyanide concentration, clinical manifestations (e.g., agitation, seizures, tachypnea, hypotension, dysrhythmias), and, most importantly, lactic acidemia confirm the diagnosis. Thiocyanate toxicity (agitation, delusions, disorientation, tremors, seizures, and coma) can occur in patients with renal insufficiency and prolonged treatment.

The starting dose of nitroprusside is 0.3 μg/kg/min. The infusion can be incrementally increased to a maximum of 10 μg/kg/min, but this rate should not be used for more than 10 minutes. Adding sodium thiosulfate to a nitroprusside infusion at a concentration of 1 g/100 mg of nitroprusside can prevent cyanide toxicity but not the accumulation of thiocyanate in the presence of renal insufficiency.

Treatment of cyanide toxicity includes discontinuation of nitroprusside and administration of sodium nitrate and sodium thiosulfate. Hemodialysis can remove thiocyanate.

XI. α_1-postsynaptic adrenergic blockers (Table 110-8) produce arterial and venous dilation. They can cause CNS side effects, including lassitude, vivid dreams, and depression. A "first dose" phenomenon (transient dizziness, palpitations, and syncope) can occur within 1 to 3 hours of the first dose.

XII. Vasodilators (Table 110-9) are not used as monotherapy because arteriolar dilation results in reflex sympathetic stimulation, activation of the renin–angiotensin system, and blunted antihypertensive effect. If used alone, these agents can precipitate myocardial ischemia in patients with underlying coronary artery disease.

XIII. Diazoxide can be used in the acute treatment of severe hypertension. A loading dose is administered by slow infusion at a rate of 15 to 30 mg/min to a total dose of 5 mg/kg. Alternatively, an intravenous (IV) bolus of 1 to 3 mg/kg can be given every 5 to 15 minutes until adequate blood pressure reduction is achieved. The bolus technique can cause hypotension. Once the blood pressure is controlled, doses can be repeated every 4 to 24 hours. Repeated administration can lead to sodium and water retention and CHF.

XIV. Trimethaphan camsylate is used for hypertensive emergencies, controlled hypotension in surgery, and for pulmonary edema in patients with pulmonary and systemic hypertension. Trimethaphan should be avoided during pregnancy. A continuous infusion is initiated at a rate of 0.5 to 1 mg/min. The dose can be increased by 0.5 to 1 mg/min every 3 to 5 minutes. Tacyhphylaxis develops within 24 to 72 hours. Administration of trimethaphan with succinylcholine and nondepolarizing neuromuscular blockers or in high doses can cause prolonged neuromuscular blockade and respiratory arrest.

TABLE 110-4. Dosing guidelines for the angiotensin-converting enzyme (ACE) inhibitors

Drug	Initial dose	Maintenance dose	Hypodynamic	Hyperdynamic
Benazepril	10 mg q.d.	20–80 mg q.d.	Reduce doses	10 mg q.d., titrate upward, divide b.i.d if response diminished at end of dosing interval
Captopril	12.5–25 mg b.i.d.-t.i.d.	25–150 mg/d divided b.i.d. or t.i.d.	Reduce doses	25 mg t.i.d., titrate upward to response
Enalapril	5 mg q.d.	10–40 mg/d divided q.d. or b.i.d.	Reduce doses	5 mg q.d., titrate upward, divide b.i.d. if response diminished at end of dosing interval
Enalaprilat	1.25 mg i.v. q6h	2.5 mg i.v. q6h	Begin 0.625 mg i.v. q6h; however, a 18q dosing interval may be required in some cases	1.25 mg i.v. q6h, titrate upward to response
Fosinopril	10 mg q.d.	20–80 mg q.d.	No change	10 mg q.d., titrate to response, divide b.i.d. if response diminished at end of dosing interval
Lisinopril	10 mg q.d.	20–40 mg q.d.	Reduce doses	10 mg q.d., titrate to response
Moexipril	7.5 mg q.d.	7.5–60 mg q.d. divided q.d. or b.i.d.	Reduce doses	7.5 mg q.d., titrate to response, divide b.i.d. if response diminished at end of dosing interval
Quinapril	10 mg q.d.	20–80 mg/d divided q.d. or b.i.d.	Reduce doses	10 mg q.d., titrate to response, divide b.i.d. if response is diminished at end of dosing interval
Ramipril	2.5 mg q.d.	2.5–20 mg/d divided q.d. or b.i.d.	Reduce doses	2.5 mg q.d., titrate to response, divide b.i.d. if response is diminished at end of dosing interval
Trandolapril	1–2 mg q.d.	2–8 mg/d divided q.d. or b.i.d.	Reduce doses	1–2 mg q.d., titrate to response, divide b.i.d. if response is diminished at end of dosing interval

q.d., every day; b.i.d., twice daily; t.i.d., three times a day; i.v., intravenous.

TABLE 110-5. Dosing guidelines for angiotensin II antagonists

Agent	Initial dose	Maintenance dose	Hypodynamic	Hyperdynamic
Losartan (CoZaar)	25–50 mg q.d.	25–100 mg/d divided q.d. or b.i.d.	Begin with 25 mg q.d., titrate to response	50 mg q.d., titrate to response, divided b.i.d. if response diminished at end of dosing interval
Valsartan (Diovan)	80 mg q.d.	80–320 mg q.d.	No change	80 mg q.d., titrate to response
Irbesartan (Avapro)	150 mg q.d.	150–300 mg q.d.	No change	150 mg q.d., titrate to response

q.d., every day; b.i.d., twice daily.

TABLE 110-6. Dosing guidelines for the alpha-2 receptor agonists

	Oral clonidine[a,b]	Transdermal clonidine[a,b]	Oral methyldopa[a,b]	Injectable methyldopa[a,b]	Oral guanabenz[a,b]	Oral guanfacine[b]
Starting dose	0.1 mg b.i.d.	one No. 1 patch weekly	250 mg b.i.d.	250 mg–1 g i.v. q6h	4 mg b.i.d.	1 mg at bedtime
Usual maintenance dose	0.3 mg b.i.d.	one No. 1–No. 3 patch weekly	500 mg-2 g/d in 2–4 doses	250 mg–1 g i.v. q6h	16 mg b.i.d.	1–3 mg q.d.
Maximal dose	2.4 mg/day	Two No. 3 patches weekly	2 g/d	250 mg–1 g i.v. q6h	32 mg b.i.d.	3 mg q.d.

[a] Dosage adjustment necessary in patients with severe renal dysfunction.
[b] Dosage adjustment may be necessary in patients with severe hepatic failure.
b.i.d., twice daily; i.v., intravenous.

TABLE 110-7. Dosing guidelines for the postganglionic inhibitors

	Guanethidine[a,b]	Guanadrel[b]
Starting dose	10 mg p.o. q.d.	5 mg p.o. b.i.d.
Usual maintenance dose	10–100 mg/d p.o.	20–75 mg/d p.o.
Maximal dose	300 mg/d p.o.	150 mg/d p.o.

[a] May need to adjust dosage in patients with creatinine clearance less than 10 ml/min.
[b] Dosage adjustment necessary in renal dysfunction patients.
p.o., orally; b.i.d., twice daily.

TABLE 110-8. Dosing guidelines for the α_1-adrenergic blockers

	Prazosin[a–c]	Terazosin[c]	Doxazosin[c]
Starting dose	1 mg b.i.d.–t.i.d.	1 mg/d	1 mg/d
Usual maintenance dose	2–20 mg/d (divided doses)	1–20 mg/d	1–16 mg/d
Maximal dose	20–40 mg/d (divided doses)	20 mg/d	16 mg/d

[a] Take the first dose at bedtime.
[b] Patients with renal failure may require smaller doses.
[c] Dosage adjustments may be necessary in patients with severe liver failure.
b.i.d., orally; t.i.d., three times daily.

TABLE 110-9. Dosing guidelines for hydralazine and minoxidil

	Hydralazine[a–c]	Minoxidil[c]
Starting dose	10 mg q.i.d. p.o.	5 mg q.d. p.o.
Usual maintenance dose	10–50 mg q.i.d. p.o.	10–40 mg/d p.o.
Maximal dose	300 mg/d p.o.	100 mg/d p.o.

[a] Take with meals (food enhances bioavailability).
[b] Dosage adjustments necessary in patients with moderate to severe renal dysfunction.
[c] Dosage adjustments may be necessary in patients with severe hepatic failure.
q.i.d., four times daily; p.o., orally.

Selected Readings

Babamoto KS, Hirokawa WT. Doxazosin: a new alpha 1-adrenergic antagonist. *Clin Pharm* 1992;11(5):415.

This review discussed the effectiveness of α_1-adrenergic antagonists in the treatment of hypertension.

Brest AN. Spironolactone in the treatment of hypertension: a review. *Clin Ther* 1986;8:568.

A discussion of the use of potassium-sparing diuretics in primary aldosteronism and congestive heart failure.

Burrell LM. A risk-benefit assessment of losartan potassium in the treatment of hypertension. *Drug Saf* 1997;16:56.

This review discussed the use of angiotensin II receptor antagonists in the treatment of hypertension.

Curry SC, Arnold-Capell P. Nitroprusside, nitroglycerin, and angiotensin-converting enzyme inhibitors. *Crit Care Clin* 1991;7:555.

A discussion of cyanide toxicity associated with nitroprusside use.

Dollery SC, ed. Clonidine. In: *Therapeutic drugs.* Vol 1. New York: Churchill Livingstone; 1991.

Discusses the use of clonidine to control reflex sympathetic activity from current drug therapy for hypertension.

Francis GS. Vasodilators in the intensive care unit. *Am Heart J* 1991;121:1875.

A review of the use of vasodilators in the critical care setting.

Gifford Jr RW. Management of hypertensive crises. *JAMA* 1991;14;266(6):829.

This review discussed the use of nitroprusside in the emergent treatment of hypertension.

Johnston CI. The place of diuretics in the treatment of hypertension in 1993: can we do better? *Clin Exp Hypertens* 1993;15(6):1239.

A discussion of the benefits and limitations of thiazide diuretics in the treatment of hypertension.

Lam AM. The choice of controlled hypotension during repair of intracranial aneurysms: techniques and complications. *Agressologie* 1990;31(6):357.

Examines the use of ganglionic blocking agents to control blood pressure during aneurysmal repair.

Maxwell RA. Guanethidine after twenty years: a pharmacologist's perspective. *Br J Clin Pharmacol* 1982;13(1):35.

This review discussed the pharmacokinetics of guanethidine during acute and long-term use.

Merhoff GC, Porter JM. Ergot intoxication: historical review and description of unusual clinical manifestations. *Ann Surg* 1974;180:773.

A report on the use of nitroprusside in the treatment of peripheral ischemia from ergotamine use.

Schuller D, Lynch JP, Fine D. Protocol-guided diuretic management: comparison of furosemide by continuous infusion and intermittent bolus. *Crit Care Med* 1997;25:1969.

This study demonstrated the effective use of an algorithm, which combines various dosing regimens of furosemide with fluid restriction, to treat patients with pulmonary edema.

Torp-Pedersen C, Kober L, Burchardt H. The place angiotensin-converting enzyme inhibition after acute myocardial infarction. *Am Heart J* 1997;134:S25.

A review of the controversies regarding which myocardial infarction patients should be treated with angiotensin-converting enzyme inhibiting agents.

Willoughby JS. Sodium nitroprusside, pregnancy and multiple intracranial aneurysms. *Anaesth Intensive Care* 1984;12(4):351.

This review discussed the use of nitroprusside in pregnancy.

111. ANTIMICROBIAL AGENTS

Erica L. Liebelt

I. General principles. This chapter reviews the use of vancomycin, imipenem, clindamycin, and the aminoglycosides. In critically ill patients, altered physiologic states may necessitate changes in the choice of antibiotic or its dosing.

II. Vancomycin. Vancomycin is effective for penicillin-sensitive, penicillin-resistant, and methicillin-resistant strains of *Staphylococcus aurerus* (MRSA) and *Staphylococcus epidermidis* as well as enterococci, penicillin-sensitive, penicillin-resistant streptococci, *Clostridium difficile,* and diphtheroids. It acts on bacterial cytoplasmic membranes and inhibits cell wall and RNA synthesis. Inappropriate use of vancomycin and cephalosporins has resulted in the development of vancomycin-resistant enterococcus or VRE (Table 111-1).

Empiric or fixed doses of 1 g every 12 hours or 500 mg every 6 hours intravenously (IV) traditionally have been used for adults with normal renal function. For *C. difficile*-mediated diarrhea, an oral dose of 125 or 250 mg every 6 hours for 5 to 7 days is recommended. Because the drug is cleared by glomerular filtration, the dose in patients with renal insufficiency should be based on the creatinine clearance.

The utility of monitoring vancomycin levels remains somewhat controversial because of lack of sufficient data relating clinical outcome or toxicity to serum vancomycin concentrations. The therapeutic range of vancomycin is 30 to 40 mg/L for peak concentrations and 5 to 10 mg/L for trough concentrations. Vancomycin levels should be monitored in patients receiving concomitant aminoglycosides, anephric patients undergoing hemodialysis, and patients with rapidly changing renal function. The "red man" or "red neck" syndrome, a nonimmunologic-mediated adverse effect associated with rapid infusion of vancomycin, is characterized by pruritus, erythema, flushing of the upper torso, angioedema, and, occasionally, hypotension. Ototoxicity rarely occurs with serum levels less than 30 mg/L and is uncommon in patients with normal renal function. Nephrotoxicity is rare with proper dosing; it occurs primarily in patients with underlying renal disease or in those on concomitant aminoglycoside therapy.

III. Carbapenems. Imipenem and meropenem are structural analogues of β-lactam antibiotics that also inhibit bacterial cell wall synthesis. They have a broad antimicrobial spectrum and are effective against a wide variety of community- and hospital-acquired organisms such as *Streptococcus* sp, *Staphylococcus* sp (except MRSA), Enterobacteriaceae, *Pseudomonas aeruginosa,* and many enteric and oropharyngeal anaerobes including *Bacteroides fragilis* and nonfragilis *Bacteroides* sp. Imipenem is combined with cilastatin, which prevents hydrolysis and inactivation of imipenem, thereby increasing its urine concentration, and inhibits the formation of nephrotoxic metabolites.

Guidelines for dosing imipenem IV are 500 mg every 6 hours for moderately severe infections caused by susceptible microorganisms or 1,000 mg every 6 to 8 hours for severe infections caused by moderately susceptible organisms. Because these agents are cleared predominantly by the kidney, patients with impaired renal function should receive a lower dose (based on the creatinine clearance). Optimal dosing in hypermetabolic patients (e.g., those with burn or sepsis) can be as high as 500 mg every 4 hours.

Common adverse effects of imipenem include nausea, vomiting, and diarrhea. The most serious complication is seizures. The risk of seizures is increased in the elderly, with large doses, and in patients with renal failure or a prior seizure.

IV. Clindamycin. Clindamycin binds to bacterial ribosomes, thereby inhibiting protein synthesis. It is active against most aerobic gram-positive bacteria (except enterococci and MRSA) as well as gram-positive and gram-negative anaerobic bacteria including *B. fragilis* and *Actinomyces* sp. Clindamycin is effective for mixed aerobic-anaerobic infections, especially surgical and gynecologic infections. It is usually

TABLE 111-1. Selected recommendations of the Hospital Infection Control Practices Advisory Committee (HICPAC) for preventing the spread of vancomycin resistance

Selected situations in which vancomycin use is appropriate

- Treatment of serious infections due to β-lactam–resistant gram-positive microorganisms
- Treatment of gram-positive infections in patients with allergies to β-lactam antimicrobials
- Prophylaxis for surgical procedures involving implantation of prosthetic materials or devices at institutions with a high rate of infections due to MRSA or MRSE

Selected situations in which vancomycin use should be discouraged

- Routine surgical prophylaxis
- Empiric antimicrobial therapy for a febrile neutropenic patent
- Treatment in response to a single blood culture positive for a coagulase-negative staphylococci, if other blood cultures drawn in the same time frame are negative
- Eradication of MRSA colonization
- Primary treatment of antibiotic-associated colitis

MRSA, methicillin-resistant *Staphylococcus aureus;* MRSE, methicillin-resistant *Staphylococcus epidermidis.* Adapted from Tablan OC, Tenover FC, Martone WJ, et al: Recommendations for preventing the spread of vancomycin resistance: recommendations of the Hospital Infection Control Practices Advisory Committee (HICPAC). *MMWR* 1994;44:1.

administered in IV doses of 1.2 to 2.7 g/d in two to four divided doses. Doses up to 4.8 g/d can be given for life-threatening infections. Although its elimination occurs primarily through hepatic metabolism, patients with liver disease can usually be given standard doses.

Clindamycin has neuromuscular blocking properties and may enhance the action of other neuromuscular blocking agents. It has been associated with the development of severe pseudomembranous colitis, which is characterized by diarrhea, abdominal pain, fever, and mucous and blood in the stool.

V. Aminoglycosides. Aminoglycosides remain first-line therapy for gram-negative sepsis, despite the availability of new extended-spectrum antibiotics. Their mechanism of action is similar to that of clindamycin. They are primarily indicated for Enterobacteriaceae and pseudomonal infections. *P. aeruginosa* is more effectively managed with tobramycin, whereas *Serratia marcescens* tends to be more effectively treated with gentamicin. Streptomycin use is limited to the treatment of enterococcal and *Mycobacterium tuberculosis* infections.

A loading dose is usually not required because steady-state aminoglycoside concentrations are achieved after only one or two doses in most people. Appropriate dosing is directly linked to renal function. Several nomograms have been developed to incorporate some measure of renal function in determining aminoglycoside dosages, although most continue to promote 8-hour dosing. Most importantly, dosing should be based on age, serum creatinine clearance, and lean body weight (LBW) or dosing body weight (DBW) if a large discrepancy is found between LBW and actual body weight (DBW = LBW + 0.40 [ABW – LBW]). When renal function is stable, creatinine clearance (CrCl) and serum creatinine (SCr) are highly correlated and SCr can be used to estimate CrCl and thus glomerular filtration rate (GFR): CrCl (ml/min) = (140–age) × LBW/72 × SCr (multiply by 0.85 for women). Maintenance doses should be based on the site of infection and on suspected infecting organisms. A usual starting dose for gentamicin and tobramycin is 1.5 mg/kg and for amikacin it is 5 mg/kg. Trough and peak aminoglycoside concentration can be determined after the patient has received the drug for three to five half-lives.

Single daily dosing (SDD) of aminoglycosides has recently become popular to maximize their clinical effectiveness, reduce the incidence of aminoglycoside toxicity, and be cost-effective. A common SDD method uses a gentamicin dose of 7 mg/kg/d and the dosage interval is adjusted using 6- to 8-hour postinfusion serum concentration and fitting this data to a nomogram.

The most common adverse effects are ototoxicity and nephrotoxicity. The risk of ototoxicity is increased with prolonged therapy (> 10 days), concomitant use of other ototoxic agents, and elevated serum drug levels. All aminoglycosides except streptomycin can cause acute tubular necrosis and renal failure. Risk factors for nephrotoxicity include preexisting renal impairment, renal hypoperfusion, and high trough drug levels.

Selected Readings

Cunha BA. Vancomycin. *Med Clin North Am* 1995;79:817.
Comprehensive review of vancomycin, including indications for use, pharmacology, and dosing.

Eng RH, Munsif AN, Yangco BG, et al. Seizure propensity with imipenem. *Arch Intern Med* 1989;149:1881.
Case series and discussion of seizures associated with imipenem.

Freeman CS, Nicolau DP, Belliveau PP, et al. Once-daily aminoglycosides: review and recommendations for clinical practice. *J Antimicrob Chemother* 1997;39:677.
Review of in vitro, animal, and clinical studies using higher dose, extended interval (once-daily) aminoglycoside regimens in selected clinical situations.

Lesar TS, Rotschafer JC, Strand LM, et al. Gentamicin dosing errors with four commonly used nomograms. *JAMA* 1982;248:1190.
A description of various predictive dosage methods for calculating gentamicin dose.

Norrby SR. Carbapenems. *Med Clin North Am* 1995;79:745.
A comprehensive review of carbapenems, including pharmacology, dosing, and adverse effects.

Soper DE. Clindamycin. *Obstet Gynecol Clin North Am* 1992;19:483.
A review of clindamycin, including pharmacology, dosing, and indications for use.

112. BETA-BLOCKER POISONING

Jeffrey R. Tucker

I. General principles. Beta-blockers were originally developed for the treatment of angina pectoris and dysrhythmias, but indications have been expanded to include a wide variety of disorders. Toxicity can result from oral, parenteral, and even ophthalmic exposure.

II. Pathogenesis. Beta-blockers act by competitively inhibiting the binding of epinephrine and norepinephrine to G-protein–coupled β-adrenergic neuroreceptors in the heart (β_1 receptors), blood vessels, bronchioles (β_2 receptors), and other organs. Binding to the beta receptors activates phosphodiesterase and increases cyclic adenosine monophosphate.

Usually, beta-blockers are rapidly absorbed after oral ingestion. Sustained-release formulations, however, may be slowly absorbed, especially after overdose. Toxicity can develop as early as 20 minutes after an overdose of an immediate-release preparation with peak effects at 1 to 2 hours. Delayed toxicity can occur with sustained-release preparations and can last for several days.

The beta-blocker dose required to produce toxicity is highly variable and depends on the sympathetic tone and metabolic capacity of the patient and the pharmacologic and pharmacokinetic properties of the specific beta-blocker. The half-life can be greatly prolonged in patients with depressed cardiac output, resulting in decreased hepatic and renal perfusion. Intrinsic heart, kidney, and liver disease as well as the concomitant use of drugs with similar activity increases the risk of toxicity.

Patients poisoned with beta-blockers possessing partial agonist activity (Table 112-1) can present with a normal heart rate or even tachycardia. Although cardioselectivity tends to be lost at high doses, the membrane-stabilizing effect, which is minimally significant at the therapeutic doses, assumes a more important role with central nervous system (CNS) toxicity and myocardial depression.

III. Clinical toxicity. Beta-blocker toxicity primarily affects the cardiovascular system and the CNS. Disturbances of cardiac rhythm and cardiac conduction can occur. Patient with severe toxicity will present with hypotension and bradycardia. Electrocardiogram (ECG) manifestations can include prolonged PR interval, intraventricular conduction delay, progressive atrioventricular block, nonspecific T-waves changes, early repolarization, and asystole. Sotalol can cause ventricular tachycardia, including torsades de pointes, ventricular fibrillation, and multifocal ventricular extrasystoles.

Central nervous system effects include lethargy, coma, and seizures. Beta-blockers with high lipid solubility (propranolol, penbutolol, metoprolol) appear more likely to cause CNS effects than those with a low lipid solubility. Bronchospasm, a relatively rare consequence of beta-blocker poisoning, usually occurs in patients with preexisting reactive airway disease. Hypoglycemia is an infrequent complication of beta-blocker toxicity. It appears to be more common in diabetics, children, and uremic patients and is caused by the blockade of hyperglycemic effects of catecholamines. CNS toxicity has been reported in the absence of significant cardiovascular toxicity or hypoglycemia.

IV. Evaluation. Beta-blocker poisoning should be suspected in patients who suddenly develop bradycardia, hypotension, or seizures, particularly when bradycardia is resistant to usual doses of chronotropic drugs. Evaluation should begin with a complete set of vital signs, continuous cardiac monitoring, and a 12-lead ECG. Physical examination should focus on the cardiovascular, pulmonary, and neurologic systems. Vital signs and physical examination should be repeated frequently. Laboratory evaluation of symptomatic patients should include complete blood count, electrolytes, blood urea nitrogen, creatinine clearance, and glucose level. Arterial blood gases and a chest radiograph should also be assessed in patients with abnormal vital signs or altered level of consciousness.

TABLE 112-1. Pharmacologic and pharmacokinetic properties of β-adrenergic blocking agents

	Adrenergic receptor blocking activity	Intrinsic sympathomimetic activity	Lipid solubility	Extent of absorption (%)	Absolute oral bioavailability (%)	Half-life (h)	Protein binding (%)	Clearance (ml/min)	Metabolism/excretion
Acebutolol	β_1[a]	+	Low	90	20–60	3–4	26	615	Hepatic, renal excretion 30%–40%, nonrenal 50%–60%
Betaxolol	β_1[a]	0	Low	≅100	89	14–22	≈50	NA	Hepatic; >80% recovered in urine
Bisoprolol	β_1[a]	0	Low	≥90	80	9–12	≈30	NA	≈50% excreted unchanged in urine, remainder as inactive metabolites
Esmolol	β_1[a]	0	Moderate	NA	NA	0.15	55	170 ml/min/kg	Rapid metabolism by esterases in cytosol of red blood cells
Metoprolol, long-acting	β_1[a]	0	Moderate	95	40–50	3–7	12	1,100	Hepatic, renal excretion <5% unchanged
Carteolol	β_1, β_2	++	Low	80	85	6	23–30	NA	50%–70% unchanged in urine
Nadolol	β_1, β_2	0	Low	30	30–50	20–24	30	200	Urine unchanged

Continued.

Penbutolol	β_1, β_2	+	High	≈100	≈100	5	80–98	NA	Hepatic (conjugation and oxidation); renal excretion of metabolites
Pindolol	β_1, β_2	+++	Moderate	95	≈100	3–4	40	400	Urinary excretion of metabolites (60%–74%) and unchanged drug (35%–40%)
Propranolol, long-acting	β_1, β_2	0	High	90	30	3–5	90	1,000	Hepatic; <1% excreted unchanged in urine
Sotalol	β_1, β_2	0	Low	No data	90–100	12	0	150	Not metabolized; excreted unchanged in urine
Timolol	β_1, β_2	0	Low to moderate	90	75	4	10	660	Hepatic; urinary excretion of metabolites and unchanged drug
Carvedilol	$\beta_1, \beta_2, \alpha_1$	0	High	NA	25–35	6–10	95–98	NA	Hepatic (aromatic ring oxidation and conjugation), 16% renal excretion
Labetolol	β_1, α_1	0	Moderate	100	30–40	5–5.8	50	2,700	55%–60% excreted in urine as conjugates or unchanged drug

[a] Inhibits β_2 receptors (bronchial and vascular) at higher doses.
[b] In elderly hypertensive patients with normal renal function, $t_{1/2}$ is variable (7–15 h).
NA, not applicable (available intravenously only); 0, none; +, low; ++, moderate; +++, high.

V. Management. Advanced life support measures should be instituted as necessary. An intravenous (IV) line should be established in all patients. Those with altered mental status should have a bedside glucose determination or empiric administration of dextrose. The administration of naloxone and thiamine should also be considered. Hypotension should initially be treated with IV fluids. Seizures should be treated with benzodiazepines and barbiturates. Invasive cardiovascular monitoring should be considered in patients with hemodynamic instability.

Activated charcoal and gastric lavage are the preferred methods for gastric decontamination. Syrup of ipecac use is contraindicated because of the potential rapid onset of hemodynamic compromise or seizure and obtundation after a beta-blocker overdose. Atropine has been recommended before lavage to block vagal tone and potential cardiovascular depressant effects. Whole-bowel lavage can be used for gut decontamination in sustained-release preparations.

Many drugs have been used to treat hypotension and bradycardia from beta-blocker toxicity. Glucagon is the most consistently effective agent. An initial IV bolus of 3 to 10 mg for adults (children 0.05 mg/kg) is followed by an continuous infusion of 1 to 10 mg/h (children 0.07 mg/kg/h). The dose is titrated to the patient's response and a large dose may be necessary. Glucagon appears to act by stimulating the adenyl cyclase enzyme system through a nonadrenergic receptor. Glucagon should be reconstituted in a solution of 5% dextrose in water or preservative-free saline rather than the phenol diluent provided by the manufacturer because of concerns about phenol toxicity in large doses.

Other agents used in the treatment of bradycardia, hypotension, and heart block include atropine, isoproterenol, epinephrine, norepinephrine, dopamine, dobutamine, and calcium (Chapter 113). The efficacy of these agents has been variable and inconsistent, frequently requiring very high doses to raise blood pressure and heart rate. The simultaneous use of multiple agents can be effective when a single agent fails. Ventricular tachydysrhythmias induced by sotalol have been treated with lidocaine, isoproterenol, magnesium, and cardioversion-defibrillation.

Electrical cardiac pacing may be needed if bradycardia, hypotension, and heart block fail to respond to pharmacologic therapy, or if ventricular tachydysrhythmias associated with a prolonged QT interval are difficult to control. In severe overdoses, the pacemaker may not capture and if capture occurs, the increased heart rate may not increase blood pressure. In such cases, intraaortic balloon pump counterpulsation and extracorporeal circulatory bypass pumps have been successfully used for cardiovascular support.

Selected Readings

Adlerfliegel F, Leeman M, Demaeyer P, et al. Sotalol poisoning associated with asystole. *Intensive Care Med* 1993;19:57.

A case report and discussion of sotalol overdose with prolonged QT interval and asystole.

Buiumsohn A, Eisenberg ES, Jacob H, et al. Seizures and intraventricular conduction defect in propranolol poisoning. *Ann Intern Med* 1979;91:860.

A case report and discussion of the lipid solubility of propranolol, which allows it to cross the blood-brain barrier and can cause seizures along with cardiovascular toxicity.

Frishman W. Clinical pharmacology of the new beta-adrenergic blocking drugs. 1. Pharmacodynamic and pharmacokinetic properties. *Am Heart J* 1979;98:663.

A discussion of the important pharmacodynamic properties of the beta-blockers: beta-blocking potency, cardioselectivity, partial agonist activity, membrane-stabilizing activity, and intrinsic sympathomimetic activity.

Frishman W, Jacob H, Eisenberg E, et al. Clinical pharmacology of the new beta-adrenergic blocking drugs. Part 8. Self-poisoning with β-adrenoceptor blocking agents: recognition and management. *Am Heart J* 1979;98:798.

A review of the clinical knowledge regarding management and diagnosis of beta-blocker toxicity (circa 1979).

Frishman WH. Beta-adrenergic blockers. *Med Clin North Am* 1988;72:37.

An extensive review of the pharmacology, indications, and adverse effects of beta-blockers.

Gwinup GR. Propranolol toxicity presenting with early repolarization, ST changes and peaked T waves on EKG. *Ann Emerg Med* 1998;17:171.

A case report of an atypical presentation of propranolol toxicity with ST elevation, early repolarization, and peaked T waves as opposed to the most common presentation of bradycardia and hypotension.

Hohnloser SH, Woosley Rl. Sotalol. *N Engl J Med* 1994;331:31.

A review article on sotalol, a β-adrenergic blocker, with a unique property of prolongation of the QT interval (class III antiarrhythmic).

Laake K, Kittang E, Refstad SO, et al. Convulsions and possible spasms of the lower oesophageal sphincter in a fatal case of propranolol intoxication. *Acta Med Scand* 1981;210:137.

A case report and brief discussion of noncardiac effects of propranolol such as seizures and esophageal spasm.

Taboulet P, Cariou A, Berdeaux A, et al. Pathophysiology and management of self-poisoning with beta-blockers. *J Toxicol Clin Toxicol* 1993;31:531.

A review article containing an excellent overview of the pharmacologic management of beta-blocker toxicity.

Weinstein RS. Recognition and management of poisoning with beta-adrenergic blocking agents. *Ann Emerg Med* 1984;12;1123.

An overview of beta blocker toxicity with a focus on effective management and electrocardiographic changes.

113. CHANNEL BLOCKER POISONING

Richard Y. Wang

I. General principles. The three most common calcium channel blockers (CCB) are diltiazem, nifedipine, and verapamil. They are used to treat a variety of conditions, including angina, hypertension, dysrhythmias, congestive heart failure, Raynaud's syndrome, and migraine headaches. All three agents decrease coronary vascular resistance, increase coronary blood flow, and decrease myocardial oxygen demand. Diltiazem and verapamil can slow atrioventricular nodal conduction and decrease contractility. Nifedipine does not appear to affect myocardial conduction and contractility at therapeutic doses. Amlodipine, felodipine, israpidine, nicardipine, nimodipine, nisoldipine) are dihydropyridine derivatives similar to nifedpine. Effects of bepridil and mibefradil are also similar to nifedpine.

II. Pharmacology. Calcium channel blockers prevent extracellular calcium from entering into cardiac and smooth muscle through L-type, calcium-specific membrane channels. Mibefradil also blocks T-type calcium channels; bepridil also has sodium-channel blocking activity. Because calcium influx is necessary for muscle contraction, CCBs cause vasodilation and decreased cardiac contractility. Verapamil and diltiazem also decrease sinus node discharge and conduction through the atrioventricular node.

Immediate-release preparations are well absorbed and have an onset of action within 30 minutes of ingestion. Sustained-release preparations, available for diltiazem, nifedipine, and verapamil, have delayed onset and prolonged duration of toxicity in the overdose setting. The smallest doses resulting in toxicity in adults are 720 mg for verapamil, 420 mg for diltiazem, and 50 mg for nifedipine.

III. Clinical manifestations. Cardiovascular toxicity is the primary manifestation of CCB poisoning. Hypotension, bradycardia, atrioventricular block, and asystole have all been reported after overdoses of verapamil and diltiazem. A compensatory tachycardia is not associated with the hypotension caused by these agents because of their primary negative inotropic and chronotropic effect. Verapamil and diltiazem can also cause high-grade atrioventricular blockade or sinus arrest accompanied by a junctional escape rhythm.

Nifedipine overdose typically results in hypotension and tachycardia. Cardiac conduction disorders are seen less commonly. Bepridil overdose can cause a prolonged QT interval and torsades de pointes.

Noncardiac manifestations of CCB toxicity include nausea, vomiting, lethargy, confusion, hyperglycemia, metabolic acidosis, noncardiogenic pulmonary edema, ileus, and mesenteric ischemia. Seizures can occur after verapamil overdose.

Chronic toxicity occurs primarily in the elderly. Hypotension and sinus arrest have been reported. Underlying liver disease and the combined use of other cardiac medications can exacerbate CCB toxicity.

IV. Differential diagnosis. Hypotension, conduction disorders and altered mental status can also be seen in myocardial disease, cerebrovascular accident, anaphylaxis, hypovolemic shock, renal failure-induced hyperkalemia, and poisoning by other agents. Cardiac glycoside toxicity presents with more pronounced gastrointestinal symptoms and hyperkalemia. Delayed cardiac conduction, hypotension, mental status changes, vomiting, and hypoglycemia are seen with β-adrenoreceptor blocker toxicity. Antiarrhythmic, clonidine, quinine, chloroquine, organophosphate, tricyclic antidepressant, opioid, and sedative-hypnotic poisoning should also be considered.

V. Management. Asymptomatic patients presenting after an acute overdose of a non–sustained-release preparation require 4 to 6 hours of observation before medical clearance. Those with a sustained-release preparation overdose require 12 to 24 hours of observation. All patients with hypotension, bradycardia, or atrioventricular block from CCBs require admission to an intensive care setting.

Gastrointestinal decontamination should be performed as soon as possible. Activated charcoal is most useful if given early, but can be effective as late as 4 hours after ingestion of sustained-release preparations. Multiple dose-activated charcoal and whole bowel irrigation is reserved for sustained-release overdoses. Gastric lavage should be reserved for patients who present early after a life-threatening ingestion; many sustained-release preparations will not fit through an orogastric lavage tube.

Symptomatic hypotension should be treated initially with intravenous (IV) crystalloid fluid challenge. When hypotension is caused by bradycardia or atrioventricular blockade, atropine and electrical pacing should also considered; however, they are often ineffective. Other modalities for the treatment of hypotension and shock from CCB overdose include calcium, glucagon, vasopressors, amrinone, and insulin. The initial dose of calcium in adults is 10 ml of 10% calcium chloride or 30 ml of 10% calcium gluconate. This should be infused no faster than 1 to 2 ml/min. Calcium chloride provides three times as much calcium ion as calcium gluconate but it is more tissue toxic if extravasation occurs. The serum calcium concentration should be monitored when repeated doses of calcium therapy are administered. Direct-acting vasopressors (e.g., norepinephrine, epinephrine) should be used to treat hypotension when calcium salts are ineffective.

Calcium salts, atropine, and isoproterenol can be used initially to treat symptomatic bradycardia. Glucagon can reverse myocardial depression as well as bradycardia. The IV loading dose of glucagon is 2 to 10 mg; this is followed by a maintenance infusion with the dose per hour equal to the minimally effective loading dose. Glucagon treatment may be limited by its availability and induction of emesis. Amrinone can be used if the aforementioned therapy is not successful in maintaining an adequate inotropic response. A loading dose of 1 mg/kg of amrinone is followed by a maintenance infusion of 3 to 6 mg/kg/min.

A new treatment being evaluated for patients with refractory hypotension from CCB toxicity is high-dose insulin infusion. In experimental models, this treatment was more effective in increasing myocardial contractility than calcium chloride, epinephrine, or glucagon. The protocol used in patients with CCB toxicity is as follows: insulin (1 to 2 IU/kg) and glucose (25 g) boluses followed by infusions of insulin (0.2 to 1.0 IU/kg/h), glucose (20% dextrose in water to maintain euglycemia), and potassium (adjusted to maintain a normokalemic state) infusions.

Intraaortic balloon pump or cardiac bypass pump support should be considered for patients with refractory hypotension from CCB toxicity. Most patients recover fully if vital signs can be supported while the drug is endogenously metabolized and eliminated.

Selected Readings

Alousi AA, Canter JM, Fort DJ. The beneficial effect of amrinone on acute drug-induced heart failure in the anesthetized dog. *Cardiovasc Res* 1985;19:483.

This study demonstrated that amrinone improved myocardial contractility during calcium channel blocker toxicity.

Bower JO, Mengle HAK. The additive effects of calcium and digitalis: a warning with a report of two deaths. *JAMA* 1936;106:1151.

These cases demonstrated the concern for administering calcium in the setting of cardiac glycoside toxicity.

Frierson J, Bailly D, Shultz T, et al. Refractory cardiogenic shock and complete heart block after unsuspected verapamil-SR and atenolol overdose. *Clin Cardiol* 1991; 14:933.

This case report showed the successful use of intraaortic balloon counterpulsation to improve cardiac output and blood pressure in the setting of a mixed calcium channel and β-adrenoreceptor blocker overdose.

Gay R, Angeo S, Lee R, et al. Treatment of verapamil toxicity in intact dogs. *J Clin Invest* 1986;77:1805.

This study verified that increased serum calcium concentration improved inotropy and blood pressure in calcium channel blocker toxicity.

Kline JA, Leonva E, Raymond RM. Beneficial myocardial metabolic effects of insulin during verapamil toxicity in the anesthetized canine. *Crit Care Med* 1995;23:1251.
This study reported on high-dose insulin, showing improved survival when compared with calcium, epinephrine, or glucagon.

Ramoska EA, Spiller HA, Myers A. Calcium channel blocker toxicity. *Ann Emerg Med* 1990;19:196.
The limited efficacy of atropine alone in the treatment of bradycardia from calcium channel blocker toxicity was described in this article.

Ramoska EA, Spiller HA, Winter M, et al. A one-year evaluation of calcium channel blocker overdoses: toxicity and treatment. *Ann Emerg Med* 1993;22:196.
This analysis reported the various cardiac manifestations and treatments in patients with calcium channel blocker toxicity.

Roberts D, Honcharik N, Sitar DS, et al. Diltiazem overdose: pharmacokinetics of diltiazem and its metabolites and effect of multiple dose charcoal therapy. *J Toxicol Clin Toxicol* 1991;29:45.
This case report indicated that the beneficial effect of multiple dose-activated charcoal therapy is not from enhancing serum drug clearance, but to limiting further drug absorption from the gut.

Schoffstall JM, Spivey WH, Gambone JM, et al. Effects of calcium channel blocker overdose-induced toxicity in the conscious dog. *Ann Emerg Med* 1991;20:1104.
This study demonstrated the disparate hemodynamic effects of the calcium channel blocking agents in toxicity.

Tenebein M. Position statement: whole bowel irrigation. American Academy of Clinical Toxicology, European Association of Poisons Centers and Clinical Toxicologists. *J Toxicol Clin Toxicol* 1977;35:753.
This review discussed the role of whole bowel irrigation therapy in patients with overdoses of sustained-release formulations.

Tom PA, Morrow CT, Kelen GD. Delayed hypotension after overdose of sustained release verapamil. *J Emerg Med* 1994;12:621.
A case report demonstrating the marked delayed onset of effect that can occur from the ingestion of sustained-release formulations of calcium channel blocking agents.

Walter FG, Frye G, Mullen JT, et al. Amelioration of nifedipine poisoning associated with glucagon therapy. *Ann Emerg Med* 1993;22:1234.
This case report provided information on the effectiveness of glucagon in reversing nifedipine-induced hypotension.

Wolfe LR, Spadafora MP, Otten EJ. Use of amrinone and glucagon in a case of calcium channel blocker overdose. *Ann Emerg Med* 1993;22:1225.
Amrinone was demonstrated to be successful in the management of calcium channel blocker poisoning in this case report.

Zaritsky AL, Horowitz M, Chernow B. Glucagon antagonism of calcium channel blocker-induced myocardial dysfunction. *Crit Care Med* 1988;16:246.
This study demonstrated glucagon to improve calcium channel blocker-induced myocardial depression.

114. CHOLINERGIC AGENTS

Erica L. Liebelt

I. General principles. Cholinergic poisoning can result from exposure to drugs that directly stimulate cholinergic (muscarinic) receptors (e.g., bethanechol, pilocarpine, and urecholine) and to agents that inhibit acetylcholinesterase (e.g., organophosphate and carbamate insecticides), and carbamate drugs (edrophonium, neostigmine, physostigmine, pyridostigmine, and tacrine). Nerve agents such as GA (Tabun), GB (Sarin), GD (Soman), GF, and VX are similar in structure and function to the organophosphorus insecticides and cause similar toxicity.

II. Pharmacology and pathophysiology. The neurotransmitter, acetylcholine, and its receptors are found in the central nervous system (CNS), muscarinic sites in the parasympathetic nervous system, and nicotinic sites in the sympathetic and parasympathetic ganglia and at the neuromuscular junction. Effects of organophosphates and carbamates are predominantly caused by accumulation of acetylcholine at synapses, resulting in sustained depolarization. Organophosphates can irreversibly inhibit acetylcholinesterase and cause toxicity lasting for days to months, until adequate amounts of the enzyme regenerate. Carbamates reversibly inhibit this enzyme and have a shorter duration of action; symptoms persisting more than 12 to 24 hours suggest continued absorption (inadequate decontamination).

III. Clinical presentation. Effects usually begin minutes to hours after dermal, pulmonary, or oral exposure. Onset can be delayed with lipophilic organophosphates (fenthion and chlorfenthion) and those requiring hepatic metabolism to increase their toxicity (parathion). Signs and symptoms of acetylcholinesterase inhibition can be divided into muscarinic, nicotinic, and CNS effects (Table 114-1); they are described by the mnemonics DUMBELS (diarrhea, urination, miosis, bronchospasm, emesis, lacrimation, salivation) and SLUDGE (salivation, lacrimation, urination, defecation, emesis). Death usually results from respiratory failure, which is caused by respiratory muscle weakness, CNS depression, bronchospasm, and bronchorrhea.

Two additional types of organophosphate toxicity have been described. An intermediate syndrome can occur 24 to 96 hours after the initial cholinergic crisis; it lasts 4 to 18 days. This syndrome is characterized by paralysis of proximal limb muscles, neck flexor muscles, motor cranial nerves, and respiratory muscles without prominent muscarinic findings. Organophosphorus ester-induced delayed neurotoxicity (OPIDN) is a peripheral neuropathy that develops 1 to 3 weeks after acute exposure and can continue to worsen for several months. It appears to be mediated by a specific "neurotoxic esterase" in peripheral neurons.

IV. Laboratory evaluation. Studies that should be obtained in severe poisonings include electrocardiogram, arterial blood gases, chest x-ray, electrolytes, glucose, amylase, creatine kinase, and renal and liver function tests. Acute organophosphate poisoning can be classified based on the degree of depression of red blood cell (RBC) cholinesterase activity, a surrogate marker for acetylcholinesterase activity: mild (20% to 50% of baseline), moderate (10% to 20% of baseline), and severe (< 10% of baseline). The diagnosis is usually confirmed retrospectively because most facilities cannot measure cholinesterase enzyme activity on an immediate basis. Because of wide interindividual variability, significant depression of RBC cholinesterase activity can occur but still fall within the "normal" range. Plasma cholinesterase activity is a sensitive but less specific indicator of exposure; it can be depressed in some medical conditions and with chronic exposure, or it can be genetically deficient. No specific tests for OPIDN are available other than electromyography and nerve conduction studies coupled with the history of exposure.

V. Management. Symptomatic patients should be admitted to an intensive care unit. Aggressive dermal and gastrointestinal decontamination and supportive care with attention to adequate ventilation, prevention of aspiration, and control of respiratory secretions is essential.

TABLE 114-1. Signs and symptoms of cholinesterase poisoning

Muscarinic
Salivation
Lacrimation
Bronchorrea/bronchoconstriction
Urination
Vomiting/diarrhea
Bradycardia
Miosis
Nicotinic
Muscle fasciculations
Muscle weakness
Muscle paralysis
Tachycardia
Hypertension
Central nervous system
Excitability
Confusion
Agitation
Lethargy
Coma
Seizures
Death

VI. Antidotal therapy. Atropine is the primary treatment for serious cholinergic poisonings. It is the only treatment necessary for receptor agonist poisoning. Adult doses should begin with an intravenous (IV) dose of 1 to 2 mg in mild to moderate cases and 2 to 5 mg in severe cases. Pediatric dosing starts at 0.02 to 0.05 mg/kg. Atropine should be administered every 10 to 30 minutes until excessive muscarinic signs subside. Pupils dilate early and should not be used to assess the response to atropine. In organophosphate poisoning, cumulative daily doses in the range of 100 mg are commonly required; a continuous drip may be easier to administer and titrate. In general, more atropine is required during the first 24 hours, with doses decreasing dramatically as pralidoxime takes effect.

Pralidoxime (2-PAM; Protopam) specifically reactivates acetylcholinesterase by reversing phosphorylation of the active site on this enzyme. It will regenerate acetylcholinesterase at muscarinic, nicotinic, and CNS sites, whereas atropine only acts at muscarinic sites. It is indicated only for moderate or severe organophosphate poisoning. The initial adult dose is 1 g IV over 30 minutes and then repeated in 30 minutes if little or no response is seen. The initial pediatric dose is 25 to 50 mg/kg IV (maximum 1 g). Repeated boluses of 0.5 to 1.0 g IV can be administered every 6 to 8 hours if symptoms persist or recur. Alternatively, it can be given by continuous infusion (500 mg/h of a 2.5% solution).

Diazepam should also be used for the treatment of seizures. Because seizures are particularly common after exposure to nerve agents, high-dose benzodiazepines (diazepam 0.2–0.4 mg/kg) should be administered at the first sign of CNS toxicity in this setting.

Selected Readings

Coye MJ, Barnett PG, Midtling JE, et al. Clinical confirmation of organophosphate poisoning by serial cholinesterase analyses. *Arch Intern Med* 1987;147:438.

A case series describing agricultural workers with organophosphate pesticide exposure that supports the use of sequential postexposure plasma cholinesterase analyses to confirm the diagnosis of organophosphate poisoning in the absence of baseline values.

deKort WL, Kiestra SH, Sangster B. The use of atropine and oximes in organophosphate intoxications: a modified approach. *J Toxicol Clin Toxicol* 1988;26:199.
This article contains a discussion of the prolonged use of oxime therapy and the limited use of atropine therapy in organophosphate poisoning.

Johnson MK. Organophosphates and delayed neuropathy—is NTE alive and well? *Toxicol Appl Pharmacol* 1990;102:385.
A review of the effects of organophosphates on neuropathy target esterase (NTE) and its relationship to polyneuropathy.

Kiss Z, Fazekas T. Arrhythmias in organophosphate poisonings. *Acta Cardiol* 1979; 5:323.
A review of arrhythmias associated with organophosphate poisoning, noting QT prolongation, ST and T-wave changes, and ventricular arrhythmias.

Lifshitz M, Rotenberg M, Sofer S, et al. Carbamate poisoning and oxime treatment in children: a clinical and laboratory study. *Pediatrics* 1994;93:652.
A retrospective series of children with carbamate poisoning demonstrates that oxime therapy will not exacerbate cholinergic symptoms.

Lotti M. Treatment of acute organophosphate poisoning. *Med J Aust* 1991;154:51.
This article reviews the methods of diagnosis and treatment of organophosphate and carbamate poisoning.

Lotti M, Becker CE, Aminoff MJ. Organophosphate polyneuropathy: pathogenesis and prevention. *Neurology* 1984;34:658.
This review describes the pathogenesis and clinical presentation of delayed organophosphate-induced polyneuropathy.

Medicis JJ, Stork CM, Howland MA, et al. Pharmacokinetics following a loading plus a continuous infusion of pralidoxime compared with the traditional short infusion regimen in human volunteers. *J Toxicol Clin Toxicol* 1997;35:227.
This study showed that a loading dose followed by continuous infusion of pralidoxime maintains therapeutic concentrations longer than the traditional bolus infusion in healthy volunteers.

Senanayake N, Karalliedde L. Neurotoxic effects of organophosphorus insecticides: an intermediate syndrome. *N Engl J Med* 1987;316:761.
This report describes a characteristic constellation of delayed neurotoxic effects in patients with particular organophosphate poisoning denoted as the intermediate syndrome.

Sidell FR, Borak J. Chemical warfare agents. II. Nerve agents. *Ann Emerg Med* 1992;21:865.
This review summarizes the clinical effects of nerve agent exposure and describes the management and treatment strategies for emergency medical personnel.

Taluri J, Roberts J. Organophosphate poisoning. *Ann Emerg Med* 1987;16:193.
This article reviews the physiology, models of poisoning, clinical presentation, laboratory findings, diagnosis, and treatment of organophosphate exposure.

115. COCAINE POISONING

Jeffrey R. Tucker

I. General principles. Illicit forms of cocaine include the hydrochloride salt and its alkalinization products, freebase and crack. Cocaine hydrochloride is water-soluble, readily absorbed from any mucosal surface, and can be administered intravenously (IV). Freebase and crack are insoluble in water but can be smoked. In the case of "body packers" (people who attempt to smuggle cocaine by ingesting wrapped packet of cocaine) and "body stuffers" (those who swallow or conceal loosely wrapped cocaine in body cavities when encountered by law enforcement agents), massive overdose can occur from rupture or leakage of the packets.

II. Pathogenesis. Cocaine promotes the release of neurotransmitters (e.g., dopamine and norepinephrine) while also blocking their reuptake in the central and sympathetic nervous system. Cocaine is also a local anesthetic that blocks initiation and conduction of nerve impulse by decreasing axonal membrane permeability to sodium ions; at high doses, this class 1 antiarrhythmic effect contributes to cardiotoxicity. Cocaine is rapidly metabolized by liver esterases and plasma cholinesterase and by nonenzymatic hydrolysis. Only small amounts are eliminated as unchanged drug in urine. Patients with pseudocholinesterase deficiency can be at greater risk of toxicity because of their reduced capacity for metabolism through the pseudocholinesterase pathway. After IV injection or inhalation, a subjective euphoric response occurs in 3 to 5 minutes, with a cardiovascular response peaking in 8 to 12 minutes and lasting approximately 30 minutes. After nasal insufflation (snorting), a euphoric effect occurs within 15 to 20 minutes after exposure; cardiovascular changes and plasma levels peak within 20 to 60 minutes; and effects last several hours. Time to onset, time to peak effect, and duration of effect are somewhat longer following ingestion. Effects can be markedly delayed and prolonged following packet ingestion.

III. Clinical presentation. Toxicity has been demonstrated in all organ systems. Signs and symptoms of acute poisoning include elevated pulse, blood pressure, respirations, and temperature, the magnitude of which is roughly proportional to the degree of toxicity. Patients with mild poisoning can have normal or nearly normal vital signs. Other manifestations include anxiety, agitation, euphoria, headache, tremors, twitching, nausea, vomiting, diaphoresis, mydriasis, and pallor.

Patients with moderate poisoning can manifest mild to moderately increased vital signs, confusion, hallucinations, hyperactivity, clonus, increased muscle tone, abdominal cramps, and brief tonic-clonic seizures. Tea-colored urine should alert the physician to the possibility of rhabdomyolysis and potential renal failure.

Patients with severe poisoning have markedly abnormal vital signs with malignant hyperthermia, tachydysrhythmias, and status epilepticus or coma with flaccid paralysis. Other manifestations include apnea, cyanosis, and Cheyne-Stokes respirations. Laboratory abnormalities include leukocytosis, hypokalemia, and hyperglycemia. Finding cocaine and metabolites in the urine supports the diagnosis.

Cardiovascular collapse, bradycardia, and hypotension are preterminal events.

Complications can be acute or occur hours to days after actual cocaine use. Cerebrovascular complications include cerebrovascular accidents, subarachnoid or intracerebral hemorrhage, and cerebral vasculitis. Cardiovascular complications include myocardial, bowel, and kidney ischemia; infarction; skin necrosis; and aortic dissection. Cerebral and renal vasculitis and cardiomyopathy have been reported. Pulmonary infarcts, barotrauma; eosinophilia with granuloma formation, and noncardiogenic pulmonary edema can occur. Inhalational exposure can result in cough, hemoptysis, reactive airway disease, pneumonitis ("crack lung"), and barotrauma (e.g., pneumothorax, pneumomediastinum).

Chronic nasal use can result in rhinitis, epistaxis, and septal perforation. Systemic manifestations of chronic use include anorexia, weight loss, insomnia, formication, impotence, depression, paranoia, and psychosis.

IV. Evaluation. Evaluation should focus on the cardiac, pulmonary, and neurologic systems. Continuous electrocardiographic monitoring and frequent monitoring of vital signs, including core body temperature, are essential. Patients with moderate to severe toxicity should have the following: an electrocardiogram and chest x-ray study; analysis of complete blood count, electrolytes, glucose, blood urea nitrogen, creatinine, arterial blood gas, urinalysis, creatine, and phosphokinase; and qualitative toxicologic analysis of blood and urine. Urine screening can detect cocaine metabolites for as long as 3 days after exposure.

Standard protocols for ruling out myocardial infarction and ischemia should be followed in patients with chest pain of potential cardiac origin. Patients with a persistent or severe headache, abnormal neurologic examination, or prolonged seizures require computed tomography scan and lumbar puncture to rule out subarachnoid hemorrhage. Occult infections (e.g., endocarditis, hepatitis, pneumonia, epidural abscess) should be excluded in those with hyperthermia, particularly injection drug users.

V. Treatment. Advanced life support measures should be instituted as necessary. Supplemental oxygen, dextrose (25 g IV), and thiamine (100 mg IV) should be administered to patients with altered mental status, seizures, or coma. Agitation, anxiety, and seizures can be treated with a benzodiazepine, such as midazolam (2–5 mg IV), diazepam (2–10 mg IV), or lorazepam (1–4 mg IV). Status epilepticus must be treated aggressively with IV benzodiazepines; early paralysis and short-acting barbiturates (amobarbital, thiopental, pentobarbital) should employed in refractory cases. Vecuronium (0.08–0.1 mg/kg) or pancuronium (0.06–0.1 mg/kg) are the preferred paralytic agents. Paralysis, along with aggressive cooling measures, is also indicated in patients with severe hyperthermia.

Moderate hypertension and tachycardia usually respond to benzodiazepine sedation. Severe hypertension is best treated with titratable IV agents, such as phentolamine (1–2 mg per dose), nitroglycerin, and nitroprusside. Dysrhythmias should be treated according to standard advanced cardiac life support (ACLS) protocols. Treatment of ventricular dysrhythmias should also include sodium bicarbonate. Labetalol, esmolol, and propranolol can worsen coronary artery vasoconstriction and should not be given to patients with concomitant chest pain. Myocardial ischemia should otherwise be treated as usual. Adjunctive therapy with benzodiazepines is recommended. Phentolamine can be effective in reducing myocardial oxygen demand and improving coronary blood flow. Hypotension requires active fluid resuscitation. If vasopressor therapy is indicated, a direct-acting drug (e.g., norepinephrine) is preferred because cocaine depletes neurotransmitters and prevents their reuptake. Other complications are treated in standard fashion.

Activated charcoal (1 g/kg orally) should be given to all those who ingest cocaine. Asymptomatic body packers or stuffers should be treated with multiple-dose charcoal plus laxatives or whole-bowel irrigation. Close observation with IV access and continuous ECG monitoring is necessary. Endoscopic removal of intact packets must be performed with caution because packet rupture can occur. If signs or symptoms of cocaine toxicity are present or if intestinal obstruction occurs, immediate surgical intervention is indicated.

Selected Readings

Gay GR, Inaba DS, Sheppard CW, et al. Cocaine history, epidemiology, human pharmacology and treatment. A perspective on a new debut for an old girl. *J Toxicol Clin Toxicol* 1975;8:149.

Excellent discussion about historical usage of cocaine.

Hollander JE. The management of cocaine-associated myocardial ischemia. *N Engl J Med* 1995;333:1267.

An excellent review article on the management of cocaine-associated chest pain.

Hollander JE, Hoffman US. Cocaine induced myocardial infarction: an analysis and review of the literature. *J Emerg Med* 1992;10:169.

Identification of a group of young individuals at risk for myocardial infarction.

Isner JM, Estes M, Thompson PD, et al. Acute cardiac events temporally related to cocaine abuse. *N Engl J Med* 1986;315:1438.

A report of seven patients with cardiac toxicity associated with nonintravenous use of cocaine.

Lange HA, Cigarroa RG, Flores ED, et al. Potentiation of cocaine-induced coronary vasoconstriction by beta-adrenergic blockade. *Ann Intern Med* 1990;112:897.

Randomized, double-blind, placebo trial in cardiac catherization laboratory showing effects of β-adrenergic blockade.

McCarron MM, Wood JD. The cocaine body packer syndrome. *JAMA* 1983;250:1417.

A prospective study of 75 body packers.

Mouhaffel AH, Madu EC, Satmary WA, et al. Cardiovascular complication of cocaine. *Chest* 1995;107:1426.

A concise review of the cardiovascular complication of cocaine.

Pollack CV, Biggers DW, Carlton FB, et al. Two crack cocaine body stuffers. *Ann Emerg Med* 1992;21:1370.

A discussion about the controversies regarding the management of cocaine body stuffers.

Roth D, Alarcon FJ. Fernandez JA, et al. Acute rhabdomyolysis associated with cocaine intoxication. *N Engl J Med* 1988;319:673.

A description of a group of cocaine-intoxicated patients with rhabdomyolysis and renal failure.

Spivey WH, Euerle B. Neurologic complication of cocaine abuse. *Ann Emerg Med* 1990; 19:1422.

A concise review of the neurologic complication of cocaine abuse.

116. CYCLIC ANTIDEPRESSANT POISONING

Richard Y. Wang

I. General principles. Cyclic antidepressants are used for endogenous depression, enuresis, migraine headaches, chronic pain control, smoking cessation, and cocaine detoxification. Toxic effects predominantly involve the central nervous system (CNS) and the cardiovascular system.

The tricyclic antidepressants (TCAs) include amitriptyline, nortriptyline, imipramine, desipramine, clomipramine, and doxepin. They block postsynaptic receptors for histamine, dopamine, acetylcholine, serotonin, and norepinephrine; inhibit the reuptake of biogenic amine neurotransmitters; and have local anesthetic or quinidinelike membrane effects. These agents can cause cardiac conduction disturbances and they have a negative inotropic effect. Polycyclic antidepressants, which have similar activity, include amoxapine, bupropion, nefazodone, and trazodone.

The selective serotonin reuptake inhibitors (SSRIs), another class of cyclic antidepressants, include fluoxetine, paroxetine, sertraline, citalopram, and fluoxetine. These agents block some serotonin receptors, inhibit the reuptake of serotonin at others, and enhance the release of serotonin presynaptically. Mirtazepine and venlafaxine are nonselective serotonin reuptake inhibitors; they also inhibit norepinephrine reuptake.

II. Clinical manifestations. The onset of symptoms following TCA overdose is rapid. Early manifestations include tachycardia and mild hypertension, and anticholinergic effects. The progression of toxicity can be precipitous. Peak toxicity usually occurs within 4 to 6 hours of ingestion and includes abnormal mentation, seizures, hypotension, dysrhythmias, and conduction disorders. The SSRIs are likely to cause sedation only. Other agents tend to cause more CNS than cardiovascular toxicity. Bupropion can cause seizures, even in therapeutic dosing. Seizures are usually brief but status epilepticus can occur without any prodrome, particularly with amoxapine, loxapine, or bupropion.

Sinus tachycardia is usually the presenting dysrhythmia. Aberrancy and ventricular tachycardia develop with increasing toxicity and the overall QRS axis shifts rightward. Initially, TCAs cause the terminal 40 msec of the frontal plane QRS complex to shift rightward (130 to 270 degrees); this is typically manifest as a widened S wave in leads I and aVL and an R wave in aVR. Repolarization abnormalities, intraventricular conduction delays, ventricular dysrhythmia, high-grade atrioventricular block, profound bradycardias, and asystole may ensue. Trazodone can cause marked prolongation of the QTc interval and torsades de pointes ventricular tachycardia.

Administration of two SSRIs—a SSRI and a MAO inhibitor—or a SSRI and a TCA with strong serotonergic effects (e.g., clomipromine) can induce the serotonin syndrome. This syndrome results in altered mentation, autonomic dysfunction, and neuromuscular irritability. Patients may develop hyperthermia, rhabdomyolysis, and multisystem organ failure in severe cases.

III. Differential diagnosis. Many substances have toxicity similar to the cyclic antidepressants. The phenothiazines, particularly thioridazine and mesoridazine, have anticholinergic effects and can cause prolongation of the QRS duration and QTc interval. The atypical antipsychotics (e.g., risperidone, olanzapine) can cause sedation, myoclonus, and cardiac effects. Hypokalemia, hypocalcemia, and the type IA and IC antidysrhythmic agents can increase the QRS duration. β-Adrenoreceptor blockers (especially, propanolol) can cause seizures and conduction disorders.

IV. Evaluation. The physical examination should focus on evaluating the level of consciousness, respiratory function, and cardiovascular status. All patients should have cardiac and oxygen saturation monitoring. Patients with abnormal vital signs should have routine laboratory studies, and an arterial blood gas study, electrocardiogram (ECG), and chest radiograph. Because rhabdomyolysis can occur, most frequently with seizures, creatinine kinase levels should be followed. Frequent ECGs are necessary and should be done any time the patient has a change in status. Quantitative drug levels serve only to confirm an overdose. Poor correlation is found between toxicity and serum concentrations.

V. Management. Patients with cyclic antidepressant overdose require immediate evaluation, cardiac and oxygen saturation monitoring, stabilization, and gastrointestinal decontamination. If the patient remains asymptomatic after a 6-hour period of observation, toxicity is unlikely. Asymptomatic means normal ECG, vital signs, and mental status. All patients with clinical manifestations of toxicity should be admitted to a monitored bed. Patients with depressed mental status or hypoventilation should be immediately intubated to prevent respiratory acidosis and subsequent deterioration of their condition.

Gastrointestinal decontamination should include activated charcoal. Syrup of ipecac is contraindicated. Patients should be given multiple doses of activated charcoal until they awake because some cyclic antidepressants undergo enterohepatic circulation that can prolong toxicity.

Prevention of seizures and their aggressive treatment are paramount because seizures lead to acidemia and acidemia exacerbates cardiotoxicity. Benzodiazepines, barbiturates, neuromuscular blocking agents, and general anesthetics may be necessary for seizure control. Phenytoin use is controversial and physostigmine is contraindicated in patients with seizures, coma, or cardiac conduction disturbances. Paralyzed patients should continue to receive anticonvulsants.

Hypotension is initially treated with intravenous (IV) crystalloid fluid boluses. A sodium bicarbonate infusion (150 mEq in 1 liter of 5% dextrose in water solution) should also be given, particularly when hypotension is associated with acidemia or in the presence of conduction disorders (i.e., QRS > 100 msec in the limb leads) and ventricular dysrhythmias. KCl (20–40 mEq/L) is added to the infusion to prevent hypokalemia resulting from alkalemia. The infusion should be titrated to maintain a blood pH of 7.45 to 7.55. A combination of a bicarbonate infusion and hyperventilation may be more useful than either alone, although hyperventilation is recommended for patients who cannot tolerate either a fluid or sodium load (e.g., renal insufficiency, pulmonary edema). Intermittent boluses of sodium bicarbonate (1–2 mEq/kg, IV) may be necessary, in addition to increasing the infusion rate, to achieve the desired pH. A bicarbonate bolus should also be given in the event of seizures (caused by the resultant lactic acidosis) and for ventricular dysrhythmias.

Persistent hypotension requires the addition of direct-acting vasopressor agents (e.g., norepinephrine, epinephrine) and then inotropic agents (e.g., dobutamine). Lidocaine therapy should be used when ventricular dysrhythmias are not responsive to sodium bicarbonate. Type IA and IC antidysrhythmics are contraindicated for use in this setting. Electric countershock therapy may be of limited value in treating these dysrhythmias because of persistent drug effects.

Treatment of the serotonin syndrome is supportive and should include aggressive rapid cooling. Sedation, paralysis, and intubation may be necessary. Therapy with nonspecific serotonin receptor antagonists (e.g., oral cyproheptadine, 4–8 mg every 8 hours) may shorten the duration of the clinical manifestations.

Selected Readings

Beaubein AR, Carpenter DC, Mathieu JF, et al. Antagonism of imipramine poisoning by anticonvulsants in the rat. *Toxciol Appl Pharmacol* 1976;38:1.

This article discussed the inability of phenytoin to decrease the incidence of tricyclic antidepressant-induced seizures.

Boehnert M, Lovejoy FH. Value of the QRS duration versus the serum drug level in predicting seizures and ventricular arrhythmias after an acute overdose of tricyclic antidepressants. *N Engl J Med* 1985;313:474.

The study demonstrated the important clinical significance of the QRS duration in association with arrhythmias and seizures from tricyclic antidepressant toxicity.

Buchman AL, Dauer J, Geiderman J. The use of vasoactive agents in the treatment of refractory hypotension in tricyclic antidepressant overdose. *J Clin Psychopharmacol* 1990;10:409.

This review discussed the various vasoactive agents that can be used in the treatment of tricyclic antidepressant poisoned patients.

Callaham M, Schumaker H, Pentel P. Phenytoin prophylaxis of cardiotoxicity in experimental amitriptyline poisoning. *J Pharmacol Exp Ther* 1988;245:216.
This study demonstrated phenytoin did not reverse tricyclic antidepressant-induced ventricular tachydysrhythmias and did increase their incidence.

Connolly SJ, Mitchell LB, Swerdlow CD, et al. Clinical efficacy and electrophysiology of imipramine for ventricular tachycardia. *Am J Cardiol* 1984;53:516.
This study showed the effects of tricyclic antidepressants on cardiac conduction to resemble class I antiarrhythmic agents.

Lheureux P, Vranckx M, Leduc D, et al. Flumazenil in mixed benzodiazepine/tricyclic antidepressant overdose: in a placebo-controlled study in the dog. *Am J Emerg Med* 1992;10:184.
This study demonstrated flumazenil to increase the incidence of seizures in the setting of benzodiazepine and tricyclic antidepressant toxicity.

Martin TE. Serotonin syndrome. *Ann Emerg Med* 1996;28:520.
A clinical review on serotonin syndrome.

Nattel S, Mittleman M. Treatment of ventricular tachyarrhythmias resulting from amitriptyline toxicity in dogs. *J Pharacol Exp Ther* 1984;231:430.
An article showing the benefits of sodium bicarbonate and hyperventilation in reversing tricyclic antidepressant-induced conduction defects.

Newton RW. Physostigmine salicylate in the treatment of tricyclic antidepressant overdosage. *JAMA* 1975;231:941.
This report demonstrated the increased incidence of seizures and peripheral cholinergic manifestations from the use of physostigmine in tricyclic antidepressant poisoned patients.

Pentel PR, Benowitz NL. Efficacy and mechanism of action of sodium bicarbonate in the treatment of desipramine toxicity in rats. *J Pharmacol Exp Ther* 1984;230:12.
A study showing that acidosis increased the effects of tricyclic antidepressant-induced cardiotoxicity.

Sasyniuk BI, Jhamandas V. Mechanism of reversal of toxic effects of amitriptyline on cardiac Purkinje fibers by sodium bicarbonate. *J Pharmacol Exp Ther* 1984;232:387.
This study demonstrated increased extracellular sodium concentration to reverse the effects of tricyclic antidepressants on the action potential.

Tokarski GF, Young MJ. Criteria for admitting patients with tricyclic antidepressant overdose. *J Emerg Med* 1998;6:121.
This article discussed the application of a clinical algorithm to determine hospital admission versus discharge in tricyclic antidepressant overdosed patients.

Vohra J, Burrows G, Hunt D, et al. The effect of toxic and therapeutic doses of tricyclic antidepressant drugs on intracardiac conduction. *Eur J Cardiol* 1975;3:219.
This study demonstrated impaired intracardiac conduction in patients with tricyclic antidepressant poisoning.

Wolfe TR, Caravati EM, Rollins DE, et al. Terminal 40-ms frontal plane QRS axis as a marker for tricyclic antidepressant overdose. *Ann Emerg Med* 1989;18:348.
This study showed the association of the rightward axis shift of the terminal 40 msec of the QRS complex with tricyclic antidepressant toxicity.

117. CYCLOSPORINE

Erica L. Liebelt

I. General principles. Cyclosporine is an immunosuppressive drug used to prevent solid organ allograft rejection, graft-versus-host disease, and to treat selected patients with autoimmune diseases. It blocks cytokine synthesis and receptor expression needed for T-lymphocyte activation. As a result, the activation and proliferation of helper and cytotoxic T cells, essential for the alloantigen rejection process, are disrupted. Cyclosporine also inhibits various ATP-dependent cellular export proteins, which may account for its ability to inhibit cellular multidrug resistance.

II. Pharmacokinetics. Oral cyclosporine (Neoral and Sandimmune) has a relatively low bioavailability. Because of this low fractional absorption and significant first-pass metabolism, oral cyclosporine doses are two to three times larger than intravenous (IV) doses to achieve equivalent circulating concentrations. Any factor affecting gastric emptying (metoclopramide) and intestinal transit time (diarrhea) can influence the rate and extent of cyclosporine absorption from the gut.

Cyclosporine is lipophilic and, thus, distributes widely throughout body tissues, concentrating in the liver, kidneys, and especially fat, producing higher cyclosporine concentrations than in the serum. It is highly bound to lipoproteins rather than to albumin. Because of the differential distribution into erythrocytes, plasma, and leukocytes, whole blood cyclosporine concentrations are two to three times higher than serum or plasma concentrations. It persists in body tissue weeks to months after discontinuation and does not readily penetrate the blood–brain barrier. The volume of distribution is not altered in patients with hepatic or renal failure.

Cyclosporine is extensively metabolized by hepatic cytochrome P-450 enzymes, with more than 90% excreted as metabolites into the bile and eliminated in the feces. Various factors can alter the rate of cyclosporine metabolism (e.g., hepatic function, patient age, and interactions with other drugs). Cyclosporine clearance in pediatric transplant recipients is significantly faster than in adults. The mean elimination half-life varies from 7 to 24 hours, depending on the type of transplant and concurrent disease states. Patients with liver failure have relatively long cyclosporine elimination half-lives (averaging 20 hours) and require lower doses.

III. Drug interactions. Drugs that induce or inhibit the hepatic cytochrome P-450 enzyme system can have significant effects on cyclosporine concentrations. Those that increase cyclosporine concentrations include ketoconazole, fluconazole, erythromycin, diltiazem, nicardipine, and cimetidine. Naringenin, a compound in grapefruit juice, causes an increase in both parent and metabolite cyclosporine levels by increasing its bioavailability.

IV. Drug monitoring. When monitoring patients on cyclosporine therapy, it is important to understand that therapeutic 12-hour trough concentrations vary with the analytical methods used to measure cyclosporine concentrations, the sample matrix (plasma, serum, or whole blood), and factors that can affect blood concentrations. A precise cyclosporine concentration versus response relationship for both therapeutic and toxic effects has been difficult to define because many confounding patient factors affect acute rejection rates and creatinine levels, including the use of other immunosuppressants, preservation time, and the use of various cyclosporine drug analysis techniques (Table 117-1).

V. Toxicity. Cyclosporine has been demonstrated to be nephrotoxic in both the acute and chronic settings. It is dose-related and manifested as renal insufficiency (rising creatinine level). The mechanism of this toxicity appears to be an interference of prostaglandin synthesis in renal cortical tissue, which increases thomboxane A_2 concentrations, and causes intrarenal vasoconstriction. Cyclosporine-associated hypertension is another common toxic effect probably caused by the nephrotoxic effects of the drug and renal vasoconstriction.

TABLE 117-1. Cyclosporine 12-hour trough concentration ranges for various analytic methods

Transplant	Sample matrix	Analytic method[a]	Target range (ng/ml)
Kidney	Blood	HPLC	150–250 (day 0–day 120) 100–200 (after day 120)
	Blood	P-FPIA or P-RIA[b]	200–800
	Blood	M-RIA or M-FPIA	150–400
	Serum/plasma	P-FPIA	100–250
Liver	Blood	HPLC	150–300
		M-RIA or M-FPIA	150–400
		P-FPIA	400–800
Heart	Blood	HPLC	150–300
		M-RIA or M-FPIA	150–400
Bone marrow	Serum/plasma	P-FPIA or P-RIA[b]	100–250

[a] HPLC, high-performance liquid chromatography; M-RIA monoclonal radioimmunoassay; M-FPIA, monocional fluorescence polarization immunoassay; P-FPIA, polyclonal fluorescence polarization immunoassay; P-RIA, polyclonal radioimmunoassay.
[b] No longer available.

Cyclosporine also causes hepatotoxicity (transaminase and bilirubin elevations) and is likely related to the inhibition of bile secretion pathways. Neurotoxicity has been reported to occur at very high blood concentrations, low cholesterol levels, low magnesium levels, and in liver transplant recipients. Reported effects include encephalopathy, seizures, headache, visual disorders, white-matter changes, and coma.

Cyclosporine overdoses have been documented with both the oral and intravenous preparations. In general, both acute and chronic toxicity seem to be limited, except in infants and neonates. The most common signs and symptoms after intentional overdoses and overdoses caused by therapeutic dosing errors are hypertension, tachycardia, tremor, nausea and vomiting, and drowsiness. In addition, gingivitis, gastric discomfort, hepatic enzyme elevations, mild renal dysfunction, and burning sensations in the mouth, feet, and face have also been reported. In the pediatric population, more serious toxicity such as oliguric renal failure, metabolic acidosis, and respiratory depression can occur. Cyclosporine blood levels in such patients may not correlate with clinical toxicity.

VI. Treatment. Treatment for cyclosporine toxicity includes decreasing the dose or stopping the drug. In an acute oral overdose, activated charcoal is probably indicated, especially if a large amount is ingested or there are co-ingestants. However, cyclosporine's large molecular weight and limited oral bioavailability can minimize the effect of charcoal. Treatment options for parenteral overdose are limited because of cyclosporine's large volume of distribution. Blood exchange transfusion has been reported in the setting of neonatal cyclosporine overdose, although this modality has its limitations because of the above-mentioned reasons. Hemodialysis and hemoperfusion are not effective in removing cyclosporine.

Selected Readings

Arellano F, Monka C, Krupp PF. Acute cyclosporin overdose. A review of present clinical experience. [Published erratum appears in *Drug Saf* 1991;6:338.] *Drug Saf* 1991;6:266.

Summary of toxic effects on 27 patients with oral or parenteral overdosage of cyclosporine and suggested guidelines for management.

DeGroen PC, Aksamit AJ, Rakela J, et al. Central nervous system toxicity after liver transplantation: the role of cyclosporine and cholesterol. *N Engl J Med* 1987; 317:861.

A case series of patients with cyclosporine-associated central nervous system toxicity associated with low cholesterol levels.

Honcharik N, Anthone S. Activated charcoal in acute cyclosporin overdose. *Lancet* 1985;1:1051.

A case report describing the effects of activated charcoal on acute oral cyclosporine overdose.

Kahan BD. Cyclosporine. *N Engl J Med* 1989;321:1725.

A comprehensive review of cyclosporine, including pharmacology and toxic effects.

Kokado Y, Takahara S, Ishibashi M, et al. An acute overdose of cyclosporine. *Transplantation* 1989;47:1096.

A case report describing the hepatotoxic effects of an acute oral overdose of cyclosporine.

Ptachcinski RJ, Venkataramanan R, Burckart GJ. Clinical pharmacokinetics of cyclosporin. *Clin Pharmacokinet* 1986;11:107.

A detailed review of the pharmacology and therapeutic monitoring of cyclosporine.

Rush DN. Cyclosporine toxicity to organs other than the kidney. *Clin Biochem* 1991;24:101.

A detailed review of cyclosporine toxicity to multiple organs.

Thompson CB, June CH, Sullivan KM, et al. Association between cyclosporin neurotoxicity and hypomagnesaemia. *Lancet* 1984;2:1116.

A case series of bone-marrow transplant recipients with cyclosporine neurotoxicity associated with hypomagnesemia.

118. DIGITALIS POISONING

Jeffrey R. Tucker

I. General principles. Cardiac glycosides (CGs) are naturally occurring substances whose medicinal benefits have been recognized for more than 200 years. They are found in a variety of plants (e.g., bay laurel or *Nerium oleander,* purple foxglove or *Digitalis purpurea,* squill or *Urginea maritima*) and in the skin secretions of Bufo toads (e.g., the Colorado river toad). Digoxin is the primary CG used in medicine today.

II. Pathogenesis. Toxicity is an exaggeration of a therapeutic action. CGs inhibit the sodium-potassium adenosine triphosphatase (Na-K-ATPase) pump. Inhibition of the pump causes changes in intracellular sodium and calcium and a positive inotropic effect. Toxic cardiac effects include increased vagal tone, increased automaticity, and depressed atrioventricular (AV) conduction. Digoxin is primarily eliminated by renal excretion. Clearance of digoxin is reduced in renal failure, resulting in increased serum concentrations. Commonly accepted therapeutic levels of digoxin are 0.8 to 2.0 ng/ml.

Increased end-organ sensitivity to the effects of CGs is seen in the elderly and in patients with cardiomyopathy, myocardial ischemia, electrolyte disturbances (hypokalemia, hypomagnesemia, and hypercalcemia), renal dysfunction, hepatic disease, hypothyroidism, and chronic obstructive pulmonary disease. Increased digoxin levels can result from concomitant therapy with drugs such as amiodarone, cyclosporine, erythromycin, neomycin, propafenone, quinidine, and tetracycline, and verapamil.

III. Clinical presentation. Manifestations of poisoning include gastrointestinal, central nervous system, and visual effects, as well as cardiotoxicity. Those with chronic intoxication may present with complaints that mimic more common illnesses, such as influenza or gastroenteritis, and not be recognized as signs of poisoning.

Gastrointestinal symptoms include anorexia, nausea, vomiting, and abdominal pain. Fatigue, weakness, and dizziness are common complaints. Neuropsychiatric manifestations include confusion, delirium, depression, hallucinations, headache, lethargy, vertigo, and seizures. Cloudy, blurred, and diminished vision, and yellow-green halos or images appearing washed in yellow (xanthopsia) are the most common visual symptoms.

Cardiac manifestations are common and frequently life threatening. Arrhythmias frequently associated with CG toxicity include ventricular premature beats, supraventricular tachycardia with a conduction block, junctional tachycardia, sinus bradycardia, AV nodal blocks, ventricular tachycardia, and ventricular fibrillation. Tachycardia (enhanced automaticity) with variable AV block (impaired conduction), accelerated junctional rhythm (regularization of atrial fibrillation), and fascicular tachycardia are highly suggestive of CG toxicity.

Acute poisoning of the Na-K-ATPase pump can result in markedly elevated serum potassium levels. In contrast, hypokalemia and hypomagnesemia are commonly seen in chronic intoxication, presumably because of concomitant diuretic use.

IV. Evaluation. Physical examination should focus on the vital signs and evaluation of cardiac, gastrointestinal, and neurologic symptoms. Ancillary testing should include an electrocardiogram; evaluation of serum electrolytes, calcium, and magnesium; renal function tests; oxygen saturation or arterial blood gas analysis; and a serum digoxin level. A chest radiograph may also be indicated. Serial serum digoxin and potassium concentrations should be obtained, particular following acute overdose. Drug levels should be interpreted in the overall clinical context and not relied on as the sole indicator of the presence or absence of chronic toxicity. An elevated digoxin level supports the diagnosis. However, some patients can develop toxicity at therapeutic levels and other can be asymptomatic despite toxic levels. A level obtained before distribution is complete (within 6 hours of administration) will be higher than tissue levels and not predictive of toxicity.

V. Management. Meticulous attention to supportive care and a search for correctable conditions (e.g., hypoxia, hypoventilation, hypovolemia, hypoglycemia, and electrolyte disturbances) are essential. All patients should have continuous cardiac monitoring. Advanced life support measures should be instituted as necessary. Activated charcoal should be administered to patients with recent ingestions. Pretreatment with atropine has been recommended prior to gastric intubation because this procedure can cause vagal stimulation and bradycardia.

Atropine can be used for AV block. Because of concerns about pacer-induced ventricular fibrillation, antidotal therapy with digoxin-specific antibody Fab fragments (Digibind) is recommended in patients unresponsive to atropine. Fab fragments can also reverse ventricular tachyarrhythmias, other conduction disturbances, myocardial depression, and hyperkalemia. Phenytoin has classically been the antiarrhythmic of choice for ventricular tachyarrhythmias because it increases the ventricular fibrillation threshold and enhances conduction through the AV node. Intravenous administration of magnesium has been shown to counteract ventricular irritability from digitalis toxicity. Lidocaine is also acceptable. Fab fragments are now considered the treatment of choice for any patient with hemodynamic instability or life-threatening ventricular dysrhythmia. Antiarrythmic therapy is still recommended as a temporizing measure. Electrical cardioversion can precipitate ventricular fibrillation and should be performed with extreme caution. A low energy setting should be used.

Supplemental potassium may be beneficial in chronic digitalis toxicity when diuretic-induced hypokalemia is a factor. Potassium should not be routinely administered to the acutely poisoned patient because hyperkalemia may ensue. Fab fragments are the treatment of choice for patients with hyperkalemia secondary to acute intoxication, which can initially be treated with intravenous glucose, insulin, and sodium bicarbonate. Calcium can enhance digitalis cardiac toxicity and should be avoided.

The dose of Fab fragment is based on the estimated body load of digoxin. The body load is equal to the amount (mg) of an acute ingestion or, in chronic intoxication, the serum digoxin level (ng/ml) multiplied by 5.6 times the body weight (kg) and divided by 1,000. One vial of Fab (40 mg) will bind 0.6 mg of digoxin. The number of vials required can be calculated by dividing the total body burden by 0.6. Patients with acute poisoning have a much higher body load than those with chronic poisoning. If the amount of an acute ingestion is unknown, empiric therapy should begin with 5 to 10 vials. If the serum level is not yet known but chronic intoxication is highly likely, empiric therapy should begin with 1 to 2 vials. If cardiac arrest is imminent or has occurred, the dose can be given as a bolus. Otherwise, it should be infused over 30 minutes. A precipitous drop in serum potassium, the emergence of supraventricular tachydysrhythmias previously controlled by digoxin, and worsening of congestive heart failure in a patient dependent on digoxin for inotropic support are potential complications of Fab fragment therapy. Allergic reactions are rare. Recurrence of toxicity days after treatment is possible.

Selected Readings

Antman EM, Wenger TL, Butler VP, et al. Treatment of 150 cases of life-threatening digitalis intoxication with digoxin-specific Fab antibody fragments: final report of a multi-center study. *Circulation* 1990;81:1744.

A multicenter study of Fab fragment in which 90% of patients had a treatment response.

Bismuth C, Gaultier M, Conso F, et al. Hyperkalemia in acute digitalis poisoning: prognostic significance and therapeutic implications. *Clin Toxicol* 1973;153:153.

A study demonstrating the prognostic importance of hyperkalemia. Patients with potassium above 5.5 mEq/L had 100% mortality.

Fisch C, Knoehel SB. Digitalis cardiotoxicity. *J Am Coll Cardiol* 1985;5:91A.

Excellent review of the most electrophysiologic mechanism for digitalis induced arrhythmias.

French JH, Thomas RG, Siskind AP, et al. Magnesium therapy in massive digoxin intoxication. *Ann Emerg Med* 1984;13:562.

A case of recurrent ventricular fibrillation that failed to respond to lidocaine or phenytoin, but responded to magnesium infusion.

Ingelfinger JA, Goldman P. The serum digitalis concentration—does it diagnose digitalis toxicity? *N Engl J Med* 1976;294:867.

A discussion of the importance and limitations of the serum digitalis levels and the significance of clinical information such as renal function, serum potassium, and cardiac impairment in the diagnosis of digitalis toxicity.

Kelly RA, Smith TW. Recognition and management of digitalis toxicity. *Am J Cardiol* 1992:69:108G.

A discussion of the recognition and management of the factors leading to increase risk of toxicity in certain patients.

Kirk MA. Digitalis: therapeutics and poisoning. In: Irwin RS, Cerra FB, Rippe JM, eds. *Intensive care medicine,* 4th ed. Philadelphia: Lippincott–Raven; 1998.

A comprehensive review with extensive reference list.

Leikin J, Vogel S. Graff J, et al. Use of Fab fragments of digoxin-specific antibodies in the therapy of massive digoxin poisoning. *Ann Emerg Med* 1985;14:175.

Early case report of massive digoxin poisoning with multiple arrhythmias not responsive to lidocaine which did respond to the administration of Fab fragments.

Lewis RP. Clinical use of serum digoxin concentrations. *Am J Cardiol* 1992:69:97G.

A discussion of the use and the limitations of the digoxin concentrations as well as the technical problem with the serum assay.

Mahdyoon H, Battilana G, Rosman H, et al. The evolving pattern of digoxin intoxication: observations at a large urban hospital from 1980 to 1988. *Am Heart J* 1990;120:1189.

A retrospective review of the hospitalized patients with heart failure and of the difficulty in making the diagnosis of digoxin toxicity.

Smith TW. Digitalis: mechanisms of action and clinical use. *N Engl J Med* 1988;318:358.

An excellent discussion about sodium and calcium effects on the excitation-contraction coupling and the mechanism of action of digitalis.

Smith TW, Butler VP, Haber E, et al. Treatment of life-threatening digitalis intoxication with digoxin-specific Fab antibody fragments: experience in 26 cases. *N Engl J Med* 1982;307:1357.

Initial report of 26 patients successfully and safely treated with digoxin-specific Fab fragments.

Taboulet P, Baud FJ, Bismuth C, et al. Acute digitalis intoxication—is pacing still appropriate? *J Toxicol Clin Toxicol* 1993;31:261.

A retrospective study comparing the outcome of cardiac pacing against Fab fragments. Results favor fragments, but are not statistically significant.

Woolf AD, Wenger T, Smith TW, et al. The use of digoxin-specific Fab fragments for severe digitalis intoxication in children. *N Engl J Med* 1992;326:1739.

Recommendation for the use of Fab fragments based on its use in 29 children and adolescents. Data support the idea that adolescents are more sensitive to the effects of digitalis than younger children.

119. HYDROCARBONS

Richard Y. Wang

I. General principles

A. Aliphatic hydrocarbons, also known as petroleum distillates, include gasoline, naphtha, lighter fluid, mineral spirits, kerosene, and fuel oil. Toxicity can occur by ingestion, inhalation, and dermal absorption. Following ingestion of an aliphatic hydrocarbon, the major potential toxicity is chemical pneumonitis from aspiration.

B. Halogenated hydrocarbons are aliphatic hydrocarbons that contain atoms of chlorine, bromine, fluorine, or iodine. These agents are found in solvents, degreasers, dry cleaning agents, refrigerants, aerosol propellants, and fumigants. Toxic effects can involve the liver and kidneys as well as the central nervous system (CNS) and the heart. Exposures occur most commonly through inhalation. Carbon tetrachloride is metabolized to free radicals, which causes centrilobular hepatic necrosis. Methylene chloride is metabolized to carbon monoxide, which contributes to its toxicity.

C. Aromatic hydrocarbons are agents with one or more benzene rings. They include benzene, toluene, xylene, phenol, and styrene. They are common constituents of glues, paint, paint removers, lacquers, degreasers, and adhesives. CNS depression is the primary effect of acute exposures. Toxicity most often results from intentional inhalation for recreational purposes.

D. Terpenes, which are derived from plants, include compounds such as turpentine, pine oil, and camphor.

II. Clinical manifestations

A. Aliphatic hydrocarbons. Symptoms of aspiration typically begin within 30 minutes of ingestion; they include coughing, gasping, and choking. Patients who do not have respiratory symptoms within 6 hours of ingestion are unlikely to become symptomatic. Respiratory toxicity can progress and peak in the first 24 to 48 hours. Tachypnea with grunting respirations, nasal flaring, retractions, cyanosis, wheezing, rhonchi, and rales may be present. In severe cases, pulmonary edema and hemoptysis can occur. Arterial blood gases may demonstrate hypoxemia from ventilation-perfusion mismatch and early hypocarbia, which progresses to hypercarbia and acidosis. Chest radiograph abnormalities, typically bibasilar infiltrates, occur in up to 75% of exposures, appearing within 2 hours in 88% of patients and by 12 hours in 98%. Symptoms usually resolve in 2 to 5 days. Radiographic abnormalities can persist for several days to weeks. Fever secondary to chemical pneumonitis is common within the first 48 hours. The persistence of fever beyond 48 hours suggests a bacterial infection.

Gastrointestinal symptoms, such as oropharyngeal irritation, nausea, vomiting, and abdominal pain are common. CNS effects can range from dizziness and confusion to somnolence and, rarely, coma and seizures. They usually occur only in patients with severe aspiration or large intentional ingestions. Peripheral neuropathy has been reported after chronic exposure to the aliphatic hydrocarbons. Cardiovascular toxicity is uncommon, but syncope, dysrhythmias, and sudden death after gasoline siphoning have been reported. Dermatologic manifestations appear as burns and include erythema and blister formations. Parental administration of petroleum distillates has caused local cellulitis, thrombophlebitis, and necrotizing myositis, with resultant compartment syndromes.

B. Halogenated hydrocarbons. CNS effects can range from dizziness, headache, confusion, euphoria, and ataxia to seizures, lethargy, coma, and apnea. Fatal cardiac dysrhythmias have also been reported. Carbon tetrachloride can cause hepatoxicity. Early symptoms include nausea, vomiting, abdominal pain, and diarrhea. Clinical hepatitis generally occurs on days 2 to 4, with fever, elevated liver function test, prolonged prothrombin time, liver tenderness and enlargement, and jaundice. Early fatalities can result from respiratory depression or cardiac dysrhythmias. More commonly, death occurs as the result of hepatorenal failure. Methylene chloride exposure can cause light-headedness, headache, lethargy, syncope, irritability, gait disturbance, stupor, and coma. Carboxyhemoglobin fractions can range from 8% to 50%; elevated levels may not be evident until several hours after exposure.

C. Aromatic hydrocarbons. CNS effects are similar to those described for aliphatic and halogenated hydrocarbons. Long-term exposure to benzene can result in bone marrow depression, which can progress to aplastic anemia. Chronic toluene inhalation is associated with peripheral neuropathy and renal dysfunction. Renal tubular acidosis, electrolyte disturbances (e.g., hypokalemia, hypophosphatemia, hypocalcemia, hyperchloremia), and rhabdomyolysis can occur.

D. Terpenes. Ingestion of terpenes can cause gastrointestinal irritation and CNS depression. In severe exposures, coma or seizures can result. Turpentine ingestion has been associated with hemorrhagic cystitis with dysuria and hematuria occurring 12 hours to 3 days following exposure.

III. Diagnostic evaluation. The identity of the agent(s) involved, the amount, time and route of exposure, and the nature and progression of symptoms should be documented. The physical examination should focus on the vital signs and the respiratory, CNS, cardiovascular, and gastrointestinal systems. In symptomatic patients or those who ingested agents with systemic toxicity, pulse oximetry or arterial blood gas analysis, chest radiography, complete blood count, electrolyte, blood urea nitrogen, creatinine, glucose, liver function tests, creatine kinase, urinalysis, and carboxyhemoglobin measurement may be indicated.

IV. Management. Treatment involves supportive care and monitoring for respiratory depression and cardiac dysrhythmias. Patients with ingestions who remain or become asymptomatic after 6 hours of observation and have a normal chest radiograph (2 hours or more after exposure) can be discharged. Patients with persistent symptoms; abnormal chest films, arterial blood gases, or pulse oximetry; and suicidal intentions should be hospitalized.

Oxygen is indicated for patients with respiratory symptoms or an elevated carboxyhemoglobin level. Bronchospasm should be treated with selective (β_2) bronchodilators because of the potential for myocardial sensitization to catecholamines to occur. Continuous positive airway pressure, high frequency jet ventilation, and extracorporeal membrane oxygenation may be necessary to maintain adequate oxygenation. Chemical pneumonitis is managed supportively. Steroids have not been shown to be beneficial in this setting and prophylactic antibiotics are not recommended. Antibiotics should be given only to patients with documented bacterial pneumonia (e.g., Gram's stain or culture of sputum or tracheal aspirate) or worsening chest radiograph, leukocytosis, and fevers persisting more than 48 hours.

Gastric decontamination is recommended only for recent ingestions of potentially toxic amounts of halogenated, aromatic, or terpene hydrocarbons: 0.3 ml/kg for carbon tetrachloride, 5 ml/kg for pine oil, and 1 to 2 ml/kg for other agents. Gastric aspiration is the preferred method. Activated charcoal should also be given. If cutaneous exposure has occurred, contaminated clothing should be removed immediately and the skin cleansed with soap and water.

N-acetylcysteine may prevent carbon tetrachloride-induced hepatotoxicity by scavenging free radicals. The oral dosage is 140 mg/kg (loading) and then 70 mg/kg every 4 hours until hepatotoxicity resolves.

Selected Readings

Anas N, Namasonthi V, Gisnburg CM. Criteria for hospitalizing children who have ingested products containing hydrocarbon. *JAMA* 1981;246:840.

This study observed patients who presented and remained asymptomatic after 6 to 8 hours of observation and who did not develop subsequent toxic manifestations.

Bass M. Sudden sniffing death. *JAMA* 1970;212:2075.

This case report described an intoxicated volatile substance user who suddenly died on exertion.

Brown J, Burke B, Dajani AS, et al. Experimental kerosene pneumonia: evaluation of some therapeutic regimens. *J Pediatr* 1974;84:393.
This study demonstrated that early antibiotic administration did not prevent infection and promoted the growth of more resistant bacterial strains.

Daffner RH, Jimenez JP. The double gastric fluid level in kerosene poisoning. *Pediatr Radiol* 1973;106:383.
This report described the "double bubble" sign on the abdominal radiograph.

Gerarde HW. Toxicological studies on hydrocarbons. IX. The aspiration hazard and toxicity of hydrocarbons and hydrocarbon mixtures. *Arch Environ Health* 1963;6:329.
This study demonstrated the main determinants of aspiration potential for hydrocarbons to be viscosity, surface tension, and volatility.

Gurwitz D, Kattan M, Levison H, et al. Pulmonary function abnormalities in asymptomatic children after hydrocarbon pneumonitis. *Pediatrics* 1970;62:78.
This study demonstrated that most patients with hydrocarbon aspiration have no significant sequelae despite having minor pulmonary function abnormalities.

Hansbrough JF, Saputa-Sirvent R, et al. Hydrocarbon contact injuries. *J Trauma* 1985;25:250.
This report demonstrated hydrocarbon-induced dermatitis and full thickness burns.

James FW, Kaplan S, Benzing G. Cardiac complications following hydrocarbon ingestion. *Am J Dis Child* 1971;121:431.
This report described the cardiovascular manifestations associated with a hydrocarbon exposure.

Larsen F, Leira HL. Organic brain syndrome and long term exposure to toluene: a clinical psychiatric study of vocationally active printing workers. *J Occup Med* 1988;30:875.
This article contains an analysis of pathologies on computed tomography scan, electroencephalogram, and neuropsychiatric testing in patients chronically exposed to solvents.

Marks MI, Chicoine L, Legere G, et al. Adrenocorticosteroid treatment of hydrocarbon pneumonia in children—a cooperative study. *J Pediatr* 1972;81:366.
This study showed that early steroid administration did not prevent or limit pulmonary inflammatory response from hydrocarbon injury.

Meadows R, Verghese A. Medical complications of glue sniffing. *South Med J* 1996;89:455.
This review discusses the acute and chronic manifestations associated with glue sniffing.

Press E. Cooperative kerosene poisoning study: evaluation of gastric lavage and other factors in the treatment of accidental ingestion of petroleum distillate products. *Pediatrics* 1962;29:648.
This study demonstrated an increased incidence of pulmonary complications when vomiting occurred after kerosene poisoning.

Rinsky RA, Smith AB, Hornung R, et al. Benzene and leukemia: an epidemiologic risk assessment. *N Engl J Med* 1987;316:1044.
This study showed an association between long-term benzene exposure and leukemia.

Wolfsdorf J, Kundig H. Kerosene poisoning in primates. *S Afr Med J* 1972;46:619.
This study demonstrated the lack of pulmonary toxicity from hydrocarbon exposure when aspiration did not occur.

120. ISONIAZID POISONING

Erica L. Liebelt

I. General principles. Isoniazid (INH) is primarily used for the treatment of tuberculosis. INH overdose is most common in the American Indian population in Alaska and in the Southwest, where the prevalence for tuberculosis and suicide rates are high. It is seen in urban areas where large of populations of Southeast Asian and other Third World country immigrants live.

II. Pharmacology. Isoniazid is rapidly and completely absorbed after oral administration, with peak concentrations normally occurring within 1 to 2 hours. INH is widely distributed throughout the body with a volume of distribution approximating that of total body water (0.6 L/kg). Most INH is metabolized in the liver within 24 hours by acetylation to acetylisoniazid and by hydrolysis to isonicotinic acid and hydrazine. Genetic variation in acetylation significantly alters plasma concentration, elimination half-life, and toxicity. The elimination half-life is 0.5 to 1.5 hours in rapid acetylators and 2 to 4 hours in slow acetylators. Slow acetylators may have a higher percentage of the parent drug metabolized to hydrazine, a potential hepatotoxin.

The usual therapeutic dose of INH is 5 mg/kg/d for adults and 10 mg/kg/d for children up to a maximum of 300 mg/d. An acute ingestion of 1.5 to 3 g in adults is potentially toxic and 6 to 10 g can cause severe poisoning. In patients with preexisting seizure disorders, seizures have occurred with doses as low as 14 mg/kg/d.

III. Pathophysiology. The neurologic toxicity of INH is caused by its effects on γ-aminobutyric acid (GABA) and, possibly, glutamate concentrations in the brain. GABA is the primary inhibitory neurotransmitter, whereas glutamate is an excitatory neurotransmitter. The enzyme *L*-glutamic acid decarboxylase (GAD) converts glutamic acid to GABA with the active form of vitamin B_6, pyridoxal 5′ phosphate, acting as coenzyme. Isoniazid decreases GABA synthesis by (a) lowering pyridoxine concentrations in the body through the formation of isoniazid-pyridoxine hydrazones, (b) competitively inhibiting the conversion of pyridoxine to pyridoxal 5′ phosphate, and (c) inactivating pyridoxal phosphate-containing enzymes (Fig. 120-1). Metabolic acidosis results from lactic acidosis secondary to seizure activity and interference with nicotinamide-adenine dinucleotide (NAD)-mediated conversion of lactate to pyruvate. Hyperglycemia results from blockage of specific steps in the Krebs' cycle that require NAD and from stimulation of glucagon secretion. INH-induced hepatitis may be caused by the covalent binding of hydrazine metabolites to liver macromolecules. Increased acetylhydrazine or hydrazine concentrations in slow acetylators may be responsible for the increased incidence of hepatotoxicity in this cohort.

IV. Clinical presentation. Effects appear 30 minutes to 2 hours after acute overdose. Nausea, vomiting, dizziness, slurred speech, blurred vision, and visual hallucinations (bright colors, spots, strange designs) are among the first symptoms. Lethargy, stupor, and coma can rapidly develop, followed by tonic-clonic seizures and hyperreflexia or areflexia. In severe cases, cardiovascular and respiratory collapse can result in death. Metabolic abnormalities include severe metabolic acidosis, hyperglycemia, glycosuria, ketonuria, and hyperkalemia. The triad of metabolic acidosis refractory to sodium bicarbonate therapy, seizures that are refractory to anticonvulsants, and coma suggests INH overdose. Other toxins to consider in the differential diagnosis of intractable seizures include theophylline, amoxapine, maprotiline, cyanide, organophosphate insecticides, fluoride, and carbon monoxide.

Hepatotoxicity from chronic exposure is usually manifest by elevated serum aminotransferase concentrations within the first few months of therapy. Slow acetylators, increased age, alcohol consumption, and rifampin coadministration can increase the risk of this form of toxicity. Peripheral neuropathy, related to pyridoxine deficiency, usually occurs within 3 to 35 weeks of initiating therapy and can be prevented by coadministration of pyridoxine in high-risk patients.

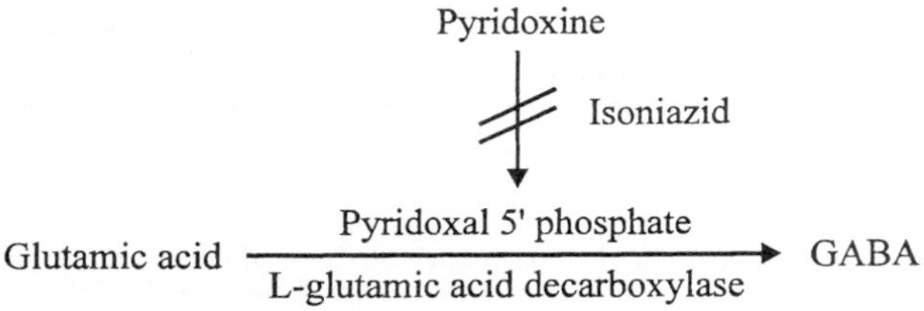

Pyridoxine

Isoniazid

Glutamic acid → GABA (Pyridoxal 5' phosphate / L-glutamic acid decarboxylase)

FIG. 120-1. Role of isoniazid (INH) in the reduction of γ-aminobutyric acid (GABA) synthesis. Pyridoxal 5′ phosphate acts as a coenzyme with *L*-glutamic acid decarboxylase to form GABA from glutamic acid. The INH blocks the conversion of pyridoxine to pyridoxal 5′ phosphate, resulting in decreased GABA formation and a decreased seizure threshold.

V. Management. The management of acute overdose includes protection of the airway, support of respirations, treatment of seizures, correction of metabolic acidosis, and minimization of drug absorption. Gastrointestinal decontamination should be carried out with activated charcoal—orally or by gastric tube, depending on the mental status of the patient. Laboratory evaluation should include blood for glucose, electrolytes, arterial blood gas with pH and bicarbonate, and renal function.

Seizure activity should be treated with a combination of benzodiazepines (diazepam) and pyridoxine. Diazepam has been shown to potentiate the action of pyridoxine. Treatment of metabolic acidosis should be guided by arterial blood gas and electrolyte measurements. In most cases, intravenous sodium bicarbonate will not fully correct acid-base abnormalities until pyridoxine has been administered. Hemodialysis or hemoperfusion should be considered in patients with intractable acid-base abnormalities, persistent seizures, and liver or renal failure.

VI. Antidotal therapy. Pyridoxine or vitamin B_6 is considered the antidote for neurologic toxicity. Pyridoxine has been shown to reverse coma as well as terminate seizure toxicity. Pyridoxine also prevents recurrent seizure activity and contributes to the resolution of metabolic acidosis. A dose of pyridoxine equal to the amount of INH ingested should be given at the first sign of neurologic toxicity. If the amount ingested is not known, at least 5 g of parenteral pyridoxine should be given. In patients without seizure activity, pyridoxine can be administered intravenously over 30 minutes. It should be given as a bolus over 3 to 5 minutes in those with seizure activity; it can be repeated until the INH dose is exceeded, seizures stop, or consciousness is regained.

Selected Readings

Bredemann JA, Krechel SW, Eggers GWN. Treatment of refractory seizures in massive isoniazid overdose. *Anesth Analg* 1990;71:554.

A discussion of the pathophysiology of isoniazid-induced seizures and pyridoxine therapy as well as use of thiopental infusion for refractory seizures.

Brent J, Vo N, Kulig K, et al. Reversal of prolonged isoniazid-induced coma by pyridoxine. *Arch Intern Med* 1990;150:1751.

Three case reports and discussion on the effectiveness of pyridoxine in reversing isoniazid-induced coma.

Chin L, Sievers ML, Laird HE, et al. Evaluation of diazepam and pyridoxine as antidotes to isoniazid intoxication in rats and dogs. *Toxicol Appl Pharmacol* 1978;45:713.

Basic science evidence to support the concomitant use of pyridoxine and diazepam in preventing isoniazid-induced seizures and coma.

Dickinson DS, Bailey WC, Hirschowitz BI, et al. Risk factors for isoniazid (INH)-induced liver dysfunction. *J Clin Gastroenterol* 1981;3:271.

A prospective review of risk factors for isoniazid-induced liver dysfunction, suggesting slow acetylators seem to be at increased risk.

Konigshausen TH, Altrogge G, Hein D, et al. Hemodialysis and hemoperfusion in the treatment of most severe INH poisoning. *Vet Hum Toxicol* 1979;21(Suppl):12.

A discussion of two cases of isoniazid poisoning treated with hemodialysis and hemoperfusion.

Wason S, Lacouture PG, Lovejoy FH. Single high-dose pyridoxine treatment for isoniazid overdose. *JAMA* 1981;246:1102.

A review of clinical outcomes of patients treated with high-dose pyridoxine therapy versus little or no pyridoxine, demonstrating pyridoxine's beneficial effects in terminating seizures and lessening coma.

121. LITHIUM

Jeffrey R. Tucker

I. **General principles.** Lithium is the drug of choice for the treatment and prevention of manic-depressive or bipolar disorders. It is also used in some patients with unipolar depression and schizophrenia. Lithium carbonate is available as a 300-mg (~ 8 mEq) tablet or capsules or a 450-mg (~ 12 mEq) sustained-release preparation.

II. **Pathogenesis.** Lithium is rapidly absorbed from the gastrointestinal tract, with peak levels in 2 to 4 hours with standard preparations. Absorption may be delayed more than 4 to 12 hours with sustained-release preparations and after an overdose. The initial volume of distribution is 0.3 to 0.4 L/kg, but redistribution to intracellular tissue leads to a final volume of 0.7 to 1 L/kg. Slow distribution explains why initial serum lithium levels can be very high with few or no signs of toxicity.

Lithium is eliminated almost completely by renal excretion. It is filtered at the glomerulus, with more than 80% reabsorbed in the proximal tubule against a concentration gradient that does not distinguish lithium from sodium. Dehydration or sodium depletion will lead to increased lithium reabsorption and possible toxicity.

The exact mechanisms of lithium's therapeutic and toxic effects remain unknown. Effective serum lithium concentrations for acute mania are considered to be 0.8 to 1.25 mEq/L and serum levels for prophylaxis against recurrent bipolar illness are 0.75 to 1 mEq/L. Careful monitoring is essential because of the low toxic-to-therapeutic ratio. Drug levels drawn prior to complete distribution (within 10 to 12 hours after the last dose) do not accurately correlate with tissue levels and clinical effects or toxicity.

III. **Clinical presentation.** Lithium intoxication can follow an acute overdose or can result from chronic accumulation, because of either an increase in dosage or a decrease in lithium elimination by the kidneys. Acute lithium toxicity could result from an acute ingestion of at least 1 mEq/kg (~ 40 mg/kg lithium carbonate). Chronic toxicity typically results from a decrease in lithium elimination by the kidneys. Most serious toxicity occurs in patients with chronic intoxication.

Lithium toxicity primarily involves the central nervous and gastrointestinal systems. Gastrointestinal effects include nausea, vomiting, abdominal cramps, and diarrhea. Neurologic toxicity usually develops gradually, can worsen even as serum lithium levels are falling, and can persist for days to weeks after cessation of therapy, in part because of slow movement of lithium into and out of intracellular brain sites. Signs of mild to moderate toxicity include lethargy, memory impairment, fine tremor, confusion, agitation, coarse tremor, hyperreflexia, dysarthria, and nystagmus. Severe toxicity can result in delirium, coma, and seizure. Permanent sequelae (e.g., encephalopathy, choreoathetosis, nystagmus, and ataxia) have been described.

Nonspecific electrocardiographic (ECG) changes (e.g., U waves and flat, biphasic, or inverted T waves) can be seen with therapeutic as well as overdoses. Life-threatening dysrhythmias are rare, although sinus and junctional bradycardia, sinoatrial, and first-degree atrioventricular block have been reported.

Effects on renal function include impaired urinary concentrating ability, nephrogenic diabetes insipidus, and a salt-losing nephritis. These effects, which usually correct within several weeks after stopping therapy, are believed to be dose-related.

Metabolic abnormalities associated with lithium use include hypercalcemia, hypermagnesemia, nonketotic hyperglycemia, transient diabetic ketoacidosis, and goiter.

IV. **Evaluation.** The history should include the type and amount of lithium preparation ingested, time of ingestion, and presence of symptoms. It is important to distinguish between chronic intoxication, acute overdose, and acute overdose in a patient using lithium chronically. The physical examination should focus on the vital signs, neurologic function, and cardiovascular status. Tests should include serum electrolytes, glucose, blood urea nitrogen, creatinine, and ECG. After an acute overdose, lithium levels should be repeated at frequent intervals until a peak is observed. Elevated levels should be repeated until they fall below the toxic range and the patient is asymptomatic. Levels drawn after acute toxicity cannot be used reliably to predict toxicity or to guide therapy. The severity of chronic intoxication generally correlates well with the serum lithium level. Mild neurotoxic effects can occur even with levels below 1.5 mEq/L in patients on chronic therapy. Steady-state levels of 1.5 to 3.0 mEq/L are associated with mild or moderate toxicity. Severe poisoning and death can result from serum levels higher than 3 to 4 mEq/L.

V. Treatment. Initial management should be the assessment and stabilization of the airway, oxygen and assisted ventilation as indicated, and insertion of an intravenous line. In patients with altered mental status, consider administration of dextrose, naloxone, and thiamine. Seizures should be treated with benzodiazepines and barbiturates. Hypovolemia should be treated with intravenous fluids. Cardiac arrhythmias do not usually require treatment but should respond to the usual agents.

After acute ingestion, gastric decontamination should be done to reduce absorption of lithium. Activated charcoal does not bind lithium and should be given only for co-ingestants. Most patients have spontaneous vomiting so inducing emesis is unlikely to be helpful. Gastric lavage should be considered in patients who are obtunded or comatose. Whole bowel irrigation may be useful, especially for an acute overdose of sustained-release tablets. Preliminary evidence in animals and human volunteers suggests that sodium polystyrene sulfonate (Kayexalate) binds lithium and may enhance its elimination.

Intravenous fluid is effective in restoring and maintaining effective renal lithium elimination. After a saline bolus (10–20 ml/kg), the patient can be started on maintenance fluids to maintain an adequate urine output of 1 to 3 ml/kg/h. No evidence indicates that excessive hydration increases lithium elimination.

Hemodialysis is the most efficient method to enhance the elimination of lithium, with clearance rates of 100 to 150 ml/min. Indications for hemodialysis are not well established. Patients with severe toxicity and those with renal failure should undergo dialysis. Patients with chronic serum levels exceeding 3.5 to 4 mEq/L and those with acute poisoning and peak levels exceeding 9 to 10 mEq/L should also be considered for hemodialysis. Serum lithium levels often rebound after hemodialysis because of redistribution from intracellular tissue compartments. Hemodialysis should be repeated frequently until the serum level drawn 6 to 8 hours after the last dialysis is 1 mEq/L or less.

Selected Readings

Amdisen A. Clinical features and management of lithium poisoning. *Med Toxicol* 1988; 3:18.

An excellent review of the difficult aspects of the diagnosis and management of acute and chronic lithium toxicity.

Apte SN, Langston JW. Permanent neurological deficits due to lithium toxicity. *Ann Neurol* 1983;13:453.

A case series of two lithium toxic patients with permanent deficits in memory and ataxia.

Bellomo R, Kearly Y, Parkin G, et al. Treatment of life-threatening lithium toxicity with continuous arterio-venous hemofiltration. *Crit Care Med* 1991;19:836.

A case report of a patient successfully treated with an alternative technology to increase lithium elimination.

Clendenin NJ, Pond SM, Kaysen G, et al. Potential pitfalls in the evaluation of the usefulness of hemodialysis for the removal of lithium. *J Toxicol Clin Toxicol* 1982;19:341.

Discussion of calculation of lithium clearance and potential for error due to the method measuring lithium concentration: whole blood, serum or red cells.

Groleau G. Lithium toxicity. *Emerg Med Clin North Am* 1994;12:511.

An excellent review of the pathogenesis and clinical presentation of lithium toxicity.

Jaeger A, Sauder P, Kopfersehmitt J, et al. When should dialysis be performed in lithium poisoning? A kinetic study in 14 cases of lithium poisoning. *J Toxicol Clin Toxicol* 1982;31:429.

A study on lithium kinetics of 14 patients suggests that the decision regarding hemodialysis can be made within 8 to 12 hours from admission.

Mitchell JE, MacKenzie TB. Cardiac effects of lithium therapy in man: a review. *J Clin Psychiatry* 1982;43:47.

A review of the cardiac effects of lithium, focusing on electrocardiographic changes, conduction defects, and structural abnormalities of the heart.

Price LH, Henninger GR. Lithium in the treatment of mood disorders. *N Engl J Med* 1994;331:591.

A review of the history, pharmacology, clinical indications, and toxicity of lithium therapy.

Roberge RJ, Martin TG, Schneider SM. Use of sodium polystyrene sulfonate in a lithium overdose. *Ann Emerg Med* 1993;22:1911.

A case report of the first use of sodium polystyrene sulfonate for the treatment of lithium toxicity.

Simard M, Gumbiner B, Lee A, et al. Lithium carbonate intoxication: a case report and review of the literature. *Arch Intern Med* 1989;149:36.

A detailed review of the common adverse effects of lithium.

Smith SW, Ling LJ, Halstenson CE. Whole-bowel irrigation as a treatment for acute lithium overdose. *Ann Emerg Med* 1991;20:536.

A study in human volunteers that suggests that whole-bowel irrigation is an effective method of decontamination for sustained-release lithium.

Thornnley-Brown D, Galla JH, Williams PD, et al. Lithium toxicity associated with a trichobezoar. *Ann Intern Med* 1992;116:739.

A case report of elevated lithium toxicity not responsive to hemodialysis because of bezoar formation.

Tomaszewski C, Musso C, Pearson JR, et al. Prevention of lithium absorption by sodium polystyrene sulfonate in volunteers. *Ann Emerg Med* 1992;21:1308.

A study of human volunteers showing that sodium polystyrene sulfonate decreases the absorption of lithium.

Weinstein MR, Goldfield MD. Cardiovascular malformations with lithium use during pregnancy. *Am J Psychiatry* 1975;132:529.

Infants exposed to lithium appear to have an increased risk of cardiovascular anomalies. The authors caution against the use of lithium in pregnant women.

122. LOCAL ANESTHETICS

Richard Y. Wang

I. General principles. This chapter focuses on the nonparenteral, nonsubcutaneous use of local anesthetics in the management of postoperative or postprocedural pain, a common problem in the intensive care unit. When used for this purpose, local anesthetics can be administered in a single injection or as a continuous infusion nerve block. Blocks can be central, thoracic, or peripheral. Agents marketed in the United States are listed in Table 122-1.

II. Pharmacology. All local anesthetics inhibit nerve conduction by interfering with transit of sodium ions into the nerve cell. Systemic absorption of relatively low doses of local anesthetics is generally benign; effects include analgesia, anticonvulsant activity, mild sedation, antiarrhythmic activity, and mild increases in blood pressure, cardiac output, and peripheral vascular resistance. Absorption of greater amounts can result in serious toxicity such as confusion, respiratory depression, hallucination, seizures, hypertension, hypotension, arrhythmias, myocardial depression, and methemoglobinemia.

III. Pharmacokinetics. Local anesthetics are categorized as either ester or amide derivatives, which is significant because of their different routes of metabolism. In addition, patients who are allergic to an ester derivative are potentially allergic to (and should not be given) other esters but not to amide derivatives, and vice versa. The ester-types are predominantly hydrolyzed by plasma pseudocholinesterase and the amides are biotransformed in the liver. Clearance of ester agents can be reduced and, hence, the effects of these agents enhanced by the relative deficiency of plasma cholinesterase in neonates and infants younger than 6 months. Various factors have been assessed for their contribution to augmented risk for local anesthetic toxicity, predominantly for lidocaine. In general, weight, gender, race, parturition status, and renal disease have a minor impact. Low cardiac output states are associated with reduced drug clearance and volume of distribution, whereas cirrhosis is associated with reduced clearance and increased volume of distribution. Neonates exhibit an unchanged or reduced clearance and increased volume of distribution and half-life for anesthetics. Some studies demonstrate reduced clearance, increased half-life, and faster systemic absorption after epidural and subarachnoid administration in the elderly, whereas others do not.

IV. Dosing recommendations. Dosing guidelines and indications for use of local anesthetics, both approved and not approved by the US Food and Drug Administration are provided in Table 122-2. If analgesia is inadequate at the upper limit of the suggested dosing range, consider the addition of epinephrine or a systemic opioid, testing of the catheter, or abandoning the technique. Infusion rates should be reduced in pediatric patients at risk for seizures.

TABLE 122-1. Systemic local anesthetics available in the United States

Esters
Chloroprocaine (Nesacaine)
Procaine (Novocain)
Tetracaine (Pontocaine)
Amides
Mepivacaine (Carbocaine)
Etidocaine (Duranest)
Bupivacaine (Marcaine, Sensorcaine)
Ropivacaine (Naropin)
Lidocaine (Xylocaine)

TABLE 122-2. Local anesthetic dosing recommendations for FDA-approved and nonapproved indications

Drug	Concentration (%)	Volume (ml)	Total dose (mg)
Chloroprocaine			
FDA-approved procedures			
Mandibular	2	2–3	40–60
Infraorbital	2	0.5–1	10–20
Brachial plexus	2	30–40	600–800
Digital	1	3–4	30–40
Pudendal	2	10/each side	400
Paracervical	1	3/each of 4 sites	up to 120
FDA-nonapproved procedures			
IVRA upper limb	0.5	40	200
IVRA lower limb	0.5	60	300
Epidural	3	5/increment to T_4 block	150/increment
		20–30/h[a]	600–900/h[a]
Tetracaine			
FDA-approved procedures			
Spinal	1	0.5–1.5	5–15
FDA-nonapproved procedures			
Brachial plexus	0.25	4	10
Sciatic/femoral	0.25	4	10
Intercostal	0.25	4	10
Caudal	0.1–0.25	0.5–1.5/space	0.5–3.75/space
	0.25	15–20	37.5–50
			2 mg/kg[b]
Epidural	0.25	6–14	15–35
	0.5	3–10	15–50
Mepivacaine			
FDA-approved procedures			
Cervical, brachial, intercostal, pudendal	1	5–40	50–400
	2	5–20	100–400
		0.4/kg[b]	8/kg[b]

Transvaginal (paracervical + pudendal)	1	Up to 30 (both sides)	Up to 300 (both sides)
Paracervical	1	Up to 20 (both sides)	Up to 200 (both sides)
Caudal and epidural	1	15–30	150–300
	1.5	10–25	150–375
		0.73/kg[b]	11/kg[b]
	2	10–20	200–400
Therapeutic (pain)	1	1–5	10–50
	2	1–5	20–100
FDA-nonapproved procedures			
Epidural	2	10/h[a]	200/h[a]
Etidocaine			
FDA-approved procedures			
Peripheral nerve	1	5–40	50–400
Peridural	1	10–30	100–300
	1.5	10–20	150–300
Caudal	1	10–30	100–300
Retrobulbar	1	2–4	20–40
	1.5	2–4	30–60
Maxillary	1.5	1–5	15–75
FDA-nonapproved procedures			
Intercostal	0.5	30–60	150–300
	1	3/space	30/space
Thoracic epidural	1.5	4/h[a]	60/h[a]
Brachial plexus	0.5	20–30	100–150
	0.75	20–30	150–225
Celiac plexus	0.25	40	100
Prilocaine			
FDA-nonapproved procedures			
IVRA upper limb	0.5	40	200
	1	20–40	300–400
Epidural	2	20	400
Brachial plexus	1.5	30	450
Sciatic/femoral	1	25–35	250–350
	1.5	20–30	300–450
Peripheral nerve			5–7/kg[b,c]

Continued

TABLE 122-2. *Continued.*

Drug	Concentration (%)	Volume (ml)	Total dose (mg)
Lidocaine			
FDA-approved procedures			
IVRA	0.5	10–60	50–300
Brachial plexus	1.5	15–20	225–300
Intercostal	1	3/space	30/space
Paravertebral	1	3–5	30–50
Pudendal (each side)	1	10	100
Paracervical (each side)	1	10	100
Cervical	1	5	50
Lumbar	1	5–10	50–100
Epidural (thoracic)	1	20–30	200–300
(lumbar)	1	25–30	250–300
Caudal (obstetrical)	1	20–30	250–300
(surgical)	1.5	15–20	225–300
FDA-nonapproved procedures			
Interpleural			2.1/min[a]
Intercostal	2	5/space	100/space
	1.5/1[a,d]	0.2/kg/0.1/kg/h[a,d]	3/kg/1/kg/h[a,d]
Epidural	1.5	5/increment to T_4 block	75/increment
	2	15–20	300–400
	2/0.4[a,d]	8–15/0.5–1 per min[a,d]	160–300/2–4/min[a,d]
	1.5/0.75[a,d]	10/1h[a,d]	150/75/h[a,d]
Caudal			5–7/kg[b]
	1.5[b]	0.73/kg[b]	11/kg[b]
Brachial plexus	1[b]	10[b]	100[b]
Intraarticular	0.5	20	100
Spinal	2	2.5–3	
			1.2/inch of body height
			100
	1	1/0.5–1 increment to block	10/5–10 increment to block
Sciatic/femoral	1[b]	1/y of age[b]	10/y of age[b]

Bupivacaine			
FDA-approved procedures			
Epidural	0.75	10–20	75–150
	0.5	10–20	50–100
	0.25	10–20	25–50
Caudal	0.5	15–30	75–150
	0.25	15–30	37.5–75
Peripheral nerve	0.5	5 to max. 80	25 to max. 400
	0.25	5 to max. 160	12.5 to max. 400
Retrobulbar	0.75	2–4	15–30
Sympathetic	0.25	20–50	50–125
Intraarticular	0.25	20–40	50–100
	0.5	20–30	100–150
	0.75	20	150
FDA-nonapproved procedures			
Caudal	0.75	0.3/kg	2.2/kg
	0.25[b]	1.2/kg[b]	3/kg[b]
	0.5[b]	0.75/kg[b]	3.7/kg[b]
			1.5–2.5/kg[b]
	0.125	1/kg	1.25/kg
Sciatic/femoral	0.25[b]	5–10[b]	12.5–25[b]
	0.25/0.125[a,d]	30/6 per h[a,d]	75/7.5/h[a,d]
	0.5	0.6/kg	3/kg
	0.375	45	169
	0.25–0.5/0.25–0.5[a,d]	10–20/2–4/h[a,d]	25–100/5–20/h[a,d]
	0.25/0.25[a,d]	10/7/h[a,d]	25/17.5/h[a,d]
Peripheral nerve			1.5–2.5/kg[b]
Intercostal	0.25	3/h[a]	7.5/h[a]
	0.5/0.5[a,d]	10/5–7/h[a,d]	50/25–35/h[a,d]
	0.75/0.25[a,d]	20–28/5–9h[a,d]	150–210/12.5–22.5/h[a,d]
	0.5	12 q8h	60 q8h
	0.5/0.5[a,d]	20/0.1/kg/h[a,d]	100/0.5/kg/h[a,d]
	0.5/0.5[a,d]	30/3/h[a,d]	150/15/h[a,d]
	0.5/0.5[a,d]	20/5–10/h[a,d]	100/25–50/h[a,d]

Continued

TABLE 122-2. *Continued.*

Drug	Concentration (%)	Volume (ml)	Total dose (mg)
Brachial plexus	0.25[b]	10[b]	25[b]
	0.25–0.5/0.25–0.5[a,d]	10–20/2–4/h[a,d]	25–100/5–20/h[a,d]
Lumbar plexus	0.5/0.25[a,d]	0.4/0.14/h[a,d]	2/kg/0.35/kg/h[a,d]
Spinal	0.125	6–10	7.5–12.5
	0.5	4	20
	0.5	2.5	12.5
	0.25/0.125[a,d]	1.5/1.5/h[a,d]	3.75/1.875/h[a,d]
	0.25	0.5	1.25
Epidural	0.25–0.375/NA[a,d]	0.5–1/0.5–1/h[a,d]	1.25–3.75/1.25–3.75/h[a,d]
	0.25/0.25 or 0.125[a,d]	12–15/7 or 12/h[a,d]	
	0.166[a]	1–6/h[a]	30–37.5/15–17.5/h[a,d]
	0.125[a]	10/h[a]	1.66–9.96/ha
	0.25/0.25[a,b,d]	0.5/kg/0.08/kg/h[a,b,d]	12.5/h[a]
			1.25/kg/0.2/kg/h[a,b,d]
	0.5/0.5[a,d]	20–25/8/h[a]	
	0.1–0.5[a]	4–18/h[a]	100–125/40/h[a,d]
	0.5	0.5/kg[b]	0.4–90/h[a]
			2.5/kg[b]
			2–2.5/kg/0.4–0.5/kg/h[b,e]
	0.75/0.75/0.25[a,d]	7/4/h/4/h[a,d]	2–2.5/kg/0.2–0.25/kg/h[b,f]
	0.25/0.125[a,d]	10/10/h[a,d]	
	0.2/0.2[a,d]	5/3–5/h[a,d]	
	0.25/0.125[a,d]	10/7/h[a,d]	52.5/30/h/10/h[a,d]
	0.5/0.5[a,d]	20–30/8/h[a,d]	25/12.5/h[a,d]
	0.975	16	10/6–10/h[a,d]
	0.5/0.5[a,b,d]	0.2/kg/0.2/h/kg[a,b,d]	25/8.75/h[a,d]
			10.–150/40/h[a,d]
	0.25/0.25[a,b,d]	0.05/kg/segment/0.1/kg/h[a,b,d]	156
	0.125[b]	0.75/kg[b]	1/kg/1/kg/h[a,b,d]
	0.125–0.25[a]	0.1–0.4/kg/h[a]	0.125/kg/segment/0.25/kg/h[a,b,d]

	0.5/0.25[a,d]	6/3/h[a,d]	
	0.125[a]	5/h[a]	0.9375/kg[b]
	0.5/0.125[a,d]	8/7.5/h[a,d]	0.25–0.5/kg/h[a]
	0.1[a]	3–6/h[a]	30/7.5/h[a,d]
	0.25/0.25[a,d]	10–20/7/h[a,d]	6.25/h[a]
	0.1/0.1[a,d]	5/5/h[a,d]	40/9.375/h[a,d]
			3–6/h[a]
			25–50/17.5/h[a,d]
			5/5/h[a,d]
	0.5/0.8[a,d]	6/15/h[a,d]	30/12/h[a,d]
	0.5/0.5[a,d]	9/5/h[a,d]	45/25/h[a,d]
	0.25/0.25[a,d]	10/3–10/h[a,d]	25/7.5–25/h[a,d]
	0.5/0.125[a,d]	10/15/h[a,d]	50/18.75/h[a,d]
Interpleural	0.25[a]	5/h[a]	12.5/h[a]
			1.5/kg
	0.25[a,b]	0.5/kg/h[a,b]	1.25/kg/h[a,b]
	0.25	10–20	25–50
	0.5	20	100
	0.5/0.25[a,d]	20/8/h[a,d]	100/20/h[a,d]
	0.5/0.25[a,d]	15–20/5–10/h[a,d]	75–100/12.5–25/h[a,d]
	0.375/0.375[a,d]	20/6/h[a,d]	75/22.5/h[a,d]
	0.375	20 q4h	75 q4h
	0.25	20–40	50–100
	0.5	20–30	100–150
	0.5	21	105
	0.25[a]	0.125/kg/h[a]	0.3125/kg/h[a]
	0.5	0.4/kg q6h	2/kg q6h
	0.25	20 q4h	50 q4h
	0.5	20 q4h	100 q4h
	0.5a	10/h[a]	50 h[a]
	0.5/0.25[a,d]	20/10/h[a,d]	100 25/h[a,d]
	0.25	10 q8h	25 q8h
	0.375	20 q6h	75 q6h

Continued

TABLE 122-2. *Continued.*

Drug	Concentration (%)	Volume (ml)	Total dose (mg)
	0.375	20	75
	0.25[a,b]	0.5–1/kg/h[a,b]	1.25–2.5/kg/h[a,b]
Ropivacaine			
FDA-approved procedures			
Epidural anesthesia	0.5	15–30	75–100
	0.75	15–25	119–188
	1.0	15–20	150–200
Major nerve block	0.50	35–50	175–250
Peripheral nerve block	0.50	1–40	5–200
Epidural pain management	0.5	5–15	25–75
	0.2	6–10/h[a]	12–20/h[a]

IVRA, intravenous regional anesthesia; NA, not available; q4h, every 4 hours; q8h, every 8 hours.
[a] Continuous infusion.
[b] Pediatric dose.
[c] Maximum dose = 600 mg, not recommended ≤ 6 months of age.
[d] Loading dose/maintenance dose.
[e] Older infants, toddlers, children.
[f] Neonates.

V. Drug interactions. The combined use of local anesthetics and sedative-hypnotic agents can enhance central nervous system (CNS) and respiratory depression. Similarly, myocardial depression and dysrhythmias may be observed when local anesthetics are used in conjuction with type Ia antiarrhythmics (e.g., quinidine). Decreased cholinesterase activity from either anticholinesterase agents (e.g., organophosphate insecticides, neostigmine) or altered endogenous activity (genetic variation, pregnant women, infants, hepatic disease) will prolong the effects of ester derivatives. Increased plasma lidocaine concentrations can occur with the use of cimetidine.

Selected Readings

Barash PG, Kopri VA, Langou R, et al. Is cocaine a sympathetic stimulant during general anesthesia? *JAMA* 1980;243:1437.

This study demonstrated that topical administration of cocaine did not cause significant changes in cardiovascular functions.

Berkowitz A, Rosenberg J. Femoral block with mepivacaine for muscle biopsy in malignant hyperthermia patients. *Anesthesiology* 1985;62:651.

This report demonstrated the safe use of mepivacaine for cutaneous nerve blocks in patients susceptible to malignant hyperthermia.

Bigler D, Hjortso NC, Edstrom H, et al. Comparative effects of intrathecal bupivacaine and tetracaine on analgesia, cardiovascular function and plasma catecholamines. *Acta Anaesthesiol Scand* 1986;30:199.

This study demonstrated intrathecal tetracaine to cause systemic hypotension from sympathetic blockade.

Grant SA, Hoffman RS. Use of tetracaine, epinephrine, and cocaine as a topical anesthetic in the emergency department. *Ann Emerg Med* 1992;21:987.

This review discussed the pharmacology and efficacy of the topical preparation tetracaine, adrenaline, and cocaine (TAC).

Hall AH, Kulig KW, Rumack BH. Drug- and chemical-induced methaemoglobinaemia. *Medical Toxicology* 1986;1:253.

This article discussed the various causes of methemoglobinemia, including the local anesthetic agents.

Jatlow P, Barash PG, Van Dyke C, et al. Cocaine and succinylcholine sensitivity: a new caution. *Anesth Analg* 1979;58:235.

This study demonstrated prolonged duration of cocaine in patients with low dibucaine numbers (atypical cholinesterase), documented succinylcholine sensitivity, or both.

Johnson WT, De Stigter T. Hypersensitivity to procaine, tetracaine, mepivacaine, and methylparaben: report of a case. *J Am Dent Assoc* 1983;106(1):53.

This report describes an allergic reaction to local anesthetic agents.

Kellet PB, Copeland CS. Methemoglobinemia associated benzocaine-containing lubricant. *Anesthesiology* 1983;59:463.

This report discussed methemoglobinemia induced by benzocaine use.

Mofenson HC, Caraccio TR, Miller H, et al. Lidocaine toxicity from topical mucosal application. *Clin Pediatr* 1983;22:190.

A discussion of lidocaine-induced seizures from its topical administration.

Moore PA. Bupivacaine: a long-lasting local anesthetic for dentistry. *Oral Surg* 1984;58:369.

This review discussed the benefits of bupivacaine over other local anesthetics.

Orlinsky M, Hudson C, Chan L, et al. Pain comparison of unbuffered versus buffered lidocaine in local wound infiltration. *J Emerg Med* 1992;10:441.

This study demonstrated less pain when lidocaine is mixed with sodium bicarbonate prior to local wound infiltration.

Prescott LT, Adjepon-Yamoah KK, Talbot RG. Impaired lignocaine metabolism in patients with myocardial infarction and cardiac failure. *BMJ* 1976;1:939.

This study showed increased serum lidocaine concentrations in patients with congestive heart failure during lidocaine therapy.

Skidmore RA, Patterson JD, Tomsick RS. Local anesthetics. *Dermatol Surg* 1996; 22:511.

This review discussed the pharmacokinetics and adverse effects associated with the local anesthetic agents.

Southorn P, Vasdev GMS, Chantigian RC, et al. Reducing the potential morbidity of an unintentional spinal anaesthetic by aspirating cerebrospinal fluid. *Br J Anaesth* 1996;76:467.

This report described central nervous system toxicity resulting from the inadvertent contamination of the cerebral spinal fluid with the local anesthetic during spinal anesthesia.

123. METHYLXANTHINE POISONING

Erica L. Liebelt

I. General principles. Theophylline is the methylxanthine of most clinical importance, although caffeine and theobromine, with similar clinical toxicity, may also be encountered in poisoning (Table 123-1). Intentional overdoses and iatrogenic misadventures (miscalculation of dose, change in frequency of administration, lack of serum drug level monitoring, overdosing of a patient in whom chronic illness or an unrecognized drug-to-drug interaction leads to reduced clearance of theophylline) account for most theophylline poisonings.

II. Pathophysiology. The pathophysiology of theophylline remains incompletely understood, although three primary mechanisms have been postulated: inhibition of cyclic guanosine monophosphate (cGMP) or adenosine monophosphate (cAMP) activity, adenosine receptor antagonism, and β-adrenergic stimulation secondary to elevated levels of circulating plasma catecholamines.

Theophylline is metabolized by the mixed function oxidase system in the liver. Many drugs, chemicals, and medical conditions affect the steady-state serum concentration and elimination half-life of theophylline. Drugs or conditions increasing serum theophylline concentration include erythromycin, fluoroquinolones, antacids, beta-blockers, cirrhosis, and congestive heart failure. At therapeutic doses, the elimination half-life of theophylline varies widely with the age of the patient. It averages 4.5 to 5 hours in healthy adults, is shorter in children and smokers, and longer in infants, the elderly, and those with heart, liver, and pulmonary disease.

III. Clinical toxicity. Cardiac, central nervous system (CNS), gastrointestinal, and musculoskeletal symptoms as well as metabolic derangements characterize theophylline toxicity. Sinus tachycardia is invariably present but supraventricular tachycardia and ventricular arrhythmias can also occur. In mild theophylline poisoning, mild hypertension can occur, whereas in severe theophylline poisoning, hypotension with a widened pulse pressure is seen. Seizures are also characteristic of severe theophylline poisoning. They are usually multiple and typically recalcitrant to conventional anticonvulsants. Seizures after theophylline intoxication are associated with a high frequency of permanent neurologic disability and a mortality rate that approaches 50% in elderly patients.

Gastrointestinal effects consist of vomiting, diarrhea, and hematemesis. Skeletal muscle tremor, a common feature, can include myoclonic jerks. Metabolic acidosis, hypokalemia, hyperglycemia, hypophosphatemia, hypomagnesemia, and hypercalcemia are the primary metabolic disturbances accompanying acute theophylline intoxication.

The clinical presentation varies depending on whether the poisoning occurs through a single ingestion (acute intoxication), chronic overmedication (chronic intoxication), or acute on therapeutic intoxication (where the patient has maintained serum theophylline concentrations in the therapeutic range but then ingests a single toxic dose). After acute overdose, mild clinical intoxication (nausea, vomiting, tachycardia) occurs with theophylline concentrations of 20 to 40 μg/ml; with levels greater than 70 μg/ml, life-threatening events (intractable seizures and severe cardiac arrhythmias) can appear. Metabolic abnormalities are seen more commonly with acute intoxications. In chronic intoxication, no correlation is seen between serum theophylline concentration and the appearance of life-threatening events, although age appears to be a significant risk factor. Serious toxicity can occur even with theophylline concentrations in the therapeutic or mildly toxic range. Toxicity is typically delayed and prolonged after ingestions of sustained-release formulations.

IV. Evaluation. The physical examination should focus on the cardiovascular and neuromuscular systems. Cardiac rhythm and oxygen saturation should be monitored. Laboratory tests should include serum theophylline concentration, serum electrolytes, arterial blood gas, anion gap, blood urea nitrogen, creatinine, calcium,

TABLE 123-1. Xanthine derivatives

Common name	Chemical name
Aminophylline	Theophylline ethylenediamine
Caffeine	1,3,7-Trimethyl xanthine
Dyphylline	7-(2,3-Dihydroxypropyl) theophylline
Enprofylline	3-Propyl xanthine
Oxtriphylline	7-Choline theophylline
Pentoxifylline	Dimethyl-1-(5-oxyhexyl) xanthine
Theobromine	3,7-Dimethyl xanthine
Theophylline	1,3-Dimethyl xanthine

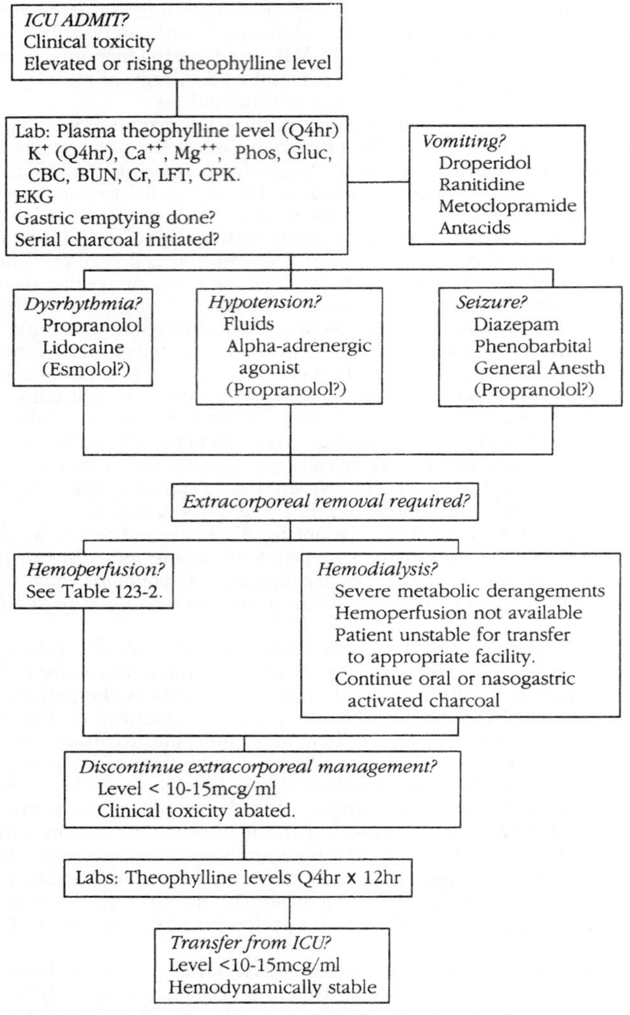

FIG. 123-1. Management of theophylline poisoning.

TABLE 123-2. Indications for hemodialysis/hemoperfusion

Acute toxicity
Peak serum theophylline concentration > 80–100 µg/ml
Peak serum theophylline concentration > 60–80 µg/ml and intractable vomiting
Theophylline concentration > 70 µg/ml 4 hours after ingestion of sustained-release preparation
Seizures or cardiac arrhythmias or hypotension and theophylline concentration > 40 µg/ml
Chronic toxicity
Age > 60 years or < 6 months and theophylline concentration > 40 µg/ml
Age < 60 years or > 6 months and theophylline concentration > 60 µg/ml
Patients with respiratory failure, congestive heart failure, or liver disease

magnesium, phosphorus, glucose, creatine phosphokinase, complete blood count, and electrocardiogram. Theophylline concentrations should be obtained every 1 to 2 hours until a peak or plateau and subsequent decline has been observed. Urine should be evaluated frequently for evidence of myoglobinuria, particularly in patients who develop seizures.

V. Management. The management of theophylline intoxication involves decreasing systemic absorption, enhancing elimination, and providing supportive care (Fig. 123-1). Supportive care should focus on airway protection, correction of cardiovascular abnormalities, and maintenance of normal blood pH. In patients who present after large ingestions of sustained-release preparations, gastric emptying should be considered because of the propensity for these tablets to coalesce. Oral-activated charcoal is highly effective at reducing the absorption of theophylline and should be administered to all patients with recent ingestions.

Multiple-dose activated charcoal greatly enhances the elimination of theophylline and can be as effective as hemodialysis. Aggressive antiemetic therapy (e.g., droperidol, metoclopramide, ondansetron, and histamine antagonists) may be necessary in order for the patient to tolerate charcoal. Cimetidine, however, should be avoided because it impairs theophylline clearance.

In severely intoxicated patients, rapid removal of theophylline using hemodialysis or hemoperfusion is imperative (Table 123-2). A nephrologist should be involved early in these cases. Charcoal hemoperfusion has traditionally been considered the extracorporeal removal method of choice for theophylline toxicity. However, hemodialysis, which has also been accepted as an alternative method of extracorporeal drug removal, offers some advantages over hemoperfusion; specifically, it is more readily performed, more widely available, and has a lower risk of bleeding diathesis.

Adenosine can be used to treat hemodynamically significant supraventricular tachycardia. Lidocaine is the recommended treatment for ventricular arrhythmias with hemodynamic compromise. Phenylephrine or norepinephrine may be more efficacious than dopamine as a vasopressor agent for hypotension.

Seizures should be treated aggressively with high doses of benzodiazepines. Phenytoin is unlikely to be effective. Thiopental or pentobarbital may be necessary for prolonged seizures. Neuromuscular blockade should also be considered for refractory seizures because of potential morbidity resulting from rhabdomyolysis, hyperthermia, and acidosis.

Hypokalemia results from the intracellular shift of potassium rather than from decreased total body potassium content. Treatment is best accomplished by lowering the theophylline concentration. Aggressive potassium replacement can result in hyperkalemia when toxicity resolves.

Selected Readings

Amitai Y, Lovejoy FH. Characteristics of vomiting associated with acute sustained release theophylline poisoning: implications for management with oral activated charcoal. *J Toxicol Clin Toxicol* 1987;25:539.

A case series of patients with protracted vomiting from acute theophylline toxicity and limiting ability to tolerate oral charcoal, suggesting the need for aggressive antiemetic therapy.

Olson KR, Benowitz NL, Woo OF, et al. Theophylline overdose: acute single ingestion versus chronic repeated overmedication. *Am J Emerg Med* 1985;3:386.

A case series of patients with acute and chronic theophylline intoxication demonstrating different clinical and metabolic characteristics between the two groups.

Shannon M. Life-threatening events after theophylline overdose: a 10-year prospective analysis. *Arch Intern Med* 1999;159:989.

Most comprehensive series of patients with theophylline intoxication demonstrating that chronic overmedication results in significantly more morbidity and mortality.

Shannon M. Predictors of major toxicity after theophylline overdose. *Ann Intern Med* 1993;119:1161.

A prospective series of 249 patients demonstrating that major toxicity was associated with peak theophylline concentration greater than 100 mg/L after acute intoxication and age more than 60 years (regardless of theophylline concentration) after chronic overmedication.

Shannon M, Lovejoy FH. The influence of age vs. peak serum concentration on life-threatening events after chronic theophylline intoxication. *Arch Intern Med* 1990;150:2045.

A case series of patients with chronic theophylline intoxication demonstrating that peak theophylline concentration was unable to predict which patients would have seizures or arrhythmias.

Shannon MW. Comparative efficacy of hemodialysis and hemoperfusion in severe theophylline intoxication. *Acad Emerg Med* 1997;4:674.

A 10-year prospective observational study demonstrating comparable efficacy of hemodialysis and hemoperfusion in reducing the morbidity of severe theophylline intoxication.

124. MONOAMINE OXIDASE INHIBITOR POISONING

Jeffrey R. Tucker

I. General principles. Monoamine oxidase inhibitors (MAOIs) have been used in the treatment of depression since the 1950s. Current indications include neurotic illness with depressive features, treatment-resistant depression, atypical depression, eating disorders, anxiety, and phobia. Available agents include isocarboxazid (Marplan), phenelzine (Nardil), and tranylcypromine (Parnate). The antitumor agent procarbazine (Matulane) also inhibits MAO. Selegiline (Eldepryl), used in the treatment of dementia and Parkinson's disease, selectively inhibits MAO-B.

II. Pathogenesis. Monoamine oxidase is a flavin-containing enzyme located in the mitochondrial membranes of almost all tissues. Two distinct molecular types of MAO have been identified: MAO-A and MAO-B. Monoaminergic neurons contain predominantly MAO-A, whereas serotonergic neurons contain MAO-A and MAO-B.

Monoamine oxidase is involved in the regulation of catecholamine metabolism. Neuronal MAO inactivates, by oxidative deamination, epinephrine, norepinephrine, dopamine, and 5-hydroxytryptophan (5-HT). Hepatic MAO, along with catechol-O-methyl transferase, inactivates endogenous (adrenal), ingested or parenterally administered monoamines. MAO present in the gut wall also contributes to the inactivation of dietary monoamines such as tyramine. Inhibition of MAO prevents these functions.

When given by mouth, MAOIs are readily absorbed. Maximal MAO inhibition occurs within days but maximal antidepressant effects do not occur for 2 to 3 weeks. Their biologic activity is prolonged because they irreversibly inactivate MAO. Two weeks may be required for the normal activity of MAO to be restored after withdrawal of these agents.

III. Clinical presentation

A. Acute toxicity. Acute overdose is characterized by a delay in onset of clinical toxicity for as long as 24 hours after ingestion. Toxicity begins with manifestations of neuromuscular hyperactivity such as agitation, tremors, hyperreflexia, and myoclonus. Manifestations of more advanced toxicity include altered mental status; increased pulse, blood pressure, and temperature; and rhabdomyolysis. Severe toxicity is characterized by seizures, central nervous system depression, respiratory depression, rigidity, hyperpyrexia, hypotension, cardiovascular collapse, and death.

B. Chronic toxicity. Patient with chronic toxicity may manifest tremors, insomnia, hyperhidrosis, agitation, hypomanic behavior, hallucinations, confusion, and seizures.

C. Drug and dietary interactions. A sympathomimetic reaction can occur following exposure to monoamines such as amphetamines, cocaine, dopamine, epinephrine, isoproterenol, norepinephrine, phenylephrine, and tyramine. Foods with high tyramine content include aged cheeses; aged, pickled, putrefied, or smoked fish and meats; red wine; and yeast. Manifestations include headache, hypertension, tachycardia, diaphoresis, agitation, hypertonicity, hyperreflexia with myoclonus, rigidity, seizure, and coma. Effects begin 30 to 90 minutes after exposure. The duration of effect is variable but often resolves with a few hours. The serotonin syndrome can result from the interaction between MAOIs and drugs with serotoninergic activity (e.g., meperidine, dextromethorphan, fluoxetine, sumatriptan, and venlafaxine). The reaction is characterized by rapid onset of disorientation, muscular rigidity, severe hypertension or hypotension, coma, seizures, and death. Other adverse drug interactions have been reported with theophylline, levodopa, sulfonylureas, and imipramine.

IV. Evaluation. The physical examination should focus on assessing the cardiovascular status, mental status, and neuromuscular activity. Patients with abnormal vital signs or neuromuscular hyperactivity should have an electrocardiogram, complete blood count, serum electrolytes, blood urea nitrogen, creatinine, glucose and creatinine phosphokinase, and a urinalysis. Patients with moderate to severe toxicity should also have an arterial blood gas analysis, coagulation profile, liver function tests, and chest x-ray study. Those with evidence of rhabdomyolysis should have serum calcium, magnesium, and phosphate levels evaluated. MAOIs are generally not detectable by routine toxicology testing.

V. Treatment. Avoidance of iatrogenic drug and dietary interactions is critical in the care of patients on MAOIs who are hospitalized for any reason. Patients with suspected MAOI overdose require extended observation in a monitored setting because of the potential for delayed toxicity. Continuous cardiac monitoring should also be instituted. Treatment should focus on stabilization of abnormal vital signs and control of neuromuscular hyperactivity. Decontamination with activated charcoal is recommended in patients with recent ingestions.

Agitation, neuromuscular hyperactivity, and seizures can lead to hyperpyrexia and other complications such as metabolic acidosis, disseminated intravascular coagulation (DIC), rhabdomyolysis, and neurologic morbidity. Aggressive control with benzodiazepines, barbiturates, and pharmacologic paralysis is appropriate. Seizures may require large doses of benzodiazepines or phenobarbital. Phenothiazines and butyrophenones should be avoided in the treatment of agitation. Routine cooling measures should be used for the treatment of hyperthermia. Reliance on antipyretic agents is inappropriate for patients who have pharmacologically induced temperature elevations. The use of dantrolene and bromocriptine for the treatment of hyperpyrexia and neuromuscular hyperactivity caused by MAOI overdose is controversial.

Severe hypertension is most safely treated with a rapidly reversible agent such as intravenous nitroprusside or nitroglycerin. Longer acting agents have also been recommended, but should be used with caution because hypertension is often followed by severe hypotension.

Resuscitation of the hypotensive patients begins with volume replacement. Pressors may be necessary in refractory cases. A direct-acting agent (e.g., norepinephrine) is preferred to indirect-acting agents (e.g., dopamine), which require the release of intracellular amines.

Cardiac arrhythmias are generally a premorbid sign; when present, they should be treated with lidocaine, procainamide, or phenytoin. Bretylium causes release of stored catecholamine and should be avoided in the treatment of arrhythmias.

Patients with severe or symptomatic hypertension after drug or dietary interactions should be treated with a rapidly acting oral agent such as nifedipine or a parenteral agent such as labetalol, nitroprusside, nitroglycerin, or phentolamine. Mild hypertension may respond to benzodiazepine.

Patients with the serotonin syndrome have been successfully treated with nonselective 5-HT antagonists such as cyproheptadine, methysergide, haloperidol, and propanolol. Cyprohepatadine and methysergide must be administered orally, whereas haloperidol and propanolol can be given intravenously. The initial dose of cyprohepatidine is 4 to 8 mg. A response is typically noted within 2 hours.

Selected Readings

Asch DA, Parker RM. The Libby Zion case. *N Engl J Med* 1988;318:771.

A case of unknown monoamine oxidase inhibitor adverse drug reaction which had a significant impact on medical education.

Ciraulo DA, Shader RI. Fluoxetine drug-drug interactions. I. Antidepressants and antipsychotics. *J Clin Psychopharmacol* 1990;10:48.

A brief review about the potential for drugs interaction between selective serotonin reuptake inhibitors and monoamine oxidase inhibitors.

Clary C, Mandos L, Schweizer E. Results of a brief survey on the prescribing practices for monoamine oxidase inhibitor antidepressants. *J Clin Psychiatry* 1990;51:226.

Recent survey about the prescribing practice of psychiatrists and the infrequent use of monoamine oxidase inhibitors.

Fallon B, Foorte B, Walsh BT, et al. Spontaneous hypertensive episodes with monoamine oxidase inhibitors. *J Clin Psychiatry* 1988;49:163.

Two case reports and a review of unexplained hypertensive reactions to monoamine oxidase inhibitors with no known dietary or medication interactions.

Feighner JP, Boyer WF, Tyler DL, et al. Adverse consequences of fluoxetine–monoamine oxidase inhibitor combination therapy. *J Clin Psychiatry* 1990;51:222.

Clinical series of patients treated with monoamine oxidase inhibitors and fluoxetine who developed serotonin syndrome.

Kaplan RF, Feinglass NG, Webster W, et al. Phenelzine overdose treated with dantrolene sodium. *JAMA* 1986:255:642.

Discusses the use of dantrolene for the hypermetabolic response of monoamine oxidase inhibitor overdose.

Linden CH, Rumack BH, Strehilke C. Monoamine oxidase inhibitor overdose. *Ann Emerg Med* 1984;13:1137.

A case report of the typical findings of monoamine oxidase inhibitor overdose and a review of the literature.

Martin TG. Serotonin syndrome. *Ann Emerg Med* 1996;28:520.

An excellent review of this new serotonin syndrome with a discussion of its pathophysiology and the clinical manifestation.

Murphy DL, Sunolerland T, Cohen RM. Monoamine oxidase inhibiting antidepressants: a clinical update. *Psychiatr Clin North Am* 1984;7:549.

An excellent review about the efficacy of monoamine oxidase inhibitors and the important drug and food interaction that exists with the unique antidepressants.

Pope HG, Jones JM, Hudson JL, et al. Toxic reactions to the combination of monoamine oxidase inhibitors and tryptophan. *Am J Psychiatry* 1985;142:491.

Presentation of eight case of neurologic toxicity with the combination of monoamine oxidase inhibitor and L-tryptophan.

Sauter D, Linden CH. Monoamine oxidase inhibitor toxicity. In: Irwin RS, Cerra FB, Rippe JM, eds. *Intensive care medicine,* 4th ed. Philadelphia: Lippincott–Raven; 1998.

Comprehensive review with extensive reference list.

Thorp M, Toombs D, Harmon B. Monoamine oxidase inhibitor overdose. *West J Med* 1997;166:275.

A case report with an extensive table of adverse monoamine oxidase inhibitor drug interactions.

Tolelson GD. Monoamine oxidase inhibitors: a review. *J Clin Psychiatry* 1983;44:280.

A review of monoamine oxidase inhibitors with a focus on the mechanism of action, clinical indications and drug interactions.

125. NEUROLEPTIC AGENTS

Richard Y. Wang

I. General principles. Neuroleptics, also known as antipsychotic agents and major tranquilizers, are primarily used in the therapy of schizophrenia, the manic phase of bipolar disorders, and agitated behavior. They are also used as preanesthetics and to treat nausea, vomiting, headaches, and hiccups. Neuroleptics primarily act by binding to and blocking type 2 dopamine receptors in the central nervous system (CNS). They also have variable affinity for α-adrenergic, histamine, muscarinic, serotonergic, and other dopaminergic receptors. Toxic effects include anticholinergic syndrome, extrapyramidal syndromes, neuroleptic malignant syndrome, and central nervous and cardiovascular system depression.

II. Clinical manifestations

A. Toxicology. Toxicity following overdosage results from exaggerated pharmacologic activity; it includes CNS and cardiovascular depression and agitated delirium. CNS depression is usually evident within 1 to 2 hours, and maximal severity is apparent within 6 hours of ingestion. Seizures, neuromuscular agitation, loss of sweating ability, and hypothalamic dysfunction can cause hyperthermia.

Cardiovascular effects include hypotension, cardiac conduction disturbances, tachyarrhythmias, and bradyarrhythmias. Conduction disturbances include all degrees of atrioventricular (AV) block, bundle-branch, and fascicular block, and nonspecific intraventricular conduction delay. Electrocardiographic changes (e.g., prolonged PR and QT intervals, ST-segment depression, T-wave abnormalities, and increased U waves) may be seen within several hours of overdose. Thioridazine, mesoridazine, and pimozide are responsible for the most fatal poisonings because of their greater cardiotoxicity. Although neuroleptic malignant syndrome is an idiosyncratic reaction and rarely occurs following acute overdose, hypertension, hyperthermia, and hypertonia have been described. Early deaths are caused by arrhythmias, shock, aspiration, and respiratory failure. Later complications include cerebral and pulmonary edema, disseminated intravascular coagulation, renal failure, and infection.

B. Adverse effects. Unintended effects may occur early or late during the course of therapy and can be the result of interactions with other drugs. Extrapyramidal side effects are common, resulting from the interference with dopaminergic function in the basal ganglia. Common with low-milligram, high-potency agents, they can occur early (hours to days), at an intermediate stage (days to months), or late (> 3 months) in the course of therapy. Early extrapyramidal syndromes include acute dystonia; intermediate syndromes include akathisia and parkinsonism; and late disorders include tardive dyskinesia and focal perioral tremor.

C. Acute dystonic reactions are characterized by abrupt onset, an intermittent and repetitive nature, normal physical examination except for muscular findings, a history of recent drug use, and rapid response to anticholinergic drug therapy. Muscle contractions may be focal at the onset and then spread to contiguous muscles. Patients remain alert and oriented. Muscles of the eye, face, tongue, neck, and torso can be involved. Although these reactions are rarely life-threatening, those involving the tongue, jaw, and neck can result in upper airway compromise, impaired respiratory mechanics, and death.

Symptoms of akathisia include feeling restless, jittery, and tense, and difficulty in sitting still. Examination may reveal agitation and motor hyperactivity with semipurposeful limb movements, especially of the legs and feet.

Drug-induced parkinsonism is indistinguishable from other causes of this syndrome except for the history of drug exposure. It is characterized by increased motor tone, decreased motor activity, tremors, and postural instability. Tremors typically occur in the forearm and hand, are present at rest, worsen with agitation or excitement, and disappear with sleep. Examination may also reveal a shuffling gait cogwheel rigidity, limited upward gaze and positive glabellar, snout, and sucking reflexes.

D. Differential diagnosis. Poisoning by alcohols, antiarrhythmics, anticholinergics, anticonvulsants, antihistamines, opioids, and sedative-hypnotic agents can cause CNS and cardiovascular effects similar to those resulting from a neuroleptic overdose. Acute dystonic reaction can be confused with seizures, cerebrovascular accidents, encephalitis, tetanus, hypocalcemia, and strychnine poisoning.

III. Management

A. Overdose. Patients with protracted hypotension, CNS depression or agitation, seizures, or arrhythmias should be admitted to an intensive care setting. Hypotension should be treated with intravenous fluids initially, and then with direct-acting vasopressors (e.g., norepinephrine, phenylephrine). Sinus and supraventricular tachycardias rarely require treatment. Ventricular tachycardia should be treated with lidocaine or electrical cardioversion, depending on hemodyanmic stability. Sodium bicarbonate (1–2 mEq/kg) infusion is recommended for patients with wide QRS complexes. Type Ia, Ic, and II antiarrhythmics are to be avoided. Symptomatic bradyarrhythmias should be treated with atropine, epinephrine, dopamine, and isoproterenol. Seizures can be treated with benzodizepines or short-acting barbiturates. The effectiveness of phenytoin for phenothiazine-induced seizures has not been established and is not recommended for seizure management. Activated charcoal is indicated for gastrointestinal decontamination. Repeated dose therapy may be of potential benefit in symptomatic patients. Most patients with neuroleptic poisoning recover completely within several hours to days, depending on the severity of toxicity.

B. Extrapyramidal syndromes. Acute dystonic reactions are managed with anticholinergic agents. Benztropine mesylate (Cogentin, 1–2 mg) or diphenhydramine (Benadryl, 50–100 mg) administered parentally can be used. On resolution of the immediate symptoms, the anticholinergic agent should be continued for another 48 to 72 hours. Benzodiazepines can be used as adjunctive therapy if the anticholinergic agents are not effective. Sedation with benzodiazepines may be beneficial for akathisia. Neuroleptic-induced parkinsonism can be treated with either benztropine, biperiden, diphenhydramine, or trihexyphenidyl. Long-term treatment with these agents is needed for patients who require continued neuroleptic therapy. Amantadine (100–400 mg/d orally) is also effective and has fewer side effects.

Selected Readings

American College of Neuropharmacology–Food and Drug Administration Task Force. Neurologic syndromes associated with antipsychotic drug use. *N Engl J Med* 1973; 289:20.

This is a discussion of the movement disorders associated with the use of neuroleptic agents.

Arita M, Surawicz B. Electrophysiologic effects of phenothiazines on canine cardiac fibers. *J Pharmacol Exp Ther* 1973;184:619.

This study demonstrated increased sodium concentration to reverse thioridazine-induced repolarization abnormalities, but not the depolarization effects.

Buckley NA, Whyte IM, Dawson AH. Cardiotoxicity more common in thioridazine overdose than with other neuroleptics. *Clin Toxicol* 1995;33:199.

This case series analysis demonstrated thioridazine to be associated with increased frequency of arrhythmias and cardiac conduction disorders when compared with other neuroleptic agents.

Gupta J, Lovejoy FH. Acute phenothiazine toxicity in childhood: a five-year survey. *Pediatrics* 1967;39:771.

This report discussed the manifestations of phenothiazine toxicity in children.

Hale PW, Poklis A. Cardiotoxicity of thioridazine and two stereoisomeric forms of thioridzine 5-sulfoxide in the isolated perfused rat heart. *Toxicol Appl Pharmacol* 1986;86:44.

This study demonstrated thioridazine's metabolite, mesoridazine, to be more arrhythmogenic than the parent compound.

Huston JR, Bell GE. The effect of thioridazine and chlorpromazine on the electrocardiogram. *JAMA* 1966;198:134.
This article reported the electrocardiographic effects of neuroleptics to be similar to the type Ia antidysrhythmic agents.

Landmark K, Glomstein A, Oye I. The effect of thioridazine and promazine on the isolated contracting rat heart. *Acta Pharmacol Toxicol* 1969;27:173.
This study demonstrated thioridazine to have a dose-dependent negative chronotropic effect.

Langslet A. ECG changes induced by phenothiazine drugs in the anesthetized rat. *Acta Pharmacol Toxicol* 1970;28:258.
This ex vivo study demonstrated phenothiazine-induced, dose-dependent cardiac conduction disorders.

Nierenberg D, Disch M, Manheimer E, et al. Facilitating prompt diagnosis and treatment of the neuroleptic malignant syndrome. *Clin Pharmacol Ther* 1991;50:580.
This review discussed the factors contributing to neuroleptic malignant syndrome.

Rosebush PI, Stewart T, Mazurek MF. The treatment of neuroleptic malignant syndrome: are dantrolene and bromocriptine useful adjuncts to supportive care? *Br J Psychiatry* 1991;159:709.
This study demonstrated supportive therapy to be more beneficial than dantrolene or bromocriptine in the treatment of neuroleptic malignant syndrome.

Rosenberg MR, Green M. Neuroleptic malignant syndrome. *Arch Intern Med* 1989;149:1927.
This review discussed the delayed therapeutic effects of dopaminergic agents used in the treatment of neuroleptic malignant syndrome.

Rupniak NM, Jenner P, Marsden CD. Acute dystonia induced by neuroleptic drugs. *Psychopharmacology* 1986;88:403.
This review discussed the cause and occurrence of dystonia during drug therapy.

Shalev A, Hermesh H, Munitz H. Mortality from neuroleptic malignant syndrome. *J Clin Psychiatry* 1989;50:18.
This review discussed the factors attributed to the decrease in mortality from neuroleptic malignant syndrome.

Vassallo SU, Delaney KA. Pharmacologic effects on thermoregulation: mechanisms of drug-related heatstroke. *J Toxicol Clin Toxicol* 1989;27:199.
This review discussed the supportive management of neuroleptic malignant syndrome.

126. NEUROMUSCULAR BLOCKING AGENTS

Erica L. Liebelt

I. General principles. Neuromuscular blocking agents (NMBAs) are used to (a) facilitate intubation and airway control, (b) decrease oxygen consumption requirements, and (c) improve patient compliance with mechanical ventilation refractory to sedatives. NMBAs are structurally similar to acetylcholine and categorized as nondepolarizing or depolarizing, depending on the specific action at the neuromuscular junction.

Nondepolarizing or competitive NMBAs compete with acetylcholine at its receptor sites on the motor endplate to prevent depolarization and contraction of skeletal muscle fibers. In addition, they block presynaptic receptors, which can prevent positive feedback and decrease the production of acetylcholine. Examples include pancuronium, vecuronium, atracurium, rocuronium, and *d*-tubocurarine.

Succinylcholine, the prototypical depolarizing NMBA, acts similar to acetylcholine at the endplate receptor, causing persistent depolarization of the postjunctional membrane, resulting initially in transient muscle fasciculation with subsequent paralysis. Paralysis occurs because succinylcholine is not metabolized as rapidly as acetylcholine and the depolarized membrane remains unresponsive to additional impulses. Succinylcholine is used primarily for rapid sequence intubation and is less suitable for prolonged use because an unpredictable duration of neuromuscular blockade can develop. Rocuronium is a comparable short-acting, nondepolarizing NMBA that is used for rapid sequence intubation.

II. Pharmacology. Each NMBA has characteristic pharmacologic properties that make them more or less useful for specific patients and clinical situations (Table 126-1). The time to onset of paralysis for each drug, which is determined by dose, distribution and redistribution kinetics, and receptor sensitivity, generally occurs within 3 to 5 minutes. Elimination varies by route of metabolism and excretion. Despite similar plasma concentrations and dosing techniques, intensity and duration of neuromuscular blockade vary from patient to patient because of altered pharmacokinetics and pharmacodynamic responses. Clearance of these drugs can be altered by hypo- and hyperdynamic physiologic states.

III. Dosing guidelines. Dosing should be individualized and based on lean body weight (Table 126-2). Longer-acting NMBAs (pancuronium and vecuronium) are usually administered by intermittent bolus as needed to achieve clinical goals. Intermittent bolus therapy is impractical for prolonged therapy with shorter-acting NMBAs such as atracurium or rocuronium. Continuous infusion of NMBAs may reduce required daily dosages compared with intermittent bolus therapy. Infusion rates should be titrated based on individual response because of varying patient response, physiologic state, and use of adjuvant drugs.

Guidelines for NMBA dosage reduction for patients with renal and hepatic dysfunction have not been clearly established. Because of pancronium's primary renal clearance, a reduction in dosing up to 50% may be required for patients with renal dysfunction or biliary obstruction. Maintenance infusions of vecuronium may need to be reduced by 50% in patients with cholestasis and hepatic dysfunction. Dose reduction of atracurium in patients with renal and hepatic dysfunction is not required. Elderly patients with decreased renal and hepatic function and alterations in body composition may require smaller daily doses of NMBAs.

Hyperdynamic patients (e.g., those with burns) may exhibit decreased sensitivity to competitive neuromuscular blockers which starts as early as 1 week after injury, peaks at 15 to 40 days after injury, and lasts many months. They may have dose requirements of NMBAs 2.5 to 5.0 times the normal dose. Increases in dosage requirements have also been described for critically ill patients receiving prolonged continuous infusions of NMBAs, possibly because of changes in the neuromuscular junction causing drug resistance.

TABLE 126-1. Pharmacology summary of selected neuromuscular blockers

Drug	Onset	Duration	Metabolism	Elimination
Depolarizing				
Succinylcholine	0.5–1 min	4–6 min	Plasma cholinesterases	10% unchanged in urine
Nondepolarizing				
Long-acting				
Pancuronium	2–3 min	30–60 min	30–40% by liver	60% unchanged drug and metabolites in urine, 11% in bile
Intermediate-acting				
Vecuronium	2–5 min	20–40 min	Spontaneous deacetylation and liver metabolism, active metabolites	20% unchanged drug in urine, 45% unchanged drug, and 25% metabolites in bile
Atracurium	3–5 min	20–35 min	Ester hydrolysis and Hofmann elimination in plasma	Unchanged drug and metabolites in urine and bile
Short-acting				
Mivacurium	3–5 min	15–30 min	Ester hydrolysis by plasma and cholinesterase in plasma	Unchanged drug and metabolites in urine and bile
Rocuronium	1 min	30–60 min	Deacetylation and liver metabolism, inactive metabolite	Primarily biliary excretion, 33% unchanged drug in urine

TABLE 126-2. Dosing guidelines for selected neuromuscular blockage agents

Drug	Single/intermittent dose	Continuous infusion	
		Loading dose	Maintenance dose
Succinylcholine	1–2 mg/kg	N/A	N/A
Rocuronium	0.8 mg/kg	N/A	N/A
Pancuronium	0.1–0.2 mg/kg every 1–3 hrs	.03–0.1 mg/kg	.06–0.1 mg/kg/hr
Vecuronium	0.1–0.2 mg/kg every 1 hr	0.1 mg/kg	.05–0.1 mg/kg/hr
Atracurium	0.5 mg/kg	0.5 mg/kg	0.4–1.0 mg/kg/hr

IV. Prolonged paralysis and drug interactions. Prolonged muscle weakness and paralysis can occur with intermittent or short-term NMBA dosing regimens as well as with continuous infusions. Persistent paralysis for a few hours or days after termination of long-term treatment with NMBA may be caused by drug overdose or delayed elimination of parent or metabolites in the presence of organ dysfunction. A second pattern of neuromuscular dysfunction is manifest by an acute quadriplegic myopathy and weakness that may last for several weeks to months. This dysfunction may result from a variety of factors (organ dysfunction, metabolic factors, concomitant drug therapy) altering the pharmacokinetics of NMBAs.

Concomitant drug use can affect the degree and duration of neuromuscular blockade. Aminoglycosides can prolong NMBA effects by decreasing the amount of acetylcholine release by nerve impulses and stabilizing postjunctional membranes. Cardiovascular agents such as beta-blockers, calcium channel blockers, procainamide, furosemide, and quinidine can also potentiate neuromuscular blockade. Corticosteroids can potentiate steroid myopathy. Chronic anticonvulsant therapy can cause resistance to neuromuscular blocking effects.

Train-of-four (TOF) peripheral nerve stimulation is a method used to monitor neuromuscular blockade. Routine use of TOF may decrease the incidence and severity of prolonged paralysis by allowing for its early detection and subsequent dosing adjustments.

Selected Readings

Ali HH, Savarese JJ. Monitoring of neuromuscular function. *Anesthesiology* 1976;45:216.
An excellent review of the pathophysiology of neuromuscular blockade and monitoring of neuromuscular function.

Fiamengo SA, Savarese JJ. Use of muscle relaxants in intensive care units. *Crit Care Med* 1991;19:1457.
A succinct review of complications and adverse effects of neuromuscular relaxants and the need for monitoring with peripheral nerve stimulators.

Gooch JL, Suchyta MR, Balbierz JM, et al. Prolonged paralysis after treatment with neuromuscular junction blocking agents. *Crit Care Med* 1991;19:1125.
A case series of ICU patients with prolonged paralysis after treatment with neuromuscular blocking agents, demonstrating neurogenic atrophy based on electrodiagnostic and muscle pathology findings.

Larijani GE, Gratz I, Silverberg M, et al. Clinical pharmacology of the neuromuscular blocking agents. *Drug Intelligence and Clinical Pharmacy* 1991;25:54.
A review of the physiology of neuromuscular transmission and pharmacology of common neuromuscular blocking agents.

Watling SM, Dasta JF. Prolonged paralysis in intensive care unit patients after the use of neuromuscular blocking agents: a review of the literature. *Crit Care Med* 1994;22:884.
A review of prolonged neuromuscular blockade caused by vecuronium and atracurium and proposed causes for this phenomenon based on case reports and studies in literature.

127. NONSTEROIDAL ANTIINFLAMMATORY DRUGS

Jeffrey R. Tucker

I. General principles. Nonsteroidal antiinflammatory drugs (NSAIDs) include aspirin, other salicylicates, and a variety of other aspirinlike drugs. NSAIDs have analgesic, antipyretic, and antiinflammatory activity. Therapeutic effects and gastrointestinal and renal side effects are caused by inhibition of cyclooxegenase and prostaglandin synthesis. Aspirin is the only NSAID with significant antiplatelet activity.

II. Pathophysiology

A. Salicylates. Absorption can continue for 24 hours after an acute overdose because of delayed dissolution of tablets or formation of gastric concretions. Following single therapeutic doses, salicylate is metabolized in the liver to the inactive metabolites. The remaining 10% of the dose is excreted unchanged in the urine. When serum concentrations exceed 20 mg/dl, the metabolism becomes saturated and elimination changes from first-order to zero-order kinetics and the half-life increases from about 2.5 hours to as long as 40 hours. Renal excretion of salicylate then becomes the most important route of elimination.

Following overdose, direct stimulation of the respiratory center in the medulla by toxic salicylate concentrations results in a respiratory alkalosis. The accumulation of salicylate in cells causes uncoupling of mitochondrial oxidative phosphorylation, which leads to the characteristic increased anion gap metabolic acidosis.

B. NSAIDs. Nonsalicylate NSAIDs are rapidly absorbed following ingestion; they have small volumes of distribution and are highly protein-bound. In contrast to salicylates, the metabolism of most nonsalicylate NSAIDs is not saturable and elimination follows first-order kinetics.

III. Clinical presentation

A. Salicylates. Salicylate poisoning can occur with acute as well as chronic overdose. Severity should be assessed by direct evaluation of clinical manifestations and acid-base status rather than by the serum salicylate level or the Done nomogram. Mild poisoning is defined by the presence of alkalemia (serum pH > 7.4) and alkaluria (urine pH < 6). Signs and symptoms include nausea, vomiting, abdominal pain, diaphoresis, headache, tinnitus, and tachypnea. Moderate poisoning is defined by a normal or alkaline serum pH and aciduria (urine pH < 6). Gastrointestinal tract and neurologic symptoms are more pronounced. Arterial blood gas and electrolyte analysis reveals combined respiratory alkalosis and metabolic acidosis with an increased anion gap. Severe poisoning is defined by the presence of acidemia and aciduria. Signs and symptoms include coma, seizures, respiratory depression, shock, or noncardiogenic pulmonary edema. Because of gastrointestinal, renal, and insensible fluid losses, dehydration is invariably present and often underestimated.

B. Other NSAIDs. Metabolic acidosis, coma, seizures, hepatic dysfunction, hypotension, and cardiovascular collapse are relatively common after phenylbutazone overdose. Other nonsalicylate NSAIDs rarely cause severe poisoning. Typical findings after acute overdose include nausea, vomiting, abdominal pain, headache, confusion, tinnitus, drowsiness, and hyperventilation. Symptoms usually last several hours. Tonic-clonic seizures and muscle twitching has been reported after mefenamic acid overdose.

IV. Evaluation

A. Salicylates. Initial laboratory evaluation should include arterial blood gases, electrolytes, glucose, blood urea nitrogen, and creatinine level, and urinalysis. In patients with moderate to severe poisoning, further evaluation should include determinations of serum calcium, magnesium, and ketones; liver function tests; complete blood cell count; coagulation studies; and an electrocardiogram and chest radiograph. Because patients often confuse aspirin and acetaminophen, toxicology testing should be done for both substances. Serial salicylate levels should be performed to assess the efficacy of decontamination and elimination therapies.

B. Other NSAIDs. The diagnostic evaluation of patients with acute NSAID overdose is the same as for salicylates. Evaluation of acid-base, electrolyte, and renal parameters is particularly important. Additional ancillary testing is dictated by clinical severity.

V. Management

A. Salicylates. Resuscitative measures should be instituted as necessary. If endotracheal intubation and mechanical ventilation are instituted, hyperventilation is essential to prevent acidemia and the resultant increased tissue penetration of salicylic acid into the central nervous system (CNS). Noncardiac pulmonary edema should be treated with intubation and positive end-expiratory pressure (PEEP) rather than diuretics. Because CNS hypoglycemia can occur despite a normal serum glucose, obtain a finger stick blood sugar or empirically treat with $D_{50}W$ in patients with altered mental status.

Further therapy is directed at limiting absorption, correcting dehydration and metabolic abnormalities, and enhancing elimination. Gastrointestinal tract decontamination should be performed in all patients with intentional overdoses and in those with accidental ingestions of greater than 150 mg/kg. It may be effective for as long as 24 hours following overdose and in patients with spontaneous vomiting, because of delayed absorption and concretion formation. Activated charcoal—the preferred therapy—should be given to all patients. Gastric lavage and endoscopy may have a role in patients with large ingestions and rising drug levels despite charcoal therapy. The administration of multiple-dose charcoal to enhance salicylate elimination should also be considered but the clinical efficacy of this therapy is debatable.

Initial fluid therapy should be intravenous 5% dextrose in normal saline or 5% dextrose in one-half normal saline with one ampule (50 mEq) of sodium bicarbonate and potassium (10–20 mEq/L) with 1 to 3 L given over the first 1 to 2 hours. Electrolyte abnormalities should be corrected.

Salicylate elimination can be enhanced by urinary alkalinization and diuresis and extracorporeal removal. Indications for urinary alkalinization include systemic symptoms, acid-base abnormalities, or salicylate levels greater than 30 mg/dl after an acute overdose. The goal is to achieve a urine pH of 7.5 or greater and a urine output of 2 to 4 ml/kg/h (Table 127-1). Acetazolamide should not be used to alkalinize the urine because it can cause a concomitant systemic acidosis, which may promote tissue distribution of salicylate and result in clinical deterioration. Alkali therapy should be withheld if the serum pH is greater than 7.55. Hemodialysis is indicated in patients with severe poisoning and in those with moderate poisoning who fail to respond to alkaline diuresis. It is essential for a successful outcome in those with coma, seizures, cerebral or pulmonary edema, or renal failure.

TABLE 127-1. Alkaline diuresis therapy of salicylate poisoning: fluid and electrolyte therapy[a]

Grade	Intravenous Solution	$NaHCO_3$ (amp/L)	Potassium (mEq/L)
Mild	D_5NS	1	20
Moderate	D_5½NS	2	40
Severe	D_5W	3	60

[a] Initial treatment should include hydration with 1 to 3 L of a saline solution containing dextrose (see text).

D_5NS, 5% dextrose in normal saline; D_5½NS, 5% dextrose in one-half normal saline; D_5W, 5% dextrose in water; $NaHCO_3$, 50 mEq sodium bicarbonate per 50 ml ampule (8.4%).

B. Other NSAIDs. The treatment of nonsalicylate NSAID poisoning is supportive and symptomatic. Advanced life support measures and invasive monitoring may be required in severe cases. Renal function should be monitored carefully in patients with abnormal urinalysis, underlying renal disease, or advanced age. Gastrointestinal tract decontamination with activated charcoal is recommended for patients who present within 4 hours of a significant ingestion.

Selected Readings

Balali-Mood M, Proudfoot AT, Critchley JAJH, et al. Mefenamic acid overdose. *Lancet* 1981;1354.

A case series of mefenamic acid overdose that showed a high number of patients with neurologic toxicity such as seizures and muscle twitching.

Brenner BE, Simon RR. Management of salicylate intoxication. *Drugs* 1987;24:335.

A review article on salicylate toxicity with a discussion of the different bedside tests for salicylates.

Duffens KR, Smilkstein MJ, Bessen HA, et al. Falsely elevated salicylate levels due to diflunisal overdose. *J Emerg Med* 1987;5:499.

A case report and discussion of the cross-reactivity of diflunisal with the immunoassay and colormimetric assay for salicylates.

Dugandzic RM, Tiemey MG, Dickinson GE, et al. Evaluation of the validity of the Done nomogram in the management of acute salicylate intoxication. *Ann Emerg Med* 1989;18:1186.

A retrospective study of 55 acute salicylate intoxications which demonstrated management decisions should be based on the clinical presentation and serum salicylates level.

Gabow PA, Anderson RJ, Potts DE, et al. Acid base disturbances in the salicylate intoxicated adult. *Arch Intern Med* 1978;138:1481.

A retrospective study of 67 adults with salicylate toxicity focusing on acid-base disturbances. The presence of acidemia in this group correlated with neurologic symptoms.

Hall AH, Smolinske SC, Conrad FL, et al. Ibuprofen overdose: 126 cases. *Ann Emerg Med* 1986;15:1308.

A retrospective review of 126 ibuprofen overdose cases in adults and children. Ibuprofen toxicity in most cases was benign, but 2 children had seizures and one child died.

Hill JB. Experimental salicylate poisoning: observations on the effects of altering blood pH on tissue and plasma salicylate concentrations. *Pediatrics* 1971;47:658.

An experimental model that demonstrated the importance of acid base on the distribution of salicylates. Acidemia facilitates salicylate distribution into the brain.

Johnson D, Eppler J, Giesbrecht E, et al. Effect of multiple-dose activated charcoal on the clearance of high-dose intravenous aspirin in a porcine model. *Ann Emerg Med* 1995;26:569.

An animal model showing no benefit of multiple-dose activated charcoal in the clearance of high-dose aspirin.

Linden CH, Townsend PL. Metabolic acidosis after acute ibuprofen overdosage. *J Pediatr* 1987;111;922.

Two case reports and a discussion of the increased anion gap after acute ibuprofen overdose.

McGuigan MA. A two-year review of salicylate deaths in Ontario. *Arch Intern Med* 1987;147:510.

A retrospective study of salicylate deaths that demonstrated specific management difficulties such as establishing the diagnosis, administering activated charcoal, and using hemodialysis.

Notarianni L. A reassessment of the treatment of salicylate poisoning. *Drug Saf* 1992; 7:292.

A review article focusing on the recent developments in salicylate toxicity including the discouragement of forced diuresis to enhance elimination.

Smith M. The metabolic basis of the major symptoms in acute salicylate intoxication. *Clin Toxicol* 1968;1:387.

The classic paper on the effects of salicylates on metabolism and the clinical symptoms.

Smolinske SC, Hall AH, Vandenberg SA, et al. Toxic effects of nonsteroidal anti-inflammatory drugs in overdose: an overview of recent evidence on clinical effects and dose-response relationships. *Drug Saf* 1990;5:253.

The clinical effects and toxicity of 26 different nonsteroidal antiinflammatory drugs are discussed.

Veltri JC, Rollins DE. A comparison of the frequency and severity of poisoning cases for ingestion of acetaminophen, aspirin, and ibuprofen. *Am J Emerg Med* 1988; 6:104.

Data from the American Association of Poison Control Center regarding exposure to analgesics revealed that the majority of patients had a low rate of serious effects.

Wortzman DJ, Grunfeld A. Delay absorption following enteric-coated aspirin overdose. *Ann Emerg Med* 1987;16:434.

A case report of delayed toxicity following an overdose of sustained-release salicylate preparation.

128. OPIOIDS

Richard Y. Wang

I. General principles. Opioids, also known as narcotics, bind to specific receptors in the central nervous system (CNS) to produce analgesia, euphoria, and sedative effects. All opioids have the same overall physiologic effect as morphine, the prototype of this group. However, some differences exist among these agents.

II. Semisynthetic and synthetic opioids

A. Heroin has two to five times the analgesic potency of morphine, with similar effects on the CNS. The drug can be administered intravenously (IV) or intranasally and can be mixed with other drugs of abuse (e.g., cocaine for speedballing). The incidence of pulmonary edema among heroin overdose patients is reportedly 50% to 67% and results in death in 3% to 9% of these cases. The onset of pulmonary edema is usually immediate but many clinicians recommend admission, observation, or both for 24 hours.

B. Fentanyl has a potency approximately 200 times that of morphine. It is sometimes abused by hospital personnel. The transdermal depot delivery system allows for prolonged absorption and prolonged duration of action.

C. Meperidine is equal in potency to morphine but it has an increased propensity for dysphoric and hallucinogenic episodes as well as the ability to produce CNS excitation, tremors, muscle twitching, mydriasis, and seizures with toxic dose. Seizures are caused by the accumulation of the metabolite normeperidine. Repetitive meperidine use, acute ingestion of a large amount, or decreased renal clearance produces a high ratio of normeperidine to meperidine with potential metabolite toxicity.

D. Diphenoxylate, a meperidine congener, is used with atropine (Lomotil) to decrease gut motility in diarrhea. This drug appears to be particularly toxic to children, with as few as 0.5 to 6 tablets causing serious symptoms and 1.2 mg/kg being potentially fatal. Lomotil overdose often results in mild to moderate anticholinergic activity in addition to the opiate effects. Symptoms arising from a toxic ingestion can be delayed up to 30 hours, owing to the anticholinergic-induced reduction in gastrointestinal tract motility.

E. Methadone is used for detoxification or maintenance of an opiate addict. It is frequently diverted from legal channels, accounting for most acute opiate overdoses in certain areas of the United States. As little as 40 to 50 mg can cause coma and respiratory depression in nondependent adults. Methadone has a much longer duration of action than morphine with an average half-life of 25 hours.

F. Propoxyphene, which is structurally related to methadone, is available alone or in combination with aspirin or acetaminophen. The clinical course following an overdose can be rapidly progressive with seizures and respiratory arrest. Propoxyphene and its metabolite norpropoxyphene appear to be cardiotoxic and can cause nonspecific ST- and T-wave abnormalities, widened QRS complexes with idioventricular rhythm, ventricular bigeminy, and bundle-branch block.

III. Clinical manifestations. Coma, respiratory depression, and miosis are the hallmarks of opiate intoxication. Pulmonary edema can complicate the course of an opiate overdose and is especially prevalent following heroin, codeine, methadone, and propoxyphene overdose. It is usually apparent within 2 hours of parenteral heroin use but can occur up to 24 hours following methadone ingestion. In most patients, the lungs are initially clear to auscultation. Significant pulmonary findings beyond 24 to 48 hours suggest aspiration or bacterial pneumonia. Talc, a common contaminant of street heroin, can produce pulmonary granulomatosis when injected chronically. Seizures could be caused by brain abscess, intracranial hemorrhage, or other CNS pathology as well as proconvulsant opioid (e.g., meperidine, propoxyphene, pentazocine) or adulterant (e.g., local anesthetic) effects.

Hypotension may be present in patients with coma and respiratory acidosis or arrest. Acute changes in the electrocardiogram have been noted with heroin and propoxyphene overdose. Nonspecific ST-segment and T-wave changes, atrioventricular blocks, atrial fibrillation, prolonged QT intervals, and ventricular dysrhythmias can occur. These cardiovascular findings can result from metabolic derangements associated with hypoxia, a direct effect of the abused agent, or toxicity of an adulterant (e.g., quinine) found in street drugs. Rhabdomyolysis and renal failure, resulting from prolonged coma, can be a complication of the clinical course of an acute overdose.

IV. Evaluation. Evaluation should focus on the neurologic, pulmonary, and cardiovascular systems. All patients should have oxygen saturation measurements. Those with abnormal vital signs should have arterial blood gas analysis, chest radiograph, and electrocardiogram. Routine laboratory testing and toxicology screening tests may also be appropriate. Because prescription opioid preparations often contain acetaminophen or aspirin, levels of these drugs should be determined in all patients with oral overdoses. Not all opioids are detected by urine drug assays. Opioid serum levels are usually not warranted because they are not helpful in the therapeutic plan.

V. Management. Advanced life support measures should be instituted as necessary. Naloxone can reverse the respiratory depression of opiate intoxication and may obviate the need for tracheal intubation and mechanical ventilation. The initial dose is 2 to 10 mg, administered by the intravenous, intramuscular, intralingual, endotracheal, or intraosseous routes. Smaller amounts (0.1–0.4 mg) should be administered to opiate-dependent patients to prevent the precipitation of withdrawal symptoms. Repeat doses or a continuous infusion of naloxone may be required because it has a shorter half-life than most opioids. A continuous naloxone infusion is indicated in patients who respond to the initial bolus and then relapse. The infusion is administered at a rate of two thirds of the initially effective bolus dose per hour with half of the bolus dose repeated 15 minutes after the infusion is started. Long-acting opioid antagonists (e.g., nalmefene, naltrexone) are not recommended for use to reverse opioid toxicity because of the difficulty in titrating to clinical effect and the potential for precipitating prolonged withdrawal states.

Patients who require antagonist therapy for reversal of respiratory depression caused by an oral overdose, those with recurrent toxicity after IV use, and children who ingest any amount of Lomotil should be observed in an intensive care unit for at least 24 hours. In contrast, patients who remain asymptomatic for several hours following treatment for an IV overdose are unlikely to develop delayed complications and can be discharged.

Selected Readings

Dauberstein JL, Kaufman DM. A clinical study of an epidemic of heroin intoxication and heroin-induced pulmonary edema. *Am J Med* 1971;51:704.

This report described the occurrence of pulmonary edema with heroin toxicity.

Goldfrank K, Weisman RS, Errick JK, et al. A dosing nomogram for continuous infusion intravenous naloxone. *Ann Emerg Med* 1986;15:566.

This study determined the dosing protocol for naloxone infusion.

Hodding FC, Jann M, Ackerman IP. Drug withdrawal syndromes: a literature review. *West J Med* 1980;133:383.

A discussion of the manifestations of various drug withdrawal syndromes, including opioid.

Kaiko RF, Foley KM, Grabinski PY, et al. Central nervous system excitatory effects from meperidine in cancer patients. *Ann Neurol* 1983;13:180.

This report described seizures with the chronic use of meperidine in patients with renal insufficiency.

Langston JW, Ballard P, Tetrud JW, et al. Chronic parkinsonism in humans due to a by-product of meperidine-analog synthesis. *Science* 1983;219:979.

This report described the occurrence of the "frozen addict" syndrome from the drug contaminant—1-methyl-4-phenyl-1,2,3,6-tetrahydropyridine (MPTP).

Lund-Jacobsen H. Cardio-respiratory toxicity of propoxyphene and norpropoxyphene in conscious rabbits. *Acta Pharacol Toxicol* 1978;42:171.

This study demonstrated seizures resulting from propoxyphene and its metabolite, norpropoxyphene.

MacDonald KL, Rutherford GW, Friedman SM, et al. Botulism and botulism-like illness in chronic drug abusers. *Ann Intern Med* 1985;102:616.

This report described the occurrence of botulism in intravenous drug users.

Manfredi PL, Ribeiro S, Chandler SW, et al. Inappropriate use of naloxone in cancer patients with pain. *J Pain Symptom Manage* 1996;11:131.

An analysis of the precipitation of pain syndromes when naloxone was administered to cancer patients with misdiagnosed opioid toxicity.

Martin WR, Hecker J, Clark R, et al. China White epidemic: an eastern United States emergency department experience. *Ann Emerg Med* 1991;20:158.

This report described epidemic deaths in heroin users from the use of a fentanyl analogue.

McCarron MM, Challoner KR, Thompson GA. Diphenoxylate-atropine (Lomotil) overdose in children: an update (report of eight cases and review of the literature). *Pediatrics* 199;87:694.

A report on the marked delayed onset of effect from Lomotil ingestion in children.

Nightingale SL. Important new safety information for tramadol hydrochloride. *JAMA* 1996;275:1224.

This report described seizures from both therapeutic dosing and overdose of tramadol.

Stork CM, Redd JT, Fine K, et al. Propoxyphene-induced wide QRS complex dysrhythmia responsive to sodium bicarbonate-a case report. *J Toxicol Clin Toxicol* 1995;33:179.

This case report described electrocardiographic abnormalities from a propoxyphene overdose that reversed with sodium bicarbonate treatment.

Utecht MJ, Facinelli Stone A McCarron MM. Heroin body packers. *J Emerg Med* 1993;11:33.

This report described the prolonged duration of effect from ruptured heroin packets.

Wiley J, Wiley CC, Torrey SB, et al. Clonidine poisoning in young children. *J Pediatr* 1990;116:654.

A report on the ability of naloxone to reverse the central nervous system depressant effects of clonidine in some patients.

129. PESTICIDE POISONING

Erica L. Liebelt

I. General principles. This chapter focuses on the toxicity and treatment interventions for selected pesticides. The organophosphates are covered in Chapter 114. Initial management includes limiting further chemical absorption by the patient and protection of rescue personnel. Clothing should be removed and the skin washed with soap and water to eliminate residue following topical exposures. No specific antidotal therapy or elimination enhancement techniques are available for most of the compounds, making aggressive supportive care the mainstay of therapy.

II. Organochlorines. Organochlorine compounds are used as insecticides, soil fumigants, solvents, and herbicides. Examples are endrin, dieldrin, aldrin, chlordane, dichlorodiphenyl trichloroethane (DDT), and lindane. Systemic toxicity can occur by ingestion, dermal absorption, or inhalation; it is characterized primarily by central nervous system (CNS) dysfunction. Some agents (kelthane, perthane, and lindane) are likely to cause CNS sedation more than excitation, whereas another (eldrin) can cause hyperthermia and decerebrate posturing. Seizures can occur without a prodrome. Ingestion can result in vomiting and diarrhea. Cardiac dysrhythmias have been reported.

Multiple doses of activated charcoal or cholestyramine should be administered to interrupt enteric circulation and enhance elimination. Seizures can be managed with benzodiazepines and barbiturates.

III. Anticoagulants. Anticoagulants used as rodenticides include warfarin and the newer superwarfarin agents (brodifacoum, difenacoum, and indanedione derivatives). The superwarfarins are approximately 100 times more potent than warfarin and have a much longer half-life. Anticoagulants inhibit vitamin K 2, 3-epoxide reductase and, to a lesser extent, vitamin K reductase. Vitamin K is the active coenzyme responsible for activation of clotting factors II, VII, IX, and X as well as anticoagulant factors proteins C and protein S.

The primary toxic manifestation of these compounds is development of a coagulopathy which can present as cutaneous bleeding, soft tissue ecchymosis, gingival bleeding, epistaxis, and hematuria.

Vitamin K_1 (phytonadione) is the only form of vitamin K that is effective for treatment. It can be given orally, subcutaneously, intramuscularly, and intravenously. Treatment duration will be highly variable and must be titrated to clinical and laboratory response. Patients with life-threatening bleeding should also be treated with fresh frozen plasma.

IV. Strychnine. Strychnine is used as an animal pesticide. It is also found as an adulterant in illicit drugs such as cocaine and heroin. Strychnine competitively antagonizes postsynaptic glycine receptors at the spinal cord, reducing neuromuscular inhibition and resulting in contraction of both flexor and extensor muscle groups.

The onset of strychnine toxicity is rapid, usually within 15 to 30 minutes after exposure. Facial muscle spasms result in risus sardonicus (the "sardonic smile") and trismus. Opisthotonos, abdominal muscle contractions, and tonic movements resemble seizures, although mental status is preserved, making true seizures highly unlikely. Strychnine toxicity usually resolves within 12 to 24 hours. No specific elimination enhancement treatment modalities exist.

Benzodiazepines and barbiturates are the agents of choice in terminating muscle contractions. Termination of muscle contractions is important in preventing or reversing lactic acidosis, rhabdomyolysis, hyperthermia, and respiratory depression. Nondepolarizing muscle blockers may be required for refractory convulsions.

V. Sodium monofluoroacetate (SMFA; Compound 1080). SMFA is used primarily to exterminate rodents and larger mammals. This compound, which is structurally similar to acetate, enters the tricarboxylic acid cycle, inhibits metabolic enzymes, and halts cellular respiration. Initial symptoms of nausea and vomiting are followed by agitation, seizures, coma, ventricular arrhythmias, and hypotension. Laboratory abnormalities include metabolic acidosis and hypocalcemia with QT interval prolongation.

Seizures can be treated with benzodiazepines or barbiturates. Hypocalcemia and prolonged QT intervals may require calcium and magnesium supplementation.

VI. Aluminum and zinc phosphide. These insecticides and rodenticides are commonly used as solid fumigants and grain preservatives. Phosphine is slowly released when phosphides react with moisture in an enclosed environment. Inhalation of phosphine gas results in eye and mucous membrane irritation and rapid onset of pulmonary symptoms including cough and dyspnea. Oral ingestion of phosphides causes profound gastrointestinal (GI) symptoms, including nausea, vomiting, and abdominal pain. Pulmonary edema and respiratory failure can be delayed for several hours after oral exposure to phosphides. Fatalities are related to cardiovascular collapse. The diagnosis is suggested by a decaying fish odor. Magnesium therapy should be considered in patients with arrhythmias or hypomagnesemia.

VII. Methyl bromide. Methyl bromide is a colorless gas used primarily as a fumigant to control for nematodes, insects, rodents, fungi, and weeds. It is one of the most widely used pesticides in California. Symptoms can be delayed 6 hours or longer after exposure. Mild toxicity is characterized by dizziness, headache, confusion, weakness, nausea, vomiting, and dyspnea; it mimics viral symptoms. Skin irritation and burns can occur under clothes and rubber gloves where gas is trapped. Significant exposure can result in tremor, myoclonus, and behavioral changes as well as pulmonary edema, seizures, and coma. Fatalities result from pulmonary and CNS toxicity. Serum bromide levels are not helpful in determining the severity of exposure, but they can confirm it.

VIII. N, N-Diethyl-m-toluamide (DEET). DEET is the active ingredient in numerous commercial insect repellents. Anaphylactic reactions have been reported with cutaneous application. Most poisonings result from the application of concentrated DEET preparations or repeated application of lower concentration preparations. Toxicity may also follow ingestion. Systemic manifestations include anxiety, behavioral changes, tremors, lethargy, ataxia, confusion, seizures, and coma.

IX. Paraquat. Paraquat is a contact herbicide. It is extremely toxic when ingested. Following absorption, paraquat is selectively taken up by alveolar cells of the lung where it is reduced to a free radical. Paraquat radicals react with oxygen to form superoxide radicals which then cause lipid peroxidation and cellular destruction. Patients who ingest more than 40 mg/kg usually die within hours to a few days from multiple organ failure including acute respiratory distress syndrome, cerebral edema, myocardial necrosis, and hepatic and renal failure. Patients who ingest 20 to 40 mg/kg may die from pulmonary fibrosis, which progresses over a period of days to weeks. Paraquat is extremely corrosive to mucous membranes and can cause mouth, throat, and GI burns.

Multiple doses of activated charcoal or Fuller's earth (1–2 g/kg) should be continued until evidence of adsorbent in the stool is seen. Oxygen should only be used when absolutely necessary and at the minimal level possible. Excessive oxygen supplementation can increase the formation of paraquat free radicals and worsen pulmonary toxicity. Hemoperfusion may be helpful if performed soon after ingestion.

X. Diquat. Diquat is a herbicide that is structurally similar to paraquat. Unlike paraquat, it spares the pulmonary system. Toxicity is manifested by GI symptoms, CNS dysfunction, and renal failure. Brainstem infarctions can occur.

Selected Readings

Cohn WJ, Boylan JJ, Blanke RV, et al. Treatment of chlordecone (Kepone) toxicity with cholestyramine. *N Engl J Med* 1978;298:243.

A clinical study demonstrating increased elimination of chlordecone with administration of cholestyramine in poisoned industrial workers.

Edmunds M, Sheehan TM, Van't Hoff W. Strychnine poisoning: clinical and toxicological observations on a non-fatal case. *J Toxicol Clin Toxicol* 1986;24:245.

A case report and general discussion of strychnine poisoning and its management.

Egekeze JO, Oehme FW. Sodium monofluoroacetate (SMFA, compound 1080): a literature review. *Vet Hum Toxicol* 1979;21:411.

A review of sodium monofluoroacetate describing the pathophysiology, toxicity, and treatment.

Hine CH. Methyl bromide poisoning: a review of ten cases. *J Occup Med* 1969;11:1.

A case series of patients describing sources and clinical toxicity of methyl bromide.

Katona B, Wason S. Superwarfarin poisoning. *J Emerg Med* 1989;7:627.

A review article describing clinical toxicity of superwarfarin compounds including a suggested approach to the management of patients with intentional and unintentional rodenticide ingestions.

Oransky S, Roseman B, Fish D, et al. Seizures temporally associated with use of DEET insect repellent in New York and Connecticut. *MMWR* 1989;38:678.

A report of four children and one adult who developed seizures—all had cutaneous exposure to DEET.

Pond SM. Manifestations and management of paraquat poisoning. *Med J Aust* 1990;152:256.

An excellent review of pathophysiology, clinical toxicity, and management of paraquat poisoning.

Telch J, Jarvis DA. Acute intoxication with lindane (gamma benzene hexachloride). *Can Med Assoc J* 1982;126:662.

A case report and discussion of the association between cutaneous use of lindane and seizures.

Wilson R, Lovejoy FH, Jaeger RJ, et al. Acute phosphine poisoning aboard a grain freighter: epidemiologic, clinical, and pathological findings. *JAMA* 1980;244:148.

A case series of patients who developed acute phosphine poisoning; contains a description of the clinical presentation and epidemiology of these poisonings.

130. PHENCYCLIDINE AND HALLUCINOGENS

Jeffrey R. Tucker

I. **General principles.** Phencyclidine (PCP) is a dissociative anesthetic that produces a variety of alterations in consciousness and behavior, with hallucinations occurring in approximately 10% of users. In contrast, hallucinogens such as lysergic acid diethylamine (LSD) and methylenedioxymethamphetamine (MDMA) can intensify or distort sensory perception and commonly evoke hallucinations.

II. **Pathogenesis**

A. **Phencyclidine.** Phenyl-cyclohexyl-piperidine (PCP) is a synthetic compound chemically related to ketamine. It decreases pain perception and can produce anesthesia. It is a stimulant-type street drug used to obtain a "high." PCP acts on multiple chemical sites in the brain; the resulting clinical effects are unpredictable. Several analogs of PCP are occasionally used as street drugs. PCP is well absorbed from the gastrointestinal (GI) tract and from the lungs. It is commonly added to marijuana or tobacco, which is then smoked. PCP has a large volume of distribution and concentrates in the brain, lungs, and liver. The main route of PCP elimination is oxidative metabolism.

B. **Hallucinogens.** The psychedelic hallucinogens are either synthetic indoleamines (derivatives of tryptamine), phenethylamines (derivatives of amphetamines), or plant products called organics. Derivatives of tryptamine include lysergic acid (LSD or "acid"), dimethyltryptamine (DMT), morning-glory seeds (*Ipomoea* and Rivea genera), *psilocybe* and other mushroom species (psilocybin, psilocin), and toad skin secretions (bufotenin). Derivatives of phenethylamines include methylenedioxymethamphetamine (MDMA), dimethoxymethylamphetamine (DOM), dimethoxyamphetamine (DMA), methylenedioxyethamphetamine (MDEA), and the peyote cactus *Lophophora williamsii* (mescaline). The clinical effects produced by different agents are very similar.

Hallucinogenic drugs cause two major groups of symptoms. The first is related to their mind-altering effects; the second results from physiologic effects. Homicide, self-destructive behavior, and accidental injuries can occur, and acute or chronic psychosis may be precipitated by the psychedelic experience. Hallucinogens are readily absorbed from the GI tract following ingestion. Severe toxicity can result from intravenous injection.

III. **Clinical presentation**

A. **PCP.** Manifestations of PCP toxicity include alterations in sensorium, behavioral disturbances, motor rigidity, autonomic instability, and alterations in vital signs. Hypertension and nystagmus are hallmarks of PCP intoxication, occurring in approximately 57% of cases. Nystagmus can be horizontal, vertical, or even rotatory. Rhabdomyolysis is another common complication.

Four major pattern of toxicity have been described: (a) coma, (b) organic catatonic syndrome, (c) toxic psychosis, and (d) acute brain syndrome. Minor patterns, which represent mild toxicity, include (a) lethargy or stupor, (b) bizarre behavior, (c) violent behavior, (d) agitation, and (e) euphoria. Patients may experience more than one pattern during an episode of intoxication.

B. **Hallucinogens.** Psychedelic effects, known to users as a "trip" or "tripping," are characterized by changes in sensory perception. They include euphoria or dysphoria; an increase in the intensity of sensory perception; distortions of time, place, and body image; visual hallucinations; synesthesias (i.e., "seeing sounds" and "hearing colors"); illusions; loss of spatial sense; and feelings of unreality. Physiologic effects that commonly accompany psychedelic ones include facial flushing, mild tachycardia, mild to moderate hypertension, dilated pupils, nausea, vomiting, and diarrhea. Significant or life-threatening autonomic effects are rare and usually occur only after large overdoses. Manifestations include stupor or coma, bradycardia or tachycardia, shock or hypertension, malignant hyperthermia, seizures, muscle rigidity, and coagulopathy. Dark urine may be the first sign of rhabdomyolysis.

IV. Evaluation. The physical examination should focus on the vital signs, sensorium, behavior, motor signs, and autonomic findings. The temperature should be taken as quickly as possible. Laboratory tests and radiographs should be obtained as clinically indicated. Severely ill patients should have arterial blood gases (ABG) to rule out metabolic acidosis. A computed tomography head scan should be obtained in comatose patients or if head trauma or intracerebral bleeding is suspected. Patients with significant toxicity require serum chemistries, including a complete blood count, electrolytes, blood urea nitrogen, creatinine, glucose, creatine phosphokinase, coagulation profile, ABG, urinalysis, and serum transaminases. Patients with altered mental status should have a bedside fingerstick blood sugar.

V. Treatment. Treatment is aimed at counteracting cerebral stimulation and providing supportive care. Advanced life-support measures should be instituted as necessary. Activated charcoal is indicated for recent ingestions. No specific antidote exists for PCP or hallucinogen intoxication. Diazepam is the sedative of choice for patients with agitation, seizures, and hyperthermia. Haloperidol (5–10 mg orally, intravenously, or intramuscularly; repeated as necessary) has been found to be effective in improving the overall toxic effects of PCP. Some physicians prefer diazepam because haloperidol can produce malignant neuroleptic syndrome. The standard recommendation of "talking down" patients with the psychedelic pattern of intoxication is often impractical and can be ineffective for severely disturbed or uncommunicative patients. Naloxone is not recommended unless the patient has respiratory depression. Intravenous (IV) fluids should be administered to correct dehydration, electrolyte imbalances, or marked acidosis and to maintain brisk urine output. Intravenous labetalol is recommended for hypertensive urgencies and IV nitroprusside for hypertensive emergencies. Dysrhythmias can be treated as usual. For patients with hyperthermia, aggressive cooling measures are necessary. Paralytic agents may be necessary. Rhabdomyolysis should be treated in the usual fashion.

Selected Readings

Abraham HD, Aldridge AM. Adverse consequences of lysergic acid diethylamide. *Addiction* 1993;88:1327.

An article about the recent rise of lysergic use and the adverse effect associated with it.

Burns RS, Lerner SE. Perspective: acute phencyclidine intoxication. *J Toxicol Clin Toxicol* 1976;9:477.

An extensive discussion about the acute effects phencyclidine toxicity.

Callaway CW, Clark RF. Hyperthermia in psychostimulant overdose. *Ann Emerg Med* 1994;24:68.

An excellent review article about the current understanding of the treatment of hyperthermia in overdose patients.

Javitt DC, Zukin SR. Recent advances in the phencyclidine model of schizophrenia. *Am J Psychiatry* 1991;148:1301.

An excellent discussion of the clinically relevant interaction of phencyclidine (PCP) binding and dose range of PCP effects.

Klepfisz A, Racy J. Homicide and LSD. *JAMA* 1973;223:429.

A case report about a psychotic event associated with lysergic acid (LSD) use.

Lytttle T, Goldstein, Gartz J. Bufo toads and bufotenine fact and fiction surrounding an alleged psychedelic. *Journal of Psychedelic Drugs* 1996;28:267.

An extensive discussion about the current understanding of Bufo toad and bufotenine.

McCann UD, Slate SO, Ricaurte GA. Adverse reactions with 3, 4-methylenedioxymethamphetamine (MDMA; "Ecstasy"). *Drug Saf* 1996;15;107.

An excellent review about acute and chronic complication of MDMA use.

McCarron MM, Phencyclidine and Hallucinogens. In: Irwin RS, Cerra FB, Rippe JM. Intensive Care Medicine, 4th ed. Philadelphia: Lippincott–Raven; 1999.

Comprehensive review with extensive reference list.

McCarron MM, Schuleze BW, Thompson GA, et al. Acute phencycholine intoxication: incidence of clinical findings in 1,000 cases. *Ann Emerg Med* 1981;10:237.

A large clinical review of 1,000 patients which showed that the typical findings of hypertension and nystagmus were present in 57% of the patients.

Patel R, Das M, Palazzolo M, et al. Myoglobinuric acute renal failure in phencyclidine overdose: report of observation in eight cases. *Ann Emerg Med* 1980;9:549.

A report of the clinical findings in eight patients with myoglobinuric acute renal failure.

Ricaurte GA, Forno LS, Wilson MA, et al. 3, 4-methylenedioxymethamphetamine selectives damage central serotonergic neurons in nonhumans primates. *JAMA* 1988;260:51.

Experimental models of monkeys demonstrate the selective neurotoxicity of MDMA.

Schultes RE. Hallucinogens of plant origin. *Science* 1969;163:245.

A discussion about the diverse types of hallucinogens present throughout the plant kingdom.

Ulrich R, Patten. The rise, decline and fall of LSD. *Perspect Biol Med* 1991;34:561.

An excellent review article about the historical importance of lysergic acid (LSD) as therapeutic agent and as a psychedelic agent.

131. SEDATIVE-HYPNOTIC POISONING

Richard Y. Wang

I. General principles. Sedative-hypnotic agents include benzodiazepines, barbiturates, nonbenzodiazepine–nonbarbiturate sedatives, and some muscle relaxants. They are used to treat anxiety, depression, panic disorders, insomnia, musculoskeletal disorders, seizures, and alcohol withdrawal, and as an adjunct to anesthesia. γ-Hydroxybutyrate (GHB), originally used for anesthesia induction, is now illegal in the United States. It is abused for its euphoric effects and sometimes used to facilitate date rape. Most sedative–hypnotics act by facilitating the action of γ-aminobutyric acid, an inhibitory central nervous system (CNS) neurotransmitter.

II. Clinical manifestations

- **A. Benzodiazepine** overdoses produce slurred speech, lethargy, ataxia, nystagmus, and coma. Loss of deep tendon reflexes and apnea are unusual in isolated benzodiazepine overdose, except with a massive overdose. Cardiac arrest and pulmonary edema from pure benzodiazepine overdose is rare. Paradoxical reactions can occur; they include tremulousness, apprehension, insomnia, anxiety, agitation, hallucinations, and manic responses.
- **B. Barbiturates** produce sedation within 30 minutes of ingestion, which can progress to coma, respiratory collapse, hypotension, and hypothermia. Bullous skin lesions can develop over pressure points in patients with prolonged coma. The lesions are tense, surrounded by erythema, and the bullous fluid has detectable amounts of barbiturate. Barbiturates suppress brain electrical activity and full recovery has been reported after an isoelectric tracing on an electroencephalograph.
- **C. Chloral hydrate** toxicity includes gastrointestinal irritation, CNS depression, and cardiac tachydysrhythmias. Delayed manifestations of toxicity include dermal exfoliation, renal tubular necrosis, and hepatotoxicity.
- **D. Ethchlorvynol** poisoning results in altered sensorium, nystagmus, respiratory depression, coma, seizures, and noncardiogenic pulmonary edema. The breath or gastric aspirate may have a characteristic odor of a new plastic shower curtain.
- **E. Glutethimide** is unique because of the fluctuating level of CNS depression and anticholinergic effects associated with poisoning.
- **F. Meprobamate** toxicity includes CNS depression, respiratory depression, seizures, hypotension, and dysrhythmias. Carisprodol (Soma), a commonly used muscle relaxant, is metabolized to meprobamate. Meprobamate can form gastric concretions, resulting in progressive, cyclic, or prolonged toxicity.
- **G. Baclofen** poisonings is manifest by CNS depression, seizures, apnea, bradycardia, hypotension, and hypothermia.
- **H. γ-Hydroxybutyrate** (GHB) was originally used as an anesthetic induction agent and subsequently misused for its euphoric effects and to facilitate date rape. It is illegal to possess GHB in the United States. Its precursor, γ-butyrolactone (GBL) is a street drug that causes similar, but more prolonged toxicity. Symptoms of GHB toxicity occur rapidly and death has resulted from its combined use with opioids. Drowsiness, euphoria, hallucinations, delirium, nausea, vomiting, hypothermia, clonic activity of the limbs, seizures, and coma may be seen. Recovery from pure GHB poisoning appears to be rapid, with return of consciousness within a few hours of ingestion.

III. Evaluation. The physical examination should focus on evaluating the level of consciousness, respiratory function, and cardiovascular status. All patients should have cardiac and oxygen saturation monitoring. Patients with abnormal vital signs should have routine laboratory studies, and an arterial blood gas, electrocardiogram, and chest radiograph. Patients with prolonged deep coma are at risk for rhabdomyolysis and should have a creatine kinase measured.

Thin-layer chromatography and gas chromatography-mass spectrometry of the urine can confirm the presence of these agents. Quantitative serum barbiturates assays are also available. Qualitative urine immunoassays for benzodiazepines only detect agents that are metabolized by the oxazepam pathway. A negative qualitative benzodiazepine screen does not rule out the presence of a benzodiazepine, but rather indicates a failure to detect one.

IV. Management. The most important aspect of management is support for airway and breathing. Early airway protection is imperative because up to 40% of patients may aspirate. Intubation is recommended if patients cannot protect their airway or are hypoventilating.

Flumazenil (Romazicon), a competitive inhibitor of benzodiazepines at their CNS receptor sites, can reverse the sedative effects of benzodiazepine. Variable response on respiratory rate has been noted in several clinical trials. Flumazenil should be used with caution in patients who are benzodiazepine tolerant because of the potential for causing withdrawal seizures. Other patients at risk for seizures from flumazenil therapy include those with polypharmacy overdoses in whom reversal of benzodiazepine effect may unmask the epileptogenic effects of drugs such as cyclic antidepressants, isoniazid, and cocaine. Patients iatrogenically oversedated by benzodiazepines during medical procedures may benefit from flumazenil treatment. The initial dose of flumazenil, given intravenously (IV), is 0.05 to 0.2 mg followed by 0.1 to 0.2 mg every minute until 1 to 2 mg has been administered. Failure to respond to 2 mg suggests that benzodiazepines are unlikely to have caused the coma.

Activated charcoal is the method of choice for gastrointestinal decontamination. Gastric lavage may also be of benefit in patients who are comatose. Multidose, activated charcoal can enhance the elimination of barbiturates and be effective for other sedative-hypnotic agents. Alkaline diuresis with a sodium bicarbonate infusion can also enhance the elimination of phenobarbital.

Hypotension should initially be treated with crystalloids and then with vasopressors such as dopamine and norepinephrine. Hypotension refractory to supportive care is an indication for hemoperfusion or hemodialysis.

β-Adrenoreceptor blockers (e.g., propranolol 1 mg IV) are recommended for the treatment of tachydysrhythmias caused by choral hydrate poisoning if standard therapeutic agents (e.g., lidocaine) fail. Hemodialysis should be considered in patients with refractory dysrhythmias.

Symptomatic bradycardia caused by baclofen can be successfully treated with atropine.

Selected Readings

Berg MJ, Berlinger WG, Goldberg MJ, et al. Acceleration of the body clearance of phenobarbital by oral activated charcoal. *N Engl J Med* 1982;307:642.

This study demonstrated repeat doses of activated charcoal to decrease the half-life of intravenously administered phenobarbital.

Beveridge AW, Lawson AAH. Occurrence of bullous lesions in acute barbiturate intoxication. *BMJ* 1965;1:835.

This report describes the presence of bullous skin lesions in barbiturate poisoned patients.

Frenia ML, Schauben JL, Wears RL, et al. Multiple dose activated charcoal compared to urinary alkalinization for the enhancement of phenobarbital elimination. *Clin Toxicol* 1996;34:169.

This study demonstrated repeat dose activated charcoal to decrease elimination phenobarbital half-life more than urinary alkalinization.

Garnier R, Gueraulte E, Muzard D, et al. Acute zolpidem poisoning—analysis of 344 cases. *J Toxicol Clin Toxicol* 1994;32:391.

This survey described the low incidence of respiratory depression from zolpidem overdose alone.

Glauser FL, Smith WR, Caldwell A, et al. Ethchlorvynol (Placidyl) induced pulmonary edema. *Ann Intern Med* 1976;84:46.

This study demonstrated the direct toxic effects of ethchlorvynol on lung tissue.

Graham SR, Day RO, Lee R, et al. Overdose with chloral hydrate: a pharmacological and therapeutic review. *Med J Aust* 1988;149:686.

This review described the cardiac dysrhythmias associated with chloral hydrate toxicity and its treatment.

Hansen AR, Kennedy KA, Amber JA, et al. Glutethimide poisoning: a metabolite contributes to morbidity and mortality. *N Engl J Med* 1975;292:250.

This report attributed the enterohepatic recirculation of active metabolites to the fluctuating levels of consciousness in glutethimide toxicity.

Norman TR, Graham BD. Plasma concentrations of benzodiazepines. *Prog Neuropsychopharmacol Biol Psychiatry* 1984;18:115.

This review discussed how quantitative measurement of sedative hypnotic levels is not useful or necessary in overdoses.

Paul S, Marangos PJ, Skolnick P. The benzodiazepine GABA-chloride ionophore receptor complex. *Biol Psychiatry* 1981;16:213.

The mechanism of action of sedative hypnotic is discussed.

Schwartz HS. Acute meprobamate poisoning with gastrotomy and removal of a drug containing mass. *N Engl J Med* 1976;295:1177.

This report described the potential for meprobamate to form bezoars and the need for their removal by surgery.

Serfay M, Masterton G. Fatal poisonings attributed to benzodiazepines in Britain during the 1980s. *Br J Psychiatry* 1993;163:386.

This report described fatalities from benzodiazepine poisoning to be uncommon and associated with combined overdoses.

Shubin H, Weil MH. The mechanism of shock following suicidal doses of barbiturate, narcotics and tranquilizer drugs. *Am J Med* 1965;36:853.

The contributing factors to sedative hypnotic-induced hypotension are discussed.

Spivey WH. Flumazenil and seizures: analysis of 43 cases. *Clin Ther* 1992;14:292.

This survey demonstrated the various causes of seizures associated with flumazenil use.

132. SYMPATHOMIMETIC POISONING

Erica L. Liebelt

I. General principles. Sympathomimetic agents are catecholamine analogs that stimulate the sympathetic nervous system. Although amphetamines are US Food and Drug Administration (FDA) schedule II substances, other sympathomimetics are found in over-the-counter cough and cold preparations and in topical ophthalmic vasoconstrictor and nasal decongestant solutions (Table 132-1). Amphetamines are currently only approved for treating hyperkinetic behavior disorders in children, short-term weight reduction, and narcolepsy. Sustained-release preparations with effects lasting 12 to 24 hours are available.

Commonly abused sympathomimetics include dextroamphetamine, methamphetamine, designer amphetamine derivatives (phenylethylamines) such as MDMA or Ecstasy (3, 4-methylenedioxymethamphetamine), and the over-the-counter anorexiants ephedrine and phenylpropanolamine (PPA). STP or DOM (2, 5-dimethoxy-4-methylamphetamine) and MDA (3-methoxy-4, 5-methylene-deoxyamphetamine) were also popular in the 1960s and 1970s.

The prescription anorexiants dexfenfluramine and fenfluramine (prescribed with phentermine as "Fen-phen") were withdrawn from the market several years ago when their use was associated with pulmonary hypertension and valvular heart disease. Following the Persian Gulf War and relief efforts in Somalia in the mid-1990s, the practice of chewing the leaves of *Catha edulis* or "khat," a plant containing the sympathomimetic cathinone and indigenous to northern Africa, spread to the United States.

II. Pharmacology. Sympathomimetics, primarily norepinephrine and dopamine, both promote the release and block the reuptake of central nervous (CNS) and sympathetic neurotransmitters. The phenylethylamines also inhibit serotonin reuptake, which may account for their hallucinogenic effects. PPA is a selective peripheral α-adrenergic agonist that can cause the release of stored norepinephrine from presynaptic neurons. Like clonidine, the imidazoline decongestants (e.g., clonidine) are central α_2 adrenergic agonists, which decrease sympathetic outflow from the CNS. Because they also have peripheral α-agonist activity, clinical effects are variable and depend on the dose and underlying level of sympathetic activity.

The crystallized form of methamphetamine ("ice") can be smoked. Abuse of Ritalin or methylphenidate has occurred via the nasal insufflation of crushed tablets.

Smoking and intravenous (IV) injection of amphetamines produces almost instantaneous effects. Effects occur a few minutes after insufflation and about 30 minutes following ingestion.

Sympathomimetics are weak bases. In an acid urine, they exist primarily in an ionized state and cannot be reabosrbed in the distal renal tubules. Thus, their elimination is enhanced. The plasma half-lives of amphetamines vary from 7 to 34 hours (depending on urine flow and urine pH), whereas the half-lives of PPA, ephedrine, and pseudoephedrine are significantly shorter, ranging from 2 to 4 hours.

III. Clinical presentation. CNS effects, which include anxiety, restlessness, nervousness, agitation, confusion, delirium, hyperactivity, and muscle fasciculations, can progress to rigidity, seizures, and coma. Severe hyperpyrexia is seen in serious and fatal poisonings. Cardiovascular effects include palpitations, tachyarrhythmias, and hypertension. Other sympathomimetic effects include nausea, vomiting, and mydriasis. Death can result from hyperthermia, cerebrovascular accidents, myocardial infarction, and cardiac arrhythmias.

Patients who have ingested large amounts of PPA typically present with nervousness, tremulousness, anxiety, headache, and mild hypertension. Severe hypertension with reflex bradycardia can occur, although combination products or multiple drugs can produce tachycardia. Hypertensive crises with resulting intracerebral hemorrhage or vasospasm and infarction have been reported.

TABLE 132-1. Sympathomimetic Agents

Generic Name	Common Name
Nonprescription over-the-counter agents	
Phenylpropanolamine	Dexatrim, Comtrex, Allerest
Pseudoephedrine	Sudafed, Novafed
Ephedrine	Primatene, Bronkaid
Propylhexedrine	Benzedrex Inhaler
Desoxyephedrine	Vicks Inhaler
Imidazolines	
Naphazoline	Clear Eyes, Naphcon, Privine
Oxymetazoline	Afrin, Dristan
Tetrahydrozoline	Murine, Visine
Zylometazoline	Otrivin
Prescription (DEA schedule II or III) agents	
Amphetamines	
Methylphenidate	Ritalin
Amphetamine	Adderall
Dextroamphetamine	Dexedrine, Adderall
Phentermine	Fastin, Ionamin

DEA, Drug enforcement agency

Imidazolines produce a toxidrome similar to that seen in narcotic and clonidine poisoning. Ingestions of as little as 2 to 5 ml of topical eye decongestants in a toddler can cause significant toxicity. Symptoms include lethargy, which can progress to coma and alternate with agitation and hyperactivity. Effects on vital signs are variable—initial hypertension and bradycardia can be followed by hypotension and bradycardia.

Drug interactions between sympathomimetics and monoamine oxidase inhibitors can result in life-threatening hypertension, hyperthermia, and vasomotor instability. Use of certain amphetamines with other serotonergic agents can produce the serotonin syndrome—altered mental status, myoclonus, muscle rigidity, and hyperthermia.

IV. Management. Advanced life support measures should be instituted as necessary. All patients should have continuous cardiac monitoring. Temperature must be monitored frequently to detect the development of hyperthermia. Gastrointestinal decontamination can be undertaken with activated charcoal for recent ingestions. It should also be considered hours after the ingestion of sustained-release formulations. Symptomatic patients should have an electrocardiogram and measurement done of electrolytes, blood urea nitrogen, creatinine, glucose, and creatine phosphokinase. A urinalysis with positive dipstick for blood in the absence of red blood cells suggests myoglobinuria. Emergent head computed tomography imaging should be performed on patients with prolonged or focal seizures or coma.

Seizures and CNS excitation should be treated with benzodiazepines (e.g., diazepam and midazolam). Patients with extreme agitation and acute psychosis can be treated with haloperidol or droperidol in conjunction with benzodiazepines. However, neuroleptic agents should be used cautiously because they lower the seizure threshold, alter temperature, and can exacerbate the existing symptoms. Control of excessive muscular activity by sedation and paralysis is extremely important in preventing and treating hyperthermia and rhabdomyolysis. Hyperthermia should also be treated aggressively with external cooling measures and hydration. No indication is seen for dantrolene or bromocriptine therapy for amphetamine-induced hyperthermia. Rhabdomyolysis should be treated with IV fluids to maintain adequate urine output.

Hypertensive emergencies should be treated with IV nitroprusside or alpha-blockers (e.g., phentolamine) in conjunction with benzodiazepines to control agitation. Acid diuresis is not recommended for enhanced elimination because of adverse metabolic consequences such as systemic acidemia and precipitation of renal failure in patients with myoglobinuria.

Patients with hypertension, seizures, arrhythmias, hyperthermia, altered mental status, or hypotension should be hospitalized in an intensive care unit. Patients with mild tachycardia and anxiety can be observed for 6 hours in the emergency department providing they were exposed only to short-acting agents and all signs and symptoms have resolved before discharge.

Selected Readings

Cho AK. Ice: a new dosage form of an old drug. *Science* 1990;249:631.

A review of the history, pharmacology, abuse patterns, and clinical effects of methamphetamine.

Derlet RW, Rice P, Horowitz Z, et al. Amphetamine toxicity: experience with 127 cases. *J Emerg Med* 1989;7:157.

This retrospective review of 127 cases of amphetamine toxicity discusses toxic clinical symptoms, management, and outcomes.

Ginsberg MD, Hertzman M, Schmidt-Nowara W. Amphetamine intoxication with coagulopathy, hyperthermia, and reversible renal failure: a syndrome resembling heatstroke. *Ann Intern Med* 1970;73:81.

A case report and discussion on similarities of amphetamine intoxication with heatstroke.

Jerrard DA. "Designer drugs": a current perspective. *J Emerg Med* 1990;8:733.

A comprehensive review of "designer drugs" including amphetamines.

Kase CS, Foster TE, Reed JE, et al. Intracerebral hemorrhage and phenylpropanolamine use. *Neurology* 1987;37:399.

Two case reports and discussions of intracerebral hemorrhage associated with phenylpropanolamine use.

Klein-Schwartz W, Gorman R, Oderda GM, et al. Central nervous system depression from ingestion of non-prescription eyedrops. *Am J Emerg Med* 1984;2:217.

Case reports and review of clinical effects and outcomes of ingestion of imidazoline eyedrops.

Liebelt EL, Shannon MW. Small doses, big problems: a selected review of highly toxic common medications. *Pediatr Emerg Care* 1993;9:292.

This review includes discussion of clinical toxicity of imidazolines in children.

Pentel P. Toxicity from over-the-counter stimulants. *JAMA* 1984;252:1898.

A review of over-the-counter stimulants, including phenylpropanolamine, ephedrine, and pseudoephedrine.

Scandling J, Spital A. Amphetamine-associated myoglobinuric renal failure. *South Med J* 1982;75:237.

A case report and discussion of myoglobinuric renal failure after amphetamine ingestion.

Swenson RD, Golper TA, Bennet WM. Acute renal failure and rhabdomyolysis after ingestion of phenylpropanolamine-containing diet pills. *JAMA* 1982;248:1216.

Case reports and discussion on association of phenylpropanolamine ingestion, acute renal failure, and rhabdomyolysis.

133. SYSTEMIC ASPHYXIANTS

Jeffrey R. Tucker

I. General principles. Systemic asphyxiants prevent the transport and release of oxygen by hemoglobin and myoglobin or block its cellular utilization.

A. Cyanide. Cyanide salts are used in electroplating, metal cleaning and extraction, and in laboratory and photographic processes. Cyanide is also liberated from cyanogens, cyanogenic glycosides (e.g., bitter cassava, peach pits), nitriles, sodium nitroprusside, and synthetic materials through spontaneous or thermal decomposition, hepatic metabolism, or reactions with acids.

Cyanide binds to the ferric (Fe^{3+}) ion of mitochondrial cytochrome oxidase and disrupts electron transport and oxidative phosphorylation. This results in anaerobic metabolism with lactic acidosis. Detoxification is accomplished by the enzyme rhodanese (sulfur transferase), which catalyzes complexing of cyanide with sulfur to form the less toxic thiocyanate.

B. Hydrogen sulfide. Hydrogen sulfide (H_2S) is a colorless, irritating gas with a sulfur or rotten egg odor. It occurs naturally in natural gas, volcanic gas, hot springs, sewer gas, and swampy soils; it is a product of many industrial and manufacturing processes. The mechanism of toxicity is the same as for cyanide.

C. Methemoglobinemia. Methemoglobin is hemoglobin with the iron oxidized to the ferric (Fe^{3+}) state rather than in the normal ferrous (Fe^{2+}) state. It is unable to bind and transport oxygen. Normally, 1% or less of total hemoglobin exists as methemoglobin. Exposure to drugs and chemicals that are direct oxidants or have oxidizing metabolites can result in higher methemoglobin fractions (methemoglobinemia). Aniline, amino-, nitro-, and nitroso derivatives, antimalarials, dapsone, local anesthetics, nitrates, nitrites, phenazopyridine, and sulfonamides are common offenders. Two physiologic mechanisms prevent this from occurring: reduction (inactivation) of hemoglobin-oxidizing compounds and reduction of methemoglobin back to hemoglobin by nicotinamide adenine dinucleotide (NADH)- and nicotinamide adenine dinucleotide phosphate (NADPH)-dependent methemoglobin reductases. Oxidation and precipitation of hemoglobin protein, resulting in Heinz body hemolytic anemia, can accompany methemoglobinemia.

II. Clinical presentation

A. Cyanide. Life-threatening symptoms can occur within seconds of hydrogen cyanide gas inhalation and within 30 minutes of cyanide salt ingestion. They may not occur until several hours after the ingestion of other cyanide compounds. Signs and symptoms of poisoning are caused by hypoxia. Early manifestations include giddiness, headache, anxiety, tachycardia, hyperpnea, hypertension, and palpitations. Later effects include shock, increased anion gap metabolic acidosis, dysrhythmias, coma, seizures, pulmonary edema, respiratory failure, and death.

B. Hydrogen sulfide. Manifestations of poisoning are similar to those of cyanide. Irritant effects such as tearing, rhinitis, throat pain, and cough may also be present. H_2S is known for its rapid "knockdown effect": exposure to high concentrations typically causes sudden collapse. A history of potential exposure; rapid onset and progression of symptoms; rotten egg odor of the clothes, breath, or freshly drawn blood; and black discoloration of the patient's silver coins and jewelry are diagnostic clues.

C. Methemoglobinemia. Methemoglobin fractions of approximately 15% (1.5 g/dl) produce central cyanosis. Patients usually appear much less ill than would be expected with a similar degree of cyanosis from a cardiac or respiratory cause. With increasing levels, manifestations of hypoxia occur. Cyanosis unresponsive to 100% oxygen and a dark or chocolate brown color of freshly drawn blood support the diagnosis. An arterial oxygen saturation gap, a difference between the oxygen saturation calculated from the Po_2 and that measured by co-oximeter, indicates that an abnormal hemoglobin such as carboxyhemoglobin, sulfhemoglobin, or methemoglobin is present. The oxygen saturation measured by pulse oximetry will be falsely elevated but less than the calculated one.

III. Examination. Examination should focus on vital signs and respiratory, cardiovascular, and central nervous system (CNS) function. Symptomatic patients should have continuous cardiac monitoring and pulse oximetry; testing of electrolytes, blood urea nitrogen, creatinine, glucose, arterial blood gases; and electrocardiogram and chest x-ray studies.

Increased serum lactate, venous Po_2 (>40 mm Hg), and oxygen saturation and decreased difference (<20%) between arterial and central venous oxygen saturation support the diagnosis of cyanide poisoning. An elevated whole blood cyanide level is confirmatory. An elevated blood sulfide level has been used to confirm the diagnosis of H_2S poisoning. A quantitative methemoglobin level, measured by co-oximetry confirms the diagnosis of methemoglobinemia. Examining a peripheral blood smear and monitoring the hematocrit, reticulocyte count, and plasma free hemoglobin may be helpful.

IV. Treatment. Standard advanced life-support measures and decontamination procedures should be instituted as necessary. Supplemental oxygen should be administered to all symptomatic patients. Seizures should be treated with anticonvulsants in addition to antidotal therapy. Severe metabolic acidosis should be treated with sodium bicarbonate. Hyperbaric oxygen therapy should be considered in patients unresponsive to other measures.

A. Cyanide. The Lilly Cyanide antidote kit containing amyl nitrite, sodium nitrite, and sodium thiosulfate is the only cyanide antidote currently available in the United States. Nitrites promote the formation of methemoglobin which is thought to bind cyanide and promote its release from cytochrome oxidase; thiosulfate provides additional substrate for detoxification. Amyl nitrite can be inhaled for 30 seconds of each minute as a first-aid measure; place a broken pearl between two sheets of gauze and over the nose and mouth using a fresh one every few minutes. Once intravenous (IV) access is established, administer IV nitrite (300 mg over several minutes) followed by IV sodium thiosulfate (12.5 g over several minutes). Additional nitrite dosing should be titrated to the clinical response. Adverse effects of sodium nitrite include hypotension and excessive methemoglobin.

B. Hydrogen sulfide. Amyl and sodium nitrite therapy may also be useful in patients with hydrogen sulfide poisoning who have not regained consciousness. Dosing and precautions are the same as for cyanide poisoning.

C. Methemoglobinemia. Methylene blue, the antidote for methemoglobinemia, is a cofactor for NADPH-dependent methemoglobin reductase and markedly increases its activity. Asymptomatic or mildly symptomatic patients with a methemoglobin fraction of 30% or less may not require such therapy; the methemoglobin fraction will return to normal in 24 to 72 hours. Those with higher methemoglobin fractions or manifestations of ischemia should be given IV methylene blue (0.1 to 0.2 mg/kg of a 1% solution over 5 minutes). Additional doses, up to a total of 7 mg/kg, may be necessary. Methylene blue is ineffective in patients with glucose-6-phosphate dehydrogenase (G-6-PD) deficiency and is contraindicated in patients with G-6-PD deficiency caused by hemolysis. Exchange transfusion may be necessary in such patients and in those with very high methemoglobin fractions.

Selected Readings

Baud FJ, Barriot P, Toffis V, et al. Elevated blood cyanide concentrations in victims of smoke inhalation. *N Engl J Med* 1991;325:1761.

A clinical study demonstrating that an elevated lactate level is sensitive indicator for cyanide toxicity.

Hall AH. Systemic asphyxiants. In: Irwin RS, Cerra FB, Rippe JM, eds. *Intensive care medicine,* 4th ed. Philadelphia: Lippincott–Raven; 1999.

A comprehensive review with extensive reference list.

Hall AH, Kulig KW, Rumack BH. Drug- and chemical-induced methaemoglobinaemia: clinical features and management. *Medical Toxicology* 1986;1;253.

A review article about the different forms of methemoglobinemia: physiologic, congenital, and acquired.

Hall AH, Rumack BH. Clinical toxicology of cyanide. *Ann Emerg Med* 1986;15:1067.

An excellent review article about the sources, clinical presentation, and treatment of cyanide toxicity.

Hall AH, Rumack BH, Schaffer MI, et al. Clinical toxicology of cyanide: North American clinical experiences. In: Bailantyne B, Marrs TC, eds. *Clinical and experimental toxicology of cyanides.* Bristok, UK: Wright; 1987:312.

An excellent discussion of cyanide deaths in North America, including the 1982 famous Chicago tampering incident.

Hoidal CR, Hall AH, Robinson MD, et al. Hydrogen sulfide poisoning from toxic inhalations of roofing asphalt fumes. *Ann Emerg Med* 1986;15:826.

Two cases of inhalation of roofing asphalt fumes show the rare but potential devastating effects from hydrogen sulfide gas.

Kirk MA, Gerace R, Kulig KW. Cyanide and methemoglobin kinetics in smoke inhalation victims treated with the cyanide antidote kit. *Ann Emerg Med* 1993;22:1413.

Administration of sodium nitrite was safe for smoke inhalation patients in the presence of concomitant carbon monoxide in seven patients.

Kurt TL, Day LC, Reed WS, et al. Cyanide poisoning from glue-on nail remover. *Am J Emerg* 1991;9:271.

A case report involving acetonitrile, which is metabolized to cyanide with the potential for delayed toxicity.

Park CM, Nagel FL. Sulfhemoglobinemia: clinical and molecular aspects. *N Engl J Med* 1984;310:1579.

A review articles which discuss the confusion and difficulty in distinguishing sulfhemoglobinemia and methemoglobinemia.

Peters JW. Hydrogen sulfide poisoning in a hospital setting. *JAMA* 1981;246:1588.

A case report and investigation about how not to clean a drain full of plaster of paris sludge with 90% sulfuric acid.

Pollack ES, Pollack CV. Incidence of subclinical methemoglobinemia in infants with diarrhea. *Ann Emerg Med* 1994;24:652.

A prospective study showing that 64% of infants aged less than 6 months of age with diarrhea had elevated methhemoglobin levels.

Schnapp LM, Cohen NH. Pulse oximetry: uses and abuses. *Chest* 1990;98:1244.

An excellent discussion about the benefits and limitations of pulse oximetry and how dyshemoglobinemias can affect the results.

Trapp W. Massive cyanide poisoning with recovery: a Boxing-day story. *Can Med Assoc J* 1970;102:517.

An interesting case report involving successful treatment of a cyanide victim.

Way JL, End E, Sheehy MH, et al. Effects of oxygen on cyanide intoxication. IV. Hyperbaric oxygen. *Toxicol Appl Pharmacol* 1972;22;415.

A laboratory investigation that showed no benefit of hyperbaric oxygen on cyanide poisoned mice.

134. WITHDRAWAL SYNDROMES

Richard Y. Wang

I. General principles. A variety of agents including antidepressants, ethanol, benzodiazepines, other sedative–hypnotic agents, opioids, and some antihypertensive and cardiovascular drugs can produce withdrawal syndromes on abrupt discontinuation of chronic use. This chapter focuses on the effects of withdrawal from ethanol, benzodiazepines, and opioids—the three drugs most commonly causing withdrawal syndromes in patients in the intensive care unit (ICU). Manifestations and management of nonbenzodiazepine sedative–hypnotic withdrawal are similar to that for ethanol and benzodiazepines.

II. Ethanol. Withdrawal symptoms occur when the baseline serum ethanol level decreases significantly. In the chronic alcoholic, signs of withdrawal are commonly present even when the ethanol level is 100 mg/dl or greater.

Acute tremulousness usually begins 6 to 8 hours after reduction in ethanol intake. Patients usually complain of nausea, vomiting, anorexia, and insomnia. The physical examination reveals mild central nervous system (CNS) and autonomic hyperactivity such as tachycardia, mild hypertension, hyperreflexia, irritability, and a resting tremor. These symptoms peak at about 24 to 36 hours, and most patients recover uneventfully in a few days. Approximately 25% of these patients go on to more serious withdrawal states, including delirium tremens.

Ethanol withdrawal seizures occur between 7 and 48 hours after cessation or relative abstinence from drinking. Withdrawal symptoms can precede the seizures or the seizure may herald the onset of ethanol withdrawal. They are short, generalized, tonic-clonic events, which are usually isolated. Status epilepticus or recurrent seizure activity lasting longer than 6 hours is distinctly uncommon in ethanol withdrawal and suggests another diagnosis.

Alcohol hallucinations are predominantly visual and associated with tremulousness. A subset of hallucinating patients does not demonstrate any other symptoms of withdrawal. Known as "alcohol hallucinosis," it begins within 8 to 48 hours of cessation of drinking. It is characterized by auditory hallucinations. In most cases, symptoms last 1 to 6 days, although they can persist for months and come to resemble chronic paranoid schizophrenia.

The hallmark of delirium tremens is a significant change in mental status associated with dramatic autonomic and CNS hyperactivity. The onset of delirium tremens is rarely seen before 48 to 72 hours after cessation or reduction in drinking, and can be delayed as long as 5 to 14 days. These patients manifest disorientation, global confusion, hallucinations, and delusions. Speech is unintelligible and psychomotor agitation present. Autonomic disturbances are present and cardiac dysrhythmias can occur. With early recognition, ICU monitoring, and aggressive treatment, mortality rates have decreased significantly.

The differential diagnosis of ethanol withdrawal includes other causes of a hyperadrenergic state. These include hypoglycemia, withdrawal from other sedative–hypnotic agents, and toxicity from sympathomimetic drugs (e.g., cocaine, amphetamine).

Achievement of adequate sedation is the cornerstone of successful treatment of ethanol withdrawal. Benzodiazepines have proved the most effective agents for this purpose. Diazepam, chlordiazepoxide, and lorazepam are the most commonly used parenteral agents. Therapy with intravenous (IV) benzodiazepine is titrated to the desired effect (sleepy but arousable) by the use of frequent boluses until withdrawal symptoms subside. Oral benzodiazepine therapy should be instituted simultaneously and is the preferred route once symptoms have been controlled. Barbiturates (e.g., pentobarbital, phenobarbital) are an alternative class of cross-tolerant sedative–hypnotic agents that can be used to treat ethanol withdrawal. Agents that are not recommended because of adverse effects or lack of controlled trials demonstrating their efficacy include paraldehyde, ethanol, neuroleptics, and sympatholytics.

Patients with ethanol withdrawal seizures should be sedated with benzodiazepines or barbiturates. No evidence indicates that phenytoin has any therapeutic efficacy in the treatment or prevention of ethanol withdrawal seizures. Because status epilepticus is uncommon in ethanol withdrawal, an evaluation for traumatic injuries and infection is necessary in those with this condition.

Volume resuscitation, correction of electrolyte abnormalities, and vigilance in the diagnosis and treatment of coexisting medical and surgical disorders are vital in reducing morbidity and mortality.

III. Benzodiazepines. Withdrawal from benzodiazepines can be as severe as withdrawal from barbiturates or ethanol. Iatrogenic-induced benzodiazepine withdrawal has resulted from the use of flumazenil in benzodiazepine-dependent patients.

Benzodiazepine withdrawal is also characterized by CNS excitation and autonomic hyperactivity. Mild early manifestations of withdrawal include anxiety, apprehension, irritability, dysphasia, and insomnia. Somatic complaints commonly include nausea, palpitations, tremor, diaphoresis, and muscle twitching. More severe signs include vomiting, tachycardia, postural hypotension, fasciculations, hallucinations, seizures, and hyperthermia.

Treatment strategies for benzodiazepine withdrawal are similar to those used for ethanol withdrawal. Reinstitution of the drug at a dose that relieves withdrawal symptoms followed by slow taper over a period of 2 to 4 weeks minimizes symptoms and effects the desired decrease in CNS tolerance. A long-acting benzodiazepine with active metabolites (e.g., diazepam, chlordiazepoxide) is preferred. Barbiturates can also be used in the treatment of benzodiazepine withdrawal. Blocking peripheral manifestations of withdrawal with β-adrenergic antagonists or clonidine may obscure early warnings of impending delirium and cloud the assessment of sedation adequacy achieved with concurrent cross-tolerant medications.

IV. Opioids. Unlike withdrawal from sedative–hypnotic agents, opioid withdrawal is not life-threatening (except in neonates). Withdrawal symptoms usually appear about the time of the next expected dose. Withdrawal from heroin begins 4 to 8 hours after the last dose, whereas withdrawal from methadone is delayed until 36 to 72 hours after the last dose. Opioid withdrawal can be precipitated in the opioid-dependent patient with the administration of opioid antagonists (e.g., naloxone) and opioid agonists–antagonists (e.g., pentazocine, nalbuphine, butorphanol).

Early manifestations of opioid withdrawal include mydriasis, lacrimation, rhinorrhea, diaphoresis, yawning, piloerection, anxiety, and restlessness. Myalgias, vomiting, diarrhea, anorexia, abdominal pain, and dehydration accompany more severe withdrawal. Fever, seizures, and altered mental status cannot be attributed to opioid withdrawal.

Treatment of opioid withdrawal includes the use of cross-tolerant opioid replacement (e.g., methadone) and sympatholytic therapy (e.g., clonidine). Methadone can be given in a dose of 10 to 20 mg orally or intramuscularly every hour until sedation is achieved. The total amount required for initial control can be given subsequently on a daily basis in a single or divided dose. Benzodiazepines are not cross-tolerant with opioids. Their role is limited to the management of significant anxiety associated with opioid withdrawal. Patients with dehydration from gastrointestinal fluid loss should be rehydrated.

Selected Readings

Blum K, Eubanks JD, Wallace JE, et al. Enhancement of alcohol withdrawal convulsions in mice by haloperidol. *Clin Toxicol* 1976;69:427.

This study demonstrated that haloperidol lowered seizure threshold in an alcohol withdrawal model.

Desmond MM, Schwanecke RP, Wilson GS, et al. Maternal barbiturate utilization and neonatal withdrawal symptomatology. *J Pediatr* 1972;80:190.

Neonatal barbiturate withdrawal symptoms are described.

Fultz JM, Senay EC. Guidelines for the management of hospitalized narcotics addicts. *Ann Intern Med* 1975;82:815.

A methadone withdrawal regimen is proposed in this article.

Gold MS, Redmond DE, Kleber HD. Clonidine blocks acute opiate withdrawal symptoms. *Lancet* 1978;2:599.
This study demonstrated the efficacy of clonidine for opioid withdrawal.

Isbell H, Faser HF, Wikler A, et al. An experimental study of the etiology of "rum fits" and delirium tremens. *Quart J Stud Alcohol* 1953;16:1.
This study demonstrated alcohol withdrawal to be associated with the cessation of drinking.

Malpas TJ, Darlow BA, Lennox R, et al. Maternal methadone dosage and neonatal withdrawal. *Aust NZ J Obstet Gynaecol* 1995;35:175.
This report described seizures as one of the manifestations of neonatal opioid withdrawal syndrome.

Martin PR, Bhushan CM, Kapur BM, et al. Intravenous phenobarbital therapy in barbiturate and other hypno-sedative withdrawal reactions. *Clin Pharmacol Ther* 1979;26:256.
This study described the use of parenteral phenobarbital in the management of sedative hypnotic withdrawal.

Rathlev N, Donofrio G, Fish S, et al. The lack of efficacy of phenytoin in the prevention of recurrent alcohol-related seizures. *Ann Emerg Med* 1994;23:513.
This study demonstrated phenytoin did not protect against alcohol withdrawal seizures.

Ritson B, Chick J. Comparison of two benzodiazepines in the treatment of alcohol withdrawal: effects in symptoms and cognitive recovery. *Drug Alcohol Depend* 1986;18:329.
This study demonstrated lorazepam to be less effective than diazepam in the treatment of alcohol withdrawal.

Tavel ME. A new look at an old syndrome: delirium tremens. *Arch Intern Med* 1962; 109:129.
This analysis demonstrated good supportive care to decrease mortality associated with delirium tremens.

Thompson WL, Johnson AD, Maddrey WL, et al. Diazepam and paraldehyde for treatment of severe delirium tremens: a controlled trial. *Ann Intern Med* 1975; 82:175.
This study demonstrated the benefit of parenterally administered diazepam for delirium tremens.

Victor M, Adams RD. The effect of alcohol on the nervous system. *Research Publications—Association for Research in Nervous and Mental Diseases* 1953;32:526.
This classic paper described the manifestations of ethanol withdrawal.

Victor M, Brausch C. The role of abstinence in the genesis of alcoholic epilepsy. *Epilepsia* 1967;8:1.
This report analyzed the nature of alcohol withdrawal seizures.

Woods JH, Winger G. Current benzodiazepine issues. *Psychopharmacology* 1995; 118:107.
This review discussed factors contributing to benzodiazepine dependency.

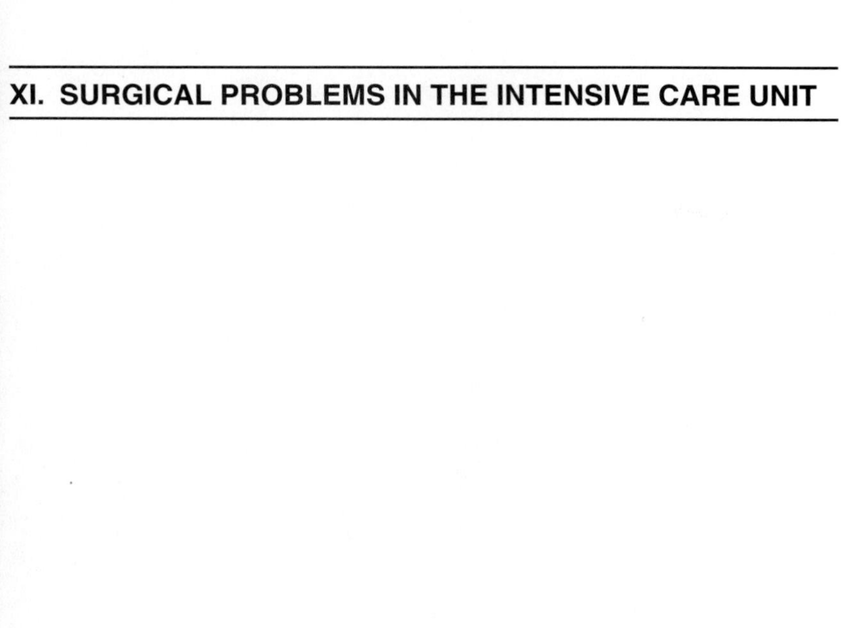

XI. SURGICAL PROBLEMS IN THE INTENSIVE CARE UNIT

135. EPISTAXIS

Freda D. McCarter, Fred A. Luchette, and Jack L. Gluckman

I. General principles. Epistaxis is a common clinical problem. It is usually mild and self-limited. However, epistaxis can become a severe and life-threatening emergency. An understanding of the anatomic blood supply to the nose is essential to rendering appropriate management.

The internal and external carotid arteries supply blood to the nose. The internal carotid gives rise to the anterior and posterior ethmoidal arteries. These intracranial vessels pierce the cribiform plate to supply blood to the superior portion of the nasal passages. The anterior ethmoidal artery supplies the anterior superior septum and the anterolateral nasal wall. The posterior ethmoidal artery supplies the posterior—superior and the posterolateral nasal wall.

The external carotid artery gives rise to the facial and internal maxillary arteries, which supply the cutaneous and mucosal surfaces of the nasal passage. The superior labial artery, as a terminal branch of the facial artery, supplies the nasal floor and inferior septum. Most nasal blood flow is derived from the terminal branches of the internal maxillary artery. The largest and most important of these terminal branches is the sphenopalatine artery which perfuses the posterior septum and the lateral nasal walls. Posterior epistaxis usually originates from the sphenopalatine artery and anterior bleeding usually originates from Kisselbach's plexus, a region where the internal and external blood supply anastomose.

II. Pathogenesis. Blunt trauma is the most common cause of epistaxis. Iatrogenic injury is common in the intensive care setting. Feeding and nasogastric tubes abrade and irritate the nasal passages. Nonhumidified oxygen delivered through a nasal cannula dries the mucosa. Primary and secondary coagulopathies are also important considerations in the pathogenesis of epistaxis.

Preexisting conditions can increase the risk of epistaxis. Abuse of cocaine and nasal decongestants desiccates the mucosa. Preexisting bony or cartilaginous deformities (e.g., severe septal deviation) cause airflow turbulence and irritation. Minor trauma and dryness in patients with atherosclerosis or hypertension results in brisk persistent bleeding that is difficult to control because the systolic pressure is elevated and the diseased vessels are noncompressible. The incidence of posterior epistaxis is higher in these patients.

III. Diagnosis. A distinction between anterior and posterior epistaxis must be established by physical diagnosis to provide appropriate management. The airway is a priority in unstable patients and intubation may be required to assure airway protection. Gastric decompression will evacuate aspirated blood and minimize aspiration.

In stable patients with epistaxis, a careful history and a thorough physical examination should be performed. The history must include any previous episodes of epistaxis, evidence of coagulopathy, and use of anticoagulants. Vital signs should be monitored. All nasal tubes are removed to permit complete visualization of the mucosa. The examination is carried out under good lighting with a nasal speculum and suction. Posterior bleeding may require nasal endoscopy for adequate visualization. In the face of diffuse bleeding, the vasoconstrictive properties of topical cocaine or neosynephrine with lidocaine can enhance visualization and subsequent treatment. Complete blood count and coagulation studies should be obtained.

IV. Treatment. Prevention is important. Nasal tubes should be rotated and inspected on a regular basis. Humidified oxygen and facemasks are essential to prevent mucosal desiccation. Hypertension and coagulopathies should be treated immediately.

The mainstay of treatment for direct control of bleeding is cautery, nasal packing, and arterial ligation or embolization. Most nosebleeds occur on the anterior septum at Kisselbach's plexus. In most cases, external digital pressure for 5 to 10 minutes can achieve hemostasis. Cautery, also a reasonable way to achieve hemostasis, can be done with silver nitrate or electrocautery. Care must be taken not to perforate the septum.

If cautery is insufficient to achieve hemostasis, then packing is necessary. Packing should be placed anteriorly or posteriorly with respect to the location of the bleeding. Commercial nasal packing impregnated with vasoconstrictive agents or hemostatic agents is widely available. However, petroleum gauze is a satisfactory alternative. Posterior bleeding presents a challenge with respect to effective packing. A Foley catheter is a reasonable alternative to posterior gauze packing. After appropriate local anesthesia is applied, the catheter is inserted into the nose and the balloon is inflated in the posterior nasal cavity with 10 to 20 ml of saline. The catheter is then secured to the ala with an umbilical clamp. Packing can be removed when coagulation defects or others causes of bleeding have been addressed.

If epistaxis is recurrent or long-term hemostasis is not achieved with sufficient packing, arterial ligation or embolization is necessary. Posterior nasal bleeding is controlled by ligation of the internal maxillary artery. Anterior bleeding is abated by the ligation of the ethmoidal arteries. In the case of diffuse bleeding, both the internal maxillary artery and ethmoidal artery should be ligated. Angiographic embolization of the internal maxillary is an alternative to ligation. The ethmoidal arteries arise from the internal carotid, and embolization should not be attempted. Deciding between surgical ligation and embolization should be done individually. Either procedure requires a stable patient and the appropriate ancillary staff. Both procedures result in a high rate of hemostasis.

Selected Readings

Elahi MM, Parnes LS, Fox AJ, et al. Therapeutic embolization in the treatment of intractable epistaxis. *Arch Otolarngol Head Neck Surg* 1995;121:65.

This reference provides a review of arterial embolization.

Strong EB, Bell DA, Johnson LP, et al. Intractable epistaxis: transantral ligation vs. embolization: efficacy review and cost analysis. *Otolarngol Head Neck Surg* 1995; 113:674.

This reference provides insight in the cost-effectiveness of ligation and embolization.

Viducich RA, Blanda MP, Gerson LW. Posterior epistaxis: clinical features and acute complications. *Ann Emerg Med* 1995;25:592.

This reference provides a review of posterior epistaxis and its complications.

136. ESOPHAGEAL PERFORATION AND ACUTE MEDIASTINITIS

M. Ryan Moon, Robert M. Mentzer, and Fred A. Luchette

I. Esophageal perforation

A. Etiology. The esophagus can be subjected to a variety of pathophysiologic stresses that can result in rupture, including increased wall tension from instrumentation, foreign bodies, high intraluminal pressures from retching, or blunt or penetrating trauma. Generally, the causes of esophageal perforation can be grouped into spontaneous perforations and penetrating injuries. Penetrating injuries can be categorized as intraluminal or extraluminal.

1. **Spontaneous rupture.** Spontaneous rupture occurs secondary to an increase in intraluminal pressure that is greater than the esophagus can tolerate. The normal esophagus can be subjected to very high pressures with retching against a closed glottis or upper esophageal sphincter, as in Boerhaave's syndrome. The diseased esophagus can be much more susceptible to perforation from smaller increases in luminal pressure, such as erosions secondary to esophageal cancer or other inflammatory lesions. Other potential causes include tuberculosis, Barrett's esophagus, idiopathic eosinophilic esophagitis, and necrosis secondary to sclerotherapy or banding for esophageal varicies.
2. **Extraluminal perforation.** Common causes of extraluminal perforations include penetrating trauma and surgical procedures. Any penetrating injury in the proximity of the esophagus should be examined to exclude injury, because early diagnosis reduces morbidity. Cervical spine procedures, pneumonectomy, laparoscopic Nissen fundoplication, aortic surgery, and even tube thorocostomy have been shown to have a small but real risk of esophageal perforation. Primary esophageal surgery, either resection or modification, carries a risk of perforation or leak. Anastomotic leak from esophagectomy occurs in approximately 9% of patients undergoing transhiatal resection and in 3% to 5% with intrathoracic anastomosis.
3. **Intraluminal perforation.** Most esophageal injuries occur as a result of instrumentation with intraluminal force, in the normal or diseased esophagus as well as in the pathologic esophagus. The maneuvers required to dilate or examine the strictured esophagus can lead to tension on the leading edge of the stricture, the point most likely to rupture. The cervical esophagus is most often injured at the cricopharyngeus muscle, most commonly occurring with rigid instrumentation. Esophageal atresia has been associated with perforation during feeding tube placement. Other less common causes of esophageal perforation include transesophageal echocardiography, attempted endotracheal intubation, or foreign body ingestion. Chemical injury from drug ingestion or burns from alkali or strong acids can also be associated with perforation, typically if the injury causes full-thickness necrosis. In these instances, the esophageal wall is the weakest, whereas the mucosa is sloughing or scar is developing, and instrumentation should be avoided.

B. Clinical presentation. Free perforation of the esophagus into the mediastinum results in the extrusion of aerobic and anaerobic organisms as well as air into the surrounding tissues. As swallowing continues, esophageal contents are expelled, resulting in subcutaneous emphysema into the facial planes and chest wall. Patients typically present with increasing pain, fever, dysphagia, and odynophagia. Tachycardia is often an early sign of mediastinitis. Hoarseness and cervical tenderness are hallmarks of cervical esophageal injury. Thoracic perforations may present with a septic response and respiratory distress. Proximal injuries usually involve the right chest and pleura, whereas distal injuries violate the left pleura. The pain associated with thoracic esophageal perforation can be precordial, epigastric, or even referred to the scapular region. These symptoms progress over the course of hours (<12 hours) and early diagnosis and intervention can lead to a less complicated course.

C. Diagnosis. Although a chest x-ray study may show signs of mediastinal air or associated hydropneumothorax, contrast esophagram is the most sensitive test and it is generally well tolerated. Water-soluble contrast should be avoided because of the potential for pulmonary complications, and because barium contrast gives a higher resolution of small leaks. Computed tomography (CT) has been shown to be both sensitive and specific when the patient's condition precludes performance of an esophagram. Characteristic findings on CT include extraluminal air, periesophageal fluid, wall thickening, and extraluminal contrast. Direct examination with esophagoscopy provides little value in the diagnosis of esophageal perforations because instrumentation can further damage the esophagus and smaller injuries can be missed.

D. Treatment. Treatment of esophageal perforation depends on the time interval between perforation and therapy, esophageal pathology, and injury magnitude. For injuries diagnosed within 12 hours of perforation, optimal treatment includes primary closure of the wound with drainage of the region. Additional support of the repair can be provided to minimize postoperative leaks using parietal pleura, intercostal muscle, an omental patch, or latissimus dorsi muscle flap. If the injury is diagnosed late (>12 hours) or if inflammation is extensive, generous drainage is undertaken and the esophagus is diverted. Broad-spectrum antibiotic coverage should be provided. Esophagectomy may be indicated in patients with obstructing carcinoma in the acute setting, but mortality rates are higher than with elective resection. Perforations limited to the mediastinum without extension into the pleural space can be treated expectantly with antibiotics and hyperalimentation. Esophageal stents, irrigation with fibrin glue, and endoscopic clipping have recently been reported as successful nonsurgical types of management. Nonsurgical approaches can be considered provided the general principles of minimizing soilage, controlling drainage, and nutritional support are maintained. However, most cases usually require surgical intervention.

II. Acute mediastinitis. Acute mediastinitis is a serious and often life-threatening infection involving the deep structures of the mediastinum. It is most commonly associated with sternotomy and intrathoracic procedures. Cervical and thoracic esophageal perforation can lead to acute mediastinitis as well, often seen with delayed diagnosis. Infections from adjacent structures should be considered, including primary pulmonary infections, tracheal injuries, and peridontal disease. Although superficial wound infections are seen in approximately 4% of patients, only 1% to 2% develop deep infection involving the mediastinum. Recent studies have demonstrated a serious infection rate of 1.3% with a 90-day postoperative mortality rate of 11.8% in patients undergoing coronary artery bypass grafting. Factors associated with an increased risk of infection include obesity, duration of surgery, prolonged cardiopulmonary bypass, emergent operations, reoperations, use of bilateral internal mammary artery grafts, and diabetes mellitus. The risk of developing acute mediastinitis in the immunocompromised orthotopic heart transplant recipient is almost four times greater than observed in other sternotomy patients.

A. Clinical presentation. Typically, mediastinitis is manifested by fever, pain, or tachycardia. The pain can be localized to the chest or radiate to the neck, and it may be pleuritic. Infections generally occur from 3 days to 4 weeks postoperatively, but can present up to 3 months later. Increasing sternal pain with drainage is common, and sternal instability is frequently a hallmark finding.

B. Diagnosis. A delay in both diagnosis and aggressive treatment results in a marked increase in morbidity and mortality. The chest x-ray film may show mediastinal air tracking in the tissue planes of the neck or an air stripe between the leaves of the sternum. A retrosternal air pocket may be seen on the lateral view. CT scans may be of limited value in postoperative patients because the natural tissue planes have been disrupted and mediastinal air may already be present. Studies have suggested that CT scans are only diagnostic after 14 days postoperatively.

C. Treatment. The primary goal of treatment for mediastinitis is to control the infection and evaluate its source. In cases related to esophageal perforation, persistent soilage from the esophagus must be controlled. Any collections of fluid or necrotic tissue should be drained or debrided, respectively. Urgent thoracotomy may be indicated to disrupt pleural loculations. Early exploration may only require irrigation and sternal rewiring. More often, the sternum will require debridement of the bone edges to achieve bleeding margins. Any loculations with purulence should be addressed and irrigation catheters may be used to minimize recurrent loculations and clear infarction.

If a radical sternal debridement is required, an omental pedicle flap or pectoralis major muscle flap can be used. For larger defects, a rectus femoris flap can be used for closure. Early wound closure is clearly a benefit to the patient's morbidity, mortality, and length of hospitalization. However, some studies have shown that, despite adequate closure, many patients experienced persistent postoperative pain and sternal instability.

Selected Readings

Bueker A, Wein BB, Neuerburg JM, et al. Esophageal perforation: comparison of use of aqueous and barium-containing contrast media. *Radiology* 1997;202:683.

A nice comparison of two modalities used to diagnose esophageal perforation.

Lee S, Mergo PJ, Ros PR. The leaking esophagus: CT patterns of esophageal rupture, perforation, and fistulization. *Crit Rev Diag Imaging* 1996;37:461.

This study provides radiographic features for the diagnosis of esophageal pathology.

Millano CA, Kesler K, Archibald H, et al. Mediastinitis after coronary artery bypass graft surgery. Risk factors and long-term survival. *Circulation* 1995;92:2245.

A good review of the risk factors and associated morbidity and mortality of mediastinitis after coronary artery bypass surgery.

Unite D'Hygiene Et De Lutte Cotre l'Infection. Risk factors for deep sternal wound infections after sternotomy: a prospective, multicenter study. *J Thorac Cardiovasc Surg* 1996;111:1200.

An excellent review of risk factors associated with the development of mediastinitis after sternotomy.

137. DIAGNOSIS AND MANAGEMENT OF INTRAABDOMINAL SEPSIS

Freda D. McCarter and Fred A. Luchette

I. General principles. Intraabdominal sepsis is not uncommon in the intensive care setting (ICU). Its presentations and causes are varied. It can present as an uncomplicated appendicitis or as a case of overwhelming sepsis. Two important groups compriseost of the patients encountered in the ICU. The first group includes the postoperative patient. These patients may have undergone an emergent or an elective procedure, and the suggestion of intraabdominal infection is higher. The efficacy of prophylactic antibiotics has decreased the occurrence of postoperative infections, but has not totally eradicated the phenomenon. The second group of patients present insidiously, and diagnosis is often challenging. These patients may have been in the ICU for a period of time with another set of unrelated problems. They may develop diverticulitis, cholecystitis, pseudomembranous colitis, or pancreatitis. Clinical findings and the presence of an ileus without evidence of nosocomial infection elsewhere may be the only clue to diagnosis. Regardless of the group or presentation, the diagnosis of intraabdominal sepsis must be made as soon as possible to institute appropriate intervention and therapy.

II. Pathogenesis. Intraabdominal sepsis can result either from spontaneous causes or from contamination of the abdomen by a perforated viscus. Abscess formation is common and typically contains mixed flora. Aerobic, anaerobic, and facultative gram-negative organisms are the common pathogens. Facultative and aerobic gram-negative organisms (e.g., *Escherichia coli*) release endotoxin and endotoxin-associated proteins. Endotoxin is rapidly absorbed by the peritoneum into the systemic circulation. The systemic effects include tachycardia, fever, and peripheral vasodilation, which all contribute to a decline in cardiac output and blood pressure. Cytokines and leukocyte-derived inflammatory mediators give rise to this response. Bacterial synergy can also suppress the host defense mechanism and facilitate bacterial proliferation. Notably, *Bacteroides fragilis* produces a polysaccharide capsule that inhibits complement activation and leukocyte migration (Table 137-1).

III. Diagnosis. History and physical examination may provide sufficient evidence to diagnose intraabdominal sepsis. Classic clinical findings include fever, leukocytosis, and localized abdominal pain or tenderness. The evolution of symptoms and pain should be ascertained, as well as the character of the pain. Hypotensive vitals signs may indicate hypovolemia or impending septic shock. Physical examination should be thorough and complete with attention directed toward localization of the disease process.

Plain radiographs may be helpful in securing a diagnosis. Air, an excellent contrast media, may identify a mechanical bowel obstruction, an extraluminal mass effect, pneumatosis cystoides, or a perforated viscus as pneumoperitoneum. Chest x-ray study may reveal a basal pneumonia, which can account for the referred pain to the abdomen. A complete blood count, electrolytes, and hepatic profile are essential. Leukocytosis is common in intraabdominal sepsis. Serum amylase and bilirubin provide insight into possible causes originating in the pancreas or gallbladder. Elevation of liver enzymes is indicative of conversion from normal hepatic protein synthesis to the synthesis of the acute-phase reactants associated with sepsis.

In the absence of physical or radiographic findings, abdominal computed tomography (CT) scan or ultrasound may be helpful. CT scanning is the best modality for identifying intraabdominal pathology. It also allows for accurate diagnostic aspiration and drainage of abscesses. Unfortunately, this imaging study requires transportation of the critically ill patient to the radiology suite, whereas ultrasound is portable and can be done at the bedside. This advantage over CT scan has to be weighed against the lower sensitivity of ultrasound in identifying intraabdominal

TABLE 137-1. Bacteria commonly encountered in intraabdominal infections

Facultative gram-negative bacilli	Obligate anaerobes	Facultative gram-positive cocci
Escherichia coli	*Bacteroides fragilis*	Enterococci
Klebsiella species	*Bacteroides* sp	*Staphylococcus* sp
Proteus species	*Fusobacterium* sp	*Streptococcus* sp
Enterobacter species	*Clostridium* sp	
Morganella morganii	*Peptococcus* sp	
Other enteric gram-negative bacilli	*Peptostreptococcus* sp	
Aerobic gram-negative bacilli	*Lactobacillus* sp	
Pseudomonas aeroginosa		

abscesses. Bowel gas, body habitus, and suboptimal visualization of the retroperitoneum also limit the diagnostic capabilities of ultrasound.

IV. Management. All patients suspected of intraabdominal sepsis should be resuscitated with crystalloid as necessary, and food should be withheld until a diagnosis is made. Surgical consultation is essential. Some forms of intraabdominal sepsis (e.g., spontaneous bacterial peritonitis and salpingitis) respond to antibiotics. However, most cases of intraabdominal sepsis require drainage. Localized collections are preferentially drained by percutaneous access, which can be accomplished with either CT or ultrasound guidance by an experienced interventional radiologist. Diffuse peritonitis mandates operative management. In this case, exploratory surgery is essential to control the primary pathology. Perforated bowel must be resected and necrotic tissue must be debrided. Drainage or evacuation of abscess cavities is paramount. A planned second-look laparotomy may be necessary to achieve complete evacuation.

Antibiotics are as important as abscess drainage in the management of intraabdominal sepsis. Antimicrobial agents are begun as soon as the diagnosis of intraabdominal sepsis is suggested; they should be active against enteric gram-negative facultative and obligate anaerobic bacilli. Upper gastrointestinal tract perforations release smaller amounts of pathogens than the lower gastrointestinal tract. Gram-positive aerobic and gram-negative anaerobic organisms predominate in the stomach, duodenum, and jejunum. In contrast, gram-negative facultative organisms predominate in the distal small bowel. Colonic perforations contaminate the peritoneal cavity with high densities of gram-negative facultative and obligate anaerobes. Nephrotoxic and ototoxic complications have removed aminoglycosides from their status as the "gold standard" in the management of intraabdominal infections. β-lactam antibiotics in combination with metronidazole, clindamycin, or β-lactamase inhibitors have been shown to be as effective as aminoglycosides in community-acquired cases of peritoneal sepsis, as have quinolones. Antibiotic regimens should be reevaluated after culture results are conclusive. Appropriate change in therapeutic agents should be made to ensure that antimicrobial coverage is optimal. Enterococci are low level pathogens, and antienterococcal therapy should be instituted only if culture are positive in a second site (ie., blood, catheter tips).

Selected Readings

Cerra FB. Multiple organ failure syndrome. *Dis Mon* 1992;26:816.
This article provides insight into intraabdominal sepsis as a contributing factor to the multiple organ failure syndrome.

Johnson WC, Gerzof SG, Robbins AH, et al. Treatment of abdominal abscesses: comparative evaluation of operative drainage versus percutaneous catheter drainage guided by computed tomography or ultrasound. *Ann Surg* 1981;194:510.
Different drainage methods are compared and their efficacy discussed.

Lee MI, Saini S, Brink JA. Treatment of critically ill patients with sepsis of an unknown cause: value of percutaneous cholecystomy. *Am J Surg* 1991;156:1163.
This article provides insight into the underlying problem of acalculous cholecystitis.
Onderdonk AB, Bartlett JG, Loule T, et al. Microbial synergy in experimental intra-abdominal abscess. *Infect Immun* 1976;13:22.
This reference explores microbial synergy in the development of intraabdominal abscesses.

138. ACUTE PANCREATITIS

M. Ryan Moon, Fred A. Luchette, and Michael L. Steer

I. Definition, classification, and pathology. Pancreatitis is an inflammatory disease of the pancreas that is clinically defined as a process of rapid onset, usually associated with pain and alterations in exocrine function. With successful treatment, complete resolution can be expected. Mild pancreatitis is associated with interstitial edema, a mild infiltration of inflammatory cells, and evidence of intrapancreatic or peripancreatic fat necrosis. In contrast, severe pancreatitis is usually associated with acinar cell necrosis that can be focal or diffusely distributed throughout the gland. In addition, thrombosis of intrapancreatic vessels, vascular disruption with intraparenchymal hemorrhage, and abscess formation may be noted.

II. Etiology. In developed countries, alcoholism and biliary tract disease account for 70% to 80% of all episodes of acute pancreatitis. Another 10% to 20% of patients have idiopathic pancreatitis, and the remaining 5% to 10% develop pancreatitis in association with operative procedures (common duct exploration, cardiopulmonary bypass, transplantation), endoscopic retrograde cholangiopancreatinography (ERCP), hyperparathyroidism, penetrating ulcers, renal failure, or scorpion bites.

A. Biliary tract disease. The onset of pancreatitis associated with biliary tract stones is related to the passage of stones through the terminal biliopancreatic duct and into the duodenum. Studies suggest that acute pancreatitis is triggered by obstruction of the pancreatic duct by the stone, or from edema and inflammation associated with stone passage. The pancreas synthesizes and secretes a large array of potentially harmful digestive enzymes, and the pathologic appearance of the pancreas during an acute attack suggests that an autodigestive injury has occurred.

B. Ethanol abuse. Most patients with ethanol-associated pancreatitis develop their first clinical attack of pancreatitis after many years of abuse. This cause of pancreatitis is more common among men, and the mean duration of consumption of ethanol before the first attack is 11 to 18 years. The mechanism by which alcohol leads to pancreatic injury is unclear. Some studies suggest a direct toxic, druglike effect on acinar cells or, alternatively, induction of ductal hypertension secondary to stimulation of both exocrine secretion and sphincteric contraction.

III. Clinical presentation and physical examination. Symptoms of acute pancreatitis include abdominal pain, nausea, and vomiting. Patients with acute pancreatitis typically appear anxious and ill. Tachycardia, tachypnea, and hypotension are common. The pain, usually localized to the epigastrium, is rapid in onset and constant, and patients often move around in search of a more comfortable position—unlike those with peritonitis caused by a perforated viscus who remain motionless. Abdominal examination reveals tenderness and both voluntary and involuntary guarding, which can be limited to the epigastrium or diffusely present throughout the abdomen. Distension is common, bowel sounds are often diminished or absent, and flank ecchymosis (Grey-Turner's sign) or other evidence of retroperitoneal bleeding (Cullen's sign) may be noted.

IV. Laboratory tests. Significant losses of intravascular fluid can cause the hematocrit, hemoglobin, blood urea nitrogen, and serum creatinine to rise. Hypoalbuminemia is common, but the serum electrolytes remain normal unless vomiting has been significant. The white blood cell count is usually elevated because of the pancreatic inflammatory process, and the serum glucose level is commonly elevated because of the combined effects of elevated circulating catecholamines and decreased insulin release. A mild rise in serum bilirubin, probably secondary to a nonobstructive cholestasis, is frequently seen even in nonbiliary pancreatitis. Some patients can develop hypocalcemia that is out of proportion to the degree of hypoalbuminemia, which is a poor prognostic sign.

A. Amylase. The serum amylase is usually elevated during an attack of pancreatitis, but the magnitude of the rise does not depend on the severity, because as many as 10% of patients with near normal amylase levels may have lethal pancreatitis. Amylase can be synthesized at extrapancreatic sites (salivary glands, fallopian tube, lung) or produced by nonpancreatic tumors (lung, prostate, ovary). Some patients with disorders that might be confused with acute pancreatitis may also have hyperamylasemia, including acute cholecystitis, perforated gastric or duodenal ulcers, small bowel obstruction, intestinal ischemia, or infarction. Approximately 0.5% of individuals have macroamylasemia, in which amylase is bound to an abnormal circulating protein and subsequently is not cleared by the kidney. In this setting, measurement of urinary amylase levels can be helpful because these levels are usually low. Additionally, amylase clearance can be reduced in advanced renal disease, which can lead to a spurious elevation. The urine amylase level may remain elevated long after serum amylase levels have returned to normal, which may prove useful in patients who are first seen several days after an acute attack of pancreatitis and who are found to have normal serum amylase activity.

B. Radiologic diagnosis. Routine chest radiographs and abdominal films will show nonspecific findings, such as basilar atelectasis, left-sided pleural effusion, paralytic ileus, and calcifications. Ultrasonography is usually limited by the presence of intestinal gas in the upper abdomen during the early stages of acute pancreatitis. Computed tomography (CT) is the most useful imaging modality because it can define gross features of the pancreas and peripancreatic organs without being limited by gas-filled loops of bowel. Dynamic CT, performed by rapidly imaging the pancreas during bolus injection of contrast material can define areas of necrosis (no enhancement).

V. Prognosis. Most patients with acute pancreatitis have a relatively mild self-limited attack that resolves with only supportive treatment. However, 5% to 10% of patients in most series have a severe attack that is associated with considerable morbidity and a mortality rate that can approach 40%. Certain clinical features have been identified that are associated with a poor prognosis: age more than 60 years, a "first attack," postoperative pancreatitis, hypocalcemia, and the presence of either Grey Turner's or Cullen's sign. Investigators in New York and Glascow evaluated large groups of patients with pancreatitis and identified clinical and laboratory features that are available during the initial 48 hours of an attack. These criteria, referred to as the Ranson criteria, are listed in Table 138-1. The presence of fewer than three of the Ranson criteria is associated with mild pancreatitis, little morbidity, and a mortality rate of less than 1%. In contrast, many patients with three or more of these signs have severe pancreatitis, with a 34% incidence of septic complications and a mortality rate that, with seven to eight

TABLE 138-1. Ranson's prognostic signs

On admission
Age > 55 years
White blood cell count > 16,000/mm^3
Blood glucose > 200 mg/dl
Lactate dehydrogenase > 350 IU/L
Glutamic oxaloacetic transaminase > 250 I.U./L
During initial 48 hours
Hematocrit decrease > 10%
Blood urea nitrogen rise > 5 mg/dl
Serum Ca^{2+} < 8 mg/dl
PaO_2 < 60 mm Hg
Base deficit > 4 mEq/L
Fluid sequestration > 6 L

prognostic signs, can reach 90%. The morbidity of an individual attack is also closely related to the presence of peripancreatic fluid collections demonstrable by CT, with a 61% incidence of late pancreatic abscess in those patients with two or more peripancreatic fluid collections, and a 12% to 17% incidence in those with one fluid collection or inflammation confined to the pancreas or peripancreatic fat.

VI. Treatment. During the early stages of acute pancreatitis, efforts should be made to confirm the diagnosis, control the pain, and support fluid and electrolyte needs. The pain of pancreatitis is often difficult to control and narcotic medications are commonly required. The early stage of severe pancreatitis is characterized by major fluid and electrolyte losses. Repeated emesis and poor fluid intake can lead to hypochloremic alkalosis. Leakage of intravascular fluid into the inflamed retroperitoneum, pulmonary parenchyma, and soft tissues elsewhere in the body can contribute to hypovolemia. Hemodynamic parameters can resemble those of septic shock (i.e., a hyperdynamic state) and necessitate care in an intensive care setting. Mechanical ventilatory support may be needed. Meticulous management of fluid and electrolytes is essential, and assessment may be aided with the use of a Swan-Ganz catheter to monitor ventricular filling pressures, and an indwelling urethral catheter to monitor urine output. The role of prophylactic antibiotics is unclear, but recent studies have indicated that patients with severe gallstone-induced pancreatitis may benefit. Nasogastric decompression has not been shown to alter the morbidity or mortality of pancreatitis, yet many clinicians believe it improves patient comfort.

A. Role of surgery and endoscopy in gallstone pancreatitis. Most patients with biliary tract stone-induced pancreatitis recover quickly and uneventfully as the offending stone is either passed into the duodenum or migrates away from the ampulla of Vater by moving proximally in the duct. Based on current data, patients with mild pancreatitis should not undergo either early surgical or endoscopic intervention, because these measures do not alter the course of the disease. However, early intervention is warranted (surgical or endoscopic) for patients with severe gallstone pancreatitis. Recent studies have demonstrated a lower morbidity, most likely by reducing the incidence of associated cholangitis. Because recurrence of gallstone pancreatitis is high, most clinicians recommend some form of treatment prior to discharge from the hospital. This can be done by laparoscopic or open cholecystectomy combined with surgical or endoscopic duct clearance, or endoscopic sphincterotomy with duct clearance.

VII. Local complications. Patients with uncomplicated pancreatitis usually recover uneventfully within 1 to 2 weeks. In contrast, patients with severe pancreatitis frequently have one or more of the local complications of pancreatitis. Ultrasound and CT can be used to diagnose and define accurately the extent of acute fluid collections and pseudocysts. Both techniques can be used to follow disease progression and to determine the presence or absence of a wall, which distinguishes a pseudocyst from an acute fluid collection. Dynamic contrast-enhanced CT is the most accurate means of identifying and quantitating areas of pancreatic necrosis, whereas ERCP is helpful in determining if fluid collections communicate with the main pancreatic duct. It can also be used to localize the point of duct rupture in patients with either pancreatic ascites or pancreatic-pleural fistulas. Extraintestinal gas on ultrasound or CT suggests either pancreatic abscess or necrosis, but this finding is noted only occasionally. More often, patients with either infected necrosis or abscess are found to have poorly enhanced areas on dynamic CT or fluid collections on ultrasound in a clinical setting of suspected sepsis.

VIII. Management. Acute pancreatic and peripancreatic fluid collections are defined as fluid collections in or near the pancreas that occur early in the course of acute pancreatitis and lack a wall of granulation or fibrous tissue. They generally require no specific treatment. Attempts to drain these collections either by percutaneously placed catheters or by early surgical intervention should be discouraged.

Pancreatic necrosis represents an area of nonviable pancreatic tissue that can be diffuse or focal and that is typically associated with peripancreatic fat necrosis. Pancreatic necrosis can either be sterile or infected. Sterile necrosis, particularly when it involves large portions of the pancreas, has been treated by surgical necrectomy combined with postoperative lavage of the peripancreatic area. However, considerable controversy surrounds this area of management, because surgical intervention can be associated with significant morbidity and can cause secondary infection of the inflamed but previously sterile pancreas. Because the absence of infection does not guarantee that recovery is possible without debridement, aggressive surgical intervention should be considered in a patient with pancreatic necrosis and a deteriorating clinical course. Infected necrosis (r) MDNM is always an indication for surgical intervention whether it is detected by the presence of extraintestinal gas on CT examination or by fine-needle aspiration of an area of pancreatic necrosis. Organisms recovered in areas of infected pancreatic necrosis are usually those present in the gastrointestinal tract (*Klebsiella* spp., *Pseudomonas* spp., *Escherichia coli, Enterococcus* spp., *Proteus* spp.). Percutaneous drainage of these areas with indwelling catheters is almost always unsuccessful. Patients typically require repeated surgical debridement and drainage. The mortality rate for untreated or inadequately treated infected pancreatic necrosis may approach 100%.

Pancreatic pseudocyst is a collection of peripancreatic fluid rich in digestive enzymes that is enclosed by a nonepithelialized wall of fibrous or granulation tissue. It is round or ovoid in shape, and is usually not present prior to 4 to 6 weeks from the onset of pancreatitis. Pancreatic pseudocysts can be asymptomatic, or can cause symptoms related to local tenderness or to obstruction of adjacent organs (e.g., the stomach, duodenum, and bile duct). On occasion, pseudocysts can contribute to the progression of pancreatitis by causing pancreatic duct obstruction. Treatment of chronic pseudocysts is needed only for those that become symptomatic, and even those greater than 6 cm in diameter can be observed safely. Several methods of treating pseudocysts have been proposed, including internal surgical drainage (cystogastrostomy, cystoduodenostomy, Roux-y-cystojejunostomy), endoscopic drainage (cystogastrostomy, cystoduodenostomy), and percutaneous drainage (aspiration followed by administration of somatostatin and catheter drainage). However, percutaneous drainage has been associated with recurrence after aspiration or infection after catheter drainage. In healthy surgical candidates, internal surgical drainage would be an appropriate first choice for the treatment of symptomatic pseudocysts, whereas an attempt at endoscopic drainage would be appropriate for poor surgical risk patients.

Bacteria may be present in a pseudocyst as a result of contamination. When pus is present, however, the lesion should be referred to as a "pancreatic abscess," which always requires some form of intervention. These abscesses may be more approachable to percutaneous drainage when compared with infected necrosis, simply because of the liquid consistency of the collection.

Leakage of pseudocysts into the peritoneal cavity or chest leads to the development of pancreatic ascites or pancreatic-pleural fistula, respectively. Although patients with pancreatic ascites or pleural fistulas may respond to nonoperative therapy (bowel rest, parenteral nutrition, somatostatin), such attempts are usually unsuccessful and some form of intervention is needed. An ERCP should be performed to identify the site of duct disruption which can be treated by distal pancreatectomy if located in the pancreatic tail. Alternatively, anastomosis of a Roux-y loop of jejunum to the site of rupture, particularly if it in the head or neck of the gland, may be preferable. Recent studies have suggested that endoscopically placed stents can be used to prevent leakage from the duct, and this nonoperative approach might be useful in the management of these complications.

Selected Readings

Bradley EL, Allen K. A prospective longitudinal study of observation versus surgical intervention in the management of necrotizing pancreatitis. *Am J Surg* 1991;161:19. *A convincing study showing evidence that selected cases of sterile pancreatic necrosis may be successfully treated without surgical intervention.*

Neoptolemos JP, Carr-Locke DL, London NJ, et al. Controlled trial of urgent endoscopic retrograde cholangiopancreatography and endoscopic sphincterotomy versus conservative treatment for acute pancreatitis due to gallstones. *Lancet* 1988;2:979.

These investigators make a case that early aggressive ERCP with sphincterotomy provides an effective alternative treatment in the management of severe gallstone-induced pancreatitis.

Ranson JHC, Balthazar E, Caccavale R, et al. Computed tomography and the prediction of pancreatic abscess in acute pancreatitis. *Ann Surg* 1985;201:656.

This article demonstrates the value of computed tomography in the diagnosis of pancreatitis as well as its ability to identify patients with increased risk of developing associated local complications.

Ranson JHC, Rifkind KM, Roses DF, et al. Prognostic signs and the role of operative management in acute pancreatitis. *Surg Gynecol Obstet* 1974;139:69.

An excellent review of the multiple indicators of severe pancreatitis as well as the role of early operative intervention and its effects on prognosis.

Sainio V, Kemppainen E, Puolakkainen P, et al. Early antibiotic treatment in acute necrotizing pancreatitis. *Lancet* 1995;346:663.

A persuasive discussion supporting a role for antibiotics use in severe pancreatitis, showing a reduction in mortality.

Vitas GJ, Sarr MG. Selected management of pancreatic pseudocysts: operative versus expectant management. *Surgery* 1992;111:123.

A nice review of criteria for operative and expectant management of pancreatic pseudocysts.

139. MESENTERIC ISCHEMIA

M. Ryan Moon, Fred A. Luchette, and Peter E. Rice

I. General principles. Mesenteric ischemia encompasses a broad spectrum of pathophysiologic changes resulting from inadequate oxygen delivery to the gut. These changes range from subtle and reversible mucosal injury to frank transmural infarction of the intestine. Arterial embolization (50%) and thrombosis (25%) account for the majority of mesenteric ischemic cases, followed by nonocclusive hypoperfusion (20%) and venous thrombosis (5%). The clinical presentation varies widely as well, ranging from no signs or symptoms to the classic presentation of pain out of proportion to physical findings. The constellation of pathophysiologic changes associated with mesenteric ischemia, combined with concurrent comorbid factors, can subsequently lead to multiple organ failure and nosocomial infection, two leading causes of mortality in the intensive care unit.

II. Etiology

A. Nonocclusive ischemia. Critically ill patients are susceptible to a functional derangement of arteriolar tone in the mesenteric bed. Cardiac disease, congestive heart failure, pericardial tamponade, or cardiogenic shock can lead to the release of vasoconstrictive mediators, with subsequent shunt of blood flow away from mesenteric circulation. Pharmocologic agents such as digitalis, propranolol, α-adrenergic agents, or arginine vasopressin, as well as circulating inflammatory mediators secondary to sepsis, trauma, or burns, can also lead to mesenteric hypoperfusion. Most cases of nonocclusive mesenteric ischemia are clinically unapparent. However, some cases can proceed to clinically evident ischemia and infarction, with a mortality rate that approaches 70%.

B. Occlusive ischemia. Occlusive mesenteric ischemia results from acute embolism or thrombosis of the superior mesenteric artery or thrombosis of the mesenteric veins. Embolic events are usually secondary to atrial fibrillation, valvular disease, myocardial infarction, or cardiomyopathy, whereas thrombotic arterial occlusion is typically an acute event superimposed on chronic atherosclerotic disease. Thrombosis of one or more vessels can be precipitated by hypercoagulable states, collagen vascular disease, hematologic disorders, or diabetes mellitus. Mesenteric venous occlusion, a rare entity, is usually associated with hypercoagulable states, cancer, and myeloproliferative disorders.

III. Pathophysiology. The splanchnic circulatory bed receives approximately 25% of the cardiac output. Precapillary arterioles serve as resistance vessels that regulate local blood flow. Postcapillary venules and veins serve as capacitance vessels; they can autotransfuse blood from the splanchnic bed to the systemic circulation during hypovolumia or shock. Reduction in perfusion pressure during normal autoregulation will lead to compensatory dilation of the resistance arterioles, thereby preserving local blood flow to the intestine. However, this local regulation can be overcome by different metabolites produced by focally ischemic intestine.

How mesenteric ischemia leads to injury is incompletely understood. Hypoxia can cause depletion and net hydrolysis of adenosine triphosphate (ATP), resulting in profound acidosis. Reperfusion can lead to the accumulation of toxic oxygen metabolites, such as hydroxyl, hydrogen peroxide, and superoxide. Infiltration and adherence of neutrophils to injured tissue subsequently leads to the release of proteases and more toxic metabolites. Regardless of the mechanism, intestinal ischemia can lead to increased permeability to various substances, with the systemic release of several proinflammatory mediators, including endotoxin and cytokines.

IV. Pathology. After superior mesenteric arterial occlusion, the intestine becomes spastic and aperistaltic. Necrosis begins in the mucosa, and full-thickness infarction can occur after 8 to 10 hours of severe ischemia. Mucosal injury, which can be visible after only 10 minutes of ischemia, consists of the appearance of glandular cells and epithelial separation from the basement membrane. The villi are exquisitely susceptible to ischemic injury; after prolonged ischemia, necrosis can proceed through all layers of the intestine, producing submucosal edema and hemorrhage. Hypoperfusion without complete arterial occlusion produces these same histologic changes, but over a longer period of time. Mucosal injury without full-thickness damage may be reversible with reperfusion; however, reperfusion may lead to increased mucosal injury, and can potentially produce more extensive necrosis of villi and crypts than ischemia alone.

V. Diagnosis

A. Clinical presentation and diagnosis. The presentation of mesenteric ischemia can range from subtle signs and symptoms to severe abdominal pain and gastrointestinal bleeding. Diagnosis rests heavily on possessing a high index of suspicion. Care must be taken not to overlook critically ill patients with masked symptoms or those who represent high-risk patients with cardiac disease, hypotension, sepsis, or hemorrhage. Severe abdominal pain is the most common presenting symptom. In contrast to arterial embolization, nonocclusive or thrombotic ischemia can present with chronic or progressive abdominal pain. Pain may be absent in up to 25% of patients, and bloody diarrhea, abdominal distension, mental status changes, or tachycardia may be the only clues to the diagnosis. Although peritonitis and acidosis usually implies transmural infarction, the absence of such findings does not exclude mesenteric ischemia. The severity of signs and symptoms often does not correlate with the extent of mucosal injury. Peripheral blood leukocyte counts, amylase, alkaline phosphatase, lactate dehydrogenase, and aspartate transferase concentrations all may be elevated, but these tests are neither sensitive nor specific. The radiographic finding of "thumbprinting" caused by submucosal bowel edema is considered the hallmark of bowel ischemia, but invariably indicates advanced disease. Computed tomography (CT) may demonstrate venous gas and occluded arterial vessels, but absence of these findings does not exclude the diagnosis. In cases of mesenteric venous thrombosis, CT with an intravenous contrast medium may demonstrate clot within the vessel.

B. Vascular imaging. Arteriography is considered the "gold standard" for the diagnosis of mesenteric ischemia, because it can differentiate between occlusive and nonocclusive types of insult and can distinguish between embolization and thrombosis of the superior mesenteric artery. However, atherosclerotic disease in the superior mesenteric or celiac arteries does not necessarily correlate with acute ischemia unless embolus can be demonstrated. Nonocclusive ischemia is suggested by vasoconstriction or "pruning" of smaller mesenteric vessels, and by impaired filling of intramural vessels, but these findings do not reveal any information about the extent of intestinal injury.

C. Endoscopy and laparoscopy. Endoscopic evaluation is the diagnostic method of choice in patients in whom colonic rather than small bowel ischemia is suspected, such as those with predominantly left-sided abdominal pain and bloody diarrhea, or those who have recently undergone abdominal aortic surgery. Acute injury is manifested by hyperemic mucosa alternating with pale areas and areas with petechial hemorrhage. Subacute injury appears as ulcerations with submucosal hemorrhage, whereas more severe injury demonstrates pseudomembranes with exudates. Frank intestinal gangrene appears black or green through the endoscope. Only those patients with grossly necrotic mucosa are at significant risk for perforation and, accordingly, are the only patients who require surgical exploration. Patients with lesser degrees of injury at the time of the initial colonoscopy should be followed with repeat endoscopic examinations. The degree of histologic mucosal injury often does not correlate with the endoscopic appearance of the mucosa. Furthermore, abnormal endoscopic findings cannot always predict transmural viability because only the mucosa can be evaluated. In most cases, mesenteric ischemia occurs in the part of the gastrointestinal tract supplied by the superior mesenteric artery (small intestine and right colon). Although the small intestine is beyond the reach of the conventional endoscope, it is possible to evaluate the right colon, which is also supplied by the superior mesenteric artery. The recent enthusiasm for laparoscopic surgery has produced several reports of the use of this new methodology to diagnose mesenteric ischemia. Unfortunately, a negative laparoscopic examination may not exclude the diagnosis, because transmural infarction is a late finding and the mucosa is not visible by laparoscopy.

VI. Management. The most challenging aspect of the management of patients with suspected mesenteric ischemia is establishing the diagnosis before irreversible infarction occurs. The early use of mesenteric angiography seems prudent when the clinical presentation makes the diagnosis of superior mesenteric artery embolization likely. With evidence of peritonitis, however, transmural infarction probably already is present and delaying definitive surgery to perform an angiogram may be unwise. If angiography reveals occlusion of the superior mesenteric artery without collateral circulation—a finding suggestive of an acute event (rather than chronic occlusion)—urgent surgery for vascular reconstruction and possible bowel resection is mandated. If the arteriogram reveals nonocclusive ischemia, intraarterial papaverine can be infused to reverse vasoconstriction. In such cases, however, management should be aimed at aggressive medical therapy to maximize perfusion and oxygen delivery to the mesenteric circulation. Measures to improve mesenteric perfusion include intravascular volume loading, the use of inotropic agents, treatment with angiotensin-converting enzyme inhibitors (to block mesenteric vasospasm induced by angiotensin II), and discontinuing digoxin (implicated as a mesenteric vasoconstrictor). Invasive hemodynamic monitoring in the intensive care unit is recommended to evaluate the effectiveness of ongoing therapy, as is frequent monitoring of blood lactate levels and arterial pH. All medications that cause mesenteric vasoconstriction (e.g., digitalis or vasopressin) should be discontinued.

The abdomen should be reexamined frequently and angiograms repeated. If abdominal findings progress despite maximal medical therapy, exploratory laparotomy is indicated to resect infarcted bowel. Patients who present with left-sided abdominal pain and bloody diarrhea can be managed differently, because ischemic colitis is the most likely diagnosis. A history of recent aortic surgery should prompt immediate evaluation for colonic ischemia in this setting. Endoscopy rather than angiography is the diagnostic method of choice; repeat endoscopic examinations may be necessary to monitor ongoing or progressive ischemia to determine if and when surgery is required. Only gross mucosal necrosis puts the patient at risk and mandates surgery. Nevertheless, the endoscopic findings should be interpreted in the clinical context; the presence of acidosis, leukocytosis, or peritoneal signs should prompt exploration regardless of the appearance of the mucosa.

Selected Readings

Haglund U. Systemic mediators released from the gut in critical illness. *Crit Care Med* 1993;21:S15.

A good overview of the numerous systemic mediators that can affect the morbidity and mortality associated with mesenteric ischemia.

Harward TRS, Smith S, Seeger JM. Detection of celiac axis and superior mesenteric artery occlusive disease with use of abdominal duplex scanning. *J Vasc Surg* 1993; 17:738.

This study analyzes the use of noninvasive imaging in cases of mesenteric ischemia and provides evidence of its potential diagnostic value.

Kaleya RN, Boley SJ. Acute mesenteric ischemia. *Crit Care Clin* 1995;11:(2)479.

A great review of the topic.

Kaleya RN, Sammartano RJ, Boley SJ. Aggressive approach to intestinal ischemia. *Surg Clin North Am* 1992;72:157.

This article provides an overview of the management of mesenteric ischemia.

140. ABDOMINAL COMPARTMENT SYNDROMES

Arthur Williams, Fred A. Luchette, and Dietmar H. Wittmann

I. **General principles.** The abdominal cavity is a compartment with a containing wall with limited compliance. Elevated intraabdominal pressure (IAP) can profoundly impair blood flow and organ function. Once a critical volume threshold has been reached, small increments in tissue volume lead to exponential increases in intraperitoneal pressure which, in turn, leads to cardiac, pulmonary, and renal decompensation; organ failure; and even death, if not reversed promptly.

II. **Definitions.** Compartment syndrome is a condition in which increased pressure within a confined anatomic space adversely affects the function and viability of the tissues within. Abdominal compartment syndrome is defined as a sustained increase in pressure within the abdominal wall, pelvis, diaphragm, and retroperitoneum that adversely affects the function of the organs and tissue within and adjacent to the abdominal cavity. This condition usually requires operative decompression. Abdominal hypertension is a sustained increase in IAP that may or may not require operative decompression. Normal abdominal pressure is below 10 mm Hg. Mild abdominal hypertension, defined as pressures in the range of 10 to 20 mm Hg, is usually not clinically significant. Moderate abdominal hypertension is defined as sustained pressures of 21 to 35 mm Hg for which operative intervention may be required. Severe abdominal hypertension is sustained pressures greater than 35 mm Hg for which operative decompression is always warranted.

III. **Causes.** Table 140-1 lists a wide variety of causes of increased intraabdominal pressure. Most abdominal hypertension is caused by peritoneal, mesenteric, or retroperitoneal edema impinging on the fascial envelope of the abdominal compartment. The peritoneum comprises a total surface area of 1.8 m^2, which is approximately equivalent to the entire surface area of the skin. Small increases, therefore, in peritoneal thickness can harbor an enormous amount of fluid. This capacity for edema can quickly outstrip the compensatory elasticity of the abdominal fascia and diaphragm and lead to compromise.

IV. **Measurement of intraabdominal pressure.** Direct measurements of IAP rely on an intraperitoneal catheter connected to a pressure transducer to take direct measurements. This is the preferred method for most experimental studies. However, less invasive indirect measurements rely on pressure transduction to the inferior vena cava, the stomach, or, most commonly, the bladder. The bladder behaves as a passive diaphragm when its volume is between 50 and 100 ml. To determine the IAP transvesiclely, 50 to 100 ml of sterile saline is instilled into the empty bladder through a Foley catheter. The tubing of the drainage bag is clamped and a 16-gauge needle is advanced through the aspiration port and connected to a pressure transducer or manometer. The recordings obtained in this manner correlate well with direct measurements in the range of 5 to 70 mm Hg.

V. **Signs, symptoms, and consequences of elevated IAP.** Clinically, the patient with increased IAP presents with a tense abdominal wall, shallow respirations, low urinary output, and increased central venous pressure. Patients requiring mechanical respiration have increased ventilatory pressures. Cardiac output initially rises slightly as venous return from intraabdominal veins begins to increase, but quickly diminishes as pressures rise above 10 mm Hg. This decrease in preload is caused by blood pooling in the lower extremities and a functional narrowing of the vena cava as it enters the chest. Additionally, afterload is increased and ventricular function is decreased as intraabdominal pressure is transmitted to the thoracic cage and negatively impacts on cardiac compliance and filling. Pulmonary function is impaired through a decrease in diaphragmatic excursion, resulting in atelectasis, pneumonia, and ventilation-perfusion mismatch. The addition of positive end-expiratory ventilation to maintain alveolar patency only worsens the intrathoracic pressure and cardiac output. Renal function is impaired through the

TABLE 140-1. Causes of abdominal hypertension

Peritonitis
Trauma, burns
Fluid overload—hemorrhage or septic shock
Retroperitoneal hematoma
Peritoneal operative trauma
Bowel edema, reperfusion injury, acute pancreatitis
Ileus, bowel obstruction
Intraabdominal mass
Abdominal closure under tension
Ascites, intraabdominal fluid collection
Laparoscopic abdominal insufflation

decrease in cardiac output, the compression of both renal inflow and outflow, and the direct compression of the kidney parenchyma causing a "renal compartment syndrome." Similar consequences ensue for liver and splanchnic blood flow with a likely decrease in protein production and possible increase in bacterial translocation. Fortunately, all of these consequences can be reversed with early abdominal decompression.

VI. Therapeutic decompression. Nonoperative decompression is reserved for those patients with abdominal distension caused by ascites. Operative decompression involves opening the abdominal cavity in the operating room under optimal conditions. This entails correcting intravascular fluid deficits, temperature, and coagulation abnormalities. Incidences of postdecompression decompensation have been reported when the systemic vascular resistance (SVR) falls markedly after decompression, outstripping the increase in cardiac output. Therefore, all patients should be monitored carefully and volume resuscitated prior to decompression. Use of vasoconstrictors after decompression may be of benefit to prevent the sudden drop in SVR.

After decompression, the abdomen can be reapproximated by a variety of methods. Simply closing the skin with a temporary closure may be sufficient in certain situations. However, the skin can act as a nonelastic envelope and may not result in sufficient decompression. Synthetic fascial materials that are sutured to the fascial edges, which can be reapproximated slowly, provide the best solution. Moist dressings are applied to prevent both wound desiccation and bacterial proliferation. The abdomen is reclosed when the fascia can be reapproximated without undue tension.

Selected Readings

Barnes GE, Laine GA, Giam PY, et al. Cardiovascular responses to elevation of intra-abdominal hydrostatic pressure. *Am J Physiol* 1985;248:R209.

Explains precisely the hemodynamic effects of abdominal compartment syndrome (ACS).

Burch JM, Moore EE, Moore FA, et al. The abdominal compartment syndrome [Review]. *Surg Clin North Am* 1996;76:833.

A concise, yet elegant review of the subject matter.

Kron IL, Harman PK, Nolan AP. The measurement of intraabdominal pressure as a criteria for abdominal re-exploration. *Ann Surg* 1984;199:28.

One of the first articles to advocate operative intervention for intraabdominal pressure above 25 mmHg.

Smith PC, Tweddell JS, Bessey PQ. Alternative approaches to abdominal wound closure in severely injured patients with massive visceral edema. *J Trauma* 1992;32:16.

A handy and well thought-out review of a difficult problem.

Wittmann DH, Aprahamian C, Bergstein JM. A burr-like device to facilitate temporary abdominal closure in planned multiple laparotomies. *Eur J Surg* 1993;159:75.

A practical technique for temporary closure of the abdominal wound.

141. NECROTIZING FASCIITIS AND OTHER SOFT TISSUE INFECTIONS

Arthur Williams, Fred A. Luchette, and David H. Ahrenholz

I. **General principles.** The skin is the largest organ of the human body. Any break in the skin can allow colonization of organisms within hours and infection if the organisms are capable of invading the surrounding viable tissue. Local factors predisposing to infection include tissue edema, hematoma, ischemia, and foreign body. Systemic factors include diabetes mellitus, cirrhosis, collagen vascular disease, malignancy, malnutrition, advanced age, trauma, neutropenia, atherosclerosis, and steroid use.

II. **Terminology (Table 141-1).** Cellulitis is a nonpyogenic infection characterized by spreading erythema and edema. This condition is usually adequately treated by antibiotics against gram-positive organisms with elevation and warm compresses used to resolve the tissue edema. Generally, surgical intervention is not required. An abscess forms at the subcutaneous level and usually resolves with simple incision and drainage. Antibiotics are reserved for those patients with an underlying chronic disease state or who have evidence of a poorly localized infection. Necrotizing fasciitis is the generic term used to describe an infection that spreads along the fascia. This typically results after a deep puncture, abscess, or surgical procedure, allowing bacterial access to the fascial plane where there is minimal resistance to lateral bacterial spread. Aggressive surgical debridement in combination with parenteral antibiotics is warranted. Muscular infection, when caused by *Clostridium perfringens,* can set up a life-threatening situation. Necrotizing muscular infections mandate surgical exploration and require radical debridement of infected and necrotic tissue until healthy, bleeding, viable tissue is reached, which may include amputation. Hyperbaric oxygen can be helpful but it should not be substituted for early, aggressive surgical debridement.

III. **Pathogens associated with skin infections.** Superficial group A β-hemolytic *Streptococcus pyogenes* can induce either a marked cellulitis (erysipelas) or a dermal ulceration similar to impetigo. Spread to the dermal lymphatics (streptococcal lymphangitis), causing the red streaks seen clinically, can ultimately lead to septicemia. In the preantibiotic era septicemia resulted in significant mortality and often required amputation. Fascial infection with streptococcus can lead to widespread fascial involvement underneath apparently normal appearing skin. Ultimately, patchy dermal necrosis and cutaneous erythema appear. Streptococcal myositis is typically caused by anaerobic streptococci after major trauma. Some strains of *S. pyogenes* elaborate a potent exotoxin capable of stimulating host cytokine release, leading to profound cardiovascular collapse, known as toxic shock syndrome.

Staphylococcus aureus is a less invasive organism. Infection typically results in an inflammatory exudate (pus) and is usually relegated to the subcutaneous space. Staphylococcal muscular infection (pyomyositis) usually results from hematogenous spread to areas of muscular injury or hematoma.

Clostridium infection is associated with significant muscular infections. These gram-positive, spore-forming, obligate anaerobes release potent exotoxins in ischemic muscle, leading to myonecrosis and severe systemic involvement. However, not all clostridial infection involves myonecrosis. Both subcutaneous and clostridial fasciitis are characterized by a thin, brownish drainage, musky odor, and abundant gas production, but have minimal systemic toxicity and morbidity and mortality are uncommon.

Oral flora and enteric flora are responsible for infection in contaminated wounds from bites or in the perineal region, which can develop into significant life- or limb-threatening infections.

IV. **Infections responding to antibiotics.** Most superficial infections respond to antibiotic therapy alone. *S. pyogenes* cellulitis will respond to penicillin or cephalosporin

TABLE 141-1. Terminology of soft tissue infections

Tissue Level	Term	Common Pathogen	Treatment
Epidermis/ dermis	Cellulitis	*Streptococcus pyogenes*	Antibiotics, heat, elevation
Subcutaneous tissue	Abscess	*Staphylococcus aureas*	Antibiotics plus incise and drain[a]
Fascia	Necrotizing fasciitis	Mixed flora	Antibiotics plus surgical debridement
Muscle	Myonecrosis	*Clostridium perfringens*	Antibiotics plus radical debridement or amputation

[a]Antibiotics for poorly localized infections.

therapy; however, resistance is emerging. Needle recovery of organisms or skin biopsy is unlikely and unnecessary for most patients.

Human bite wounds result in mixed oral flora, with *Eikenella corrodens* often recoverable. This pathogen is usually sensitive to penicillin or cephalosporin, but resistant to dicloxacillin. *Pasteurella multocida* is often isolated from dog bites. Infection from this organism can be treated with penicillin, cephalosporins, or tetracycline and does not require surgical debridement.

Subcutaneous infection or abscess usually resolves after simple incision and drainage. Antibiotics are reserved for patients with decreased host defenses or evidence of surrounding cellulitis.

V. Infections requiring surgical debridement. Superficial infections do not usually require significant surgical therapy. Exceptions include deep infection into the subcutaneous space in diabetics or infections involving the tendon or joint space. Also, hidradenitis supportiva of the axilla or groin that does not respond to antibiotic therapy initially may require complete surgical excision of the gland-bearing skin with subsequent skin grafting or healing from secondary intention. Clostridial abscess or localized subcutaneous clostridial infection, which induces a watery brown, musky discharge with soft tissue gas, will respond to localized surgical debridement and parenteral antibiotics.

A. Necrotizing fasciitis. Necrotizing fasciitis can result from a single causative organism after a minor wound or chronic ulcer or it can be polymicrobial, as seen with intravenous drug users. Perineal infection commonly results from enteric organisms. In children, varicella infection can be complicated by streptococcal necrotizing fasciitis.

The pathogenesis of necrotizing fasciitis stems from the few barriers to lateral spread of organisms at the fascial level. Perineal necrotizing fasciitis usually results from neglected or inadequately treated perineal infection (Fournier syndrome). Other predisposing conditions include diabetes, intravenous drug use, granulocytopenia, and alcoholism.

Diagnosis of these deep, soft tissue infections relies on a high index of suspicion and a low threshold is seen for surgical treatment of them. Streptococcal necrotizing fasciitis is usually fulminant in nature, beginning with wound erythema, fever, edema, and watery drainage. Pain, tachycardia, and leukocytosis follow. Dermal necrosis and thrombosis of cutaneous blood vessels cause blistering and cyanosis. Blood cultures may be positive. Other organisms present similarly but are usually more indolent. Plain radiographs occasionally demonstrate soft tissue gas. Computed tomography scanning or magnetic resonance imaging can demonstrate fascial thickening, soft tissue fluid, or gas. Needle aspiration may recover infected fluid but its absence is not diagnostic. In equivocal cases, bedside biopsy with frozen section analysis can be helpful.

The mainstay of treatment is early surgical debridement. Preparation of hypovolemic patients for surgery is critical and extensive radiologic investigations unwarranted in the face of spreading infection. Initial antibiotic therapy should be broad spectrum against facultative and anaerobic enteric organisms. The antibiotic regimen can be tailored to the intraoperative culture results. When the skin is edematous but viable, minimal debridement is necessary. Wound drainage with secondary healing is usually all that is necessary. A subset of patients will require extensive subcutaneous debridement to viable margins, necessitating soft tissue coverage and skin grafting for wound closure. Perineal infections may require a diverting colostomy; however, good local wound care in a dedicated setting usually eliminates this procedure. Aggressive nutritional support is invariably required. The mortality rate approaches 25% to 80%, depending on comorbid conditions.

B. Myonecrosis. Nonclostridial myonecrosis is the end result of untreated necrotizing fasciitis. No unique signs or symptoms exist and mortality remains high.

Clostridial myonecrosis is the most virulent soft tissue infection if allowed to go unchecked. Traumatic, contaminated wounds allow entry of soil organisms such as *Clostridia* when these wounds are inadequately debrided or mistakenly closed. Also, bacteria can inoculate surgical wounds after operation on the gastrointestinal tract.

The pathogenesis relies in traumatic, ischemic injury to produce an anaerobic environment for the clostridial spores to germinate and release a variety of exotoxins. Local gas production worsens the ischemia and the infection spreads with startling rapidity. Rarely, the spores can lie dormant and produce infection in acutely contused areas of previous infection.

Diagnosis relies on clinical assessment of systemic toxicity, confusion, marked pain, woody edema, and gram-positive rods in a Gram's stain. Soft tissue gas is present in 40% of cases. Sudden cardiovascular collapse can ensue from the elaborated exotoxins. Treatment involves wide surgical debridement, high dose parenteral penicillin therapy and aggressive fluid replenishment. Wound packing and supportive care follow surgical debridement. Hyperbaric oxygen suppresses toxin formation but does not inactivate circulating toxins. Emergency limb amputation may be required. The emphasis on early aggressive debridement has decreased the mortality rate to 25%.

Selected Readings

Ahrenholz DH. Necrotizing soft tissue infections. *Surg Clin North Am* 1988;68:199.
An excellent, concise review of diagnosis and management.

Jones J. *Investigation upon the nature, cause and treatment of hospital gangrene as it prevailed in the Confederate armies, 1861–65.* New York: US Sanitary Commission Surgical Memoirs of the War of the Rebellion; 1871.
This text chronicles the devastating consequences of infection in the preantibiotic era.

Kaiser RE, Cerrra FB. Progressive necrotizing surgical infections—a unified approach. *J Trauma* 1981;21:349.
Findings from this clinical series of patients advocates early surgical debridement as the primary treatment with antibiotics as adjunctive therapy to minimize morbidity and mortality.

Nowak E. Flesh-eating bacteria: not new, but still worrisome [News]. *Science* 1994; 264:1665.
A look behind the news headlines of the dreaded "flesh-eating bacteria."

Simmons RL, Ahrenholz DH. Infections of the skin and soft tissue, In: Howard RJ, Simmons RL, eds. *Surgical infectious diseases,* 3rd ed. Norwalk, CT: Appleton and Lange; 1994:625.
A textbook with in-depth coverage of soft tissue infections.

142. PRESSURE SORES: PREVENTION AND TREATMENT

Arthur Williams, John Kitzmiller, and Fred A. Luchette

I. Epidemiology. In an acute care setting, pressure sores account for 3% to 11% of admissions. As the geriatric segment of the population continues its rapid growth, residents in chronic care facilities are the highest risk group for the development of pressure sores. Patients with spinal cord injury and patients in the intensive care unit often have multiple risk factors for the development of this difficult problem.

II. Pathophysiology. Pressure sores form as the end result of unrelieved pressure exerted on tissue over bony prominences. Normal arterial capillary blood pressure closes at 32 mm Hg and virtually all weight-bearing prominences are subject to this critical pressure while in the supine position. Prolonged exposure to ischemia results in tissue necrosis; however, differing tissues exhibit different sensitivities to ischemia. Muscle has much poorer tolerance to hypoxia than skin or subcutaneous tissue, which explains the "tip of the iceberg" phenomenon in patients with pressure sores. Studies have shown that ischemic necrosis can be prevented with intermittent restoration of blood flow. Complicating the ischemic skin breakdown in critically ill patients are other factors such as poor nutrition, hypotension, impaired mobility and sensation, and contamination with stool or urine.

III. Prevention. Prevention of pressure sores begins with education and dedicated care. The tenents of prevention include pressure reduction over bony prominences, alteration of weight-bearing surfaces, good skin hygiene, and adequate nutrition. Pressure dispersion techniques include foam mattress, air mattress, low air loss beds, air-fluidized beds, and oscillating support surfaces. These resources, which should be tailored toward the patient at high risk for developing pressure sores, can be cost-effective. Patients with acute traumatic injuries and a decreased level of consciousness should be removed from backboards and cervical collars as soon as safely possible.

IV. Wound classification and management. Wounds are classified as follows:

Grade 1: Nonblanchable erythema of the skin with the lesion being limited to the epidermis and dermis.
Grade 2: Full thickness ulceration of the skin extending through to the subcutaneous adipose tissue.
Grade 3: Ulceration extending to the underlying muscle.
Grade 4: Ulceration extending through muscle and involving bone.

Management strategies entail identification, debridement, wound dressings, pressure dispersion, and maximization of overall health status. Most grade 1 and 2 ulcers respond well to these measures. For grade 3 and 4 ulcers, wet to moist dressings are initially recommended to provide optimal wound environment for healing; however, an occlusive hydrocolloid dressing can be used as an alternative in a well-debrided wound with minimal dead space. Deeper ulcers also respond better if air-fluidized pressure dispersion is used. With appropriate care, up to 80% of pressure sores will heal without surgery.

V. Operative treatment. Because of the high recurrence rate for primary flap closure, surgical closure is reserved for patients whose wounds have plateaued in healing despite maximal conservative (including nutritional) therapy. Surgery is almost never necessary for the ambulatory patient. At operation, all devitalized tissue is removed and bony prominences reduced. A variety of muscular advancement flaps are used, depending on the wound location. Care is taken to avoid hematoma formation and tension on the closure.

Postoperatively, it is critical to avoid compression on the flap vascular pedicle and to minimize tension or shearing forces. A special air or fluid mattress is important for the first 3 weeks. Gradually, a program of weight bearing is used throughout the following 6 to 8 weeks. The greatest challenge is to minimize future risks of pressure sore development in the patient.

Selected Readings

Dansereau JG, Conway H. Closure of decubitus in paraplegics. *Plast Reconstr Surg* 1964;33:474.
An early article with sound principles that still apply.

Inman KJ, Sibbald WJ, Rutledge FS, et al. Clinical utility and cost-effectiveness of an air suspension bed in the prevention of pressure ulcers. *JAMA* 1993;269:1139.
Provides a solid argument for the cost-effectiveness of air mattress technology.

National Pressure Ulcer Advisory Panel. *Pressure ulcer treatment: clinical practice guideline.* Bethesda, MD: US Department of Health and Human Services 1994:15.
The government's approach to pressure ulcer management with useful statistics.

143. PAIN MANAGEMENT IN THE CRITICALLY ILL

Freda D. McCarter, Fred A. Luchette, and Donald S. Stevens

I. General principles. Pain is a prevalent problem in the intensive care unit. Ineffective analgesia is usually a consequence of inadequate drug administration. Because many patients are intubated and unable to communicate, nursing staff is left to administer *pro re nata* [PRN (as needed)] analgesia. This can result in patients remaining in pain for prolonged periods of time. Some more common reasons for inadequate pain treatment is fear of depressing spontaneous breathing, inducing opioid dependence, or precipitating cardiovascular instability.

II. Pathogenesis. Acute pain begins in the skin or deeper tissues. Locally released algogens sensitize or stimulate peripheral nociceptors. This signal is propagated along the nociceptor fibers of the dorsal horn of the spinal cord. An amplified or attenuated signal is then transmitted to pain-specific areas in the structures of the deep brain or the cerebral cortex, which responds by reflex sympathetic discharge and hypothalamic stimulation. This increased sympathetic discharge results in tachycardia, increased stroke volume, increased cardiac work, and increased myocardial oxygen consumption, whereas the reflex hypothalamic stimulation leads to increased release of catabolic stress hormones and decreased synthesis of anabolic hormones.

III. Diagnosis. The location, severity, and quality of the patient's pain should be ascertained whenever possible and should correlate with the area of wounding. If the pain is located in a nonsurgical or a noninjured area, secondary sources (e.g., chronic pain or intraoperative malpositioning) should be explored. The patient should be asked to quantify the pain whenever possible. In patients who are unable to communicate, the only manifestation of increased pain may be systemic signs of sympathetic stimulation. These include restlessness, sweating, tachycardia, lacrimation, pupillary dilation, and hypertension.

IV. Treatment. Management should be targeted at interrupting pain conduction in any one of various levels along the nociceptor pathway. Different analgesic techniques can be used to disrupt nociception transmission at the periphery, the spinal cord, or the entire nervous system. The risk and expected advantages to the patient must be considered prior to selecting a particular level.

Peripheral analgesic techniques include nonsteroidal antiinflammatory drugs (NSAIDs), local anesthetic infiltration, and peripheral nerve blocks. NSAIDs interfere with the production of prostaglandins. Ketorolac is the only form of parenteral NSAID available in the United States. It can be added to an opioid regimen to provide additional pain relief without compromising respiratory drive. As with all NSAIDs, ketorolac can cause peptic ulceration, nausea, and inhibition of platelet function. It should not be administered in patients with renal failure or for more than 5 days.

Local anesthetic techniques can also be useful in the management of pain in certain circumstances. In hernia studies, local anesthesia was reported to have a greater effect on the severity of postoperative pain than spinal or general anesthesia. Intercostal nerve blocks are effective in providing analgesia for thoracic injuries. Disadvantages of this method include the risk of pneumothorax, the need for repeated injections, and the risk of systemic toxicity. Paravertebral blocks can be administered once or by continuous infusion through an indwelling catheter; they have the advantage of providing analgesia over several dermatomes. Interpleural analgesia can be used to manage several types of pain in the thorax and abdomen. Inaccurate catheter placement has been a major problem with this route. Contraindications to interpleural analgesia are fibrosis of the pleura, blood or fluid in the pleural space, or recent thoracic infection.

Spinal cord analgesic techniques include transcutaneous electric nerve stimulation (TENS), subarachnoid conduction blockade, and epidural conduction blockade.

TENS uses high frequency, low intensity stimulation through skin electrodes to control postoperative pain. It is associated with a reduced rate of nausea, vomiting, atelectasis, and ileus. Conduction blockade through subarachnoid or epidural catheter placement can be accomplished with anesthetics or opioids. Local anesthetics block afferent nerve transmission, whereas opioids downregulate nociceptive signals. Continuous epidural anesthesia with local anesthetics allows for prolonged analgesia, but hypotension secondary to sympathetic blockade is a common side effect. Hypotension can usually be alleviated with expansion of the intravascular volume prior to anesthetic administration. The most common side effects of epidural opioid anesthesia are nausea, pruritis, and urinary retention. These problems can be treated with appropriate medication for the symptom. Respiratory depression is the most serious side effect of epidural opioids. The incidence of respiratory depression is low—1% of patients at most. Respiratory depression peaks at 1 hour after administration and again at 6 to 12 hours. Sedation occurs first, prior to respiratory depression. Clinically significant respiratory depression should be treated with divided doses of an opioid antagonist, such as naloxone.

Systemic anesthetic techniques include inhalation agents, sedatives, and opioids. Inhalational agents have a limited role in treating critically ill patients, but occasional use during painful bedside procedures may be beneficial. Sedatives (e.g., benzodiazepines, barbiturates, phenothiazines, and butyrophenones) can be given in conjunction with opioids. These drugs, which have no analgesic properties, should be administered for anxiolysis, sedation, or amnesia. Carefully monitor respiratory effort, because these drugs can depress consciousness and ventilation. Systemic opioid analgesia can be administered intramuscularly, subcutaneously, transdermally, or intravenously. Doses must be carefully considered. In alert patients, patient-controlled analgesia (PCA) may be considered. PCAs have a programmed lock-out interval, which prevents the danger of overdosing.

Selected Readings

Benedetti UC, Bonica J, Bellucci G. Pathophysiology and therapy of postoperative pain: a review. *Adv Pain Res Ther* 1984;7:373.

This article provides a scientific approach to pain management.

Puntillo KA, Wilkie DJ. *Pain in the critically ill.* Gaithersburg, MD: Aspen Press; 1991.

Here is a complete review of pain pathophysiology and management in the critically ill patient.

Ready LB, Edwards TW. IASP Task Force on Acute Pain. *The management of acute pain: a practical manual.* Seattle: IASP Publications; 1992.

This reference provides an excellent review of postoperative pain management.

Sriwatankul K, Weis OF, Alloza JL. Analysis of narcotic usage in the treatment of postoperative pain. *JAMA* 1983;250:926.

An analysis of narcotic efficacy and dosage.

144. OBSTETRIC PROBLEMS IN THE INTENSIVE CARE UNIT

M. Ryan Moon, Fred A. Luchette, and Jonathan F. Critchlow

I. General principles. The management of the acutely ill pregnant patient presents challenges to the intensive care unit team because of the disease states unique to pregnancy, concurrent anatomic changes in the mother, and the altered cardiopulmonary physiology of mother and fetus. This chapter primarily focuses on surgical issues; see Chapter 45 for respiratory issues.

II. Maternal–fetal physiology. A number of hemodynamic changes occur during pregnancy to increase oxygen delivery to the placenta during gestation and delivery. Cardiac output increases during the first trimester and peaks in the second trimester to almost 50% above normal. This is accomplished by an increase in heart rate and stroke volume and by a decrease in systemic vascular resistance. During later pregnancy, assuming the supine position causes caval compression by the gravid uterus, which can markedly decrease venous return. During labor, uterine contraction increases venous return but also markedly increases afterload; the latter effect can be detrimental to patients with underlying cardiac disease.

Blood volume increases in the first trimester and peaks at 140% of the nonpregnant state by the third trimester. Both red cell mass and total blood volume increase, but because red cell mass does not increase at the same rate as plasma volume, a modest dilutional anemia is present because of excess extracellular water. Hematocrits of 30% to 35% and serum albumin concentrations of 3.0 to 3.5 are considered normal in pregnancy.

Marked changes in the lung, ventilatory control, and respiratory mechanics also occur. Chronic compensated hyperventilation with a resultant P_aCO_2 of 30 to 35 mm Hg results from increases in respiratory rate and tidal volume. Pregnancy is associated with small decreases in total lung volume and functional residual capacity. In early pregnancy, tidal volume increases by 30% but later may decrease as the diaphragm rises because of the upward shift of intraabdominal contents.

Fetal oxygen delivery is a function of arterial oxygen content, the flow of blood through the uterine arteries, placental transfer, and the special attributes of fetal hemoglobin. Uterine blood vessels are usually maximally dilated. Uterine blood flow, thus, is not self-regulating but is directly related to maternal blood pressure. Alkalosis, diminished maternal cardiac output or blood pressure, uterine contractions, or increased sympathetic tone can adversely affect blood flow to the placenta. Despite the relative inefficiency of placental oxygen transfer, the greater oxygen affinity of fetal hemoglobin affords the fetus a blood oxygen content very close to that of maternal blood, even though the P_aO_2 is substantially lower.

III. Radiation exposure. Radiography is often essential in the diagnosis and management of the critically ill patient; in pregnant women, however, radiation exposure to the fetus is of concern. The risk of fetal death, malformation, or later childhood malignancies depends on gestational age at the time of exposure and the amount of radiation delivered. In the first weeks of pregnancy, radiation doses of 10 cGy can cause fetal death. During the first 12 weeks of gestation, the fetus is vulnerable to developmental abnormalities. Exposures greater than 5 to 10 cGy should be avoided. The acceptable level of radiation exposure is probably much higher beyond 15 weeks gestation. A chest roentgenogram exposes the maternal lungs to approximately 0.5 cGy and the shielded fetus to much less exposure. A single film of the pelvis yields less than 1 cGy to the fetus. Abdominal computed tomography (CT) scans deliver between 5 and 10 cGy to the fetus. Plain films necessary for diagnosis are safe and should be obtained without undue concern over fetal exposure. Although CT scans have been done on pregnant patients without obvious sequelae, the role of CT scanning, especially in early pregnancy, remains controversial.

IV. Hypertensive disorders of pregnancy. Preeclampsia is defined as hypertension occurring after the 20th week of pregnancy with proteinuria (>2 g/d) and peripheral edema. Preeclampsia occurs in 10% of all pregnancies and is common in nulliparous women; it can be associated with acute renal, cardiac, or pulmonary failure, and disseminated intravascular coagulation (DIC). Eclampsia is defined as the onset of seizures unrelated to a known seizure disorder or anatomic focus.

Arteriolar constriction leads to a generalized increase in peripheral vascular resistance, which diminishes circulating blood volume and flow to essential organs, and to microangiopathy. Circulating albumin concentrations and plasma oncotic pressures are also lower in preeclampsia than during normal pregnancy. Renal function is impaired by decreased renal blood flow, endothelial cell swelling, and fibrin deposition in glomeruli. In preeclampsia, hyperreflexia commonly results from central nervous system irritability. In eclampsia, grand mal seizures occur, probably secondary to hypertensive encephalopathy, cerebral vasospasm, and cerebral edema. A particular combination of end-organ abnormalities, termed the HELLP syndrome (hemolysis; elevated liver (enzymes); low platelets), affects 2% to 12% of severely preeclamptic patients. Typical early manifestations include nonspecific malaise, weight gain, and right upper-quadrant discomfort. Hypertension may be absent in as many as 50% of patients in the early stages of the syndrome. The liver is primarily involved, with fibrin deposits leading to areas of necrosis and occasional subcapsular hematoma formation. The diagnosis is made by documentation of hemolysis on peripheral smear and elevated circulating lactate dehydrogenase, elevated liver function test values, and a platelet count less than 100,000 cells/mm^3.

A. Management. Because the definitive treatment of preeclampsia is delivery, most patients must be stabilized and then have delivery shortly thereafter. If the fetus is very immature, stabilization and observation, if possible, are the best approaches. Bedrest and vigorous intravenous (IV) fluid therapy should be initiated. Blood pressure should be controlled with vasodilators. In the absence of pulmonary edema, diuretics should be avoided, as they can further decrease circulating blood volume and blood flow to the uterus. Although somewhat controversial, $MgSO_4$ remains the most commonly used prophylactic anticonvulsant and it helps to decrease uterine tone. Eclamptic seizures are best treated with IV diazepam (5–10 mg). Intravenous $MgSO_4$ is used by some, although others would immediately begin therapy with phenytoin (10 mg/kg IV over 20 minutes). Despite being potentially teratogenic in early pregnancy, phenytoin seems to have little effect on the developed fetus.

Treatment of HELLP syndrome is similar to that given for severe preeclampsia. Patients should be stabilized, coagulation profiles checked and corrected, and the fetus evaluated for well-being and maturity. Fetuses greater than 35 weeks or with mature lungs should be prepared for delivery, which can be accomplished vaginally in most cases. Fetal immaturity carries the risk of DIC, acute renal failure, or rupture of subcapsular hematoma with expectant management. Bedrest, IV fluids, and antihypertensives are essential.

V. Hemorrhage. Blood loss at the time of delivery is a normal phenomenon. A 500-ml blood loss is expected with a vaginal delivery; it can increase to 1 L during a routine cesarean section.

A. Antepartum hemorrhage. Placenta previa, which involves areas of the placenta overlying the cervical os, occurs at a rate of 1 out of 200 pregnancies. The severity of the condition can be graded by ultrasound according to the amount of placental tissue that impinges on or covers the cervical os. Bleeding is painless and usually occurs as multiple sporadic bleeds from the lower uterine segment through the os. Any digital examination should be performed with great care in the operating room; however, severe hemorrhage is relatively rare. In these cases, immediate cesarean section is indicated. If the fetus is matured beyond 35 weeks, delivery should be accomplished without delay if bleeding persists. Patients with less developed fetuses should be managed expectantly to allow for further fetal maturation.

Placental abruption is the premature separation of the placenta from the uterus. The anatomic location and severity of abruption can lead to hemorrhage, which can either be contained or be visible through the os. Abruption can occur in up to 1 of 100 pregnancies, with a maternal mortality rate of several percent, and a fetal mortality rate of 25% to 40%. Most patients present with pain, which increases with contractions. External bleeding is inconsistent. Because most of the blood loss may be intrauterine, the degree of maternal volume depletion may not correlate with observed blood loss even in patients who present with vaginal bleeding. A predelivery diagnosis of abruption is most often made on clinical grounds and by excluding placenta previa. Ultrasound can easily identify placenta previa, but may not accurately diagnose an abruption.

Treatment of abruption includes resuscitation and stabilization with fluids. Fetal monitoring is essential because there is a high incidence of fetal distress. Because of the risk of fetal abruption-induced DIC, coagulation studies should be made and factors repleted as needed. Some form of DIC occurs in 15% to 30% of cases. Emergent cesarean section is indicated for maternal or fetal distress.

Treatment of patients with refractory bleeding involves vigorous repletion of clotting factors, especially platelets, and removal of all placental fragments. Heparin therapy is not useful and can be harmful. On occasion, hysterectomy or even hypogastric artery ligation or embolization may be necessary to control severe bleeding.

B. Postpartum hemorrhage. Significant bleeding only occurs in 2% to 5% of pregnancies. Conditions that inhibit adequate contraction of the uterus are the most common reasons; they include retained clot, overdistension of the uterus, lacerations, idiopathic uterine atony, and use of certain drugs, such as terbutaline or $MgSO_4$. Compression and massage of the uterus may be all that is necessary to stimulate adequate contraction. Oxytocin can be administered as a continuous infusion to increase contractions; intramuscular injections of ergonovine are also effective. However, care must be used with ergonovine because it has been implicated in cases of intracerebral hemorrhage. Postpartum bleeding that continues after oxytocic therapy must be treated surgically. If the uterus contracts and bleeding persists, other sources of bleeding must be explored (e.g., lacerations, retained placental fragments, and coagulopathy). Angiographic transcatheter embolization therapy occasionally may be of benefit.

VI. Trauma. Trauma complicates 6% to 7% of all pregnancies, although fewer than 1% of pregnant women require hospitalization. Maternal injury has been associated with an increased incidence of premature labor, spontaneous abortion, abruptio placentae, fetomaternal hemorrhage, and intrauterine fetal demise. Fetal death from trauma exceeds that of maternal death by three- to ninefold.

Increased blood volume that accompanies gestation may improve tolerance for hemorrhage but can significantly delay the appearance of signs of bleeding until severe shock is manifested. Because fetal well-being is dependent on uterine blood flow, moderate decreases in maternal cardiac output and blood pressure that are insufficient to cause maternal shock, can be detrimental to the fetus. Upward displacement of the uterus and bladder make these organs more susceptible to injury.

Most maternal injuries during pregnancy result from blunt trauma, with automobile accidents being the most common. Serious injuries do not seem to carry a higher mortality in pregnant women when compared to nonpregnant women. Uterine rupture carries an incidence of less than 1% of all cases of maternal trauma. However, maternal death rates approach 10% with this entity, usually secondary to coexisting injuries, and fetal loss is almost universal. Abruption carries a greater risk to the fetus than to the mother.

A. Management. The initial resuscitation and primary survey of the injured pregnant woman should follow guidelines outlined by the American College of Surgeons Committee on Trauma, Advanced Trauma Life Support Program. Because of increased vascularity of nasal passages, nasotracheal intubation should be done with caution. If possible, the pregnant woman should be transported and cared for lying on the left side to improve venous return. The pneumatic antishock garment (PASG) can have deleterious effects on blood volume by compressing the uterus against the inferior vena cava, especially in late pregnancy.

Blood should be sent for standard tests, including blood typing, Rh screening, and the Kleihaur-Betke test. Rh immunization should be given within 72 hours to Rh-negative mothers sustaining more than the most trivial trauma. During the first trimester, 50 μg of Rh immune globulin should be administered. The dose should be increased to 300 μg in more advanced pregnancy. Additional doses may be necessary in cases where large volumes of fetomaternal hemorrhage or continued fetal blood are seen in serial Kleihaur-Betke assays.

Both mother and fetus should have continuous monitoring. Maternal blood pressure, heart rate, hematocrit, and arterial P_aCO_2 are not predictive of fetal survival. Fetal heart rate, while not predictive of fetal outcome, may allow for earlier detection of fetal distress. Increased uterine contractions (>8/h) are often seen as an early warning of impending placental abruption. The definitive therapy rendered the pregnant trauma victim should mirror that given to those who are not pregnant. Because of the increased vascularity around the uterus, pelvis fractures should be aggressively stabilized. Special consideration should be given to cesarean section in situations of fetal distress and in states of refractory maternal shock. Removal of the fetus may be lifesaving to the child and mother, and the increased venous return following delivery may improve resuscitation efforts.

Selected Readings

Barton JR, Sibai BM. Care of the pregnancy complicating HELLP syndrome. *Obstet Gynecol Clin North Am* 1991;18(2):165.

A nice review of the diagnosis and management of the individual entities (i.e., hemolysis, elevated liver enzyme, and low platelets) making up this illness of pregnancy.

Brent RL. The effects of embryonic and fetal exposure to x-ray, microwaves, and ultrasound: counseling the pregnant and nonpregnant patient. *Semin Oncol* 1989;16:347.

This article covers the risks of various types of radiation exposure on the unborn.

Cunningham FG, Pritchard JA. How should hypertension during pregnancy be managed? *Med Clin North Am* 1984;68:505.

An excellent overview of the diagnosis and management of the hypertensive diseases of pregnancy.

Drost RF, Rosemary AS, Sherman HF, et al. Major trauma in pregnant women: maternal/fetal outcome. *J Trauma* 1990;30:576.

This is a good synopsis of the fetal and maternal morbidity and mortality associated with trauma.

Kaunitz AM, Hughes JM, Grimes D, et al. Causes of maternal mortality in the United States. *Obstet Gynecol* 1985;65:605.

A good review article on the many causes of maternal morbidity and mortality in the United States.

XII. SHOCK AND TRAUMA

145. SHOCK: AN OVERVIEW

Kevin M. Dwyer and Arthur L. Trask

I. Definition. Shock is a systemic disorder affecting multiple organ systems. Perfusion can be decreased, either universally (as in hypotension), or it can be limited to maldistribution (as in septic shock). A modern definition of shock is "a syndrome initiated by acute systemic hypoperfusion, leading to tissue hypoxia and vital organ dysfunction." Early diagnosis and treatment of shock is essential to restore cellular perfusion.

II. Classification

A. Hypovolemic shock. Hypovolemic shock occurs with the loss of an adequate circulating fluid volume. It is often the first consideration in the resuscitation of a patient with hypoperfusion, and it is often a component with other forms of shock. Physical findings include cold, clammy skin; tachycardia; decreased urinary output; tachypnea; and, ultimately, hypotension. Hypovolemic shock is further stratified into four classes (Table 145-1).

Hypovolemic shock could be secondary to hemorrhage or nonhemorrhagic volume depletion. Blood loss can be external or internal. Nonhemorrhagic hypovolemic shock occurs because of overall volume fluid loss, usually from all fluid compartments. Overall volume depletion occurs with excessive gastrointestinal, urinary, or evaporative losses. Examples are vomiting, fistulas, and diarrhea for gastrointestinal losses; diabetes and diabetes insipidus for urinary losses; and evaporative losses with fever, burns, or abdominal surgery. Compartment fluid shifting, such as with small bowel obstruction, can also present as hypovolemia.

B. Obstructive shock. Obstructive forms of shock are those in which the underlying lesion is a mechanical obstruction to normal cardiac output with a decrease in systemic perfusion. An example is cardiac tamponade, with clinical signs that include jugular venous distention, pulses paradoxis, and muffled heart tones. Other examples are tension pneumothorax and pulmonary or air embolism.

C. Cardiogenic shock. Cardiogenic shock is caused by pump failure from factors such as extensive myocardial infarction, reduced cardiac contractility (cardiomyopathy, sepsis induced cardiac depression), aortic stenosis or dissection, ventricular filling abnormalities (mitral stenosis), acute valvular failure, or cardiac dysrhythmias.

D. Distributive shock. Septic shock is the classic example of distributive shock. Septic shock is manifest by a decrease in systemic vascular resistance and cardiac filling, but an increase in cardiac output. Despite the increase in cardiac output, with an increase in oxygen delivery, evidence supports a tissue oxygen deficit at the cellular level. Other examples of this form of shock are hyperthyroidism, anaphylaxis, and severe liver dysfunction. Neurogenic shock results in autonomic dysfunction, wherein occurs abnormal blood flow distribution caused by a fall in peripheral vascular tone.

E. Endocrine shock. In the intensive care setting, hypothyroidism, hyperthyroidism, and hypoadrenalism can lead to poor tissue perfusion. Finally, increasing evidence exists of adrenal insufficiency in the critically ill with unexplained hypotension, which may be partly caused by adrenal suppression or dysfunction.

F. Monitoring and diagnosis in shock

1. Vital signs. The diagnosis of shock was originally based on abnormalities in a patient's physiologic variables or vital signs. Although global vital signs may not fully reflect end-organ perfusion, they are the foundation in screening for shock. Alterations in heart rate are common in shock. Tachycardia is most common and in shock it is related to intravascular volume loss. The heart rate increases as volume decreases to maintain cardiac output, which functions until the rate increases to more than 130 beats/min, at which time

TABLE 145-1. Classification of hypovolemic shock

Hypovolemic Shock	Class I	Class II	Class III	Class IV
Blood loss (ml)	Up to 750	750–1500	1500–2000	≥2000
Blood volume (%)	Up to 15%	15%–30%	30%–40%	≥40%
Pulse rate	<100	>100	>120	140+
Blood pressure	Normal	Normal	Decreased	Decreased
Capillary refill	Normal	Decreased	Decreased	Decreased
Respiratory rate	14–20	20–30	30–40	>35
Urinary output (ml/h)	30+	20–30	5–15	<5
Mental status	Slightly anxious	Anxious	Confused	Lethargic
Fluid replacement	Crystalloid	Crystalloid	Crystalloid + blood	Crystalloid + blood

the rate may interfere with ventricular filling. Patients who are on beta-blocker therapy, have a pacemaker, or have spinal cord injuries may not be able to increase their heart rate sufficiently to increase their cardiac output in response to shock. Unless the aforementioned conditions exist, bradycardia in the critically ill is indicative of severe physiologic derangement and pending cardiovascular collapse and demands immediate attention.

Hypotension is a hallmark of shock yet it can occur late in shock. Even with a normal blood pressure, tissue perfusion can be significantly decreased. Hypotension is caused by hypovolemia, systemic vasodilation, or decreased myocardial contractility. Mean arterial pressure (MAP) is the most consistent measure.

MAP = diastolic blood pressure (DBP)
+ (systolic blood pressure (SBP) – DBP)/3

In many cases, the patient's temperature is elevated in shock. This may suggest the presence of an infection, which should be considered as a cause of shock. However, in the critically ill, there are many causes of fever not due to infection. Hypothermia suggests severe physiologic derangement and has a significant impact on a patient's survival in shock. It should be avoided and corrected rapidly.

Kidney function is an important predictor of the presence of shock as inadequate renal blood flow results in decreased urine output. Oliguria is one of the earliest signs of inadequate tissue perfusion. Pulse oximetry uses the differential light absorption characteristics of oxyhemoglobin and deoxyhemoglobin in cutaneous vessels to calculate the percentage of hemoglobin (Hgb) in the blood that is saturated with oxygen. It provides an early warning of hypoxemia and is a standard monitor in the intensive care unit (ICU).

2. **Invasive hemodynamic monitoring.** The Swan-Ganz pulmonary artery catheter measures pulmonary artery systolic and diastolic blood pressure, pulmonary artery occlusion (wedge) pressure (PAOP), central venous pressure (CVP), and cardiac output (CO). A patient's pressure, flow, and volume status can then be assessed through the measured and calculated variables (Table 145-2).

   Intracardiac filling pressure measurements (e.g., CVP and PAOP) are used to estimate intravascular volume or preload. Preload, by the Frank-Starling law, is defined in terms of myocardial fibril length at end-diastole. Left ventricular end-diastolic volume (LVEDV) is assumed proportional to myofibril length and end-diastolic pressure (LVDEP). In the absence of valvular disease and pulmonary hypertension, LVDEP equals left atrial

TABLE 145-2. Hemodynamic variables

Variable	Unit	Normal Range
Measured variables		
Systolic blood pressure	Torr	90–140
Diastolic blood pressure	Torr	60–90
Systolic pulmonary artery pressure	Torr	15–30
Diastolic pulmonary artery pressure	Torr	4–12
Pulmonary artery occlusion pressure	Torr	2–12
Central venous pressure	Torr	0–8
Heart rate	Beats/min	60–100
Cardiac output	L/min	5–7
Right ventricular ejection fraction	(Fraction)	0.40–0.60
Calculated variables		
Mean arterial pressure	Torr	70–105
Mean pulmonary artery pressure	Torr	9–16
Cardiac index	L/min/m^2	2.8–4.2
Stroke volume	ml/beat	Varies
Stroke volume Index	ml/beat m^2	30–65
Systemic vascular resistance index	dyne • sec • cm^{-5}	1,600–2,400
Pulmonary vascular resistance index	dyne • sec • cm^{-5}	250–340
Left ventricular stroke work index	g • m/m^2	43–62
Right ventricular stroke work index	g • m/m^2	7–12
Coronary perfusion pressure	Torr	>60
Right ventricular end-diastolic work index	ml/m^2	60–100
Body surface area	M^2	Varies

pressure and PAOP is equal to left atrial pressure. Therefore, in a perfect system, PAOP reflects LVEDV. In the critically ill, intracardiac compliance is highly variable and PAOP is not an accurate measure of LVEDV. However, the trend of the measurement is valuable in assessing overall volume status and its response to therapy. The optimal PAOP is that value which maximizes cardiac output, oxygen delivery, and oxygen consumption. In a compliant right ventricle, CVP can also be used to assess volume status with less accuracy.

Coronary perfusion pressure (CPP) should be maintained above 50 mm Hg.

$$CPP = DBP - PAOP$$

Vascular resistance [systemic vascular resistance (SVR) and the pulmonary vascular resistance index (PVRI) is characterized by the following formulas.

$$SVRI\ (dynes \cdot sec \cdot cm^{-5}) = (MAP - CVP)\ (79.9)/CI$$
$$PVRI + (MPAP - PAOP)\ (79.9)/CI$$

Increased SVRI is seen in obstructive, hypopvolemic, late septic, and cardiogenic shock. Decreased SVRI is common in distributive shock states. Increased PVRI is seen in patients with acute respiratory distress syndrome, increased intraabdominal pressure, or mitral and aortic stenosis.

The ventricular stroke work indices [left ventricular stroke work index (LVSWI) and right ventricular stroke work index (RVSWI)], which describe how much work ventricles perform, can identify patients with poor cardiac function.

$$LVSWI\ (in\ g \cdot m/m^2) = (MAP - PAOP)\ (SVI)\ (0.0136)$$
$$RVSWI\ (in\ g \cdot m/m^2) = (MPAP - CVP)\ (SVI)\ (0.0136)$$

When evaluating decreased stroke work, consider it may be caused by decreased vascular volume (decreased SVI), increased vascular resistance (increased MAP or MPAP), or decreased contractility.

Volumetric pulmonary artery catheters, introduced in the 1980s, can give an accurate measure through thermistor determination of right ventricular ejection fraction (RVEF). The RVEF is used to calculate right ventricular end-diastolic volume index (RVEDVI) (RVEDVI = SVI/RVEF).

Estimates of preload are far more accurate using RVEDVI than is the use of CVP and PAOP, particularly in patients on positive end-expiratory pressure (PEEP) and with increased intraabdominal pressure.

Continuous cardiac output catheters, which were introduced in the 1990s, continuously measure mixed venous oxygen saturation, and soon will measure right ventricular volume also.

G. Oxygen transport assessment. One of the goals of adequate tissue perfusion is whether oxygen transport (delivery) to the tissues is sufficient to meet the demand for oxygen (consumption) at the cellular level. If oxygen demand (amount of oxygen required by the tissues) exceeds oxygen delivery, the cells adapt by switching to anaerobic metabolism. This results in the development of lactic acidosis and eventual cellular death. The goal, therefore, is to augment oxygen delivery so that oxygen consumption can meet tissue oxygen demands.

To assess oxygen transport, the amount of oxygen content of the blood needs to be known. Oxygen exists in blood either mostly as bound to hemoglobin (98%) or dissolved in plasma (<2%). The pulmonary end-capillary oxygen ($Cc'O_2$) content is the highest content of oxygen possible.

$$Cc'O_2 = (1.39 \times Hgb \times 1.0) + (PAO_2 \times 0.0031)$$

Artery oxygen content is calculated as follows:

$$CaO_2 = (1.39 \times Hgb \times SaO_2) + (PaO_2 \times 0.0031)$$

The pulmonary artery is the best source of true mixed venous oxygen content (CvO_2).

$$CvO_2 = (1.39 \times Hgb \times SvO_2) + (PvO_2 \times 0.0031)$$

If Hgb is 15 g/dl, and SvO_2 is 75%, then CvO_2 = 15 ml O_2/dl blood.

The arteriovenous oxygen content difference ($Ca - vO_2$) represents the amount of oxygen extracted by the tissues and organs.

$$Ca - vO_2 = CaO_2 - CvO_2 = 20 \text{ ml } O_2/dl - 15 \text{ ml } O_2/dl = 5 \text{ ml } O_2/dl$$

The amount of oxygen delivered to the tissues (DO_2) and the oxygen consumption (VO_2) is the arteriovenous oxygen content difference times the cardiac index (CI).

$$DO_2 = CI \times CaO_2 \times 10 \text{ dl/L } (600 \text{ ml } O_2/min/m^2 \text{ with Hgb of 15 g/dl, CI of 3 L/min/m}^2)$$

$$VO_2 = CI \times Ca - vO_2 \times 10 \text{ dl/L } (150 \text{ ml } O_2/min/m^2 \text{ with Hgb of 15 g/dl, CI of 3 L/min/m}^2)$$

The oxygen extraction ratio or the oxygen utilization coefficient (OUC) characterizes the balance between delivery and consumption.

$$OUC = VO_2/DO_2 = 0.25$$

An OUC more than 0.25 suggests an inadequate oxygen supply to meet the demand, frequently seen in shock.

H. Shock resuscitation adequacy. Continuous Svo_2 measurement through fiberoptic catheters correlates well with oxygen extraction ratios. It is a sensitive but nonspecific indicator of oxygen transport. Increases in $o_2$sat, Hgb, and CI result in an increase in Svo_2. Uncompensated increases in oxygen consumption result in a decrease in Svo_2. By itself, Svo_2 does not reflect the oxygen transport adequacy of nonperfused vascular beds. However, a low Svo_2 (<0.065) always indicates inadequate delivery of oxygen to meet its consumption. A high Svo_2 (>0.78) implies a maldistribution of peripheral blood flow. This is often associated with high-flow states such as cirrhosis, sepsis, pregnancy, and inflammation.

Oxygen debt forces cells to switch to anaerobic metabolism to make adenosine triphosphate via glycolysis. The by-products of glycolysis are hydrogen ion (H^+), pyruvate, and lactate. Accumulation of these products results in acidosis, injury, and eventual cellular death. Measurements of pH, base deficit, and serum lactate are all used to assess the presence of shock. Base deficit is the amount of base, in micro moles per liter required to titrate whole blood to normal pH. The presence of an elevated base deficit correlates with the presence and severity of shock. It helps guide fluid resuscitation and helps determine the time to terminate operative procedures (damage control) to facilitate resuscitation in the ICU. Sodium bicarbonate infusion alters its effectiveness.

Elevated lactate levels require a careful assessment of the patient's general perfusion and organ function. Serum lactate levels elevate as a result of two processes:

1. Excess production of lactate from ongoing anaerobic metabolism.
2. Decreased lactate metabolism caused by hypoperfusion or dysfunction of the liver or kidneys.

Some intensivists stress the importance of normalizing serum lactate levels in the management of the patient in shock. Others feel that normalizing the base excess is a more satisfactory goal. A smaller number believe that super levels of oxygen delivery and oxygen consumption should guide the resuscitation. We believe each practitioner must follow the logic which most works for him or her.

III. Treatment principles. Survival of the shock syndrome depends on prompt diagnosis and the initiation of treatment. Diagnosis and treatment of the underlying cause of shock is essential to successful resuscitation. For the tissues to receive adequate oxygen, the oxygen content of the blood should be optimized. Patients in shock have increased oxygen requirements and minute ventilation and may experience respiratory fatigue. They usually have mental status changes, which can further decrease their ventilation. Frequently, these patients have primary or secondary (acute respiratory distress syndrome), pulmonary failure, further decreasing good gas exchange. Many of these patients need to be intubated and mechanically ventilated. If not, they at least require supplemental oxygen and close observation.

Increasing the intravascular hemoglobin content can easily enhance oxygen delivery. A patient who is in shock and anemic should receive transfusion. No ideal hemoglobin level has proved to increase survival. Certainly, those critically ill patients with profound anemia (Hgb <7) should receive transfusions to increase their oxygen content. Too much hemoglobin (>15) can lead to a decrease in cardiac output and sludge capillaries. Most clinicians believe that a hemoglobin between 9 and 11 is beneficial to a patient in shock.

A goal of resuscitation would be to maximize cardiac index and thereby, oxygen delivery. Tachycardia is the physiologic response that temporarily can increase perfusion. Therapy directed to maximizing preload, decreasing afterload, and enhancing contractility should result in an increased cardiac index and enhanced oxygen delivery to the tissues.

Almost every shock state has a diminished preload. Infusion of a balanced salt solution is the initial treatment of choice. The amount will be determined by the patient's size and deficit, but an initial 20 ml/kg is standard. Endpoints are a reduction in heart rate and an increase in blood pressure, urine output, and oxygen delivery. Crystalloid infusion is just as efficacious as infusion of colloid for resuscitation. Because colloid solutions are much more expensive, their use in resuscitation is not warranted. Resuscitation should proceed through large-bore intravenous catheters, either peripherally or centrally, as needed. Care must be taken in large volume resuscitation to avoid hypothermia; therefore, use blood and fluid warmers as needed. The Trendelenburg position offers no benefit to resuscitation of patients in shock.

In cardiogenic shock, afterload reduction may enhance perfusion. A vasodilator (e.g., nitroprusside) is ideal because it is short acting and can be titrated easily. It should not be started in patients with inadequate preload, and it should be used cautiously in patients with coronary artery disease as it can cause coronary steal. An intraaortic balloon counterpulsion pump is often used for patients with poor myocardial function after myocardial infarction as an afterload reducer. These patients all need a pulmonary catheter to guide therapy.

Once preload is optimized, cardiac contractility can be enhanced to increase cardiac output as necessary. Dopamine in low doses ("renal dose," 3 μg/kg/min) may enhance splanchnic perfusion to a degree as well as have a mild β-stimulatory effect. As the dose is increased, the cardiac effect increases until at 10 μg/kg/min α-adrenergic stimulation is noted. Dobutamine has a pure β_1 effect, will not cause vasoconstriction, and may lead to splanchnic vasodilation. Its enhancement of cardiac output in many patients may be primarily caused by an increase in heart rate. Norepinephrine is a profound vasoconstrictor with some β_1 effects. It is a safe pressor to use only when a patient is volume resuscitated. Amrinone is a phosphodiesterase III inhibitor that is useful in the treatment of congestive heart failure because it increases stroke volume. Its side effects are vasodilation and hypotension.

IV. Summary. The goal in shock resuscitation is to enhance cellular perfusion and, thereby, oxygen and substrate delivery to the cells. Oxygen delivery will then exceed the oxygen demand created at the cellular level. Oxygen delivery must be sufficient so that oxygen consumption is not "flow dependent" and the cellular oxygen demand is met.

Selected Readings

Bone RC. The pathogenesis of sepsis. *Ann Intern Med* 1991;115:457.
An excellent review of septic shock.

Burchell SA, Yu M, Takiguchi SA, et al. Evaluation of a continuous cardiac output and mixed venous oxygen saturation catheter in critically ill surgical patients. *Crit Care Med* 1997;25:388.
Discusses continuous monitoring and oxygen transport.

Chang MC, Meredith JW. Cardiac preload, splanchnic perfusion, and their relationship during resuscitation in trauma patients. *J Trauma* 1997;42:577.
A good reference on preload and perfusion.

Cheatham ML, Chang MC, Safcsak K, et al. Right ventricular end-diastolic volume index and pulmonary artery occlusion pressure vs cardiac index in patients on positive end-expiratory pressure. *Crit Care Med* 1994;22;A98.
Evaluation of the effectiveness of invasive monitors during positive end-expiratory pressure.

Committee on Trauma. *Advanced trauma life support program for physicians.* Chicago: American College of Surgeons; 1993.
Applicable definition of shock and its management in trauma.

Davis JW, Shackford SR, Mackersie RC, et al. Base deficit as a guide to volume resuscitation. *J Trauma* 1988;28:1464.
Reference on using base deficit as an endpoint of resuscitation.

Gentilello LM. Advances in the management of hypothermia. *Surg Clin North Am* 1995;75:243.
A review on the disadvantages and management of hypothermia.

Hinshaw LB, Cox BG. *The fundamental mechanisms of shock.* New York: Plenum Press; 1972:13.
The classic reference on shock.

Mizock BA, Falk JL. Lactic acidosis in critical illness. *Crit Care Med* 1992;20:80.
Discussion of the use of lactic acidosis as a monitor of organ perfusion.

Nelson LD. Assessment of oxygenation: oxygenation indices. *Respiratory Care* 1993; 38:631.
Good reference on oxygen transport physiology.

Richer M, Rovert S, Lebel M. Renal hemodynamics during norepinephrine and low-dose dopamine infusions in man. *Crit Care Med* 1996;24:1150.
Good reference on balancing the effect of pressure.

Shoemaker WC, Appel PL, Kram HB, et al. Prospective trial of supranormal values of survivors as therapeutic goals in high-risk surgical patients. *Chest* 1988;94:1176.
The classic reference on supranormal oxygen transport and its effectiveness.

Swan HJC, Ganz W, Forrester J, et al. Catheterization of the heart in man with use of a flow-directed balloon-tipped catheter. *N Engl J Med* 1970;283:447.
The classic reference on the introduction of pulmonary catheters.

Velanovich V. Crystalloid versus colloid fluid resuscitation a meta-analysis of mortality. *Surgery* 1989;105:65.
An informative article on crystalloid versus colloid fluid resuscitation.

146. HEMORRHAGE AND RESUSCITATION

Kevin M. Dwyer and Arthur L. Trask

I. General principles. Exsanguination is second only to central nervous system injuries as the cause of death in trauma. Control of hemorrhage is second in importance only to adequate ventilation in trauma resuscitation.

Hemorrhagic shock alone has been shown to result in a multitude of responses that can lead to organ injury and multiple organ dysfunction. It is the tissue injury during reperfusion that is most severe. This reperfusion injury and the degree of organ damage will depend on both the severity and the duration of shock.

II. Hemostasis. The first step in resuscitation of hemorrhagic shock is to stop the hemorrhage. The only way to save a patient from exsanguination is to stop the bleeding and then restore vascular volume and oxygen-carrying capability. The cornerstone of trauma care is to attend to the injured patient promptly, establish adequate ventilation and oxygenation, stop obvious external bleeding, and transfer quickly to definitive trauma care. It has been shown that a patient with major hemorrhage (gunshot wound to the torso) has better survival when taken immediately to a trauma center (scoop and run) then have infusion of crystalloid solution. Rapid infusion of crystalloid can dilute the remainder of the blood volume or coagulation factors and increase hemorrhage prior to surgical hemostasis. The establishment of fluid resuscitation is not detrimental in all cases, however. It is necessary for the head-injured and multiple-injured patients and those patients with long transport times. However, the concept of rapid transfer to definitive care at a trauma center is paramount for all severely injured patients.

III. Fluid resuscitation. Restoration of vascular volume and blood flow begins as hemostasis is being achieved. In cases of a moderate amount of blood loss, vascular volume is maintained by shifting of the interstitial and the intracellular fluid to the vascular space. Crystalloid infusion will help restore vascular volume as well as institial and intracellular fluid. Once hemorrhage becomes severe and a critical decrease in red cell mass occurs, transfusions of packed red blood cells must commence. In practice, if a patient is hypotensive and unresponsive to 2 L of crystalloid infusion, or if the patient is initially responsive but continues to cycle into hemodynamic instability, blood should be transfused. This could be cross-matched blood, type-specific blood, or O-negative blood, depending on what is available.

Crystalloid infusion is the frontline fluid used to resuscitate patients in hemorrhagic shock. For years, debate has centered on the use of crystalloids or colloid solutions for resuscitation. Proponents of colloid infusion maintain that colloid solutions require less fluid for resuscitation because colloids remain intravascular and would attract the interstitial and intracellular fluid into the vascular space. Much less edema would occur after resuscitation and, perhaps, less organ damage with crystalloid infusion. Those who believe in resuscitation with crystallod solution point out that the hemorrhagic shock patients have a loss of integrity of their vascular membrane. Colloids may leak out into the interstitium and actually make the edema worse, causing organ failure. In practice, edema and organ damage are mostly related to shock and not to what fluid is used for resuscitation. Crystalloid solutions are much less expensive and readily available. Lactate Ringer's solution is standard and normal saline is used if blood transfusion is necessary.

Hypertonic saline has received much attention as a resuscitative fluid since the mid-1970s. The role of hypertonic saline in the intensive care unit is questionable. Because hypertonic saline infusion can raise blood pressure faster, overall less fluid would be necessary for the prehospital setting. Blood transfusions, being the ideal choice for hemorrhage resuscitation, carry a small but significant risk of deadly infectious diseases (e.g., human immunodeficiency virus and hepatitis). Much research has been directed at producing hemoglobin solutions to replace blood.

IV. Endpoints of resuscitation. Many patients who are resuscitated to a normal blood pressure still do poorly with cyclic hypotension and experience organ failure. Other endpoints of adequate resuscitation have been sought to define when a patient is resuscitated. These include a normal cardiac output, measurement of adequate oxygen delivery and consumption, and supernormal resuscitation. The degree of acidosis, secondary to lactate production from anaerobic metabolism and its correction, is currently used as the best obtainable endpoint of resuscitation. Although it correlates fairly well with resuscitation, a small percentage of patients go on to organ failure. Many authors believe that devices that actually test the oxygen tension of individual organs (e.g., the stomach) lead to a more accurate, although less practical, assessment of resuscitation. Irreversible shock is the point where, despite aggressive efforts for resuscitation, the patient goes on to organ failure and death. This endpoint should never be assumed.

V. Correction of coagulopathy Patients who have received large amounts of fluids and blood should have a coagulation panel to include prothrombin time (PT), activated partial thromboplastin time (aPTT), and platelet count. When suspicion of a consumptive coagulopathy exists, a complete disseminated intravascular coagulation (DIC) panel should be done, which includes fibrinogen, *d*-dimer, and fibrin split products (FSP). The bleeding patient with thrombocytopenia, hypofibrinogenemia, and elevated FSP and *d*-dimer should be considered to have DIC. Thromboelastography (TEG) is a simple test that provides a rapid and comprehensive analysis of coagulation status and can replace the DIC panel. It has been used extensively in cardiac and transplant surgery.

Prolonged hypotension, hypothermia, dilution with massive infusion of fluid, and massive transfusion with packed red blood cells that do not contain coagulation factors can lead to a coagulopathy. Correction primarily involves aggressive resuscitation, stopping the hemorrhage, and **rewarming**. Once this is begun, replacement of specific products may become necessary. A bleeding patient, with a PT or aPTT 1.5 times normal will need transfusion of fresh frozen plasma (FFP). Fibrinogen counts less than 100 will need cryoprecipitate or FFP. Patients with platelet count below 20,000 always need platelet transfusions. Patients with platelet counts below 60,000 with intracerebral hemorrhage (<90,000) or a liver laceration may need platelet transfusion. Each unit of platelets, now more often single-donor platelets, raises the count at least 5,000. Other treatments include ε-aminocaproic acid for primary fibrinolysis, 1-deamino-[8-D-arginine] vasopressin for uremia, and vitamin K for malnutrition and liver failure. Congenital hemophiliac's need replacement of specific factors.

Selected Readings

Bickell WH, Wall MJ, Pepe PE, et al. Immediate versus delayed fluid resuscitation for hypotensive patients with penetrating torso injuries. *N Engl J Med* 1994;331:1105.
The classic reference to the principle of hemostasis first and scoop and run.

Davis JW, Shackford SR, Mackersie RC, et al. Base deficit as a guide to volume resuscitation. J Trauma 1988;28:1464.
The basic reference on using base deficit as an endpoint of resuscitation.

Faringer PD, Mullins RJ, Johnson RL, et al. Blood component supplementation during massive transfusion of AS-1 cells in trauma patients. *J Trauma* 1993;34:481.
A good reference on massive transfusions.

Ivatury RR, Simon RJ, Havriliak D, et al. Gastric mucosal pH and oxygen delivery and oxygen consumption indices in the assessment of adequacy of resuscitation after trauma: a prospective randomized study. *J Trauma* 1995;39:128.
Reference to the use of endorgan perfusion for endpoints of resuscitation.

Kaufmann CR, Dwyer KM, Crews JD, et al. Usefulness of thromboelastography in assessment of trauma patient coagulation. *J Trauma* 1997;42:716.
An excellent reference on the use of thromboelastography in trauma.

Mattox K, Maningas PA, Moore EE, et al. Prehospital hypertonic saline/dextran infusion for posttraumatic hypotension: the USA multicenter study. *Ann Surg* 1991; 213:482.
Reference as to the use of hypertonic saline.

Peitzman AB, Billiar TR, Harbrecht BG, et al. Hemorrhagic shock. *Curr Probl Surg* 1995;32:927.
A good overall review and reference on hemorrhagic shock.

Poole GV, Meridith JW, Pennell T, et al. Comparison of colloids and crystalloids in resuscitation from hemorrhagic shock. *Surg Gynecol Obstet* 1982;154:577.
The classic review of use of colloids versus crystalloids in resuscitation.

Sauaia A, Moore FA, Moore EE, et al. Epidemiology of trauma deaths: a reassessment. *J Trauma* 1995;38:185.
General reference on trauma.

Shires GT, Barber AE, Illner HP. Current status of resuscitation: solutions including hypertonic saline. *Adv Surg* 1995;28:133.
A good reference to resuscitative fluids.

Waxman K. Shock: ischemia, reperfusion, and inflammation. *New Horizons* 1996; 4(2):153.
Reference to second paragraph and expansion of theory.

Winslow RM. Blood substitutes in development. *Exp Opin Invest Drugs* 1996;5:1443.
Good reference on blood substitutes.

147. TRAUMA: AN OVERVIEW

Kevin M. Dwyer and Arthur L. Trask

I. General principles. Traumatic injury has reached epidemic proportions; it is the leading cause of death for persons aged less than 45 years and is the third leading cause of death for all ages, exceeded only by cardiovascular disease and cancer. Injury prevention is the most important method of dealing with this medical problem.

The intensive care of traumatic injury is highlighted in this section. Traumatic injury patients who require intensive care comprise a high proportion of the total intensive care unit bed utilization in the world today.

II. Trauma care systems. A trauma care system is a comprehensive, organized approach to the management of the injured patient. Without this organized systematic approach, the intensivists responsible for the care of the trauma patients would be overwhelmed because of lack of data prior to the patient's arrival in their unit. Figure 147-1 illustrates the components of the trauma system (Fig. 147-1). A key point of quality trauma management is the team approach, with prearranged communication flow of data as the patient moves through the system. Performance improvement (previously known as quality improvement) is essential to making the care better and the outcomes more efficient and effective.

Suggested Readings

American College of Surgeons Committee on Trauma. *Advanced trauma life support course for doctors.* Chicago: American College of Surgeons; 1997.

Physicians throughout the world also recognize the trauma care course that was developed by the Committee on Trauma as the standard.

American College of Surgeons Committee on Trauma. *National Trauma Data Bank.* Chicago: American College of Surgeons; 1999.

Although yet to be accepted by every trauma center, the American College of Surgeons is hoping that its National Trauma Data Bank will eventually be fed data from throughout the United States and, ultimately, the world.

American College of Surgeons Committee on Trauma. *Resources for optimal care of the injured patient: 1999.* Chicago: American College of Surgeons; 1999.

This optimal care document is the worldwide standard recognized as the guideline for trauma care systems.

Trunkey DD, Blaisdell FW. Care of the surgical patient. In: *Scientific American surgery.* Section IV: Trauma. New York: Scientific American Inc.; 1999.

This section remains an excellent current reference on trauma management.

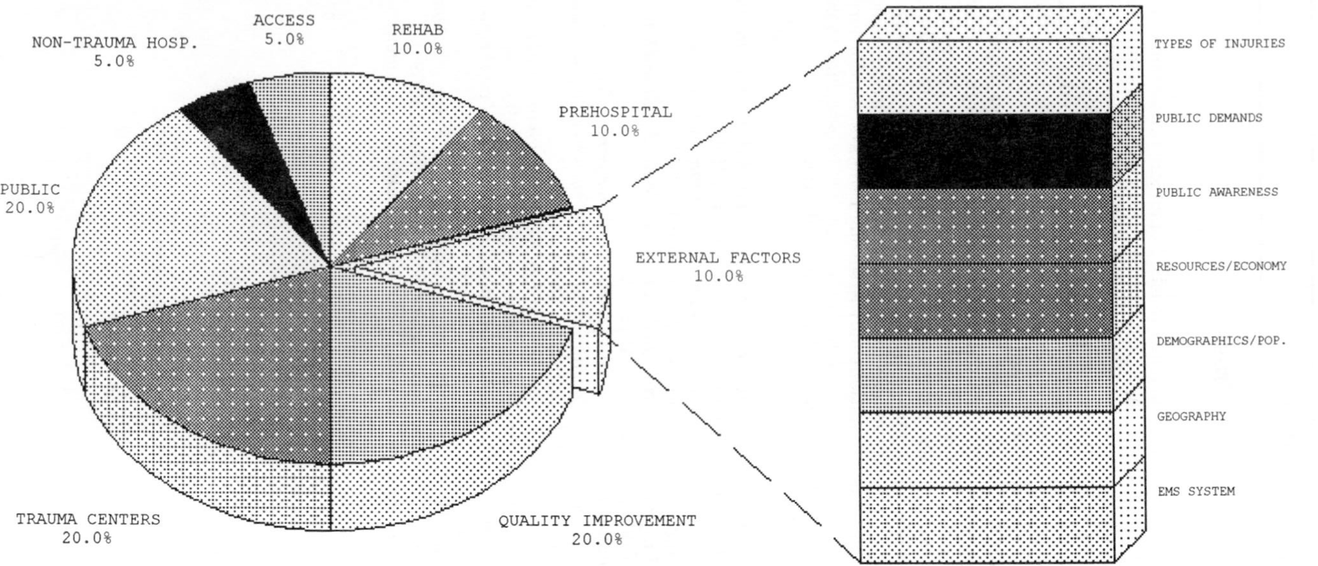

FIG. 147-1. Components of the trauma system.

148. CRITICAL CARE OF PATIENTS WITH TRAUMATIC BRAIN INJURY

Kevin M. Dwyer and Arthur L. Trask

I. General principles. Every year, 150,000 trauma deaths occur in the United States with about half of them related to brain injury. The outcome of brain trauma is related to the extent of the initial brain injury coupled with secondary damage caused by ischemia from hypotension and hypoxia. The medical care team, from the time of injury to management in the intensive care unit (ICU), should focus on the prevention of secondary brain injury.

In 1960, Lundberg described intracranial pressure (ICP) in the normal and abnormal states. The management of increased ICP is the hallmark of aggressive treatment of severe brain injury. In 1974, Jennett and Teasdale described the clinical measure that came to be known as the Glascow Coma scale (GCS) (Table 148-1). It is the universally excepted simple method of identifying and stratifying patients with brain injuries. Computed tomography (CT) revolutionized the care of these patients with by enabling the quick identification of severe brain injury and surgically treatable lesions. Early diagnosis and aggressive treatment of severe brain injury enable improved outcome as shown in a landmark study in 1977 by Becker and others. Management of severe brain trauma continues to evolve, but clearly, expedient management of airway, hypoxia, hypotension, and rapid transport to a capable facility is essential.

II. National guidelines for the management of severe head injury. A joint venture of the Brain Trauma Foundation, The American Association of Neurological Surgeons, and the Joint Section on Neurotrauma and Critical Care produced these national guidelines in 1995. The guidelines were based on three levels of clinical certainty, supported by clinical research.

Standards: Represent accepted principles of patient management that reflect a "high degree" of clinical certainty.

Guidelines: Represent a particular strategy or range of management strategies that reflect a moderate degree of clinical certainty.

Options: Are there remaining strategies for patient management for which there is unclear clinical certainty?

The following topics are mentioned with their level of certainty as assessed by the panel of neurologic surgeons:

Management of blood pressure (guideline). Ample evidence is seen that early postinjury hypotension increases the morbidity and mortality from severe brain injury.

Indications for intracranial pressure monitoring (standard). Patients with severe head injury (GCS < 8 and CT abnormalities) are at high risk for elevated ICP > 20. Treatment modalities for elevated ICP carry risks. ICP monitoring is essential for proper use of interventions to protect the brain from further injury.

Intracranial pressure monitoring technology (guideline). The ventriculostomy is the most effective and reliable method of measuring ICP. Infrequent complications include hemorrhage, infection, malposition, and malfunction. Intraparenchymal monitors should be used if the ventriculostomy cannot be placed (collapsed ventricles).

Cerebral perfusion measurement (option). Cerebral perfusion pressure [CPP = mean arterial pressure (MAP) – ICP] should be monitored and maintained above 70 mm Hg.

Hyperventilation (guideline). Maintain an arterial P_{CO_2} no lower than 30 to 35 mm Hg in severe traumatic brain injury for the first several days, with exceptions for lower values only for acute deteriations or elevated ICP refractory to all

TABLE 148-1. Glasgow Coma Scale

Eye opening response	**E**
Spontaneous	4
To voice	3
To pain	2
None	1
Best verbal response	**V**
Oriented	5
Confused conversation	4
Inappropriate words	3
Incomprehensible sounds	2
None	1
Best motor response	**M**
Obeys commands	6
Localizes pain	5
Withdraws to pain	4
Flexor response	3
Extensor response	2
None	1
Score	**E + V + M = 3–15**

other treatments. Recent evidence of cerebral ischemia has curtailed the use of prolonged, aggressive hyperventilation (P_{CO_2} of 25).

Mannitol (guideline). Mannitol effectively controls elevated ICP after severe brain injury. Effective doses are boluses between 0.25 and 1.0 g/kg. Optional guidelines are as follows:

Mannitol can be used prior to initial CT scan in patients with signs of transtentorial herniation (fixed, dilated pupils).

Serum osmolality should be kept below 320 mOsm because of the potential for renal failure.

Mannitol can be followed by furosemide for patients with congestive heart failure.

Barbiturates (standard). Barbiturates lower brain metabolism. They can lower increased ICP in a hemodynamically stable patient who is refractory to other treatments. It is associated with a reduced mortality in this setting, but should not be used prophylactically.

Steroids (standard). No benefit is seen of steroid use in brain injury, and they should not be used.

Acute resuscitation and ICP (option). No studies exist that show the benefit of aggressive management of potentially increased ICP prior to monitoring. However, evidence does suggest that prevention of secondary brain injury improves outcome. Early intubation, treatment of hypotension, and adequate sedation should be initiated in the severely brain injured patient.

Nutritional support (guideline). Caloric replacement should begin within 72 hours after injury. A nonparalyzed patient should receive 140% of resting metabolic expenditure; at least 15% of the calories should be provided by proteins.

Prophylactic anticonvulsants (standard). The use of phenytoin or carbamazepine can prevent early posttraumatic seizures (< 7 days). Risk factors for seizures include a GCS less than 10, cerebral contusion, depressed skull fracture, subdural or epidural hematoma, penetrating head wound, or a seizure. No evidence supports the use of anticonvulsants to prevent late seizures in blunt head injury.

III. Pathology and pathophysiology of traumatic brain injury

A. Skull fractures. The cranial vault, basal skull, and facial bones offer some protection to the brain but can fail in the event of **high-energy** impact. Skull fragments and bone can be driven into the brain from a depressed skull fracture. The basilar skull is much more substantial and requires much more impact before fracture. However, many cranial nerves are at risk along the base of the brain. A transverse fracture through the petrous portion of the temporal bone can disrupt the seventh or eight cranial nerve. A fracture through the frontal skull base can injure the optic or the olfactory nerve, which is the most frequently injured cranial nerve. The facial bones can be fractured along the many pillars and struts of the face. Airway protection is a primary concern with extensive facial injuries and cervical spine extension injuries are common. Clear discharge from the nose or blood from the auditory canal may be from a cerebrospinal fistula.

B. Extracerebral hematoma. Tears in the dural arteries (e.g., the middle meningeal) can produce an epidural hematoma. This is a rapidly expanding mass that can encroach on the brain causing coma and death. The patient may present with a normal GCS, but progress to death in a few hours.

A subdural hematoma usually forms from disruptions of the venous sinuses or bridging veins beneath the dura. These lesions can also expand, although usually much slower, and are more frequently associated with parenchymal damage. Subarachnoid hemorrhage occurs frequently after head injury. Spontaneous subarachnoid hemorrhage from an intracranial aneurysm rupture may be the precipitating cause of a subsequent traumatic event.

C. Parenchymal injuries. Disruption of the brain substance can occur from direct injury, a countercoup injury, acceleration–deceleration forces, or from differential shearing force injuries of both the neuropil and its vascular network. The frontal and temporal poles are often injured as the brain decelerates against the anterior and inferior walls of their fossa. Deeper contusions occur in well-defined locations. These include the corpus callosum, the superior cerebella peduncle, and midbrain. These are visible deep contusions, but much more global injury occurs to the brain from axonal shear and disruption. Cerebral contusions can grow to produce a secondary mass effect, distortion of the cerebral axis and shift, and ultimately herniation. The second CT scan frequently is worse as the contusion gains more edema with age and the total shear injury becomes more apparent.

D. Brain edema. Edema formation is the early response of the brain to injury. It contributes to brain mass, causing vasoconstriction, and can lead to herniation. Vasogenic edema occurs adjacent to contusions. Cytotoxic edema can form in response to ischemia. A late hydrostatic form can occur if venous drainage capacity is overwhelmed. Hypoosmolar states can exacerbate brain edema and need to be avoided.

IV. Secondary brain injury. A secondary brain injury can occur after traumatic brain injury from ischemia and infarction. This is caused by a loss of autoregulation and carbon dioxide vasoreactivity combined with systemic hypotension. Secondary brain injury can also be caused by the formation of noxious influences that evolve from the brain's response to injury. These include free radical formation and lipid peroxidation, inappropriate neurotransmitter release that kills large populations of surrounding neurons, and inflammatory reactions to released cellular content. Avoidance of hypoxia and hypotension will decrease the effects of secondary brain injury.

V. Initial radiologic examination and surgical triage. After initial resuscitation, assessment, and management of life-threatening conditions in the multiple injured patient, those with suspected head injury need a prompt CT scan of the head. The unresponsive patient also needs full trauma radiologic assessment, including a cervical spine and chest x-ray study. Brain injuries detected by CT scan fall into three categories:

1. Lesions that require immediate surgical intervention: Epidural and subdural hematomas greater than 1 cm and a midline shift, open depressed skull fractures, and closed depressed skull fractures deeper than 1 cm.
2. Nonsurgical lesions associated with the development of intracranial hypertension: Multiple contusions are frequent in patients with low GCS scores.
3. Traumatic injuries that most likely will not lead to increased ICP: Linear skull fractures, small subanachnoid hemorrhage (SAH), and tiny subdural hematomas.

VI. Management of severe traumatic brain injury in the critical care setting. The management of severe brain injury requires close monitoring in the critical care unit with invasive devices, such as ICP monitors, Swan-Ganz catheters, and jugular venous saturation catheters. Patients with a GCS less than 8 with a CT scan that reveals a brain injury, need ICP monitoring and aggressive fluid management. A standardized approach, such as a protocol, for management of the patient with severe brain injury involving both the neurosurgeon and intensivist may lead to better outcomes.

The care of the severely brain injured patient begins at the moment the injury is addressed at the scene. The patient often needs early endotracheal intubation by experienced prehospital providers to maintain oxygenation. Systolic blood pressure needs to be supported with saline and blood as necessary. The patient is quickly assessed and other life-threatening injuries are treated. Radiographic examination should include a chest x-ray study, lateral cervical spine radiograph, and a CT scan of the head to triage the patient to the operating room or the ICU.

Resuscitation continues in the ICU. Direct invasive monitoring is necessary, with placement of arterial line, central venous pressure, an ICP monitor, preferably a ventriculostomy, and, if necessary, a pulmonary artery catheter and a jugular bulb venous saturation monitor. Anticonvulsants are administered routinely to suppress any potential seizure activity.

VII. Control of intracranial hypertension. Uncontrolled ICP is the single most common condition associated with death in the severely brain-injured patient. Periodic CT scans need to be performed to confirm the absence of a surgical lesion. ICP elevation needs to be treated with a predetermined, expedient, systematic approach.

Patients with a GCS less than 8 need to be intubated and placed on a ventilator. The patient needs to be sedated and paralyzed for intubation to avoid ICP elevations. When the patient is suctioned, lidocaine can be instilled down the endotracheal tube to prevent gagging. If the patient is normotensive, the head of the bed can be placed at 30 degrees. Mild hyperventilation (P_{CO_2} 30–35 mm Hg) will reduce the increased brain blood volume, but avoid ischemia produced by lower levels of P_{CO_2}. Use of a jugular bulb saturation monitor may help avoid this ischemia. Complete sedation and paralysis may be necessary. Drainage of cerebrospinal fluid with a ventriculostomy is an efficient way of decreasing ICP. Complications such as ventriculitis, plugging, and overdrainage are uncommon. The drain needs to be placed at the level of the base of the head to accurately measure ICP. Intermittent bolus mannitol (0.5–1.0 g/kg body weight given intravenously) is the next step used to help decrease ICP that is persistently elevated. **Caution: avoid serum osmality levels greater than 320,** which can produce serious systemic complications.

A. Cerebral perfusion pressure. The concept of maintaining CPP (CPP = MAP – ICP) recognizes the need to avoid brain ischemia in severe brain injury. The injured brain suffers from cerebral vasoparalysis and a significant incidence of measured vasospasm after trauma can increase ischemia. Maintenance of adequate blood pressure to a CPP of approximately 70 mm Hg is desirable to overcome these forces.

Maintenance of CPP of 70 mm Hg requires normovolemia or hypervolemia. CVP or pulmonary wedge pressure monitoring is required. Large volumes of saline may be necessary. If volume resuscitation is adequate, as determined by central pressures, and the CPP is still low, vasopressors should be considered. Systemic hypertension may be necessary with sharply elevated ICPs.

A newer global form of monitoring cerebral perfusion is with a jugular bulb venous oxygen saturation monitor. This is placed directly in the internal jugular vein and fed to the base of the skull. It measures brain oxygen extraction. This measurement has greatest utility in ventilator management. In the setting of an elevated ICP, more aggressive hyperventilation may be attempted as long as the jugular venous saturation remains above threshold (55%). If jugular venous desaturation occurs, an intervention to improve perfusion (e.g., less ventilation) or increasing CPP would be required.

If the patient's ICP still does not respond, then pentobarbital coma may be considered to reduce brain metabolism. The use of a pentobarbital coma requires pulmonary catheter monitoring because it can cause myocardial depression, vasodilation, and resultant poor organ perfusion. The following dose is recommended: 10 mg/kg body weight over 30 minutes, with 5 mg/kg every hour for 3 hours, and a maintenance dose of 1 mg/kg/h. The endpoint is gauged by achievement of burst suppression on electroencephalography.

Salvage surgical procedures (e.g., lobe removal or calvarial and dural opening) have been proposed. The decision for these procedures is based on survivability and brain viability.

VIII. Additional considerations in the management of severe traumatic brain injury

A. Cervical spine. A negative lateral cervical spine x-ray study does not rule out spinal instability in an unconscious patient. The patient needs to be maintained in a cushioned hard collar. If a good clinical examination of the patient is not achieved in 48 hours, then further evaluation of the cervical spine should be considered. This can be done with a full series with flexion extension views under fluoroscopy. A complete CT scan of the cervical spine from the skull base to T1 can reasonably exclude serious spinous injury.

B. Pulmonary aspiration is common with brain-injured patients. Good pulmonary toilet and prevention of hypoxia and additional episodes of aspiration are essential. Initially, nasogastric suctioning is required. If gastric feedings are initiated, the stomach should be monitored for residual volume. Acute respiratory distress syndrome is common in brain and other trauma. Although positive end-expiratory pressure (PEEP) may elevate ICP slightly, the maintenance of adequate oxygenation takes precedence.

C. Cardiovascular circulating endogenous cathecholamines are elevated with severe brain trauma. In addition, the management of severe brain trauma requires infusion of large volumes of fluid as well as vasopressors. This puts a tremendous load on the heart. The patient with known or suspected cardiovascular disease may progress to heart failure. These patients must be monitored with pulmonary artery catheters.

Brain trauma patients in general are hypercoagulable; they frequently develop deep venous thrombosis and are at risk for pulmonary embolus. Bedrest, sedation, and chemical paralysis can increase this risk. These patients must have pneumatic compression devices in place. Subcutaneous or low molecular weight heparin is contraindicated in the early course because of the increased risk of rebleeding in the injured brain. Some patients with severe injuries to the brain stem can develop a coagulopathy and it should be anticipated and treated. This is an ominous clinical manifestation with a poor prognosis for brain recovery.

D. Endocrine and metabolic systems. It is essential to maintain a normal to elevated serum osmolality in the management of the severely brain injured patient. Normal saline or Ringer's lactated is the fluid of choice for maintenance of volume. Brain injury can cause the syndrome of inappropriate secretion of antidiuretic hormone later in its course, retaining water and diluting plasma electrolytes. Water restriction is the treatment for mild hyponatremia, but not at the expense of CPP. This syndrome needs to be distinguished from the cerebral salt wasting syndrome, which is thought to be caused by a brain-secreted naturetic peptide. These patients are usually hypovolemic and fluid restriction would be dangerous. Salt and volume replacement is the treatment in these cases.

Diabetes insipidus, secondary to loss of antidiuretic hormone, can also occur in the severely injured brain. This can be indicative of a hypothalmus or pituitary stalk injury, or unfortunately, brain death. Severe dehydration from water loss through uncontrolled urine can occur rapidly. The treatment is resuscitation of fluid volume and, when the diagnosis is certain, intravenous desmopressin acetate.

Glucose is usually avoided in resuscitation and maintenance fluids to prevent lactate formation in the brain. However, the patient with multiple trauma, including a severely injured brain, is hypermetabolic and requires early nutrition within 48 hours, preferably via the gastrointestinal tract.

E. Musculoskelatal system and skin. Because the severely brain inured patient is at high risk to develop bed sores, prevention techniques should be initiated early. Prolonged use of neuromuscular blocking agents leads to neuropathies and myopathies. They should only be used when absolutely necessary and stopped as soon as possible.

IX. Management of the postacute survivors with severe brain injury. Once ICP in a severe brain injury has returned to normal and is stable, sedation and paralytics can be withdrawn. If the ICP remains normal, then the monitor can be removed. Physical medicine and physical, occupational, and speech therapy all need to be part of the rehabilitation phase. Many of these patients will need early tracheostomy for airway protection and ventilator weaning. The swallowing reflex may be compromised and early testing for dysfunction and feeding tube gastrostomy placement is indicated.

Aggressive, immediate management of the severe traumatic brain-injured patients along these guidelines should reduce mortality rates to below 30% and improve functional outcome.

Selected Readings

Becker DP. Common themes in head injury. In Becker DP, Gudeman SK, eds. *Textbook of head injury.* Philadelphia: WB Saunders; 1989.

An excellent overview reference.

Bullock R, Chestnut RM, Clifton G, et al. *Guidelines for the management of severe head injury.* New York: Brain Trauma Foundation; 1995.

This is the "gold standard" for the management of traumatic brain injury which has been approved by the Congress of Neurological Surgeons and the American Association of Neurologic Surgeons.

Clifton GL, Robertson CS, Hodge S, et al. The metabolic response to severe head injury. *J Neurosurg* 1984;60:687.

The future of traumatic brain injury management clearly depends on improved understanding of the brain's metabolism and the aberrations caused by injury.

Rosner MJ, Daughton SD. Cerebral perfusion pressure management in head injury. *J Trauma* 1990;30:933.

A key article on the newer strategy for managing brain injury.

149. SPINAL CORD TRAUMA

Kevin M. Dwyer and Arthur L. Trask

I. General principles. Vertebral column fracture and spinal cord injury cause substantial morbidity and mortality. Although not as frequent as head trauma, an estimated 10,000 traumatic spinal cord injury cases occur every year in the United States. The prevalence of spinal cord injuries is, in descending order, cervical, thoracic, lumbar, and sacral. The mechanism of injury can be blunt or penetrating. The goal of treatment of spinal cord injury is to preserve residual neurologic function and aid recovery, stabilize hemodynamic and pulmonary function, and restore spinal alignment and stability.

II. Neurologic grading scales The Frankel classification is simple and widely used. This grading system assesses the extent of motor and sensory injuries, but does not take into account the significance of bowel or bladder function (Table 149-1).

III. Specific neurologic syndromes

A. Brown–Sequard syndrome. This is an ipsilateral motor and posterior column function loss and contralateral loss of spinothalamic tract function approximately two segments below the level of the injury.

B. Central cord syndrome. This syndrome results from hyperextension injury, often in patients with preexisting spondylosis. It classically presents with upper extremity weakness out of proportion to the lower extremity weakness. Prognosis is generally favorable.

C. Anterior cord syndrome. A result of flexion or anterior compression of the cord, motor and lateral column functions are lost, with characteristic preservation of posterior column function. Prognosis is not as good as in the central cord syndrome.

D. Conus medullaris syndrome. This syndrome results from a thoracolumbar junction (usually T11-L1) fracture or injury with a combination of upper and lower motor neuron deficits. It appears much like a spinal cord injury but usually without preservation of sexual and sphincter function.

E. Cauda equina syndrome. Resembling a peripheral nerve injury or a lumbar plexus injury, this syndrome has a more favorable outcome than the conus injury.

IV. Acute management of spinal cord injury. All persons sustaining major blunt trauma must be deemed by medical personnel to have a spinal cord injury until such is proved otherwise. Any motor or sensory signs, pain, incontinence, or external sign of trauma should especially alert medical personnel to the possibility of spine fracture and spinal cord injury. **Immobilize the spine with a cervical collar in combination with a rigid spine backboard.**

Spinal shock and respiratory muscle failure should be considered for patients with cervical or high thoracic injuries, which can cause a "sympathectomy" syndrome consisting of hypotension and bradycardia because of unopposed vagal tone. Fluid support, appropriate hemodynamic monitoring, and pressors may be necessary. If the patient shows signs of spinal cord injury, the high-dose methylprednisolone protocol outlined by the National Spinal Cord Injury Study II is recommended:

Give within 8 hours of injury: 30 mg/kg intravenous (IV) methylprednisolone over 1 hour; then 5.4 mg/kg/h for the next 23 hours.

Appropriate gastritis or ulcer prophylaxis should be given. No steroid is infused in cases of penetrating injury because of possible visceral involvement and sepsis.

V. Cervical traction. Do not place patients under cervical traction until appropriate radiographic studies are obtained in the emergency department. Significant risks of increasing neurologic deficits exist. **Only** a physician trained in spinal fracture management should apply traction.

TABLE 149-1. The Frankel grading system for spinal cord injury

A: Complete neurologic injury
B: Incomplete: preserved sensation only
C: Incomplete: nonfunctional motor
D: Incomplete: functional motor
E: Complete recovery (abnormal reflexes allowed)

VI. Medical management of spinal cord-injured patients. Several medical problems are frequently associated with a vertebral fracture or spinal cord injury. Some are related to the systemic effect of spinal cord injury and others to the paralysis and prolonged immobilization.

VII. Cardiovascular. Early recognition and treatment of neurogenic shock is essential. This usually occurs after cervical or upper thoracic injury. The combination of hypotension and bradycardia can cause secondary neurologic injury, as well as pulmonary, renal, and cerebral insults, which is especially true in the multisystem trauma patient. A baseline electrocardiogram should be obtained and a central venous catheter inserted to allow proper monitoring and fluid resuscitation. Unstable patients should also have an arterial line placed. Symptomatic bradycardia is treated with IV atropine (0.2–1.0 mg) as necessary. Pressors may be necessary to maintain adequate perfusion pressures. Dopamine is the usual drug of choice, starting with dose range of 3 to 5 μg/kg/h and increasing as necessary.

VIII. Pulmonary. Pulmonary problems are those most commonly faced by a patient with acute spinal cord injury, especially those in the cervical area. Any involvement of the phrenic nerve accentuates the problem. Other concurrent thoracic or pulmonary injuries complicate the problem. Aggressive suctioning, possibly intubation, and therapeutic bronchoscopy may be necessary.

IX. Thromboembolic. Spinal cord-injured patients are susceptible to thromboembolic problems. Unless absolutely contraindicated, both low-dose heparin (5,000 U subcutaneously twice daily) and lower extremity pneumatic compressive devices are used. Consideration should be given for prophylactic vena cava filter placement for patients with high lesions and for those who are likely to have a long immobilization period.

X. Gastrointestinal and nutritional considerations. A nasogastric or orogastric tube should be inserted initially to prevent gastric distension and possible perforation. An H_2 receptor antagonist or sucralfate is used as a gastritis prophylaxis. After stabilization, nutritional support is essential with 150% of the basal caloric requirement. Pancreatitis and cholecystitis can occur, especially in patients with cervical and high thoracic cord injuries. Proper monitoring and anticipation of these problems will keep the complication rate low.

XI. Genitourninary. Careful observation for urinary tract infection is essential. Removal of the indwelling catheter, with intermittent catheterization is the goal.

XII. Cutaneous and musculoskeletal. Constant positioning and steady pressure of greater than 1 to 2 hours can cause a decubitus formation. This problem is best treated by prevention. Kinetic treatment beds and meticulous daily skin care are essential.

Early mobilization of joints with physical therapy will help prevent contractures. Heterotopic bone formation can further complicate this injury and as yet no reliable prophylaxis or treatment protocol has been established to prevent it.

XIII. Conclusion. Numerous neurologic and systemic complications can occur in the face of a spinal cord injury. The goal of treatment continues to be early spine immobilization, stabilization of hemodynamic and pulmonary status, and prevention of medical complications.

Selected Readings

Bracken MB, Shepard MJ, Collins WF, et al. A randomized controlled trial of methylprednisolone or naloxone in the treatment of acute spinal-cord injury: results of the second National Acute Spinal Cord Injury Study. *N Engl J Med* 1990;322:1405.
Principle reference for the use of steroids with spinal cord injury.

Frankel HL, Hancock DO, Hysolop G, et al. The value of postural reduction in the initial treatment of closed injuries of the spine with paraplegia and tetraplegia. *Paraplegia* 1969;31:179.

Gilbert J. Critical care management of the patient with acute spinal cord injury. *Crit Care Clin* 1987;3:549.

Green BA, Green KL, Klose KL. Kinetic therapy for spinal cord injury. *Spine* 1983;8:722.

150. ABDOMINAL TRAUMA

Kevin M. Dwyer and Arthur L. Trask

I. General principles. Abdominal trauma occurs in 20% of civilian injuries requiring operation and one half of all preventable deaths are related to inappropriate management of abdominal trauma.

II. Diagnostic methods. Clinical findings indicative of abdominal trauma include abdominal contusions, pain, tenderness, absent bowel sounds, or unexplained hypotension. Physical examination can be misleading. Peritoneal signs are absent in 40% of patients with significant intraabdominal injuries. Physical findings are unreliable for patients with an abnormal sensorium secondary to head trauma, spinal cord injury, or intoxication. A variety of diagnostic approaches have been developed for abdominal trauma.

A. Mandatory exploration. Abdominal exploration is required in patients with anterior abdominal gunshot wounds because visceral injury is present in more than 90% of cases. For patients with stab wounds, the presence of peritoneal signs, hemodynamic instability, or evisceration of abdominal contents, exploration is necessary. Unexplained hypotension with physical signs of abdominal trauma may warrant exploration.

B. Local exploration of stab wound can identify fascial penetration and the need for laparotomy.

C. Diagnostic peritoneal lavage. Diagnostic peritoneal lavage (DPL) is used to evaluate patients with blunt trauma and also for patients with stab wounds. DPL is positive in blunt trauma when gross blood is returned or the lavage fluid contains more than 100,000/ml red blood cells (RBC), bilirubin or amylase concentration higher than plasma, or bacteria or food particles. A white blood cell count of more than 500/ml is no longer considered an absolute indication for laparotomy, but is suggestive of a hollow viscous injury. A DPL for a stab wound is considered positive with 5,000 to 20,000 RBC/ml. DPL has high sensitivity for most injuries, although it can miss early hollow viscus, retroperitoneal, and diaphragmatic injuries.

D. Computed tomography (CT). Traditionally, CT does not have the sensitivity for finding an injury that DPL has. However, with the evolution of spiral CT, its sensitivity is improving. CT has the advantage of defining the severity of organ injury, thereby selecting good candidates for nonoperative management. CT can be particularly helpful with retroperitoneal injuries and in patients with pelvic fractures. CT can still miss intestinal and pancreatic injuries. Both CT and DPL evaluate the abdomen at a single point in time, and a repeat procedure may be necessary for evolving or missed lesions.

E. Serial observation. The serial observation technique can be used for some blunt trauma and superficial stab wound patients with normal mentation.

F. Ultrasonography and laparoscopy. Abdominal ultrasound is accurate in detecting intraabdominal blood (94% to 96%) in experienced hands; it is fast, portable, and noninvasive. Laparoscopy is accurate in finding peritoneal or diaphragmatic penetration from stab wounds or tangential gunshot wounds.

III. Specific injuries

A. Spleen. The spleen is commonly injured in both blunt and penetrating trauma. Patients may have left upper quadrant pain and tenderness, left shoulder pain, lower left rib fractures, and hemodynamic instability.

Both DPL and CT scanning are accurate in finding a splenic injury. DPL should be considered in unstable patients, whereas CT scanning can identify stable patients for nonoperative management.

Asplenic patients are at increased risk for sudden and often lethal systemic bacterial infection. This syndrome termed "overwhelming postsplenectomy infection" (OPSI) is usually caused by encapsulated organisms such as *Strep-*

tococcus pneumoniae. The incidence of OPSI is 1% after splenectomy, with a greater risk in the pediatric age group. Therefore, nonoperative management, which is used in well over half of the splenic injuries seen is preferred. It has a 95% success rate. The success rate is higher in children because of a thickened splenic capsule. Hemodynamically stable children and adults with nonhemorrhaging spleens and no evidence of other injuries needing laparotomy can be observed closely. The incidence of delayed rupture is higher in older patients. Angiography with embolization can be considered for stable patients with extravasation of dye.

Patients undergoing nonoperative management should be closely monitored, usually in an intensive care unit (ICU) for 48 to 72 hours, with serial hematocrits and abdominal examination. Progressive healing occurs over 6 weeks.

For patients who do have a splenectomy, pneumococcal vaccination is given to them after splenectomy and prior to discharge or 2 weeks postoperatively. Long-term prophylactic antibiotics may be effective in preventing OPSI in children.

B. Liver and porta hepatis. The liver is the most commonly injured organ in abdominal trauma. The mortality rate is 11% from exsanguination or associated head injury. Classification of injury is from I to V, going from minor tears to major lobar disruptions and avulsion from the inferior vena cava. Early deaths are from hemorrhage and late deaths from intraabdominal sepsis and multiorgan failure.

Nonoperative management of liver trauma in hemodynamically stable patients is indicated in blunt trauma patients in whom the CT scan does not show active bleeding and no other injuries requiring surgery. Angiography with embolization can be used to stop arterial hemorrhage. The patients should be watched closely for 48 to 72 hours. Operative therapy should proceed for patients who are hemodynamically unstable, develop peritonitis, or require continuous blood transfusions. Complications of liver injury include bleeding, both early and late (traumatic hemobilia); bile leakage; and intraabdominal infection. Traumatic hemobilia results from erosion of an injured blood vessel into a biliary duct. The triad of right upper quadrant abdominal pain, jaundice, and gastrointestinal hemorrhage occur in only one third of these patients. Control of hemobilia is by selective embolization.

Bile leakage occurs in 25% of patients with major hepatic injuries. Symptoms are hyperbilirubinemia and signs of infection. Treatment is with closed drainage at surgery or CT scanning with guided percutaneous drainage. These biliary fistula usually close spontaneously in 2 to 3 weeks in the absence of distal obstruction. Hemobilia, an arterial biliary fistula, is a rare but deadly complication of hepatic trauma. *Abscesses* occur in 10% of patients with liver injuries. The likelihood of infection increases with the grade of liver injury, number of transfusions, use of sump drains, concomitant bowel injury, and perihepatic packing. Aggressive diagnosis and drainage, either CT scan-guided or by exploration, is imperative to decrease mortality.

Traumatic injuries to the porta hepatis are uncommon; they are mostly found with penetrating trauma and have a 50% mortality rate from hemorrhage. Injuries to the gall bladder are treated with cholecystectomy. Injuries to the extrahepatic ducts require primary repair or bowel anastomosis.

C. Small intestine. The small intestine is the most commonly injured organ in penetrating abdominal trauma. Diagnosis of small bowel injury in blunt trauma is difficult, and physical findings may be delayed until the patient is septic. Patients with abdominal wall bruising, especially from a seat belt, should arouse suspicion. Patients with lumbar chance fractures also have a high degree of small bowel (as well as pancreatic and duodenal) injuries. DPL is diagnostic in approximately 95% of patients with intestinal injury. Findings on CT scan of small bowel injury include free air, free fluid without a solid organ injury, and, to a lesser degree, thickened bowel wall and mesenteric hematoma. CT can miss a small bowel injury and close follow-up is warranted. Peritonitis on physical examination warrants exploration.

D. Duodenum. Duodenal injuries are uncommon but have a high (17%) mortality rate. Most are caused by penetrating trauma; the more complex the injury, the greater (10 times) the mortality rate. Early death is from exsanguination from surrounding vessels, and late death is from sepsis. Delay in diagnosis, which increases the rate of sepsis, occurs 30% of the time. Perforation is often retroperitoneal, with a delay in physical findings. DPL can be unreliable and the subtle signs on CT scan of retroperitoneal air or extravasation of contrast can be missed. Upper gastrointestinal contrast studies (UGI) may be useful.

A duodenal intramural hematoma,a rare injury from blunt trauma, is more common in children. It manifests as a partial or complete obstruction of the duodenum. Diagnosis is by UGI. Treatment is nasogastric suction and parental nutrition until the hematoma absorbs and the obstruction is relieved.

E. Pancreas. Pancreatic injuries are also unusual; they are associated with hemorrhage and are more common in penetrating trauma. The delayed mortality and morbidity rates are high, especially if extensive damage has occurred, if the pancreatic duct is involved, and if the duodenum is also involved (21% of the time).

The diagnosis of pancreatic trauma is done at the time of surgery or in the setting of blunt trauma, by CT scan. Hyperamylasemia is absent in 30% of blunt pancreatic injury, and is nonspecific when it is present. Because a CT scan can miss some pancreatic injuries, close surveillance is necessary.

F. Colon and rectum. Colon injuries, common in penetrating trauma, are diagnosed at laparotomy. Knife wounds to the flank can injure the colon; these can be found at laparotomy or with CT scanning with oral and colonic contrast. Blunt injuries to the colon are rare and as with small bowel injuries can be missed by CT scan and DPL. The rectum may be injured with pelvic fractures, pelvic gunshot wounds, and perineal trauma. Any suspicion of rectal injury warrants proctosigmoidoscopy to avoid a missed injury and pelvic sepsis.

G. Genitourinary. Blunt trauma accounts for 80% of renal injuries. Gross or marked microscopic hematuria warrants further evaluation with an abdominal CT scan. CT scan also enables diagnose of renal trauma with penetrating flank wounds. Many blunt renal injuries can be observed unless a renal pedicle injury has occurred with ongoing hemorrhage or thrombosis. Most penetrating renal injuries are explored. A one-shot, intravenous pyelogram to define the noninjured kidney function should be attempted prior to exploring a renal hematoma.

Postoperative renal failure can be associated with renal trauma but is more likely related to the severity and length of shock. Complications of renal trauma include delayed hemorrhage, abscess, and urinoma. Adequate drainage is used to treat the latter two complication. Urinary leak should be suspected with azotemia and a normal glomerular filtration rate.

The bladder is the most frequently injured organ in patients with pelvic fractures. Most patients with bladder injuries have gross hematuria. Retrograde cystogram is required for diagnosis. Extraperitoneal injuries need catheter drainage only because up to 80% close within 10 days. Intraperitoneal ruptures need surgical repair. Ureteral injuries are rare and occur in penetrating trauma.

The urethra can also be injured in pelvic fractures. It is mainly a risk in male patients. Physical signs are blood at the meatus, scrotal hematoma, and a high riding prostate on rectal examination, although these may be absent. Injuries are diagnosed by retrograde urethrogram prior to insertion of urinary catheter. Treatment is delayed repair and suprapubic drainage of the bladder.

Vaginal tears can occur with penetrating trauma and pelvic fracture. They need to be identified to avoid major infections. Injuries to male genitalia should be debrided conservatively and repaired.

The uterus is rarely injured unless the patient is pregnant. Pregnant patients need to be evaluated by obstetric ultrasound to look for fetal viability, placenta abruptio, and uterine injuries. A vaginal examination should also be done to check for blood. Patients with viable pregnancies should be watched with uterine or fetal monitoring for several hours once all other injuries are identified.

H. Major vascular injuries. Early death from abdominal injuries is from hemorrhage. Injuries to the abdominal aorta and its major branches, the inferior vena cava, the root of the mesentery, and large parenchymal disruptions require expedient exploration. The patient in shock from abdominal hemorrhage needs immediate control of the hemorrhage, control of contamination from hollow viscous injuries, ongoing resuscitation, and rewarming. Vascular repair should only be done for organ viability in this situation. The abdomen should then be packed and the skin quickly closed. The patient is taken to the ICU for resuscitation, rewarming and correction of coagulapathy. This is called *damage control.* The patient can be returned to the operating room for definitive repair once resuscitation is complete.

Patients such as these can develop abdominal compartment syndrome after fascial closure, or even with just skin closure. Symptoms include a distended, tense abdomen with decreasing urine output and increasing airway pressures. Diagnosis can be suggested by increasing peak airway pressures and made by an elevated (>30 ml H_2O) bladder pressure. Decompression is necessary for organ viability.

I. Pelvic fractures. Pelvic fracture is the third most common injury in motor vehicle crash fatalities, and open pelvic fractures carry a 50% mortality rate. Hemorrhage is the leading cause of death, and sepsis the leading cause of delayed death. Pelvic fractures are identified by instability on physical examination and by x-ray study. Evaluation for bladder, rectal, and urethral injuries may be necessary.

High-grade injuries require aggressive resuscitation, early control of hemorrhage, and massive transfusion. Hemorrhage from unstable fractures can be slowed by application of an external fixator. Continued hemorrhage may be amenable to embolization via angiography. Concurrent abdominal hemorrhage needs to be ruled out early with a supraumbilical DPL or a CT scan if the patient is hemodynamically stable.

Patients with major pelvic fractures need management in the ICU, often with central monitoring. Up to 15% of these patients can develop acute respiratory distress syndrome secondary to shock and other injuries. Prophylaxis for deep venous thrombosis is essential. Once hemorrhage is controlled, subcutaneous aqueous or low molecular weight heparin should be started. Placement of an inferior vena caval filter should be considered in patients with very severe pelvic fractures or those associated with other lower extremity fractures.

Suggested Readings

Asensio JA, Feliciano DV, Britt LD, et al. Management of duodenal injuries. *Curr Probl Surg* 1993;11:1021.

A good review.

Burch JM, Martin R, Richardson RJ, et al. Evolution of the treatment of the injured colon in the 1980s. *Arch Surg* 1991;126:97.

A good review.

Burgess AR, Eastridge BJ, Young JWR, et al. Pelvic ring disruptions: effective classification system and treatment protocols. *J Trauma* 1990;30:848.

Excellent classification of pelvic fractures.

Henneman PL, Marx JA, Moore EE, et al. Diagnostic peritoneal lavage: accuracy in predicting necessary laparotomy following blunt and penetrating trauma. *J Trauma* 1990;30:1345.

A good reference on diagnostic peritoneal lavage.

Holdsworth RJ, Irving AD, Cuschieri A. Postsplenectomy sepsis and its mortality rate: actual versus perceived risks. *Br J Surg* 1991;78:1031.

An informative report on postsplenectomy sepsis and its mortality rate.

Husmann DA, Morris JS. Attempted nonoperative management of blunt renal lacerations extending through the corticomedullary junction: the short-term and long-term sequelae. *J Urol* 1990;143:682.

A good lead paper on nonoperative management.

McKenney MG, Martin L, Lentz K, et al. 1,000 consecutive ultrasounds for blunt abdominal trauma. *J Trauma* 1996;40:607.

A research reference on ultrasound use in trauma.

Moore EE, Mattox KL, Feliciano DV. *Trauma.* Norwalk, CT: Appleton & Lange, 1991.

A general and statistical reference.

Mucha Jr P, Welch TJ. Hemorrhage in major pelvic fractures. *Surg Clin North Am* 1989;68:757.

A good reference on management of pelvic fracture hemorrhage.

Pachter HL, Knudson M, Esrig B, et al. Status of nonoperative management of blunt hepatic injuries in 1995: a multicenter experience with 404 patients. *J Trauma* 1996;40:31.

A discussion of the nonoperative management of blunt hepatic injuries.

Smith JS, Cooney RN, Mucha P. Nonoperative management of the ruptured spleen: a revalidation of criteria. *Surgery* 1996;120:745.

A reference on the current management of the injured spleen.

Wisner DH, Chun Y, Blaisdell FW. Blunt intestinal injury. *Arch Surg* 1990;125:1319.

A good review of blunt intestinal injury.

Wisner DM, Wold RC, Frey CF. Diagnosis and treatment of pancreatic injuries. *Arch Surg* 1990;1250:1109.

A good review of pancreatic injuries.

151. BURN MANAGEMENT

Kevin M. Dwyer and Arthur L. Trask

I. General principles. In the United States, more than 100,000 thermally injured patients are hospitalized each year and 12,000 die. The care of the burn patient has progressed; before World War II, the average burn size associated with a 50% mortality rate [median lethal dose (LD_{50})] in healthy adults was 30% total body surface area (TBSA) and now the LD_{50} ranges from 65% to 75% TBSA. The three major of causes of death in burn victims are cardiopulmonary complications, uncontrolled infection, and the development of multiple organ failure.

II. Classification of thermal injury. The three most important predictive variables of survival in thermal injury are the patient's **age,** the **size** and **depth** of the burn, and concomitant inhalation injury. Burns are classified in Table 151-1.

The most commonly used system of estimating burn size is the rule of nines, whereby each portion of the body is divided into multiples of nine. The head and neck are 9%, the anterior and posterior torso are 18% each, each thigh is 9%, each lower leg is 9%, each arm is 9%, and the perineum is 1%. This is relatively accurate for adults; however, for infants and younger children, the TBSA proportions are different as the head takes up a much larger percentage. Most burn centers use the Lund-Browder chart to determine burn percentage more accurately for all age groups. The percentage of the body that has been burned (and depth) is important to estimate how much fluid is required in resuscitation.

III. Volume resuscitation: pathophysiology and management. Thermal injury induces a metabolic stress response and causes a major fluid shift. Multiple vasoactive mediators are released, altering the permeability of the vascular endothelium with leakage of intravascular fluid into the interstitium. These vasoactive mediators include kinins, serotonin, histamine, prostaglandins, and oxygen radicals. Edema rapidly accumulates in the burn wound and also in the nonburned tissues to a lessor extent. The edema in the nonburned tissues is related to the vascular permeability and the severe hypoproteinemic state that occurs both with leakage of proteins out of the vascular space and with the hypermetabolic response. With the loss of fluid, vasoconstriction follows, and unless this fluid loss is corrected, burn shock ensues and hypoperfusion, organ failure, and death occur.

The goal of volume resuscitation is first to correct the hypoperfusion and, once corrected, to try not to overhydrate with subsequent formation of pulmonary edema, although evidence indicates that under resuscitation leads to the formation of pulmonary edema (acute respiratory distress syndrome) more than does overhydration does.

A number of different fluid resuscitation regimens are available. One popular regimen is the Parkland formula; another is the modified Brooke formula (Table 151-2). With both formulas, it is important to begin the hydration early and provide half the 24-hour total over the first 8 hours. Regardless of the regimen used, the key is to monitor the endpoints of resuscitation, namely pulse, blood pressure, urine output (0.5–1.0 ml/kg/h), and acidosis. If the endpoints are not being met, then the fluid resuscitation needs to be more aggressive. Approximately 20% of patients will be overhydrated, particularly with the Parkland formula. If the urine output is greater than 2 ml/kg/h, then the rate of infusion can be decreased by 25%. It is important to test the urine for glucose, as a glucose osmotic diuresis can mimic the output of a well-hydrated patient. Decreasing the infusion in this case may underresuscitate the patient.

Of patients, 10% or more may not respond as expected to fluid hydration; their urine output will remain low and they will continue to manifest signs of shock. These patients are typically older, have underlying medical conditions, had a delay in the initiation of resuscitation, and may have a concomitant inhalation injury. These patients may need a pulmonary arterial catheter to guide resusci-

TABLE 151-1. Burn classification

Depth	Color	Texture	Symptoms	Healing
First-degree—epidermis	Red, pink	Moist	Painful	1 week, no scar
Second-degree—upper dermis	Pink	Moist	Painful	2 weeks, no scar; superficial blisters
Deep lower dermis	Lighter		No pain	Destroyed 3 weeks, no scar or no blisters; cutaneous nerves; skin grafting
Third-degree—entire dermis	Milky white		No pain	Dry skin; grafting, tanned leather

tation. These catheters are not put in routinely because of the risk of serious infections. Because of the increasing evidence that oxidants play a role in early and late tissue damage, antioxidant use is under intense study and may be added to early resuscitation.

Both regimens switch to colloids and D_5W on the second day. The patient's vascular integrity should improve somewhat after 24 hours. The colloid is to help counterbalance to some extent the loss of protein and the oncotic pressure. The goal is a serum albumin level between 2 and 2.5 g/dl. Burn wounds have a great insensible evaporative water loss, with the accumulation of sodium in the extracellular space. After 24 hours of resuscitation, D_5W is used to balance this effect. Hydration can also proceed orally at this time.

By the third postburn day, the vascular integrity usually returns to normal and patients begin to mobilize all of the fluid they have received. Urine output is brisk. Hypokalemia must be avoided, as potassium is dumped with this diuresis and also moves from the intravascular space to the intracellular space. Hemoglobin levels should also be monitored at least biweekly as red cell survival is decreased in patients with significant burn injury. Patients with burn injuries may also be victims of traumatic injury with subsequent blood loss. The decision for blood transfusion should be based on hemodynamic and physiologic criteria and not on an absolute hemoglobin level.

IV. Smoke inhalation injury. An inhalation injury significantly increases the mortality rate of these patients, regardless of burn size. Patients with inhalation injuries may require up to 50% more fluid for adequate resuscitation.

Any patient burned in a closed space should be treated as having a smoke inhalation injury. Patients may have a burned face, singed nasal hairs, and cough up soot. Severe injuries can present with hoarseness and respiratory distress. Any patients with suspected inhalation injury need to be assessed quickly. If evi-

TABLE 151-2. Fluid resuscitation regimens

First 24 Hours	Second 24 Hours
Parkland lactated Ringers, 4 ml/kg/%/burn/24 h 50% over the first 8 h	D_5W, 2 ml/kg/%burn plus plasma, 0.3–0.5 ml/kg/%/burn
Modified Brooke lactated Ringers, 2 ml/kg/%/burn/24 h 50% over the first 8 h	D_5W, 1–2 ml/kg/%burn, plus plasma, 0.3–0.5 ml/kg/%burn

dence is seen of an inhalation injury, the patient should undergo endotracheal intubation and mechanical ventilation. Bronchoscopy can be used to diagnose inhalation injury and to see if the injury involves the lower airways. A xenon ventilation-perfusion scan can also be used to diagnose the extent of a lower respiratory injury. Healing time for patients with lower respiratory injury is longer.

Patients with inhalation injury receive humidified oxygenated air and frequent suctioning of copious secretions. Bronchodilators may be necessary. Positive end-expiratory pressure is also frequently used to maintain the patency of the alveoli. Prophylactic antibiotics are not recommended as they can select out antibiotic-resistant bacteria. Steroids are not indicated in inhalation injury; they can lead to increased mortality.

V. Escharotomy. Circumferential burns of the extremities can lead to compromise of the vascular supply once resuscitation and resultant burn edema begins. Escharotomy may be necessary early in the course of treatment for limb salvage.

VI. Metabolic and nutritional considerations. The hypermetabolic response that occurs after a thermal injury is greater than that observed after any form of trauma or sepsis. The magnitude of the response parallels the severity of the burn to a maximum of a burn size of 60%. An increase in temperature of 2°F to 3°F occurs with this response. Patients are kept in a warm environment to help decrease the total energy expenditure.

A major thermal injury is characterized by increased muscle proteolysis, lipolysis, and gluconeogenesis. Burn wounds use glucose in greatly increased quantities. Severe loss of nitrogen, which also occurs, needs to be replaced to fight the muscle wasting and to enhance the immune system. This replacement is absolutely necessary to fight infection and for wound healing. Burn patients need two to three times the basal energy expenditure.

Significant burn injuries require 2 g/kg protein. Of calories, 50% to 60% should be glucose and the calorie-to-nitrogen ratio should approach 100:1. All attempts should be made to feed the patient enterally as enteral feeding decreases the risk of infection.

VII. Infection and immunity. Patients with significant burns are a high risk of infection and this can cause late deaths. The lungs and the burn itself are the most common sites and the foci for fatal infection. Other sites of infection include central lines and Foley catheters. A strong belief exists that the intestine may be a source of unexplained bacteremia via bacterial translocation, the risk of which *may be* decreased by enteral feedings.

A. Burn wound sepsis. Burn victims develop multiple defects in their immune system that predisposes them to an increased risk of infection. This immunocompromised state combined with loss of the skin barrier in the burn wound can lead to severe burn wound infections. Topical antimicrobials (e.g., silver sulfadiazine or mafenide acetate) as well as local wound care, which help decrease the amount of burn wound infections, should be adhered to. However, they cannot eradicate burn wound sepsis.

The early signs of burn wound sepsis are diffuse or focal discoloration of the burn, purulent fluid from the wound, and too rapid eschar separation. If not treated at the earliest possible time, systemic sepsis will develop. Diagnosis is by biopsy of the wound. Systemic antibiotics are started if infection is suspected, and altered or stopped once burn biopsies and blood culture results are obtained. If burn wound sepsis is present, total excision of the infected burn is indicated. These patients usually require a tremendous amount of fluid to overcome the vasodilation and the amount of fluid lost in surgery. They also require multiple blood transfusions with surgical excisions. Most burn centers practice early excision of the eschar and grafting to prevent the occurrence of burn wound sepsis.

B. Pneumonia. Pneumonia is emerging as a frequent cause of infectious death in burn victims as the incidence of burn wound sepsis decreases. Burn victims are susceptible to pneumonia because of their immunocompromised state and their immobility and inability to clear secretions. An inhalation injury greatly increases the risk of pneumonia, as does the size of the burn. Prevention is by maintaining good pulmonary toilet. Antibiotics should not be used prophylactically in burn patients. Once strong evidence of pneumonia is seen, antibiotic therapy should be directed by the results of the Gram's stain, culture of the sputum or bronchoscopy specimen, and the local biograms.

VIII. Electrical injury. Electrical injuries are divided into high- or low-voltage injuries. Low-voltage injuries present as thermal burns with injuries to the tissue from the outside in. High-voltage injuries may present with little injury to the skin, but significant injuries to the muscle, vasculature, and bone underneath. The pattern of injury can travel through many different body areas, depending on the path of the charge.

Patients with electrical injuries must be monitored for cardiac arrythmias. They may have fracture of their spine and precautions must be followed. Fluid resuscitation must be begun quickly; frequently, these patients require a much higher volume of fluid because of underlying tissue injury. Myonecrosis will lead to myoglobinuria, which can lead to renal failure. These patients need to maintain a high urine output of 100 ml/h, and mannitol may be added once resuscitation is well underway. Early escharotomy and fasciotomy may be necessary for limb salvage. Areas of myonecrosis must be carefully looked for with imaging scans, if necessary. Necrotic muscle must be removed to avoid sepsis. Intra-abdominal injuries are not infrequent.

This chapter is based on the chapter by Deitch EA, Rutan RL, Rutan TC. Burn management. In: Irwin RS, Cerra FB, Rippe JM, eds. *Intensive care medicine* 4th ed. Philadelphia: Lippincott–Raven; 1999.

Selected Readings

Herndon DN, Curreri PW, Abston S, et al. Treatment of burns. *Curr Probl Surg* 1987; 24:341.

An excellent and credible review.

Pruitt Jr BA. Advances in fluid theory and the early care of the burn patient. *World J Surg* 1978;2:139.

A classic on the fluid management of burns.

Shirani KZ, Pruitt BA, Mason AD. The influence of inhalation injury and pneumonia on burn mortality. *Ann Surg* 1987;205:92.

This article emphasizes the importance of inhalation injury and its effects on outcome.

Wilmore DW, Aulick LH. Metabolic changes in burned patients. *Surg Clin North Am* 1978;58:1173.

Another classic reference.

152. THORACIC TRAUMA

Kevin M. Dwyer and Arthur L. Trask

I. General principles. Thoracic injury is the primary cause of death in 25% of trauma patients. Most mortality occurs within minutes of injury because of disruption of the great vessels, heart, or the tracheobronchial tree. Of the survivors, only 15% need surgical intervention, yet the cost of treating nonoperative chest injury is high. Guidelines as established by the American College of Surgeons Committee on Trauma in the Advanced Trauma Life Support course should be followed in the evaluation and resuscitation of thoracic trauma.

In the patient with chest trauma, four injury patterns in this category constitute an immediate threat to life: tension pneumothorax, massive hemothorax, open pneumothorax, and flail chest or pulmonary contusion. *Tension pneumothorax* presents with respiratory distress along with any of the following: (a) tracheal deviation away from the affected side, (b) decreased or absent breath sounds on the affected side, (c) distended neck veins and hypotension. Treatment involves immediate needle decompression in the second intercostal space, mid-clavicular line followed by tube thoracostomy.

Massive hemothorax presents similarly to a tension pneumothorax but with earlier signs of hypovolemic shock. Initial treatment involves fluid resuscitation and tube thoracostomy.

Open pneumothorax is caused by a full-thickness loss of the chest wall and creation of a sucking chest wound (air sucked into the chest during inspiration causing a pneumothorax. Early treatment is coverage of the wound and tube thoracostomy.

Flail chest or pulmonary contusion is secondary to massive chest wall injury with multiple rib fractures and underlying lung injury with impaired gas exchange. Treatment involves maintaining oxygenation and ventilation.

II. Indications for urgent surgical intervention

A. Bleeding. An immediate return of more than 1,500 ml of blood is an indication for thoracotomy. Continuing blood losses from the chest tube at a rate of more than 250 ml/h with a penetrating injury requires an urgent exploration. Continuous losses in blunt trauma that require an operation are unusual and may be more indicative of coagulopathy, hypothermia, or intraabdominal bleeding through a disrupted diaphragm.

B. Cardiovascular collapse. Loss of vital signs in the emergency department is an indication for immediate thoracotomy. Patients who undergo cardiac arrest in the field but arrive with some signs of life, agonal respiration, or cardiac activity may be candidates for emergency department thoracotomy (EDT) also. Patients with a penetrating chest injury who arrive with no vital signs benefit the most (up to 20%) with EDT. Of those patients with penetrating cardiac injuries who undergo cardiac arrest in the emergency department, EDT may save up to 50%. Minimal chance for survival with EDT is seen for patients with a blunt injury with prehospital arrest, and many authors discourage its use. EDT allows treatment of chest injuries (cardiac lacerations, pulmonary laceration, and tamponade) and aids in resuscitation with cardiac massage and aortic cross-clamping.

C. Massive air leak. Continuous flow of air through a chest tube with an inability to ventilate, oxygenate, or reexpand the lung indicates a major injury to the airways. The chest tube apparatus should be checked for leaks, and then the tube placed on water seal to minimize the leak. Smaller tidal volumes and minimal mechanical airway pressure may help. Urgent bronchoscopy, possibly selective intubation of the uninjured bronchus, and operative repair are required.

D. Tamponade. Violation of the cardiac chambers or intrapericardial great vessels can result in the accumulation of fluid in the pericardial sac, and quickly lead to tamponade. Cardiac tamponade obstructs cardiac outflow and decreases venous return, leading to hypotension, tachycardia, decreased pulse pressure, distended neck veins, pulses paradoxis, and equalization of pressures in the cardiac chambers. In the trauma patient with hypovolemia, these signs can vary and Beck's triad of hypotension, tachycardia, and muffled heart tones are present only one third of the time. The diagnosis is made by mechanism of injury, clinical impression, and ultrasonography, if available immediately. Patients in extremis will be diagnosed by immediate thoracotomy and they can be decompressed with pericardotomy. Patients with hypotension who are diagnosed without thoracotomy can undergo pericardiocentesis or a pericardial window to stabilize their vital signs enroute to the operating room for full exploration and injury repair.

E. Bronchovenous air embolism. Air embolism occurs when an adjacent bronchus and pulmonary vein are disrupted and air passes into the left atrium through a traumatic bronchovenous fistula. The air then impedes left ventricular filling and can move into and obstruct the coronary arteries, causing an infarction. This usually happens to a patient with a penetrating injury who is initially stable, but suffers cardiovascular collapse with intubation and positive pressure ventilation. Treatment is placement in a Trendelenberg position, immediate thoracotomy, hilar cross-clamping, and aspiration of air from the left ventricle and aortic root. Results are extremely poor.

III. Diagnostic valuation

A. Chest radiograph. An early chest x-ray study is essential for most trauma patients and for all trauma patients with chest trauma. An anterioposterior, supine film is obtained after the primary survey; an upright film can only be obtained in a stable patient with a cleared cervical spine. The chest x-ray film needs to be evaluated for pneumo- and hemothorax; pneumomediastinum; fractured ribs, vertebrae, and clavicle; endotracheal and catheter position; widening of the mediastinum (> 8 cm), and the integrity of the aortic knob and diaphragm.

B. Computed tomography (CT). Contrast CT scanning with the new helical scanners is used to evaluate the great vessels in a blunt chest injury. These new CT scans of the chest at 5-mm cuts are the screening tool of choice for detecting suspected aortic injury. In some centers, three-dimensional reconstruction of helical CT images is sufficiently accurate to replace angiography. In most centers, aortic arch angiography is still the standard for diagnosing a disruption of the thoracic aorta.

C. Ultrasound. Transthoracic ultrasound of the pericardium should be performed as part of the evaluation of the abdomen for fluid in blunt trauma. It also is effective in identifying a pericardial effusion in penetrating trauma. Transesophageal echocardiography (TEE) has been used to visualize the heart, pericardial space, and thoracic great vessels; in experienced hands, a descending aortic injury can be detected as well. Echocardiography is used to evaluate cardiac function and injury in blunt trauma.

D. Angiography. Angiography is essential for all stable patients with clinical or radiographic evidence of a major vascular injury. In addition, all patients with penetrating injuries in the thoracic outlet and the root of the neck, or with a gunshot wound that traverse the mediastinum should undergo angiography.

IV. Management of specific injuries

A. Chest wall and pleural space

1. **Rib fractures.** The number of rib fractures in adults correlates with the severity of pulmonary injury and shock. Rib fractures in children are of greater significance as their ribs are more elastic. First rib fractures are occasionally associated with injuries to the subclavian vessels and brachial plexus, particularly if lateral or posterior displacement has occurred.
2. **Flail chest.** Flail chest occurs when a blunt injury causes a portion of the chest wall to lose bony continuity with the thorax, and this portion has paradoxical inward movement on inspiration. This is usually caused by multiple fractures of a segment of ribs or of the costal cartilages on both sides with a floating sternum. This can lead to ineffective ventilation with decreased vital capacity and

atelectasis. The most important factor is the severity of the underlying pulmonary contusion. The treatment of flail chest is excellent analgesia, vigorous pulmonary toilet, and selective use of mechanical ventilation for pulmonary failure.

3. **Sternal fracture.** Most sternal fractures are caused by the chest striking the steering wheel or dash. Now, more are associated with the shoulder harness, especially in older women. The severity of the underlying injuries is related to mechanism, with more serious injuries associated with not wearing the shoulder belt.
4. **Scapular fracture and scapulothoracic dissociation.** The scapula is a strong bone that is well protected by muscle. It takes tremendous force to break it and the likelihood of other injuries, mostly head and chest wall is high. Scapulothoracic dislocation occurs when the muscular and neurovascular structures of the arm and shoulder are torn from the chest wall. Perfusion must be restored, although neurologic function rarely returns.
5. **Traumatic asphyxia.** Protracted crush injuries of the chest and upper abdomen result in asphyxia syndrome presenting with cyanosis, petechial hemorrhages, and edema of the head, neck and chest, and conjunctivae. It is thought to be caused by severe venous hypertension secondary to compression of the superior vena cava. Neurologic symptoms such as disorientation, visual disturbances, and seizures frequently occur.
6. **Pnemothorax.** Air in the pleural space usually comes from alveolar rupture or a lacerated lung from shear or a fractured rib. Bronchial ruptures and open wounds also lead to a pneumothorax. Treatment is with a large chest tube (36–40 Fr). A pneumothorax seen only on CT scan can be watched if not mechanically ventilated.
7. **Tension pneumothorax.** A pneumothorax that is caused by a one-way leak of air rapidly expands into a tension pneumothorax. Patients who receive positive pressure ventilation are at higher risk. The air causes the lung to collapse and the mediastinum to shift with loss of cardiac output. Clinical signs are as previously mentioned and the treatment is immediate needle decompression and tube thoracostomy.
8. **Open pneumothorax.** As discussed, a chest wall defect can result in a sucking chest wound, with accumulation of intrapleural air under tension. A petrolatum gauze dressing with one side open to allow air egress, followed by a tube thoracostomy is the treatment of choice. Operative repair can be done later.
9. **Hemothorax.** Blood in the pleural cavity from blunt trauma is usually from rib fractures, chest wall bleeding, or small lung operations. Massive hemothorax (> 1,500 ml) from blunt trauma usually presents in cardiovascular collapse. Penetrating chest injuries with severe hemorrhage more likely will require surgery. Drainage of a hemothorax is necessary to avoid a trapped space and non-reexpansion of the lung.

B. Lung

1. **Contusion.** Pulmonary contusion results from direct force on the lung from a blow to the chest wall or by a missile effect. It is characterized by intraalveolar edema and hemorrhage with consolidation. The affect of ineffective gas exchange reaches its peak between 18 and 36 hours, and may require mechanical ventilation. The appearance on chest x-ray film also lags behind the clinical course. Patients generally improve in 72 hours unless pneumonia or acute respiratory distress syndrome (ARDS) follows. The treatment for flail chest also applies here as well as trying to avoid excessive fluid infusion, if possible. A severe unilateral contusion may require one lung ventilation.
2. **Laceration.** Lung laceration present with a hemopneumothorax. Tube toracostomy will reexpand the lung and most lacerations will seal. Persistent major air leaks and bleeding may require surgery and resection.
3. **Acute respiratory distress syndrome.** ARDS, as a consequence of trauma, can occur with or without fat embolism. Fat embolism is characterized by diffuse pulmonary infiltrates, neurologic dysfunction, and petechial rash occur-

ring 24 to 72 hours after long bone fracture or its manipulation. The diagnosis is made by criteria as other tests such as fat globules in the blood, urine or bronchoalveolar lavage are sensitive or specific. Treatment is supportive as for any severe case of ARDS.

C. Trachea and major bronchi. Patients with cough, hemoptysis, and cervical emphysema after a penetrating chest wound may have an intrathoracic tracheal injury. It is rare for this injury to occur with a blunt blow to the upper chest. Orotracheal intubation should be expedient, and preparation for a surgical airway should commence if endotracheal intubation is unsuccessful. Bronchoscopy should performed early in the management.

Symptoms of major bronchial injuries have been described, and associated great vessel and cardiac injuries are frequent in penetrating trauma. Blunt disruptions, which are caused by shearing forces, are usually within 2 cm of the carina. Early bronchoscopy followed by surgical repair is indicated.

D. Heart

1. **Blunt cardiac injury.** Contusion of the myocardium results from direct compression of the heart by blunt trauma to the chest wall. The true incidence is unknown, and the measurement of creatine kinase isoforms and echocardiography add little to the clinical course. Outside of a very few patients who present with cardiac failure, the most important complication is arrhythmia, which usually occurs in the first 24 hours. Patients with a normal initial electrocardiogram (ECG) do not manifest arrhythmia. Therefore, only patients who have an abnormal ECG need to be monitored—usually for just 24 hours. Echocardiography and other studies should be reserved for patients with heart failure, new valvular incompetence, or suspected pretraumatic myocardial infarction.

   Blunt cardiac rupture is rarely seen as most patients hemorrhage rapidly. Some who make to the hospital usually present with cardiac tamponade with rupture of a low pressure chamber (right atrium 50%).

   Blunt valvular injuries, which are rare, usually occur in the aortic, mitral, or tricuspid valve.

2. **Penetrating cardiac injury.** Penetrating injuries to the heart are usually from an anterior wound in an area bounded by the clavicles, the midclavicular lines, and the upper abdomen. The heart can be reached from the neck, axilla, and back. Knife wounds can present with tamponade because of the smaller hole, whereas gun shot wounds usually present in arrest from exsanguination. Transthoracic ultrasound is warranted with a suspected cardiac injury. A pericardial effusion needs further evaluation with a pericardial window. When diagnosed by EDT, the tamponade can be relieved and the wound secured for repair in the operating room.

E. Great vessels. Disruption of the thoracic aorta is the second leading cause of death from blunt trauma. It is caused by rapid deceleration that triggers shearing forces at fixed points in the aorta. The most common site of rupture is just distal to the origin of the left subclavian artery at the ligamentum arteriosum. Of these patients, 70% to 85% die immediately. Those that survive have the aorta's adventia intact as a contained rupture; 40% of these patients may free rupture in 24 hours. An aortic tear is suggested from the mechanism of injury, severity of chest trauma, and findings on chest x-ray film. Of those, 85% with aortic rupture will have a widened medastinum; an indistinct aortic knob is also a suspicious finding. Other findings include an apical cap, left pleural effusion, rightward displacement of the trachea and the esophagus, loss of aortopulmonary window, and displacement down of the left mainstem bronchus; 2% will have a normal chest x-ray finding. Further screening for stable patients is by helical CT scan and no evidence of vessel injury or periaortic blood excludes aortic rupture. Angiography is still the standard for diagnosis. Patients with disruption should be placed on beta-blockers and the wound repaired.

Injuries to the branches of the arch of the aorta are unusual; more than 90% are caused by penetrating injuries. Symptoms of injuries include exsanguinating hemorrhage, loss of pulse in an upper extremity, base of the neck hematoma, symptoms of a stroke, or decreased consciousness without a head injury. Mediastinal hematomas on chest x-ray film also demand evaluation. Angiography is the procedure of choice for patients not hemorrhaging. Operative repair is for wall rupture, while dissection may be treated with heparinization.

1. **Diaphragm.** Injuries to the diaphragm can be easily missed and the mortality rate of strangulation of delayed visceral herniation is 20%; 50% are missed on initial radiographic evaluation. Most of the injuries are caused by penetrating trauma, and with any suspicion that a penetrating wound may have caused the injury, the diaphragm should be further evaluated with diagnostic peritoneal lavage, a contrast gastrointestinal study, laparoscopy, or laparotomy. Blunt injuries to the diaphragm, which are unusual, are usually large rents; 80% are associated with other severe injuries and many are discovered on exploration of the abdomen.
2. **Esophagus.** Esophageal injuries almost always result from penetrating trauma. They must be sought early as delay leads to overwhelming mediastinal sepsis, and cannot be primarily repaired. Evaluation is by endoscopy, followed by a contrast esophagography, if not seen on endoscopy. Blunt injuries are very rare, usually in the distal esophagus, and are associated with subcutaneous and mediastinal air.

F. Critical care. Antibiotics are used in the treatment of suspected esophageal injuries, pneumonia, empyema, and thoracoabdominal injuries. Controversy surrounds the use of prophylactic antibiotics. A meta-analysis supports the use of prophylactic antibiotics for tube thoracostomy for the short term in penetrating trauma.

Pain control is essential to avoid pulmonary failure and increased mortality and morbidity. Although intravenous narcotics can be effective, their depressant effect can further retard ventilation and pulmonary toilet. Regional anesthesia with an epidural catheter, intercostal blocks, or extrapleural instillation is essential, especially for patients with multiple fractures, advanced age, or underlying pulmonary disease.

G. Late sequelae of thoracic injury. Initial failure to drain the pleural space after chest trauma occurs in 15% of all patients with hemothorax. Retained blood clots become difficult to drain, and can progress to an empyema. If not drained after two attempts with tube thoacostomy, drainage via the video-assisted thorascopic surgery is effective. Empyema complicates up to 3% to 5% of admissions for chest trauma. A retained hemothorax is the greatest risk factor, and diaphragm rupture is another. Diagnosis may require CT scanning. Tube thoracostomy is the treatment with thoracotomy for patients who remain systemically ill and need better drainage.

Injury to the thoracic duct will lead to a chylothorax. Therapy is with tube thoracostomy and either parental or medium chain triglyceride enteral feeding to decrease lymphatic flow. If the leak does not seal in 2 to 3 weeks, surgical ligation may be necessary.

1. **Tracheoesophageal fistula (TEF)** results either from a dehiscence of an airway-digestive tract repair or from a missed disruption of the distal membranous trachea that erodes into the esophagus. The patient usually coughs with swallowing, and the diagnosis is by esophagogram or endoscopy. Treatment is surgical.
2. **Tracheoinnominate fistula (TIF)** occurs with the erosion of a tracheostomy tube through the trachea into the innominate artery. Patients usually exsanguinate into their lungs. The use of new low-pressure cuff tracheostomy tubes has greatly reduced the incidence of this complication.

Selected Readings

Baumgartner F, Sheppard B, de Virgilio C, et al. Tracheal and main bronchial disruptions after blunt chest trauma: presentation and management. *Ann Thorac Surg* 1990;50:569.

Cachecho R, Grindlinger GA, Lee VW. The clinical significance of myocardial contusion. *J Trauma* 1992;33:68.

Committee on Trauma. *Advanced trauma life support program for physicians.* Chicago: American College of Surgeons; 1997.

Fabian TC, Richardson JD, Croce MA, et al. Prospective study of blunt aortic injury: multicenter trial of the American Association for the Surgery of Trauma. *J Trauma* 1997;42:374.

Fallon WF, Wears RL. Prophylactic antibiotics for the prevention of infectious complications including empyema following tube thoracostomy for trauma: results of meta-analysis. *J Trauma* 1992;33:110.

Kshettry VR, Bolmon RMI. Chest trauma: assessment, diagnosis, and management. *Clin Chest Med* 1994;15:137.

Mackersie RC, Karagianes TG, Hoyt DB, et al. Prospective evaluation of epidural and intravenous administration of fentanyl for pain control and restoration of ventilatory function following multiple rib fractures. *J Trauma* 1991;31:443.

Mattox KL. Indications for thoracotomy: deciding to operate. *Surg Clin North Am* 1989;69:47.

Mattox KL, Wall MJ, Pickard LR. Thoracic trauma: general considerations and indications for thoracotomy. In: Feliciano DV, Moore EE, Mattox KL, eds. *Trauma.* Stamford, CT: Appleton & Lange; 1996:345.

Miller W, Bennett EVJ, Root HD, et al. Management of penetrating and blunt diaphragmatic injury. *J Trauma* 1984;24:403.

Mirvis SE, Shanmuganathan K, Miller BH, et al. Traumatic aortic injury: diagnosis with contrast-enhanced CT—five-year experience at a major trauma center. *Radiology* 1996;200:413.

Pate JW. Tracheobronchial and esophageal injuries. *Surg Clin North Am* 1989;69:111.

Ziegler DW, Agarwal NN. The morbidity and mortality of rib fractures. *J Trauma* 1994;37:975.

153. COMPARTMENT SYNDROMES

Kevin M. Dwyer and Arthur L. Trask

I. Definition. The muscles of the extremities are divided into compartments, each having its own nerve and blood supply, which are delineated by a tough layer of noncompliant fascia. A compartment syndrome occurs when increased interstitial pressure within a myofascial compartment compromises capillary perfusion and, hence, neuromuscular function. Compartment syndromes almost always result from an increase in the volume of the muscle as a result of edema caused by mechanical or ischemic injury. Compartment syndromes can be chronic or acute, but only the acute syndrome is limb- and, occasionally, life-threatening.

II. Pathophysiology. The common mechanism of clinical events that cause compartment syndrome is the elevation of pressure leading to impaired tissue perfusion. This is usually caused by interstitial edema fluid, although bleeding can cause it as well.

III. Clinical presentation. Although compartment syndromes can occur in the buttock, thigh, foot, forearm, and hand, they occur mostly in the leg. This is because the muscle bulk is large in the leg and its fascial compartments are relatively small and noncompliant. Most compartment syndromes occur as the result of long bone fractures, muscle contusion, or the reestablishment of perfusion after acute ischemia. Crush injuries, common in earthquakes and explosions, are frequently associated with compartment syndromes. Compartment syndromes can be iatrogenic (e.g., a cast applied too tightly). Other predisposing factors in the critical care setting can contribute to the development of compartment syndromes. These include malignant hyperthermia, neuroleptic seizures, tetany, or profound shock with massive edema.

IV. Diagnosis. The key findings of compartment syndrome in the alert patient are pain, tenderness, hypoesthesia, weakness, and tenseness. The pain is severe, worsens, and is out of proportion to what is expected for the condition. Pain is induced or exacerbated by passive stretch of the muscles in that compartment. Hypoesthesia is secondary to compression of the sensory nerve in that compartment. The muscle strength gets weaker and finally the compartment is tense and tender on palpation. The diagnosis is much more difficult in sedated, obtunded, or unconscious patients. The loss of a pulse or capillary refill occurs late in compartment syndrome and is indicative of extensive neuromuscular damage. Therefore, an objective test is used to measure compartment pressure to confirm it in the obtunded patient in the right clinical setting. This can be done by nerve conduction studies, which are accurate but require highly trained individuals, and false–positive results are seen in those patients with primary nerve injuries. Direct measurement of compartment pressures is the most practical and widely used objective test to document the presence of a compartment syndrome. The fastest and easiest measurement method is using a strain gauge transducer–amplifier attached to a monitor. All four leg compartments should be assessed quickly and repeatedly.

Disagreement exists to what is the pressure above which compartment syndrome is present. Most agree that compartment pressures below 30 mm Hg are within normal limits; between 30 and 60 mm Hg they are of concern; and above 60 mm Hg they are always associated with neuromuscular death. What is most important is a decision based on the clinical information and the natural progression of the disease process. A compartment pressure of 35 mm Hg in a delayed revascularization of the leg will only increase and demands fasciotomy. An asymptomatic patient 48 hours after injury with the same pressure may not need fasciotomy, only close follow-up.

V. Management. It is critical that the developing compartment syndrome be recognized early, because neuromuscular dysfunction is fully reversible when promptly treated. Once compartment syndrome is recognized, fasciotomy should be performed immediately. Permanent damage to nerves and muscles occurs in 6 to 12 hours. Of amputations done after trauma, 75% were associated with a delay in performing fasciotomy or an inadequate fasciotomy. Preoperatively, all constrictive dressings to the leg should be removed; the leg should not be elevated as elevation can worsen arterial inflow.

The surgical fasciotomy should remove all the potentially constricting layers of soft tissue around the swollen muscle groups to relieve compartmental hypertension, assure that arterial perfusion is adequate, and debride all obviously necrotic muscle. The fascia is the most constricting layer, and a complete incision of the fascia is the most important step. A complete incision of the skin may also be necessary, as the skin may be constricting as well.

The most generally accepted technique uses a medial calf incision to decompress the superficial and deep posterior compartments and a lateral incision to decompress the anterior and lateral compartments. This technique allows all the compartments to be fully inspected for dead muscle. When acute arterial insufficiency and compartment syndrome coexist, fasciotomy should be done first, as the delay for a lengthy arterial anastomosis can lead to irreversible myonecrosis. If, after a fasciotomy, the patient develops the metabolic sequelae of massive myonecrosis (metabolic acidosis, hyperkalemia, and myglobinuria), immediate amputation may be lifesaving.

After fasciotomy, the wounds should be left open and covered with moist, sterile dressings. The leg is elevated and passive range of motion begun. Wounds usually can be closed in a week, either primarily or with split-thickness skin graft.

VI. Complications. Complications of a neglected compartment syndrome include ischemic neuropathy, myonecrosis, and fibrosis resulting in contractures. Permanent loss of function can occur, and persistent pain, weakness, and parasthesias can lead to late amputation. Severe shock can occur with the reperfusion of dead or severely compromised muscle as mentioned. Myoglobinemia peaks 3 hours after circulation is restored and, combined with the hypoperfusion of shock, is the leading cause of renal failure. The release of large amounts of intracellular potassium can lead to arrhythmias and cardiac arrest. Laboratory findings consistent with rhabdomyolysis are hyperkalemia, hyperphosphatemia, metabolic acidosis, and a markedly elevated creatine kinase level. Myoglobin in the serum and the urine can be measured, although the results usually take time. Tea-colored urine is characteristic of myoglobinuria, although treatment should be initiated well before this sign.

Aggressive intravascular volume resuscitation is the mainstay of rhabdomyolysis treatment. Effective urine flow of 100 ml/h is established by volume loading plus mannitol and alkalizing the urine to 6.5 (to prevent precipitation of myoglobin) with a cautious infusion of sodium bicarbonate. Symptomatic hyperkalemia needs to be treated with intravenous injection of calcium, glucose, insulin, and sodium bicarbonate, supplemented with the use of exchange resins and dialysis, as necessary. Amputation of the offending extremity may be lifesaving if symptoms are severe and persistent. These patients need to be supported by dialysis and most patients avoid renal failure if the compartment syndrome is aggressively managed in the acute setting.

Selected Readings

Hyde GL, Peck D, Powell DC. Compartment syndromes. Early diagnosis and a bedside operation. *Am Surg* 1983;49:563.
An excellent review article.

Mubarak SJ, Owen CA, Hargens AR, et al. Acute compartment syndromes: diagnosis and treatment with the aid of the wick catheter. *J Bone Joint Surg Am* 1978;60:1091.
This reference is still of value today.

Perry MO. Compartment syndromes and reperfusion injury. *Surg Clin North Am* 1988;68:853.
A valuable review of this subject.

Santangelo ML, Usberti M, Di Salvo E, et al. A study of the pathology of the crush syndrome. *Surg Gynecol Obstet* 1982;154:372.
This article provides a lucid review of the effects of crush.

154. SEPSIS

Paul E. Marik and Joseph Varon

I. General principles and definitions. In recent decades, the reported incidence of sepsis in the United States has increased dramatically, with an estimated 500,000 new episodes of sepsis each year. Despite the use of antimicrobial agents and advanced life supportive care, the mortality rate of the patients with sepsis has remained consistently between 30% and 40% over the last two decades. A wide variety of definitions have been applied to sepsis, including sepsis syndrome, severe sepsis, septicemia, and septic shock. In 1991, the American College of Chest Physicians and Society of Critical Care Medicine developed a new set of terms and definitions to define sepsis in a more precise manner. The term "systemic inflammatory response syndrome" (SIRS) was coined to describe the systemic response to a wide variety of insults. It is characterized by two or more of the following clinical manifestations: (a) a body temperature of more than 38°C or less than 36°C; (b) a heart rate of more than 90 beats/min; (c) tachypnea, as manifested by a respiratory rate of more than 20 breaths/min; (d) an alteration of the white blood cell count of greater than 12,000 cells/mm^3, less than 4,000 cells/mm^3, or the presence of greater than 10% immature neutrophils.

When the systemic inflammatory response syndrome is the result of a confirmed infectious process, it is termed "sepsis." Severe sepsis is defined as sepsis plus either organ dysfunction or evidence of hypoperfusion or hypotension.

Septic shock, a subset of severe sepsis, is defined as sepsis-induced hypotension, persisting despite adequate fluid resuscitation, along with the presence of hypoperfusion abnormalities or organ dysfunction.

II. Pathogenesis and clinical features of sepsis. The clinical manifestations of sepsis are the result of an excessive host response to infectious agents, uncontrolled by natural inhibitors. The initial phase of sepsis is characterized by the production of proinflammatory humoral mediators, which include the cytokine network, as well as the complement, coagulation, and fibrinolytic systems. In addition, neutrophils, mononuclear cells, endothelial cells, and other cells of the host defense system are activated. Tumor necrosis factor-α (TNF-α) is the first proinflammatory cytokine that is released, followed by interleukin-1 (IL-1), interleukin-6 (IL-6), and interleukin-8 (IL-8). TNF-α and IL-1 are the most important proinflammatory cytokines; they are biologically closely related, act synergistically, and are largely responsible for the development of the systemic inflammatory response and secondary tissue damage in patients with sepsis.

Sepsis results in a decrease in systemic vascular resistance and generalized blood flow maldistribution. The effective intravascular volume is reduced, which is a major factor leading to circulatory instability. Multiple factors are responsible for the decreased intravascular volume, including an increase in venous capacitance and venous pooling, a generalized increase in microvascular permeability, increased insensible losses, and poor fluid intake. In more than 90% of patients who have been aggressively "volume loaded" to assure the absence of hypovolemia, cardiac output is normal or elevated. Despite the high cardiac output, clinical and experimental studies have demonstrated that sepsis is characterized by biventricular systolic dysfunction (depressed ejection fraction) and diastolic dysfunction (altered chamber compliance). The cardiac output and indices of ventricular function normalize as patients recover from the septic insult, whereas ventricular function remains depressed (despite inotropic agents) in the nonsurvivors.

The initial symptoms of sepsis are nonspecific and include malaise, tachycardia, tachypnea, fever, and sometimes hypothermia. Although most patients with sepsis have an elevated white blood cell count, some patients present with a low white blood cell count, which generally is a poor prognostic sign. Other clinical manifestations include altered mental status, hypotension, respiratory alkalosis, metabolic acidosis, hypoxemia with acute lung injury, thrombocytopenia, consumptive coagulopathy, proteinuria, acute tubular necrosis, intrahepatic cholestasis, elevated transaminases, hyperglycemia, and hypoglycemia. The manifestations of sepsis can sometimes be subtle, particularly in patients who are very young, elderly, or with chronic debilitating or immunosuppressing conditions. These patients may present with normothermia or hypothermia. An altered mental state or an otherwise unexplained respiratory alkalosis may be the presenting feature of sepsis. The most common primary focus of infection and the spectrum of implicated pathogens in patients with sepsis are listed in Tables 154-1 and 154-2.

III. Management. The management of patients with severe sepsis is based largely on treating or eliminating the source of infection and using appropriate antimicrobial agents and hemodynamic and other physiologic supportive measures. The choice of antibiotics is largely determined by the source or focus of infection, the patient's immunologic status, and whether the infection is nosocomial or community-acquired. (See Chapter 111 for choice of antimicrobial agents). Although antimicrobial therapy should be targeted against specific microorganisms, in most cases, empiric therapy is started as soon as the diagnosis of sepsis is suggested. Initial empiric management often requires more than one antibiotic to cover the most likely potential pathogens. Once a pathogen is isolated, monotherapy is adequate for most infections. The indications for double antimicrobial therapy include, suspected or proved *Pseudomonas aeruginosa* infections, enterococcal infections, the treatment of febrile-neutropenic patients, and severe intraabdominal infections. In patients with culture-negative sepsis, continuation of the initial empiric combination is warranted. Additional antibiotics or a change in antibiotics may be required in the patients with culture-negative sepsis who do not appear to be responding to the initial empiric regimen.

The primary aim of the initial phase of resuscitation is to achieve an adequate perfusion pressure; a mean arterial pressure of 70 to 80 mm Hg is recommended. Few data suggest that increasing cardiac output to achieve "supra-normal" levels of oxygen delivery improves the outcome of patients with sepsis; indeed, this approach may be harmful. Aggressive volume resuscitation is considered the best initial therapy for the cardiovascular instability of sepsis. Fluid requirements for the initial resuscitation of patients with septic shock are frequently large, with up to 10 L of crystalloid or 4 L of colloid being required in the first 24 hours. The choice of crystalloid or colloid (or both) for resuscitation of septic patients remains controversial.

Those patients who remain hypotensive or display evidence of end-organ dysfunction despite adequate fluid resuscitation are likely to benefit from the use of vasoactive agents. Although the benefit of pulmonary artery catheterization in this setting remains unproved, this procedure allows for the rational titration of fluid and vasoactive drug therapy. Dopamine has traditionally been the vasoactive drug of choice in patients with sepsis. However, dopamine may not be the ideal drug. In sepsis, chronotropic sensitivity to β_2-adrenergic stimulation is increased and tachycardia and tachydysrhythmias can limit the use of dopamine. In addition, dopamine has been demonstrated to cause an uncompensated increase in oxygen requirements with a maldistribution of blood flow in vital tissue beds. However, the combination of dobutamine and norepinephrine has been demonstrated to increase both the cardiac output and peripheral vascular resistance and to improve indices of tissue oxygenation in patients with severe sepsis. The use of dobutamine in isolation can cause or potentiate hypotension due to β_2-mediated vasodilation, particularly in vol-

TABLE 154-1. The most common primary focus of infection in patients with sepsis

Respiratory tract	25%
Intraabdominal/pelvis	25%
Bacteremia	15%
Urinary tract	10%
Skin	5%
Intravascular catheter	5%
Unknown/other	15%

TABLE 154-2. The microbiology of sepsis in the "nonimmunocompromised" host

Categories	
Gram-negative	25%
Gram-positive	25%
Mixed gram-negative/positive	20%
Fungal (Candida) only	3%
Anaerobes	2%
Unknown	25%
Gram-negative bacteria	
Escherichia coli	25%
Klebsiella or *Citrobacter* spp	20%
Pseudomonas aeruginosa	15%
Enterobacter spp	10%
Proteus spp	5%
Other gram-negative	25%
Gram-positive bacteria	
Staphylococcus aureus	35%
Enterococcus spp	20%
Coagulase-negative staphylococcus	15%
Streptococcus pneumoniae	10%
Other gram-positive bacteria	20%

ume underresuscitated patients. Phosphodiesterase inhibitors and vasopressin can be considered for patients who respond poorly to exogenous catecholamines; however, limited data exist on the use of these agents in sepsis. Adrenal insufficiency should always be suspected in patients who fail to respond to catecholamines.

To improve the outcome of patients with sepsis, a number of adjunctive therapeutic approaches have been tested, including high-dose corticosteroids, inhibitors of prostaglandin synthesis, antiendotoxin therapy, and anticytokine therapy. To date, none of these approaches have resulted in a survival benefit for patients with sepsis.

Selected Readings

Cronin L, Cook DJ, Carlet J. Corticosteroids treatment for sepsis: a critical appraisal and meta-analysis of the literature. *Crit Care Med* 1995;23:1430.

A meta-analysis and review of the use of corticosteroids in sepsis.

Hinshaw LB. Sepsis/septic shock: participation of the microcirculation: an abbreviated review. *Crit Care Med* 1996;24:1072.

This paper reviews the microcirculatory changes in sepsis.

Imm A, Carlson RW. Fluid resuscitation in circulatory shock. *Crit Care Clin* 1993;9:313.

An excellent review on fluid resuscitation.

Lynn WA, Cohen J. Adjunctive therapy for septic shock: a review of experimental approaches. *Clin Infect Dis* 1995;20:143.

An excellent review of the adjunctive and novel agents that have been used to treat sepsis.

Marik PE, Varon J. The hemodynamic derangements in sepsis: implications for treatment strategies. *Chest* 1998;114:854.

This paper reviews the cardiovascular changes and oxygen metabolism in sepsis.

Parrillo JE, Parker MM, Natanson C. Septic shock in humans: advances in understanding of pathogenesis, cardiovascular dysfunction and therapy. *Ann Intern Med* 1990;113:227.

An excellent review of the pathophysiologic changes in sepsis, with particular reference to the cardiovascular system.

Rudis MI, Basha MA, Zarowitz BJ. Is it time to reposition vasopressors and inotropes in sepsis? *Crit Care Med* 1996;24:525.

An overview of the role of vasoactive drugs in sepsis.

155. MULTIPLE ORGAN DYSFUNCTION SYNDROME

Joseph Varon and Paul E. Marik

I. General principles and definitions. With the widespread use of advanced technology for organ support, patients rarely die from their presenting disease but rather from its pathophysiologic consequences, namely, the sequential dysfunction and failure of several organ systems. This syndrome has been called "multi-organ dysfunction syndrome" (MODS). MODS has been defined as "the presence of altered organ function in an acutely ill patient such that homeostasis cannot be maintained without intervention." Earlier terminology such as "multiple organ system failure" (MOSF) and "multi-system organ failure (MSOF)" should be avoided as it has become increasing apparent that MODS is not an "all-or-nothing" condition, but rather a continuum of dynamically changing organ failure. Additional definitions commonly used in conjunction with MODS include the "systemic inflammatory response syndrome" (SIRS), the "compensatory antiinflammatory response syndrome" (CARS), and the "mixed antagonists response syndrome" (MARS).

In the United States, MODS develops during 15% of all intensive care unit (ICU) admissions and is responsible for up to 80% of all ICU deaths. It is interesting that the progressive dysfunction of organ systems can occur in a predictable manner. During the first 72 hours of the original insult, respiratory failure commonly occurs. This is followed by hepatic failure (5–7 days), gastrointestinal bleeding (10–15 days), and finally renal failure (11–17 days), in the typical case. The extent to which an individual organ is likely to be damaged in patients with MODS is variable.

II. Pathophysiology. The pathophysiologic process leading to MODS has not been well defined. However, several hypotheses exist as to the mechanisms that initiate and perpetuate MODS. Among them, the most commonly cited include:

A. Gut hypothesis—the motor of MODS. This is currently the most popular theory to explain the development of MODS in critically ill patients. Splanchnic hypoperfusion is a common finding following multiple trauma, sepsis, shock, or thermal injuries. The gut is highly susceptible to diminished tissue perfusion and oxygenation as it has a higher critical oxygen requirement (DO_2) than the whole body and other vital organs, and the mucosal counter-current microcirculation renders the villi particularly vulnerable to ischemia. Gut mucosal ischemia increases gut permeability, alters gut immune function, and increases translocation of bacteria. Because of hepatic dysfunction, these bacterial toxins escape into the systemic circulation and activate the host's inflammatory response, which leads to tissue injury and organ dysfunction. Increased intestinal mucosal permeability can, therefore, be central to the development of MODS. Indeed, Doig et al. demonstrated an excellent relationship between increased intestinal permeability on admission to the ICU and the subsequent development of MODS.

B. Endotoxin-macrophage hypothesis. In patients with MODS, infection with gram-negative microorganisms is relatively common, so that endotoxin has been proposed as a key mediator in this clinical syndrome. In this hypothesis, after the initial event (i.e., sepsis, pancreatitis, trauma), MODS develops as a result of the production and liberation of cytokines and other mediators by endotoxin-activated macrophages. Indeed, experimental endotoxemia has been associated with systemic microvascular thrombosis which, in turn, leads to organ ischemia and injury.

C. Tissue hypoxia-microvascular hypothesis. Inadequate cellular oxygen supply can occur as a consequence of macro- and macrovascular changes. Protracted hypovolemia, anemia, hypoxemia, and myocardial failure will result in a decrease in tissue oxygen delivery. Tissue hypoxia will result in organ dysfunction and eventually cell death.

D. Integrated hypothesis. In most patients with MODS, the development of this syndrome cannot be traced to a single cause. In these patients, MODS can be viewed as the effect of impaired host defenses and inappropriate host regulation of inflammatory responses.

III. Diagnostic criteria and scoring systems. At least 20 scoring systems used to diagnose and quantify the severity of MODS have been described. These scoring systems differ appreciably, making it extremely difficult to compare the results from different research groups. In 1994, the European Society of Intensive Care Medicine organized a consensus meeting to create the *Sepsis-related Organ Failure Assessment* (SOFA) score to describe and quantitate the degree of organ dysfunction or failure over time in groups of patients and individual patients. The SOFA score was constructed using simple physiologic measures of dysfunction in six organ systems. The elements of the SOFA scoring system are depicted in Table 155-1. The SOFA score was not designed to predict outcome, but rather to describe and quantitate the sequence of complications in critically ill patients. Using similar physiologic variables to those used in the SOFA score, Marshal et al. developed the *Multiple Organ Dysfunction score* (MODS).

IV. Management. The management of the patient with MODS remains a formidable challenge. Despite advances in critical care therapeutics, the mortality rate of multiple organ failure remains unchanged since the syndrome was characterized more than two decades ago. At the present time, no modalities can actively reverse established organ failure; hence, the treatment of these patients consists of metabolic and hemodynamic support until the process reverses itself or death occurs. An increasing emphasis is being placed on prevention of organ dysfunction, including maintenance of tissue oxygenation, nutrition, and infection control.

The primary goal in the management of any critically ill patient must be to prevent the occurrence of a single organ failure and, when possible, specific corrective therapy of all identifiable risk factors for the development of MODS. The importance of maintaining adequate tissue perfusion in the high risk patients has been increasingly recognized. The level of perioperative tissue oxygen debt has been related to the postoperative incidence of MODS and patient outcome. Failure of the gut barrier function is central to the gut hypothesis. Gastric intramucosal acidosis or hypercarbia can serve as a marker of the adequacy of splanchnic perfusion. "Splanchnic resuscitation" should be initiated early to prevent or reverse intramucosal acidosis or hypercarbia. The institution of early enteral nutrition may be important in maintaining the gut mucosal barrier function and in preventing the development of MODS. Experimental models have demonstrated that total parenteral nutrition results in increased bacterial translocation. In addition, glutamine-supplemented enteral diet decreases bacterial translocation.

To reduce the risk of autoinfection with gut organisms, some authors have recommended the use of "selective decontamination of the digestive tract" (SDD) to prevent bacterial translocation. This method involves the use of nonabsorbable and intravenous antibiotics. Despite the publication of more than 50 controlled trials, it remains a controversial subject, with widely disparate views on the role of this technique. The published data seem to show some evidence that SDD can reduce acquired infection during intensive care. Most individual studies, however, have shown no effect on mortality, although meta-analyses suggest a 10% overall reduction.

V. Prognosis. Depending on the organs involved, MODS carries a mortality rate that varies from 30% to 100%. It is clear, however, that the greater the number of organs failures that occur and their duration, the less likely is the patient to survive MODS. Table 155-2 depicts ICU survival rates as a function of the total number of failing organ systems.

TABLE 155-1. The SOFA Score

Sofa Score	1	2	3	4
Respiration				
Pao/Fio mm Hg	< 400	< 300	< 200 with respiratory support	< 100
Coagulation				
Platelets × $10^3/mm^3$	< 150	< 100	< 50	< 20
Liver				
Bilirubin mg/dl	1.2–1.9	2.0–5.9	6.0–11.9	> 12
Cardiovascular				
Hypotension	MAP < 70 mm Hg	Dopamine ≤ 5 or dobutamine any dose	Dopamine > 5 or epinephrine ≤ 0.1 or norepinephrine ≤ 0.1	Dopamine > 15 or epinephrine > 0.1 or norepinephrine > 0.1
Central nervous system				
Glasgow Coma score	13–14	10–12	6–9	< 6
Renal				
Creatinine mg/dl or urine output	1.2–1.9	2.0–3.4	3.5–4.9 or < 500ml/d	> 5.0 or < 200 ml/d

TABLE 155-2. Intensive care unit survival rates as a function of the number of failing organ systems

Number of Organ Systems Failing	Mortality (%)
0	1
1	7
2	26
3	48
4	70
5	83

Selected Readings

Bone RC, Grodzin CJ, Balk RA. Sepsis: a new hypothesis for pathogenesis of the disease process. *Chest* 1997;112:235.
This article reviews the definitions and pathophysiology of sepsis, and the various terms used to describe multiple organ dysfunction syndrome (SIRS, MODS, CARS, and MARS).

Cerra FB. Multiple organ failure syndrome. *Dis Mon* 1992;38:843.
An excellent in-depth review of multiple organ dysfunction syndrome.

Deitch EA. Multiple organ failure. *Adv Surg* 1993;26:333.
A good review on the proposed mechanisms of multiple organ dysfunction syndrome.

Doig CJ, Sutherland LR, Sandham JS, et al. Increased intestinal permeability is associated with the development of multiple organ dysfunction syndrome in critically ill ICU patients. *Am J Respir Crit Care Med* 1998;158:444.
This study demonstrates the association between increased intestinal permeability and the development of multiple organ dysfunction syndrome.

Knaus WA, Wagner DP. Multiple systems organ failure: epidemiology and prognosis. *Crit Care Clin* 1989;5:221.
This article reviews the relationship between the number of organs failing and overall mortality.

Marshall JC, Cook DJ, Christou NV, et al. Multiple organ dysfunction score: a reliable descriptor of a complex clinical outcome. *Crit Care Med* 1995;23:1638.
This article describes the multiple organ dysfunction score and its relationship to mortality.

Pastores SM, Katz DP, Kvetan V. Splanchnic ischemia and gut mucosal injury in sepsis and the multiple organ dysfunction syndrome. *Am J Gastroenterol* 1996;91:1697.
An excellent review on the role of the gut in multiple organ dysfunction syndrome.

Ramsay G, van Saene RH. Selective decontamination in the intensive care and surgical practice; where are we? *World J Surg* 1998;22:164.
An overview of the role of selective decontamination of the gastrointestinal tract in the intensive care unit.

Vincent JL, Moreno R, Takala J, et al. The SOFA (Sepsis-related Organ Failure Assessment) score to describe organ dysfunction/failure. On behalf of the Working Group on Sepsis-Related Problems of the European Society of Intensive Care Medicine. *Intensive Care Med* 1996;22:707.
This article describes the sepsis-related organ failure assessment scoring system.

XIII. NEUROLOGIC PROBLEMS IN THE INTENSIVE CARE UNIT

156. AN APPROACH TO NEUROLOGIC PROBLEMS IN THE INTENSIVE CARE UNIT

David A. Drachman

I. General principles. Neurologic problems present in the intensive care unit (ICU), either as primary neurologic problems or as neurologic complications secondary to medical or surgical disorders. Only a few common neurologic *situations* occur in the ICU, although they can be caused by many *diseases:*

1. Depressed state of consciousness, coma
2. Altered mental function
3. Required support of respirations or other vital functions
4. Monitoring: increased intracranial pressure (ICP), respirations, consciousness
5. Determination of brain death
6. Prevention of further damage to the central nervous system (CNS)
7. Management of seizures or status epilepticus
8. Evaluation of a neurologic change occurring in a known medical disease
9. Management of medical disease developing during neurologic illness

Primary neurologic problems in the ICU include myasthenia gravis, the Guillain-Barré syndrome, head trauma, or stroke. These patients represent the minority of neurologic problems seen in the ICU. Neurologic complications of medical disease, which are far more common, include (a) impaired consciousness following cardiopulmonary resuscitation; (b) development of delirium; or (c) the occurrence of focal neurologic deficits in a patient with multisystem disease.

II. Indications for neurologic consultation in the ICU.

A. Depressed state of consciousness. Depressed consciousness, ranging from lethargy to coma, raises many questions: Is there a focal brainstem lesion or diffuse cerebral involvement? Is there an anatomic lesion or a metabolic disorder? Have vital brainstem functions been impaired? Is intracranial pressure increased? The most common primary neurologic causes of depressed consciousness include head trauma, intracranial hemorrhage, and inapparent seizures. The secondary conditions seen most often are metabolic-anoxic, drug intoxication, or diabetic acidosis. It is crucial to establish whether depressed consciousness has resulted from intrinsic brainstem damage, increased intracranial pressure, toxins, widespread anoxic ischemia, or other less common causes. It is particularly important to identify rapidly the component(s) that may be treatable.

Examination of the patient with depressed consciousness includes evaluation of mental status, cranial nerve functions, motor functions and coordination, reflexes, sensation, and vascular integrity, supplemented by appropriate laboratory studies. Detailed evaluation of memory and cognitive function is rarely possible in lethargic patients, and is impossible when stupor or coma are present. The physician's job is to estimate the responsiveness of the patient, including vital functions, respiratory pattern, opening the eyes, response to painful stimuli, and speech. Cranial nerve evaluations include vision (e.g., blink to threat), pupillary size and response, corneal reflexes, cough, 'Doll's eyes' responses, and, if absent, ice water caloric response. Facial movements to pain, and gag reflex are tested. Motor function is evaluated by observing all limbs for spontaneous movement, symmetry, and adventitious movements. A pinch or another noxious stimulus may help evaluate purposeful defensive movements. Decerebrate (four-limb extensor) or decorticate (upper limbs flexor, lower limbs extensor) rigidity is observed, and tone is assessed for spasticity or rigidity. Deep tendon reflexes are checked, and grasp, suck, snout, and plantar reflexes are evaluated. Pain is often the only testable sensation; withdrawal from pinprick in the feet must be distinguished from an extensor plantar response. Vascular status is evaluated by listening for bruits over the carotid, subclavian, and vertebral arteries.

This examination reveals the patient's state of consciousness, integrity of brainstem reflexes, and the presence of focal neurologic deficits. Neurodiagnostic and imaging studies often help in the analysis of comatose patients in the ICU despite the obstacles to obtaining them.

Management of patients with depressed consciousness depends on determining the cause and on applying the appropriate techniques for eliminating toxins, reducing intracranial pressure, and maintaining vital functions.

B. Altered mental function. In the awake patient, many disorders can affect mental function, producing patterns of confusion, delirium, aphasia, dementia, or isolated memory impairment. The physician must decide if the abnormal mentation is a recent change or is longstanding. Did the change develop abruptly after surgery or cardiac arrest; is it improving, worsening, or stable?

Confusion and delirium often result from metabolic and toxic disorders, and they are commonly reversible. Persistent aphasia and isolated memory impairment suggest focal anatomic damage to the brain. Dementia cannot be evaluated in patients with depressed consciousness, confusion, or delirium. In patients with a clear sensorium, it can indicate either reversible (drug-induced, depression-related) conditions or irreversible damage (diffuse anoxia or ischemia).

Recent change of mental status in the ICU requires prompt investigation by an experienced neurologist as early as possible.

C. Support of respiration and other vital functions. Respiratory support is needed for neurologic patients with loss of brainstem control of respiration or with impairment of effective transmission of neural impulses to respiratory muscles. Brainstem lesions produce characteristic respiratory patterns, depending on the site of damage (e.g., central neurogenic hyperventilation, Cheyne-Stokes or periodic breathing, or apnea).

Transmission of respiratory impulses can be impaired at the cervical spinal cord, anterior horn cells, peripheral nerves, neuromuscular junctions, or muscles of respiration. Cervical traumatic injuries, amyotrophic lateral sclerosis, the Guillain-Barré syndrome, myasthenia gravis, and muscular dystrophy each interfere with breathing at different levels; some conditions are transitory (Guillain-Barré syndrome) or treatable (myasthenia gravis), with complete recovery if respiration is successfully maintained.

D. Monitoring intracranial pressure and state of consciousness. Head trauma, subarachnoid hemorrhage, and stroke may require neural monitoring. Lethargic patients should be observed for increased intracranial pressure caused by cerebral edema, intracranial (subdural, epidural, intracerebral) hemorrhage, or both. Once uncal or tonsillar herniation with brainstem compression occurs, the secondary brain injury may far outweigh the initial damage. Methods for monitoring ICP and assessing consciousness with the Glasgow Coma scale are described elsewhere (Chapter 148 and Appendix).

E. Determination of brain death. Death of the brain and brainstem is equivalent to death of the patient. Brain death is specifically a determination that the brain *and* the brainstem are already dead—not a prediction of unlikely useful recovery. The mnemonic *CADRE* is useful to remember the criteria for brain death: **C**oma, **A**pnea, **D**ilated, fixed pupils, **R**eflex (brainstem) absence, and **E**lectroencephalographic (EEG) silence.

F. Preventing further damage to the CNS. In stroke, thrombolytic treatment can reverse the ischemic process and neuroprotective agents may prevent further damage. Spinal cord compression by tumor requires radiation therapy to avoid cord transection. Cerebral ischemia, anoxia, hemorrhage, increased ICP, spinal cord compression, and other acute disorders require prompt institution of treatment.

G. Managing status epilepticus. Status epilepticus threatens lasting deficits or death if not controlled. Patients with continuous seizures that cannot be promptly arrested must be treated in the ICU; therapy ranging up to general anesthesia or artificial ventilation may be required.

H. Evaluating neurologic disease in severe medical illness. Patients in the ICU with myocardial infarctions, subacute bacterial endocarditis, cardiac arrhythmias, pneumonia, renal disease, and so on may develop neurologic changes during treatment for the medical problem. The neurologic findings, whether from the underlying disease or coincidental, require the attention of a neurologist.

I. Managing severe medical disease in neurologic illness. Patients with chronic neurologic disorders often develop unrelated medical illness: myocardial infarcts occurring in demented patients or septicemia in patients with multiple sclerosis. Early recognition of a change in the neurologic patient's condition is often critical to a successful outcome.

J. Prognostic and ethical considerations. When severe damage involves the brain, physicians and families often need guidance regarding the probable outcome. Three critical questions need answering: Will the patient survive? Has irreversible brain damage occurred? What is the likely degree of residual disability? The most important consideration is often whether irreversible damage has affected crucial brain areas, rather than the level of consciousness. The probability of neurologic recovery declines with age, size and location of the lesion, and duration of the deficit. Some reported statistical guidelines are of value in estimating recovery (e.g., Levy D, Caronna J, Singer B, et al.).

Selected Readings

Levy D, Caronna J, Singer B, et al. Predicting outcome from hypoxic-ischemic coma. *JAMA* 1985;253:1420.

An excellent summary of the features that predict survival and function following hypoxic-ischemic coma.

Plum F, Posner JB. *The diagnosis of stupor and coma,* 3rd ed. Philadelphia: FA Davis; 1982.

A classic review of the neurologic aspects of impaired consciousness.

Ropper A. *Neurological and neurosurgical intensive care,* 3rd ed. New York: Raven Press; 1993.

A multiauthor book with detailed discussions of many aspects of neurologic intensive care.

Wanzer S, Federman D, Adelstein S, et al. The physician's responsibility toward hopelessly ill patients: a second look. *N Engl J Med* 1989;320:844.

A thoughtful approach to end-of-life issues in patients with terminal illness.

157. EVALUATING THE PATIENT WITH ALTERED CONSCIOUSNESS IN THE INTENSIVE CARE UNIT

Majaz Moonis, Kevin J. Felice, and David A. Drachman

I. General principles. Many diseases lead to acute impairment of consciousness, including some that are potentially life threatening but treatable if recognized early. Evaluating the patient with an altered level of consciousness must be systematic and efficient. The approach to the patient with impaired consciousness includes (a) rapid determination of the type of mental status change; (b) administration of life support measures when needed; (c) obtaining a detailed history, physical examination, and ancillary studies to determine precisely the cause of the nervous system disorder; and (d) initiation of definitive treatment based on this assessment. This chapter defines altered states of consciousness and presents an approach to bedside evaluation of the comatose patient.

II. The patient who appears unconscious. These patients lie mostly motionless, with their eyes closed, seemingly unaware of their environment. The causes of this condition include normal sleep, depressed consciousness, and brain death, whereas the locked-in state and psychogenic coma can also simulate unconsciousness. Patients with the locked-in state are motionless because they are paralyzed, but preservation of consciousness exists and can be confirmed by communicating through a preserved movement (e.g., eye blink) and by demonstrating electroencephalographic (EEG) reactivity (e.g., alpha waves that attenuate with eye opening). Patients in psychogenic coma also have clinical and EEG evidence of wakefulness. This diagnosis should be considered in the seemingly unconscious patient who exhibits active resistance, rapid closure of the eyelids, pupillary constriction to visual threat, fast phase of nystagmus on oculovestibular or optokinetic testing, and avoidance of self-injury.

A. Depressed consciousness. If brain dysfunction is mild, the patient may be described as *lethargic,* hypersomnolent, or drowsy. In this state, wakefulness is achieved following a modest level of sensory stimulation; the patient becomes oriented and makes appropriate responses, then slips back to unconsciousness. *Obtundation* refers to the patient who is mentally dulled when aroused by modest stimulation, reflecting a greater degree of brain dysfunction. *Stuporous* patients can be aroused only with vigorous noxious stimulation; during the transient arousal, they may display purposeful movements (e.g., ward off painful stimuli or remove intravenous lines) but lack normal content of consciousness. Patients in *coma* cannot be aroused and are unresponsive to vigorous sensory stimulation. Although the patient usually lies motionless, movements such as stereotyped, inappropriate postures (e.g., decerebration, decortication) and spinal cord reflexes (e.g., triple flexion and Babinski responses) can occur.

B. Brain death. Brain death is the irreversible destruction of the brain, with the resulting total absence of all cortical and brainstem function, although spinal cord reflexes may remain. It is not to be confused with incomplete brain damage with poor prognosis. In brain death, pupils are midposition and round, and no inspiratory effort (i.e., central apnea) is made, even when arterial carbon dioxide tension (P_{CO_2}) is raised to levels that should stimulate respiration. Sedating medications, drug intoxications, metabolic disturbances, hypothermia, and shock should be excluded as complicating conditions in determining brain death.

III. The patient who appears awake and alert but is confused or noncommunicative

A. Acute confusional state. Patients with *confusion* are easily distracted by environmental stimuli, and poor attention span impairs recall and recent memory. Repeated prompting may be required for a response. *Delirium* is a type of confusional state in which psychomotor and autonomic overactivity occur and often visual hallucinations as well. Hyperexcitability can alternate with periods of relative lucidity or with periods of depressed consciousness. *Nonconvulsive seizures* can present as an acute confusional state; important signs that are suggestive of this diagnosis are episodic staring, eye deviation or nystagmoid jerks, facial or hand clonic activity, and automatisms.

B. Receptive aphasia. The patient is awake and alert but unable to comprehend written or verbal commands. Speech production is fluent but often with paraphasias—inappropriately substituted words or nonsensical jargon during spontaneous speech or when the patient is asked to name objects. Patients with *global aphasia* show no evidence of comprehension and are unable to communicate either by writing or speaking.

C. Akinetic mutism. In these patients, brainstem function is intact and sleep–wake cycles may be present, but little evidence is seen of cognitive function. These patients may open their eyes to auditory stimulation or track moving objects, but only a paucity of spontaneous movement occurs. A similar but more severe state of brain injury is the *persistent vegetative state,* which usually follows prolonged coma. Complex subcortical responses are absent, but decorticate or decerebrate posturing and other rudimentary subcortical responses (e.g., yawn, cough) are seen.

IV. Localization of brain dysfunction in the patient with altered consciousness. Table 157-1 provides a guideline to anatomic localization of brain dysfunction associated with various states of altered consciousness. The importance of localization cannot be overstated because an accurate anatomic diagnosis is critical to arriving at the exact cause of the patient's condition.

V. Diagnostic approach to the patient with altered consciousness. The history is critical in determining the cause of the patient's condition, and efforts to locate family members, witnesses, and medication lists are almost always fruitful. For example, knowledge of preexisting cerebral dysfunction (e.g., dementia, multiple sclerosis, mental retardation) is important in determining the degree of depressed consciousness or confusion expected for a specific systemic derangement (e.g., hyponatremia, sepsis, drug intoxication). A reliable account of the tempo of loss of consciousness is important. For example, truly sudden coma in a healthy person suggests drug intoxication, intracranial hemorrhage, meningoencephalitis, or an unwitnessed seizure. In general, *focal neurologic signs* suggest a structural cause of altered consciousness, although focal weakness or partial motor seizures sometimes occur in metabolic encephalopathies. Other falsely localizing signs include sixth nerve palsies caused by transmitted increased intracranial pressure and visual field cuts caused by compression of the posterior cerebral artery. Conversely, a nonfocal examination does not invariably indicate toxic-metabolic encephalopathy. Meningoencephalitis, subarachnoid hemorrhage, bilateral subdural hematomas, or thrombosis of the superior sagittal sinus can cause symmetric neurologic dysfunction. With these important caveats in mind, Table 157-2 presents a classification of causes associated with altered consciousness.

TABLE 157-1. Localization of brain dysfunction in patients with apparent change in consciousness

Clinical State	Area of Dysfunction
Depressed consciousness	
Drowsiness	Reticular activating system (RAS)
Stupor/coma	RAS and bilateral cerebral hemispheres
Acute confusional state	Bilateral cerebral hemispheres
Receptive aphasia	Dominant temporoparietal lobes
Akinetic mutism	Bilateral frontal lobes
Persistent vegetative state	Bilateral cerebral hemispheres

TABLE 157-2. Classification of causes of altered consciousness based on most common clinical presentation

1. Depressed consciousness or acute confusional state without focal or lateralizing neurologic signs, and without signs of meningeal irritation
   - Metabolic disorders: hepatic failure, uremia, hypercapnia, hypoxia, hypoglycemia, diabetic hyperosmolar state, hypercalcemia, thiamine or cobalamine deficiency, hypotension, severe anemia.
   - Drug intoxications or poisoning: opiates, alcohol, barbiturates, tricyclic antidepressants, amphetamines, anticholinergics, other sedatives, carbon monoxide, heavy metal toxins
   - Infectious and other febrile illnesses: septicemia, pneumonia, rheumatic fever, connective tissue diseases
   - Nonconvulsive status epilepticus or postconvulsive delirium
   - Situational psychoses: intensive care unit, puerperal, postoperative, or posttraumatic psychoses; severe sleep deprivation can be complicating factor
   - Abstinence states (i.e., withdrawal states): alcohol (delirium tremens), barbiturates, benzodiazepines
   - Space-occupying lesions: bilateral subdural hematoma, midline cerebral tumors (e.g., lymphoma, glioma), abscess
   - Hydrocephalus
2. Altered consciousness with signs of meningeal irritation[a]
   - Infectious disorders: meningoencephalitis (bacterial, viral, fungal, parasitic)
   - Subarachnoid hemorrhage: brain contusion, ruptured aneurysm, or other vascular malformation
   - Rheumatologic conditions: meningeal granulomatous disorders (e.g., sarcoid, Wegener's granulomatosis)
3. Altered consciousness with focal or lateralizing neurologic signs
   - Space-occupying lesion: neoplasm, hemorrhage, inflammatory process (e.g., abscess, autoimmune, encephalitis)
   - Cerebral ischemia or infarction: stroke, hypertensive encephalopathy

[a]Meningismus is often absent in deeply comatose patients with meningeal inflammation.

VI. Ancillary tests. A computed tomographic (CT) or magnetic resonance imaging (MRI) scan without contrast demonstrates intracranial hemorrhage and hydrocephalus; contrast enhancement may be required for suspected infectious or neoplastic masses. The CT scan does not reliably rule out inflammation, subarachnoid blood, or early ischemia. The diagnosis of toxic-metabolic encephalopathy requires identification of a metabolic derangement or other abnormality sufficient to explain the clinical state. It is not always logistically possible to perform magnetic resonance imaging on patients with altered consciousness who are medically unstable, but this technology demonstrates early ischemia and encephalitis and provides excellent images of the posterior fossa. The cerebrospinal fluid must be examined if meningoencephalitis or subarachnoid hemorrhage is suspected. Of all the tests available to patients in the intensive care unit, only an EEG provides a physiologic marker of brain function. EEG is critical to the diagnosis of nonconvulsive status epilepticus and may be helpful in the diagnosis of early cerebral infarction (focal slowing), psychogenic coma (normal), locked-in state (normal), and brain death (presence of electrocerebral silence, although this is not a requirement).

VII. Initiation of emergency treatment. Definitive treatment of altered consciousness depends on the underlying cause, but urgent therapeutic interventions may be required in life-threatening conditions or to prevent further central nervous system insult. Meticulous attention to fluid replacement, oxygenation, suctioning, positioning, nutrition, corneal protection, and bowel and bladder care are essential. Sedating drugs confound the accurate monitoring of the patient's neurologic condition and should be avoided whenever possible.

Selected Readings

Adams RD, Victor M, Ropper AH. *Principles of neurology,* 6th ed. New York: McGraw-Hill; 1997.
A lucid and comprehensive review on disorders of consciousness (Chapter 17) and acute confusional states (Chapter 20).

Felice KJ, Schwartz WJ, Drachman DA. Evaluating the patient with altered consciousness in the intensive care unit. In: Irwin RS, Cerra FB, Rippe JM, eds. *Intensive care medicine,* 4th ed. Philadelphia: Lippincott–Raven; 1999.
The full length version of this chapter.

Fisher CM. The neurological examination of the comatose patient. *Acta Neurol Scand* 1969;45(Suppl 36):1–56.
Insightful account of important neurological signs.

Plum F, Posner JB. *Diagnosis of stupor and coma,* 3rd ed. Philadelphia: FA Davis; 1980.
Classic monograph, with original investigations on stupor and coma.

158. METABOLIC ENCEPHALOPATHY

Paula D. Ravin

I. General principles

A. Metabolic encephalopathy describes any process affecting global brain function by altering its biochemical function. The most common cause of altered mental status in the intensive care unit (ICU) setting, it is also one of the most treatable. The patients most at risk for developing metabolic encephalopathy are those with single or multiple organ failure, the elderly (aged >60 years), those receiving multiple central nervous system (CNS) toxic agents, and those with severe nutritional deficiencies. Other risk factors include infection, temperature dysregulation, chronic degenerative neurologic or psychiatric diseases, and endocrine disorders. Metabolic encephalopathy should be suspected when an altered cognitive status is seen in the absence of focal neurologic signs or an obvious anatomic lesion (e.g., a head injury) is present. In mild cases, it is easily mistaken for fatigue or psychogenic depression, whereas more severe cases can develop into coma and are life threatening.

B. Mental changes can start as mild confusion with intermittent disorientation and difficulty attending to questions. *Delirium* can occur with heightened arousal, alternating with somnolence, often worse at night, and fluctuating throughout the day. Progressive *lethargy* can lead to *stupor* and *coma*. This course may be punctuated by focal or generalized *seizures* and postictal somnolence (Table 158-1).

Disorders that can be confused with metabolic encephalopathy include brain tumors, encephalitis, meningitis, closed head trauma, and brainstem cerebrovascular events. Table 158-2 outlines some of the cardinal differences between brainstem stroke and metabolic encephalopathy. Most focal neurologic findings are not attributable to metabolic causes and other sources must be sought.

II. Evaluation. The clinical examination should evaluate the patient's level of arousal, posture in bed, breathing pattern, vital signs, and behavioral fluctuations that may suggest metabolic encephalopathy (Table 158-3):

1. Behavioral changes: Early signs include lack of attention, decreased spontaneous speech and mild confusion.
2. Cranial nerve examination: Small, responsive pupils are the rule in metabolic encephalopathy with preserved ocular movements or "Bell's phenomenon," with the eyes slightly deviated upward and outward as if the patient were asleep.
3. Changes in the respiratory pattern: Periodic respirations with hyperventilation followed by brief periods of apnea or hypopnea are usually seen in metabolic disturbance, whereas other central neurogenic respiratory patterns generally occur with brainstem dysfunction or structural lesions.
4. Abnormal motor activity: Tremors, myoclonus, asterixis, choreoathetosis, rigidity, and generalized muscle spasms are common in metabolic disorders, often in combination and sometimes changing over the course of the disorder.
5. Reflex examination: Hyperreflexia and extensor plantar responses are seen.
6. Sensation: Sensory responses are unreliable, especially when the patient's level of arousal waxes and wanes.
7. Abnormal autonomic responses: Occult sepsis should be ruled out before looking for other metabolic causes.
8. Seizures: These occur most often at the beginning of metabolic derangement and can be difficult to control until the underlying problem is corrected.
9. Laboratory investigations: These are crucial in defining any metabolic encephalopathy and include blood glucose, electrolytes, blood gases, hepatic function panel, ammonia, blood urea nitrogen (BUN), and creatinine. Serum and urine osmolality, cerebrospinal fluid (CSF) analysis, serum magnesium and

TABLE 158-1. Patient profile in metabolic encephalopathy

Gradual onset over hours
Progressive if untreated
Waxing and waning level of consciousness
Patient treated with multiple CNS acting drugs
Patient with organ failure, postoperative state, electrolyte disturbance, endocrine disease
No evidence of brain tumor or stroke on neurologic examination—usually nonfocal (except hypoglycemia)
Sometimes heralded by focal or generalized seizures
Increased spontaneous motor activity—restlessness, asterixis, myoclonus, tremors, rigidity
Abnormal blood chemistries, blood gases, anemia
Usually normal CNS imaging studies
Generalized EEG abnormalities—slowing, triphasic waves
Gradual recovery once treatment is initiated

CNS, central nervous system; EEG, electroencephalogram.

phosphate levels, and specific hormone levels may also be needed. A toxicology screen includes barbiturates, opiates, benzodiazepines, caffeine, salicylates, theophylline, and alcohol. With a sudden change in mental status, a bolus of 25 g of glucose should be administered intravenously (IV) before other tests are drawn.

10. Electroencephalogram (EEG): The EEG is slow in metabolic encephalopathy but can also exhibit frontal high voltage activity. The EEG can exclude status epilepticus when in doubt.

TABLE 158-2. Signs and symptoms of brainstem cerebrovascular accident vs. metabolic encephalopathy

	Brainstem CVA	Metabolic encephalopathy
Patient profile	Known vascular disease Hypercoagulable state Acute onset (< 8 h) Age usually > 50 y	Organ failure Subacute onset (> 8 h) except low BS Any age, often > 60 y
Motor involvement	Hemiplegic or paraplegic	Moving all limbs, except low BS
Sensory involvement	Unilateral facial sensory change or loss	Absent
Mental status	Obtunded or agitated	Waxing and waning
Pupils	May have Horner's or small, fixed, dilated pupil	Normoactive
Eye movements	Dysconjugate Skew deviation CN III, IV, or VI pareses	Conjugate Midline
Respirations	Apneustic Central hyperpnea	Normal Hyperpneic with brief apnea (12–30 sec)

CVA, cerebrovascular accident; BS, blood sugar; CN, cranial nerve.

TABLE 158-3. Evaluation for metabolic encephalopathy

Neurologic examination
- Mental status
- Pupillary responses
- Oculomotor responses
- Respiratory pattern
- Motor activity, strength
- DTRs, plantar responses

Initial laboratory studies
- Blood sugar, electrolytes, lactate dehydrogenase, aspartate aminotransferase, alanine aminotransferase, SGPT, ammonia, blood urea nitrogen, creatinine clearance, white blood cells, differential, hemoglobulin, hematocrit, blood gases

Electroencephalogram

Neuroimaging
- Head computed tomography scan or magnetic resonance imaging

± Lumbar puncture, toxin screens, serum and urine osmolality, psychiatric examination

DTR, deep tendon reflexes.

11. Neuroimaging: Cranial computed tomography (CT) or magnetic resonance imaging (MRI) is often critical when a rapid deterioration occur in mental status without focal signs or obvious metabolic causes; however, these studies may not identify an early brainstem stroke.
12. Lumbar puncture: This procedure is indicated when subarachnoid hemorrhage or infection is suspected in the setting of fever, headache, or meningismus.

III. Etiology

A. Causes of metabolic encephalopathy. Drugs and toxins lead all other causes of metabolic encephalopathy at a frequency of approximately 50%; hepatic, renal, and pulmonary failure rank second in frequency (~12%); and endocrine or electrolyte disturbances third (8%). Hyperthermia and thiamine deficiency (Wernicke's encephalopathy) both cause petechial lesions in specific areas of the brain. These also appear in cardiac bypass surgery, subacute bacterial endocarditis, and hypoglycemia. Metabolic encephalopathy in these settings can cause permanent deficits.

B. Hepatic failure. Blunting of affect or lethargy occurs early; mania or agitated delirium is seen in 10% to 20% of cases. It is usually caused by portacaval shunting of neurotoxic substances. A direct correlation exists between elevation of serum transaminases and more impaired cognitive state. The EEG may show triphasic waves or slowing of background. Prolonged or repeated bouts of hepatic encephalopathy can lead to acquired hepatocerebral degeneration with permanent basal ganglia dysfunction.

C. Reye's syndrome. This disorder occurs in children from 1 to 10 years, starting 4 to 7 days after a viral infection such as chicken pox or influenza A or B *and* exposure to aspirin. The initial events are irritability, vomiting, headache, and blurred vision, with progression to agitated delirium with combativeness and stupor. The morbidity and mortality are now approximately 10% to 20%. Poor outcome factors include age less than 1 year and serum ammonia levels more than five times normal and prothrombin time of more than 20 seconds.

D. Renal failure. Encephalopathy can occur acutely, with chronic *renal insufficiency* or chronic *dialysis.* The clinical picture does not correlate with BUN or creatinine levels; it starts with delirium, hyperventilation, increased motor activity, and finally, obtundation.

A motor component is prominent with an admixture of movements producing "twitch-convulsive" like fasciculations. Generalized convulsions are frequent at the onset with metabolic acidosis and low serum bicarbonate.

Acute *dialysis disequilibrium syndrome* is seen in children undergoing large exchanges of dialysate and water intoxication in 30 to 60 minutes. Dialysis dementia is insidious with postdialysis lethargy, asterixis, myoclonus, dysphasia, and progressive decline in cognitive function.

E. **Pulmonary failure.** Encephalopathy occurs with a combination of hypercarbia and hypoxemia, and appears with a rapid increase in P_{CO_2} over baseline. The prognosis is good if there is no concomitant cerebral ischemia.

F. **Hypoglycemic encephalopathy.** The most common cause is accidental overdose of oral hypoglycemic agents. Insulin reactions occur at glucose levels below 40 mg/dl; focal neurologic signs (e.g., hemiparesis, cortical blindness, or dysphasia) are common and shift rapidly. Generalized convulsions appear at glucose levels below 30 mg/dl followed by postictal coma.

Treatment is a bolus of one ampule of 50% glucose, delivered quickly when a rapid change in level of arousal occurs to avoid permanent deficits from hypoglycemia.

G. **Hyperglycemic encephalopathy.** This condition is accompanied by hypokalemia, hypophosphatemia, hyperosmolality, and ketoacidosis or lactic acidosis with serum glucose levels greater than 300 mg/dl. Neurologic changes match abnormalities of serum osmolality and the rate at which it is corrected.

Too rapid correction of hyperosmolality by IV hydration results in cerebral water intoxication and increased intracranial pressure.

H. **Other electrolyte disturbances.** Mild to moderate *hyponatremia* (120–130 mEq/L) is evidenced by confusion or delirium with asterixis and multifocal myoclonus. Seizures occur with serum sodium less than 110 mEq/L or decreases faster than 5 mEq/L/h to 120 mEq/L. Common causes of hyponatremia are syndrome of inappropriate antidiuretic hormone secretion, excess volume expansion with hypotonic IV solutions, and renal failure with decreased glomerular filtration rate. Too rapid correction of hyponatremia can result in central pontine myelinolysis with flaccid quadriparesis, dysphagia, and dysarthria evolving over several days. Hypernatremia is seen less often, usually in children with severe diarrhea and inadequate hydration or diabetes insipidus and depressed consciousness.

Metabolic acidosis is often related to organ failure, drug intoxication, or volume depletion.

I. **Pancreatic failure.** Waxing and waning cognitive function can be seen in the setting of repeated bouts of pancreatitis, with secondary seizures caused by hyperglycemia, hypocalcemia, and hypotension.

J. **Endocrine disorders.** *Hypoadrenalism* often occurs following withdrawal of exogenous steroids, septicemia, surgery, or pituitary damage. It is evidenced by decreased muscle tone and reflexes. Hyperadrenalism can produce lethargy, depression, and coma or agitated delirium and frank psychosis. Correction of the adrenal imbalance may result in neurologic recovery days to weeks later.

Hypothyroidism can produce "myxedema madness" with hypothermia, pretibial edema, coarse hair and facies, pseudomyotonic reflexes (delayed relaxation of the knee jerk), and behavioral changes. Hyperthyroidism can manifest as a "thyroid storm" or as an "apathetic" form with recent weight loss, atrial fibrillation, congestive heart failure, and proximal myopathy.

Hypopituitarism can be caused acutely by pituitary hemorrhage or radiation and surgery resulting in multiple endocrine deficiencies.

Hyperparathyroidism often starts with asthenia and vague personality changes, evolving into delirium or coma when calcium levels exceed 15 mg/dl, as is seen in secondary hypercalcemia from bone lesions and renal failure. Hypocalcemia causes depressed consciousness in parallel with lowered levels of calcium (<4.0 mEq/L) with tetany as a hallmark.

IV. **Conclusions.** Metabolic encephalopathy is one of the most common neurologic disorders seen in the ICU setting. The features that distinguish most metabolic encephalopathies are (a) a nonfocal examination in patients with altered states of consciousness, (b) increased motor activity, (c) intact pupillary and ocular reflexes, and (d) laboratory abnormalities supporting the clinical picture. Many patients in the ICU already suffer from chronic organ failure and encephalopathy, making them more susceptible to minor perturbations in their neurologic state.

Selected Readings

Ayus JC, Krothapalli RK, Arieff AI. Treatment of symptomatic hyponatremia and its relation to brain damage: a prospective study. *N Engl J Med* 1987;317:1190.
Clarifies the treatment regimen and critical nature of sodium correction and the brain.

Fishbain DA, Rotundo D. Frequency of hypoglycemic delirium in a psychiatric emergency service. *Psychosomatics* 1988;29(3):346.
Enlightening treatise highlighting this underdiagnosed problem.

Hattori S, Mochio S, Isogai Y, et al. Central pontine myelinolysis followed by frequent hyperglycemia and hypoglycemia: report of an autopsy case. *Brain Nerve* 1989; 41:795.
A description of the clinical presentation of central pontine myelinolysis.

Hurwitz ES. Reye's syndrome. *Epidemiol Rev* 1989;11:249.
Current understanding of Reye's syndrome and a review of the literature.

Kaminski HJ, Ruff RL. Neurologic complications of endocrine diseases. *Neurol Clin* 1989;7:489.
Good overview of neuroendocrinology.

Laursen H, Westergaard G. Enhanced permeability to horseradish peroxidase across cerebral vessels in the rat after portacaval anastamosis. *Neuropathol Appl Neurobiol* 1979;3:29.
A scientific description of hepatic failure and neurotoxicity.

Plum F, Posner JB. The physiologic pathology of signs and symptoms of coma. In: Plum F, ed. *The diagnosis of stupor and coma,* 3rd ed. Philadelphia: FA Davis; 1980:33.
The classic reference on depressed consciousness states.

Raskin NH, Fishman RA. Neurologic disorders in renal failure. *N Engl J Med* 1976;294: 143, 204.
A good review article on neurologic disorder in renal failure.

Sheridan PH, Sato S. Triphasic waves of metabolic encephalopathy versus spike-wave stupor. *J Neurol Neurosurg Psychiatry* 1986;49(1):108.
Describes the differences between metabolic encephalopathy and status epilepticus seen on the encephalogram.

Victor M. Neurologic disorders due to alcoholism and malnutrition. In: Baker AB, Baker LH, eds. *Clinical neurology.* Philadelphia: Harper & Row; 1983:24.
A concise review of the clinical spectrum of alcoholism and neurologic disease.

159. GENERALIZED ANOXIA/ISCHEMIA OF THE NERVOUS SYSTEM

Majaz Moonis and Carol F. Lippa

I. General principles. The brain tolerates oxygen deprivation poorly. Anoxia resulting from respiratory failure from any cause is better tolerated than when the primary event is cardiac arrest. In the latter condition, anaerobic metabolism ensues within 5 minutes. In these injuries, excess glutamate release results in activation of the excitotoxic cascade, calcium influx into neurons and cell death.

II. Diagnosis. In a comatose patient without focal findings, anoxic encephalopathy is suggested by the circumstances preceding the loss of consciousness (cardiac arrest, hanging, status asthmaticus, status epilepticus) and exclusion of other causes of coma. Both for management and for prognosis, it is important to identify whether the primary event leading to coma was cardiac (ischemic anoxia) or pulmonary (hypoxic). The latter carries a better prognosis. Blood gases at the time of the event provide useful corroboration. A PaO_2 less than 30 mm Hg often results in coma.

The neurologic examination is usually nonfocal, although occasionally soft lateralizing neurologic signs have been documented. A computed tomography scan of the brain is useful in ruling out structural lesions, such as a brainstem stroke. Blood glucose, liver function tests including ammonia, blood urea nitrogen, and creatinine should be obtained to rule out hypoglycemia or other causes of metabolic encephalopathy. A toxic screen should be obtained in all cases where the primary cause of coma is not clear. An immediate electroencephalogram (EEG) is indicated if nonconvulsive status epilepticus is suspected.

III. Clinical course and prognosis. Many patients with severe anoxia die within 72 hours or evolve into a persistent vegetative state. The shorter the duration of hypoxia, especially in younger patients, the better the chance of a functional recovery. Comatose patients who sustain prolonged anoxia rarely recover unless signs of improvement occur within the first few days. After 48 hours, if two of three brainstem signs (pupillary response, corneal responses, and "Dolls eyes") are not present, the chances of functional neurologic recovery approach zero. Other signs indicating a poor prognosis include generalized edema on delayed neuroimaging scans and a deterioration of the background EEG rhythm.

A rare delayed sequela may be seen 3 to 30 days after the initial recovery from an anoxic event, especially following carbon monoxide poisoning; a late functional decline occurs, with irritability, lethargy, and increased muscle tone. Pathologically, widespread demyelination is found. Most patients survive this second insult. Intention myoclonus is another delayed consequence. If necessary, this can be distinguished from seizures by the absence of corresponding EEG changes.

The outcome of anoxic encephalopathy is determined by several factors, the most important being the time before effective circulation is reestablished. If consciousness is maintained during the hypoxic episode, prognosis for recovery is excellent. Total anoxia, if reversed within 4 minutes, carries the same prognosis. Overall, patients with an out-of-hospital cardiac arrest have a 50% chance of awakening. Complete recovery occurs in 80% of cases, if the coma resolves within 24 hours. Recovery can occur after much longer periods of coma in children.

Out of hospital cardiac arrest time (AT) plus the cardiopulmonary resuscitation (CPR) time determine the total time to reestablish blood blow. When AT is less than 6 minutes and CPR time is less than 30 minutes, moderate recovery is possible. However, AT longer than 6 minutes carries a poor prognosis for meaningful recovery.

A. Favorable prognostic indicators include:

- Recovery of multiple brainstem responses within 48 hours of arrest (pupillary, corneal, and oculovestibular).
- Return of purposeful motor movements within 24 hours (localization of pain).
- Young age (children may do well even beyond this time period).

- Primary pulmonary event leading to the coma.
- Hypothermia at AT (cold water drowning).

B. Poor prognostic indicators in patients with persistent coma after 72 hours include:

- The absence of pupillary responses or motor response to pain on the third day
- Certain abnormal EEG patterns including alpha coma or burst suppression.
- Patients with absent cortical N20 response after 72 hours of coma usually fail to recover, although somatosensory evoked potentials have limited prognostic utility. If the cortical N20 responses can be elicited, however, the chances of improvement are increased to 25%.
- Although not part of a routine investigation, CSF in patients showing a neuron-specific enolase of more than 24 ng/ml at 24 hour or a creatine kinase-BB more than 50 U/L at 48 to 72 hours usually indicates failure to recover.

IV. Treatment. Adequate oxygenation ($Pa{O_2}$ over 100 mm Hg) and blood pressure (90 to 110 mm Hg) should be maintained. Patients should be kept slightly hypovolemic and the head of the bed elevated to 30 degrees. Underlying causes such as toxin or drug ingestion should be treated. Cardiac arrhythmias should be controlled. A diligent search for infections should be done and treated appropriately. Patients should not be allowed to become hyperthermic. All other toxic, metabolic, or structural causes of comas should be ruled out. Vital signs, hematocrit, electrolytes, blood sugar, and serum osmolarity should be maintained within the normal range. Seizures occur in 25% cases; if they are present, fosphenytoin at 20 phenytoin equivalents can be given intravenously or intramuscularly. In contrast to other agents, it has a low risk of inducing hypotension at this stage where patients may have hemodynamic instability. Alternatively, phenytoin in the same doses can be given with careful blood pressure and cardiac monitoring. If serious acute underlying cardiac arrhythmias exist, intravenous phenobarbital is preferred. If seizures are controlled, a delayed EEG is done after 48 hours. If persistent seizures occur, continuous EEG monitoring may be required. Status epilepticus should be treated using established protocols. Both persistent nonconvulsive status and myoclonic status are very poor prognostic indicators.

No role exists for use of steroids or high-dose barbiturates, and hyperosmolar agents are seldom helpful in anoxic or hypoxic coma. Controlled hyperventilation with a $P{CO_2}$ of 25 to 28 mm may be effective in the short term to avoid impending herniation. Once coma begins to lighten, early mobilization should be the goal to prevent other complications.

V. Brain death. The criteria for brain death are defined in Chapters 156 and 172. Total absence of electrocerebral activity, not associated with sedative hypnotic drugs or hypothermia, is helpful in confirming brain death in difficult cases. Similarly, a brain scan showing absence of blood flow is strongly suggestive of brain death. Many institutions have specific brain death protocols that should be followed when determining brain death.

Selected Reading

Abramson NS, Safar P, Detre KM. Neurological recovery after cardiac arrest. Effect of duration of ischemia. *Crit Care Med* 1985;14:930.

A useful paper that reviews the relationship between the duration of cerebral ischemia and clinical outcome in anoxic encephalopathy.

Chatrian GE. Coma, other states of altered responsiveness and brain death. In: Daly DD, Pedley AT, eds. *Current practice of clinical electroencephalography,* 2nd ed. Philadelphia: Lippincott–Raven; 1990:425.

Electroencephalogram patterns and their prognostic significance in coma.

Garcia JH. Morphology of cerebral ischemia. *Crit Care Med* 1988;16:979.

A review of various sequelae of anoxic encephalopathy.

Lewy DE, Bates D, Caronna JJ, et al. Prognosis in non-traumatic coma. *Ann Intern Med* 1981;94:293.

A landmark paper on the prognosis in nontraumatic coma.

Plum F, Posner JB. *Multifocal, diffuse and metabolic brain diseases causing stupor and coma in the diagnosis of stupor and coma.* Philadelphia: FA Davis; 1982;177.
A classic work that reviews anoxic encephalopathy.
Simon RP. Hypoxia versus ischemia. *Neurology* 1999;52:7.
A thoughtful discussion on the prognostic outcome between the two types of cerebral anoxia.
Wijdicks EF, Parisi JE, Sharbrough FW. Prognostic value of myoclonus status in comatose survivors of cardiac arrest. *Ann Neurol* 1994;35:239.
A brief paper that assesses the different types of seizure activity in anoxic encephalopathy and prognostic implications of the various seizure types.
Zandbergen EGJ, de Haan RJ, Stoutenbeek CP et al. Systemic review of early prediction of poor outcome in anoxic-ischemic coma. *Lancet* 1998;352:1808.
A summary of the literature concerning reliable indicators of death or a vegetative state following acute anoxia.

160. STATUS EPILEPTICUS

Catherine A. Phillips

I. Definition and classification. *Status epilepticus,* called simply "status" in this chapter, is traditionally defined as a seizure, or sequential seizures, lasting 30 minutes or longer without recovery between attacks. A more practical definition is continuous seizure activity lasting 5 minutes or longer, or two or more seizures with incomplete recovery of consciousness between them. In status, seizures of a few minutes' duration may be followed by prolonged unconsciousness leading to the next seizure. Clinical manifestations of seizure activity may consist only of nystagmus or twitching of the face or a limb, or may be evident only on electroencephalography (EEG).

Myoclonic status is repetitive, asynchronous myoclonus with variable clouding of consciousness, usually in the setting of severe encephalopathy such as cerebral anoxia; patients are usually comatose. Simple partial status epilepticus is continuous or repetitive focal seizures without loss of consciousness. This includes epilepsia partialis continua, with continuous localized clonic seizure activity that does not generalize and in which consciousness is maintained.

Nonconvulsive status (e.g., absence or complex partial status) is a confusional state of 30 minutes or more. In absence status, consciousness varies with subtle myoclonic facial movements and automatisms of face and hands. Complex partial status involves either a series of complex partial seizures, separated by a confusional state, or a prolonged state of partial responsiveness and semipurposeful automatisms.

II. Etiology. Symptomatic status—status caused by a neurologic or metabolic insult—is more common than idiopathic status. Stroke caused more than 25% of the cases in one series. Decreasing antiepileptic medication, alcohol or other drug withdrawal, anoxia, metabolic disorders (electrolyte abnormalities, hypo- or hyperglycemia, uremia, sepsis), and drug toxicity can cause status. Viral encephalitis from Epstein-Barr syndrome or herpes simplex virus can have an abrupt onset heralded by status epilepticus.

III. Prognosis and sequelae. The cause of status is an important factor influencing mortality. Anoxia has the highest mortality rate, followed by hemorrhage, tumor, metabolic disorders, and systemic infection. Status caused by alcohol withdrawal and antiepileptic drug discontinuation, and idiopathic status have lower mortality rates. The duration of status and the patient's age also affect prognosis: in one study, status lasting more than 60 minutes had a mortality rate of 32%, compared with 2.7% for status lasting fewer than 60 minutes. Patients aged more than 70 years have a much higher mortality rate. Overall, status has a mortality rate between 7% and 25%. Status may also cause intellectual deterioration, permanent neurologic deficits, and chronic epilepsy.

IV. Initial assessment and medical management. Status epilepticus is a medical emergency. This discussion concentrates on generalized tonic–clonic status epilepticus—the most common form of status with the most severe neurologic sequelae.

A. Diagnosis. Patients with generalized tonic–clonic status usually do not convulse continuously and observation is necessary to determine that generalized seizures occur without recovery of consciousness. In nonconvulsive or focal motor status, the diagnosis requires 30 minutes of continuous clinical (or electrical) seizure activity. When status epilepticus presents with a change in mental status only, an EEG is required for confirmation.

B. Initial management and medical stabilization. For generalized status, the initial assessment and treatment should begin within 5 minutes of onset of seizure activity (Table 160-1).

The history should include any information on a preexisting chronic seizure disorder and antiepileptic drug use. The examination should focus on signs of systemic illness (e.g., uremia, hepatic disease, infection), illicit drug use, evi-

TABLE 160-1. Management protocol for generalized status epilepticus in adults

1. If diagnosis is uncertain, observe recurrence of generalized seizures without subsequent recovery of consciousness.
2. Assess cardiopulmonary status; establish airway, administer O_2, initiate cardiac monitoring.
3. Start intravenous (IV) line with normal saline.
4. Draw blood for complete blood count and differential, glucose, blood urea nitrogen, creatinine, electrolytes, calcium, antiepileptic drug levels, toxin screen; perform bedside glucose determination.
5. Give glucose (D_{50}) 50 ml and thiamine 100 mg IV if hypoglycemia present.
6. Monitor respirations, blood pressure, ECG, oximetry, and, if possible, EEG.
7. Give lorazepam (0.1 mg/kg) IV bolus, <2 mg/min, if patient is actively seizing.
8. Immediately start phenytoin (20 mg/kg) IV, ≤ 50 mg/min, with slower rate if hypotension develops.
9. Give additional boluses of phenytoin (5 mg/kg), to a maximum of 30 mg/kg, if patient is still seizing.
10. If status continues after phenytoin infusion is completed, immediately start phenobarbital (20 mg/kg) IV ≤ 100 mg/min; intubation is necessary either before or during phenobarbital infusion.
11. If status persists, induce coma with short-acting barbiturate
    a. During induction, continuous EEG to monitor for control of seizures and level of anesthesia is needed.
    b. Pentobarbital: 5 mg/kg IV load, given slowly; give additional 5 mg/kg boluses as necessary to produce burst-suppression pattern is present.
    c. Maintenance infusion of 0.5–5 mg/kg/h.
    d. Monitor EEG hourly once burst-suppression pattern is present.
    e. Stop pentobarbital at 12 hours; if seizures recur, resume infusion for 24 hours, then stop again; continue this process as necessary.

ECG, electrocardiogram; EEG, electroencephalogram.

dence of trauma, or focal neurologic abnormalities. After blood has been obtained, glucose is administered. Hypoglycemic status is rare but easily reversible, and it can cause irreversible central nervous system (CNS) damage if untreated. Because glucose can precipitate Wernicke-Korsakoff syndrome in individuals with marginal nutrition, thiamine should be given. Subsequent intravenous (IV) infusions should consist of saline solution, as some antiepileptic drugs precipitate in glucose solutions. Hyperthermia caused by status should be treated with alcohol sponge baths, cooling blankets, or ice packs. Oxygenation must be maintained. Metabolic acidosis often develops early in status but usually resolves spontaneously once seizures stop; treatment with bicarbonate is usually not necessary. Blood pressure must be carefully monitored; if hypotension occurs, the brain is vulnerable to inadequate perfusion. Pharmacologic intervention for the seizures can exacerbate hypotension. When a metabolic disorder causes status, pharmacologic intervention alone is not effective. Systemic and CNS infections must be excluded; lumbar puncture is often necessary, although leukocytosis, fever, and cerebrospinal fluid pleocytosis may be caused by status itself. A contrast-enhanced head computed tomography scan may demonstrate a structural cause of status, but should be done after the patient has been stabilized and status terminated. Magnetic resonance imaging is preferred but is often not practical in the emergent setting.

V. Pharmacologic management. If seizures persist, IV benzodiazepines are started; if seizures have stopped temporarily or if prolonged stupor is present between attacks, intravenous phenytoin should be started and benzodiazepines may not be necessary. Phenobarbital is as effective as the combination of benzodiazepines and phenytoin for initial therapy, but CNS depression is a major side effect.

A. Benzodiazepines. Diazepam is extremely effective but has a brief duration of action (10–25 minutes); lorazepam is equally effective with a much longer duration of action (2–24 hours). The onset of lorazepam's action is less than 3 minutes, which is rapid enough for the treatment of status. Both benzodiazepines have essentially the same cardiac, respiratory, and CNS depressant side effects. Lorazepam should be given 0.1 mg/kg IV at 2 mg/min; the dose may be repeated if needed, up to a total of 0.2 mg/kg. The dose of diazepam is 0.15 mg/kg, with an additional 0.1 mg/kg if necessary. (*Respiratory depression and apnea can occur abruptly with doses as small as 1 mg.*) Previous administration of sedative drugs (e.g., barbiturates) and increasing age potentiate cardiorespiratory side effects. Hypotension may be partially caused by the propylene glycol solvent in IV diazepam and lorazepam. Rectal diazepam is an alternative; for adults, 7.5 to 10 mg of the IV preparation or 0.2 mg/kg of the rectal gel, is administered per rectum; significant respiratory depression has not been reported with the rectal administration. Absorption of these agents by intramuscular (IM) administration is delayed and incomplete, and this route is unsuitable for treating status.

B. Phenytoin. *Phenytoin* IV is very effective in status (it should *not* be given IM). A 20 mg/kg load is given at 50 mg/min, with an additional 10 mg/kg if the initial load is not effective. Hypotension, electrocardiographic changes and respiratory depression can occur, partly from the propylene glycol diluent. Cardiac monitoring should be performed and the drug given more slowly (25 mg/ min) in elderly patients or in those with a history of cardiac arrhythmias, compromised pulmonary function, or hypotension. The most common adverse effect is hypotension. *Fosphenytoin,* a water-soluble prodrug of phenytoin, is rapidly converted to phenytoin. Fosphenytoin has greater aqueous solubility than phenytoin and propylene glycol is not needed as a diluent. It may be used IV or IM, is nonirritating,, and rapidly and completely absorbed by either route. Therapeutic phenytoin concentrations are attained in 10 minutes with rapid IV infusion and in 30 minutes with slower IV infusion or IM injection. Fosphenytoin should be considered when IV access is not available or phenytoin infusion is poorly tolerated at the infusion site. Fosphenytoin is dosed in "phenytoin equivalents" (PE) units, which are the same as for phenytoin (load 20 mg/kg PE); it is administered at rates up to 150 mg/min PE.

C. Phenobarbital. If status persists 10 minutes after phenytoin is given, IV phenobarbital should be given (10 mg/kg) as an initial dose, then repeated if seizures continue (up to 20 mg/kg). Phenobarbital can be administered up to 100 mg/min. *Respiratory depression is a major side effect,* especially if benzodiazepines have been used, and it is imperative to monitor respirations and ensure an adequate airway.

D. Refractory status epilepticus. If status continues after full loading doses of phenytoin and phenobarbital, a drug-induced coma with barbiturates is indicated. Patients must be intubated and pentobarbital is used most commonly, although thiopental and methohexital have been used successfully. Phenobarbital is not used for this purpose because it causes very prolonged coma. Cardiac depression is often produced and hemodynamic monitoring is required. Pressors are frequently needed. Ileus is also common. Simultaneous EEG monitoring is mandatory during induction of barbiturate coma. The pentobarbital dose must be sufficient to produce a burst-suppression EEG pattern (flat background punctuated by bursts of mixed-frequency activity). If the bursts contain electrographic seizure activity, the coma should be deepened, at times to virtual electrocerebral silence. The goal is to *terminate electrical seizure activity,* not just to produce a burst-suppression pattern. Maintenance doses of phenytoin and phenobarbital are continued and serum levels followed. Intravenous midazolam can be used for refractory status; treatment is initiated with one or two slow IV boluses of 0.1 to 0.3 mg/kg, followed by an infusion of 0.05 to 2 mg/kg/h. The half-life of midazolam can be significantly prolonged in critically ill patients, leading to drug accumulation. Tolerance to midazolam can develop in 36 to 48 hours, leading to escalating dose requirements. For this reason, if status is not terminated within 48 hours of midazolam treatment, changing to a pentobarbital infusion is recommended.

Selected Readings

DeLorenzo RJ, Towne AR, Pellock JM, et al. Status epilepticus in children, adults and the elderly. *Epilepsia* 1992;33 (Suppl 4):515.

Epidemiologic factors and determinants, including age, duration of status epilepticus, and cause, are reviewed in a retrospective study to predict outcome of status epilepticus at different ages.

Lowenstein DH, Alldredge BK. Status epilepticus. *N Engl J Med* 1998;338:970.

Reviews the current concepts in the definition, clinical features, pathophysiology, and management of status epilepticus.

Simon RP. Physiologic consequences of status epilepticus. *Epilepsia* 1985;26(Suppl 1): S58.

Reviews changes in multiple organs of the body as a result of status epilepticus, including pulmonary edema, temperature, metabolic acidosis, hormones, and so on.

Towne AR, Pellock JM, Ko D, et al. Determinants of mortality in status epilepticus. *Epilepsia* 1994;35:27.

Factors, including age, duration of seizure, cerebral vascular disease, discontinuation of antiepileptic drugs, alcohol withdrawal, trauma, and so on, as determinants of mortality in status epilepticus are addressed and discussed in detail.

Treiman DM, Meyers PD, Walton NY, et al. A comparison of four treatments for generalized convulsive status epilepticus. *N Engl J Med* 1998;339:792.

Comparison of lorazepam, diazepam followed by phenytoin, phenytoin, and phenobarbital in the treatment of generalized convulsive status epilepticus in a randomized double-blinded multicenter trial is evaluated with lorazepam being the most effective.

Working Group on Status Epilepticus. Treatment of convulsive status epilepticus. *JAMA* 1993;270:854.

Guidelines on the management of status epilepticus as recommended by an expert panel of the Epilepsy Foundation of America.

161. CEREBROVASCULAR DISEASE

Marjorie Ross, John P. Weaver, and Marc Fisher

I. General principles. Cerebrovascular disease includes stroke caused by thrombotic or embolic ischemia and intracerebral hemorrhage. Admission to the intensive care unit (ICU) setting is often warranted because of the severity of the disease or institution of newer therapies. This chapter focuses on the basic concepts needed for ICU management of cerebrovascular disease.

II. Ischemic cerebrovascular disease (ICVD)

A. Pathophysiology. ICVD is divided into carotid artery and vertebral-basilar system ischemia. Symptoms encountered in carotid system ischemia include aphasia, hemiparesis, or hemiparesthesia, whereas in vertebral-basilar system ischemia, there is disturbance of ipsilateral cranial nerve and the contralateral body function.

Three degrees of completeness can be recognized: transient ischemic attack (TIA), stroke-in-evolution, and completed stroke. A TIA is an episode of cerebrovascular dysfunction that resolves in minutes to hours. A stroke-in-evolution is a cerebrovascular event that worsens over several hours (carotid circulation) to several days (vertebral-basilar system). In a completed stroke, the deficit has been fixed for at least 24 (carotid circulation) to 72 (vertebral-basilar system) hours.

The etiology of ICVD is categorized into (a) large vessel thrombosis from atherosclerosis of carotid or vertebral-basilar arteries; (b) small vessel thrombosis, caused by lipohyalinosis of the lenticulostriate or basilar penetrating arteries, leading to a small stroke termed a “lacune”; (c) cardioembolism, commonly caused by nonvalvular atrial fibrillation, acute transmural myocardial infarction, mechanical cardiac valves, and more rarely, to patent right-to-left shunts; and (d) watershed infarction with globally diminished cerebral blood flow because of cardiac arrest or systemic hypotension, resulting most commonly in infarction between the distribution of the middle cerebral artery and both the anterior and posterior cerebral arteries.

B. Prognosis. The eventual prognosis of a completed stroke in either the carotid or vertebral-basilar distribution cannot be predicted at onset. The overall mortality rate varies from 3% to 20% in both vascular distributions. An altered level of consciousness or coma, dense hemiplegia, and conjugate eye deviation are early signs that point toward a poorer prognosis. A favorable functional outcome is seen in 20% to 70% of cases, with lacunar strokes having the best recovery.

C. Laboratory and radiologic evaluation. Early neuroimaging, which usually confirms the diagnosis, is the key in protocols for therapeutic intervention. Diffusion-weighted magnetic resonance imaging can demonstrate ischemic lesions within minutes of onset.

An electrocardiogram (ECG) should be obtained to look for rhythm disturbances or ischemic change. Echocardiography and cardiac monitoring should be considered. A contrast or transesophageal echocardiogram should also be considered in younger patients with stroke without an obvious cause.

Carotid ultrasound assesses the extracranial vessels, and can distinguish high-grade stenosis from occlusion. Transcranial Doppler ultrasound can provide information about the intracranial vessels. Magnetic resonance angiography is helpful in delineating both intra- and extracranial atherosclerosis. An erythrocyte sedimentation rate, syphilis serology, complete blood count, partial thromboplastin time, and prothrombin time should be obtained. Other blood tests to assess hypercoaguability may be helpful in selected patients.

D. Treatment. Supportive therapy for ICVD patients should begin on hospitalization. Elevated blood pressure should be observed at least 4 hours before antihypertensive therapy is initiated, unless the patient has malignant hypertension. If it remains substantially elevated, it should be carefully lowered by no more than 20% of the mean arterial pressure. Subcutaneous heparin therapy and compression boots should be considered in immobilized patients. Elevated temperature should be lowered. Oral feedings should be delayed until swallowing is well performed.

Standard therapies are directed at preventing progression of the deficit. Acute anticoagulation with heparin is considered in patients with a clear embolic source. An alternative approach is to initiate warfarin after several days. Antiplatelet therapy should be considered in patients who do not have a clear embolic source. Cerebral edema can develop, maximally, at 48 to 72 hours. We consider treating with mannitol and, in some cases, intracranial pressure monitoring to guide therapy.

New therapeutic agents are aimed at either (a) restoring impaired blood flow by dissolving the occluding thrombus or by (b) protecting against the cellular consequences of ischemia. Fibrinolytic therapy with tissue-type plasminogen activator (tPA) was shown to increase the likelihood of minimal or no disability at 3 months by 30% in patients treated in fewer than 3 hours after symptom onset. Symptomatic hemorrhage did occur in 6.4% of patients, highlighting the need for an ICU setting when instituting thrombolytic therapy. Cytoprotection with agents such as citicoline sodium (CDP-choline) may be particularly useful because of a larger therapeutic window.

III. Intracerebral hemorrhage (ICH). Nontraumatic ICH often requires management in the ICU. Most cases are caused by spontaneous (primary) ICH or rupture of saccular aneurysms and arteriovenous malformations.

A. Pathophysiology. Primary ICH is caused by extravasation of arterial blood from ruptured microaneurysms of small intracerebral arterioles. They are commonly observed along the lenticulostriate arteries, thalamoperforant arteries, and paramedian branches of the basilar artery. Continued extravasation of blood results in the formation of a hematoma, with secondary accumulation of cerebral edema, which can increase sufficiently to cause herniation. Intraventricular extension can occur and blood may be identified in the subarachnoid space. ICH can be further complicated by acute obstructive hydrocephalus caused by the intraventricular hemorrhage, or more chronic, nonobstructive hydrocephalus from poor cerebrospinal fluid resorption.

B. Diagnosis. The clinical presentation of ICH is distinctive. The onset is abrupt and neurologic deficits occur progressively over minutes to hours, and may be associated with headache and vomiting. Of patients, 44% to 72% are comatose when first seen by a physician.

The diagnosis of ICH can be made by computed tomography scan, which provides accurate information about the size and site of the hematoma as well as the degree of cerebral edema. Angiography should be considered if an underlying aneurysm or arteriovenous malformation is suspected. Lumbar puncture is contraindicated in ICH because of the risk of tentorial herniation. Testing on admission for ICH should include a coagulation profile and platelet count.

C. Treatment. The acute medical management of ICH is aimed at correction of any predisposing systemic factors to prevent further clinical deterioration. Control of hypertension is a major management problem in these cases. In response to the acute elevation of intracranial pressure (ICP) caused by the hematoma, systemic blood pressure will rise to maintain adequate cerebral perfusion pressure (CPP), which can lead to further bleeding. However, it is important to avoid unfavorable decreases in CPP, which can lead to ischemia. Therefore, the recommended goal of systolic blood pressure in the acute phase of ICH is between 110 and 160 mm Hg. Beta-blockers are the agents of choice. Vasodilators (e.g., Nipride) should be avoided because they can promote cerebral edema and elevate ICP.

Acute increases in ICP may require hyperventilation and hyperosmolar agents, such as mannitol. Treatment of ICH with steroids can be detrimental. The value of ICP monitoring in these situations remains controversial. Elevation of ICP from hydrocephalus is treated with ventriculostomy.

Surgery may be indicated for lobar ICH in which the patient continues to deteriorate, and for many cerebellar ICHs. Early surgical intervention is indicated for lesions greater than 3 cm or in smaller lesions with clinical deterioration, because of a very high untreated mortality rate. Obstructive hydrocephalus at the level of the fourth ventricle is not uncommon. Anticonvulsants are not routinely used in ICH. Prophylaxis against venous thrombosis should be accomplished with pneumatic boots.

After the patient is acutely stabilized, angiography may be performed in patients with no history of hypertension or if the bleeding is in an atypical location. This is particularly true for younger patients in whom a larger percentage of cases of ICH are caused by underlying vascular lesions, such as arteriovenous malformation or aneurysm.

The prognosis for ICH is worse for larger lesions. By location, pontine ICH has the highest mortality, followed by cerebellar and then basal gangliar ICH. Lobar ICH carries the most favorable outlook for survival and functional recovery.

Selected Readings

Bogousslavsky J, Van Melle G, Regli F. The Lausanne stroke registry. *Stroke* 1988; 19:1083.

The first registry with complete computed tomography and Doppler data on all patients, allowing correlation between clinical findings, presumed cause, and stroke location.

Borges LF. Management of nontraumatic brain hemorrhage. In: Ropper AM, Kennedy SF, eds. *Neurological and neurosurgical intensive care.* Rockville, MD: Aspen; 1988: 209.

Management of intracerebral hemorrhage in a text that is essential for all intensive care units.

Chambers BR, Norris JW, Shurvell BL, et al. Prognosis of acute stroke. *Neurology* 1987;27:221.

A helpful discussion of the prognosis of acute stroke.

Clark WM, Portland OR, Warach SJ for the Citicoline Study Group. Randomized dose response trial of citicoline in acute ischemic stroke patients. *Neurology* 1996;46 (S1):A425.

Report on a trial of citicoline, an agent with minimal risks, in acute stroke.

Dewitt LD, Wechsler LR. Transcranial Doppler. *Stroke* 1988;19:915.

An important discussion of a noninvasive technique to assess intracerebral circulation.

The National Institute of Neurological Disorders and Stroke rt-PA Stroke Study Group. Tissue PA for acute ischemic stroke. *N Engl J Med* 1995;333:1581.

The seminal work on tissue-type plasminogen activator in the treatment of acute stroke.

Omae T, Ueda K, Ogata J, et al. Parenchymatous hemorrhage: etiology, pathology and clinical aspects. In: Toule JF, ed. *Handbook of clinical neurology.* Vol 10. New York: Elsevier; 1989:287.

An excellent review on intracerebral hemorrhage.

Ott KH, Kase CS, Ojemann RG, et al. Cerebellar hemorrhage: diagnosis and treatment—a review of 56 cases. *Arch Neurol* 1974;31:160.

An excellent review on cerebellar hemorrhage, which is important because of the differences in management between cerebellar and other types of intracerebral hemorrhage.

Poungvarin N, Bhoopat W, Viniarejakul A, et al. Effects of dexamethasone in primary supratentorial intracerebral hemorrhage. *N Engl J Med* 1987;316:1229.

An important discussion of management of intracerebral hemorrhage.

162. NEURO-ONCOLOGIC PROBLEMS IN THE INTENSIVE CARE UNIT

N. Scott Litofsky and Lawrence D. Recht

I. Introduction. Neuro-oncology encompasses the care of patients with neoplasms affecting the brain, spinal cord, and peripheral nervous system that can arise either within the nervous system itself or spread from systemic malignancies. This chapter discusses the intensive care issues, which may be encountered in neuro-oncology patients, either following their surgery or as complications of their disease.

II. Elevated intracranial pressure (ICP). Elevated ICP frequently complicates the course of patients with cerebral neoplasms, which are aggressive brain tumors that often cause death because of uncontrollable elevations in ICP.

- **A. Mechanisms of elevated ICP.** The skull is a closed space including brain tissue, cerebrospinal fluid (CSF), extracellular water, and blood in vascular spaces. A perturbation of any of these components can increase ICP.
  1. **Brain parenchyma.** As the tumor grows and displaces brain parenchyma, ICP increases.
  2. **Cerebral edema.** Cerebral neoplasms produce vasogenic edema, secondary to leaky blood vessels within or adjacent to the tumor.
  3. **Hydrocephalus.** Tumors can obstruct CSF pathways (see below).
  4. **Hypercarbia.** Increased P_{CO_2} dilates cerebral vasculature; it can occur from hypoventilation, either related to seizure activity or ICP elevation, which can reduce respiratory drive.
- **B. Signs and symptoms**
  1. **Decreased level of consciousness.** As ICP increases, compression of the reticular activating system reduces the patient's level of consciousness, resulting in lethargy, obtundation, or coma.
  2. **Cognitive changes.** The patient may develop disorientation, short-term memory problems, or other cognitive deficits from elevated ICP.
  3. **Papilledema.** As increasing ICP exceeds pressure of the central retinal vein, the patient can develop swelling of the optic disks (papilledema), which can be seen with an ophthalmoscope.
  4. **Pupillary dilation.** As elevated ICP causes the brain to herniate transtentorially, compression of cranial nerve III results in unilateral pupillary dilation.
  5. **Headache.** With stretching of the dura and blood vessels from elevated ICP, the patient may experience headache, often described as "bandlike" or "pressurelike."
- **C. Management.** Mechanical and pharmacologic therapies are available to treat signs and symptoms of elevated ICP.
  1. **Head elevation.** Head elevation increases venous drainage from the brain and reduces blood volume within its vascular compartment, reducing ICP.
  2. **Lasix.** Lasix (1 mg/kg) rapidly reduces systemic circulating volume, which reduces volume in the brain.
  3. **Mannitol.** By increasing serum osmolarity, mannitol (1 g/kg initially, followed by 0.25 g/kg every 4–6 hours) draws fluid out of the brain into the vascular system, reducing brain extracellular water volume.
  4. **Hyperventilation.** Hypocarbia causes cerebral vasoconstriction, which reduces the intravascular blood volume within the brain, thus reducing ICP temporarily. At a P_{CO_2} of less than 25 mm Hg, cerebral ischemia may result. A rebound from hyperventilation can occur within approximately 24 hours, thereby negating its positive effects if used chronically. Hyperventilation requires intubation and mechanical ventilation of the patient.
  5. **Glucocorticosteroids.** Decadron (10–20 mg initially, followed by 4 mg every 6 hours or more as needed) reduces vasogenic edema and can markedly

improve symptoms of elevated ICP or mass effect in patients with cerebral neoplasms.

6. **CSF drainage.** After placement of a ventriculostomy, drainage of CSF can reduce ICP.

III. Hydrocephalus.
Increased volume of CSF under increased pressure may require urgent or emergent intensive care monitoring and treatment.

A. Etiology

1. **Subarachnoid tumor.** Carcinomatous meningitis can prevent the absorption of CSF by the arachnoid granulations. Metastatic tumors from the lung, breast, lymphoma, and leukemia are the most frequently involved systemic tumors; primary tumors behaving in this fashion include primitive neuroectodermal tumors, ependymoblastoma, and glioblastoma multiforme. Alternatively, a large "benign" tumor in the cerebellopontine angle (e.g., meningioma or vestibular schwannoma) can displace the cerebellar hemisphere, obstructing the fourth ventricle and resulting in hydrocephalus.
2. **Intraventricular tumors.** Tumors protruding into the ventricles (e.g., medulloblastoma, ependymoma, choroid plexus papilloma, intraventricular meningioma, colloid cyst and pineal region tumors) can occlude CSF pathways, thus producing hydrocephalus.
3. **Intraparenchymal tumors.** Primary or metastatic tumors in the thalamus or basal ganglia can displace brain parenchyma and occlude the foramen of Monro and third ventricle. Tumors in the pineal region may occlude the posterior third ventricle or cerebral aqueduct. Brainstem gliomas or tumors in the cerebellar hemispheres can compress the fourth ventricle.

B. Management

1. **Ventriculostomy.** In patients experiencing rapidly progressive deterioration (e.g., cerebral herniation), emergent management with a ventriculostomy to divert CSF temporarily can improve the patient's clinical picture. A neurosurgeon performs the procedure, frequently at the bedside. The ventriculostomy can also be used to monitor ICP.
2. **Tumor resection.** Resection of tumor can provide long-term treatment of hydrocephalus by decompressing the CSF pathways.
3. **Ventriculoperitoneal shunt.** Frequently, hydrocephalus related to anatomic considerations will not respond to surgical decompression alone. A permanent ventriculoperitoneal shunt is necessary to treat hydrocephalus in these cases.

IV. Seizure.
Although a seizure may not have long-term effects, if the patient has elevated ICP, a seizure can precipitate rapid deterioration. The associated hypocarbia from hypoventilation can also increase ICP substantially. Prompt intervention, therefore, is necessary, primarily to maintain an adequate airway and reduce or eliminate subsequent seizure activity.

A. Airway management.
Maintenance of an adequate airway and reestablishment of adequate ventilation is essential. Oxygen should be provided to the patient. Intubation and mechanical ventilation may be required.

B. Anticonvulsants

1. **Status epilepticus.** An effective medication to stop continuous epileptic activity acutely is lorazepam (0.1 mg/kg) given IV at less than 2 mg/min initially. The dose can be repeated if needed, up to a total of 0.2 mg/kg. If the patient is not intubated, airway and ventilatory equipment should be available. Phenytoin (20 mg/kg IV, at 50 mg/min) can be used acutely in conjunction with lorazepam.
2. **Long-term anticonvulsants.** Prophylactic anticonvulsants administered before a seizure occurs are rarely indicated unless the patient is going to surgery. Following a seizure, phenytoin and carbamazepine are most frequently used. Phenobarbital, although more sedating than phenytoin, can also be used. Carbamazepine cannot be used acutely in status epilepticus because of its availability in only an oral form.

V. Postoperative complications.
Following neurosurgical procedures, patients are observed in the intensive care unit (ICU) as required by their neurologic and medical conditions for the following intraoperative and postoperative complications.

A. Intracranial hemorrhage. Patients can bleed into the tumor bed or into the subdural or epidural spaces. Although steps are taken at surgery to prevent such complications, patients who experience significant hypertension or significant coughing and "bucking" as they emerge from anesthesia are at greater risk for such an occurrence. Postoperative hemorrhage should be suspected in a patient who fails to emerge adequately from anesthesia, who deteriorates following emergence, or who develops progressive decline in level of consciousness or focal deficits. Prompt evaluation with a computed tomography (CT) scan is indicated, with return to the operating room to remove hemorrhage as necessary. Mannitol may be required if ICP rises while awaiting definitive treatment.

B. Cerebral edema. Manipulation of the brain can lead to cerebral edema. Clinical signs can look quite similar to postoperative hemorrhage, although edema tends to occur later. Prompt treatment with mannitol and dexamethasone are indicated following a CT scan to confirm the cause of the patient's neurologic change.

C. Cerebral infarction. Vessels adjacent to the patient's tumor may be compromised during surgery. Vessels attached to tumor capsule can be injured as they are separated from it. Vessels passing through the body of the tumor may not be recognized as supplying eloquent brain. Manipulation of vessels can also cause subsequent vasospasm and cerebral ischemia. Neurologic deficit secondary to cerebral infarction will depend on the location of the tumor and the number and size of injured vessels. Cerebral infarction can also cause progressive cerebral edema. The neurologic picture may be similar to that with progressive edema from tumor or from postoperative hemorrhage. Evaluation with a CT scan is indicated for diagnosis and management of ICP, as is necessary.

D. Endocrinopathy. Endocrinopathy can result from tumors in the sella and parasellar areas or from surgery designed to treat them.

1. **Hypocortisolemia.** Low serum cortisol is frequently not observed acutely as patients are usually on glucocorticosteroids. However, after cessation of steroid treatment, a patient may experience an Addisonian crisis.
2. **Hypothyroidism.** Hypothyroidism usually does not occur for at least a week following injury to the pituitary gland or hypothalamus.
3. **Diabetes insipidus (DI).** The major endocrinopathy occurring in the ICU setting is diabetes insipidus, most commonly after craniopharyngioma or pituitary tumor resection. It usually occurs between 18 and 36 hours following surgery and is manifest by an increase in urine output greater than 200 ml/h $\times$ 2 hours consecutively, a corresponding drop in urine-specific gravity to less than 1.005, and an increase in serum sodium to greater than 147 mEq/L. Treatment with 1-deamino-[8-D-arginine] vasopressin (DDAVP) (0.25 ml) subcutaneously or intravenous is indicated when DI is recognized. One must be cautious that the patient is actually experiencing DI and is not just mobilizing surgical fluids. DI may be transient or permanent.

VI. Spinal tumors. Spinal tumors are much less common than intracranial tumors. Most patients with spinal tumors do not require ICU treatment. Exceptions include patients with spinal tumors involving the cervical spine or after transthoracic approaches to thoracic spinal neoplasms.

A. Respiratory insufficiency. Patients can have compromise of intracostal musculature or decreased diaphragmatic function with resultant inability to maintain adequate ventilation. Vital capacity should be assessed every 6 hours in these patients, as its decrement will usually be noted before respiratory insufficiency occurs. A decrease below 12 ml/kg usually requires intubation and mechanical ventilation. Once oxygen desaturation is noted, the patient decompensates rapidly.

B. Ileus. Patients with surgery on the spinal cord can experience a temporary ileus, which may require placement of a nasogastric tube not permitting the patient to consume oral substances.

C. Urinary retention. Spinal cord tumors are frequently associated with development of a neurogenic bladder. Patients often require a Foley catheter placed temporarily, which can mask the findings. Attention to urinary retention following removal of the catheter is in order. A long-term intermittent catheterization program to maintain bladder volumes less than 500 ml is necessary if urinary retention persists.

VII. Systemic complications. Frequently, patients with neuro-oncological primary problems will experience systemic complications necessitating evaluation and treatment in the ICU.

A. Deep venous thrombosis (DVT) and pulmonary embolism (PE). Patients with brain and spinal cord tumors are at risk for development of DVT and subsequent PE. Decreased movement of an extremity from a motor deficit predisposes the patient to develop DVT. Alternatively, tumors can be associated with a hypercoagulable state, which will also lead to the development of DVT. Precautions, including use of anti-embolism stockings or sequential leg compression boots, should be taken to prevent DVT from developing. Venous duplex scanning can recognize DVT before it becomes symptomatic. Once identified, treatment with anticoagulation may be problematic, especially in the immediate postoperative period. If within 2 weeks of surgery general anticoagulation is contraindicated, the patient should have placement of an inferior vena cava (Greenfield) filter to prevent PE. After 2 weeks, the judicious use of anticoagulation can be done with much less risk.

B. Cerebral infarction. Related to a hypercoagulable state or premorbid atherosclerosis, patients with neuro-oncologic disease can suffer cerebral infarction. This event should be differentiated from hemorrhage into a tumor or progressive tumor enlargement. A CT scan or magnetic resonance imaging study is essential. Issues regarding anticoagulation must be addressed.

C. Central nervous system infections. Infections in the central nervous system are uncommon in neuro-oncology patients. The likelihood of a postoperative infection in the absence of a CSF leak in a clean operative field (i.e., one that does not go through the paranasal or mastoid sinuses) is approximately 0.8%. Should CSF leak occur or if operative time is extended, the risk increases. Patients can develop wound cellulitis, a bone flap infection, or meningitis. In the presence of fever without another focus or infection or "stiff neck," lumbar puncture is essential to rule out meningitis. This complication tends to occur after 7 to 8 days and may necessitate the return of the patient from the floor to the ICU. Although bone flap infections rarely occur, they can be delayed by several months.

D. Systemic infections. Systemic infections are not uncommon; most often, they include pneumonia, urinary tract infections, or sepsis secondary to line placement. Their management does not differ in the neuro-oncology patient from any other patient in the ICU.

Selected Readings

Apuzzo MLJ, ed. *Brain surgery. Complication avoidance and management.* New York: Churchill Livingstone; 1993.

A comprehensive, two-volume textbook detailing, among other topics, avoidance and management of postoperative complications of surgery for brain tumors.

Kaye AH, Laws ER, eds. *Brain tumors.* Hong Kong: Churchill Livingstone; 1995.

A textbook with extensive descriptions of issues regarding care of brain tumor patients.

Posner JB. *Neurologic complications of cancer.* Philadelphia: FA Davis; 1995.

Definitive monograph by one of the founders of the field, covering all aspects of neuro-oncology with exhaustive references.

Vecht CJ, ed. *Neuro-oncology. Part III. Neurologic disorders in systemic cancer.* In: Vinken PJ, Bruyn GW, eds. *Handbook of clinical neurology.* Amsterdam: Elsevier; 1997.

A recent multiauthored volume in a well-known handbook series addressing neurology of cancer in a comprehensive fashion.

163. GUILLAIN-BARRÉ SYNDROME

Isabelita R. Bella and David A. Chad

I. General principles. The Guillain-Barré syndrome (GBS) is an acute inflammatory-demyelinating polyradiculoneuropathy affecting nerve roots and cranial and peripheral nerves that occurs at all ages. Patients present with an acute, flaccid paralysis with areflexia and elevated spinal fluid protein without pleocytosis. Today, it is the most common cause of rapidly progressive weakness and can be fatal because of respiratory failure and autonomic nervous system abnormalities.

II. Diagnosis

A. Clinical features. The major clinical features of GBS are rapidly evolving weakness (usually over days) and areflexia, heralded by dysesthesias of the feet, hands, or both. Weakness classically ascends from legs to arms but can start from the cranial nerves or arms and descend to the legs. In severe cases, respiratory and bulbar muscles are affected. Proximal muscle involvement is seen early in the course of the disease. Patients can become quadriparetic and respirator-dependent within a few days or can have only mild weakness of the face and limbs. Weakness typically does not progress beyond 1 month; however, progression over 6 to 8 weeks can be seen in a variant of GBS. Progression beyond 2 months is designated "chronic inflammatory demyelinating polyradiculoneuropathy" (CIDP), a disorder with a natural history different from GBS. A small percentage of patients (2% to 5%) have recurrent GBS.

Approximately two thirds of patients have an antecedent event 1 to 3 weeks prior to the onset of GBS. Often this is a flulike or diarrheal illness caused by a variety of infectious agents, including cytomegalovirus, Epstein-Barr and herpes simplex viruses, mycoplasma, chlamydia, and *Campylobacter jejuni.* It can also be associated with human immunodeficiency virus infection, Hodgkin's disease, systemic lupus erythematosus, immunization, general surgery, and renal transplantation. Lyme disease can mimic GBS.

B. Physical findings. Physical examination discloses symmetric weakness in both proximal and distal muscle groups associated with attenuation or loss of deep tendon reflexes. Objective sensory loss is usually mild. Between 10% and 25% of patients require ventilator assistance within 18 days after onset. Patients must be followed carefully with serial vital capacity measurements until weakness has stopped progressing.

Mild to moderate bilateral facial weakness often occurs in addition to bulbar difficulties. Ophthalmoparesis is unusual unless seen in the Miller Fisher variant (characterized by ophthalmoplegia, ataxia, and areflexia, with little limb weakness). Pupillary abnormalities and papilledema are rare.

Autonomic nervous system disturbances are seen in more than 50% of patients. Common findings include cardiac arrhythmias, orthostatic hypotension, and hypertension. Other changes include transient bladder paralysis, increased or decreased sweating, and paralytic ileus.

C. Laboratory features. An elevated cerebrospinal fluid (CSF) protein without an elevation in cells (albuminocytologic dissociation) is characteristic of GBS. The CSF protein may be normal within the first 48 hours but is often elevated within 1 week of onset; rarely it remains normal several weeks after the onset of GBS. The cell count rarely exceeds 10 cells/cm^3 and is mononuclear in nature. When GBS occurs as a manifestation of human immunodeficiency virus infection or Lyme disease, the CSF white cell count is generally increased (25–50 cells). The CSF glucose is always normal.

Electrodiagnostic studies typically disclose slowing (<80% of normal) of nerve conduction velocity, with prolonged distal motor and sensory latencies. The amplitude of the evoked motor responses may be reduced and is frequently dispersed. Early in the course of GBS, routine nerve conduction studies can be normal with the exception of prolonged F responses or absent H reflexes; electromyography may demonstrate only decreased numbers of motor unit potentials firing on voluntary effort. Active denervation changes may be seen several weeks later if no axon loss has occurred. Axonal variants have recently been described.

III. Pathogenesis. GBS is thought to be produced by immunologically mediated demyelination of the peripheral nervous system. It is likely that both humoral and cellular components play a role; however, the exact antigens to which the immune system response is directed have not been identified.

In recent years, the existence of an "axonal" form of GBS has become more widely recognized. The clinical syndrome of GBS may actually encompass a spectrum of pathophysiologic patterns—the traditional acute inflammatory demyelinating polyradiculoneuropathy (AIDP), an acute motor axonal neuropathy (AMAN), and acute motor sensory axonal neuropathy (AMSAN). AMSAN is generally associated with a more severe course and longer time to recovery. The varied presentations may be a result of the immune response targeting different epitopes of peripheral nerve.

IV. Pathology. Pathologic studies have usually shown endoneurial mononuclear cellular infiltration with a predilection for perivenular regions and segmental demyelination. The inflammatory process occurs throughout the length of the nerve (from the level of the root to distal nerve twigs).

V. Differential diagnosis. A number of conditions that must be differentiated from GBS include disorders of the neuromuscular junction (myasthenia gravis and botulism), disorders of peripheral nerve (tick paralysis, shellfish poisoning, toxic neuropathy, acute intermittent porphyria, diphtheritic neuropathy, and critical illness polyneuropathy), motor neuron disorders (amyotrophic lateral sclerosis and poliomyelitis), and disorders of muscle (periodic paralysis, metabolic myopathies, inflammatory myopathies, and myopathy if the patient is in intensive care).

VI. Management and treatment. Close observation for potential respiratory and autonomic nervous system dysfunction is required, preferably in an intensive care unit. Forced vital capacity (VC) and maximal inspiratory pressure should be followed. A baseline arterial blood gas should be obtained. Ropper and Kehne suggest intubation if any one of the following criteria are met: mechanical ventilatory failure with reduced expiratory VC of 12 to 15 ml/kg; oropharyngeal paresis with aspiration; falling VC over 4 to 6 hours; or clinical signs of respiratory fatigue at a VC of 15 ml/kg. Tracheostomy should be delayed as patients can improve rapidly.

Because of potential autononomic dysfunction, careful monitoring of blood pressure, fluid status, and cardiac rhythm is essential in managing patients with GBS. Hypertension can be managed with short-acting α-adrenergic–blocking agents, hypotension with fluids, and bradyarrhythmias with atropine.

Patients can be treated with plasmapheresis or intravenous immunoglobulin (IVIG). Both are equally efficacious. Plasmapheresis requires good venous access and can induce hypotension; patients with cardiovascular disease, therefore, may not tolerate the procedure well. IVIG is easier to administer but can produce side effects such flulike symptoms, headache, and malaise. It should be avoided in patients with IgA deficiency and renal insufficiency.

VII. Outcome. Most patients recover over weeks to months. Approximately 15% have no residual deficits, 65% are restored to nearly normal function, and 5% to 10% are left with severe residual weakness or numbness. Patients with the worst prognosis are those with severely low motor amplitudes on electrodiagnostic studies, presumably from axon loss. Despite close monitoring in the intensive care unit, mortality rates range from 3% to 8%. Causes of fatal outcomes include dysautonomia, sepsis, acute respiratory distress syndrome, and pulmonary emboli.

Selected Readings

Arnason BGW. Acute inflammatory demyelinating polyradiculoneuropathy. In: Dyck PJ, Thomas PK, Griffin JW, et al, eds. *Peripheral neuropathy.* Philadelphia: WB Saunders; 1993:1437.

A comprehensive chapter with a good description of the pathology.

Asbury AK, Cornblath DR. Assessment of current diagnostic criteria for Guillain-Barré syndrome. *Ann Neurol* 1990;27(Suppl):S21.

This article describes the clinical, laboratory, and electrodiagnostic criteria of Guillain-Barré syndrome.

Barohn R, Kissel J, Warmolts J, et al. Chronic inflammatory polyradiculoneuropathy. Clinical characteristics, course, and recommendations for diagnostic criteria. *Arch Neurol* 1989;46:878.

Evaluation of 60 chronic inflammatory polyradiculoneuropathy patients over a 10-year period.

Fisher CM. Unusual variant of acute idiopathic polyneuritis (syndrome of ophthalmoplegia, ataxia and areflexia). *N Engl J Med* 1956;255:57.

This article describes the Miller Fisher variant of Guillain-Barré syndrome.

French Cooperative Group on Plasma Exchange in Guillain-Barré Syndrome. Efficiency of plasma exchange in Guillain-Barré syndrome: role of replacement fluids. *Ann Neurol* 1987;22:753.

This article describes the benefits of plasma exchange if given at an early stage of the disease.

Griffin JW, Li CY, Ho TW, et al. Pathology of the motor-sensory axonal Guillain-Barré syndrome. *Ann Neurol* 1996;39:17.

An excellent article that enlightens the pathophysiology of the various forms of Guillain-Barré syndrome.

The Guillain-Barré Syndrome Study Group. Plasmapheresis and acute Guillain-Barré syndrome. *Neurology* 1985;35:1096.

This classic paper presents the benefits of plasmapheresis as seen in a large randomized trial.

Lichtenfeld P. Autonomic dysfunction in the Guillain-Barré syndrome. *Am J Med* 1971;50:772.

An excellent review of autonomic nervous system findings in Guillain-Barré syndrome.

McKhann GM, Cornblath DR, Griffin JW, et al. Acute motor axonal neuropathy: a frequent cause of acute flaccid paralysis in China. *Neurology* 1993;33:333.

This article describes a syndrome with features similar to Guillain-Barré syndrome but distinguishable from it.

McKhann GM, Griffin JW, Cornblath DR, et al. and the Guillain-Barré Syndrome Study Group. Plasmapheresis and Guillain-Barré syndrome: analysis of prognostic factors and the effect of plasmapheresis. *Ann Neurol* 1988;23:347.

This article describes the important predictive factors associated with poor outcome.

Plasma Exchange/Sandoglobulin Guillain-Barré Syndrome Trial Group. Randomised trial of plasma exchange, intravenous immunoglobulin, and combined treatments in Guillain-Barré syndrome. *Lancet* 1997;349:225.

A prospective trial comparing efficacy of certain treatment options in 383 patients.

Ropper AH. The Guillain-Barré syndrome. *N Engl J Med* 1992;326:1130.

An excellent review of Guillain-Barré syndrome.

Ropper AH, Kehne SM. Guillain-Barré syndrome: management of respiratory failure. *Neurology* 1985;35:1662.

This article suggests criteria for intubation.

Ropper AH, Wijdicks EFM, Truax BT. *Guillain-Barré syndrome.* Philadelphia: FA Davis, 1991.

An authoritative and comprehensive text on Guillain-Barré syndrome.

van der Meche FGA, Schmitz PIM, Dutch Guillain-Barré Study Group. A randomized trial comparing intravenous immune globulin and plasma exchange in Guillain-Barré syndrome. *N Engl J Med* 1992;326:1123.

First large randomized trial showing comparative efficacy of intravenous immune globulin to plasma exchange.

164. MYASTHENIA GRAVIS

Randall R. Long

I. General principles. Myasthenia gravis is an autoimmune disorder in which circulating antibodies interfere with the function of acetylcholine receptors in post-synaptic muscle membrane. As a result, muscular contraction is weakened and fatigue occurs with sustained or repeated contraction.

The prevalence of myasthenia gravis is approximately 1 in 20,000, with a 3:2 female to male predominance. The incidence among women peaks in the third decade and among men in the fifth and sixth decades.

Weakness and fatigability—the clinical hallmarks of the disease—can be mild and limited to the oculomotor muscles or can cause severe generalized weakness with respiratory failure. Ocular and bulbar muscles are most frequently affected. With myasthenic crisis, progressive weakness of bulbar and respiratory muscles results in loss of airway control and hypoventilation. Myasthenic crisis is a medical emergency that can occur acutely with systemic infection, electrolyte imbalance, and following anesthesia or use of other drugs (see below and Table 164-2).

II. Diagnosis. Myasthenia gravis should be considered for patients with unexplained weakness (particularly of ocular and bulbar muscles), muscular fatigue, and temporal fluctuation. Pupillary reflexes, sensation, and deep tendon reflexes are normal, distinguishing it from other acute and subacute paralytic illnesses. It should be considered in patients with unexplained respiratory muscle weakness or failure to wean. The diagnosis is supported by detection of antiacetylcholine receptor antibodies, a positive Tensilon test, and electrodiagnostic studies [nerve conduction studies and electromyography (EMG)].

A. Antiacetylcholine receptor antibodies. Approximately 85% of patients have serum antibodies to subunits of the acetylcholine receptor, although the antibody titer does not correlate with disease severity. The presence of the antibody strongly indicates the disease, but its absence does not exclude it, especially when only ocular manifestations are present.

B. Tensilon test. Edrophonium HCl (Tensilon) is a short-acting, parenteral cholinesterase inhibitor with peak effect within 1 minute of intravenous (IV) injection and a duration of 5 to 10 minutes. A 0.2 ml (2 mg) test dose (10 mg/ml) is given to screen for excessive cholinergic side effects (bradyarrhythmia, gastrointestinal hyperactivity, diaphoresis), which can be minimized by giving 0.5 mg atropine IV prior to the test. Electrocardiographic (ECG) monitoring is recommended. At 1 minute after the test dose, an additional 0.8 ml (8 mg) of edrophonium HCl is given. A positive test reveals transient improvement of a clear motor deficit (e.g., ptosis, ophthalmoparesis, respiratory weakness documented by measuring vital capacity). Positive responses are usually dramatic; if doubt exists, the test should be considered negative. In children, the Tensilon dose should be adjusted (0.03 mg/kg) and one fifth given as the test dose.

C. Electrodiagnostic studies. A decrement in the amplitude of a muscle action potential (>15%) after exercise or slow repetitive nerve stimulation (2–3/sec) is seen in myasthenia gravis; it is most consistently elicited from facial and proximal muscles. Conventional EMG studies are otherwise unaffected in myasthenia gravis. Single-fiber EMG, demonstrating increased jitter, is a sensitive but nonspecific marker of myasthenia gravis.

D. Chest imaging. Once the diagnosis of myasthenia gravis is established, all patients should have a chest imaging study to screen for thymic hyperplasia or thymoma.

III. Perioperative and critical care of the patient with myasthenia gravis. These patients reach the intensive care unit (ICU) setting either because of acute deterioration with respiratory compromise, or following surgery. Both situations are managed identically. *Respiratory failure* can develop rapidly; respiratory function should be monitored compulsively. Forced vital capacity (FVC), maximal inspiratory pressure (MIP), and maximal expiratory pressure (MEP), which are better indices than arterial blood gases and oximetry, should be serially charted. *An FVC less than 20 ml/kg, an MIP not as negative than –25 cm H_2O, or an MEP less than 40 cm H_2O warrant intubation*—even sooner if a clear downward trend is confirmed. Special attention should be given to respiratory toilet in patients with myasthenia gravis on cholinesterase inhibitors which can cause increased secretions.

Acute deterioration in myasthenia gravis patients warrants evaluation of contributing conditions, especially infection (Table 164-1). Medications altering neuromuscular transmission should be avoided (Table 164-2), and a warning about such medications should be on the patient's chart.

IV. Treatment of myasthenia gravis. In patients with myasthenic crisis, immunosuppressive therapy should be started if the patient is not already on it, but the effect is delayed. Plasmapheresis and IV immunnoglobulin (IVIG) are often necessary until the benefits of immunosuppression occur.

A. Plasmapheresis. Most patients demonstrate a clinical response to plasmapheresis within 48 hours, but it is short-lived unless therapy is continued intermittently. Approximately 50 ml/kg/session should be exchanged, approximating 60% to 70% of total plasma volume. Three to seven exchanges are completed at intervals of 24 to 48 hours. If increased sensitivity to cholinesterase inhibitors occurs following plasmapheresis, the dosage should be reduced accordingly.

B. Intravenous human immune globulin also produces rapid yet transient improvement in muscle strength, and is useful in myasthenic crisis or in the perioperative period, particularly for patients who cannot tolerate plasmapheresis. The customary dose is 400 mg/kg/d for 5 consecutive days. Maximal improvement occurs by approximately 7 to 10 days and persists for several weeks.

C. Corticosteroids. Corticosteroids are effective long-term therapy for most patients with a response rate greater than 80%, and many patients achieve complete remission of symptoms. I begin with 25 mg prednisone in a single daily dose, increasing by 5 mg every third day until reaching 60 mg every day. This helps avoid possible transient weakness before improvement, which is important in patients with little respiratory reserve or swallowing difficulty. Plasmapheresis or IVIG prior to corticosteroids may allow more rapid advancement of therapy. Once maximal clinical response is achieved (usually in 2 months), patients are shifted to alternate day therapy by decreasing the off-day dose and increasing the on-day dose by 10 mg once a week. The alternate day dose can then be tapered by 5 mg each month. Many patients can be maintained in remission on as little as 25 mg prednisone every other day; but *the treatment should not be stopped,* as only the rare patient remains in remission if steroids are discontinued. Azathioprine and cyclosporine are alternative agents for longer-term immune therapy, the choice based on clinical response and side effects.

D. Cholinesterase inhibition. Cholinesterase inhibitors were the mainstay of pharmacotherapy for myasthenia gravis prior to immune therapies and thymectomy, but high doses can cause *cholinergic crisis* (increased weakness from overstimulation of the neuromuscular junction). Fasciculations, diaphoresis, and diarrhea also suggest this possibility. With any doubt, discontinue anticholinesterase therapy for at least 24 hours, closely monitoring respiration and airway control. If cholinesterase inhibition is deemed necessary, it can be reinstituted IV until the patient stabilizes. Many patients show increased sensitivity to cholinesterase inhibitors after a drug holiday. Therapy, especially if given IV, should therefore

TABLE 164-1. Conditions that can contribute to interim deterioration in patients with myasthenia gravis

Intercurrent infection; occult infection should be excluded
Electrolyte imbalance (Na, K, Ca, P, Mg)
Cholinergic crisis: if any doubt, discontinue cholinesterase inhibitors
Thyrotoxicosis or hypothyroidism
Medication effects (see Table 164-2)

TABLE 164-2. Medications that can accentuate weakness in patients with myasthenia gravis

Antibiotics	Neuromuscular Blockers and Muscle Relaxants	Antiarrhythmics and Antihypertensives	Antirheumatics	Antipsychotics	Others
Amikacin	Anectine (succinylcholine)	Lidocaine	Chloroquine	Lithium	Opiate analgesics
Clindamycin	Norcuron (vecuronium)	Quinidine	D-penicillamine	Phenothiazines	Oral contraceptives
Colistin	Pavulon (pancuronium)	Procainamide		Antidepressants	Antihistamines
Gentamicin	Tracrium (atracurium)	Beta-blockers			Anticholinergics
Kanamycin	Benzodiazepines	Calcium blockers			
Lincomycin	Curare				
Neomycin	Dantrium (dantrolene)				
Polymyxin	Flexeril (cyclobenzaprine)				
Streptomycin	Lioresal (baclofen)				
Tobramycin	Robaxin (methocarbamol)				
Tetracyclines	Soma (carisoprodol)				
Trimethoprim / Sulfamethoxazole	Quinamm (quinine sulfate)				

TABLE 164-3. Cholinesterase inhibitors and dosage equivalents

		Route and Dose (mg)	
Agent	Commercial Name	Oral	Parenteral
Pyridostigmine bromide	Mestinon	60	2
Neostigmine bromide	Prostigmin	15	—
Neostigmine methylsulfate	Prostigmin	—	0.5

be resumed at a lower equivalent dose (Table 164-3). The IV infusion rate can then be gradually adjusted, depending on clinical status and side effects, until oral intake can be resumed.

E. Thymectomy. Overwhelming evidence now indicates that thymectomy favorably alters the natural history of myasthenia gravis, and should be considered early in the course except for elderly, frail patients. It remains an elective procedure, and patients in crisis should be fully stabilized before considering thymectomy. Thymectomy should be done via a sternal splitting approach that facilitates recognition and removal of all thymus tissue.

V. Conclusion. Respiratory failure is no longer a major source of morbidity or mortality for patients with myasthenia gravis. When it does occur, ventilatory support and airway control should provide the opportunity for resolution of any intercurrent contributing illnesses and rapid institution of immune therapy.

Selected Readings

Asura E. Experience with intravenous immunoglobulin in myasthenia gravis. *Clin Immunol Immunopathol* 1989;53:5170.

A landmark article outlining the use of intravenous immunoglobulin in the management of myasthenia gravis.

Drachman DB, deSilva S, Ramsay D, et al. Humoral pathogenesis of myasthenia gravis. In: Drachman DB, ed. *Myasthenia gravis: biology and treatment.* New York: New York Academy of Sciences; 1987.

An excellent analysis of the immunology of myasthenia gravis.

Howard Jr FM, Lennon VA, Finley J, et al. Clinical correlations of antibodies that bind, block, or modulate human acetylcholine receptors in myasthenia gravis. In: Drachman DB, ed. *Myasthenia gravis: biology and treatment.* New York: New York Academy of Sciences; 1987.

A detailed characterization of the strengths and limitations of antibody testing.

Johns TR. Long-term corticosteroid treatment of myasthenia gravis. In: Drachman DB, ed. *Myasthenia gravis: biology and treatment.* New York: New York Academy of Sciences; 1987.

An excellent overview of long-term immunosuppressive therapy in myasthenia gravis.

Perlo VP, Arnason B, Poskanzer D, et al. The role of thymectomy in the treatment of myasthenia gravis. *Ann NY Acad Sci* 1971;183:308.

A landmark article establishing the role of thymectomy in myasthenia gravis.

Perlo VP, Shahani B, Huggins C, et al. Effect of plasmapheresis in myasthenia gravis. *Ann NY Acad Sci* 1981;377:709.

Confirmation of earlier studies indicating a role for plasmapheresis in myasthenia gravis.

Pinching AJ, Peters DK, Newson-Davis J. Remission of myasthenia gravis following plasma exchange. *Lancet* 1976;2:1373.

A landmark article reporting the effectiveness of plasma exchange in myasthenia gravis.

Seybold ME, Drachman DB. Gradually increasing doses of prednisone in myasthenia gravis. *N Engl J Med* 1974;290:81.

A detailed look at problems associated with the introduction of corticosteroids in the treatment of myasthenia gravis.

165. MISCELLANEOUS NEUROLOGIC PROBLEMS IN THE INTENSIVE CARE UNIT

Nancy M. Fontneau and Ann L. Mitchell

I. **General principles.** This section reviews several neurologic disorders that may require or complicate care in the intensive care unit.

II. **Suicidal hanging.** Hanging is the third most common means of committing suicide. Suicidal hanging usually causes death by slow strangulation and interruption of cerebral blood flow by compression of the jugular veins or carotid arteries. Interruption of blood flow for more than a few minutes results in hypoxic-ischemic injury with neuronal death, cytotoxic and vasogenic edema, increased intracranial pressure, and altered mental status. Coma of greater than 24 hours' duration portends major neurologic dysfunction in survivors. Although some recovery is expected, dementia, amnesia, Korsakoff's syndrome, restlessness, myoclonus, and other movement disorders can result.

Management begins with cardiopulmonary resuscitation to restore adequate cerebral oxygenation. Cervical fracture should be ruled out or stabilized. Careful monitoring is indicated, with endotracheal intubation for airway obstruction from paratracheal or laryngeal trauma, or acute respiratory distress syndrome. Cardiac arrythmias and seizures are treated in the usual fashion. Raised intracranial pressure is treated with hyperventilation-induced hypocarbia, which produces reflex cerebral vasoconstriction.

III. **Electrical injuries.** Approximately 4,000 injuries and 1,000 deaths from electric shock occur annually. The severity of exterior burns, muscle necrosis, myoglobinuria and renal failure, closed head injury, and fractures depends on the voltage sustained. Alternating current is particularly problematic in that it can cause ventricular fibrillation and respiratory arrest. The tissues of the nervous system are especially vulnerable to injury, and acute or chronic neurologic sequelae are found in 25% of patients. Most common neurologic injuries involve the cervical spinal cord and peripheral nerves of the upper extremity, because the path of current most often flows through one or both arms to the ground. When current passes through the brain, patients can develop transient unconsciousness, seizures, confusion, cerebral edema, and brain hemorrhage. Patients may recover fully from their neurologic dysfunction or delayed sequelae can occur.

Management begins with cardiopulmonary resuscitation and monitoring for delayed cardiac arrhythmias. Spine and long bone fractures require stabilization. Isosmotic fluid resuscitation and alkalization of the urine help to prevent myoglobin nephropathy, similar to management in crush injuries. Debridement and fasciotomy may be necessary to prevent compartment syndrome. Extensive burns should be managed in specialized units. Tetanus prophylaxis is indicated.

IV. **Carbon monoxide poisoning.** Carbon monoxide (CO) gas is a colorless, tasteless, and odorless by-product of incomplete combustion. The atmospheric CO concentration is normally less than 0.001%, and CO concentrations of 0.1% can be fatal. CO binding to hemoglobin has a significantly longer half-life than oxygen, resulting in accumulation of carboxyhemoglobin. Clinical effects depend on the carboxyhemoglobin level as outlined in Table 165-1.

Treatment consists of administration of 100% oxygen by tight-fitting, nonrebreathing face mask, with a goal carboxyhemoglobin level of less than 5%. Hyperbaric oxygen therapy, if available, is useful for treating cerebral edema. Steroids are not useful. Of patients, 75% recover quite well; 10% to 30% develop memory impairment or extrapyramidal signs reminiscent of Parkinsonism, which results from the particular predilection for neuronal loss in the basal ganglia and substantia nigra from CO exposure.

V. **Decompression sickness.** Decompression sickness ("the bends") occurs when gases dissolved in body fluids under high atmospheric pressure come out of solu-

TABLE 165-1. Clinical effects of carbon monoxide poisoning based on carboxyhemoglobin level

Carboxyhemoglobin, %	Clinical Effects
< 10	Mild headache, dyspnea on exertion
10–20	Headache, easy fatiguability
20–30	Pounding headache, impaired dexterity, blurred vision, irritability
30–40	Weakness, nausea and vomiting, confusion or delirium, cherry red color
> 40	Tachycardia, arrhythmia
> 50	Seizures, respiratory insufficiency
> 60	Coma
60–70	Coma, death

tion under conditions of lower pressure. Situations under which decompression sickness can arise include rapid ascent of tunnel workers or scuba divers, decompression or high altitude flying with inadequate cabin pressure, and flying after scuba diving. The result is the formation of small gas bubbles in the tissues and venous blood. The bubbles can coalesce, causing local tissue ischemia or venous obstruction. Nearly 80% of patients with decompression sickness have neurologic symptoms. Focal or diffuse paresthesia is the most frequent symptom, affecting the skin and joints. Weakness of one or more limb can also occur. Visual disturbances, vertigo, headache, lethargy, paralysis, and unconsciousness are infrequent signs of small gas bubbles affecting the cerebral circulation.

Air embolism is a more severe and acute decompression illness. Overinflation of the lungs causes rupture and gas bubble formation in the pulmonary veins. Normally, the lungs filter these bubbles, but cerebral arterial embolism can result if a patent foramen ovale exists. Unconsciousness and stupor are the most common symptoms, with onset usually within 5 minutes of decompression. Most patients improve when the gas bubbles redistribute in the venous circulation. Cardiopulmonary arrest can occur.

Recompression is the definitive treatment, and the patient should be moved to the nearest decompression chamber with minimal delay. Interim management consists of placing the patient in the Trendelenberg position on the left side, and administrating 100% oxygen with air breaks to avoid pulmonary oxygen toxicity. Intubation may be needed if pulmonary edema develops. Pneumothorax or pneumomediastinum should be treated with chest tube drainage. Circulatory support with colloid and vasopressors may be required. Although steroids are often used to reduce cerebral edema in decompression sickness, no role has yet been proved for them in these cases. The National Diving Accident Network maintains a 24-hour phone consultation service to assist with diving accidents (Duke University, 919-684-2948 daytime; or 919-684-8111 24-hour emergency line).

Remarkable recovery can occur after recompression. Although recompression should be carried out as quickly as possible, treatment can be effective even after delays of up to 2 weeks. Relapse requiring repeated decompression treatment occurs in 30% to 50% of patients.

VI. Cerebral fat embolism syndrome. Cerebral fat embolism syndrome is characterized by diffuse pulmonary insufficiency with hypoxemia, neurologic dysfunction, fever, tachycardia, cutaneous petechiae, thrombocytopenia, and anemia occurring 12 to 48 hours after trauma, usually involving long bone fracture. Present pathologically are microscopic fat emboli in the gray matter, perivascular hemorrhages involving predominantly the cerebral and cerebellar white matter, and cerebral edema. Confusion, impaired consciousness, seizures, and coma are the most common neurologic symptoms. Focal neurologic signs (e.g., aphasia, hemiparesis, or decerebrate rigidity) are seen in approximately one third of patients.

Management begins with rapid immobilization of fractures, which decreases the incidence of fat embolism; attention to oxygenation; and fluid resuscitation. Computed tomography of the brain is required to rule out direct traumatic brain injury as the cause of neurologic symptoms. Raised intracranial pressure is managed by hyperventilation. Steroid therapy has not proved useful. The mortality rate can reach 10% to 20%, and permanent neurologic deficit results in 25% of patients.

VII. Hiccup. Hiccup is usually a benign self-limited condition. Prolonged hiccup can produce fatigue, sleeplessness, weight loss, difficulty in ventilation, and wound dehiscence. Troublesome hiccup is most common in patients with chest, abdomen, neck, and brainstem disorders, which damage or irritate the brainstem or phrenic, vagus, or spinal nerves. Metabolic disorders (e.g., uremia), gastroesophageal reflux disease, and toxic exposures can also result in hiccup.

Management consists of searching for and treating the underlying structural or metabolic disorder. Physical examination, appropriate radiographs, computed tomography or magnetic resonance imaging, electrolytes, glucose, blood urea nitrogen, creatinine, and a toxic screen for alcohol and barbiturates are the core studies. If central nervous system infection is suspected, lumbar puncture should be performed.

Medications and mechanical means can alleviate hiccup in most patients. Chlorpromazine (25–50 mg) can be given orally or intramuscularly three to four times a day. If this is ineffective, intravenous infusion of chlorpromazine (25–50 mg in 500 ml of normal saline) is indicated. Metoclopramide (10 mg) can be given orally four times a day; oral haloperidol (5 mg) given three times a day may also prove effective. Nonpharmacologic therapy for hiccup is effective because it alters the reflex arc responsible. Mechanical stimulation of the posterior pharynx via a red rubber catheter inserted through the nares, nasogastric intubation, and swallowing dry granulated sugar may abolish hiccup. Refractory hiccup can be treated surgically or by transcutaneous stimulation of the phrenic nerve.

VIII. Peripheral nerve disorders. Several peripheral nerve disorders are linked to the severity of the illness that makes intensive care necessary. *Critical illness polyneuropathy* is a complication of sepsis with multiple organ system failure. It is most commonly seen in patients with sepsis of greater than 2 weeks' duration and should be suspected when a patient is improving but fails to wean from the ventilator. In addition to weak respiratory muscles, the distal limb muscles are weak, tendon reflexes are reduced or absent, and sensory abnormalities are present. Except for occasional mild face weakness, cranial nerves are spared. The cause of these disorders is unclear. Diagnosis is by electromyography and nerve conduction studies. No specific treatment exists. *Compression neuropathies* also occur in the critically ill patient, and can result in significant delayed morbidity. The peroneal nerve at the fibular head and the ulnar nerve at the elbow are most commonly involved, but compression at these sites can be avoided by proper patient positioning. Additional nerves and the brachial or lumbar plexus may be compressed by hematomas resulting from trauma or from idiopathic or iatrogenic clotting disorders. Treatment is supportive in most patients, and prevention is preferred.

Selected Readings

Apfelberg DB, Masters FW, Robinson DW. Pathophysiology and treatment of electrical injuries. *J Trauma* 1974;14:453.

Pathophysiology, a treatment algorithm, and photographs of patients' electrical injuries in a helpful overview.

Bolton CF. The peripheral nervous system: effects of sepsis and critical illness. *Annals of the Royal College of Physicians and Surgeon Canada* 1986;19:371.

A fine review of clinical and electrophysiologic signs of critical illness polyneuropathy and its differential diagnosis.

Kamenar E, Burger P. Cerebral fat embolism: a neuropathological study of a microembolic state. *Stroke* 1980;11:477.

Good neuropathologic description.

McHugh TP, Stout M. Near-hanging injury. *Ann Emerg Med* 1983;12:774.
A good immediate response approach.

Melamed Y, Shupak A, Bitterman H. Medical problems associated with underwater diving. *N Engl J Med* 1992;326:30.
Excellent review of underwater diving injuries.

Min SK. A brain syndrome associated with delayed neuropsychiatric sequelae following acute carbon monoxide intoxication. *Acta Psychiatr Scand* 1986;73:80.
An excellent clinical overview.

Williamson BWA, MacIntyre IMC. Management of intractable hiccup. *BMJ* 1977;2:501.
Excellent review that includes a useful treatment algorithm.

166. SUBARACHNOID HEMORRHAGE

John P. Weaver, Marc Fisher, and Daniel F. Hanley

I. General principles. Intracranial hemorrhage secondary to the rupture of saccular aneurysms accounts for 6% to 8% of all strokes. The mortality and morbidity associated with subarachnoid hemorrhage (SAH) are significant, causing disability despite modern medical or surgical management, rehabilitation, and chronic care provided in these cases.

Subarachnoid hemorrhage is a form of stroke requiring active treatment. Management of SAH caused by a ruptured aneurysm includes early surgery to limit rebleeding, a calcium antagonist to ameliorate cerebral injury secondary to vasospasm, blood volume replacement in cases of a deficit, and circulatory control.

II. Pathogenesis. Saccular (berry) aneurysms are distinguished from other types of intracerebral aneurysms caused by trauma, vascular dissection, mycotic lesions, and those related to tumors. Of saccular aneurysms, 85% are located in the anterior circulation and 15% in the posterior circulation. Multiple aneurysms can occur in families or with systemic diseases such as polycystic kidney, Marfan's syndrome, Ehlers-Danlos syndrome, pseudoxanthoma elasticum, fibromuscular dysplasia, and coarctation of the aorta.

III. Symptoms. The clinical symptoms of intracranial aneurysms result from their expansion or rupture. Expansion can cause localized headache, facial pain, pupillary dilation and ptosis (from oculomotor nerve compression), and visual field defects (from optic nerve or chiasm compression).

A warning leak, or sentinel hemorrhage, which occurs in approximately 20% of patients, can be misdiagnosed. The physician should have a high index of suspicion for aneurysmal expansion or warning leak because such events precede major hemorrhage. Aneurysmal rupture typically produces severe headache, neck pain, nausea and vomiting, photophobia, lethargy, or loss of consciousness, reflecting the acute rise in intracranial pressure.

IV. Diagnostic evaluation Subarachnoid hemorrhage is evaluated as follows:

1. A noncontrast head computed tomography (CT) is used to identify, localize, and quantify the hemorrhage.
2. A lumbar puncture is indicated if the CT is nondiagnostic.
3. If surgery is emergent, CT angiography is the preferred study.
4. Four-vessel cerebral angiography is necessary to localize the aneurysm (or aneurysms), define the vascular anatomy, and assess vasospasm. If angiography does not reveal an aneurysm, magnetic resonance imaging and angiography can be performed to reveal aneurysms larger than 4 mm. If these studies are also negative, angiography is repeated in 2 to 3 weeks.

V. General medical management. Preoperative medical management includes bedrest, head elevation to improve cerebral venous return, pulmonary toilet, thrombophlebitis prophylaxis, antiemetics, anticonvulsant prophylaxis, and pain control. A systolic blood pressure over 160 mm Hg is managed with beta-blocking agents, which also reduce the risks of cardiac arrhythmias.

Hyponatremia can develop from hypothalamic dysfunction, causing the syndrome of inappropriate antidiuretic hormone, or to a salt-wasting diuresis, caused by an increase in circulating natriuretic peptide levels and iatrogenic volume expansion. Fluid balance, serum electrolytes, and osmolarity must be followed. Hyponatremia after SAH is treated with normal saline to support central venous pressure (CVP). Fluid restriction is rarely needed; if used, however, CVP should be monitored to minimize hypotension. Elevated intracranial pressure must be treated promptly with mannitol or ventricular cerebrospinal fluid (CSF) drainage.

Hypothalamic damage can cause cardiac dysrhythmias from excessive sympathetic stimulation; other cardiac complications can also occur with SAH.

A. Neurologic complications

1. **Rebleeding** is a serious and frequent neurologic complication of SAH, which postulated to be caused by breakdown of the perianeurysmal clot. The peak incidence of rebleeding occurs during the first day after SAH and one half to two thirds of patients die at the time of rebleeding. The antifibrinolytic agent epsilon aminocaproic acid (Amicar) can be used in patients not undergoing early surgery or at high risk of rebleeding, but it increases the risk of vasospasm.
2. **Hydrocephalus** can develop acutely within the first 24 hours after SAH because of impaired CSF resorption at the arachnoid granulations or intraventricular blood obstruction of CSF outflow. Ventricular drainage or shunting may be indicated.
3. **Cerebral vasospasm** is a major cause of morbidity and mortality. Noted angiographically in 70% of patients, vasospasm causes symptoms because of cerebral ischemia in only 36% of cases. The clinical presentation of vasospasm occurs progressively: it can be apparent as early as the third day after hemorrhage with a peak between days 4 to 12; it occurs more frequently in patients with a poor clinical condition, thick focal blood clots, or a diffuse layer of blood in the subarachnoid space. Neurologic deficits are correlated with the areas of cerebral ischemia. Vasospasm is diagnosed by angiography or noninvasively by transcranial Doppler (TCD.

VI. Hyperdynamic therapy. The current mainstay of therapy for symptomatic vasospasm is hypervolemic, hypertensive, hemodilution therapy to augment cerebral blood flow (CBF). Elevation of arterial pressure increases CBF; volume augmentation provides hemodilution, decreases viscosity, and improves cerebral microcirculation. Criteria to initiate treatment include increased TCD blood flow velocity, focal neurologic deficits, or impaired consciousness without hydrocephalus. Inotropic drugs are used to keep systolic blood pressures 20 to 40 mm Hg over pretreatment levels, and plasma volume is expanded with albumin, hetastarch, or plasmanate. Hematocrit is maintained at approximately 30. Risks of therapy include myocardial infarction, congestive heart failure, dysrhythmias, hemorrhagic infarcts, rebleeding, hyponatremia, and hemothorax.

VII. Calcium antagonists. The calcium antagonist nimodipine can ameliorate neurologic deficits caused by delayed vasospasm. Nimodipine exerts a beneficial effect by (a) decreasing postinjury intracellular calcium; (b) dilating leptomeningeal vessels; (c) improving collateral circulation to ischemic areas; (d) improving erythrocyte deformability; or (e) exerting an antiplatelet aggregating effect. The only adverse effect is mild transient hypotension. Nimodipine (60 mg) is given orally every 4 hours for 21 days from the onset of SAH. If hypotension occurs, the dose is divided in half and administered every 2 hours.

VIII. Surgical management. Current standard surgical management is craniotomy with clip occlusion of the aneurysm neck, usually within 48 hours of rupture in most noncomatose patients. The appropriate timing for surgical intervention for comatose patients is controversial. Unique problems that dictate the use of specialized techniques included vertebral-basilar system aneurysms, giant aneurysms (> 25 mm), and multiple aneurysms.

IX. Postoperative management. Angiography is performed to evaluate occlusion of the aneurysm and patency of the surrounding vessels. Treatment of intracranial hypertension may require an intracranial pressure monitor, and central venous pressure monitoring is required for hypervolemic–hypertensive therapy. The patient may be discharged from the intensive care unit when the aneurysm has been obliterated, the risk of vasospasm has passed, and other urgent medical problems have been successfully treated.

The TCD studies performed serially as a bedside test of arterial blood flow velocity (BFV), are sensitive to the onset of cerebral vasospasm; an elevated BFV often precedes ischemic complications of vasospasm. More aggressive medical treatment aimed to increase cerebral perfusion pressure and improve circulation rheology can be instituted before the onset of neurologic impairment.

X. Interventional neuroradiology. Endovascular techniques including balloon occlusion, coil technologies, angioplasty, and intraoperative arteriographic definition of vascular reconstruction are used to treat aneurysms by occluding the parent artery or by selective occlusion of the aneurysm. Early clinical reports demonstrate a relatively high success rate for aneurysm obliteration and lower morbidity and mortality than either balloon or free-coil embolization. Angioplasty can be used to treat constricted arteries during cerebral vasospasm in patients with arteriographic vasospasm without infarction and with a clipped aneurysm. Most successful angioplasties are performed in the first 48 hours after onset of major symptoms because the procedure is much less effective after cerebrovascular reserve is depleted and vascular fibrosis occurs.

Selected Readings

Biller J, Godersk JC, Adams HP. Management of aneurysmal subarachnoid hemorrhage. *Stroke* 1988;19:1300.

An excellent article describing management of SAH.

Diringer MN, Wu KC, Verbalis JG, et al. Hypervolemic therapy prevents volume contraction but not hyponatremia following subarachnoid hemorrhage. *Ann Neurol* 1992;31:543.

Fluid management following SAH.

Guglielmi G, Vinuela F, Dion J, et al. Electrothrombosis of saccular aneurysms via endovascular approach. *J Neurosurg* 1991;75:8.

Heffez DS, Passonneau JV. Effect of nimodipine on cerebral metabolism during ischemia and recirculation in the mongolian gerbils. *J Cereb Blood Flow Metab* 1985;5:523.

Calcium antagonist treatment for ischemic neurologic deficits.

Heros RC, Kistler JP. Intrancranial arterial aneurysm: an update. *Stroke* 1983;14:628.

Articles associating connective tissue and familial disease with aneurysms.

Heros RC, Kistler JP. Subarachnoid hemorrhage due to a ruptured saccular aneurysm. In Ropper AH, Kennedy SF, eds. *Neurological and neurosurgical intensive care.* Rockville, MD: Aspen Publishers; 1988:219.

A standard textbook of neurological intensive care medicine.

Jakobsson KE, Saveland H, Hillman J, et al. Warning leak and management outcome in aneurysmal subarachnoid hemorrhage. *J Neurosurg* 1996;85:995.

Article documenting the frequency of missed SAH.

Kassell NF, Sasaki T, Colohan ART, et al. Cerebral vasospasm following aneurysmal subarachnoid hemorrhage. *Stroke* 1985;16:562.

Correlation between angiography and clinical presentation of vasospasm.

Newel DW, Eskridge JM, Mayberg MR, et al. Angioplasty for the treatment of symptomatic vasospasm following subarachnoid hemorrhage. *J Neurosurg* 1989;71:654.

Interventional neuroradiology techniques for treating aneurysms and complications of aneurysm rupture.

Nichols DA, Meyer FB, Piegras DG, et al. Endovascular treatment of intracranial aneurysms. *Mayo Clin Proc* 1994;69:272.

Stebbens WE. *Pathology of the cerebral blood vessels.* St. Louis: CV Mosby; 1972:351.

The early definition of intracranial aneurysm anatomy and location.

West HH, Mani RI, Eisenberg RL. Normal cerebral arteriography in patients with spontaneous subarachnoid hemorrhage. *Neurology* 1972;27:592.

Diagnostic imaging following hemorrhage and early non-diagnostic studies.

Wilkins RM. Subarachnoid hemorrhage and saccular intracranial aneurysm: an update. *Surg Neurol* 1981;15:92.

XIV. TRANSPLANTATION

167. CRITICAL CARE OF ORGAN TRANSPLANT RECIPIENTS—INTRODUCTION

Abhinav Humar and David L. Dunn

I. General principles. The increased number of solid organ transplants during the last two decades has been paralleled by significant improvement in both patient and graft survival. This improvement has been attributed to a variety of factors: (a) the introduction in the early 1980s of a powerful immunosuppressive agent—cyclosporine A—followed almost a decade later by tacrolimus and mycophenolate mofetil; (b) the availability of antilymphocyte antibody preparations to treat rejection episodes; (c) improvements in organ preservation (e.g., use of University of Wisconsin solution); (d) thorough preoperative patient screening for existing disease processes; and (e) increasing sophistication in the postoperative intensive care of both typical and high-risk recipients. In addition, the availability of potent but nontoxic antibacterial, antifungal, and antiviral agents has allowed more effective treatment of opportunistic infections. Combined with refinements in surgical techniques, all these factors have led to the increasing success of solid organ replacement therapy.

Thus, transplantation has become the treatment of choice for many patients with end-stage failure of the kidneys, liver, endocrine pancreas, heart, lung, and most recently, the small bowel. Criteria for potential recipients have been expanded to include infants, children, and individuals thought to be at higher risk for complications (e.g., diabetic or older patients). Currently, the only patients who are excluded are those who have had malignancies that readily metastasize, those who suffer uncontrolled infections or diseases with high allograft recurrence rates, and those who are unable to withstand major surgery or who have a significantly shortened life expectancy because of disease processes unrelated to their organ dysfunction or failure.

II. Kidney. Since the first successful kidney transplant in 1954, results have dramatically improved such that it is now the treatment of choice for patients of all ages with end-stage renal disease. Current graft survival rates are excellent (87% at 1 year, 66% at 4 years). Kidney transplants improve quality of life and are less expensive, from a socioeconomic standpoint, than chronic hemodialysis. For pediatric patients with chronic renal failure, a functioning renal allograft is the only way to preserve normal growth and ensure adequate central nervous system, mental, and motor development.

III. Liver. From an essentially experimental procedure with poor results in the early 1980s, liver transplantation has progressed to become the treatment of choice for patients with acute and chronic end-stage liver disease. A dramatic improvement in graft survival occurred after the introduction of cyclosporine; the rate increased from 30% at 1 year in the early 1980s to more than 85% in the late 1990s. Liver transplants are an effective treatment for many patients, both pediatric and adult, regardless of the cause of liver failure: congenital (structural or metabolic defects), acquired (infection, trauma, intoxication), or idiopathic (cryptogenic cirrhosis, autoimmune hepatitis). Currently, no reliable means exists to substitute for a failing liver other than with a transplant. Extracorporeal perfusion, using either animal livers or bioartificial livers, may someday bridge the gap between liver failure and transplantation; clinical trials are underway.

The initial success of liver transplants led to an exponential growth in the number performed. But in the last few years the growth rate has significantly declined because of the limited number of suitable organ donors. Given the increasing disparity between the number of cadaver donors and potential recipients, recent attempts have been made to expand the donor pool. Such attempts include the use of marginal donors and innovative surgical techniques (e.g., living related transplants and split-liver transplants).

IV. Pancreas and islet cells. Primary prevention of type I (insulin-dependent) diabetes mellitus is not yet possible. Transplantation of the entire pancreas or of isolated islet cells, however, can correct the endocrine insufficiency once it occurs. At present, a pancreas transplant is the only effective option to restore continuous, near-physiologic normoglycemia. Recent evidence supports the notion that good metabolic glycemic control decreases the incidence and severity of secondary diabetic complications (neuropathy, retinopathy, vasculopathy, and nephropathy). Most pancreas transplants today are performed simultaneously with a kidney transplant in preuremic patients who have significant renal dysfunction (serum creatinine > 3.0 mg/dl) or in uremic patients who have end-stage diabetic nephropathy. However, patients with labile type I diabetes mellitus (hypoglycemic unawareness, repetitive episodes of diabetic ketoacidosis) may undergo a solitary pancreas transplant without a concomitant kidney transplant to improve their quality of life and with the intention of preventing the manifestations and progression of secondary diabetic complications. Islet transplants are undergoing intensive clinical investigation and may become a viable option within the near future.

V. Small bowel. Small bowel transplants are increasingly being performed in patients with congenital or acquired short bowel syndrome, especially if liver dysfunction occurs because of long-term total parenteral nutrition or if establishing or maintaining central venous access is difficult. If the liver disease is advanced, a combined liver–small bowel transplant should be performed. Early results are encouraging: the number of small bowel transplants will assuredly increase over the next decade.

VI. Heart. Heart transplants are the treatment of choice for patients with end-stage congenital and acquired parenchymal and vascular diseases of the heart. They are recommended after all conventional medical or surgical options have been exhausted. The field of heart transplantation experienced dramatic growth in the 1980s, thanks largely to improved immunosuppression and refinements in diagnosing and treating rejection episodes. Mechanical devices such as ventricular assist devices or the bioartificial heart now can bridge the gap between heart failure and a transplant; in the future, they may become a viable alternative to a transplant.

VII. Heart–lung and lung. Heart–lung and lung transplants are an effective treatment for patients with advanced pulmonary parenchymal or vascular disease, with or without primary or secondary cardiac involvement. This relatively new field has evolved rapidly since the first single-lung transplant with long-term success was performed in 1983. The increase in lung transplants, in large part, has occurred because of technical improvements that have resulted in fewer surgical complications. Mechanical ventilation or extracorporeal membrane oxygenation can be a temporary bridge to a transplant, but their use does not obviate the need for organ replacement.

VIII. Future of organ transplantation. Our increasing knowledge of immunobiology, the development and clinical application of a series of new immunosuppressive agents, and advances in surgical techniques and critical care have contributed to significant advances in the field of solid organ transplantation. However, although short-term results achieved after most transplants are excellent, long-term results are not as impressive. There continues to be a steady attrition of grafts after several years because of chronic graft failure. The adverse effects of immunosuppression (e.g., infection, malignancy) continue to cause patient deaths. These problems, along with the ever-increasing donor organ shortage, will be the main challenges facing the field of transplantation during the upcoming years.

Selected Readings

Barnard CN. The operation: A human cardiac transplant: an interim report of a successful operation performed at Groote Schuur Hospital, Cape Town. *S Afr Med J* 1967;41:1271.

The original report of the first successful heart transplant performed by Dr. C. Barnard.

Cooley DA. *A brief history of heart transplants and mechanical assist devices. Support and replacement of the failing heart.* Philadelphia: Lippincott–Raven; 1996.
An excellent chapter on the history of heart transplants written by a pioneer in the field.

Hamburger J, Crosnier J, Bach JF, et al. *Renal transplantation: theory and practice,* 2nd ed. Baltimore: Williams & Wilkins; 1981.
This historically relevant book provides insight into the evolution of current approaches to renal transplantation.

Kahan BD, ed. Horizons in organ transplantation. *Surg Clin North Am* 1994;74:991.
An excellent, concise look at many major topics.

Organ transplantation. Issues and recommendation. Report of the Task Force on Organ Transplantation, US Department of Health and Human Services; 1986:36.
A good outline of important issues regarding cadaver donors.

Starzl TE, Iwatsuki S, Von Thiel DH. Evolution of orthotopic liver transplant. *Hepatology* 1982;2:613.
A good historical overview.

Stratta RJ, Taylor RJ, Larsen JL, et al. Pancreas transplantation: state of the art. *Int J Pancreatol* 1995;17:1.
A recent review of the risks, benefits, and consequences.

168. CRITICAL CARE OF KIDNEY TRANSPLANT RECIPIENTS

Abhinav Humar, Rainer W.G. Gruessner, and David L. Dunn

I. General principles. Kidney transplantation has emerged as the treatment of choice for end-stage renal failure. Compared with dialysis, a successful transplant offers a better quality of life at an overall lower cost. However, despite significant improvements in patient and graft survival rates, kidney transplant recipients can develop a number of problems that require management in the critical care setting.

II. Pretransplant evaluation. One important aspect of the patient's pretransplant evaluation is obtaining information that may predict the need for perioperative intensive care unit (ICU) monitoring. Information should be sought regarding potential sources of infection as well as cardiovascular, gastrointestinal, pulmonary, neurologic, and genitourinary risk factors. If such problems are identified, then appropriate prophylactic and therapeutic measures should be initiated, thereby preventing many complications posttransplant.

III. Intraoperative and postoperative care. Intraoperative care of transplant recipients is not unlike that of other patients undergoing major surgical procedures. To decrease the incidence of acute tubular necrosis (ATN) posttransplant, a liberal hydration policy is employed intraoperatively.

Postoperatively, careful attention to fluid and electrolyte management is crucial. In patients with good initial graft function, fluid replacement can be regulated by hourly replacement of urine. Aggressive replacement of electrolytes, including calcium, magnesium, and potassium, may be necessary if patients are undergoing brisk diuresis. Patients with ATN and fluid overload or hyperkalemia may need fluid restriction, and can require hemodialysis. Monitoring for complications (surgical and medical) remains a critical task posttransplant.

IV. Surgical complications

A. Hemorrhage. Bleeding is rare after a kidney transplant; it usually occurs from unligated vessels in the graft hilum. Reexploration is seldom required.

B. Allograft thrombosis. Although the incidence of vascular thrombosis of the renal allograft is low ($< 1\%$), it is a devastating complication, usually necessitating transplant nephrectomy. Renal artery thrombosis usually presents with sudden onset of anuria. Risk factors include hypotension, multiple renal arteries, and unidentified intimal flaps. Sudden onset of graft swelling, pain, and significant hematuria characterize renal vein thrombosis. The diagnosis of vascular thrombosis is best confirmed by a Doppler ultrasound study. Although salvage of the graft is theoretically possible, its removal is usually required. Other vascular complications include aneurysms and renal vessel stenosis, but these are rare and generally are observed well after the immediate posttransplant period.

C. Urologic. Mild hematuria, which is not infrequent, is usually observed in the first 12 to 24 hours posttransplant; in most patients it resolves spontaneously. More extensive bleeding can result in retained blood clots and urinary tract obstruction, which is the most common cause of sudden cessation of urine output immediately posttransplant. Continuous bladder irrigations usually restore diuresis; if not, cystoscopy may be necessary to evacuate the clot and fulgurate the source of bleeding, which may be the ureteroneocystostomy.

Urinary leakage usually occurs secondary to technical complications or necrosis of the distal portion of the allograft ureter. Presentation usually consists of fever, clear wound drainage, tenderness over the lower abdomen, and a rising serum creatinine level. A small leak may spontaneously resolve by use of a Foley catheter, percutaneous nephrostomy tube drainage, or both. Most leaks, however, will require initial diagnosis (via a percutaneous nephrostogram and nephrostomy tube placement), followed by reexploration and ureteral reimplantation or ureteropyelostomy using a portion of the patient's own ureter.

Ureteral stenosis usually manifests several months after transplant and is thought to be secondary to rejection, ischemia, or infection or a combination of these causes. Percutaneous nephrostomy with balloon dilatation can be attempted initially, but surgical repair (e.g., reimplantation or ureteropyelostomy) often is required.

D. Wound. Fortunately, wound infection is an infrequent complication (~ 1% to 2%) after kidney transplantation. Somewhat more common, albeit still infrequent, is the development of a lymphocele in the region adjacent to the graft, which leads to pressure-related symptoms and obstruction of nearby structures (e.g., the ureter and iliac vein). Patients can present with a triad of allograft dysfunction, unilateral lower extremity edema on the side of the allograft, and hypertension. Treatment options include external drainage with sclerotherapy or internal drainage via laparoscopy or open exploration, creating a peritoneal window to link the retroperitoneal and intraperitoneal space.

V. Medical complications

A. Cardiovascular complications. The incidence of cardiac complications posttransplant depends on the level of graft function and the recipient's underlying disease and cardiac history. Correction of uremia by immediate graft function improves the cardiac index, stroke volume, and ejection fraction. Patients with diabetes, hypertension, and significant coronary disease are most likely to develop cardiac complications and may require perioperative ICU monitoring. Myocardial infarction is uncommon, occurring most frequently in recipients with preexisting risk factors. Pericarditis can occur early posttransplant, but the incidence is only 1% to 3%. It usually occurs secondary to uremia, but other causes may include infection (e.g., cytomegalovirus) and certain medications. Pericardiocentesis is mandatory if recipients develop cardiac failure, hypertension, or cardiac tamponade.

B. Pulmonary complications. Most kidney transplant recipients do not require postoperative ventilatory support unless complications such as pulmonary edema or pneumonia develop. Pulmonary edema usually is the result of fluid overreplacement intraoperatively. Fluid restriction and diuresis with intravenously administered diuretics should be implemented, followed by hemodialysis, if necessary. Another important cause of pulmonary edema in kidney transplant recipients is an adverse reaction to monoclonal anti–T-cell treatment (OKT3) for induction of immunosuppression or antirejection therapy.

Pneumonia remains one of the most common posttransplant infections, with an incidence of 10% to 25%. An aggressive approach to diagnosis is required, usually including bronchoscopy to determine the pathogen involved. If respiratory failure ensues, temporary ventilatory support may be necessary. In addition, appropriate antimicrobial or antiviral agents should be administered, and immunosuppression should be reduced or discontinued.

C. Metabolic complications. Hyperkalemia is a frequent problem perioperatively. It can develop in recipients with ATN or with poor graft function secondary to acute or chronic rejection. A potassium-binding, ion-exchange resin (e.g., Kayexalate) can be administered; recipients requiring a rapid decrease of serum potassium should receive intravenous glucose and insulin. Those who develop hyperkalemia because of poor graft function may require dialysis.

High-output diuresis immediately posttransplant can result in hypokalemia and requires appropriate potassium replacement. Other less-frequent abnormalities seen with high-output diuresis include hypomagnesemia and hypophosphatemia.

D. Infectious complications. Infections are by far the most common posttransplant problem. Mortality and morbidity have decreased in recent years because of improvement in prophylaxis, early detection, more aggressive treatment, and development of new drugs. Yet infections remain one of the leading causes of death, both early and late posttransplant. The risk of infection is greater for older recipients, for diabetic recipients, and for recipients with multiple sequential episodes of antirejection treatment.

E. Gastrointestinal complications. The incidence of gastrointestinal (GI) complications is 25%. In the upper GI tract, the most common problem is peptic ulcer disease and its associated complications such as bleeding and perforation. With the routine use of H_2 blockers and potent antacids, peptic ulcer disease has declined considerably. The most common lower GI tract complications posttransplant are colon perforation and hemorrhage. Perforation can be caused by diverticulitis, ischemic colitis, stercoral ulceration, fecal impaction, or to less common or undetermined forms of colitis.

F. Neurologic complications. Up to 30% of kidney transplant recipients develop neurologic problems. Causes may be secondary to pretransplant conditions, the patient's underlying disease, and sequelae of the transplant surgery itself. Cerebrovascular events (infarct, transient ischemic attacks, hemorrhage), albeit rare, are the most frequent complications, usually peaking in incidence during the first few months posttransplant. Other common central nervous system complications include seizures, whereas infections (bacterial and fungal meningitis and brain abscesses) generally present after the immediate posttransplant period.

Selected Readings

Balfour HH, Chage BA, Stapleton JT. A randomized, placebo-controlled trial of oral acyclovir for the prevention of cytomegalovirus disease in recipients of renal allografts. *N Engl J Med* 1989;320:1381.

One of the first studies to show the usefulness of acyclovir for the prevention of cytomegalovirus disease.

Bruno A, Adams H. Neurologic problems in renal transplant recipients. *Neurol Clin* 1988;6:305.

An excellent review of neurologic complications in kidney transplant recipients.

Fernandez-Cruz L, Targarona EM, Alcaraz ECA, et al. Acute pancreatitis after renal transplantation. *Br J Surg* 1989;76:1132.

An infrequent, but nonetheless important, complication.

Flanagan RC, Rechard CR, Lucas BA. Colonic complications of renal transplantation. *J Urol* 1988;139:503.

A good review on what can be life-threatening complications.

Goldman MH, Tilney NL, Vineyard GC, et al. A twenty-year survey of arterial complications of renal transplantation. *Surg Gynecol Obstet* 1975;141:758.

An early comprehensive review of arterial complications.

Penn I. Tumors after renal and cardiac transplantation. *Hematol Oncol Clin North Am* 1993;7:431.

A detailed review of malignancies in the renal transplant recipients.

Phillipson JD, Carpenter BJ, Itzkoff J, et al. Evaluation of cardiovascular risk for renal transplantation in diabetic patients. *Am J Med* 1986;81:630.

A useful approach to the evaluation of cardiovascular risk in diabetic renal transplant recipients.

Ramos EL. Recurrent diseases in the renal allograft. *J Am Soc Nephrol* 1991;2:109.

A comprehensive review of recurrent disease in renal transplant recipients.

Rubin RH. Infectious disease complications of renal transplantation. *Kidney Int* 1993;44:221.

A clinically useful review of posttransplant infections.

Thistethwaite Jr JR, Stuart JK, Mayes JT, et al. Complications and monitoring of OKT3 therapy. *Am J Kid Dis* 1988;11:112.

An early paper on the complications associated with the powerful immunosuppressive agent OKT3.

Troppmann C, Papalois BE, Chiou A, et al. Incidence, complications, treatment, and outcome of ulcers of the upper gastrointestinal tract after renal transplantation during the cyclosporine era. *J Am Coll Surg* 1995;180:433.

One of the very few papers on the problem of ulcers of the upper gastrointestinal tract after kidney transplants.

Waltzer WC, Frischer Z, Shabtai M, et al. Early aggressive management for the prevention of renal allograft loss and patient mortality following major urologic complications. *Clin Transplant* 1992;6:318.

A useful review of management of urologic complications.

169. CRITICAL CARE OF PANCREAS TRANSPLANT RECIPIENTS

Abhinav Humar, Scott A. Gruber, and David L. Dunn

I. General principles. A successful pancreas transplant can establish normoglycemia and insulin independence in diabetic recipients. It also has the potential to halt progression of some secondary complications of diabetes. No current method of exogenous insulin administration can produce a euglycemic, insulin-independent state akin to that achievable with a technically successful pancreas graft. Pancreas transplants are performed to improve the quality of life over that achieved by the alternative treatment—exogenous insulin administration. But as a treatment for type I diabetes, pancreas transplants have not yet achieved widespread application in all diabetics because the operative procedure is associated with complications, albeit of increasingly lower incidence, coupled with long-term side effects of immunosuppression, which together can exceed the complications caused by diabetes. Thus, pancreas transplants are preferentially performed in diabetic patients with renal failure who are also candidates for a kidney transplant and who would require immunosuppression to prevent rejection of the kidney. A pancreas transplant alone is appropriate for diabetics whose day-to-day quality of life is so poor from a management standpoint (labile serum glucose with ketoacidosis or hypoglycemic episodes; progression of severe diabetic retinopathy, nephropathy, neuropathy, or enteropathy) that chronic immunosuppression is justified to achieve insulin independence.

II. Pretransplant evaluation. Pancreas transplant procedures can be divided into three major recipient categories: (a) simultaneous cadaver pancreas-kidney (SPK) transplant; (b) pancreas transplant after a living or cadaver kidney transplant (PAK); and (c) pancreas transplant alone (PTA). All uremic type I diabetics who are candidates for a kidney transplant should be considered potential candidates for a pancreas transplant. The benefits of the pancreas transplant (insulin independence, protection of the new kidney from recurrent disease) should be weighed, on an individual basis, against the risks of the procedure (e.g., surgical complications, increased incidence of infection, malignancy).

The pretransplant evaluation does not differ substantially from that undertaken for diabetic kidney transplant recipients. Examination of the cardiovascular system is most important because significant coronary artery disease may be present without angina. Noninvasive testing may not identify such disease, so coronary angiography is performed routinely. In PTA candidates, detailed neurologic, ophthalmologic, metabolic, and renal function testing may be needed to assess the degree of progression of secondary complications. Once patients are placed on a waiting list, their medical condition should be reassessed yearly or more frequently.

III. Intra- and postoperative care

A. Surgical techniques. The initial preparation of the donor pancreas is a crucial component of a successful transplant. Examination at this time is often the best or only way to confirm suitability of the organ for transplantation. If sclerotic, calcific, or markedly discolored, the pancreas should not be used. Prior to implantation, a surgical procedure in undertaken to remove the spleen and any excess duodenum, to ligate the blood vessels at the root of the mesentery, and to perform vascular reconstruction to connect the donor superior mesenteric and splenic arteries, most commonly using a reversed segment of donor iliac artery as a Y-graft. The pancreas graft is then implanted via an anastomosis of the aforementioned arterial graft to the recipient common iliac artery and a venous anastomosis of the donor portal vein to the recipient external or common iliac vein, using an intraperitoneal approach. Generally, the kidney is placed in the left iliac fossa and the pancreas in the right iliac fossa during SPK transplantation. Once the pancreas is revascularized, a drainage procedure must be performed to handle the pancreatic exocrine secretions. Options include anastomosing the donor duodenum to the recipient bladder or to the small bowel, the latter either in continuity or to a Roux-en-Y limb.

B. Postoperative care. In general, pancreas transplant recipients do not require intensive care monitoring in the postoperative period. Laboratory values—serum glucose, hemoglobin, electrolytes, and amylase—are monitored daily, the former more frequently if normoglycemia is not immediately achieved. Nasogastric suction and intravenous fluids are continued for the first several days until bowel function returns. In the early postoperative period, regular insulin is infused to maintain plasma glucose levels less than 150 mg/dl, because chronic hyperglycemia may be detrimental to beta cells. In recipients who undergo bladder drainage, a Foley catheter is left in place for 10 to 14 days. At most centers, some form of prophylaxis is instituted against bacterial, fungal, and viral infections. Our current regimen includes ampicillin-sulbactam (5–7 days), fluconazole (5–7 days) trimethoprim-sulfamethoxazole (lifelong), and ganciclovir (3 months). In addition, many centers routinely institute some form of prophylaxis against venous thrombosis of the allograft; we use low-dose heparin during the first week.

One crucial aspect of posttransplant care is monitoring for rejection and complications (both surgical and medical). Rejection episodes can be identified by an increase in serum creatinine (in SPK recipients), a decrease in urinary amylase (in recipients with bladder drainage), an increase in serum amylase, and lastly, an increase in serum glucose levels. In cases where a kidney transplant biopsy would not be helpful (PAK or PTA), a percutaneous biopsy of the pancreas can be obtained under ultrasound or computed tomography guidance or via cystoscopy in bladder-drained allografts.

IV. Surgical and medical complications. The transplanted pancreas is susceptible to a unique set of complications because of its exocrine secretions and low blood flow. However, the incidence of graft-related complications has decreased significantly in the past decade. Factors include better preservation techniques, better surgical methods, improved prophylaxis regimens, and improved immunosuppression management.

A. Thrombosis. The incidence of thrombosis is approximately 6% for pancreas transplant cases reported to the United Network for Organ Sharing (UNOS) registry. Low-dose heparin, dextran, or antiplatelet agents are administered routinely in the early postoperative period at many centers, although the risk of postoperative bleeding is thereby slightly increased. Arterial or venous thrombosis is most common within the first several days posttransplant, heralded by an increase in blood glucose levels, an increase in insulin requirements, and a decrease in urine amylase levels. Venous thrombosis is also characteristically accompanied by hematuria, tenderness and swelling of the graft, and ipsilateral lower extremity edema. Treatment is removal of the graft.

B. Hemorrhage. Postoperative bleeding can be minimized by meticulous intraoperative control of bleeding sites. Although hemorrhage can be exacerbated by anticoagulants and antiplatelet drugs, their benefits seem to outweigh the risks. Bleeding is a much less significant cause (~1%) of graft loss than is thrombosis (~6%) according to the UNOS registry data. Significant bleeding is treated by immediate reexploration.

C. Pancreatitis. Most cases of graft pancreatitis occur early on; they are self-limited and probably are caused by ischemic preservation injury. Clinical manifestations can include graft tenderness and fever, in addition to hyperamylasemia. Treatment consists of fasting and intravenous fluid replacement. Later episodes of graft pancreatitis can be caused by reflux into the allograft duct in recipients with bladder drainage or cytomegalovirus (CMV) infection. Reflux is treated by Foley catheter drainage and, occasionally, conversion to enteric drainage; CMV infections are treated with ganciclovir.

D. Urologic complications. Urologic complications are almost exclusively limited to recipients who undergo bladder drainage. Hematuria is not uncommon in the first several months posttransplant, but it is usually transient and self-limiting. Bladder calculi can develop from exposed sutures or staples along the duodenocystostomy, which can serve as a nidus for stone formation. Recurrent urinary tract infections commonly occur concurrently. Treatment consists of cystoscopy with removal of the sutures or staples. Urinary leaks most commonly stem from the proximal duodenal cuff or the duodenal anastomosis to the bladder and typically occur during the first several weeks posttransplant. Small leaks can be successfully managed by prolonged (for at least 2 weeks) Foley catheter drainage; larger leaks require surgical intervention. Other urinary complications include chronic refractory metabolic acidosis because of bicarbonate loss, persistent and recurrent urinary tract infections, and urethritis. Along with recurrent hematuria, these complications are the major indications for converting patients from bladder drainage to enteric drainage of exocrine secretions. Eventually, 6% to 18% of recipients who undergo initial bladder drainage will require conversion to enteric drainage. For this reason, the recent trend has been to perform enteric drainage at the time of the transplant. Enteric drainage is associated with significantly fewer urinary tract infections and urologic complications, but this approach obviates the use of urinary amylase determination, which is a sensitive indicator of pancreatic allograft rejection.

E. **Infections.** Infections remain a significant problem after pancreas transplantation. Most common are superficial wound infections and intraabdominal infections, often related to graft complications such as leaks. Thanks to appropriate perioperative antimicrobial regimens (for prophylaxis against gram-positive bacteria, gram-negative bacteria, and yeast), the incidence of significant infections has decreased, although it remains approximately 10% and is associated with significant morbidity and mortality. Thus, should serious intraabdominal infection occur, whether or not associated with the above described complications, reexploration and graft removal must be strongly considered with concurrent reduction in immunosuppressive drug therapy, often such that the patient receives only low-dose corticosteroids.

Selected Readings

American Diabetes Association. Technical review: pancreas transplantation for patients with diabetes mellitus. *Diabetes Care* 1992;15:1668.

A simple review of pancreas transplants.

Gill IS, Sindhi R, Jerius JT, et al. Bench reconstruction of pancreas for transplantation: experience with 192 cases. *Clin Transplant* 1997;11:104.

An excellent technical description of the benchwork preparation of the cadaver pancreas.

Gross CR, Zehrer CL. Health-related quality of life outcomes of pancreas transplant recipients. *Clin Transplant* 1992;6:165.

An excellent paper on quality of life issues.

Kennedy WR, Navarro X, Goetz FC, et al. Effects of pancreatic transplantation in diabetic neuropathy. *N Engl J Med* 1990;322:1031.

One of the first reports of a potential benefit of pancreas transplants on the secondary complication of neuropathy.

Kuo PC, Johnson LB, Schweitzer EJ, et al. Simultaneous pancreas/kidney transplantation—a comparison of enteric and bladder drainage of exocrine pancreatic secretions. *Transplantation* 1997;63:238.

A good study comparing the two main methods for handling exocrine secretions.

Nghiem DD, Corry RJ. Technique of simultaneous pancreatoduodenal transplantation with urinary drainage of pancreatic secretion. *Am J Surg* 1987;153:405.

A good technical description of the operative procedure.

Ozaki CF, Stratta RJ, Taylor RJ, et al. Surgical complications in solitary pancreas and combined pancreas-kidney transplantations. *Am J Surg* 1992;164:546.

An excellent review of potential surgical complications.

Sutherland DER, Gruessner A. Pancreas transplantation in the United States as reported to the United Network for Organ Sharing (UNOS) and analyzed by the International Pancreas Transplant Registry. In: Cecka JM, Terasaki PI, eds. *Clinical transplants 1995.* Los Angeles: UCLA Tissue Typing Laboratory; 1996:49.

A recent report on transplant data from the international registry.

Troppmann C, Gruessner AC, Benedetti E, et al. Vascular graft thrombosis after pancreatic transplantation: univariate and multivariate operative and nonoperative risk factor analysis. *J Am Col Surg* 1996;182:285.
A comprehensive analysis of vascular complications.

USRDS 1992 Annual Data Report. VIII. Simultaneous kidney-pancreas transplantation versus kidney transplantation alone: patient survival, kidney graft survival, and post-transplant hospitalization. *Am J Kidney Dis* 1992;20 (Suppl 2):61.
An excellent report of the combined versus single organ transplant.

170. CRITICAL CARE OF LIVER TRANSPLANT RECIPIENTS

Abhinav Humar, Rainer W.G. Gruessner, and David L. Dunn

I. General principles. Liver transplantation has become the accepted treatment of choice for patients with acute and chronic end-stage liver disease. Dramatic improvements in outcome have been seen over the last 15 years, secondary to improved recipient and donor surgical techniques, improved organ preservation, better immunosuppressive drug regimens, prevention of infection, and improved care during the critical perioperative period.

II. Pretransplant evaluation. The purpose of the pretransplant evaluation is to (a) determine the appropriateness and timing of transplantation for the prospective candidate and (b) identify underlying medical problems that should be dealt with preoperatively, thus optimizing the candidate's overall condition before surgery. Intensive preoperative care is especially relevant for patients with fulminant hepatic failure or decompensated chronic hepatic failure, who may have problems involving multiple organ systems.

In the absence of absolute contraindications (active extrahepatic sepsis, extrahepatic malignancy, acquired immune deficiency syndrome (AIDS), or advanced cardiopulmonary disease), almost any disease process (acute or chronic) resulting in end-stage liver failure may be amenable to a liver transplant. Patients with chronic liver disease and decompensated cirrhosis (as indicated by spontaneous hepatic encephalopathy, refractory ascites, hepatorenal syndrome, hepatopulmonary syndrome, recurrent or refractory variceal bleeding, recurrent infection such as cholangitis or spontaneous bacterial peritonitis, intractable pruritus, and severe malnutrition) should be evaluated for a possible transplant. Patients with acute liver disease and poor prognostic indicators (Table 170-1) should also be considered. Certain patients with malignancy (e.g., small lesions identified incidentally in the cirrhotic liver) have a better prognosis after undergoing a transplant. However, patients with malignancy require preoperative radiologic investigation to ensure that the cancer has not spread outside the liver. Pretransplant care involves optimizing the patient's overall medical status and addressing problems (both related and unrelated to the liver failure) that can affect the postoperative course. The approach should be systematic, covering all major organ systems to ensure that no major problems are overlooked.

Patients with acute liver failure are generally more ill than those with chronic failure, and thus require more intensive pretransplant care. They have more severe hepatic parenchymal dysfunction, manifested by coagulopathy, hypoglycemia, and lactic acidosis. They also develop more infectious complications and exhibit a higher incidence of renal failure and neurologic complications, especially cerebral edema. Some centers use intracranial pressure monitoring to detect cerebral edema in patients with acute liver failure. Therapy (e.g., mannitol, hyperventilation, and thiopental) can then be directed to achieve an adequate cerebral perfusion pressure (>15 mm Hg). Multiple organ dysfunction syndrome is a well-described complication of fulminant hepatic failure.

III. Intraoperative care. The transplant operation itself can be divided into three phases: pre-anhepatic (mobilizing the recipient's diseased liver in preparation for its removal), anhepatic, and post-anhepatic. The anhepatic phase is characterized by decreased venous return to the heart because of occlusion of the inferior vena cava and portal vein. Many centers routinely use a venous bypass system during this time. With the recipient liver removed, the donor liver is anastomosed to the appropriate structures to place the new liver in an orthotopic position. The new liver is then reperfused, signaling the beginning of the post-anhepatic phase. The most dramatic changes in hemodynamic parameters usually occur on reperfusion, namely, hypotension and serious arrhythmias.

TABLE 170-1. Adverse prognostic indicators for patients with acute liver failure

Acetaminophen Toxicity	No Acetaminophen Toxicity
pH < 7.30	
Prothrombin time > 100 sec (INR > 6.5)	Prothrombin time > 100 sec (INR > 6.5)
Serum creatinine > 300 μmol/L (>3.4 mg/dl)	Serum creatinine > 300 μmol/L (>3.4 mg/dl)
	Age < 10 or > 40 years
	Non-A, non-B hepatitis
	Duration of jaundice before onset of encephalopathy > 7 days

INR, international normalized ratio.

IV. Postoperative care. The postoperative course can range from smooth to extremely complicated, depending mainly on the patient's preoperative status and the development of any complications. The care of all such patients involves (a) stabilization and recovery of the major organ systems (e.g., cardiovascular, pulmonary, renal); (b) evaluation of graft function and achievement of adequate immunosuppression; and (c) monitoring and treatment of complications directly and indirectly related to the transplant. Initial posttransplant care should be in a critical care unit. Patients generally require mechanical ventilatory support for the first 24 to 48 hours. Continuous hemodynamic monitoring must be maintained.

A crucial aspect of postoperative care is the repeated evaluation of graft function. With good graft function, the patient's mental status should progressively improve, the coagulation profile should normalize, hypoglycemia and hyperbilirubinemia should resolve, and serum lactate levels should clear. Serum transaminase levels will usually rise during the first 48 to 72 hours, secondary to preservation injury, and then should fall rapidly over the next 24 to 48 hours.

V. Surgical complications

A. Hemorrhage. Bleeding, which is common in the postoperative period, is usually multifactorial. It can be compounded by an underlying coagulopathy resulting from deficits in coagulation, fibrinolysis, and platelet function. Blood loss should be monitored via the abdominal drains and with serial measurement of hemoglobin and central venous pressure. If bleeding persists despite correction of coagulation deficiencies, an exploratory relaparotomy should be performed.

B. Vascular complications. The incidence of vascular complications is reported to be 8% to 12%. Thrombosis is the most common early event; stenosis and pseudoaneurysm formation occur later. Hepatic artery thrombosis (HAT) has a reported incidence of approximately 5% in adults and approximately 10% in children. After HAT, liver recipients cay be asymptomatic or they can develop severe liver failure secondary to extensive necrosis. Doppler ultrasound evaluation is the initial investigation of choice, with more than 90% sensitivity and specificity. Urgent exploration with thrombectomy and revision of the anastomosis is indicated; if the diagnosis is made early, up to 70% of grafts can be salvaged. If hepatic necrosis is extensive, a retransplant is indicated. HAT can also present in a less dramatic fashion. Thrombosis may render the common bile duct ischemic, resulting in a localized or diffuse bile leak from the anastomosis or a more chronic, diffuse biliary stricture.

Thrombosis of the portal vein is far less frequent. Liver dysfunction, tense ascites, and variceal bleeding can occur. Doppler ultrasound evaluation should establish the diagnosis. If thrombosis is diagnosed early, operative thrombectomy and revision of the anastomosis may be successful. If thrombosis occurs late, liver function is usually preserved because of the collateral veins; a retransplant is then unnecessary and attention is diverted toward relieving the left-sided portal hypertension.

C. Biliary complications. Biliary complications continue to be a significant complication after liver transplantation, occurring in 15% to 35% of cases. They manifest either as a leak or an obstruction. Leaks tend to occur early postoperatively and often require surgical repair, whereas obstruction usually occurs later and can be managed with radiologic or endoscopic techniques. Clinical symptoms of a bile leak include fever, abdominal pain, and peritoneal irritation. Ultrasound may demonstrate a fluid collection; cholangiography is required for diagnosis. Some leaks can be managed successfully by endoscopic placement of a biliary stent. If the leak does not respond to stent placement or if the patient is systemically ill, a relaparotomy is warranted.

Biliary stricture occurs later in the postoperative period and is most common at the anastomotic site, likely related to local ischemia. This process usually manifests as cholangitis, cholestasis, or both. Initial treatment involves balloon dilatation or stent placement across the site of stricture, or both. If these initial options fail, surgical revision is required.

D. Wound complications. Common problems related to the wound are infection, hematoma, and seroma. Wound hematomas can result from the presence of huge collateral veins in the abdominal wall. Wound infections will usually present after postoperative day 5. Treatment consists of opening the wound, changing the dressings, and allowing healing by secondary intention. If significant cellulitis or systemic symptoms are present, intravenous antibiotics should be administered.

E. Primary nonfunction. This is a devastating complication and the attendant mortality rate is more than 80% without a retransplant. By definition, this syndrome results from poor or no hepatic function from the time of the transplant procedure. The incidence in most centers is approximately 3% to 5%. Donor factors associated with primary nonfunction include advanced age, increased fat content of the donor liver, longer donor hospital stay before organ procurement, prolonged cold ischemia time, and reduced-size grafts. Conditions that can mimic primary nonfunction must be ruled out, such as HAT, accelerated acute rejection, and severe infection. Intravenous prostaglandin E_1 has some useful effect and should be administered to recipients with suspected primary nonfunction, at the same time they are listed for an urgent retransplant.

VI. Medical complications. A long list of medical complications can occur. Almost every major organ system can be affected. Neurologic complications generally manifest as decreased level of consciousness, seizures, or focal neurologic deficits; they are most commonly related to drugs or a poorly functioning or nonfunctioning graft. Other causes include hypoxic ischemic encephalopathy, central pontine myelinolysis, cerebral edema, and intracranial hematomas.

The pulmonary system is one of the most common sites of complications posttransplant. Infectious and noninfectious pulmonary complications occur in up to 75% of liver recipients. Noninfectious complications [e.g., pulmonary edema, pleural effusions, atelectasis, and acute respiratory distress syndrome (ARDS)] predominate in the first posttransplant week; infectious complications predominate after that. ARDS occurs in fewer than 5% of liver transplant recipients, but its associated mortality rate approaches 80%. It is most common when underlying bacterial infection is present, but other risk factors include multiple transfusions, hypertension, aspiration, and antilymphocyte therapy.

Some degree of renal dysfunction is very common, affecting almost all liver recipients. Renal failure, whether pre- or posttransplant, increases the mortality rate. Pretransplant renal problems are commonly caused by hepatorenal syndrome or acute tubular necrosis. Postoperative causes of renal dysfunction include hypovolemia, ischemic acute tubular necrosis, drug nephrotoxicity, or preexisting renal disease.

Selected Readings

Bihari DJ, Gimson AES, Williams R. Cardiovascular, pulmonary and renal complications of fulminant hepatic failure. *Semin Liver Dis* 1986;6:119.

A good review of the multiple systems that can be affected in patients with fulminant hepatic failure.

Dee GW, Kondo N, Farell ML, et al. Cardiovascular complications following liver transplantation. *Clin Transplant* 1995;9:463.
A good review of cardiovascular complications.

Gonwa TA, Klintmalm GB, Levy M, et al. Impact of pretransplant renal function on survival after liver transplantation. *Transplantation* 1995;59:361.
A good study of the negative impact of renal failure on survival.

Longnas AN, Marujo W, Stratta RJ, et al. Vascular complications after orthotopic liver transplantation. *Am J Surg* 1991;161:76.
A comprehensive review of vascular complications.

O'Connor TP, Lewis WD, Jenkins RL. Biliary tract complications after liver transplantation. *Arch Surg* 1995;130:312.
A comprehensive review of biliary complications.

O'Grady JG, Alexander GJM, Mayllar KM, et al. Early indicators of prognosis in fulminant hepatic failure. *Gastroenterology* 1989;97:439.
A landmark paper on the predictors of prognosis in patients with fulminant hepatic failure.

Plevak DJ, Southern PA, Narr BJ, et al. Intensive care unit experience in the Mayo liver transplant program: the first 100 cases. *Mayo Clin Proc* 1989;64:433.
An early, but good, paper on the intensive care problems encountered in liver transplant recipients.

Ploeg RJ, D'Alessandro AM, Knechtle SJ, et al. Risk factors for primary dysfunction after liver transplantation—a multivariate analysis. *Transplantation* 1993;55:807.
An excellent analysis of risk factors for primary nonfunction.

Poplawski SC, Gonwa TA, Goldstein RM, et al. Renal dysfunction following orthotopic liver transplantation. *Clin Transplant* 1989;3:94.
A good approach to the management of renal problems.

Starzl TE, Iwatsuki S, Von Thiel DH. Evolution of orthotopic liver transplant. *Hepatology* 1982;2:613.
A good historical overview.

Stein DP, Lederman RJ, Vogt DP, et al. Neurological complications following liver transplantation. *Ann Neurol* 1992;31:644.
A good review of neurologic complications.

171. CRITICAL CARE OF HEART, HEART–LUNG, AND LUNG TRANSPLANT RECIPIENTS

Abhinav Humar, Sara J. Shumway, and David L. Dunn

I. General principles. Since the first heart transplant in 1967, the first heart–lung transplant in 1981, and the first successful single-lung transplant in 1983, considerable progress has been made in the field of thoracic organ transplantation. Survival and quality of life have markedly improved secondary to advances in immunosuppressive drug therapy, improved selection criteria, and better medical care of recipients, especially during the crucial perioperative period.

II. Pretransplant evaluation. Candidates for a heart transplant include patients with end-stage heart failure (usually secondary to ischemic or idiopathic cardiomyopathy), intractable angina, or life-threatening ventricular arrhythmias. Much of the pretransplant evaluation is similar to that for other organ transplant recipients. Specific to heart transplantation is the need to exclude the presence of severe pulmonary hypertension, which could cause right ventricle failure posttransplant and serious chronic obstructive pulmonary disease.

Heart–lung transplants are performed almost exclusively for patients who have developed severe pulmonary vascular disease (either primary or secondary pulmonary hypertension). Single-lung transplants are performed for patients who suffer pulmonary fibrosis and chronic obstructive pulmonary disease.

III. Intraoperative care. As with other organs, cadaver donor selection criteria are important to ensure posttransplant success. A heart donor should have a normal echocardiogram and must require minimal inotropic support. Any evidence of coronary artery disease is a relative contraindication; angiography can be performed in older donors (age ≥ 45 years) to determine whether or not it is present. Lung donor criteria have been liberalized over the past several years. A PaO_2 above 100 mm Hg while the FIO_2 is 40% is desirable, without evidence of pulmonary disease, either obstructive or restrictive, based on standard physiologic testing. Whenever donor aspiration or serious infection is a possibility, however, bronchoscopy is performed. Demonstration of fungal organisms in the sputum and evidence of lobar consolidation are contraindications to use of the organ.

A heart transplant must be performed using cardiopulmonary bypass for the recipient. The diseased heart is excised along the atrioventricular groove. The new heart is placed in an orthotopic position, with anastomoses performed in the following order: left atrial, right atrial, pulmonary arterial, and aortic. Single-lung transplants are performed through a standard posterolateral thoracotomy; cardiopulmonary bypass may be necessary in selected cases. The bronchial anastomosis is performed first, followed by the pulmonary arterial and left arterial anastomoses. A telescoped bronchial anastomosis reduces the incidence of complications, and often a pedicle of vascularized omentum is wrapped around the anastomosis.

IV. Perioperative care. After heart or heart–lung transplantation, cardiac output is sustained by establishing a heart rate of 90 to 110 beats/min, using either temporary epicardial atrial pacing or low-dose isoproterenol. For recipients who may suffer transient right ventricle failure, adequate preload is important. An oximetric Swan-Ganz catheter can be helpful in monitoring pulmonary artery pressure and measuring cardiac output. Urine output and arterial blood gases must be carefully monitored. Hypotension and a low cardiac output usually respond to an infusion of fluid and to minor adjustments in inotropic support.

Cardiac tamponade can occur in heart transplant recipients; it should be considered in patients who become hypotensive with concurrent increases in central venous pressure and whose mediastinal chest tube output decreases suddenly. Serious ventricular failure posttransplant is unusual and can be related to poor donor organ selection, poor graft preservation, long ischemia time, or rarely, hyperacute rejection. Inotropes and pulmonary vasodilators can be used to manage ventricular failure, with the addition of an intraaortic balloon pump or a ventricular assist device if it seems likely that the graft will recover. In the case of very severe rejection, the only option is to list the recipient for a retransplant and proceed if and when a donor heart becomes available.

Acute failure of a transplanted lung (compared with that of a heart) is more common. Reasons include the inherent difficulty of lung preservation, unrecognized injury or trauma to the donor lung, and reperfusion edema. Lung graft failure can manifest as hypoxemia, infiltrates on radiograph, and copious secretions when reperfusion edema occurs. These patients require active diuresis. High levels of positive end-expiratory pressure can be used to maintain small airway patency; patients are kept intubated and immobile. When patients are stable, transbronchial biopsy can be performed to exclude the presence of rejection. Bronchoalveolar lavage can rule out early infection. Extracorporeal membrane oxygenation, used as a last resort, has occasionally been successful in maintaining function while antirejection therapy is administered.

V. Posttransplant complications

A. Airway complications. Airway complications occur after heart–lung or lung transplants, but are rare after heart–lung transplants because a good blood supply is maintained to the tracheal anastomosis. After solitary and double lung transplants, the bronchial anastomosis is at much greater risk for partial dehiscence, airway stenosis, or both. Hypotension, poor lung preservation, rejection, and infection can compromise blood flow to the anastomoses. The result can be ischemic necrosis and poor healing of the airway, leading to partial or total dehiscence or chronic narrowing of the bronchus.

Postoperative surveillance of the bronchial anastomosis is important. In the operating room, bronchoscopy is performed to establish the baseline appearance of the anastomosis. Frequent routine bronchoscopy is useful to survey the anastomosis for early signs of dehiscence, as well as to monitor for rejection and infection. Dehiscence usually occurs within 3 to 6 weeks posttransplant. Early signs on bronchoscopy include pallor, gray or black mucosa at the suture line, loosened sutures or knots within the airway, and herniation of tissue into the airway in case of an omental wrap. If the patient is clinically stable and the area of dehiscence is small, conservative treatment with antibiotics and serial evaluation via bronchoscopy is appropriate. Development of a bronchopleural or bronchovascular fistula requires reoperation.

Chronic stenosis can develop after initial healing. It can be managed in a variety of ways, including repeated dilations of the airway with a rigid bronchoscope or use of a metallic stent or laser photocoagulation to debride granulation tissue.

B. Rejection. A grading scale to denote the severity of heart graft rejection based on endomyocardial biopsy is used. With heart–lung transplants, it was initially thought that endomyocardial biopsy could assess lung rejection at the same time. Unfortunately, the lungs are more susceptible to rejection and are often in the process of rejection despite the presence of normal endomyocardial biopsies. Transbronchial biopsies can help diagnose lung rejection.

C. Infection. Thoracic organ transplant recipients are susceptible to bacterial, fungal, and viral infections. Infection is a particular problem in lung transplant recipients: as many as 15% to 20% of them develop some type of significant infectious disease. Fungal infections caused by Candida and Aspergillus are generally more serious than bacterial infections. Most Aspergillus infections, which are caused by the inhalation of aerosolized fungal spores, generally occur within the first 3 months posttransplant. In lung transplant recipients who suffer cystic fibrosis, infection from *Pseudomonas aeruginosa* is common. The most morbid viral infection that occurs in thoracic organ transplant recipients is caused by cytomegalovirus.

D. Graft atherosclerosis. Development of graft atherosclerosis can lead to myocardial infarction and sudden death in heart transplant recipients. Routine yearly coronary angiography is performed to permit accurate assessment of the rate of progression of coronary artery disease. Graft atherosclerosis occurs in

30% to 40% of heart transplant recipients at 3 years and in 40% to 60% by 5 years posttransplant. It remains a major obstacle to long-term survival. Immunologically mediated endothelial damage can be the stimulus for development of graft atherosclerosis. Treatment can be temporizing in the form of angioplasty for focal lesions; however, when the disease involves tapering of the distal vessels, only a heart retransplant is adequate.

E. Obliterative bronchiolitis. Obliterative bronchiolitis (OB) occurs with equal frequency after lung and heart–lung transplantation. After an initially successful lung transplant, approximately 30% of recipients develop OB. Clinically, they present with dyspnea, a clear chest radiograph, and obstructive pulmonary function tests. Histologic examination of biopsy specimens demonstrates bronchial and bronchiolar fibrosis with organization and obliteration of the bronchiolar lumen. OB appears to be a manifestation of chronic lung allograft rejection. Infections can also cause OB, especially cytomegalovirus and adenovirus. Once the diagnosis is made, therapy is support until retransplantation can be undertaken.

Selected Readings

Achuff SC. Clinical evaluation of potential heart transplant recipients. In: Baumgartner WA, Reitz BA, Achuff SC, eds. *Heart and heart–lung transplantation.* Philadelphia: WB Sanders Company; 1990:51.

An excellent chapter on the evaluation of potential heart transplant recipients.

Barnard CN. The operation: a human cardiac transplant: an interim report of a successful operation performed at Groote Schuur Hospital, Cape Town. *S Afr Med J* 1967;41:1271.

The original report of the first successful heart transplant performed by Dr. C. Barnard.

Billingham ME, Cary NRB, Hammond ME, et al. A working formulation for the standardization of nomenclature in the diagnosis of heart and lung rejection: heart rejection study group. *J Heart Lung Transplant* 1990;9:587.

An excellent summary paper on the standardization of terminology in thoracic transplantation.

Kshettry VR, Shumway SJ, Gauthier RL, et al. Technique of single lung transplantation. *Ann Thorac Surg* 1993;56:520.

A good technical paper on the techniques of single lung transplants.

Reitz BA, Wallwork JL, Hunt SA, et al. Heart-lung transplantation: successful therapy for patients with pulmonary vascular disease. *N Engl J Med* 1982;306:557.

Original report on the early success with heart–lung transplants.

Shumway SJ, Hertz MI, Maynard R, et al. Airway complications after lung and heart–lung transplantation. *Transplant Proc* 1993;25:1165.

A concise but thorough paper on airway complications after lung transplants.

Shumway SJ, Hertz MI, Petty MG, et al. Liberalization of donor criteria in lung and heart–lung transplantation. *Ann Thorac Surg* 1994;57:92.

A practical paper on the evaluation of potential heart and lung donors.

Smith CR. Techniques in cardiac transplantation. *Prog Cardiovasc Dis* 1990;32:383.

An informative paper on techniques in heart transplantation.

Starnes VA. Heart-lung transplantation: an overview. *Cardiol Clin* 1990;8:159.

A good overview of heart–lung transplantation.

Toronto Lung Transplant Group. Unilateral lung transplantation for pulmonary fibrosis. *N Engl J Med* 1986;314:1140.

Early reports on the success with unilateral lung transplants from the Toronto group.

172. CRITICAL CARE OF THE CADAVER ORGAN DONOR

Abhinav Humar, Christoph Troppmann, and David L. Dunn

I. General principles. The cadaver donor supply has not kept pace with the increased use of organ transplant therapy over the past two decades. The gap is widening between the number of available cadaver organs and the number of patients waiting for transplants. An important contributing factor is the failure to maximize the use of potential cadaver donors. In this regard, the role of physicians who care for critically ill patients is crucial. They must perform the preliminary screening tests to ascertain whether donation is possible, seek early referral to an organ procurement organization, and coordinate the approach to the donor family for obtaining consent.

II. Current status of organ donation. According to recent estimates, more than 10,000 potential brain-dead donors are found in the United States per year. In 1996, however, only 5,416 actual organ donors were used. The single most important reason for lack of organ retrieval was the inability to obtain consent. The need for public education is crucial, including more effective educational campaigns to increase awareness of the importance of organ transplants.

III. Options to increase organ availability. Mechanisms that might increase the number of available organs include (a) optimizing use of the current donor pool (e.g., multiple organ donors, marginal donors); (b) increasing the number of living donor transplants (e.g., living unrelated donors); (c) using unconventional and controversial donor sources (e.g., non-heartbeating cadaver donors, anencephalic donors); and (d) performing xenotransplants.

The cornerstone for an effective increase in the number of organ donors remains heightened public awareness and education to improve consent rates. Presumed consent laws have been implemented in many areas of the world, most notably in several countries in Europe. These laws permit organ procurement unless the potential donor has explicitly objected.

IV. Brain death. Brain death means that all brain and brainstem function has irreversibly ceased, while circulatory and ventilatory functions are maintained temporarily. The recognition of brain death became possible only after substantial advances in critical care medicine. The clinical diagnosis of brain death rests on three criteria: (a) irreversibility of the neurologic insult; (b) absence of clinical evidence of cerebral function; and, most importantly, (c) absence of clinical evidence of brainstem function. Hypothermia, medication side effects, drug overdose, and intoxication must be excluded when testing for brain death. Brain death can be diagnosed by routine neurologic examinations (including cold caloric and apnea testing on two separate occasions), coupled with prior establishment of the underlying diagnosis. In the vast majority of cases, special confirmatory tests are not necessary to diagnose brain death. Only in equivocal or questionable circumstances is it necessary to perform tests to demonstrate absence of intracranial blood flow or presence of an isoelectric encephalographic reading.

V. Organ donation process. Steps involved in successful organ donation include (a) early identification of the potential donor by the critical care physician; (b) early contact with the local or regional procurement organization; (c) completion of the preliminary screening; (d) brain death diagnosis and confirmation; (e) family notification and explanation of brain death with its legal and medical implications; (f) request for organ donation; (g) a switch in focus from treatment of elevated intracranial pressure to preservation of organ function and optimization of peripheral oxygen delivery; (h) final organ allocation; (i) certification of death; and (j) the multiple-organ procurement operation.

VI. Critical care of brain-dead organ donors. For all organ donors, core temperature, systemic arterial blood pressure, arterial oxygen saturation, and urine output need to be determined routinely and frequently. Arterial blood gases, serum electrolytes, blood urea nitrogen, serum creatinine level, liver enzymes, hemoglobin, and coagulation tests also need to be monitored regularly. The most important overall goal is to optimize organ perfusion and tissue oxygen delivery. Laboratory and clinical findings associated with adequate tissue perfusion include systolic blood pressure (100–120 mm Hg), central venous pressure (8–10 mm Hg), oxygen saturation of the arterial blood (≥ 95%), core temperature (≥ 35°C), and hematocrit (30% to 35%). The use of vasopressors should be minimized, if at all possible, because of their splanchnic vasoconstrictive effects.

A. **Cardiovascular support.** Hemodynamic instability can be marked after brain death, with wide swings between the extremes of hypotension and hypertension. Hypotension is the most common hemodynamic abnormality observed in brain-dead organ donors. The usual cause is hypovolemia resulting from a combination of vasomotor collapse after brain death and the effects of treatment protocols to decrease intracranial pressure. Until a euvolemic state is achieved, dopamine can be used temporarily.

   Hypertension can be treated with short-acting vasodilatory agents or rapidly reversible beta-blockers. Calcium channel blockers and longer acting agents must be avoided because of their negative inotropic effects.

   Tachyarrhythmias are associated with increased catecholamine release that occurs during and immediately after brain herniation. Administration of a short-acting beta-blocker is indicated to treat this problem. Use of calcium channel blockers (e.g., verapamil) must be avoided under these circumstances because of their negative inotropic effects.

B. **Respiratory maintenance.** Vigorous tracheobronchial toilet is important, with frequent suctioning using sterile precautions. At regular intervals, the lungs must be expanded by manual inflation. Preventing atelectasis facilitates oxygenation and may obviate the need for detrimental high levels of positive end-expiratory pressure. A sample of sputum should be obtained for Gram's stain and for cultures to exclude the presence of infection. The lowest F_{IO_2} capable of maintaining the Pa_{O_2} greater than 100 mm Hg should be selected.

C. **Renal function.** Maintaining adequate systemic arterial perfusion pressure and brisk urine output (>1–2 ml/kg/h), while minimizing the use of vasopressors, contributes to good renal allograft function and reduces the rate of acute tubular necrosis posttransplant. If the urine production is still insufficient (< 1 ml/kg/h) after adequate volume loading, loop or osmotic diuretics should be used. Nephrotoxic drugs should be avoided.

   Polyuria is frequent in brain-dead donors, usually secondary to diabetes insipidus. It should be suspected when urine volumes exceed 300 ml/h in conjunction with hypernatremia, elevated serum osmolality, and a low urinary sodium concentration and osmolality. Once urine output exceeds 300 ml/h because of diabetes insipidus, desmopressin (a synthetic analog of vasopressin) should be administered.

D. **Hypothermia.** After brain death, hypothermia usually ensues. Adverse effects of hypothermia include decreased myocardial contractility, hypotension, cardiac dysrhythmias, cardiac arrest, hepatic and renal dysfunction, acidosis, and coagulopathy. Donor core temperature, therefore, must be maintained at 35°C or more.

Selected Readings

Alexander JW, Vaughn WK. The use of "marginal" donors for organ transplantation. *Transplantation* 1991;51:135.
A good review on the use of less than ideal donors as a method to deal with the organ shortage.

Darby JM, Stein K, Grenvik A, et al. Approach to management of the heartbeating "brain dead" organ donor. *JAMA* 1989;261:2222.
A practical description.

Evans RW, Orians CE, Ascher NL. The potential supply of organ donors. An assessment of the efficiency of organ procurement efforts in the United States. *JAMA* 1992;267:239.
A good article on the efforts to increase organ procurement.

Guidelines for multiorgan donor management and procurement. *UNOS Update* 1993;9:14.
Useful guidelines from the national organ placement agency.

Heffron TC. Organ procurement and management of the multiorgan donor. In: Hall JB, Schmidt GA, Wood LDH, eds. *Principles of critical care.* New York: McGraw-Hill, Inc.; 1992:891.
An excellent chapter on organ procurement techniques.

Kootstra G. The asystolic, or non-heartbeating, donor. *Transplantation* 1997;63:917.
A good review.

Organ transplantation. Issues and recommendation. Report of the Task Force on Organ Transplantation, US Department of Health and Human Services; 1986:36.
A good outline of important issues concerning the availability of cadaver donors.

Starzl TE, Hakala TR, Shaw BW, et al. A flexible procedure for multiple cadaveric organ procurement. *Surg Gynecol Obstet* 1984;158:223.
A good description of the surgical technique for organ procurement.

Wijnen RMH, van der Linden CJ. Donor treatment after pronouncement of brain death: a neglected intensive care problem. *Transpl Int* 1991;4:186.
A good review.

Youngner SJ, Landefeld CS, Coulton CJ, et al. Brain death and organ retrieval: a cross-sectional survey of knowledge and concepts among health professionals. *JAMA* 1989;261:2205.
An interesting paper on opinions regarding organ procurement among non-transplant health professionals.

173. REJECTION, INFECTION, AND MALIGNANCY IN SOLID ORGAN TRANSPLANT RECIPIENTS

Abhinav Humar, Kenneth L. Brayman, and David L. Dunn

I. General principles. Today, many immunosuppressive drugs are available, and they are used at most centers in combination to achieve synergistic effects on various components of the immune system, but also to avoid drug-specific toxicities that would occur with high doses of any given agent. Significant improvements in allograft and patient survival for all organ types were achieved in the 1980s with the advent of cyclosporine A. Currently, azathioprine, cyclosporine, FK506 (tacrolimus), mycophenolate mofetil, rapamycin, and deoxyspergualin are used alone with corticosteroids or in three-drug combinations. Some centers employ antilymphocyte antibody preparations for so-called induction therapy as well.

Generally, relatively high doses of each agent are administered early posttransplant, and drug doses are progressively decreased once stable allograft function is achieved. Higher doses of the selected agents are again administered to treat rejection in addition to high-dose corticosteroids, or alternative agents are chosen. Corticosteroids generally are used in most patients, although some centers withdraw these from the regimen after 1 year of stable allograft function. In the critical care setting, drug level monitoring may be important, and interactions of these agents with other drugs must be carefully considered. Although immunosuppressive therapy effectively prevents or reverses rejection in many patients, it predisposes transplant patients to a wide variety of different types of serious infections, often caused by organisms that would not cause infection in the normal host, and to certain types of malignancies.

II. Rejection. Rejection is an immunologic response to the presence of non-self antigens. Recognition of non-self antigens (the afferent limb of the immune response) and generation of an effector response (the efferent limb) are the key components of this process. Rejection involves three broad categories: (a) hyperacute rejection, which occurs within minutes to hours posttransplant: it results from the presence of preformed recipient antidonor antibodies reacting with the allograft (pretransplant cross-match has nearly eliminated this type of rejection); (b) acute rejection, which typically occurs within days to weeks posttransplant: it involves recognition of donor antigens (primarily by T cells), and is characterized by T-cell activation and generation of a cell-mediated immune response; and (c) chronic rejection, which usually occurs months or years posttransplant: it is a gradual process characterized by progressive functional deterioration and common morphologic features, including interstitial fibrosis and progressive luminal narrowing of blood vessels (both immunologic and nonimmunologic mechanisms are thought to be involved).

A. Kidney. Acute rejection occurs in 18% to 60% of kidney transplant recipients. Those who experience acute rejection have decreased short- and long-term graft survival. The most common sign of acute rejection is a rise in the serum creatinine level. The differential diagnosis should include other possible causes such as ureteral obstruction, urinary leak, cyclosporine or tacrolimus nephrotoxicity, and hypovolemia.

Examination, initially by a duplex Doppler ultrasound study, is done to exclude other causes of an elevated creatinine level. Percutaneous renal allograft biopsy and histologic analysis of graft tissue should be done to establish the diagnosis of rejection. Acute cellular rejection is characterized by a cellular infiltrate in the interstitium, tubules, vessels, and glomeruli. Acute vascular rejection is characterized by endothelial cell swelling, intervascular coagulation, and fibrinoid necrosis of vessels.

Chronic rejection is characterized by a gradual deterioration in graft function or proteinuria occurring several months to years posttransplant. In addition to obliterative fibrosis of the small vessels, progressive interstitial fibrosis and tubular atrophy are seen. Previous acute rejection episodes significantly increase the risk of chronic rejection.

Treatment of acute rejection generally entails initial intravenous (IV) administration of high doses (~1 g) of corticosteroids. If the rejection episode does not respond within 1 to 2 days to this therapy, an anti–T-cell antibody preparation is added (OKT3, ATGAM). Attempts to treat chronic rejection with increased immunosuppression have been effective; therefore, baseline levels of immunosuppression should be maintained in this situation unless severe allograft dysfunction is observed. If end-stage renal failure recurs, retransplantation should be considered.

B. Pancreas. Acute pancreas rejection is more difficult to diagnose, compared with the kidney, because of the lack of a specific sensitive marker. Elevated serum amylase levels can be related both to rejection and to graft pancreatitis, whereas hyperglycemia is a late manifestation of acute rejection. A decrease in urine amylase levels is the most accurate signal of acute pancreas rejection, but it is only applicable to bladder-drained grafts. For a simultaneous pancreas–kidney transplant (SPK), the kidney may serve as a marker for pancreas rejection, because acute rejection can occur simultaneously in both grafts; however, so-called discordant rejection is not infrequent (25%–30% incidence). Of course, the kidney cannot serve as a marker if the pancreas is transplanted alone or in pancreas-kidney (PAK) transplants, which involve disparate donors. In these situations, percutaneous biopsy of the pancreas allograft can be performed. Findings of rejection include diffuse mononuclear cell infiltrates in the pancreatic parenchyma with ductitis, vasculitis, and necrosis. Many episodes of pancreas rejection do not respond to high-dose steroids; therefore, treatment often involves anti–T-cell antibody therapy.

C. Liver. The liver allograft differs from other commonly transplanted organs in several ways. Because of the liver's ability to abrogate the effect of circulating antidonor antibodies, hyperacute rejection of it is exceedingly uncommon, even in highly HLA-sensitized patients. Thus, a pretransplant cross-match is not a requirement for a liver transplant.

Acute rejection occurs in 50% to 70% of liver transplant recipients. Liver enzyme levels become elevated; a cholestatic picture is common. Vascular thrombosis, biliary obstruction or leak, infection, and preservation injury must be included in the differential diagnosis. A percutaneous core liver biopsy, T-tube cholangiogram, and duplex ultrasound should be obtained to ascertain the cause of liver dysfunction. The histologic features of acute rejection include activated mononuclear infiltrates in the portal spaces, along with bile ductular damage and venulitis. The most specific feature of acute rejection, when present, is endotheliitis of the portal venules and hepatic arterioles. Corticosteroids are the first-line agents in the treatment of acute hepatic rejection. A poor or incomplete histologic and enzyme response to steroids necessitates treatment with an additional agent, usually an anti–T-cell antibody preparation.

D. Heart. Acute heart rejection occurs most frequently within the first 3 months posttransplant. Percutaneous transjugular right ventricular endomyocardial biopsy allows for effective screening and early treatment of rejection episodes. Clinical signs of acute rejection can include fever, fatigue, malaise, dyspnea, and other signs of cardiac dysfunction. Accelerated coronary artery atherosclerosis in the graft is a major cause of mortality months to years posttransplant; it can represent a form of chronic rejection. The coronary arteries are affected by concentric intimal proliferation along the entire length, including the epicardial and intramyocardial regions. Congestive heart failure, ventricular arrhythmias, or myocardial infarction can be a consequence of this progressive vasculopathy.

E. Lung. Acute rejection occurs in nearly all lung transplant recipients. Prompt diagnosis and treatment are important. Transbronchial lung biopsy, with three to five samples per lung, can provide adequate tissue for histologic diagnosis. Symptoms of acute rejection include breathlessness, chest tightness, and cough.

Obliterative bronchiolitis, a manifestation of chronic lung rejection, affects approximately 50% of heart–lung transplant recipients and a somewhat smaller percentage of lung-only transplant recipients. It causes submucosal fibrosis and results in obliteration of the airways, leading to loss of lung function.

III. Infection. Infection remains a major cause of morbidity and mortality after solid organ transplants. Immunosuppression, certain medical devices, diabetes mellitus, leukopenia, uremia, cadaver allografts, and treatment of rejection episodes are all associated with decreased host immunity and increased risk for infection.

A. Bacterial infections. Bacterial infections primarily occur in the first few weeks posttransplant. The major sites are the incisional wound, respiratory tract, urinary tract, and blood stream. Perioperative systemic antibiotics decrease the risk and incidence of some infections. Intraabdominal infections predominate in liver and pancreas transplant recipients. Bacterial pneumonia is common in lung transplant recipients. For that reason, all transplant patients should receive prophylactic IV antibiotics at the time of surgery, directed against common microbes that occur as part of the endogenous microflora of the skin (all transplants), urine (kidney), bile (liver), gut (pancreas, small bowel), or upper airway (lung and heart-lung). In general, selected second- or third-generation cephalosporins or penicillins plus β-lactamase inhibitors are satisfactory.

B. Viral infections. Certain viral infections are particularly common posttransplant. Most common are infections involving the herpesvirus group; cytomegalovirus (CMV) is clinically the most important. It establishes latent infection in its host and persists throughout life. Infection has been correlated with the overall degree of immunosuppression. CMV infection usually occurs 4 to 12 weeks posttransplant or after treatment of rejection. A wide spectrum of disease manifestations can be seen during CMV infection. The infection can be subclinical or can present with a mild flulike syndrome. Leukopenia, myalgia, and malaise are usual. CMV can also present as tissue-invasive disease, resulting in interstitial pneumonitis, hepatitis, or gastrointestinal ulcerations. CMV seronegative recipients of organs from CMV seropositive donors are at highest risk. The incidence of CMV disease is reduced by use of prophylactic acyclovir or ganciclovir for 12 weeks posttransplant. Symptomatic disease is generally treated with IV ganciclovir and, if severe or life-threatening, a reduction in immunosuppression.

C. Fungal infections. Most commonly, fungal infections are caused by *Candida* spp. *Aspergillus* spp. account for a much smaller percentage but are more serious. With invasive Candida or Aspergillus infection, the mortality rate usually exceeds 20%. The standard treatment of serious posttransplant fungal infections has been amphotericin B, along with overall reduction in immunosuppression. Fluconazole, less toxic than amphotericin B, is effective against some forms of candidiasis as well as cryptococcal meningitis. Recently, liposomal amphotericin B preparations have become available and appear to be as efficacious as the standard preparation, and less nephrotoxic.

IV. Malignancy. Organ transplant recipients exhibit an increased risk for developing certain types of de novo malignancies, including nonmelanomatous skin cancers (~3–7×), lymphoproliferative disease (~20–30×), gynecologic and urologic cancers, and Kaposi's sarcoma.

A. Skin cancers. The most common malignancies in transplant recipients are skin cancers. They tend to be located on sun-exposed areas and are usually squamous cell carcinomas. Often, they are multiple and have an increased predilection to metastasize. Human papillomavirus DNA has been detected in these tumors, suggesting that immunosuppression may have a permissive effect for viral proliferation. Diagnosis and treatment are the same as for the general population. Patients are encouraged to use sunscreen liberally and to avoid significant sun exposure.

B. Posttransplant lymphoproliferative disease (PTLD). Lymphomas constitute the largest group of noncutaneous neoplasms in transplant recipients. Most (> 95%) of these lymphomas consist of a spectrum of B-cell proliferation disorders, associated with Epstein-Barr virus (EBV), known collectively as PTLD. Risk factors include degree of immunosuppression, anti–T-cell antibody therapy, tacrolimus, and primary EBV infection posttransplant.

A wide variety of clinical manifestations may be seen. Symptoms can be systemic and include fever, fatigue, weight loss, or progressive encephalopathy. Lymphadenopathy can be localized, diffuse, or absent. Intrathoracic PTLD may present with well-circumscribed pulmonary nodules, with or without mediastinal adenopathy. Abdominal pain, rectal bleeding, or bowel perforation can occur with intraabdominal involvement. Allograft involvement can occur and cause organ dysfunction. Central nervous system involvement is much more common than what occurs from lymphomas in the normal patient population.

Diagnosis is confirmed by histologic examination of tissue specimens, including in situ DNA hybridization studies to detect EBV genome. Treatment measures that have been employed include reduction of immunosuppression, IV ganciclovir or acyclovir, interferon alfa-2b, surgical extirpative therapy, or combinations of these modalities. Mortality can exceed 80%.

C. Other malignancies. A variety of other malignancies have an increased incidence in transplant recipients. Conventional treatment is appropriate for most malignancies posttransplant. A reduction in immunosuppression should occur, particularly if bone marrow suppressive chemotherapeutic agents are administered. However, allograft function should be maintained for those organs that are critical to survival (heart, liver, lung), while the risks of ongoing immunosuppression must be weighed against the benefits of organ function and the trade-off of maintenance therapy (e.g., hemodialysis, exogenous insulin, total parenteral nutrition) for other types of transplants.

Selected Readings

Basadonna GP, Matas AJ, Gillingham KJ. Early versus late acute renal allograft rejection: impact on chronic rejection. *Transplantation* 1993;55:993.

A retrospective study demonstrating the detrimental impact of late rejection episodes in kidney transplant recipients.

Brayman KL, Stephanian E, Matas AJ. Analysis of infectious complications occurring after solid-organ transplantation. *Arch Surg* 1992;127:38.

An excellent overview of infectious complications in immunosuppressed transplant patients.

Dunn DL, Najarian JS. Infectious complications in transplant surgery. In: Davis JM, Shires GT, eds. *Principles and management of surgical infection.* Philadelphia: JB Lippincott; 1991:425–464.

A good chapter on infections occurring after common transplant procedures.

Klinitmalm GB, Nevy JR, Husberg BS. Rejection in liver transplantation. *Hepatology* 1989;10:978.

A good review.

Lawrence EC. Diagnosis and management of lung allograft rejection. *Clin Chest Med* 1990;11:269.

A good review.

McMaster P. The diagnosis and treatment of pancreatic rejection. In: Dubenard JM, Sutherland DER, ed. *International handbook of pancreas transplantation.* Boston: Kluwer Academic Publishers; 1989:187.

An excellent review.

Nagano H, Tilney NL. Chronic allograft failure: the clinical problem. *Am J Med Sci* 1997;313:305.

A comprehensive review of chronic rejection.

O'Connell JB, Renlund DG. Diagnosis and treatment of cardiac allograft rejection. In: Thompson ME, ed. *Cardiac transplantation.* Philadelphia: FA Davis; 1990:147.

A good review.

Paul LC, Bendiktsson H. Chronic transplant rejection: magnitude of the problem and pathogenic mechanisms. *Transplantation Review* 1993;7:96.

A good review.

Rubin RH, Tolkoff-Rubin NE. Antimicrobial strategies in the care of organ transplant recipients. *Antimicrob Agents Chemother* 1993;37:619.

An excellent review of the medical management of infectious complications.

Sabatine MS, Auchincloss HA. Cell-mediated rejection. In: Solez R, Racusen LC, Billingham ME, eds. *Solid organ transplant rejection: mechanisms, pathology and diagnosis;* 1996:1–27.
An excellent chapter.

Solez K, Axelsen RA, Benediktsson H. International standardization of criteria for the histologic diagnosis of renal allograft rejection: the Banff working classification of kidney transplant pathology. *Kidney Int* 1993;44:411.
A landmark paper on the histologic evaluation of kidney rejection.

174. BONE MARROW TRANSPLANTATION

Karen K. Ballen and F. Marc Stewart

I. General principles. Bone marrow transplantation is considered curative therapy for many neoplastic disorders, including leukemia, lymphoma, myeloma; as well as bone marrow failure syndromes such as aplastic anemia; and genetic diseases such as thalassemia (Table 174-1). Bone marrow transplantation can also prolong survival for more common diseases such as breast and ovarian cancer. An estimated 47,000 transplants were performed worldwide in 1997. The source of stem cells can be either bone marrow (harvested from the iliac crests in the operating room), peripheral blood stem cells (collected by apheresis after stimulation with growth factors plus or minus chemotherapy), or cord blood (blood collected from the umbilical cord after the delivery of a baby). Types of transplants include autologous (using one's own stem cells) (Fig. 174-1), syngeneic (identical twin), allogeneic (family member) (Fig. 174-2), or unrelated donor (volunteer donor with similar human leukocyte antigen [HLA] type) (Fig. 174-2). The type of transplant and the source of stem cells used are complex decisions based on patient's age, medical condition, diagnosis, and the availability of a matched donor.

II. Pathogenesis. The cause of problems after transplantation are related to four main factors:

1. High-dose chemotherapy with or without total body irradiation (TBI). Side effects of the high doses of chemotherapy and radiotherapy used to prepare or condition the patient. The high doses of chemotherapy and radiotherapy, which can affect the functions of the lung, liver, heart, and kidney, can lead to problems such as interstitial pneumonitis, venoocclusive disease, cardiomyopathy, and renal failure.
2. Infection: The high doses of chemo- or radiotherapy lower the white blood cell count to essentially 0 for a period of 10 to 25 days. This prolonged period of profound neutropenia predisposes the patient to a variety of bacterial, viral, and fungal infections. For patients receiving allogeneic transplants, further suppression of lymphocyte function occurs from the transplant itself and from the use of immunosuppressive medications such as steroids, cyclosporine, and methotrexate.
3. Bleeding: The high doses of chemo- or radiotherapy also lower the platelet count. The average time for the platelet count to return above 50,000 is 2 to 4 weeks. In addition, liver damage, poor nutrition, and the use of antibiotics can also lead to an elevation in the protime, which may further exacerbate bleeding.
4. Graft-versus-host disease (GVHD). Graft-versus-host disease is a problem unique to allogeneic or unrelated bone marrow transplantation, related to the following three factors:

   - Genetic differences found between the host (patient) and the donor (graft).
   - The patient is immunocompromised (from the high doses of chemotherapy and radiation).
   - The patient is receiving cells that modulate the immune system (lymphocytes) with the transplant.

Graft-versus-host disease is more likely to occur if the patient is older, the transplant is mismatched or from an unrelated donor, and if the donor is a woman who is parous. Cyclosporine, methotrexate, and prednisone are all part of standard regimens to prevent GVHD. The bone marrow can also be depleted of lymphocytes to decrease the risk of GVHD. Acute GVHD (defined as occurring before 100 days posttransplantation) can affect the skin, liver, and intestinal tract. Patients with acute GVHD are highly immunosuppressed and require careful evaluation for infection. Empiric broad-spectrum antibiotic treatment for fever is often indicated

TABLE 174-1. Cure rates with stem cell transplantation for hematologic disease

Disease	Stem Cell Transplant	Poor Risk (%)	Good Risk (%)
Chronic myeloid leukemia	Allo	10–20	60–85
Acute myeloid leukemia	Allo	10–20	50–70
Acute lymphoblastic leukemia	Allo	10–20	30–60
Thalassemia	Allo	10–20	90
Aplastic anemia	Allo	10–20	90
Non-Hodgkins lymphoma and Hodgkin's disease (usually autologous)	Auto/Allo	10–20	40–70

even when blood counts are normal. A standard grading system exists with which to correlate survival. Chronic GVHD, which can occur months to years after transplantation, can affect the skin, liver, lung, eyes, and joints. Patients with chronic GVHD are more susceptible to infection with encapsulated organisms, viruses, and fungi.

III. Diagnosis. The diagnosis of posttransplantation problems is often difficult. The timing of the problem posttransplantation can often be helpful (Figs. 174-3 and 174-4). For instance, bacterial infections are most likely to occur in the first few weeks of transplant when the white blood count is low. Other infections such as *Pneumocystis carinii* pneumonia are more likely to occur between 30 and 180 days posttransplant. In many cases, culture results or histologic documentation (e.g., from bronchoalveolar lavage or liver biopsy) are necessary to make the diagnosis.

IV. Treatment. The treatment of the specific problems is discussed below. Treatment of transplant complications, in general, should be coordinated with the transplant physician who is knowledgeable about these complications and familiar with the history of the patient.

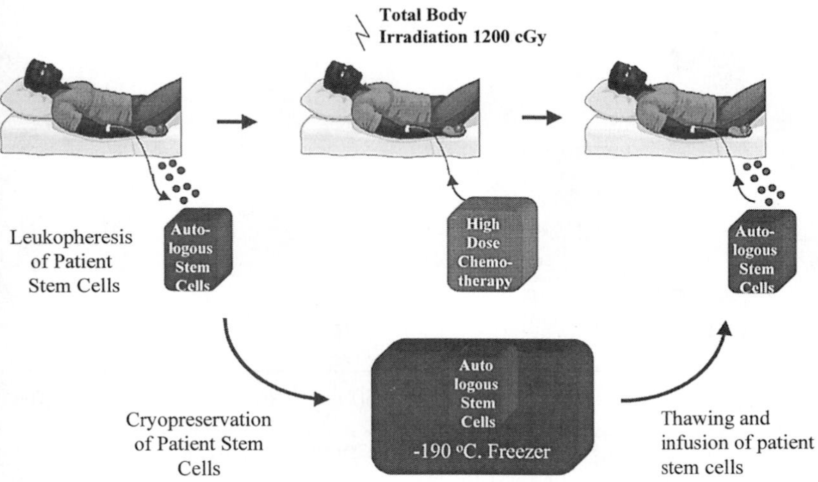

FIG. 174-1. Autologous stem cell transplantation.

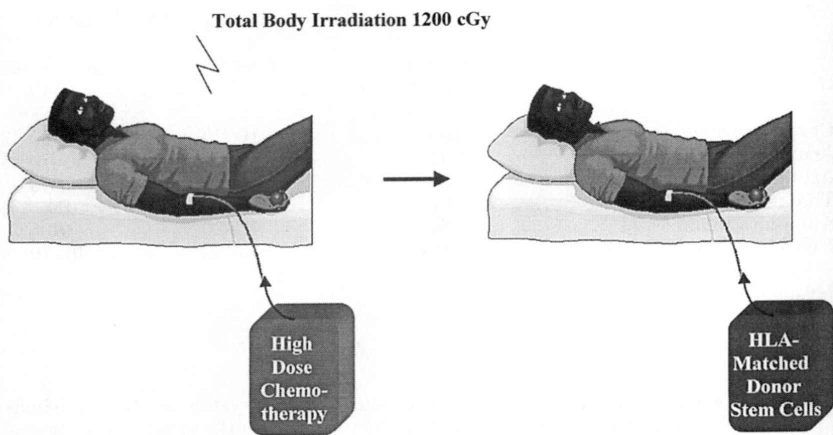

FIG. 174-2. Allogeneic stem cell transplantation.

A. **Medical complications of transplantation patients**

1. **Toxicity from chemotherapy or radiotherapy**

a. **Lung.** Several chemotherapy drugs, including BCNU and busulfan, as well as total body irradiation can lead to nonspecific pneumonitis or fibrosis in the lungs. The treatment is to rule out infectious agents and then to administer high-dose steroids—such as solumedrol (2 mg/kg/d).

b. **Liver.** The chemotherapy drugs can cause venoocclusive disease of the liver. Venoocclusive disease occurs between 1 and 4 weeks posttransplantation; it is characterized by an elevated bilirubin, weight gain, and ascites. Low-dose heparin is used in many institutions to prevent venoocclusive disease. The treatment for venoocclusive disease is usually sup-

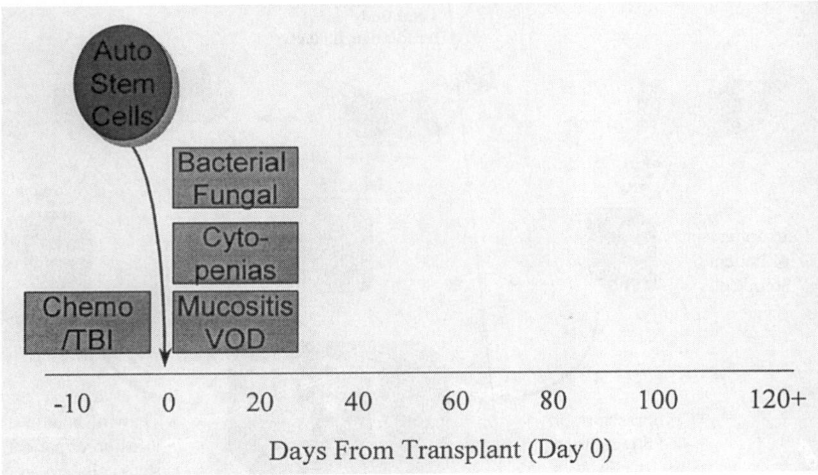

FIG. 174-3. Complications following autologous transplantation. (TBI, total body irradication; VOD, venoocclusive disease of the liver).

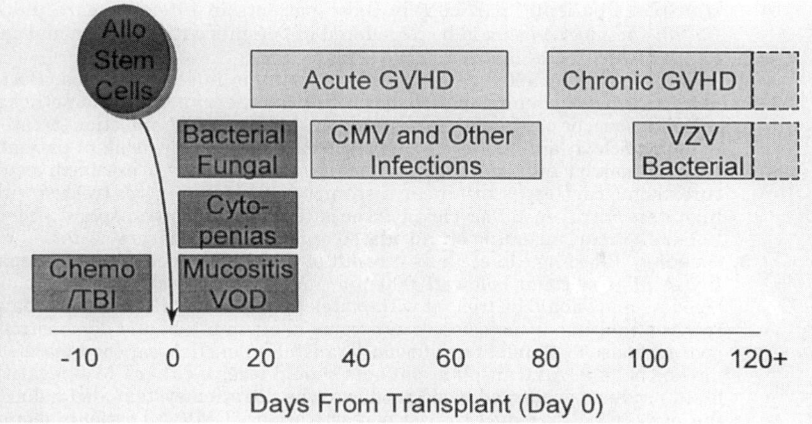

FIG. 174-4. Complications following allogeneic transplantation.(TBI, total body irradiation; GVHD, graft-versus-host disease; CMV, Cytomegalovirus; VOD, venoocclusive disease of the liver; VZV, varicella zoster virus)

portive, with care to avoid dehydration and hepatotoxins. Agents that have been used for the treatment of venoocclusive disease include thrombolytic therapy, prostaglandins, and antithrombin III, although no proven benefit to these agents exits.

c. **Heart.** High-dose cyclophosphamide occasionally can cause cardiomyopathy within a few days of receiving the drug. Treatment is supportive, including diuretics and inotropic agents, such as digoxin.

d. **Renal.** Many of the drugs used in transplant patients cause an elevation of the serum creatinine. The most common agents are the aminoglycosides, amphotericin, and cyclosporine. Cyclosporine can also contribute to the hemolytic uremic syndrome or thrombotic thrombocytopenic purpura posttransplant. The treatment is careful discontinuation of the offending agent and consideration of plasma exchange.

2. **Infection.** In the first 30 days after transplant, the most common infections are bacterial and fungal. The most likely viral infection early after transplant is herpes simplex virus. Many transplant programs, therefore, use a prophylactic regimen of antibiotics (e.g., levaquin and penicillin), antifungals (e.g., fluconazole or low-dose amphotericin), and antivirals (e.g., acyclovir). With the use of indwelling catheters, the risk of gram-positive infections such as staphylococcal and streptococcal infection is more common than gram-negative infections from *Escherichia coli* and *Pseudomonas* spp. Fungal infection is a serious infection in immunocompromised patients and may present with skin lesions (candida), sinus involvement (aspergillus or mucor), lung lesions (aspergillus or candida), or hepatitis (candida).

Fever should be treated immediately as a presumptive infection. The fever workup should consist of a careful history and physical examination, blood cultures for bacteria and fungus, urine culture, and a chest x-ray study. Antibiotics to treat gram-negative infection, including pseudomonas, should be started promptly. A common regimen is ceftazidime, with or without an aminoglycoside. If fever persists an additional 48 hours or if the central line site is red or tender, additional coverage for gram-positive infections (e.g., vancomycin) should be added. If fever persists an additional 2 to 4 days or clinical suspicion of fungus exists, amphotericin should be added as antifungal coverage. *Clostridium difficile* colitis can be a common infection in transplant patients, particularly those patients in intensive care units. *C. difficile* infection should be considered in patients with diarrhea and can be treated with oral metronidazole (Flagyl).

Between 30 and 360 days after transplant, other infections such as *Pneumocystis carinii* pneumonia (treated with trimethoprim and sulfamethoxazole, dapsone, or pentamidime) or cytomegalovirus (CMV) infection (treated with ganciclovir and γ-globulin) may become apparent. Transplant patients with pulmonary infiltrates should undergo bronchoscopy to establish a culture diagnosis. Herpes zoster can also appear at this time; it is treated with high-dose intravenous acyclovir. Even after 1 year posttransplant, infections can occur, including encapsulated organisms and herpes zoster.

3. **Bleeding.** Bleeding can occur as a result of thrombocytopenia or coagulopathy. A platelet count below 10,000/mm^3 increases the risk of spontaneous bleeding and should be treated with platelet transfusion. Patients who have received multiple transfusions can become alloimmunized and demonstrate poor response to platelet transfusion. Transfusion of HLA-matched platelets may be helpful. All transplant patients should receive either CMV-negative blood products or filtered blood products (the filtration system also reduces the load of CMV) to reduce the risk of reactivation of CMV. All patients should receive irradiated blood products to reduce the risk of transfusion-associated GVHD.

   Diffuse alveolar hemorrhage is in the differential diagnosis of pulmonary infiltrates. Bleeding can be seen on bronchoscopy. The treatment is high doses of solumedrol (e.g., 1 g/d for 3 days).

4. **Graft-versus-host disease.** Acute GVHD, which can affect the skin, liver, and intestinal tract, can be life-threatening. Skin lesions can progress from a mild rash on the palms or shoulders to grade IV GVHD with bullous changes. Local care is similar to that given a burn patient. Liver GVHD is usually associated with an elevated bilirubin and mild elevation of the alkaline phosphatase and transaminases. Intestinal GVHD can be characterized by massive diarrhea requiring fluid and electrolyte replacement. Often a biopsy of the involved site is necessary to make the diagnosis of GVHD. The initial treatment for acute GVHD is steroids (solumedrol, at 2 mg/kg/d). Patients with steroid refractory GVHD have a poor prognosis and can be treated with antithymocyte globulin, or investigational agents.

   Chronic GVHD can develop into pulmonary difficulties with bronchiolitis obliterans, skin lesions characteristic of scleroderma, liver problems, dry eyes, and dry mouth. Chronic GVHD can be treated with steroids, cyclosporine, azathioprine, or thalidomide. Patients with chronic GVHD are at high risk of infections and usually receive prophylactic antibiotics. They should be treated aggressively for fever when a high suspicion exists for fungal infection.

Selected Readings

Autologous Blood and Marrow Transplantation Registry. *ABMTR Newsletter* 1998;5:4.

Information from the Autologous Blood and Marrow Transplant Registry and the International Bone Marrow Transplant Registry, which collect statistics from more than 375 transplant centers worldwide.

Bearman SI. The syndrome of hepatic veno-occlusive disease after marrow transplantation. *Blood* 1995;85:3005.

An excellent review of the clinical features, differential diagnosis, and treatment of graft-versus-host disease.

Bilgrami S, Feingold JM, Dorsky D, et al. Incidence and outcome of *Clostridium difficile* infections following autologous peripheral blood stem cell transplantation. *Bone Marrow Transplant* 1999;23:1039.

A retrospective evaluation of 200 autologous transplant recipients, confirming a 7% incidence of Clostridium difficile.

Chao NJ, Duncan SR, Long GD, et al. Corticosteroid therapy for diffuse alveolar hemorrhage in autologous bone marrow transplant recipients. *Ann Intern Med* 1991;114:145.

A small series showing survival with the use of high doses of steroids.

Lazarus HM, Vogelsang GB, Rowe JM. Prevention and treatment of acute graft-versus-host disease: the old and the new. A report from the Eastern Cooperative Oncology Group (ECOG). *Bone Marrow Transplant* 1997;19:577.

A review article that discusses new treatment modalities for graft-versus-host disease.

Martin P, Nash R, Sanders J, et al. Reproducibility in retrospective grading of acute graft-versus-host disease after allogeneic marrow transplantation. *Bone Marrow Transplant* 1998;21:273.

This study outlines some of the difficulties in the grading system of graft-versus-host disease.

Ringden O, Remberger M, Runde V, et al. Peripheral blood stem cell transplantation from unrelated donors: a comparison with marrow transplantation. *Blood.* 1999; 94:455.

This recent study compares the engraftment times for neutrophils and platelets for two different stem cell sources—bone marrow and peripheral blood stem cells.

Schriber JR, Herzig GP. Transplantation-associated thrombotic thrombocytopenic purpura and hemolytic uremic syndrome. *Semin Hematol* 1997;34:126.

A review of the diagnosis, risk assessment, etiology, and treatment of thrombocytopenic purpura in transplant patients.

Thomas ED, Clift RA, Feiffer F, et al. Marrow transplantation for the treatment of chronic myelogeneous leukemia. *Ann Intern Med* 1986;104:155.

The classic reference describing one of the first diseases cured by bone marrow transplantation.

Wingard JR. Fungal infections after bone marrow transplant. *Biol Blood Marrow Trans* 1999;5:55.

Recent update on the biology, epidemiology, diagnosis, and treatment of fungus infections.

XV. RHEUMATOLOGIC AND IMMUNOLOGIC PROBLEMS IN THE INTENSIVE CARE UNIT

175. RHEUMATOLOGIC DISORDERS IN THE INTENSIVE CARE UNIT

David F. Giansiracusa and Leslie R. Harrold

I. General principles. Three groups of rheumatic disease patients present problems of management in the intensive care unit (ICU), including (a) rheumatologic diseases can pose problems in the execution of certain critical care procedures, such as endotracheal intubation; (b) acute rheumatologic syndromes can develop during hospitalization, and (c) prolonged immobilization itself causes problems.

II. Rheumatic diseases complicating intensive care procedures. Involvement of the cervical spine can complicate endotracheal intubations in patients with rheumatoid arthritis (RA), juvenile rheumatoid arthritis (JRA), ankylosing spondylitis (AS), or progressive systemic sclerosis. The use of fiberoptic intubation, laryngoscopy, or blind nasotracheal intubation may suffice, although a tracheostomy may be required for satisfactory tracheal cannulation.

Subluxation of the first and second cervical vertebral bodies (atlantoaxial subluxation) or a staircase cervical subluxation can occur in forced manipulation of the neck, sometimes precipitating symptoms and signs of spinal cord compression.

Patients at risk should be identified with lateral cervical spine radiographs in the flexed position that should reveal no more than 3 mm of separation between the odontoid process and the arch of the atlas. Forced neck flexion should be avoided. If neurologic symptoms of spinal cord compression develop in a patient with either atlantoaxial or staircase subluxation, computed tomography (CT) may be useful to confirm the diagnosis.

In JRA or RA, temporomandibular joint disease may limit motion of the lower jaw. Scleroderma can decrease access to the oropharynx as a result of soft tissue fibrosis. The need for nasotracheal intubation should be anticipated in all patients with limited oral apertures.

Cricoarytenoid joint disease in RA and JRA can immobilize the vocal cords in the midline position. If hoarseness is elicited, indirect laryngoscopy to evaluate mobility of the vocal cords is advisable. If the cords are immobile, inhaled corticosteroid preparations may be useful, but preparations should be made for cricothyroidotomy or tracheostomy, should the need arise to establish an emergency airway.

III. Acute rheumatic diseases in the intensive care setting

A. Gout. Definition: Gout is a disorder characterized by one or more attacks of mono- or polyarticular arthritis in the setting of prolonged hyperuricemia triggered by an inflammatory reaction to monosodium urate crystals in the joint space or nearby tissues.

1. **Pathogenesis.** Factors causing fluxes in serum urate can precipitate an acute attack (Table 175-1). An accumulation of organic acids (e.g., lactic acid, β-hydroxybutyric acid, and acetoacetic acid) can also contribute to gouty attacks. Conditions that can cause hyperuricemia and gouty arthritis are listed in Table 175-1.
2. **Clinical features.** Gouty arthritis is characterized by the sudden onset of an extremely painful arthritis involving one or more joints, is asymmetrical, and may be accompanied by fever, particularly in the case of a polyarticular involvement. The great toe is involved in more than 50% of initial attacks and in 90% of attacks at some time in the course of the disease. The other common sites of involvement include insteps, ankles, knees, wrists, fingers, and elbows. Typically, the involved area is erythematous, swollen, warm, and painful on motion and to touch.
3. **Diagnosis.** Gout is confirmed by visualization by polarized microscopy of the needle-shaped, negatively birefringent monosodium urate crystals within synovial fluid polymorphonuclear leukocytes. Because septic arthritis and gout can coexist, synovial fluid should be stained for microorganisms and cultured for bacteria.

TABLE 175-1. Factors that increase likelihood of hyperuricemia and acute gout in the critically ill patient

A. Conditions associated with increased production of uric acid
   1. Myeloproliferative disorders
   2. Lymphoproliferative disorders
   3. Chronic hemolytic anemias
   4. Multiple myeloma
   5. Severe psoriasis

B. Conditions associated with decreased renal excretion of uric acid
   1. Chronic renal disease (decreased renal function mass)
   2. Lead nephropathy (decreased fractional excretion of uric acid)
   3. Decreased effective arteriolar blood volume
      a. Congestive heart failure
      b. Sodium depletion
      c. Dehydration
      d. Diabetes insipidus
      e. Drug-induced (diuretics)
   4. Hyperlactic acidemia
      a. Hypoxemia
      b. Sepsis
      c. Shock
      d. Toxemia of pregnancy
      e. Acute alcohol intoxication
   5. Increased levels of β-hydroxybutyrate and acetoacetate
      a. Starvation
      b. Diabetic ketoacidosis
   6. Drug administration
      a. Pyrazinamide
      b. Diuretics
      c. Salicylates (low dose)
      d. Ethambutol
      e. Levodopa, α-methyldopa
      f. Cyclosporine

C. Radiocontrast dye studies

D. Surgery

4. **Treatment.** The treatment of acute gouty arthritis is listed on Table 175-2. Long-term goals (e.g., prevention of recurrent attacks, treatment of tophaceous disease or renal stones) need not be considered in the acute setting. In fact, the initiation or discontinuation of any drug that can cause acute fluxes in the serum uric acid (e.g., allopurinol, probenecid, or salicylates) may prolong an acute attack. Hyperuricemia without clinical gout need not be treated.

B. Other microcrystalline arthropathies

1. **Definition.** Other crystalline-induced syndromes can mimic gout and cause diagnostic confusion. These crystals may be composed of calcium pyrophosphate dihydrate (CPPD), calcium hydroxyapatite, or calcium oxalate.
2. **Pathogenesis.** The pathophysiology of these calcium crystal-induced arthritides involves inflammatory responses similar to that occurring in acute gout.

   The acute, self-limited form of CPPD deposition, which most closely simulates acute gout and, thus, is also known as *pseudogout,* most commonly affects the knee and can be precipitated by surgery of any type, most commonly occurring 3 days postoperatively. Severe medical illnesses (e.g., ischemic heart disease, cerebral infarction, and thrombophlebitis) can also provoke attacks of CPPD.

Patients undergoing chronic intermittent peritoneal dialysis have a high incidence of acute arthritis associated with either CPPD or calcium hydroxyapatite, whereas patients maintained on chronic hemodialysis may develop arthritis because of calcium oxalate crystals.

3. **Diagnosis.** Clinically, each of the above entities may be indistinguishable from acute gout. The diagnosis of CPPD deposition is suggested by radiographic demonstration of cartilaginous calcification of the involved joint (articular chondrocalcinosis) and is established with certainty by visualizing, under polarized microscopy, weakly positively birefringent, rhomboid-shaped crystals within synovial fluid neutrophils.

   Calcium oxalate crystals are also positively birefringent, but they are pleomorphic and bipyramidal or rodlike in shape. Smaller hydroxyapatite crystals may be definitively demonstrated by examining the synovial fluid with electron microscopy. A diagnosis of acute arthritis caused by these small crystals can be clinically presumed in the proper setting and when other diagnoses have been excluded, including joint sepsis.

4. **Treatment.** Therapeutic options for the calcium-crystalline arthropathies are identical to those for acute gout (Table 175-2).

C. Septic arthritis

1. **Definition.** Joint infection by a bacterial or fungal pathogen is the most critical diagnosis that must be established rapidly and treated appropriately in any patient who develops acute arthritis of either one or, less commonly, multiple joints. A delay in the diagnosis and treatment of this condition may lead to the destruction of articular cartilage and loss of joint function. Furthermore, a diagnosis of septic arthritis can lead to early identification of (and therapy for) the source of the septicemia, such as endocarditis.

2. **Pathogenesis.** Debilitating illnesses predispose to septic arthritis, including diabetes mellitus, alcoholism, malignancies, renal failure, system lupus erythematosus, and rheumatoid arthritis. Immunosuppressive therapy increases the risk of septic arthritis. Acute infectious arthritis can result from hematogenous spread from another site of infection, direct inoculation (e.g., from a puncture wound), or local extension (e.g., from adjacent soft tissue or bone). Septicemia is especially likely to cause infection of a diseased or prosthetic joint.

3. **Diagnosis.** Clinically, septic arthritis may be indistinguishable from the acute arthritis of other causes, such as CPPD and the other microcrystalline arthropathies. Typically, septic arthritis is acute in onset; it is monoarticular and produces swelling, tenderness, overlying erythema, warmth, and limitation of motion because of joint effusions, soft tissue swelling, and pain of the involved joint. Septic arthritis of multiple joints is well described; thus, polyarticular arthritis should not preclude consideration of infection as a cause. Accompanying fever is a variable finding; when, it may be low grade.

   Clinical suspicion remains the key to the diagnosis of septic arthritis. Because of the nature of patients in the ICU, the invasive procedures, and a large number of portals for the entry of organisms (e.g., indwelling catheters, intravenous lines), bacteremia is a concern. Any patient who develops an acutely swollen, painful joint should undergo diagnostic arthrocentesis to exclude infection unless examination of the joint indicates that the underlying process is not articular (e.g., cellulitis).

   Diagnosis of septic arthritis is confirmed by synovial fluid Gram's stains or positive cultures. Cultures should be performed both anaerobically and aerobically with special requests for fungal cultures and cultures of organisms that require a special medium for growth (e.g., *Neisseria gonorrhoeae*), if indicated. In addition to cultures, synovial fluid should be analyzed for cell count. Although leukocyte counts as low as 5,000/mm^3 occasionally are present in septic arthritis, the counts generally exceed 50,000/mm^3, and on occasion may be as high as 200,000/mm^3 with a marked neutrophil predominance.

   Although radiographs of an infected joint often appear normal early in the course of the infection, they should be obtained for evidence of osteomyelitis and as a baseline for future studies, which may show juxta-articular osteo-

TABLE 175-2. Treatment options in acute gout

Medication	Route of Administration	Dose	Side Effects	Contraindications
Adrenocorticosteroids				
ACTH	Intramuscular	40–60 IU/d for 3 days	Same as for oral prednisone	Should not be used in anticoagulated patients
Prednisone	Oral, intramuscular or intravenous	30 mg/d for 2 days, 20 mg/d for 2 days, 10 mg/d for 2 days	Sodium retention, hypokalemia, opportunistic infection, masking of signs of infection; no adrenal suppression within 1 week	Congestive heart failure underlying infection
Methylprednisolone	Intravenous	Same as for oral prednisone	Same as for oral prednisone	Same as for oral prednisone
Methylprednisolone Acetate or Triamcinolone hexacetonide	Intraarticular	20–40 mg (depends on size of affected joint)	Superimposed infection (rare)	Should not be used in anticoagulated patients
Colchicine	Oral	0.6 mg q1h until either symptomatic relief, development of gastrointestinal symptoms or a total of 10 doses[a]	Nausea, vomiting, diarrhea, abdominal pain	Serious gastrointestinal disease, hepatic failure, renal failure

	Intravenous (diluted in 20 ml saline)	2 mg initially; 1 mg q6h until dose of 4 mg[a]	Gastrointestinal toxicity rare, bone marrow suppression, severe soft tissue necrosis if extravasation occurs	Leukopenia, thrombocytopenia, poor intravenous access, renal or hepatic failure
NSAIDs				
Indomethacin	Oral	50–75 mg initially; 50 mg q8h until symptoms improve, then 25 mg until failure, resolution	Nausea, abdominal pain, gastrointestinal bleeding, peptic ulceration, headaches, confusion, seizures, renal potentiation of abnormal congestive heart failure, platelet dysfunction	Active ulcer disease, gastrointestinal bleeding, inflam- bowel disease; mental status; renal insufficiency, congestive heart failure, decreased intravascular or effective arteriolar blood volume from any cause, bleeding disorders
Other NSAIDs	Oral	High dose	As per indomethacin	As per indomethacin

[a] Dose of colchicine needs to be modified in renal and hepatic insufficiency. No colchicine should be given for next 7 days. NSAIDs, nonsteroidal antiinflammatory drugs; ACTH, adrenocorticotropic hormone; q, every.

penia, joint-space narrowing, or subchondral bone loss in later stages, particularly if diagnosis and treatment have been delayed.

4. **Treatment.** If the diagnosis of septic arthritis is either strongly suggested on clinical grounds or documented by positive Gram's stain or culture, the therapeutic approach involves (a) appropriate antibiotic therapy instituted for the presumptive or proved pathogen, (b) joint rest, and (c) adequate drainage.

   In the noncompromised patient, *Staphylococcus aureus* is the most common nongonococcal bacteria, followed by nonpneumococcal streptococci and *Streptococcus pneumoniae* (Tables 175-3 and 175-4). In the case of a prosthetic joint infection, *Staphylococcus epidermidis* is usually the causative organism, most commonly followed by *S. aureus* and *Streptococcus faecalis.* In the critically ill patient, broad-spectrum antibiotic coverage should be instituted, pending the results of cultures. In most cases, antibiotic therapy should be continued intravenously for at least 3 weeks.

   Most fungal arthritis is subacute or chronic and, thus, is not likely to represent an emergent problem in a critically ill patient. Acute arthritis has been reported to be caused by *Candida* organisms. These organisms, however, can be diagnosed by their typical appearance of synovial fluid stains, and treatment can be initiated while awaiting culture results. Treatment consists of amphotericin B administered alone, intravenously, or in combination with flucytosine, surgical drainage and debridement, and synovectomy, if necessary.

   To achieve adequate joint drainage, repeated (often daily) aspirations of synovial fluid may be necessary to relieve joint distension and remove lysosomal enzymes. If arthrocentesis cannot be frequently and adequately performed, surgical drainage or arthroscopic lavage is indicated.

   Finally, because most articular infections are the result of hematogenous spread from another site of primary infection, any patient with septic arthri-

TABLE 175-3. Antibiotic therapy of acute bacterial arthritis in the critically ill adult (known pathogen)

Organism	Antibiotic Choice	Alternatives
Staphylococcus aureus	Nafcillin 9–12 g/d (q4h) or oxacillin 9–12 g/d (q4h)	Cefazolin 4.5–6 g/d (q8h) or vancomycin 2 g/d (q12h)
Staphylococcus aureus, methicillin-resistant	Vancomycin 2 g/d (q12h)	None
Streptococcus pyogenes, Streptococcus pneumoniae	Penicillin G 12–18 million units/d (q4h)	Cefazolin or vancomycin or clindamycin 1.8 g/d (q8h)
Neisseria gonorrhoeae	Ceftriaxone 1–2 g/d (q12h)	Aztreonam, ciprofloxacin, or penicillin G
	Cefotaxime 3–6 g/d (q8h)	
Pseudomonas aeruginosa	Piperacillin 18 g/d (q4h) plus tobramycin 4–5 mg/kg/d (q8h)	Ceftazidime 6 g/d (q8h) or imipenem 2–3 g/d or aztreonam 6 g/d plus tobramycin or gentamicin or ciprofloxacin 400 mg IV (q12h)
Enterobacteriaceae	Third-generation cephalosporin plus gentamicin 4–5 mg/kg/d (q8h)	Aztreonam 3 g/d (q8h) plus gentamicin or amikacin

q, every; IV, intravenous.

TABLE 175-4. Antibiotic therapy of acute bacterial arthritis in the critically ill adult (unknown pathogen)

Gram's Stain	Presumed Organism(s)	Antibiotic(s)
Positive		
Gram-positive cocci	*Staphylococcus aureus*	Oxacillin, nafcillin, or cefazolin
Gram-positive cocci (prosthetic joint)	*Staphylococcus epidermidis, S. aureus*	Vancomycin
Gram-negative cocci	*Neisseria gonorrhoeae*	Ceftriaxone or cefotaxime
Gram-negative bacilli	*Escherichia coli, Serratia marcescens* other Enterobacteriaceae	Third-generation cephalosporin aztreonam, or ciprofloxacin
Gram-negative bacilli (thin)	*Pseudomonas aeruginosa*	Ceftazidime (or piperacillin, imipenem, or aztreonam) plus tobramycin or ciprofloxacin
Negative		
Noncompromised host	*S. aureus,*[a] Enterobacteriaceae	Third-generation cephalosporin (ceftriaxone or cefotaxime) plus vancomycin
Compromised host	*Pseudomonas aeruginosa,* Enterobacteriaceae	Imipenem (or ceftazidime, piperacillin, or aztreonam) plus tobramycin or ciprofloxacin

[a] Treatment for both gram-positive and gram-negative pathogens must be continued until cultures return.

tis without an obvious site of local inoculation should be evaluated for a primary source. Evaluation should include complete cultures from possible portals as well as blood cultures (prior to the institution of antibiotics) and other tests (e.g., echocardiogram and CT or gallium scanning) to exclude valvular vegetations or other sites of infection.

D. Hemarthrosis

1. **Definition.** In the absence of an underlying inherited disorder of coagulation, hemarthrosis in the intensive care setting is most often a complication of anticoagulation (warfarin or heparin) therapy. Hemarthrosis can also complicate severe thrombocytopenia, joint sepsis, joint trauma, and severe osteoarthritis or synovitis. Although precise criteria for hemarthrosis have not been established, the presence of a synovial fluid hematocrit in excess of 3% is generally considered diagnostic.
2. **Diagnosis.** Because hemarthrosis can be spontaneous, a history of trauma may not be present. Clinically, hemarthrosis is uniformly monoarticular and presents as a painful, swollen, and warm joint with a tense effusion on examination. A prolongation of coagulation parameters (often beyond the therapeutic range) suggests the diagnosis, but arthrocentesis is essential to confirm the diagnosis of hemarthrosis and to exclude the possibility of joint sepsis.
3. **Treatment.** Management of hemarthrosis consists of arthrocentesis. In the case of warfarin therapy, treatment consists of withholding of anticoagulants to improve clotting parameters with or without the addition of vitamin K. The temporary discomfort of hemarthrosis is often less than the risk of inducing a hypercoagulable state by the administration of vitamin K, although in the most severe cases, this may be indicated.

E. Vasculitis. Vasculitis is discussed in Chapter 178.

Selected Readings

Axelrod D, Preston S. Comparison of parenteral adrenocorticotropic hormone with oral indomethacin in the treatment of acute gout. *Arthritis Rheum* 1988;31:803.
An excellent therapeutic discussion.

Clive DM, Stoff JS. Renal syndromes associated with nonsteroidal antiinflammatory drugs. *N Engl J Med* 1984;310:563.
An excellent review of the topic.

Goldenberg DL. Infectious arthritis complicating rheumatoid arthritis and other chronic rheumatic disorders. *Arthritis Rheum* 1989;32:496.
An excellent review.

Goldenberg DL, Brandt DK, Cohen AS, et al. Treatment of septic arthritis: comparison of needle aspiration and surgery as initial modes of joint drainage. *Arthritis Rheum* 1975;18:83.
The classic paper regarding joint drainage in septic arthritis.

Goldenberg DL, Cohen AS. Acute infectious arthritis: a review of patients with nongonococcal joint infections (with emphasis on therapy and prognosis). *Am J Med* 1976; 60:369.
A classic review.

Gurley JP, Bell GR. The surgical management of patients with rheumatoid cervical spine disease. *Rheum Dis Clin North Am* 1997;23(2):317.
This and next reference are excellent discussions of establishing an airway in patients with rheumatic diseases.

Inman RD, Gallegos KV, Brause BD, et al. Clinical and microbial features of prosthetic joint infections. *Am J Med* 1984;77:47.
An excellent review.

Langford CA, Von Waes C. Upper airway obstruction in the rheumatic diseases. *Rheum Dis Clin North Am* 1997;23(2):345.
An excellent review of the topic.

McCarty DJ, ed. Crystalline deposition diseases. *Rheum Dis Clin North Am* 1988; 14(2):253.
An excellent review of the topic with 16 chapters addressing the pathophysiology, clinical, and therapeutic issues of gout and calcium-crystal-induced rheumatic syndromes.

Pioro MH, Mandell BF. Septic arthritis. *Rheum Dis Clin North Am* 1997;23(2):239.
An excellent review.

Simm LS, Mills TA. Nonsteroidal anti-inflammatory drugs. *N Engl J Med* 1980;302: 1179, 1237.
An excellent two-part review of nonsteroidal anti-inflammatory drugs.

176. ANAPHYLAXIS

Nereida A. Parada and Helen Hollingsworth

I. General principles. Anaphylaxis is the most severe and potentially fatal form of an immediate hypersensitivity reactions. The clinical features of the anaphylactic reactions are the physiologic sequelae of release of chemical mediators from tissue-based mast cells and circulating basophils and include a potential for life-threatening vascular collapse and respiratory obstruction. An *anaphylactoid reaction,* differs from anaphylactic reactions only because the chemical mediators are released by nonimmunologic mechanisms. Both will be referred to as *anaphylactic reactions.*

II. Pathophysiology

A. IgE-mediated anaphylaxis. Binding of allergenic antigen leads to bridging of adjacent IgE molecules on previously sensitized mast cells and basophils that, in turn, activates secretion of mediators of anaphylaxis (histamine, eosinophil chemotactic factor of anaphylaxis (ECF-A), and tryptase) and stimulates synthesis of kallikrein, platelet-activating factor (PAF), leukotrienes C4, D4, and E4 (LTC4, LTD4 and LTE4), products of the lipoxygenase pathway of arachidonic acid metabolism, and several cytokines. The most common substances that induce IgE antibody formation and, on subsequent challenge, provoke anaphylactic reactions (Table 176-1) are drugs, insect venoms, foods, and allergen extracts used in hyposensitization therapy.

B. Non–IgE-mediated anaphylaxis. Mast cell and basophil activation occurs through a variety of non–IgE-mediated mechanisms, including direct activation of mast cells with subsequent release of chemical mediators, cyclooxygenase inhibition, and blood product transfusion in individuals deficient in Ig-A (Table 176-2). Anaphylaxis can also be idiopathic.

C. The physiologic consequences of chemical-mediator release in anaphylaxis are (a) increased vascular permeability; (b) increased secretion from nasal and bronchiolar mucous glands; (c) smooth-muscle contraction in the blood vessels, the bronchioles, the gastrointestinal tract, and the uterus; (d) migration-attraction of eosinophils and neutrophils; (e) bradykinin generation stimulated by kallikrein substances; and (f) induction of platelet aggregation and degranulation.

III. Clinical features. The major clinical features of anaphylaxis are urticaria, angioedema, respiratory obstruction, and vascular collapse. The skin and the respiratory tract are the most commonly involved target organs, but other organs such as the heart, blood vessels, gastrointestinal tract, and genitourinary system, or other structures rich in tissue-fixed mast cells are frequently involved.

A. Urticarial eruptions are the most common manifestation of anaphylaxis. Other clinical manifestations can include (a) a sense of fright or impending doom, (b) weakness, (c) sweating, (d) sneezing, (e) rhinorrhea, (f) conjunctivitis, (g) generalized pruritus and swelling, (h) cough, (i) wheezing or breathlessness, (j) choking, (k) dysphagia, (l) vomiting, (m) abdominal pain, (n) incontinence, and (o) loss of consciousness. Profound hypotension and shock can develop as a result of significant arteriolar vasodilation, increased vascular permeability, cardiac arrhythmias, or irreversible cardiac failure, even in the absence of respiratory or other symptoms.

B. Anaphylaxis-induced fatalities most often result from involvement of the respiratory tract. Severe involvement can include (a) upper respiratory tract obstruction from laryngeal edema or (b) obstruction of small airways caused by bronchospasm, mucosal edema, and hypersecretion of mucus. The less severe respiratory symptoms include nasal congestion, profuse rhinorrhea, hypopharyngeal edema, and intense pruritus.

TABLE 176-1. Causes of IgE-mediated anaphylaxis

Type	Agent	Example
Proteins	Allergen extracts	Pollen, dust mite, mold
	Enzymes	Chymopapain, streptokinase, L-asparaginase
	Food	Egg white, legumes, milk, nuts, celery, shellfish, psyllium
	Heterologous serum	Tetanus antitoxin, antithymocyte globulin, snake antivenom
	Hormones	Insulin, ACTH, TSH, insulin, progesterone, salmon calcitonin
	Vaccines	Influenza
	Venoms	Hymenoptera
	Others	Heparin, latex, thiobarbiturates, seminal fluid
Haptens	Antibiotics	β-Lactams, ethambutol, nitrofurantoin, sulfonamides, steptomycin, vancomycin
	Disinfectants	Ethylene oxide
	Local anesthetics[a]	Benzocaine, tetracaine, xylocaine, mepivacaine
	Others	Aminopyrine, sulobromophthalein

[a] Precise mechanism not established.
ACTH, adrenocorticotropic hormone; TSH, thyroid-stimulating hormone.

TABLE 176-2. Causes of non–IgE-mediated anaphylaxis

- Complement activation
  - Blood product transfusion in IgA-deficient patient
  - Hemodialysis with cuprophane membrane
- Direct release of chemical mediators of anaphylaxis
  - Protamine[a]
  - Radiographic contrast media
  - Dextran[a]
  - Hydroxyethyl starch
  - Muscle relaxants
  - Ketamine
  - Local anesthetics[a]
  - Codeine and other opiate narcotics
  - Highly charged antibiotics, including amphotericin B
- Cyclooxygenase inhibition
  - Indomethacin
  - Acetylsalicylic acid
  - Mefenamic acid
  - Sulindac
  - Zomepirac sodium
  - Tolmetin sodium
- Other
  - Antineoplastic agents
  - Sulfiting agents
  - Exercise
  - Idiopathic recurrent anaphylaxis

[a] Precise mechanism not established.

C. **The physical examination** of a patient with anaphylactic shock often reveals a rapid, weak, irregular, or unobtainable pulse; tachypnea, respiratory distress, cyanosis, hoarseness, stridor, or dysphagia secondary to laryngeal edema; diminished breath sounds, crackles, cough, wheezes, and hyperinflated lungs from severe bronchoconstriction; urticaria; angioedema or conjunctival edema. Only a subset of these findings may be clinically evident in any given patient.

D. **Laboratory findings** in anaphylaxis include a variety of electrocardiographic abnormalities such as disturbances in rate, rhythm, repolarization, and ectopy. Biochemical abnormalities in anaphylaxis include elevation of blood histamine and tryptase levels, depression of serum complement components, and decreased levels of high molecular-weight kininogen. No diagnostic blood test is currently available.

IV. **Diagnosis and differential diagnosis**

A. **The development** of the characteristic clinical features shortly after exposure to a particular antigen or other inciting agent usually establishes the diagnosis of an anaphylactic reaction. The characteristic presentation of anaphylactic reactions includes (a) the rapid onset of pruritus, urticaria, angioedema, dizziness, dyspnea, syncope, palpitations, nausea, vomiting, abdominal pain, or diarrhea, and (b) the rapid progression of symptoms to a severe and sometimes fatal outcome. Recognition of the early signs and symptoms of anaphylaxis and prompt treatment may prevent progression to irreversible shock and death. Mild systemic reactions often last for several hours, rarely more than 24 hours. Severe manifestations (e.g., laryngeal edema, bronchoconstriction, and hypotension), if not fatal, can persist or recur for several days. Surprisingly, however, even severe manifestations can resolve within minutes of treatment.

B. **The differential diagnosis** of anaphylaxis includes (a) sudden, acute bronchoconstriction in an asthmatic, (b) vasovagal syncope, (c) tension pneumothorax, (d) mechanical upper airway obstruction, (e) pulmonary edema, (f) cardiac arrhythmias, (g) myocardial infarction with cardiogenic shock, (h) aspiration of a food bolus, (i) pulmonary embolism, (j) seizures, (k) acute drug toxicity, (l) hereditary angioedema, (m) cold or idiopathic urticaria, (n) septic shock, and (o) toxic shock.

V. **Treatment.** The treatment of anaphylaxis consists primarily of the avoidance of known precipitants. Once symptoms ensue, however, measures to support cardiopulmonary function are critical, including the aggressive use of pressors, fluid replacement, and medications to counteract the effects of released chemical mediators (Table 176-3).

A. **Supportive cardiopulmonary measures.** Oxygen saturation, blood pressure, and cardiac rhythm should be monitored closely. The maintenance of an adequate airway and ventilation is essential. Supplemental oxygen should be administered. Intubation and assisted ventilation may be necessary for laryngeal edema or severe bronchospasm. Occasionally, cricothyroidotomy is necessary because of massive laryngeal edema.

B. **Pharmacologic therapy.** The guidelines for pharmacologic therapy of anaphylaxis are listed in Table 176-3.

1. **β-adrenergic agents.** Epinephrine hydrochloride should be tried first and promptly to treat all initial manifestations of anaphylaxis. The failure to administer epinephrine or a delay in its administration may be fatal. Epinephrine acts on bronchial and cardiac beta-receptors, causing bronchial dilation and both chronotropic and inotropic cardiac stimulation. Epinephrine also stimulates α-adrenergic receptors on blood vessels, which causes vasoconstriction. Epinephrine also delays antigen absorption when infiltrated locally into an injection or sting site. Inhaled β-adrenergic agents (e.g., metaproterenol sulfate or albuterol sulfate) may also be helpful in reversing bronchoconstriction and in reducing bronchial mucus secretion.

2. **Antihistamines.** H_1 receptor-blocking antihistamines may be helpful in reversing the histamine-induced cardiopulmonary effects of vasodilatation, tachycardia, and bronchoconstriction, as well as bothersome cutaneous

TABLE 176-3. Treatment of anaphylaxis in adults

Mandatory and immediate
- General measure
  - Aqueous epinephrine (1:1,000), 0.2 to 0.5 ml SQ or IM; up to 3 doses at 1- to 5-min intervals
  - Tourniquet proximal to antigen injection or sting site
  - Aqueous epinephrine (1:1,000), 0.1 to 0.3 ml infiltrated into antigen injection or sting site
- For laryngeal obstruction or respiratory arrest
  - Establish airway: endotracheal intubation, cricothyroidotomy or tracheotomy
  - Supplemental oxygen
  - Mechanical ventilation

After clinical appraisal
- General measures
  - Diphenhydramine, 1.25 mg/kg to maximum of 50 mg, IV or IM
  - Aqueous hydrocortisone, 200 mg, or methylprednisolone, 50 mg, IV every 6 h for 24–48 h
  - Cimetidine, 300 mg, IV over 3–5 min
- For hypotension
  - Aqueous epinephrine (1:1,000), 1 ml in 500 ml of saline at 0.5–2.0 ml/min, or 1–4 μg/min, via central venous line
  - Normal saline, lactated Ringer's, or colloid volume expansion
  - Levarterenol bitartrate, 4 mg in 1,000 ml of D_5W at 2–12 μg/min IV
  - Glucagon, if patient is receiving β-blocker therapy, 1 mg/ml IV bolus or infusion or 1 mg/L of D_5W at a rate of 5–15 ml/min
- For bronchoconstriction
  - Supplemental oxygen
  - Aminophylline, only if patient *not* in shock, 5 mg/kg to maximum or 500 mg IV over 20 min, then 0.3–0.8 mg/kg/h IV
  - Metaproterenol (5%), 0.3 ml in 2.5 ml of saline, or albuterol (0.5%), 0.5 ml in 2.5 ml of saline, by nebulizer
  - Isoproterenol, if patient is refractory to other measures, 0.0375 μg/kg/min IV, increased slowly to 0.225 μg/kg/min, or 2–20 μg/min

IV, intravenously; IM, intramuscularly.

manifestations (e.g., flushing, pruritis, and urticaria). The H_2 blocker, cimetidine, has been reported to reverse refractory systemic anaphylaxis.

3. **Corticosteroids** can increase tissue response to β-adrenergic agonists as well as inhibit basophil activation and phospholipase-mediated generation of LTC4, LTD4, and LTE4. Despite the general sense that glucocorticosteroids prevent late recurrences of anaphylaxis, biphasic anaphylaxis has been reported to occur in 20% of anaphylactic reactions despite glucocorticosteroid therapy. One characteristic of patients with biphasic or protracted anaphylaxis is oral ingestion of the offending antigen. On this basis, it would be reasonable to include enteral activated charcoal and sorbitol in the therapy of such patients to reduce the absorption and duration of exposure to the antigen.

VI. Prevention of anaphylactic reactions. In view of the potential morbidity and mortality from anaphylactic reactions, prevention is of primary importance. Prevention includes obtaining a careful history to identify possible precipitants of anaphylaxis. Individuals with a history of anaphylaxis should be encouraged to wear Medic-Alert bracelets (Medic Alert Foundation, P.O. Box 1009, Turlock, CA 95380), which detail the offending precipitant(s), and to carry injectable epinephrine. Risk of anaphylaxis would be expected to increase with recurrent exposure. The time interval between exposures can also be important. Beta-blocking medication may increase the risk of developing an anaphylactic reaction and makes these reactions more refractory to treatment. Thus, patients at risk for recurrent anaphylaxis should not receive beta-blocking medication, unless no reasonable alternative exists.

VII. Management of anaphylaxis to specific precipitants

A. β-lactam antibiotic anaphylaxis. Approximately 10% of these reactions are life-threatening because of induced laryngeal edema, bronchospasm, or shock; 2% to 10% of these are fatal. Of patients who die of penicillin anaphylaxis, 75% percent have experienced previous allergic reactions to the drug. Skin testing is highly efficient in detecting IgE-mediated sensitivity and, thereby, identifying individuals at risk for developing acute allergic reactions to penicillin when both major and minor antigenic determinants are used. It does not, however, evaluate other types of sensitivity, such as serum sickness reactions, morbilliform rashes, and interstitial nephritis. Unfortunately, the minor determinant preparation is not commercially available. Cross-reactivity occurs infrequently with cephalosporins (5.4% to 16.5%) and frequently with carbapenems. Monobactams (e.g., aztreonam) do not show cross-reactivity with penicillin, but do show some cross-reactivity with the cephalosporins. In general, with a previous history of anaphylaxis, the patient should avoid the antibiotic in question. For less severe reactions and when no alternative agent is available, desensitization may be attempted in the intensive care unit setting.

B. Stinging insect venom anaphylaxis. Specific venom desensitization provides greater than 95% protection against anaphylaxis on subsequent stings. Patients should carry a kit with injectable epinephrine and be referred to an allergist for further evaluation.

C. Food anaphylaxis. The foods that cause severe reactions are peanuts, cashews, milk, filberts, walnuts, and eggs; pine nuts, soy, and shellfish also commonly do so. Of note, fatal anaphylaxis occurs most commonly in patients with asthma, in a public setting rather than in the home, and in association with delayed administration of epinephrine.

D. Radiocontrast media anaphylaxis. In patients with a history of a previous radiocontrast media anaphylactic reaction, the repeat reaction rate is reported to be 35% to 60%. Patients with a general history of allergies, whether to inhalant allergens, foods, or medications, have an increased reaction rate compared with nonallergic individuals. Low ionic contrast should be considered in at risk patients, or alternative radiographic studies (e.g., magnetic resonance imaging or ultrasound) should be contemplated. Pretreatment with corticosteroids (50 mg prednisone, 13, 7, and 1 hour prior to administration), diphenhydramine (50 mg orally or intramuscularly 1 hour prior to administration) and ephedrine (25 mg orally 1 hour prior to administration) or corticosteroids and diphenhydramine, without ephedrine may reduce the reaction rate. For an emergent procedure, it is advisable to give hydrocortisone (200 mg) intravenously immediately and repeat every 4 hours in addition to diphenhydramine until the procedure.

E. Latex-induced anaphylaxis. Patients at risk for latex allergy include those with spina bifida, a history of multiple surgeries, history of atopy, and health care workers. Latex is found in a wide spectrum of medical products: surgical gloves, Foley catheters, enema bags, rubber stoppers on medication vials and intravenous line tubing, as well as some surgical drapes and gowns. Patients with latex allergy should be cared for in latex-free operating rooms, intensive care units, and hospital rooms. Radioallergosorbent testing is available and helpful in diagnosis but may have false-negative results. A standardized skin test is not commercially available.

F. Angiotensin-converting enzyme inhibitor anaphylaxis. Severe, potentially life-threatening facial and oropharyngeal angioedema can occur in individuals with hypersensitivity to angiotensin-converting enzyme (ACE) inhibitors and angiotensin II inhibitors. Onset of angioedema usually starts within the first several hours or up to a week after beginning therapy. However, angioedema can develop after months to years of asymptomatic usage. A late onset of symptoms has been reported with the long-acting ACE inhibitors. Cross-reactivity does occur among the different ACE inhibitors, but the specific mechanism is unknown.

Selected Readings

Anderson JA. Allergic reactions to drugs and biologic agents. *JAMA* 1992; 268:2845.
Comprehensive review of drug allergies.

Bochner BS, Lichtenstein LMP. Anaphylaxis. *N Engl J Med* 1991;324:1785.
A review article that includes mechanisms, epidemiology, clinical features, and approaches to anaphylaxis prevention and therapy.

Borish L, Tamir R, Rosenwasser LJ. Intravenous desensitization to beta-lactam antibiotics. *J Allergy Clin Immunol* 1987;80:314.
Outlines desensitization protocol for β-lactam antibiotics.

Crnkovich DJ, Carlson RW. Anaphylaxis: an organized approach to management and prevention. *Journal Critical Illness* 1993;8:3,332.
A succinct review of the pathophysiology and treatment of anaphylaxis.

Greenberger PA, Patterson R. The prevention of immediate generalized reactions to radiocontrast media in high-risk patients. *J Allergy Clin Immunol* 1991;87:867.
Details the preventive management of contrast media use in emergent situations in patients with previous anaphylaxis reactions.

Hollingsworth HM, Giansiracusa DF, Parada NA. Anaphylaxis. In: Irwin RS, Cerra FB, Rippe JM, eds. *Intensive care medicine,* 4th ed. Philadelphia: Lippincott–Raven; 1999.
An in-depth discussion of critical care management of anaphylaxis.

Nichlas RA, Bernstein IL, Li JT, et al. The diagnosis and management of anaphylaxis. *J Allergy Clin Immunol* 1998;101:6.
A recent and comprehensive document that provides consensus summary statements for the treatment and management of anaphylaxis.

Roberts JR, Wuerz RC. Clinical characteristics of angiotensin-converting enzyme inhibitor-induced angioedema. *Ann Emerg Med* 1991;20:555.
Details the clinical allergic reactions to angiotensin-converting enzyme inhibitors.

Sampson HA, Mendelson L, Rosen JP. Fatal and near-fatal anaphylactic reactions to food in children and adolescents. *N Engl J Med* 1992;327:380.
A review of common food allergens and clinical manifestations.

Slater JE. Latex allergy. *J Allergy Clin Immunol* 1994;94:141.
A recent comprehensive review of the clinical features of latex allergy and treatment.

Toogood JH. Risk of anaphylaxis in patients receiving beta-blocker drugs. *J Allergy Clin Immunol* 1988;81:1.
Describes the risks of beta-blocker use in patients undergoing anaphylaxis and treatment strategy.

Valentine MD. Insect venom allergy: diagnosis and treatment. *J Allergy Clin Immunol* 1984;73:299.
A comprehensive review of venom allergy and immunotherapy.

Wong S, Dykewicz MS, Patterson R. Idiopathic anaphylaxis. *Arch Intern Med* 1990; 150:1323.
A retrospective evaluation of 175 patients with idiopathic anaphylaxis.

Zaloga GP, Delacey W, Holmboe E, et al. Glucagon reversal of hypotension in a case of anaphylactoid shock. *Ann Intern Med* 1986;105:65.
Details an anaphylaxis clinical case with response to glucagon.

177. COLLAGEN VASCULAR DISEASES IN THE INTENSIVE CARE UNIT

Leslie R. Harrold, Nancy Y.N. Liu, and David F. Giansiracusa

I. General principles. This chapter focuses on manifestations of rheumatoid arthritis, systemic lupus erythematosus, antiphospholipid antibody syndrome, systemic sclerosis, polymyositis, and dermatomyositis that may be encountered in the intensive care unit.

II. Rheumatoid arthritis

A. Definition. Rheumatoid arthritis (RA) is a chronic inflammatory disorder of unknown cause that affects synovial joints and extraarticular structures.

B. Pathogenesis. The inflammation and tissue destruction characteristic of rheumatoid arthritis appear to develop secondary to humoral and cellular-mediated immunologic processes in response to an unknown trigger.

C. Diagnosis and treatment

1. Joint disease. The diagnosis of rheumatoid arthritis is based on the presentation of articular disease. Aspects of the joint disease, cervical subluxation, tempohromandibular joint disease causing micrognathia, and cricoarytenoid arthritis, which affect intubation management, and the topic of septic arthritis are discussed in the Chapter 208 in *Intensive Care Medicine*, fourth edition. Philadelphia: Lippincott–Raven, 1999.

2. Pleural disease. Pleuritis, the most common pulmonary manifestation of rheumatoid arthritis; it can cause large pleural effusions that impair respiratory function. Pleural fluid should be examined to exclude malignancy or infection. Symptomatic RA pleural effusions are treated with nonsteroidial antiinflammatory drugs (NSAIDs), aspiration, and in some cases, surgical decortication.

3. Parenchymal lung disease. Interstitial lung disease occurs in approximately 20% to 40% of patients with RA. Symptoms include dyspnea on exertion, cough, and chest discomfort; clubbing of fingers and toes is a late manifestation. Chest radiographs reveal a fine reticular appearance; restrictive physiology and decreased diffusion capacity are characteristic findings on pulmonary function testing. Treatment is generally unsatisfactory with only 50% of patients improving with corticosteroids. Small numbers of patients reportedly have been treated with immunosuppressants, but no controlled studies have demonstrated sustained benefit.

Bronchiolitis obliterans is associated with RA. Clinical presentation includes the abrupt onset of dyspnea and a dry cough with respiratory crackles, sometimes with a midinspiratory squeak. The chest radiograph is often clear. Pulmonary function testing reveals irreversible airflow obstruction at low volumes. The prognosis is poor despite treatment with high-dose corticosteroids (with or without the addition of cytotoxic agents).

Medications used to treat RA can cause pulmonary disorders; salicylates, noncardiogenic pulmonary edema; NSAIDS (excluding nonacetylated salicylates), bronchospasm; intramuscular gold and D-penicillamine, interstitial pneumonitis; and cyclophosphamide, rarely, interstitial pneumonia and alveolar cell atypia. Methotrexate can cause hypersensitivity pneumonitis, interstitial fibrosis, and opportunistic pulmonary infection.

4. Cardiac involvement. Pericarditis is the most common cardiac manifestations. It rarely impairs left ventricular function, but constrictive pericarditis or a large pericardial effusion can severely impair cardiac filling and require pericardial aspiration and pericardiectomy. Pericardial effusions generally respond to administration of 30 to 40 mg/d of prednisone over a several week period. Rheumatoid arthritis can also cause granulomatous inflammation of the myocardium, resulting in conduction abnormalities or vasculitis, which can involve the coronary arteries and aorta. This topic is discussed in (Chapter 178, "Vasculitis in the Intensive Care Unit") as is necrotizing vasculitis.

5. **Vasculitis.** Rheumatoid vasculitis tends to occur in patients with severe deforming arthritis, subcutaneous nodules, high-titer rheumatoid factor, and Felty's syndrome. A necrotizing panarteritis affecting all layers of the involved blood vessels can also involve the skin, gastrointestinal organs, kidneys, heart, lungs, and components of the nervous system. Treatment options include high-dose corticosteroids, cytotoxic agents, and occasionally, plasmapheresis.
6. **Neurologic complications.** Arthritis of the atlantoaxial junction with erosion of the transverse ligament, fracture or erosive destruction of the odontoid, or arthritis of multiple cervical vertebral joints can cause cervical instability with resultant spinal cord compression. Destruction of the lateral atlantoaxial joints and of the foramen magnum may allow the axis to vertically sublux. Symptoms of spinal cord compression that require prompt neurosurgical evaluation include a sensation of anterior instability of the head during neck flexion, drop attacks, loss of urinary bladder and anal sphincter control, dysphagia, vertigo, hemiplegia, dysarthria, nystagmus, changes in level of consciousness, and peripheral paresthesias.

III. Systemic lupus erythematosus

A. Definition and pathogenesis. Systemic lupus erythematosus (SLE) is a multisystem disease characterized by generation of autoantibodies and immune complex vasculitis.

B. Diagnosis and treatment. The diagnosis of SLE is based on clinical and laboratory features. Severe, potentially life-threatening manifestations include renal, central nervous system, pulmonary, cardiac, and hematologic involvement.

1. **Renal.** Clinically, lupus nephritis occurs in as many as 50% of patients. Severe disease can result in rapidly progressive renal failure, congestive heart failure, and hypertension. Management of lupus nephritis depends on renal histology and functional parameters. Mesangial glomerulonephritis with normal creatinine clearance may require no specific therapy. Active nephritis with progressive azotemia requires aggressive therapy with high-dose corticosteroids (equivalent of 1 mg/kg/d of prednisone), pulse methylprednisolone (800–1,000 mg/d for 3–5 days), and/or the combination of corticosteroid therapy with cyclophosphamide (such as an intravenous pulse of cyclophosphamide 0.5 to 1.0 g/m^2/month for 6 months and then once every 3 months for 1 year beyond remission).
2. **Central nervous system.** Neuropsychiatric lupus erythematosus can cause a variety of clinical presentations, including organic brain syndromes, psychoses, affective disorders, seizures, strokes, transverse myelitis, cranial and peripheral neuropathies, movement disorders, headache, aseptic meningitis, and multiple sclerosislike syndromes. Imaging studies such as computed tomography and magnetic resonance imaging are helpful to document hemorrhage, infarcts, parenchymal disease, paracranial tumors, and abscesses. Electroencephalograms may help document seizure activity. Neuropsychologic testing may define organic and functional deficits. Corticosteroids are generally recommended in dosages ranging from doubling of the baseline dose to high-dose therapy (prednisone, 1.0–1.5 mg/kg/d, or its equivalent). In severe cases, pulse intravenous methylprednisolone (1.0 to 1.5 g/d for 3 days) or intravenous pulse cyclophosphamide can be used.
3. **Pulmonary.** Pleuritis, which occurs in approximately half of lupus patients, can cause pleural effusions that usually are small and bilateral, but massive collections can occur and require thoracentesis. Mild pleuritis usually responds to NSAIDs or low-dose corticosteroids (prednisone, 0.5 mg/kg/d, or its equivalent).

   Active lupus pneumonitis is rare. Patients present with fever, severe dyspnea, tachypnea, and hypoxemia. Chest radiographs reveal patchy alveolar infiltrates. Secondary causes such as pulmonary infection, uremic pneumonitis, and congestive heart failure must be excluded. High-dose corticosteroids and azathioprine have been used but the mortality rate remains high.

Pulmonary hemorrhage, another rare manifestation, causes acute dyspnea, tachycardia, severe hypoxemia, rales, and anemia. Hemoptysis may or may not be present. Therapy includes pulse methylprednisolone (1 g/d for 3 days) followed by high-dose oral corticosteroids (1 mg/kg/d). Cytotoxic agents should be considered in patients who fail pulse steroids or are critically ill.

Diffuse interstitial lung disease can cause dyspnea on exertion, productive cough, pleuritic pain, and rales. Chest radiographs and computerized tomography radiographs may demonstrate alveolitis and fibrosis. Pulmonary function testing reveals restriction and marked reduction in diffusing capacity without obstruction. Corticosteroids (1 mg/kg/d) may be beneficial in the prefibrotic stage.

Pulmonary hypertension, which presents as severe dyspnea on exertion and fatigue, can occur as a primary or secondary entity in SLE. Vasodilators, such as intravenous prostacyclin ($PG1_2$) may be helpful, but definitive therapy is heart/lung transplantation.

4. **Cardiac.** Pericardial disease is the most common cardiac manifestation of SLE. The presentation can include anterior or substernal chest pain that is relieved by leaning forward, dyspnea, arrhythmias, a pericardial friction rub, cardiac enlargement on chest radiograph, transient electrocardiographic changes (including ST elevation), and pericardial effusion on echocardiography. Treatment includes NSAIDs and occasionally prednisone (15–30 mg/d).

   Primary myocarditis is rare. Secondary causes of myocardial dysfunction include systemic hypertension, valvular disease, pulmonary disease, coronary artery ischemia, drug toxicity, and amyloidosis.

   Atherosclerosis is the major cause of coronary artery disease in lupus patients secondary to hypertension, hyperlipidemia, antiphospholipids, and corticosteroid use.

5. **Hematologic.** Although anemia of chronic disease is the most common form of anemia, autoimmune hemolytic anemia can be severe. Manifestations include an elevated reticulocyte count and indirect bilirubin and decreased haptoglobin levels. Most patients respond to high-dose corticosteroids (60–100 mg/d of prednisone in divided doses). If response does not occur within several weeks, other therapeutic modalities may be considered, including danazol, immunosuppressant agents, and splenectomy.

   Leukopenia, defined as a total white blood count of less than 4,500/ml, occurs in 50% to 60% of SLE patients but rarely is associated with infections or complications.

   Thrombocytopenia (i.e., platelet counts <100,000/ml) is commonly observed. Idiopathic thrombocytopenia purpura (ITP) may be the initial presentation of SLE. Therapy of severe SLE-associated ITP initially includes corticosteroid therapy in a dose of 60–100 mg/d of prednisone or its equivalent. If corticosteroids are ineffective, intravenous γ-globulin (0.4–1.0 g/d or 6–15 mg/kg/d for 4 to 7 days) may increase the platelet count rapidly.

6. **Gastrointestinal.** SLE can cause sterile peritonitis (serositis). It can also result in a small vessel vasculitis of the large or small intestine, which can cause abdominal pain and even bowel infarction. Treatment includes close observation and evaluation for bowel infarction, which may require exploratory surgery and high-dose corticosteroids for the inflammatory process.

IV. **Drug-induced lupus.** Multiple medications can potentially cause the development of lupus, usually several months after the institution of the medication. The medications that have been definitely associated with the development of lupus include methyldopa, hydralazine, procainamide, quinidine, chlorpromazine, isoniazid, and penicillamine. Symptoms of drug-induced lupus include fever, arthralgias, arthritis, pleuropericarditis, and rash. Laboratory values reveal an elevated erythrocyte sedimentation rate, mild leukopenia or thrombocytopenia, and the presence of antinuclear antibodies. Antihistone antibodies are present in 90% of drug-induced lupus patients; specific antibodies to double-stranded DNA and Smith are absent. Treatment includes discontinuing the offending medication and using NSAIDs or low-dose steroids (5–10 mg/d prednisone) to control symptoms.

V. Antiphospholipid antibody syndrome

A. Definition and pathogenesis. The antiphospholipid antibody syndrome refers to thrombotic disease affecting arteries, veins, or both in the setting of antibodies to phospholipids. The disorder can be primary or can be associated with a connective disease.

B. Diagnosis. This disorder can manifest as venous thrombosis, arterial thrombosis, recurrent fetal loss caused by thrombosis and infarction of the placenta, leg ulcers, livedo reticularis, pulmonary hypertension, migraine headaches, chorea, endocardial disease, thrombocytopenia, and Coombs' positive hemolytic anemia. Laboratory evaluation includes detection of the lupus anticoagulant and antibodies to phospholipids such as the anticardiolipin antibodies.

C. Treatment. Treatment includes antiplatelet medications and anticoagulation. In patients with arterial thromboses or severe venous thromboembolic disease, life-long anticoagulation is recommended.

VI. Systemic sclerosis

A. Definition. Systemic sclerosis (SSC) or scleroderma is a multisystem disease characterized by fibrosis and degeneration of various organs, including skin, heart, lungs, kidneys, and gastrointestinal tract.

B. Pathogenesis. Excessive synthesis of collagen by fibroblasts, increased vascular permeability, and progressive vascular narrowing in response to an unknown trigger affects skin and the viscera.

C. Diagnosis and treatment

1. **Pulmonary disease.** Pulmonary involvement in systemic sclerosis is now the primary cause of death, with a prevalence of 50% to 92%. Dyspnea, cough, and basilar crackles are the predominant clinical features of interstitial lung disease. Radiographs may reveal pulmonary fibrosis in 18% to 78% of cases. Corticosteroids with cyclophosphamide may have a role in early inflammatory stages but data currently are limited.

   Pulmonary hypertension can develop as a primary manifestation or secondary to chronic interstitial lung disease. Treatment of pulmonary hypertension includes vasodilators (e.g., nifedipine) and, potentially, a continuous infusion of prostacyclin. Heart–lung transplantation is the only definitive therapy.

2. **Cardiac.** Pericardial disease is the most common clinical manifestation of scleroderma heart disease. Pericardial effusions are usually small, although large collections (> 200 ml) can occur. Treatment with NSAIDs or low-dose corticosteroids is usually sufficient. Hemodynamic compromise requires more aggressive therapy (e.g., pericardiocentesis) and, potentially, a pericardial window.

   Focal myocardial fibrosis can involve all three layers of the heart as well as both ventricles, resulting in conduction abnormalities, including fatal ventricular arrhythmias.

3. **Renal disease.** Accelerated or malignant hypertension accompanied by signs of microangiopathic hemolytic anemia, hyperreninemia, and rapidly progressive renal failure is referred to as "scleroderma renal crisis." Up to 25% of diffuse scleroderma patients may develop the syndrome. Angiotensin converting enzyme inhibitors are the treatment of choice. Calcium channel blockers may be helpful adjuncts.

4. **Gastrointestinal disease.** Dysphagia and heartburn caused by gastroesophageal reflux frequently occur as a result of esophageal dysmotility and decreased lower esophageal sphincter pressure. Treatment includes dietary

changes (i.e., small, frequent meals), H_2 receptor antagonists, proton pump inhibitors, and motility agents (e.g., metoclopramide or cisapride).

Intestinal hypomotility and malabsorption can cause bloating, cramping, diarrhea, and constipation. Treatment includes prokinetic agents (e.g., metoclopramide and cisapride), oral antibiotics, low-residue diets, and parenteral nutrition.

5. **Raynaud's phenomenon.** Severe Raynaud's phenomenon, refractory to calcium channel blockers, can cause digital ulceration or gangrene. Treatment options include intravenous prostacyclin (up to 2 mg/kg/min for 8 hours daily for 3 days), sympathetic blocks, and sympathectomy.

VII. Polymyositis and dermatomyositis

A. Definition. Polymyositis (PM) and dermatomyositis (DM) are inflammatory diseases of skeletal muscle that present with limb girdle weakness. Skin involvement occurs in DM and visceral disease can occur in both PM and DM.

B. Pathogenesis. Skeletal muscle is damaged by a cellular immune reaction. The relationship to malignancy is controversial. A thorough physical examination and routine health screening that is specific to age and gender is recommended for persons affected with these conditions to evaluate for an associated malignancy.

C. Diagnosis and treatment

1. **Pulmonary involvement.** Interstitial lung disease, respiratory insufficiency caused by muscle weakness, and pneumonia (from aspiration, opportunistic infections, or other causes) can cause dyspnea, cough, and chest pain. Pneumonias should be treated with the appropriate antimicrobial therapy after evaluation for bacterial, mycobacterial, fungal, and pneumocystis infection. Respiratory insufficiency and interstitial lung disease are treated with supportive measures (oxygen, mechanical ventilation) and therapy is directed at the underlying myositis.
2. **Cardiac.** Myocardial inflammation can cause focal myonecrosis and patchy fibrosis of both the myocardium and conducting tissue. Significant elevations of the isoenzyme creatine kinase MB fraction should signify the possibility of ongoing myocardial inflammation. Immunosuppressant therapy for the underlying skeletal muscle involvement from PM or DM will simultaneously treat myocardial inflammation.
3. **Renal involvement.** Severe muscle necrosis can cause renal failure and metabolic abnormalities secondary to rhabdomyolysis. Therapy consists of treatment of the rhabdomyolysis and the underlying muscle disease.

VIII. Adverse effects of antirheumatic medications. For a full discussion, see Chapter 175, "Rheumatologic disorders in the intensive care unit."

Selected Readings

Balow JE, Austin HA. Renal disease in systemic lupus erythematosus. *Rheum Dis Clin North Am* 1988;16:117.
A comprehensive review of the topic.

Carette S. Cardiopulmonary manifestations of SLE. *Rheum Dis Clin North Am* 1988;14:135.
An excellent review.

Hunningshake GW, Fauci AS. Pulmonary involvement in the collagen vascular diseases. *Am Rev Respir Dis* 1979;119:471.
An excellent review.

Hurd ER. Extraarticular manifestations of rheumatoid arthritis. *Semin Arthritis Rheum* 1979;8:151.
An excellent review of extraarticular manifestations.

King Jr TE. Bronchiolitis obliterans keys to diagnosis and management. *Immunology and Allergy Practice* 1989;11:17.
An excellent discussion.

Mackworth-Young CG, Loizou S, Walport MJ. Primary antiphospholipid syndrome: features of patients with raised anticardiolipin antibodies and no other disorder. *Ann Rheum Dis* 1989;48:362.
A good discussion.

McCune JW, Globus J. Neuropsychiatric lupus. *Rheum Dis Clin North Am* 1988;14:149.
An excellent discussion.

Roschman RA, Rothenberg RJ. Pulmonary fibrosis in rheumatoid arthritis: a review of the clinical features and therapy. *Semin Arthritis Rheum* 1987;16:174.
An excellent review.

Steen VD. Scleroderma. *Rheum Dis Clin North Am* 1996;22:677.
A good overview.

178. VASCULITIS IN THE INTENSIVE CARE UNIT

Leslie R. Harrold, Nancy Y.N. Liu, and David F. Giansiracusa

I. **Definition.** The vasculitides are a group of clinicopathologic disorders in which inflammation and necrosis of blood vessel walls result in organ system abnormalities caused by thrombosis and hemorrhage. A systemic vasculitis should be considered in the patient with systemic complaints and dysfunction of any and often multiple organ systems (Table 178-1) frequently in the context of severe constitutional symptoms such as fever, malaise, and weight loss. Common complaints of patients with systemic vasculitis include cough, nausea, vomiting, abdominal pain, chest pain, weakness, paresthesias, musculoskeletal pain, and skin rashes.

This chapter addresses several forms of necrotizing vasculitis, including polyarteritis nodosa, drug-induced vasculitis, vasculitis associated with the human immunodeficiency virus (HIV), Wegener's granulomatosis, and cholesterol embolism.

II. **Polyarteritis nodosa.** Polyarteritis (PA) is a systemic necrotizing arteritis involving small and medium-sized muscular arteries that affects men twice as frequently as women, with a mean age of onset 45 years. Almost any organ can be involved, the skin, kidney, peripheral nerves, gastrointestinal (GI) tract, and joints are those organs most commonly involved.

A. **Pathogenesis.** The pathogenesis of PA is unknown. It can be a primary disorder or it can be associated with hepatic infections (hepatitis B and hepatitis C), other collagen vascular diseases (rheumatoid arthritis, systemic lupus erythematosus (SLE), and Sjögren's syndrome), as well as with malignancies, (carcinomas, lymphomas, and other myeloproliferative disorders).

B. **Diagnosis.** The diagnosis is suggested on clinical presentation and confirmed by blood vessel biopsies. Patients generally complain of malaise, weight loss, fevers, abdominal or lower extremity pain, and myalgias or arthralgias. Renal involvement, which occurs in 45% to 65% of patients, includes vasculitis of renal arteries (interlobular), hypertension, and glomerulonephritis. Peripheral neuropathy, particularly mononeuritis multiplex, occurs in 50% to 70% of cases. Central nervous system (CNS) involvement, including seizures, focal events, and altered mental status, is much less common (23%). Musculoskeletal symptoms occur in 50% of patients. Abdominal pain may be a manifestation of ischemia or thrombosis. Cutaneous lesions include nonspecific maculopapular rash, livedo reticularis, tender nodular lesions, and ulcers.

Laboratory study results such as anemia, leukocytosis, thrombocytosis, elevated erythrocyte sedimentation rate, and abnormalities of creatinine, urinalysis, transaminases, nerve conduction, and electromyograms may reflect inflammation and evidence of multisystem disease. To establish the diagnosis, histologic documentation of necrotizing vasculitis is usually required. The most accessible tissues include skin, muscle, sural nerve, and kidney. Renal biopsies usually reveal glomerulonephritis but do not help differentiate various forms of vasculitides. Arteriography usually reveals saccular or fusiform aneurysms at multiple sites.

C. **Treatment.** Currently, treatment recommendations include cyclophosphamide (2 mg/kg/d) and prednisone (1 mg/kg/d) for severe progressive systemic manifestations. For patients with less severe involvement, high-dose prednisone (60–100 mg in divided daily doses) may suffice.

III. **Hypersensitivity vasculitis.** Hypersensitivity vasculitis, which can occur in response to drugs, infectious agents, and tumor antigens, generally affects small blood vessels, capillaries, and postcapillary venules.

A. **Pathogenesis.** A hypersensitive reaction to an offending antigen results in immune complex deposition in the walls of postcapillary venules causing poly-

TABLE 178-1. Organ dysfunction occurring in systemic necrotizing vasculitis

Renal	Pneumonitis
Hypertension	Interstitial lung disease
Renal infarction	Cavitary lesion
Glomerulonephritis	Gastrointestinal
Interstitial nephritis	Cholecystitis
Skin	Bleeding
Rash, purpura	Hepatic dysfunction
Nodules	Bowel infarction
Livedo reticularis	Bowel perforation
Ulcers	Cardiac
Nervous system	Myocardial infarction
Cerebral vascular accidents	Congestive heart failure
Altered mental status	Pericarditis
Seizures	Musculoskeletal
Mononeuritis multiplex	Arthralgias
Peripheral neuropathy	Arthritis
Pulmonary	Myalgias
Pleuritis	Muscle infarction

morphonuclear leukocytic destruction of vessel walls, the so-called "leuko cytoclastic vasculitis," seen on histologic examination.

B. Diagnosis. The diagnosis is suggested by the presence of antigen or exposure t an offending drug 7 to 10 days before the clinical manifestations occur. The drug most commonly causing vasculitis include penicillin, sulfonamides, quinidine and procainamide, but virtually any drug can produce hypersensitivity vasculi tis. Table 178-2 lists drugs that frequently cause hypersensitivity vasculitis.

Cutaneous lesions, which occur in crops, include purpura on the lower extrem ities, back, or buttock regions. Systemic features, including fever, arthralgias and malaise, may be present. Other organs that can become involved include th mucosa of GI, renal glomeruli, and peripheral nerves.

C. Treatment. Because drug-induced vasculitis is usually a self-limited disease tha resolves 2 to 4 weeks after the offending agent is eliminated, discontinuation c the drug or resolution of the associated infection may be all that is required. Fo patients with severe symptoms or evidence of significant organ involvement, cor ticosteroids can be prescribed (20–60 mg/d of prednisone or its equivalent).

IV. Vasculitis associated with human immunodeficiency virus. Infection with HIV can be associated with a medium-sized vessel vasculitis similar to PA, a hypersen sitivity vasculitis, lymphomatoid granulomatosis, and primary angiitis of the CNS

A. Pathogenesis. HIV can invade into vessel walls or stimulate a humoral or cel lular immune response.

B. Diagnosis. HIV is suspected when a patient presents with a vasculitic syn drome without other potential causes for the vasculitis.

C. Treatment. Therapy should be based on the risk-to-benefit analysis of eacl patient, and can include high-dose prednisone and cyclophosphamide. Anti microbial prophylaxis during treatment has been suggested.

V. Wegener's granulomatosis. Wegener's granulomatosis is a disease of unknow cause, which is characterized by granulomatous vasculitis of the upper and lowe respiratory tract, segmental necrotizing glomerulonephritis, and systemic vas culitis of small arteries and veins. Disease with only respiratory tract involvemen is termed "limited Wegener's granulomatosis." The disease commonly affects per sons in their fourth or fifth decades of life.

A. Pathogenesis. The cause is unknown.

B. Diagnosis. Most patients present with symptoms referable to the upper res piratory tract (e.g., sinusitis, nasal obstruction, rhinitis, otitis, hearing loss

TABLE 178-2. Drugs associated with hypersensitivity vasculitis

Antibiotics	Anticonvulsants
Penicillin	Phenobarbital
Sulfonamides	Phenytoin
Tetracycline	Others
Streptomycin	Phenothiazines
Rheumatic drugs	Iodides
Aspirin	Griseofulvin
Levamisole	Propylthiouracil
Allopurinol	Antiarrhythmics
Gold	Quinidine
Phenylbutazone	Procainamide

ear pain, gingival inflammation, epistaxis, sore throat, laryngitis, and nasal septal deformity). Although only a third of patients present with symptoms of lung involvement (including cough, sputum production, dyspnea, chest pain, and hemoptysis), frequently chest radiographs are abnormal and may show nodular cavitary infiltrates or infiltrates without sharp margins. Renal manifestations may be asymptomatic, but commonly glomerulonephritis is evident at presentation. Laboratory features include a normochromic, normocytic anemia; leukocytosis and thrombocytosis; and elevation of erythrocyte sedimentation rate and C-reactive protein levels. Most patients have either cytoplasmic antineutrophil cytoplasmic antibodies or peripheral antineutrophil cytoplasmic antibody. Diagnosis is confirmed by histologic documentation of granulomatous inflammation of the lung or upper respiratory tract or histologic documentation of necrotizing vasculitis in the appropriate clinical context.

C. Treatment. Cyclophosphamide (1 to 2 mg/kg/d) is the mainstay of therapy; it is given orally with careful monitoring in order to maintain the total white blood cell count above 3,000 cells/ml or by monthly intravenous pulse. Prednisone can be added for severe disease.

VI. Cholesterol embolism. Cholesterol (athero-) embolism can produce a variety of multisystem manifestations and laboratory abnormalities that can simulate a necrotizing vasculitis. Because the most common sources of atheroemboli are atherosclerotic lesions in the aorta and in the iliac and femoral arteries, the most susceptible regions are the abdominal viscera, the kidneys, and the lower extremities.

A. Pathogenesis. Atheromatous emboli to small arteries and arterioles results in endothelial and fibroblastic proliferation, thrombosis, a foreign body giant cell response to the cholesterol crystals, and a polymorphonuclear or lymphocytic perivascular infiltration. Occasionally, a necrotizing angiitis of the small arteries occurs.

B. Diagnosis. The clinical settings in which atheroemboli most commonly occur are in the presence of an aortic aneurysm; after surgical manipulation of an atheromatous aorta or after blunt abdominal trauma; during and after angiography and intraarterial catheterization; and, spontaneously, as a complication of warfarin therapy. Patients may have cyanotic painful toes, with bluish patches and hemorrhagic areas, and potentially, ulceration or gangrene. Livido reticularis, hypertension, hematuria, leukocyturia, and proteinuria may be present. The condition can also present as a severe abdominal catastrophe with bowel infarction, peritonitis, and renal failure.

C. Treatment. The goal of treatment is supportive therapy with control of pain and blood pressure as well as increase blood flow to affected areas.

VII. For discussion of the rare entity of central nervous system vasculitis (also called isolated angiitis of the central nervous system), see Chapter 212, "Vasculitis in the Intensive Care Unit" in *Intensive Care Medicine*, fourth edition, Lippincott–Raven, 1999.

Selected Readings

Calabrese LH. Vasculitis and infection with human immunodeficiency virus. *Rheum Dis Clin North Am* 1991;17:131.
A good discussion.

Conn DL, Hunder GG. Vasculitis and related disorders. In: Kelly WH, Harris ED, Ruddy S, et al. *Textbook of rheumatology,* 3rd ed. Philadelphia: WB Saunders Co; 1989.
An excellent reference.

Conn DL, ed. Vasculitic syndromes. *Rheum Dis Clinics of N Am* 1990;16(2).
An excellent review—entire volume consisting of 17 chapters addressing different aspects of vasculitis.

Cupps TR, Fauci AS. *The vaculitides.* Philadelphia: WB Saunders; 1981: Vol. XXI in Major Problems in Internal Medicine.
The classic textbook on vasculitis.

Fan PT, Davis JA, Somer T, et al. A clinical approach to systemic vasculitis. *Semin Arthritis Rheum* 1980;9:248.
A good clinical review.

Fauci AS, Katz P, Haynes BF, et al. Cyclophosphamide therapy of severe systemic necrotizing vasculitis. *N Engl J Med* 1979;301:235.
Discusses cyclophosphamide treatment.

Fauci AS, Wolff SM. Wegener's granulomatosis: studies in eighteen patients and a review of the literature. *Medicine* 1973;52:535.
Reviews clinical presentation.

Gibson LE, Su WP. Cutaneous vasculitis. *Rheum Dis Clin North Am* 1990;16:309.
A good overview.

Niles JL. Value of tests for antineutrophil cytoplasmic autoantibodies in the diagnosis and treatment of vasculitis. *Curr Opin Rheumatol* 1993;5:18.
A good review.

Young DK, Burton MF, Herman JH. Multiple cholesterol emboli syndrome simulating systemic necrotizing vasculitis. *J Rheumatol* 1986;13:423.
A good discussion.

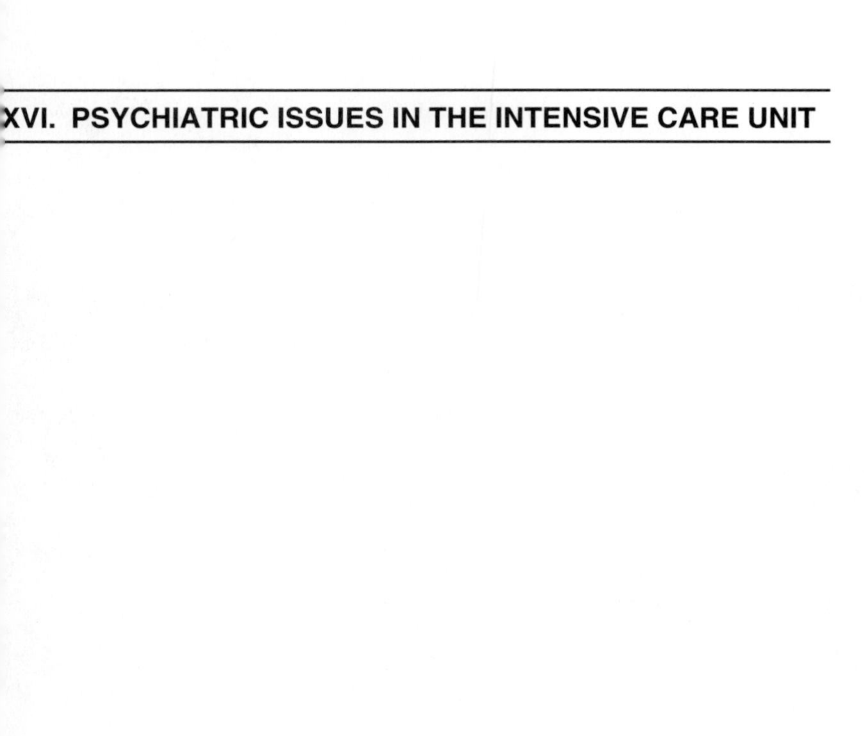

XVI. PSYCHIATRIC ISSUES IN THE INTENSIVE CARE UNIT

179. DIAGNOSIS AND TREATMENT OF AGITATION AND DELIRIUM IN THE INTENSIVE CARE UNIT PATIENT

Stephan Heckers, George E. Tesar, John Querques, and Theodore A. Stern

I. **General principles.** Agitation and delirium are common problems in the intensive care unit (ICU); they warrant evaluation and treatment of systemic and metabolic abnormalities, drug toxicity, withdrawal states, and other reversible factors.

II. **Delirium.** Also known as acute confusional state, delirium is an organic mental disorder characterized by cognitive deficits and an altered level of consciousness. It is often acute in onset and reversible within days or weeks, although some cases result in permanent cognitive dysfunction.

  A. **Clinical features.** Delirious patients exhibit inattentiveness, disorientation, and impaired short-term memory. They have alterations in perception (i.e., illusions, hallucinations) and in thought (i.e., delusions, often paranoid). Their disorganization, restlessness, and agitation can reach the point of combativeness, or they can be so quiet and slowed (i.e., psychomotorically retarded) that they are thought to have depression. These behavioral and cognitive disturbances fluctuate throughout the day and are often worse at night.

  B. **Etiology.** Delirium can be caused by a panoply of organic disturbances that cluster into four groups: (a) primary intracranial disease; (b) systemic diseases that secondarily affect the brain; (c) exogenous toxic agents; and (d) substance withdrawal. Table 179-1 lists specific entities according to this scheme and Table 179-2 lists the life-threatening causes of delirium. Table 179-3 lists common delirium-inducing drugs.

  C. **Differential diagnosis.** Delirium must be distinguished from dementia, functional psychoses (e.g., schizophrenia), secondary mania, complex partial seizures, and dissociative disorders.

III. **Agitation.** Although delirium is probably the most common cause of agitation in the ICU, many other factors that compromise a patient's ability to tolerate the ICU environment can precipitate agitation. These include:

  A. **Panic-level anxiety.** Anxiety is a prominent and expected reaction to many conditions that require intensive care, including the process of weaning from chronic ventilatory support. Extreme anxiety must be distinguished from incipient psychosis because treatments for these two conditions differ. When anxiety is the cause of agitation, education and reassurance may be beneficial.

  B. **Pain.** Often undetected because of the patient's inability to communicate effectively and undertreated for fear of promoting addiction, pain can precipitate considerable agitation.

  C. **Personality style.** Patients with rigid, obsessive, compulsive, and controlling characteristics experience the greatest difficulty coping with an ICU stay. Intolerable frustration can lead to agitation and a demand to leave the hospital against medical advice.

  D. **Poor comprehension or sensory impairment.** Mental retardation, dementia, a language barrier, or a visual or hearing impairment can compromise a patient's understanding of the need for ICU care and, thereby, precipitate agitation.

IV. **Treatment.** The cornerstone of management of the agitated or delirious patient is specific treatment for the underlying disorder(s) considered to be the causative culprit(s). This approach can involve (a) correction of metabolic and systemic abnormalities; (b) elimination of drug toxicity; and (c) treatment of drug withdrawal. Other steps, which can be instituted concurrently with these treatments or when a specific cause for delirium cannot be identified or corrected, include use of mechanical restraints and pharmacologic management with neuroleptics, benzodiazepines, and other agents. Causes of agitation other than delirium (e.g., anxiety, pain) should be treated specifically.

TABLE 179-1. Differential diagnosis of delirium

Problem	Etiologic Factors
Primary intracranial disease	Infection
	Human immunodeficiency virus encephalopathy
	Meningitis/encephalitis
	Neurosyphilis
	Neoplasm
	Seizure
	Complex partial seizure/status
	Postictal state
	Vascular
	Hypertensive encephalopathy
	Stroke
	Vasculitis
	Normal pressure hydrocephalus
Systemic diseases that secondarily affect the brain	Cardiopulmonary
	Cardiac arrest
	Shock
	Congestive heart failure
	Respiratory failure
	Endocrine/metabolic
	Acid-base disorder
	Fluid/electrolyte derangement
	Diabetic ketoacidosis
	Hypoglycemia
	Parathyroid dysfunction
	Thyroid dysfunction
	Hepatic failure/encephalopathy
	Renal failure
	Infection
	Sepsis
	Subacute bacterial endocarditis
	Neoplasm
	Paraneoplastic syndromes
	Nutritional deficiency
	Folic acid
	Vitamin B_{12} (pernicious anemia)
	Thiamine (Wernicke's encephalopathy, Wernicke-Korsakoff psychosis)
Exogenous toxic agents	Drugs of abuse
	Alcohol
	Amphetamines
	Cocaine
	Lysergic acid diethylamide
	Phencyclidine
	Nonmedicinal substances
	Carbon monoxide
	Heavy metals
	Medications (see Table 179-3)
Drug withdrawal	Alcohol
	Propanediols
	Chloral hydrate
	Meprobamate
	Sedative-hypnotic agents
	Benzodiazepines
	Barbiturates
	Narcotics

Adapted from Lipowski ZJ. Transient cognitive disorders (delirium, acute confusional states) in the elderly. *Am J Psychiatry* 1983;140:1426–1436; Ludwig, AM. *Principles of clinical psychiatry.* New York: Free Press, 1980; and Heckers S, Tesor GC, Stern TA. Diagnosis and treatment of agitation and delirium in the intensive care unit patient. In: Irwin RS, Cerra FB, Rippe JM, eds. *Intensive care medicine,* 4th ed. Philadelphia: Lippincott–Raven; 1999.

TABLE 179-2. Life-threatening causes of delirium: WWHHHIIMMP

Wernicke's encephalopathy
Withdrawal from drugs
Hypertensive encephalopathy
Hypoglycemia
Hypoxia
Intracerebral hemorrhage
Infection
Meningitis/encephalitis
Metabolic derangements
Poisoning

Adapted from Irwin RS, Cerra FB, Rippe JM, eds. *Intensive care medicine,* 4th ed. Philadelphia: Lippincott–Raven; 1999.

The pharmacologic methods used to treat delirium and to control agitation include the following agents, in addition to narcotics, propofol, and nondepolarizing muscle relaxants:

A. Oral haloperidol. In stable patients, the starting dose of this high-potency butyrophenone neuroleptic is often 2 to 5 mg three or four times daily. A lower initial dose (e.g., 0.5 mg, twice to three times daily) and gradual upward titration are advised in patients with advanced age, hemodynamic instability, or evidence of neurologic dysfunction in addition to delirium (e.g., stroke, dementia). Observation of haloperidol's effect should guide the adjustment of dosage and the frequency of administration.

B. Parenteral haloperidol. Haloperidol can be administered by the intramuscular (IM) and intravenous (IV) routes in patients whose acute agitation requires rapid treatment. The initial dose is 2 to 5 mg, depending on age, hemodynamic instability, and severity of agitation. If a calming effect does not occur within 15 to 20 minutes, the next dose should be doubled. This process of systematic dose escalation (i.e., doubling successive doses every 15 to 20 minutes) should be reserved

TABLE 179-3. Selected common delirium-inducing drugs used in the ICU

Drug Group	Agent
Antiarrhythmics	Lidocaine Mexiletine Procainamide hydrochloride Quinidine sulfate
Antibiotics	Penicillin
Anticholinergics	Atropine sulfate

Antihistamines	Nonselective
	  Diphenhydramine hydrochloride
	Histamine-2 blockers
	  Cimetidine
	  Ranitidine

Beta-blockers	Propranolol hydrochloride
Narcotics	Meperidine hydrochloride Morphine sulfate Pentazocine

Adapted from Tesar GE, Stern TA. Evaluation and treatment of agitation in the intensive care unit. *J Intensive Care Med* 1986;1:137–148; and Heckers S, Tesor GC, Stern TA. Diagnosis and treatment of agitation and delirium in the intensive care unit patient. In: Irwin RS, Cerra FB, Rippe JM, eds. *Intensive care medicine,* 4th ed. Philadelphia: Lippincott–Raven; 1999.

for the IV route and can be continued until the patient is calm. When agitation returns, the dose that ultimately tranquilized the patient should be repeated.

1. **Side effects.** In the ICU, side effects of haloperidol, whether administered orally or parenterally, are usually mild and inconsequential and are extrapyramidal and cardiovascular in nature.
   a. **Extrapyramidal effects.** The use of IV haloperidol in critically ill patients has been associated with fewer extrapyramidal effects (akathisia, dystonia, and parkinsonism) than its use IM or orally.
   b. **Cardiovascular effects.** Although haloperidol typically has trivial effects on the cardiovascular system, two potential complications can be life-threatening. First, in combination with haloperidol, propranolol has been reported to cause cardiopulmonary arrest and hypotension. Second, cardiac-conduction prolongation, premature ventricular contractions, ventricular tachycardia, torsades de pointes, and asystole can occur in some patients after the administration of haloperidol. Therefore, the corrected QT interval and serum levels of potassium, calcium, and magnesium must be monitored and normalized during high-dose haloperidol treatment.

C. **Combination of haloperidol and a benzodiazepine.** Use of a benzodiazepine in addition to haloperidol often promotes further calming. Lorazepam has been used more often than other agents for this purpose, but diazepam and midazolam are preferred when agitation is explosive.

D. **Other neuroleptics.** If IV haloperidol alone or in combination with a benzodiazepine is ineffective, use of a more sedating neuroleptic (e.g., droperidol, chlorpromazine) may be helpful. Compared with haloperidol, droperidol is less potent and more likely to produce sedation and hypotension. Chlorpromazine can cause severe orthostatic hypotension; its quinidinelike properties can increase the likelihood of cardiac arrhythmias. The risk of serious side effects is less with oral and IM administration than with IV use. Table 179-4 summarizes the pharmacologic properties of commonly used neuroleptics.

E. **Benzodiazepines.** A benzodiazepine alone is the treatment of choice when panic and severe anxiety account for agitated behavior. The continuous infusion of midazolam has been used effectively for sedation in the ICU; gradual tapering of dosage should follow prolonged use.

TABLE 179-4. Pharmacologic properties of commonly used neuroleptics

Drug	Route	Onset (Min)	Peak Effect (Min)	Active Metabolites	Starting Dose
Haloperidol	IM, IV[a]	5–20	15–45	Insignificant	*Degree of agitation*
	PO	30–60	120–240		Mild: 0.5–2 mg Moderate: 5–10 mg Severe: ≥10 mg
Droperidol	IM, IV	3–10	15–45	Insignificant	2.5–10 mg
Chlorpromazine	IM, IV[b]	5–40	10–30		25 mg
	PO	30–60	120–240		

[a] Intravenous haloperidol is not approved for routine use by the US Food and Drug Administration. Permission for its use should be requested from the hospital's formulary.
[b] Intravenous administration of chlorpromazine is more likely to cause cardiovascular disturbances (e.g., hypotension) than is intramuscular administration.
IM, intramuscular; IV, intravenous; PO, oral.
Adapted from Tesar GE, Stern TA. Rapid tranquilization of the agitated intensive care unit patient. *J Intensive Care Med* 1988;3:195–201; and Irwin RS, Cerra FB, Rippe JM, eds. *Intensive care medicine,* 4th ed. Philadelphia: Lippincott–Raven; 1999.

Selected Readings

Alexander HE, McCarty K, Giffen MB. Hypotension and cardiopulmonary arrest associated with concurrent haloperidol and propranolol therapy. *JAMA* 1984;252:87.

A report of a single case of cardiopulmonary arrest and hypotension in a woman with schizophrenia and hypertension treated with this combination of neuroleptic and beta-blocker.

Cassem NH. Psychiatric problems of the critically ill patient. In: Shoemaker WC, Ayres S, Grenvik A, et al., eds. *Textbook of Critical Care,* 2nd ed. Philadelphia: WB Saunders; 1989:1404.

A comprehensive review of the psychiatric problems commonly encountered in intensive care units, including delirium, depression, denial, fear, anxiety, and the threat to sign out.

Diagnostic and Statistical Manual of Mental Disorders, 4th ed. Washington, DC: American Psychiatric Association; 1994.

Known as DSM-IV, this "bible" of psychiatry enumerates the diagnostic criteria for the gamut of psychiatric maladies.

Hunt N, Stern TA. The association between intravenous haloperidol and torsades de pointes. *Psychosomatics* 1995;36:541.

A report of three cases of torsades de pointes in patients receiving intravenous haloperidol, as well as a review of the literature on ventricular arrhythmias associated with use of this neuroleptic.

Lipowski ZJ. Delirium (acute confusional states). *JAMA* 1987;258:1789.

A review of the clinical features, etiology, pathogenesis, and treatment of delirium.

Lipowski ZJ. Delirium in the elderly patient. *N Engl J Med* 1989;320:578.

A review of the clinical features, differential diagnosis, organic causes, and treatment of delirium, with special emphasis on the geriatric population.

Lipowski ZJ. Transient cognitive disorders (delirium, acute confusional states) in the elderly. *Am J Psychiatry* 1983;140:1426.

A discussion of the clinical features, etiology, pathogenesis, diagnosis, and treatment of delirium and related transient disorders of cognition in the elderly.

Ludwig, AM. *Principles of Clinical Psychiatry.* New York: Free Press; 1980.

This textbook of psychiatry contains a helpful chapter on organic brain syndromes, which the author refers to as the clouding-delirium-dementia-coma complex.

Tesar GE, Stern TA. Evaluation and treatment of agitation in the intensive care unit. *J Intensive Care Med* 1986;1:137.

A comprehensive review of the evaluation and management of the agitated intensive care unit patient.

Tesar GE, Stern TA. Rapid tranquilization of the agitated intensive care unit patient. *J Intensive Care Med* 1988;3:195.

A comprehensive discussion of the pharmacologic management of agitation in the intensive care unit and of the risks and benefits of neuroleptics, benzodiazepines, narcotics, and nondepolarizing muscle relaxants.

180. RECOGNITION AND TREATMENT OF ANXIETY IN THE INTENSIVE CARE UNIT PATIENT

Mark H. Pollack, Lawrence A. Labbate, John Querques, and Theodore A. Stern

I. **General principles.** Although anxiety in the intensive care unit (ICU) can be expected as a transient response to the stress of critical illness, pathologic anxiety has a negative impact on morbidity, mortality, and treatment compliance and merits timely evaluation and treatment.

II. **Definition.** Pathologic anxiety is a distressing experience of foreboding that is autonomous and persistent; it causes a level of distress beyond the patient's capacity to bear it and results in impaired function or abnormal behavior (e.g., avoidance or withdrawal).

III. **Clinical features.** Anxiety is manifested by physical, affective, behavioral, and cognitive symptoms and signs. The physical features are those associated with autonomic arousal (e.g., tachycardia, tachypnea, diaphoresis, lightheadedness). The affective component of anxiety ranges from mild edginess to terror and panic, whereas its behavioral consequences include avoidance (e.g., refusal of medical procedures) and withdrawal (e.g., demand to leave the hospital). The cognitive aspects of anxiety include worry, apprehension, and thoughts about emotional or bodily damage.

IV. **Differential diagnosis.** Anxiety in the ICU patient can be caused by a medical illness or its treatment; a primary psychiatric syndrome; or a failure to cope with the patient's critical condition.

   A. **Organic causes.** A patient's known medical illness, its complications, and its treatment should be suspected as causes of anxiety. An organic cause is suggested by anxiety that occurs in the absence of a psychologically charged situation or in conjunction with discrete physical events (e.g., supraventricular tachycardia during vasopressor treatment).

   B. **Psychiatric causes.** When primary psychopathology is the cause of anxiety in the ICU patient, the acute medical condition either exacerbates a premorbid psychiatric condition or provokes an initial episode of anxiety or panic. Anxiety can be a manifestation of delirium; substance withdrawal or intoxication; schizophrenia or its treatment with neuroleptics; or a primary anxiety disorder (e.g., panic disorder, generalized anxiety disorder, simple phobia, social phobia, posttraumatic stress disorder, obsessive-compulsive disorder).

   C. **Failure to cope.** Patients deal with the stress of hospitalization with a variety of coping strategies (e.g., rationalization, reassurance, religion, family support). Even in patients without a history of anxiety, these mechanisms can be overwhelmed in the ICU when patients regress or feel alone, the illness is sudden, or social supports are unavailable. Anxiety, fear, and feelings of vulnerability can result.

V. **Treatment.** Management of the anxious patient in the ICU involves correction of underlying organic factors and use of both pharmacologic and nonpharmacologic interventions.

   A. **Pharmacologic interventions**

      1. **Benzodiazepines.** These agents are generally considered the mainstays of anxiolytic pharmacotherapy in the ICU because of their relative safety and rapid therapeutic effects. Drug selection is determined by the clinical situation and the pharmacokinetic properties of the agent. Table 180-1 summarizes important pharmacologic properties of some commonly used benzodiazepines. For example, an acutely agitated patient requires a drug with a rapid onset of action (e.g., diazepam or midazolam). Associated with less interdose and posttreatment rebound anxiety, long-acting drugs (e.g., clonazepam) are beneficial in patients who require long-term benzodiazepine therapy.

TABLE 180-1. Pharmacologic properties of commonly used benzodiazepines

Drug	Route	Onset (Min)	Peak Effect (Min)	Active Metabolites	Starting Dose
Diazepam	IV	2–5	5–30	Nordiazepam[a]	2–5 mg
	PO	10–60	30–180		
Lorazepam	IM, IV	2–20	60–120	None	1–2 mg
	SL	2–20	20–60		0.5–1 mg
	PO	20–60	20–120		0.5–1 mg
Midazolam	IM, IV	1–2	30–40	1- and 4-hydroxy-midazolam	0.05–0.15 mg/kg

[a] Nordiazepam (desmethyldiazepam) is the active metabolite of diazepam. Its half-life is 60 to 100 hours.
IV, intravenous; PO, oral; IM, intramuscular; SL, sublingual.
Adapted from Tesar GE, Stern TA. Rapid tranquilization of the agitated intensive care unit patient. *J Intensive Care Med* 1988;3:195–201; and Pollack MH, Labbok LA, Stern TA Recognition and Treatment of Anxiety in the Intensive Care Unit Patient. In: Irwin RS, Cerra FB, Rippe JM, eds. *Intensive care medicine,* 4th ed. Philadelphia: Lippincott–Raven; 1999;2393–2401.

a. **Dose.** For many patients it is reasonable to initiate treatment with a low dose of a shorter-acting, easily metabolized agent on a fixed-dose (not as-needed) schedule (e.g., lorazepam 1 mg three or four times daily). The dosage can then be titrated to anxiolytic effect. Dosages in elderly patients should be roughly half those used in younger patients. Patients with impaired hepatic function should receive agents that have shorter half-lives and fewer (or no) active metabolites (e.g., lorazepam) to minimize drug accumulation.

b. **Route of administration.** Benzodiazepines should be administered parenterally when immediate relief of anxiety is necessary or when the oral route is unavailable. Intravenous (IV) administration of diazepam and chlordiazepoxide is preferred to the intramuscular (IM) route because IM absorption of these agents is erratic. Lorazepam, on the other hand, is well-absorbed after IM administration; it can also be given sublingually to achieve a quicker onset of action than the oral route provides. Hypotension and respiratory depression are potential risks of IV administration of benzodiazepines.

2. **Neuroleptics.** When fear and anxiety become severe and the patient is unable to reason or becomes transiently psychotic, a neuroleptic (e.g., haloperidol) is indicated. (See Chapter 179, "Diagnosis and Treatment of Agitation and Delirium in the Intensive Care Unit Patient," for a discussion of the use of neuroleptics in the ICU.)

B. **Nonpharmacologic interventions.** Clarification, education, support, appropriate reassurance, hypnosis, and behavioral strategies (e.g., relaxation techniques) can all be an important part of the management of the anxious patient. Misconceptions about illness should be identified and fears allayed.

Selected Readings

Geringer ES, Stern TA. Anxiety and depression in critically ill patients. *Problems in Critical Care* 1988;2:35.
A practical review of the manifestations, differential diagnosis, and treatment of depression and anxiety in patients with critical illness.

Tesar GE, Stern TA. Rapid tranquilization of the agitated intensive care unit patient. *J Intensive Care Med* 1988;3:195.
A comprehensive discussion of the pharmacologic management of agitation in the intensive care unit and of the risks and benefits of neuroleptics, benzodiazepines, narcotics, and nondepolarizing muscle relaxants.

181. RECOGNITION AND TREATMENT OF DEPRESSION IN THE INTENSIVE CARE UNIT PATIENT

Edith S. Geringer, John Querques, and Theodore A. Stern

I. **General principles.** More profound than the transient experience of discouragement, disappointment, sadness, grief, or despondency, major depression is a psychiatric disorder that affects mood and neurovegetative functions (e.g., sleep, appetite, concentration). Never a normal or appropriate reaction to a stressful situation, when left untreated, major depression decreases survival in general and increases morbidity and mortality from cardiac conditions. Aggressive treatment of depression in the intensive care unit (ICU) can drastically improve a patient's sense of well-being and change a demoralized, hopeless patient into an active participant in treatment.

II. **Definition.** Defined by diagnostic criteria, major depression is a syndrome characterized by a sustained period of depressed mood or anhedonia (i. e., a decrease in one's interests or drives in life) for 2 or more weeks and associated with four or more of the following eight symptoms: (a) a change in sleep pattern; (b) a sense of guilt or worthlessness; (c) a decrease in energy; (d) a decrease in concentration ability; (e) a change in appetite; (f) a change in psychomotor activity; and (g) suicidal thinking or thoughts of death. The mnemonic, SIG: E CAPS (i.e., label: energy capsules), is a helpful guide to remember these defining criteria (Table 181-1).

III. **Clinical features.** Despite the uniformity in clinical presentation these formal diagnostic criteria suggest, in actuality the manifestations of depression are myriad; they include affective, behavioral, and cognitive abnormalities (i.e., the ABCs of depression) (Table 181-2).

IV. **Differential diagnosis.** Although depression in the ICU can occur as a primary affective disorder (i.e., major depression), it can also occur as a mood disorder associated with specific organic disease or its treatment or as a psychological reaction to an acute medical illness.

   A. **Organic causes.** Various medical conditions (Table 181-3) and medications (Table 181-4) can cause depression. A thorough laboratory screen, including assessment of electrolytes, vitamin B_{12}, folate, thyroid hormones, and rapid plasma reagin reactivity, is useful when excluding these organic causes of depression, but it should be guided by results of a comprehensive history and physical examination.

   B. **Psychological reaction.** Acute medical illness, especially when critical, often threatens a patient's sense of physical integrity and of autonomy. In addition, critical illness can remind some patients of either personal or family histories of similar life-threatening circumstances. In such cases, a patient's coping strategies can falter and depression ensue.

V. **Treatment.** Management of depression includes pharmacologic treatment, psychotherapy, and electroconvulsive therapy (ECT); in the ICU, pharmacologic interventions are used most frequently. An antidepressant medication is most commonly selected because its side-effect profile best fits the patient's symptoms. Another consideration is onset of action. With the exception of psychostimulants, antidepressants take 4 to 6 weeks to achieve maximal effect; therefore, dextroamphetamine and methylphenidate, which work within days, are preferable when a quicker response is desired.

   A. **Psychostimulants.** Benign and effective, these medications are often the first agents used to treat depression in critically ill patients at the Massachusetts General Hospital. Although they can cause tachycardia, hypertension, arrhythmias, and coronary spasm, these effects are rare at the low doses (5–20 mg/d) usually used to treat depression.

   B. **Selective serotonin reuptake inhibitors (SSRIs)**

      1. **Side effects.** Compared with tricyclic antidepressants (TCAs), SSRIs are far less anticholinergic, antihistaminic, and anti-α-adrenergic and, thus, have

TABLE 181-1. Mnemonic for the eight neurovegetative features of depression—SIG: E CAPS

Sleep (increased or decreased)
Interest
Guilt (or worthlessness)
Energy
Concentration
Appetite (increased or decreased)
Psychomotor agitation or retardation
Suicidal thinking (or thoughts of death)

Adapted from Geringer LS, Stern TA: Recognition and treatment of depression in the intensive care unit patient. In: Irwin RS, Cerra FB, Rippe JM, eds. *Intensive care medicine,* 4th ed. Philadelphia: Lippincott–Raven; 1999.

fewer intolerable side effects. However, they can cause agitation, irritability, insomnia, tremulousness, diaphoresis, anorexia, nausea, vomiting, diarrhea, and sexual dysfunction. Although they also have fewer cardiovascular effects than TCAs and do not commonly cause orthostatic hypotension, two cases of bradycardia and faintness or syncope have been reported with fluoxetine use. Thus, SSRIs should be avoided in patients with sick sinus syndrome. In addition, venlafaxine (a norepinephrine and serotonin reuptake inhibitor) causes a dose-dependent increase in supine diastolic blood pressure.

2. **Drug interactions.** SSRIs are extensively metabolized by the hepatic cytochrome P-450 system; all of them, except venlafaxine and citalopram, are also inhibitors of this enzymatic pathway and, thus, raise serum levels of coadministered drugs. The interactions most likely to occur in the ICU are listed in Table 181-5. Neither fluoxetine nor fluvoxamine should ever be combined with astemizole, terfenadine, or cisapride because a lethal ventricular arrhythmia can ensue (nefazodone, an atypical antidepressant, should be avoided for the same reason). In most other cases, attention to dosage can mitigate against harmful effects of P-450 interactions.

C. Tricyclic antidepressants

1. **Side effects.** Because of their anticholinergic and anti-α-adrenergic properties, the most common adverse effects of TCAs are sedation, confusion, blurred vision, dry mouth, orthostatic hypotension, and constipation (Table 181-6). In

TABLE 181-2. Affective, behavioral, and cognitive features of depression—the ABCs

Affective symptoms
- Depressed mood
- Hopelessness
- Crying
- Irritability
- Anger
- Decreased interest

Behavioral symptoms
- Insomnia
- Anorexia
- Apathy
- Increased sleep
- Increased appetite
- Decreased energy
- Psychomotor agitation
- Psychomotor retardation
- Noncompliance
- Suicidal gesture
- Impulsivity
- Poor eye contact
- Increased or intractable pain
- Somatic preoccupation

Cognitive symptoms
- Guilty ruminations
- Decreased concentration
- Suicidal ideation
- Confusion
- Pseudodementia
- Thoughts of death

Adapted from Geringer LS, Stern TA: Recognition and treatment of depression in the intensive care unit patient. In: Irwin RS, Cerra FB, Rippe JM, eds. *Intensive care medicine,* 4th ed. Philadelphia: Lippincott–Raven; 1999.

TABLE 181-3. Selected medical conditions associated with depression

Cardiovascular
- Congestive heart failure
- Hypertensive encephalopathy

Collagen-vascular
- Systemic lupus erythematosus

Endocrine
- Diabetes mellitus
- Hypo- and hyperadrenalism
- Hypo- and hyperparathyroidism
- Hypo- and hyperthyroidism

Infectious
- Hepatitis
- Human immunodeficiency virus infection
- Mononucleosis

Metabolic
- Acid-base disorders
- Hypokalemia
- Hypo- and hypernatremia
- Renal failure

Neoplastic
- Carcinoid
- Pancreatic carcinoma

Neurologic
- Brain tumor
- Multiple sclerosis
- Parkinson's disease
- Temporal lobe epilepsy
- Stroke
- Subcortical dementia

Nutritional
- Vitamin B_{12} deficiency (pernicious anemia)
- Thiamine deficiency (Wernicke's encephalopathy)

Adapted from Geringer LS, Stern TA: Recognition and treatment of depression in the intensive care unit patient. In: Irwin RS, Cerra FB, Rippe JM, eds. *Intensive care medicine,* 4th ed. Philadelphia: Lippincott–Raven; 1999.

TABLE 181-4. Selected commonly used medications associated with depression

Acyclovir (especially at high doses)
Alcohol
Amphetaminelike drugs (withdrawal): phenylpropanolamine, fenfluramine
Anabolic steroids
Anticonvulsants (at high doses or plasma levels): carbamazepine, phenytoin, primidone
Antihypertensives: reserpine, methyldopa, thiazides, clonidine, hydralazine hydrochloride, nifedipine, prazosin
Asparaginase
Baclofen
Barbiturates
Benzodiazepines: triazolam, alprazolam, clonazepam, clorazepate, diazepam, lorazepam
Beta-blockers: atenolol, propranolol, timolol
Bromides
Bromocriptine
Carbon monoxide
Cocaine (withdrawal)
Contraceptives
Corticosteroids
Cycloserine
Dapsone
Digitalis (at high doses or in elderly patients)
Diltiazem
Disopyramide
Halothane (postoperatively)
Heavy metals
Histamine-2 receptor antagonists: cimetidine, ranitidine
Interferon-α
Isoniazid
Levodopa (especially in elderly patients)
Mefloquine
Metoclopramide
Metrizamide
Nalidixic acid
Narcotics: morphine, meperidine, methadone, pentazocine, propoxyphene
Nonsteroidal antiinflammatory drugs
Phenylephrine
Procaine derivatives: penicillin G procaine, lidocaine, procainamide
Thyroid hormones
Trimethoprim-sulfamethoxazole

Adapted from Geringer LS, Stern TA: Recognition and treatment of depression in the intensive care unit patient. In: Irwin RS, Cerra FB, Rippe JM, eds. *Intensive care medicine,* 4th ed. Philadelphia: Lippincott–Raven; 1999.

TABLE 181-5. Selected substrates and inhibitors of cytochrome P-450 isoenzymes

	1A2	2C	2D6	3A3/4
Substrates	Acetaminophen Aminophylline Haloperidol TCAs Theophylline	Barbiturates Diazepam Omeprazole Phenytoin Propranolol TCAs	Codeine Encainide Flecainide Haloperidol Hydrocodone Metoprolol Propranolol TCAs Timolol	Amiodarone Astemizole Calcium channel blockers Cisapride Diazepam Disopyramide Lidocaine Macrolide antibiotics Omeprazole Quinidine Steroids Terfenadine TCAs
Inhibitors	Fluoxetine Fluvoxamine[a] Paroxetine	Fluoxetine[a] Fluvoxamine[a] Sertraline	Fluoxetine[a] Paroxetine[a] Sertraline	Fluoxetine Fluvoxamine[a] Nefazodone[a] Sertraline

[a]Strong inhibitor.
TCA, tricyclic antidepressant.
Adapted from Geringer LS, Stern TA: Recognition and treatment of depression in the intensive care unit patient. In: Irwin RS, Cerra FB, Rippe JM, eds. *Intensive care medicine,* 4th ed. Philadelphia: Lippincott–Raven; 1999.

TABLE 181-6. Comparative properties of tricylic antidepressants

Drug	Ach Effects	Sedative Effects	OH	Target Dose Range (mg/d)	Comments
Tertiary amines					
Amitriptyline	+++	+++	+++	≥150	Most anti-cholinergic
Doxepin	++	+++	++	≥200	
Imipramine	++	++	+++	≥200	
Secondary amines					
Desipramine	+	+	+++	≥150	
Nortriptyline	++	++	+	≥100	Least OH; safest in cardiac disease
Protriptyline	+++	+	++	≥30	

Ach, anticholinergic; OH, orthostatic hypotension; +++, high; ++, moderate; +, low
Adapted from Geringer LS, Stern TA: Recognition and treatment of depression in the intensive care unit patient. In: Irwin RS, Cerra FB, Rippe JM, eds. *Intensive care medicine,* 4th ed. Philadelphia: Lippincott–Raven; 1999.

TABLE 181-7. The use of TCAs in patients with selected cardiovascular conditions

Cardiac Status	Comments	TCA of Choice (Based on Available Data)
Bundle-branch block	1. Caution advised 2. All TCAs prolong HV interval 3. Pretreatment ECG recommended in patients >50 years 4. Hospitalization/telemetric monitoring suggested at start of treatment 5. Maintain lowest effective plasma level	Nortriptyline ? Doxepin
Ventricular arrhythmia	1. TCAs possess type-I (quinidine-like) effects 2. PVCs may improve on TCAs 3. Antiarrhythmic dosage may require a decrease 4. Holter monitor suggested	Imipramine Desipramine
Orthostatic hypotension	1. All TCAs can produce further orthostatic changes that can be predicted to some degree by predrug orthostatic changes 2. Effect can occur independent of plasma levels 3. Symptoms may be minimal despite significant fall in blood pressure 4. Symptoms may decrease over time	Nortriptyline
Left ventricular dysfunction/CHF	1. Impairment of contractility is uncommon 2. CHF is very rare; it may occur secondary to heart rate increases from anticholinergic effects	All TCAs
Recent acute myocardial infarction	1. Delay use of TCAs for several weeks because of hypotension, tachycardia, and systemic effects	None
Atrial fibrillation	1. Avoid TCAs unless concurrently treated with digoxin	None
Prolonged QTc	1. Use with caution because of risk of sudden death when QTc >440 msec	Nortriptyline ? Doxepin

TCAs, tricyclic antidepressants; HV, His-ventricular; ECG, electrocardiogram; PVC, premature ventricular contraction; CHF, congestive heart failure; QTc, corrected QT interval.

Adapted from Dec GW, Stern TA. Tricylic antidepressants in the intensive care unit. *J Intensive Care Med* 1990;5:69–81; and Geringer LS, Stern TA: Recognition and treatment of depression in the intensive care unit patient. In: Irwin RS, Cerra FB, Rippe JM, eds. *Intensive care medicine,* 4th ed. Philadelphia: Lippincott–Raven; 1999.

addition, they also affect cardiac conduction and cardiac rhythm. They should be used with great caution in patients with preexisting conduction delays, in those with a corrected QT interval (QTc) of more than 440 msec, and in patients treated with other drugs that also have type-I antiarrhythmic effects. Although these agents have been used without adverse sequelae less than 6 weeks after acute myocardial infarction (MI), they are not recommended in the acute post-MI phase. The use of TCAs in patients with cardiovascular disease is summarized in Table 181-7.

D. Monoamine oxidase inhibitors. In general, phenelzine and tranylcypromine are not useful in the ICU because of the profound hypertensive crises that might result when these agents are combined with pressors.

E. Psychotherapy. Although pharmacologic treatments are the cornerstone of treatment for depressed ICU patients, psychological treatments are also important. Patients often benefit from information, clarification, reassurance, and support. One way to help patients with concerns about their future is to ask specific questions about how they believe their illness will affect their daily life. Another way of helping patients cope involves learning about their premorbid activities; this technique restores a patient's sense of identity.

F. Electroconvulsive therapy (ECT). ECT is reserved for patients with severe or delusional depression and for those who cannot tolerate or who have failed to respond to pharmacologic and talking therapies.

Selected Readings

Dec GW, Stern TA. Tricyclic antidepressants in the intensive care unit. *J Intensive Care Med* 1990;5:69.

A review of the pharmacology of tricyclic antidepressants, their major cardiovascular and neurologic effects, and the management of tricyclic antidepressant overdose.

Diagnostic and Statistical Manual of Mental Disorders, 4th ed. Washington, DC: American Psychiatric Association; 1994.

Known as DSM-IV, this "bible" of psychiatry enumerates the diagnostic criteria for the gamut of psychiatric maladies.

Ellison JM, Milofsky JE, Ely E. Fluoxetine-induced bradycardia and syncope in two patients. *J Clin Psychiatry* 1990;51:385.

A report of two cases of bradycardia—one with syncope, one with faintness—during treatment with fluoxetine.

Feighner JP. The role of venlafaxine in rational antidepressant therapy. *J Clin Psychiatry* 1994;55(Suppl A):62.

A review of the results of the preclinical and premarketing studies of venlafaxine; a discussion of the efficacy, safety, and pharmacokinetic and pharmacodynamic profiles of this serotonin and norepinephrine reuptake inhibitor.

Kaufmann MW, Murray GB, Cassem NH. Use of psychostimulants in medically ill depressed patients. *Psychosomatics* 1982;23:817.

A report of the beneficial and safe use of methylphenidate and dextroamphetamine in medically ill patients with comorbid depression.

Roose SP, Glassman AH, Giardina EGV, et al. Tricyclic antidepressants in depressed patients with cardiac conduction disease. *Arch Gen Psychiatry* 1987;44:273.

A prospective study that compared the risk of cardiac complications of imipramine and nortriptyline in depressed patients with and without cardiac conduction delays.

XVII. MORAL, ETHICAL, LEGAL, AND PUBLIC POLICY ISSUES IN THE INTENSIVE CARE UNIT

182. ETHICAL AND LEGAL ISSUES IN AN ERA OF MANAGED CARE

John J. Paris, J. Cameron Muir, and Frank E. Reardon

I. General principles. As we enter into a managed care delivery system, the ethical issues raised in the treatment of seriously ill patients are intensified. This chapter explores recent developments on several of those emerging issues: the decision-making process, do-not-resuscitate (DNR) orders, withdrawal of treatment, physician-assisted suicide, and the constraints of managed care.

II. Decision-making process. Although we have long since surpassed the era of the paternalistic physician and the passive patient, physicians, as the SUPPORT study demonstrates, continue to function independently of the preferences of critically ill patients. For many of them, "the aim of preserving life or the principle of beneficence overrides the principle of respect for autonomy." That perspective clashes with the current standard in both ethics and the law that patient preferences on withdrawal of treatment should prevail.

Good medical decision-making is not unidimensional. At a minimum, it must consider three factors: the physician, the patient, and the community. The physician must make the diagnosis, provide the prognosis, and make a recommendation. Given the recommendation, the patient or proxy then addresses the subjective values that will determine whether the proposal offers a proportionate benefit and then makes a choice.

Although the combination of patient–family choice is generally final, a third factor—society—must also be considered. With the shift in attitude from strong paternalism to the elevation of autonomy into a near absolute, individuals sometimes forget that their actions and decisions have implications for and impact on others. Consequently, society for the protection of individuals and the common good, may place constraints and limits, both positive and negative, on individual rights.

III. Responsibility for the decision. When a dispute occurs between the physician and the decision maker, the first recourse should not be to the courts but to a multidisciplinary hospital ethics committee, which would be familiar with both the medical setting and community standards. That consultative body would provide a framework for impartial but sensitive review of hard choices.

Physicians, when withholding or withdrawing life-sustaining treatment over the patient or family's objections, should not act unilaterally. All such decisions should be made in consultation with specialists, be supported by data from the literature, and have the approval of an ethics committee. Further, as the American Medical Association (AMA) "Futility Policy" guidelines indicate, if that process does not resolve the conflict, the physician should offer the family the opportunity of an outside opinion and transfer of the patient. If no physician can be found who is willing to care for the patient as the family requests, the AMA's guidelines indicate the treating physician has no further obligation to follow the family's demands for aggressive interventions.

IV. Do not resuscitate (DNR) orders. Despite the strong agreement in the ethical literature and judicial rulings that patient preferences to forgo aggressive medical interventions should be respected, the SUPPORT study reveals that physicians caring for critically ill patients are reluctant to honor such requests. This is particularly true with regard to DNR orders. The study found that, although a third of the patients preferred that cardiopulmonary resuscitation (CPR) be withheld, only 47% of the physicians accurately reported that preference and nearly half (49%) of those patients did not have a written DNR order.

Tomlinson and Brody distinguish three rationales for DNR orders: no medical benefit; poor quality of life after CPR; and poor quality of life before CPR. They adopt Blackhall's position that "Physicians have no obligation to provide, and patients and families no right to demand, medical treatment that is of no demonstrable benefit." In such cases, they too believe, the patient or family's desire for

CPR is irrelevant. The decision is entirely within the physician's technical expertise. The physician's duty is to communicate with the family and explain that the patient's physical condition is such that no intervention will reverse the dying process and, hence, none will be attempted. The most physicians should do when CPR is believed futile is to communicate that information to the patient or family so that they will understand the decision the physician has made.

V. **Withholding and withdrawal of medical interventions.** Once it is agreed that a particular medical intervention is not appropriate for a patient, either because the patient or proxy refuses it or because it is not effective in reversing or ameliorating a disease process, that intervention can be withheld or withdrawn. Universal agreement now exists, in both the ethical and legal literature, that the same justification that applies to the withholding of a treatment governs its withdrawal. From Quinlan to Cruzan, the United States Supreme Court and every state supreme court that has addressed the issue has concurred that no moral, ethical, or legal difference is seen between withholding or withdrawing medical interventions.

The moral issue facing critical care physicians involved in the withdrawal of medical interventions is to assure the patient and family that the withdrawal of treatment will not produce suffering for the patient. Physicians should take care to premedicate patients with a sedative, generally morphine, to alleviate dyspnea and pain and a benzodiazepine for anxiety. Because the goal of these medications is symptom relief, not death, they should be titrated to the intended effect.

VI. **Managed care.** America is entering a new era in medicine: managed care. Under it the health care delivery system will operate with fixed budgets, capitation, and financial risk to providers. Those institutions that miscalculate the cost or exceed budgets by providing marginally beneficial, excessively expensive treatments will prove noncompetitive in a price-sensitive market.

The threat this new system poses to the traditional way of dealing with patients in an intensive care setting is real. The autonomy-driven domination of the past three decades of medicine has led to a situation in which the patient or proxy could not only refuse an unwanted medical treatment, but could demand and would be provided, any potentially life-prolonging procedure available. It is an environment, not of community-shared values, but of subjectively chosen goals. Translated into practice, that consumer-based model of medicine is one in which the patient alone determines the worthwhileness of any potential life-prolonging treatment.

That approach to medicine, which adheres to Norman Levinsky's exhortation that physicians are to serve single-mindedly as the patient's advocate "without regard to costs or other social obligations," resulted in uncontrollable costs. The "single master" view of medicine, to use Luce's term, in which if a disagreement exists between the physician and the patient over the efficacy of a treatment, the patient's view necessarily prevailed. As Callahan notes, this led to a cultural dilemma: There is no room for professional standards and, if left unchecked, will lead to bankruptcy.

In a perceptive essay on medicine and economics written in 1984, Thurow predicted that Americans would either have to learn to say "no" to marginally beneficial high-cost medical treatments or they would revert to the marketplace as the mechanism to make that choice for them. As an egalitarian, he had hoped that society would "help physicians decide when medicine is bad medicine—not simply because it has absolutely no payoff or hurts the patient—but also because the costs are not justified by minor expected benefits." If that does not happen, he wrote, "sooner or later the United States will move toward a system of third-party controls."

Thurow's hoped-for social consensus did not happen. Given the inability to formulate publicly agreed-to constraints on individual choices, Thurow's default position, the marketplace, has come into play. Now a third party, the insurer—not the patient or physician—is determining what is to be provided.

The mechanism employed to guarantee constraint within the system, by definition, is a function of the market: financial incentives. The financial incentives—capitation, salary "withholds," and bonus arrangements—are not accidental; they are designed precisely to place the physician at financial risk for providing marginal or superfluous treatments. The ethical question at stake with regard to these "financial incentives" is not whether these incentives present a potential conflict of interest (all financial incentives, including fee-for-service, involve that danger), but whether they serve a public good. Do they help control spiraling costs? Do they reign in marginal or useless interventions? Are they effective in guaranteeing a more equitable access to the common resources? These are questions of institutional as opposed to individual claims about equity and fairness. They require a concern not only for a particular patient but for the well-being of all those affected by the plan: patients, physicians, payers, providers—and, most particularly, all the other participants in the plan.

Selected Readings

Blackhall L. Must we always use CPR? *N Engl J Med* 1987;317:1281.
A landmark article on limits for use of cardiopulmonary resuscitation.

Brody H, Campbell ML, Faber-Langedoen K, et al. Withdrawing intensive life-sustaining treatment—recommendations for compassionate clinical management. *N Engl J Med* 1997;336:652.
A clear statement on the role of comfort care management of the dying patient.

Callahan D. Necessity, futility and the good society. *J Am Geriatr Soc* 1994;42:866.
An attempt by one of the leading commentators in bioethics to put "futility" into context.

Callahan D. Shattuck Lecture: contemporary biomedical ethics. *N Engl J Med* 1980; 302:1228.
Survey of the state of biomedical ethics in 1980.

Collins J. Should doctors tell the truth? *Harpers* 1927;155:320.
A 1927 article that captures the paternalistic position that the doctor alone makes the medical decisions.

Cruzan v. Director. Missouri Dept of Health, 58 U.S. L.W. 4916 (1990).
The first United States Supreme Court opinion on withdrawal of life-sustaining treatment.

Darragh M, McCarrick PM. Managed health care: new ethical issues for all. *Kennedy Institute of Ethics Journal* 1996;6:189.
An excellent survey of ethical issues in managed care.

In re Quinlan, 70 N.J. 10, 355 A.2d 647 (1976).
The first state Supreme Court case authorizing withdrawal of a ventilator.

Lanken PN. Critical care medicine at a new crossroads: the intersection of economics and ethics in the intensive care unit. *Am J Respir Crit Care Med* 1994;149:3.
A fine analysis of the impact of managed care on critical care medicine.

Levinsky N. The doctor's master. *N Engl J Med* 1984;311:1573.
A strong statement on the physician's obligation to be an advocate for the patient in medical decision-making.

Luce J. Ethical principles in critical care. *JAMA* 1990;263:696.
A formulation of principles for critical care.

Luce JM. Physicians do not have a responsibility to provide futile or unreasonable care if a patient or family insists. *Crit Care Med* 1995;23:760.
A forceful statement by one of the nation's leading physician's on the limits of a patient's right to demand medical interventions.

Malinwoski MJ. Capitation, advances in medical technology, and the advent of a new era in medical ethics. *Am J Law Med* 1996;22:331.
A good summary of issues in managed care.

Paris JJ, Crone RK, Reardon FE. Physician refusal of requested treatment: the case of Baby L. *N Engl J Med* 1990;322:1012.
First reported case of physician refusal to provide a life-sustaining intervention.

Paris JJ, Schreiber MD, Statter M, et al. Beyond autonomy: physician refusal of life-prolonging ECMO. *N Engl J Med* 1991;325:511.
First reported case of physician refusal to continue life-prolonging technology.

Ruark JE, Raffin TA, and the Stanford University Medical Center Committee on Ethics. Initiating and withdrawing life support. *N Engl J Med* 1988;318:25.
An early report on workings of an academic medical center's ethics committee.

Smedira N, Evans BH, Grais LS, et al. Withholding and withdrawal of life-support from the critically ill. *N Engl J Med* 1990;322:309.
A set of guidelines for withdrawal of life-sustaining treatments.

The Society of Critical Care Medicine Ethics Committee. Attitudes of critical care medicine professionals concerning distribution of intensive care resources. *Crit Care Med* 1994;22:358.
A survey of attitudes of critical care providers on distribution or resources.
The SUPPORT Principal Investigators. A controlled trial to improve care for seriously ill hospitalized patients: the study to understand prognosis and preferences for outcomes and risks of treatments (SUPPORT). *JAMA* 1995;274:1591.
A landmark study of physician behavior in critical care medicine.
Thurow L. Learning to say "no." *N Engl J Med* 1984;311:1569.
A superb essay by an economist that in the absence of agreed-on societal values the marketplace will determine what medicine will be provided.
Tomlinson T, Brody H. Ethics and communication in do-not-resuscitate orders. *N Engl J Med* 1988;318:49.
An early attempt to provide guidelines on do not resuscitate orders.
Veatch RM, Spicer CM. Medically futile care: the role of the physician in setting limits. *Am J Law Med* 1992;18:15.
The best statement of the position that patient autonomy is the overriding principle in medical ethics.

APPENDIX

CALCULATIONS COMMONLY USED IN CRITICAL CARE

Mark M. Wilson

A. Fahrenheit and Celsius Temperature Conversions

°C	°F
45	113.0
44	111.2
43	109.4
42	107.6
41	105.8
40	104.0
39	102.2
38	100.4
37	98.6
36	96.8
35	95.0
34	93.2
33	91.4
32	89.6
31	87.8
30	86.0
29	84.2
28	82.4
27	80.6
26	78.8
25	77.0

°C to °F: °F = (°C × 9/5) + 32
°F to °C: °C = (°F − 32) × 5/9

B. Hemodynamic Calculations

MEAN ARTERIAL BLOOD PRESSURE (mm Hg)

= MAP
= [systolic BP + (2 × diastolic BP)]/3
= diastolic BP + 1/3 (systolic BP − diastolic BP)
Normal range: 85–95 mm Hg

FICK EQUATION FOR CARDIAC INDEX (L/min/m^2)

= CI
= CO/BSA
= oxygen consumption/(arterial O_2 content − venous O_2 content)
= [10 × $\dot{V}O_2$ (ml/min/m^2)]/[Hgb (g/dl) × 1.39 × (arterial % saturation − venous % saturation)]
Normal range: 2.5–4.2 L/min/m^2

SYSTEMIC VASCULAR RESISTANCE (dyne-sec-cm^{-5})

= SVR
= [80 × (MAP − right atrial mean BP)]/CO (L/min)
Normal range: 770–1,500 dyne-sec-cm^{-5}

PULMONARY VASCULAR RESISTANCE (dyne-sec-cm^{-5})

= PVR
= [80 × (pulmonary artery mean BP – pulmonary capillary wedge pressure)
/ CO (L/min)
Normal range: 20–120 dyne-sec-cm^{-5}

C. Pulmonary Calculations

ALVEOLAR GAS EQUATION (mm Hg)

$P_AO_2 = PIO_2 - (PaCO_2/R)$
$= [FIO_2 \times (P_{atm} - P_{H2O})] - (PaCO_2/R)$
$= 150 - (PaCO_2/R)$ (on room air, at sea level)
Normal value: ~100 mm Hg (on room air, at sea level)

ALVEOLAR–ARTERIOLE OXYGEN TENSION GRADIENT (mm Hg)

= A – a gradient
$= PAO_2 - PaO_2$
Normal values (upright): 2.5 + (0.21 × age)

ARTERIAL BLOOD OXYGEN CONTENT (ml/dl)

$= CaO_2$
= oxygen dissolved in blood + oxygen carried by hemoglobin
= [0.003 (ml O_2/dl) × PaO_2] + [1.39 × Hgb (g/dl) × % Hgb saturated with O_2]
Normal range: 17.5–23.5 ml/dl

COMPLIANCE (ml/cm H_2O)

= ΔVolume/ΔPressure
On Mechanical Ventilation:
Static respiratory system compliance = C_{st} = Tidal volume/ ($P_{plateau} - P_{end\ exp}$)
Dynamic effective compliance = C_{dyn} = Tidal volume/ ($P_{peak} - P_{end\ exp}$)

D. Electrolyte and Renal Calculations

ANION GAP (mEq/L)

$= [Na^+] - ([Cl^-] + [HCO_3^-])$
Normal range: 9–13 mEq/L

EXPECTED ANION GAP IN HYPOALBUMINEMIA

= 3 × [albumin (g/dl)]

CALCULATED SERUM OSMOLALITY (mOsm/kg)

= (2 × [Na^+]) + ([glucose]/18) + ([BUN]/2.8)
Normal range: 275–290 mOsm/kg

OSMOLAR GAP (mOsm/kg)

= Measured serum osmolality – Calculated serum osmolality
Normal range: 0–5 mOsm/kg

Na^+ CORRECTION FOR HYPERGLYCEMIA

Increase $[Na^+]$ by 1.6 mEq/L for each 100 mg/dl increase in [glucose] above 100 mg/dl

Ca^{2+} CORRECTION FOR HYPOALBUMINEMIA

Increase $[Ca^{2+}]$ by 0.8 mg/dl for each 1.0 gm/dl decrease in [albumin] from 4 g/dl

WATER DEFICIT IN HYPERNATREMIA (L)

$= [0.6 \times \text{body weight (kg)}] \times \{([Na^+]/140) - 1\}$

Na^+ DEFICIT IN HYPONATREMIA (mEq)

$= [0.6 \times \text{body weight (kg)}] \times (\text{desired plasma } [Na^+] - 140)$

FRACTIONAL EXCRETION OF SODIUM (%)

$= F_ENa$
$= \{(\text{excreted } [Na^+])/(\text{filtered } [Na^+])\} \times 100$
$= \{(\text{urine } [Na^+])/(\text{serum } [Na^+])\}/\{(\text{urine [Creat]})/(\text{serum [Creat]})\} \times 100$

CREATININE CLEARANCE (ml/min)

= (urine [Creat]) × (urine volume over 24 hours)
= {(urine [Creat (gm/dl)]) × {[urine volume (ml/d)]/1440 (min/day)]}/serum [Creat] (mg/dl)
Estimated for males = {(140 – age) × [lean body weight (kg)]}/{serum [Creat] (mg/dl) × 72}
Estimated for females = 0.85 × (estimate for males)
Normal range: 74–160 ml/min

E. Acid-Base Formulas

HENDERSON'S EQUATION FOR $[H^+]$

$[H^+]$ (nm/L) = $24 \times \{Paco_2/[Hco_3^-]\}$
Normal values: $[H^+]$ is 40 nm/L at pH of 7.40 and each 0.01 unit change in pH corresponds to an approximate opposite deviation of $[H^+]$ of 1 nm/L (over the pH range of 7.10–7.50)

METABOLIC ACIDOSIS

Bicarbonate deficit (mEq/L) = $0.5 \times$ body weight (kg) $\times (24 - [Hco_3^-])$
Expected $Paco_2$ compensation = $(1.5 \times [Hco_3^-]) + 8 \pm 2$

RESPIRATORY ACIDOSIS

Acute = $\Delta[H^+]/\Delta Paco_2 = 0.8$
Chronic = $\Delta[H^+]/\Delta Paco_2 = 0.3$

RESPIRATORY ALKALOSIS

Acute = $\Delta[H^+]/\Delta Paco_2 = 0.8$
Chronic = $\Delta[H^+]/\Delta Paco_2 = 0.17$

F. Neurologic Calculations

GLASGOW COMA SCALE

= eye score (1–4) + motor score (1–6) + verbal score (1–5)

Specific Components of the Glasgow Coma Scale:

Component	Score
Eye opening	
spontaneous	4
to speech	3
to pain	2
none	1
Motor response	
obeys commands	6
localizes	5
withdraws	4
exhibits abnormal flexion	3
exhibits abnormal extension	2
none	1
Verbal response	
oriented	5
confused, conversant	4
uses inappropriate words	3
incomprehensible sounds	2
none	1

Normal total value: 15 (range 3–15)

G. Pharmacologic Calculations

DRUG ELIMINATION CONSTANT

= Ke
= fractional elimination of drug per unit time
= $\{\ln([\text{peak}]/[\text{trough}])/(t_{peak} - t_{trough})\}$

DRUG HALF-LIFE

= $t^{1/2}$
= 0.693/Ke

VOLUME OF DISTRIBUTION (L/kg)

= Vd
= [(dose) × (fraction of active drug in circulation)]/[(area under single dose curve) × Ke]

DRUG CLEARANCE

= Vd × Ke

DRUG LOADING DOSE

= Vd × [target peak]

DRUG DOSING INTERVAL

$= \{-Ke^{-1} \times \ln ([\text{desired trough}]/[\text{desired peak}])\} + \text{infusion time (h)}$

H. Nutritional Calculations

BODY MASS INDEX

= BMI
= weight (kg)/[height (cm)]^2

RESPIRATORY QUOTIENT

= R
= CO_2 production (ml/min)/O_2 consumption (ml/min)
Normal value: 0.8

HARRIS-BENEDICT EQUATION OF RESTING ENERGY EXPENDITURE (kcal/day)

Males = 66 + [13.7 × weight (kg)] + [5 × height (cm)] – (6.8 × age)
Females = 655 + [9.6 × weight (kg)] + [1.8 × height (cm)] – (4.7 × age)

I. Severity of Illness Calculations

ACUTE PHYSIOLOGY AND CHRONIC HEALTH EVALUATION II SCORE

= APACHE II

(From Knaus WA, Draper EA, Wagner DP, Zimmerman JE: APACHE II: a severity of disease classification system. *Crit Care Med* 1985;13:818, with permission.)

PHYSIOLOGIC VARIABLE	HIGH ABNORMAL RANGE					LOW ABNORMAL RANGE			
	+4	+3	+2	+1	0	+1	+2	+3	+4
TEMPERATURE — rectal (°C)	≥41°	39°-40.9°		38.5°-38.9°	36°-38.4°	34°-35.9°	32°-33.9°	30°-31.9°	≤29.9°
MEAN ARTERIAL PRESSURE — mm Hg	≥160	130-159	110-129		70-109		50-69		≤49
HEART RATE (ventricular response)	≥180	140-179	110-139		70-109		55-69	40-54	≤39
RESPIRATORY RATE — (non-ventilated or ventilated)	≥50	35-49		25-34	12-24	10-11	6-9		≤5
OXYGENATION: A-aDO$_2$ or PaO$_2$ (mm Hg) a. FIO$_2$ ≥0.5 record A-aDO$_2$	≥500	350-499	200-349		<200				
b. FIO$_2$ <0.5 record only PaO$_2$					PO$_2$ >70	PO$_2$ 61-70		PO$_2$ 55-60	PO$_2$ <55
ARTERIAL pH	≥7.7	7.6-7.69		7.5-7.59	7.33-7.49		7.25-7.32	7.15-7.24	<7.15
SERUM SODIUM (mMol/L)	≥180	160-179	155-159	150-154	130-149		120-129	111-119	≤110
SERUM POTASSIUM (mMol/L)	≥7	6-6.9		5.5-5.9	3.5-5.4	3-3.4	2.5-2.9		<2.5
SERUM CREATININE (mg/100 ml) (Double point score for acute renal failure)	≥3.5	2-3.4	1.5-1.9		0.6-1.4		<0.6		
HEMATOCRIT (%)	≥60		50-59.9	46-49.9	30-45.9		20-29.9		<20
WHITE BLOOD COUNT (total/mm3) (in 1,000s)	≥40		20-39.9	15-19.9	3-14.9		1-2.9		<1
GLASGOW COMA SCORE (GCS): Score = 15 minus actual GCS									
[A] Total ACUTE PHYSIOLOGY SCORE (APS): Sum of the 12 individual variable points									
Serum HCO$_3$ (venous-mMol/L) [Not preferred, use if no ABGs]	≥52	41-51.9		32-40.9	22-31.9		18-21.9	15-17.9	<15

B AGE POINTS:
Assign points to age as follows:

AGE(yrs)	Points
≤ 44	0
45-54	2
55-64	3
65-74	5
≥ 75	6

C CHRONIC HEALTH POINTS
If the patient has a history of severe organ system insufficiency or is immuno-compromised assign points as follows:

a. for nonoperative or emergency postoperative patients — 5 points
   or
b. for elective postoperative patients — 2 points

DEFINITIONS
Organ Insufficiency or immuno-compromised state must have been evident **prior** to this hospital admission and conform to the following criteria:

LIVER: Biopsy proven cirrhosis and documented portal hypertension; episodes of past upper GI bleeding attributed to portal hypertension; or prior episodes of hepatic failure/encephalopathy/coma.

CARDIOVASCULAR: New York Heart Association Class IV.

RESPIRATORY: Chronic restrictive, obstructive, or vascular disease resulting in severe exercise restriction, i.e., unable to climb stairs or perform household duties; or documented chronic hypoxia, hypercapnia, secondary polycythemia, severe pulmonary hypertension (>40mmHg), or respirator dependency.

RENAL: Receiving chronic dialysis.

IMMUNO-COMPROMISED: The patient has received therapy that suppresses resistance to infection, e.g., immuno-suppression, chemotherapy, radiation, long term or recent high dose steroids, or has a disease that is sufficiently advanced to suppress resistance to infection, e.g., leukemia, lymphoma, AIDS.

APACHE II SCORE

Sum of A + B + C

A APS points ________

B Age points ________

C Chronic Health points ________

Total APACHE II ________

From ref. 1, with permission.

SUBJECT INDEX

Page numbers followed by *t* indicates tabular material.

D

N